The Complete
Mental Health
Directory

2008
Sixth Edition

The Complete Mental Health Directory

A Comprehensive
Source Book for
Individuals and Professionals

A Sedgwick Press Book

Grey House Publishing

PUBLISHER:	Leslie Mackenzie
EDITOR:	Richard Gottlieb
EDITORIAL DIRECTOR:	Laura Mars-Proietti
PRODUCTION MANAGER:	Karen Stevens
MEDICAL EDITOR:	Nada Stotland, MD
PRODUCTION ASSISTANTS:	Erica Irish, Karynn Ketiinq, Alicia Miles, Erica Schneider
MARKETING DIRECTOR:	Jessica Moody

Grey House Publishing, Inc.
185 Millerton Road
Millerton, NY 12546
518.789.8700
FAX 518.789.0545
www.greyhouse.com
e-mail: books @greyhouse.com

First edition printed 1999
Sixth edition printed 2008

Biennial
Spine title: The complete mental health directory
    v.27.5
"A comprehensive source book for individuals and professionals"
Includes indexes
ISSN: 1538-0556

1. Mental health services—United States—Directories.

RA790.6.C625
362—dc21
ISBN: 978-1-59237-285-0   softcover

2001-233121

Table of Contents

Article: *Developments and Controversies in Mental Health*
Introduction

SECTION ONE
Adjustment Disorders 1
Alcohol and Substance Abuse & Dependence..9
Anxiety Disorders 30
Attention Deficit/Hyperactivity Disorder (ADHD)...............................45
Asperger's Syndrome...61
Autistic Disorder 65
Bipolar Disorders 84
Cognitive Disorders 93
Conduct Disorder 99
Depression 104
Dissociative Disorders 117
Eating Disorders 122
Facticious Disorder 134
Gender Identification Disorder 137
Impulse Control Disorders..140
Obsessive Compulsive Disorder 146
Paraphilias (Perversions) 154
Personality Disorders..157
Post Traumatic Stress Disorder..164
Psychosomatic (Somatizing) Disorders 171
Schizophrenia...175
Sexual Disorders 186
Sleep Disorders 191
Suicide 194
Tic Disorders..200

Each of the above chapters includes a description and the following sections:
*Association & Agencies; Books; Periodicals & Pamphlets; Research Centers;
Support Groups & Hot Lines; Video & Audio; Web Sites*

Pediatric & Adolescent Issues 206

SECTION TWO: Associations & Organizations

Mental Health Associations & Organizations

National 216

State 228

SECTION THREE: Government Agencies

Government Agencies

Federal 270

State 275

SECTION FOUR: Professional & Support Services

Professional Support & Services

Accreditation & Quality Assurance 305

Associations 307

Books

General 330

Adjustment Disorders 355

Anxiety Disorders 362

Asperger's Syndrome 364

Attention Deficit & Hyperactivity Disorder (ADHD) 365

Autistic Disorder 366

Cognitive Disorders 366

Conduct Disorder 367

Depression 368

Dissociative Disorders 370

Eating Disorders 371

Factitious Disorders 372

Gender Identification Disorder 372

Impulse Control Disorder 373

Obsessive Compulsive Disorder 373

Personality Disorders 374

Post Traumatic Stress Disorder 376

Psychosomatic (Somatizing) Disorders 380

Schizophrenia 381

Sexual Disorders 382

Suicide 382

Pediatric & Adolescent Issues 383

Conferences & Meetings 392

Consulting Services 395

Periodicals & Pamphlets 396

Testing & Evaluation 409

Training & Recruitment 412

Video & Audio...424
Web Sites..427
Workbooks & Manuals....................................431
Directories & Databases 434

SECTION FIVE: Publishers
Publishers..441

SECTION SIX: Facilities
State 448

SECTION SEVEN: Clinical Management
Management Companies...................................480
Software Companies 499
Information Services.......................................516

SECTION EIGHT: Pharmaceutical Companies
Manufacturers A-Z..523
Drugs A-Z..525

INDEXES
Disorder Index 530
Entry Index 549
Geographic Index...584

Introduction

This sixth edition of *The Complete Mental Health Directory* is a unique reference directory with comprehensive coverage of 27 specific mental health disorders, from Adjustment Disorders to Tic Disorders, plus coverage of conditions as they relate to the Pediatric and Adolescent population. In addition to specific disorder resources, this reference includes Professional Services, Publishers, Facilities, Clinical Management and Pharmaceutical Companies.

The Complete Mental Health Directory offers valuable information for those suffering from a mental condition, their families and support systems, as well as mental health professionals. It combines, in a single volume, disorder descriptions written in clear, layman's terms and a wide variety of resources, including Associations, Publications, Support Groups, Web Sites, State Agencies and Facilities. Here's where you'll find where to go and who to ask – for the most diagnosed mental health disorders in the country.

Again this year, Dr. Nada Stotland, Professor of Psychiatry and Obstetrics & Gynecology at the Rush Medical Center in Chicago and President of the American Psychiatric Association, worked with us to assure accuracy of disorder descriptions and resources. You'll find the latest in recommended treatments, the most valuable publications on each disorder, and an up-to-the-minute list of pharmaceuticals used to treat mental health conditions.

Praise for *The Complete Mental Health Directory:*

> " . . . provides information useful for public, academic and professional collections."
> *ARBA*

In addition to the 4,739 listings in *The Complete Mental Health Directory*, an article written by Dr. Stotland, **Developments and Controversies in Mental Health** follows this Introduction and discusses the reality of mental illnesses, the culpability of those who commit crimes while suffering from a mental illness, the risks of psychiatric medications, and the question of substance abuse – is it a disease or moral weakness? Following this article, a list of **Mental Disorders by Diagnostic Category** helps patients and professionals be better educated about categorical diagnoses, symptoms and treatments.

The Complete Mental Health Directory is organized into eight sections.

SECTION ONE: Disorders

This section consists of 26 chapters dealing with specific mental health disorders from Adjustment Disorders to Tic Disorders. Each chapter begins with a description, written in clear, accessible language and includes symptoms, prevalence and treatment options. Many disorder descriptions include information on specific syndromes within a general category; you will find, for example, Panic Disorder and Social Anxiety Disorder addressed within the Anxiety Disorder chapter.

Following the descriptions are specific resources relevant to the disorder, including Associations, Books, Agencies, Periodicals, Pamphlets, Support Groups, Hot Lines, Resource Centers, Audio & Video Tapes, and Web Sites.

SECTIONS TWO & THREE: Associations, Organizations, Government Agencies
More than 1,000 National Associations, and Federal and State Agencies are profiled in these sections that offer general mental health services and support for patients and their families. Listings include name, address, phone, fax, e-mail, web site and key executives

SECTION FOUR: Professional Support & Services
This section provides resources that support the wide range of professionals in the mental heath field. Included are specific chapters on Accreditation and Quality Assurance, Associations, Conferences and Meetings, Training and Recruitment, Workbooks and Manuals, and other categories.

SECTION FIVE: Publishers
This section lists major publishers whose main focus is health care or mental health issues. This material is suitable for both professionals in the mental health industry as well as patients and their network community.

SECTION SIX: Facilities
This section lists major facilities and hospitals, arranged by state, that provide treatment for persons with mental health disorders.

SECTION SEVEN: Clinical Management
Here you will find products and services that support the Clinical Management of mental health, including Directories and Databases, Management Companies, and Information Services, that offer patient, medical, and marketing information.

SECTION EIGHT: Pharmaceuticals Companies
The current information in this section profiles the pharmaceutical companies that manufacture drugs to treat mental health disorders. Arranged in two ways, first by companies with complete contact information, and second by medication with generic names, the condition it treats, and the company that manufactures it.

INDEXES
> **Disorder Index** lists all entries, and additional topics relevant to mental health.
> **Entry Index** is an alphabetical list of all entries.
> **Geographic Index** lists entries by state, making it easy to gather statewide resources.

This data is also available as **The Complete Mental Health Directory – Online Database.** Using powerful search and retrieval software, this interactive Online Database quickly accesses the information in the print version, searchable by dozens of criteria. Visit www.greyhouse.com for a free search.

Developments and Controversies in Mental Health

By Nada L Stotland, MD, MPH

Developments in mental health have created more controversy than those in any other area of medicine. Psychiatric medications and other treatments are misunderstood. Psychiatric disorders and treatments are stigmatized. There are concerns about whether psychiatric diagnoses are being applied to too many people-especially children-and about the effects of psychiatric medications on children and pregnant women. There are differences of opinion about the use of psychiatric expertise in legal cases. Most health insurance does not offer equal coverage of mental, as compared with other medical disorders. Following are questions and answers about controversial issues in mental health.

Are mental illnesses real?

We have increasing evidence from brain scans and other tests that mental illnesses are associated with very real changes in the brain. It is not only mental health professionals who consider mental illnesses real and serious. Psychiatry is part of the required curriculum of every medical school; it is a medical specialty fully recognized by the entire medical community. The American Psychiatric Association researches and publishes the Diagnostic and Statistical Manual of Mental Disorders (DSM), now in its fourth edition, which is used throughout the country to make the diagnoses that are vital to fitting a treatment program to an individual needing mental health care. The criteria for making diagnoses are developed by complete reviews of the medical literature followed by field trials to see how useful the diagnoses are in the real world. Each edition requires many years of background work, and new editions are needed because knowledge in mental health, as in every other field, grows over time. Diagnoses in the DSM are based mostly on signs and symptoms that are clear, observable, and definite. They are closely linked to responses to treatment. The DSM also makes allowances for the ways the signs and symptoms of mental illnesses can vary from culture to culture. The DSM also includes a category, "Mental Disorders Secondary to a Medical Condition." The brain is a part of the body, and it is no surprise that a number of general medical conditions can cause problems with thinking, feeling, and behavior. For example, an excess of thyroid hormones tends to make an individual jumpy and overactive, while a deficit of thyroid hormones tends to decrease an individual's energy and activity, in a way that can easily be confused with clinical depression. Brain tumors and metastases of cancers from other parts of the body can cause depression and changes in personality. People with liver or kidney failure become confused and disoriented. Everybody should have a family doctor or primary care physician, and it is a very good idea to check with that physician when mental symptoms appear.

Should people with mental illnesses be held responsible for crimes they commit?

The DSM states clearly that diagnoses of mental disorders should not replace criminal responsibility. There is no good evidence that psychiatric medications cause people to commit suicide or homicide. There are times, however, when untreated psychotic illness so contorts people's perceptions of reality and ability to think that they are driven to commit crimes; for example, a person may be convinced that people around him are really aliens trying to kill him, or that God has ordered her to break the law in some way. In these cases, the person's mental state should be taken into account during criminal proceedings.

Are psychiatric diagnoses a substitute for normal responses to the ups and downs of life? Are they applied too readily? Are too many psychiatric medications prescribed?

Any illness can be more or less serious. Some people 'tough it out' when treatment could prevent great suffering and disability. Others run to the doctor for every minor symptom. Either response can be a problem. The cardinal rule is that no diagnosis should be given until the individual with symptoms has had a thorough examination and until all factors contributing to the symptoms have been identified. There is no evidence that people will flock to mental health care providers just because care is available; people go when they are in trouble and need help. Like most other medications, such as antibiotics, psychiatric medications can be both underused and overused. Most people with mental disorders are still going untreated. At the same time, some people are prescribed medication without having had a thorough examination. One of the biggest controversies is about attention deficit/hyperactivity disorder (ADHD) in children. There is a distinct difference between ADHD and the activities of a child without the disorder. A child with ADHD interrupts other children constantly, is so fidgety that others can't concentrate, and disrupts the classroom. ADHD makes it difficult for a child to make friends and to learn in school. Examination of a child must include a complete evaluation of the family and school setting, to make sure that the child is not simply reacting to a difficult situation of some kind. Prescribing a medication should never be the first or automatic response when there are concerns about a child's behavior.

What is 'screening' for mental disorders?

Screening is a technique used in many areas of medicine. A simple, quick, inexpensive test or observation is used to identify individuals who may be at risk of a particular condition, be it high blood pressure, diabetes, tuberculosis, depression, anxiety, or alcohol dependence. Screening, by definition, does not result in a diagnosis-it should lead to a proper evaluation by an expert. Screening has saved many lives. In the case of children, teachers and pediatricians or family practitioners do informal screening all the time; is a child able to see the blackboard, hear the teacher, pay attention, interact normally with other children? Unless there is evidence of child abuse, concerns are relayed only to the child's parents or guardians, who then make any decisions about how to proceed.

What do psychiatric medications do?

The function of psychiatric medications is to restore people to their own best levels of emotions and behaviors. An antidepressant will not make a person who is not depressed any happier. Antipsychotic medications diminish or eliminate the hallucinations and delusions and confusion that make life miserable for people with schizophrenia and similar diseases. Lithium and anticonvulsants keep people with bipolar, or manic-depressive, ill-

ness from the terrible highs and lows that disrupt their lives and those of their families. Medication for ADHD helps a child to concentrate and sit still when s/he wants to—-it is not a sedative.

How long does a person have to take psychiatric medication? Is it addictive?

The effects of psychiatric medications are generally reversible—-that is, when an individual stops taking them, their thoughts and feelings go back to the way they were before the medication was started. That does not mean that medications have to be taken forever. The time period a medication is prescribed is related to the natural course of the disease. Major depressive episodes, for example, last about nine months. After this time, the medication can be stopped-unless the individual has had repeated bouts of illness and prefers to stay on medication to prevent more episodes. People with chronic, lifelong diseases benefit from taking medication for longer periods of time. Among psychiatric medications, only benzodiazepines, or minor tranquillizers, have the potential to be addictive. An addiction means that you have to take more and more to get the same effect.

Are psychiatric medications safe?

All medications can have side effects. These differ from person to person; medication may have to be changed until the best 'fit' is found. Patients must be followed carefully after any medication is prescribed; writing a prescription and making a follow-up appointment months later is not acceptable Lithium and older antidepressants, 'tricyclics,' can be fatal if large overdoses are taken; blood levels have to be measured on a regular basis. Medications should be tapered off rather than stopped abruptly, to give the brain and the rest of the body time to readjust. Recently the Food and Drug Administration has issued warnings about the use of antidepressants by children and pregnant women. These warnings are controversial. The studies that led to concerns about a relationship between antidepressant medication and suicidality have serious scientific flaws, and did not distinguish between thoughts of suicide, which are very common, and actual suicide. They did not address the problem that untreated depression is a very real and common cause of suicide. Studies of the effects of newer medications taken during pregnancy on the baby have been generally reassuring, but some new reports link particular antidepressants to cardiac and behavioral abnormalities in a small fraction of babies. However, untreated depression poses risks for mothers and babies as well, and discontinuing antidepressant medication during pregnancy results in a very high rate of relapse. Since this field is changing almost weekly, and since the possible dangers of medication must be weighed against the dangers of depression itself, professionals, pregnant patients, and families need to look for the latest research, and take each woman's history and circumstances into account, when making treatment decisions.

Are all mental health professionals equally qualified?

Each category of mental health care professional has its own training and licensing requirements, and requirements can differ from state to state as well. Counselors (marital, family, school, occupational) generally have a bachelor's or master's degree in counseling. Professional social workers have to complete a two-year master's degree program. Some psychologists stop at the master's degree level, but most have PhD or PsyD (Doctor of Psychology) degrees; to be licensed, they generally must complete some on-the-job training as well. Psychiatrists are medical doctors who complete four year residencies in psychiatry after graduating from medical school. They may also take a national examination in order to become certified by the American Board of Psychiatry and Neurology. Psychologists have special expertise in research and psychological testing as well as in the performance of psychotherapy. Psychiatrists have full medical training and can prescribe medications as well as doing psychotherapy.

Are psychiatric treatments dangerous, even barbaric, as they are sometimes depicted in the entertainment media?

Every kind of medical care has evolved over time, but the perception of psychiatric treatment sometimes gets stuck in the 1930s or 1950s. During the Civil War, amputations were often performed without anesthesia. In the 1930s, electroconvulsive ('shock') therapy was performed without anesthesia. Neither of these treatments is performed without anesthesia today. Electroconvulsive therapy, or ECT, can save the lives of people with depression

so severe that they cannot eat, sleep, speak, or move. It is applied in low doses, to only one side of the brain, so that aftereffects are minimal in most cases. It is performed only with patients' consent.

What are the rights of people with mental illnesses?

Psychiatry is unique among medical specialties in that psychiatrists are not only allowed, but required, to treat some people against their will. Psychiatric disorders can interfere with a person's ability to make sound judgments, and the purpose of psychiatric treatment is to restore the ability to make judgments and take control of one's life. When an individual is suicidal or homicidal, the state requires that that person, and others, be protected until the symptoms can be effectively treated. This can be done on an emergency basis, but further hospitalization requires a legal proceeding in which the individual can be represented by a lawyer. The number of people in mental hospitals has fallen drastically over the last few decades; often there are not enough inpatient beds to serve those who need and wish to have hospital care.

Are alcoholism and substance abuse diseases or moral weaknesses?

Ultimately, all competent adults must take responsibility for their own behaviors. However, there is clear evidence that some people are genetically vulnerable to dependence on alcohol or other substances, and that alcoholism and substance abuse are associated with observable changes in brain structure and function that make it much more difficult for the individual to abstain. Alcohol and substance abuse often occur along with other mental disorders; the chances of success are much greater if both, rather than only one or the other, are treated.

Are mental health care professionals anti-religion?

It is the ethical obligation of mental health care professionals to respect the values and beliefs of their clients-not to be judgmental. Most people who have struggled with mental illnesses report that their religious faith was a major factor in their recovery. Some people feel that the neutrality of mental health professionals can undermine religious values that are important to them and that the role of prayer is underestimated in traditional mental health treatment. In response, groups of therapists specifically aligned with one religion or another have developed faith-based treatments.

Are mental illnesses curable?

One of the most important developments in mental health care is the concept that our goal should be recovery—-helping people reach their full psychological and social potential—-rather than just the reduction of symptoms. It is important for patients and their treating professionals to work assertively toward that goal, by combining medication and psychotherapy, augmenting treatment with occupational therapy and social skills training when necessary, and trying different medications, doses, and combinations.

Does psychotherapy work, and, if so, how?

The easiest psychotherapies to study are those based on a specific plan, often called 'manual-based' psychotherapies: cognitive-behavioral therapy and interpersonal therapy. Cognitive-behavioral therapy focuses on the negative thoughts associated with an individual's symptoms: 'There is no hope for me,' 'nobody likes me,' 'something bad is going to happen to me,' and on the ways the individual behaves in response to those thoughts. First, these thoughts are identified, and then the individual and therapist examine them to determine whether they are fully realistic. The therapist and individual develop homework for the individual to do, to practice replacing the unrealistic negative thoughts with more realistic, optimistic thoughts, and to develop behaviors that reflect optimism. Interpersonal psychotherapy focuses on relationships in the individual's current life. There is strong evidence that both these types of therapy are effective for mild to moderate depression and for some kinds of anxiety disorders. The traditional psychotherapy is psychodynamic psychotherapy, which was developed from psychoanalysis as described by Sigmund Freud and his followers. Psychodynamic psychotherapy focuses on the individual's inner psychological conflicts and their relationships to childhood experiences. Since it is not structured like the newer psychotherapies, it has been more difficult to study scientifically. However, there is increasing evidence of its effectiveness in relieving symptoms. It also helps people understand themselves better. Brain imaging techniques allow us to see that effective psychotherapy has much the same effect in the brain as effective medication therapy.

Which is better, psychotherapy or medication?

Studies indicate that a combination of psychotherapy and medication produces the best results. Optimally, the same health care professional should provide both, but circumstances often require that treatment is 'split.' Many health care plans require primary care physicians to prescribe medication, and cover psychotherapy by social workers and psychologists, but not by psychiatrists. In those cases, it is very important for the two professionals to share information about the treatment on a regular basis.

Mental Disorders by Diagnostic Category

Adjustment Disorders

Alcohol and Substance Abuse & Dependence

Anxiety Disorders
    Dissociative Disorders
    Generalized Anxiety Disorder
    Obsessive Compulsive Disorder
    Post-traumatic Stress Disorder
    Social Anxiety Disorder

Mental Disorders usually Diagnosed in Childhood/Adolescence
    ADHD
    Autistic Disorder
    Asperger's Syndrome
    Conduct Disorder
    Tic Disorders

Cognitive Disorders

Eating Disorders

Factitious Disorder

Impulse Control Disorders

Mood Disorders
    Bipolar Disorders
    Depression
    Dysthymic Disorder
    Major Depression
    Postpartum Depression & Premenstrual Dysphoric Disorder

Personality Disorders

Psychotic Disorders
    Brief Psychotic Disorder
    Delusional Disorders
    Schizoaffective Disorder
    Schizophrenia

Somatoform Disorders
    Hypochondria
    Somatization Disorder

Sexual & Gender Identity Disorders
    Gender Identity Disorder
    Paraphilias

Sleep Disorders

User's Guide

Below is a sample listing illustrating the kind of information that is or might be included in an Association entry, with additional fields that apply to publication and trade show listings. Each numbered items of information is described in the paragraphs on the following page.

---

1. **12345**

      2.   **Association of the Mentally Ill**
      3.   29 Simmons Street
           Philadelphia, PA 15201

                    4.   234-555-1111
                    5.   234-555-1112
                    6.   800-555-1113
                    7.   TDD: 234-555-1114
                    8.   Info@association-mh.com
                    9.   www.association-mh.com

10.   William Lancaster, Executive Director
         Monty Spitz, Marketing Manager
         Kathleen Morrison, Medical Consultant

11.   Association for Mental Health is funded by the Mental Health Community Support Program. The purpose of the association is to share information about services, providers and ways to cope with mental illnesses. Available services include referrals, professional seminars, support groups, and a variety of publications.

12.   1 M *Members*

13.   *Founded*: 1984

14.   Bi Monthly

15. $59.00

16.   110,000

User's Key

1. **Record Number:** Entries are listed alphabetically within each category and numbered sequentially. The entry number, rather than the page number, are used in the indexes to refer to listings.

2. **Title:** Formal name of association or publication. Where names are completely capitalized, the listing will appear at the beginning of the section. If listing is a publication or trade show, the publisher or sponsoring organization will appear below the title.

3. **Address:** Location or permanent address of the association.

4. **Phone Number:** The listed phone number is usually for the main office of the association, but may also be for the sales, marketing, or public relations office as provided.

5. **Fax Number:** This is listed when provided by the association.

6. **Toll-Free Number:** This is listed when provided by the association.

7. **TDD:** This is listed when provided by the association. It refers to Telephone Device for the Deaf.

8. **E-mail:** This is listed when provided by the association.

9. **Web Site:** This is listed when provided by the association and is also referred to as an URL address. These web sites are accessed through the Internet by typing http://before the URL address.

10. **Key Executives**: Lists key contacts of the association, publication or sponsoring organization.

11. **Description:** This paragraph contains a brief description of the association, their purpose and services.

12. **Members:** Total number of association members.

13. **Founded:** Year association was founded.

14. **Frequency:** If listing is a publication.

15. **Subscription Price:** If listing is a publication.

16. **Circulation**: If listing is a publication.

Adjustment Disorders

Introduction

The experience of stress in life is inevitable and begins in utero. When we are faced with a painful event or situation, we do our best to cope, get through it, and move on. How we cope and how long it takes vary according to the stressful situation and the resources the individual brings to it. In most situations, we respond appropriately to the stressful event or situation and show an adaptive response.

Adjustment Disorders are maladaptive reactions to a stressful event or situation. The adjustment is to a real event or situation (e.g.,the breaking up of a relationship, being laid off), and the disorder signifies that the reaction is more extreme than would be warranted considering the stressor, or it keeps the individual from functioning as usual.

SYMPTOMS

• The development of emotional or behavioral symptoms is in response to an identifiable stressor except bereavement within three months of the appearance of the stressor;
• The emotions or behaviors are significant either because the distress is more extreme than would normally be caused by the stressor, or because the emotions or behaviors are clearly impairing the person's social, school, or work functioning;
• If the symptoms persist for less than six months after the stressor ends, the disorder is considered acute; if symptoms persist for longer than six months, the disorder is considered to be chronic.
• Adjustment Disorders are divided into several subtypes:

• **Depressed Mood** - predominant mood is depression, with symptoms such as tearfulness, hopelessness, sadness, sleep disturbances;
• **Anxiety** - predominant symptoms are edginess, nervousness, worry, or in children, fears of separation from important attachment figures;
• **Anxiety and Depressed Mood** - chief manifestations are a combination of depression and anxiety;
• **Disturbance of Conduct** - predominant symptoms are conduct which involves either a violation of other people's rights (e.g., reckless driving, fighting), or the violation of social norms and rules.

ASSOCIATED FEATURES

Many commonplace events can be stressful (e.g., first day of school, changing jobs). If the stressor is an acute event (like an impending operation), the onset of the disturbance is usually immediate but may not last more than six months after the stressor ends. If the stressor or its consequences continue (such as a long-term illness), the Adjustment Disorder may also continue. Whatever the nature of the event, it caused the person to feel overwhelmed. A person may be reacting to one or many stressors; the stressor may affect one person or the whole family. The more severe the stressor, the more likely that an Adjustment Disorder will develop. If a person is already vulnerable, e.g., is suffering from a disability or a mental disorder, an Adjustment Disorder is more likely.

The diagnosis of an Adjustment Disorder is called a residual category, meaning that other possible diagnoses must be ruled out first. For example, symptoms that are part of a personality disorder and become worse under stress are not usually considered to be Adjustment Disorders unless they are new types of symptoms for the individual.

There are three questions to consider in diagnosing Adjustment Disorder: How out-of-proportion is the response to the stressor? How long does it go on? To what extent does it impair the person's ability to function in social, workplace, and school settings?

The emotional response may show itself in excessive worry and edginess, excessive sadness and hopelessness or a combination of these. There may also be changes in behavior in response to the stressful event or situation, with the person violating other people's rights or breaking agreed-upon rules and regulations. The emotional response and the changes in behavior persist, even after the stressful event or circumstances have ended. Finally, the response significantly affects the person's normal functioning in social, school or work settings.

Adjustment Disorders increase the risk of suicidal behavior and completed suicide, and they also complicate the course of other medical conditions (for example, patients may not take their medication, eat properly, etc).

PREVALENCE

Men and women of all ages, as well as children, can suffer from this disorder. In outpatient mental health centers the diagnosis of Adjustment Disorder ranges from five percent to twenty percent.

TREATMENT OPTIONS

Anyone who is experiencing one or more stressful events or circumstances and feels overwhelmed or markedly distressed and cannot function normally, should seek help. A psychiatrist or other mental health professional should make an evaluation including a referral for physical examination if necessary. Treatment prescribed is often psychotherapy and, depending on the circumstances, can include individual, couple, or family therapy. Medication is sometimes prescribed for a few weeks or months. In most instances long-term therapy will not be necessary and the person can expect marked improvement within 8 to 12 sessions.

Associations & Agencies

2 **Alive Alone**
1112 Champaign Drive
Van Wert, OH 45891
419-238-7879
E-mail: alivealone@bright.net
www.alivealone.org

Kay Bevington, Founder

Self-help network of parents who have lost child/children. Provides education and publications to promote communication and healing, assists in resolving grief, and develops the means to reinvest lives for a positive future.

Year Founded: 1988

3 **At Health**
14241 NE Woodinville-Duvall Road
Suite 104
Woodinville, WA 98072-8564

360-668-3808
888-284-3258
Fax: 360-668-2216
E-mail: support@athealth.com
www.athealth.com

Providing trustworthy online information, tools, and training that enhance the ability of practitioners to furnish high quality, personalized care to those they serve.

4   AtHealth.Com
14241 NE Woodinville-Duvall Road
#104
Woodinville, WA 98072-8564
360-668-3808
888-284-3258
Fax: 360-668-2216
E-mail: support@athealth.com
www.athealth.com

Providing trustworthy online information, tools, and training that enhance the ability of practitioners to furnish high quality, personalized care to those they serve.

5   Bereaved Parents of the USA
PO Box 95
Park Forest, IL 60466
708-748-7866
Fax: 708-748-7866
E-mail: jbgoodrich@sbcglobal.net
www.bereavedparentsusa.org

Beverley Hurley, President
John Goodrich, National Contact

Designed to aid and suport bereaved parents and their families who are struggling to survive their grief after the death of a child.

6   Center For Mental Health Services
PO Box 42557
Washington, DC 20015-4800
866-889-2647
800-789-2647
Fax: 240-221-4295
E-mail: info@mentalhealth.org
www.mentalhealth.samhsa.gov

A Kathryn Power, MEd, Director
Edward B Searle, Deputy Director

Information about resources, technical assistance, research, training, networks, and other federal clearing houses, and fact sheets and materials.

7   Center for Family Support (CFS)
333 7th Avenue
9th floor
New York, NY 10001-5004
212-629-7939
Fax: 212-239-2211
E-mail: jortiz@cfsny.org
www.cfsny.org

Steven Vernickofs, Executive Director

An agency that continues to develop new programs to serve families and individuals with their care needs. They currently offer services throughout the New York City region including: New Jersey, Long Island and the Lower Hudson Valley.

8   Center for Loss in Multiple Birth (CLIMB)
PO Box 91377
Anchorage, AK 99509
907-222-5321
E-mail: climb@pobox.alaska.net
www.climb-support.org

Jean Kollantai, Founder

Support by and for parents who have experienced the death of one or more of their twins or higher multiples during pregnance, birth, in infancy, or childhood. Newsletter, information on specialized topics, pen pals, phone support.

9   First Candle/SIDS Alliance
1314 Bedford Avenue
Suite 210
Baltimore, MD 21208
410-653-8226
800-221-7437
Fax: 410-653-8709
E-mail: info@firstcandle.org
www.firstcandle.org

Deborah M Boyd, Executive Director
Laura L Reno, Director Marketing/Public Affair

National nonprofit health organization uniting parents, care givers and researchers nationwide with government, business and community service groups to advance infant health and survival. With help from a national network of member and partner organizations, we are working to increase public participation and support in the fight against infant mortality.

10   Grief Recovery After Substance Passing (GRASP)
C/O Patricia Wittberger
1088 Torrey Pines Road
Chula Vista, CA 91915
843-705-2217
Fax: 619-397-3493
E-mail: mom@jennysjourney.org
www.grasphelp.org

Patricia Wittberger, Contact

Support and advocacy group for parents who have suffered the death of a child due to substance abuse. Provides opportunity for parents to share theri greif and experiences without shame or recrimination.

Year Founded: 2002

11   National Association for the Dually Diagnosed (NADD)
NADD Press
132 Fair Street
Kingston, NY 12401-4802
845-331-4336
800-331-5362
Fax: 845-331-4569
E-mail: info@thenadd.org
www.thenadd.org

Dr. Robert Fletcher, Founder/CEO
Donna Nagy, President

Not-for-profit membership association established for professionals, care providers and families to promote understanding of and services for individuals who have developmental disabilities and mental health needs.

12 National Mental Health Consumer's Self-Help
1211 Chestnut Street
Suite 1207
Philadelphia, PA 19107
215-751-1810
800-553-4539
Fax: 215-636-6312
E-mail: info@mhselfhelp.org
www.mhselfhelp.org

Joseph Rogers, Executive Director
Susan Rogers, Director of Special Projects

Funded by the National Institute of Mental Health Community Support Program, the purpose of the Clearinghouse is to encourage the development and growth of consumer self-help groups.

13 National Mental Health Consumers' Self-Help Clearinghouse
1211 Chestnut Street
Suite 1207
Philadelphia, PA 19107
215-751-1810
800-553-4539
Fax: 215-636-6312
E-mail: info@mhselfhelp.org
www.mhselfhelp.org

Joseph Rogers, Executive Director

A national consumer technical assistance center that has played a major role in the development of the mental health consumer movement.
Year Founded: 1986

14 National Organization of Parents of Murdered Children
100 E 8th Street
Suite 202
Cincinnati, OH 45202
513-721-5683
888-818-7662
Fax: 513-345-4489
E-mail: natlpomc@aol.com
www.pomc.org

Dan Levey, President
Ann Reed, VP

Provides self help groups to support persons who survived the violent death of someone close, as they seek to recover. Newsletter, and court accompaniment also provided in many areas. Offers guidelines for starting local chapters. Parole Block Program and Second Option Service also available.
Year Founded: 1978

15 SAMHSA's National Mental Health Information Center
US Department of Health and Human Services
PO Box 42557
Washington, DC 20015
240-221-4021
800-789-2647
Fax: 240-221-4295
TDD: 866-889-2647
www.mentalhealth.samhsa.gov

A Kathryn Power MEd, Director
Edward B Searle, Deputy Director

Provides information about mental health via a toll-free telephone number, this web site, and more than 600 publications. Developed for users of mental health services and their families, the general public, policy makers, providers, and the media.

16 Save Our Sons And Daughters (SOSAD)
2441 W Grand Blvd
Detroit, MI 48208-1210
313-361-5200
Fax: 313-361-0055
E-mail: sosadb@aol.com

Clementine Barfield, Contact

Crisis intervention and violence prevention program that provides support and advocacy for survivors of homicide or other traumatic loss.
1987 pages

17 Survivors of Loved Ones' Suicides (SOLOS)
PO Box 592
Dumfries, VA 22026-0592
703-580-8958
E-mail: solos@1000deaths.com
www.1000deaths.com

Christine Smith, President
Betsy Beasley, VP

Organization to help provide support for the families and friends who have suffered the suicide loss of a loved one.

18 Tender Hearts
Triplet Connection
PO Box 429
Spring City, UT 84662
435-851-1105
Fax: 435-462-7466
E-mail: tc@tripletconnection.org
www.tripletconnection.org

Janet L Bleyl, President
Cheryl L Newcomb, Chairman

Network of parents who have lost one or more children in multiple births. Information on selection reduction. Newletter, information and referrals, phone support and pen pals.

19 The M.I.S.S. Foundation
PO Box 5333
Peoria, AZ 85385-5333
623-979-1000
888-455-6577
Fax: 623-979-1001
E-mail: info@missfoundation.org
www.missfoundation.org

Joanne Cacciatore MSW C.T., Founder
Mary E Geitz, VP

Offers emergency and on-going support for families suffering from the loss of a child. Provides information, referrals, phone support, newsletter, pen pals, literature, advocacy and online chat room support. Information on local group development.
Year Founded: 1995

20 Triplet Connection
PO Box 429
Spring City, UT 84662

435-851-1105
Fax: 435-462-7466
www.tripletconnection.org

Janet L Bleyl, President
Cheryl L Newcomb, Chairman

Network of parents who have lost one or more children in multiple births. Information on selection reduction. Newletter, information and referrals, phone support and pen pals.

Year Founded: 1983

21   UNITE Inc Grief Support
PO Box 65
7600 Central Avenue
Drexel Hill, PA 19026
888-488-6483
E-mail: administrator@unitegriefsupport.org
www.unitegriefsupport.org

Barbara Bond-Moury, Chairperson
Joanne Porreca, Administrator

Support for parents grieving miscarriage, stillbirth and infant death. Also provides support for parents through subsequent pregnancies. Group meetings, phone help, newsletter, annual conference. Offers group facilitator and grief counselor training programs. Professional in advisory roles.

Year Founded: 1975

Books

22   Consumer's Guide to Psychiatric Drugs
New Harbinger Publications
5674 Shattuck Avenue
Oakland, CA 94609-1662
510-652-2002
800-748-6273
Fax: 510-652-5472
E-mail: customerservice@newharbinger.com
www.newharbinger.com

Helps consumers understand what treatment options are available and what side effects to expect. Covers possible interactions with other drugs, medical conditions and other concerns. Explains how each drug works, and offers detailed information about treatments for depression, bipolar disorder, anxiety and sleep disorders, as well as other conditions. *$16.95*

340 pages ISBN 1-572241-11-X

23   Don't Despair on Thursdays: the Children's Grief-Management Book
ADD WareHouse
300 NW 70th Avenue
Suite 102
Plantation, FL 33317
954-792-8100
800-233-9273
Fax: 954-792-8545
E-mail: sales@addwarehouse.com
www.addwarehouse.com

Children are sure to be comforted by the friendly manner and sensitivity that this book imparts as it explains the grief process to children and helps them understand that grieving is a normal response. For children ages 4-10. *$18.95*

61 pages Year Founded: 1996 ISBN 0-933849-60-5

24   Don't Feed the Monster on Tuesdays: The Children's Self-Esteem Book
ADD WareHouse
300 NW 70th Avenue
Suite 102
Plantation, FL 33317
954-792-8100
800-233-9273
Fax: 954-792-8545
E-mail: sales@addwarehouse.com
www.addwarehouse.com

Strikes right at the heart of the basic elements of self-esteem. It presents valuable information to children that will help them understand the importance of their self worth. A friendly book that children ages 4 to 10 will love. *$18.95*

55 pages Year Founded: 1991 ISBN 0-933849-38-9

25   Don't Pop Your Cork on Mondays: The Children's Anti-Stress Book
ADD WareHouse
300 NW 70th Avenue
Suite 102
Plantation, FL 33317
954-792-8100
800-233-9273
Fax: 954-792-8545
E-mail: sales@addwarehouse.com
www.addwarehouse.com

This book explores the causes and effects of stress and offers children techniques for dealing with everyday stress factors. Bold and colorful cartoons project a blend of sensitivity and broad humor. Ages 4-10. *$18.95*

48 pages Year Founded: 1988 ISBN 0-933849-18-4

26   Don't Rant and Rave on Wednesdays: The Children's Anger-Control Book
ADD WareHouse
300 NW 70th Avenue
Suite 102
Plantation, FL 33317
954-792-8100
800-233-9273
Fax: 954-792-8545
E-mail: sales@addwarehouse.com
www.addwarehouse.com

A book that will delight both children and adults. Explains the causes of anger and offers methods that can help children reduce the amount of anger they feel. Gives effective techniques to help young people control their behavior even when they are angry. Ages 5-12. *$18.95*

61 pages Year Founded: 1994 ISBN 0-933849-54-0

27   Drug Therapy and Adjustment Disorders
Mason Crest Publishers
370 Reed Road
Suite 302
Broomall, PA 19008
610-543-6200
866-627-2665
Fax: 610-543-3878
E-mail: dtaylor@masoncrest.com
www.masoncrest.com

Adolescents are among those who suffer from adjustment disorders, many without knowing what it is or how it affects their lives. This book offers information on the advances in the development of antidepressants with fewer side effects and how their more selective effect on the neurotransmitters of the brain has led to their use in treatment for adjustment disorders.

ISBN 1-590845-80-9

28 **Preventing Maladjustment from Infancy Through Adolescence**
Sage Publications
2455 Teller Road
Thousand Oaks, CA 91320
805-499-9774
800-818-7243
Fax: 800-583-2665
E-mail: info@sagepub.com
www.sagepub.com

Examines the theoretical and historical issues of prevention with children and youth, and delineates those factors which place the individual at risk. Hardcover $109.00 & Paperback $51.95

156 pages Year Founded: 1987 ISBN 0-803928-68-8

29 **Stress Response Syndromes: Personality Styles and Interventions**
Jason Aronson-Rowman & Littlefield Publishers
200 Park Avenue South
Suite 1109
New York, NY 10003
212-529-3888
Fax: 212-529-4223
E-mail: custerv@rowman.com
www.aronson.com

Incorporation of the most recent advances in the understanding and treatment of stress response syndromes to date. Describes the general characteristics, including signs and symptoms, and elaborates on treatment techniques that integrate cognitive and dynamic approaches. *$43.00*

451 pages ISBN 0-765703-13-0

30 **Transition from School to Post-School Life for Individuals with Disabilities**
Charles C Thomas Publisher
PO Box 19265
Springfield, IL 62794-9265
217-789-8980
800-258-8980
Fax: 217-789-9130
www.ccthomas.com

Designed to assist professionals in developing and implementing transition services for students with disabilities. Specifically, this book focuses on the importance of assessment in transition planning and targets the various domains that should be included in any achool-to-work transition assessment. advocates a transdisciplinary school-based approach to transition assessment that involves not only school-based professionals in the assessment process but community agency representatives as well. Available in paperback for $41.95. *$61.95*

300 pages Year Founded: 2004 ISBN 0-398074-80-1

31 **Treatment of Stress Response Syndromes**
American Psychiatric Publishing
1000 Wilson Boulevard
Suite 1825
Arlington, VA 22209-3901

703-907-7322
800-368-5777
Fax: 703-907-1091
E-mail: appi@psych.org
www.appi.org

A comprehensive clinical guide to treating patients with disorders related to loss, trauma and terror. Author Mardi J Horowitz, MD, is the clinical researcher who is largely responsible for modern concepts of posttraumatic stress disorder (PTSD). In this book he reveals the latest strategies for treating PTSD and expands the coverage to include several related diagnoses. *$27.50*

134 pages Year Founded: 2003 ISBN 1-585621-07-2

32 **When A Friend Dies**
Free Spirit Publishing
217 Fifth Avenue North
Suite 200
Minneapolis, MN 55101-1299
612-338-2068
Fax: 612-337-5050
E-mail: help4kids@freespirit.com
www.freespirit.com

The death of a friend is a wrenching event for anyone at any age. Teenagers especially need help coping. This compassionate book answers questions grieving teens often have, like 'How should I be acting?''Is it wrong to go to parties and have fun?' and 'What if I can't handle my grief on my own?' The author has seen her children suffer from the death of a friend, and she knows what teens go through. Also recommended for parents and teachers of teens who have experienced a painful loss. *$9.95*

128 pages

Periodicals & Pamphlets

33 **National Association for the Dually Diagnosed: NADD Newsletter**
NADD Press
132 Fair Street
Kingston, NY 12401-4802
845-331-4336
800-331-5362
Fax: 845-331-4569
E-mail: info@thenadd.org
www.thenadd.org

Dr. Robert Fletcher, Executive Director

Bi-monthly publication designed to promote interest of professional and parent development with resources for individuals who have the coexistence of mental illness and mental retardation.

ISSN 1065-25-74

34 **Treatment of Children with Mental Disorders**
National Institute of Mental Health
6001 Executive Boulevard
Room 8184
Bethesda, MD 20892-9663
866-615-6464
Fax: 301-443-4279
TTY: 301-443-8431
E-mail: nimhinfo@nih.gov
www.nimh.nih.gov

Ruth Dubois, Assistant Chief

A short booklet that contains questions and answers about therapy for children with mental disorders. Includes a chart of mental disorders and medications used.

Support Groups & Hot Lines

35 Compassionate Friends
PO Box 3696
Oak Brook, IL 60522-3696
630-990-0010
877-969-0010
Fax: 630-990-0246
E-mail: nationaloffice@compassionatefriends.org
www.compassionatefriends.org

Kitty Edler, President
Gloria Horsley, Vp

For parents suffering the loss of a child.

36 Friends for Survival
PO Box 214463
Sacramento, CA 95821
916-392-0664
www.friendsforsurvival.org

Marilyn Koenig, Contact

Assists family, friends, and professionals following a suicide death.

37 National SHARE Office
St. Joseph Health Center
300 1st Capitol Drive
Saint Charles, MO 63301-2893
636-947-6164
800-821-6819
Fax: 636-947-7486
E-mail: share@nationalshareoffice.com
www.NationalSHAREOffice.com

Mandy Murphey Brown, President
Susan Pundmann, Executive Director

Pregnancy and infant loss support.

38 Parents of Murdered Children
100 East Eighth Street
Suite 202
Cincinnati, OH 45202
513-721-5683
888-818-7662
Fax: 513-345-4489
E-mail: natlpomc@aol.com
www.www.pomc.com

Parents supporting parents who have suffered the loss of a murdered child.

39 Rainbows
2100 Golf Road
Suite 370
Rolling Meadows, IL 60008
847-952-1770
Fax: 847-952-1774
E-mail: info@rainbows.org
www.rainbows.org

Suzy Yehl Marta, Founder/President

An international, not-for-profit organization that fosters emotional healing among children grieving a loss from a life-altering crisis. Rainbows provides training and curricula for ages 4 through adults: Sunbeams: Preschool edition;

Rainbows: Elementary Edition; Spectrum: High School Edition; Kaleidoscope: College age/Adult Edition; Prism: Single/Stepparent Edition and Silver Linings: Community Crisis response Editions.

40 Survivors of Loved Ones' Suicides (SOLOS)
PO Box 592
Dumfries, VA 22026-0592
703-580-8958
E-mail: solos@1000deaths.com
www.1000deaths.com

For the families and friends who have suffered the suicide loss of a loved one.

Web Sites

41 www.1000deaths.com
Survivors of Loved Ones' Suicides

Group for those who have suffered a suicide loss.

42 www.DivorceNet.com
DivorceNet

Legally oriented, searchable site.

43 www.alivealone.org
Alive Alone

Self-help network of parents who have lost an only child or all of their children. Provides education and publications to promote communication and healing, assists in resolving grief, and develops the means to reinvest lives for a positive future.

44 www.athealth.com
At Health

Provides information and tools to enhance practititioners quality for those whom they serve.

45 www.bereavedparentsusa.org
Bereaved Parents' Network

Designed to aid and suport bereaved parents and their families who are struggling to survive their grief after the death of a child. Information and referrals, newsletter, phone support, conferences, support group meetings. Assistance and guidelines in starting groups.

46 www.cfsny.org
Center for Family Support

Agency devoted to the development of mentally retarded children.

47 www.climb-support.org
Center for Loss in Multiple Birth

Support by and for parents who have experienced the death of one or more of their twins or higher multiples during pregnance, birth, in infancy, or childhood. Newsletter, information on specialized topics, pen pals, phone support.

48 www.compassionatefriends.org
Compassionate Friends

Organization for those having lost a child.

49 www.counselingforloss.com
Counseling for Loss and Life Changes

Look under articles for reprints of writings and links.

50   **www.cyberpsych.org**
      CyberPsych

Hosts the American Psychoanalyists Foundation, American Association of Suicideology, Society for the Exploration of Psychotherapy Intergration, and Anxiety Disorders Association of America. Also subcategories of the anxiety disorders, as well as general information, including panic disorder, phobias, obsessive compulsive disorder (OCD), social phobia, generalized anxiety disorder, post traumatic stress disorder, and phobias of childhood. Book reviews and links to web pages sharing the topics.

51   **www.death-dying.com**
      Death and Dying Grief Support

Information on grief and loss.

52   **www.divorceasfriends.com**
      Bill Ferguson's How to Divorce as Friends

Useful information on how to eliminate the anger usually associated with divorce.

53   **www.divorcecentral.com**
      Surviving the Emotional Trauma of Divorce

Offers helpful advice and suggestions on what to expect emotionally, and how to deal with the emotional effects of divorce.

54   **www.divorceinfo.com**
      Divorce Information

Simply written and covers all the issues.

55   **www.divorcemag.com**
      Divorce Magazine

The printed magazine's commercial site.

56   **www.divorcesupport.com**
      Divorce Support

Covers all aspects of divorce.

57   **www.friendsforsurvival.org**
      Friends for Survival

Assisting anyone who has suffered the loss of a loved one through suicide death.

58   **www.grasphelp.org**
      Grief Recovery After A Substance Passing

Support and advocacy group for parents who have suffered the death of a child due to substance abuse. Provides opportunity for parents to share theri greif and experiences without shame or recrimination. They will provide information and suggestions for those wanting to start a similar group elsewhere.

59   **www.griefnet.org**
      GriefNet

Useful information on coping with loss.

60   **www.mhselfhelp.org**
      National Self-Help Clearinghouse

Encouraging the development and growth of consumer self-help groups.

61   **www.misschildren.org**
      Mothers in Sympathy and Support

Help for mothers suffering the loss of a child.

62   **www.missfoundation.org**
      MISS Foundation

Offers emergency and on-going support for families suffering from the loss of a child. Provides information, referrals, phone support, newsletter, pen pals, literature, advocacy and online chat room support. Information on local group development. Local support group listings online.

63   **www.nationalshareoffice.com**
      National SHARE Office

Pregnancy and infant loss support.

64   **www.planetpsych.com**
      PlanetPsych.com

Learn about disorders, their treatments and other topics in psychology. Articles are listed under the related topic areas. Ask a therapist a question for free, or view the directory of professionals in your area. If you are a therapist sign up for the directory. Current features, self-help, interactive, and newsletter archives.

65   **www.pomc.com**
      Parents of Murdered Children

Help for anyone who has suffered the loss of a murdered child.

66   **www.psychcentral.com**
      Psych Central

Personalized one-stop index for psychology, support, and mental health issues, resources, and people on the Internet.

67   **www.psycom.net/depression.central.grief.html**
      Grief and Bereavement

Helpful information for those grieving from the loss of a loved one.

68   **www.rainbows.org**
      Rainbows

Group for grieving parents and children.

69   **www.realtionshipjourney.com**
      Relationship and Learning Center

Articles on divorce, among other articles.

70   **www.safecrossingsfoundation.org**
      Safe Crossings Foundation

For children facing a loved one's death.

71   **www.sidsalliance.org**
      First Candle/SIDS Alliance

For those who have suffered the loss of an infant through SIDS.

72   **www.spig.clara.net/guidline.htm**
      Guidelines for Separating Parents

Useful information that helps to decrease the stress associated with separation.

73 www.thenadd.org
National Association for The Dually Diagnosed:
NADD

Provides conferences, educational services and training materials for those with mentally retarded children.

74 www.tripletconnection.org
Tender Hearts

Network of parents who have lost one or more children in multiple births. Information on selection reduction. Newletter, information and referrals, phone support and pen pals.

75 www.unitegriefsupport.org
UNITE

Support for parents grieving miscarriage, stillbirth and infant death. Also provides support for parents through subsequent pregnancies. Group meetings, phone help, newsletter, annual conference. Offers group facilitator and grief counselor training programs. Professional in advisory roles.

76 www.utexas.edu
Life after Loss: Dealing with Grief

Six page overview for college students.

77 www.widownet.org
WidowNet

Help for someone suffering the loss of a spouse.

Directories & Databases

78 After School And More
Resources for Children with Special Needs
116 E 16th Street
5th Floor
New York, NY 10003
212-677-4650
Fax: 212-254-4070
E-mail: info@resourcenyc.org
www.resourcenyc.org

The most complete directory of after school programs for children with disabilities and special needs in the metropolitan New York area focusing on weekend and holiday programs. *$25.00*

ISBN 0-967836-57-3

79 Camps 2008
Resources for Children with Special Needs
116 E 16th Street
5th Floor
New York, NY 10003
212-677-4550
Fax: 212-254-4070
E-mail: info@resourcenyc.org
www.resourcenyc.org

Our guide includes profiles of more than 300 day camps, recreation, tutoring, and travel programs, museums, nature experience and summer employment in New York City, sleep away programs in the northeast, and travel programs throughout the U.S. that serve both special and mainstream children. *$25.00*

1 per year Year Founded: 2006 ISBN 0-967836-57-3

Alcohol/Substance Abuse & Dependence

Introduction

Substance abuse and addictive disorders are among the most destructive mental disorders in America today, contributing to a host of medical and social problems and to widespread individual suffering. Alcohol, a drug that is widely available and socially approved, is the most abused of all substances, and alcohol addiction is a pervasive mental disorder. Like all addictive disorders, alcohol addiction is characterized by repeated use despite repeated adverse consequences, and by physical and psychological craving.

Alcohol addiction can be treated, but successful recovery is dependent on acceptance by the patient that he or she has an illness; it is this acceptance that is often the greatest stumbling block to treatment.

Relapse is common for several reasons: lack of acceptace of a diagnosis; genetic vulnerability; and social factors. Although many people relapse, it takes about three tries at treatment before the results are fairly permanent, and most people do eventually respond to treatment.

Scientific understanding of how alcohol works on the body and the brain, and the underlying physiology of addiction, has advanced remarkably in recent years. Successful treatment very often requires involvement by the patient in some form of self-help group, such as Alcoholics Anonymous or another 12-step program.

The substances referred to in this section include: amphetamines; marijuana; cocaine (and its purer derivative, crack); hallucinogens, such as LSD; inhalants, such as butane gas or cleaning fluid; opioids, such as morphine, heroin, or codeine; and benzodiazepines like Valium and Zanax. Caffeine and nicotine, both of which have the potential for abuse and dependence, are not included.

SYMPTOMS

Alcohol and Substance Abuse Symptoms
• Repeated use resulting in inability to fulfill fundamental obligations at work, school, or home, e.g., repeated absences, poor work performance, family neglect;
• Repeated use, resulting in dangerous situation, e.g., driving or operating a machine while impaired;
• Repeated alcohol and substance-related legal problems, e.g., arrests for disorderly conduct;
•)Continued use despite persistent social or interpersonal problems worsened by the effects of substance abuse;
• Alcohol abuse can occur without tolerance, as in binge drinking, a particular problem for young people on college campuses and elsewhere.

Alcohol and Substance Dependence Problems
• Alcohol or substance is often taken in greater amounts or for a longer period than intended;
• Repeated wish or unsuccessful attempts to control use;
• A great deal of time is taken to get and use alcohol or substance or to recover from its effects;
• Important social, work, or recreational activities are missed because of use;
• Use continues in spite of the person knowing about the persistent psychological or physical problems it causes, e.g., depression induced by cocaine or continued drinking.

Tolerance:
• Need for increased amounts of alcohol or the substance to achieve desired effect;
• Diminished effects with continued use of the same amount of alcohol or substance.

Withdrawal:
• Characteristic withdrawal syndrome, prolonged taking and then stopping/reducing alcohol or substance causing physical and mental symptoms;
• Same or a related substance is taken to avoid/alleviate the withdrawal symptoms.

ASSOCIATED FEATURES

Frequently, alcohol abuse and dependence occur together with dependence on other substances, and alcohol may be used to counteract the ill effects of these substances. Depression, anxiety, and sleep disorders are common in alcohol dependence.

Typically, accidents, injuries and suicide accompany alcohol dependence, and it is estimated that half of all traffic accidents involve alcoholic intoxication. Absenteeism, low work productivity and injuries on the job are often caused by alcohol dependence. Alcohol is also the most common cause of preventable birth defects, including fetal alcohol syndrome, according to the American Psychiatric Association.

Women and men tend to have different drinking patterns. Society is more tolerant of male drunkeness than of female; women tend to drink alone and in secret and are more susceptible to medical complications of alcoholism. Alcohol abuse severely damages organ systems including the brain, the liver, the heart, and the digestive tract.

Genetics has a considerable influence on a person's propensity for substance abuse disorders, and such disorders are associated with significant changes in the brain.

Many individuals with substance or alcohol-use disorders take more than one substance and suffer from other mental symptoms and disorders as well. Individuals with a wide variety of mental disorders sometimes abuse drugs as an attempt to medicate themselves. Forty-seven percent of people with Schizophrenia have drug abuse/disorders. People with Antisocial Personality Disorder often abuse substances, including amphetamines such as cocaine. Substance-related disorders can also lead to other mental disorders. Use of the synthetic hallucinogen Ecstasy is associated with acute and paranoid psychoses, and the prolonged use of cocaine (a stimulant) can lead to paranoid psychosis with violent behavior. Substance use and the effects on an individual's employment and relationships, as well as legal difficulties, can precipitate anxiety and mood disorders. Intravenous substance abuse is associated with a high risk of HIV infections and other medical complications.

Chronic drug and alcohol abuse can lead to difficulty in memory and problem solving, and impaired sexual functioning.

Childhood sexual abuse is strongly associated with substance dependence and with a number of other mental symptoms and disorders.

PREVALENCE

Alcohol dependence and abuse are among the most prevalent mental disorders in the general population. One community study in the US found that about eight percent of the adult population had alcohol dependence and about five percent had alcohol abuse at some time in their lives. Approximately six percent had alcohol dependence or abuse during the preceding year.

There are large cultural differences in attitudes toward substances. In some cultures, mood altering drugs, including alcohol, are well accepted; in others they are strictly forbidden.

Those between the ages of 18 and 24 have a high prevalence for abuse of all substances. Early adolescent drug and alcohol use is associated with a slight but significant decline in intellectual abilities. Substance related disorders are more common among males than females. The lifetime prevalence of use of any drugs (aside from alcohol) in the US is 11.9 percent; in males it is twice as high as in females. About thirteen percent of the general population is estimated to use cannabis (marijuana); about seven to nine percent of 18 to 25 year-olds have used amphetamines at least once; eight to 15.5 percent of 26 to 34 year-olds have used hallucinogens like LSD at least once. Inhalants have been used at least once by five percent of the population. Inhalants are used mainly by boys between eight and 19 years old, and especially by 13 to 15 year-olds.

TREATMENT OPTIONS

Diagnosis and treatment of alcohol dependence has improved as understanding of the physiology of addiction has advanced. But successful treatment still relies on acceptance by the patient that he or she has an illness, as well as support from other people who have gone through the same process. For this reason, medical treatment is most often successful when it is accompanied by involvement in a support group, for both the patient and family members; these may include Alcoholics Anonymous (AA) and Al-Anon, 12-step spiritual programs that have gained popularity over the years. Local groups can be found in almost every community by looking in the phone book. Recently, similar groups have formed that do not emphasize spirituality, as these do, but rely on group support for sobriety.

There is a growing controversy over the need for people who have had an alcohol problem to abstain completely from alcohol for the rest of their lives, one of the central beliefs of AA. Some researchers and clinicians are arguing that it is possible for some former alcoholics to resume controlled social drinking. AA, in the past, has discouraged members from using psychotropic medications; this is often counterproductive. Most alcohol treatment programs have been developed for men. Successful programs for women are less confrontational and include arrangements for child care.

Treatment for alcoholism has been hospital-based in the past, but has increasingly moved to the outpatient setting.Hospital treatment is necessary for withdrawal when alcohol use has been heavy and steady. Delirium tremens, a consequence of very heavy drinking, can be fatal.

Medical treatment of alcohol dependence may include

Anabuse, a drug that makes an individual violently ill if alcohol is used. Group or hospital-based treatment may also be useful, and psychotherapy can help the patient more effectively deal with underlying conflicts and interpersonal problems.

Denial of illness and ambivalence about abstinence can make treatment difficult. A patient's cravings can be overwhelmingly intense, and the individual's social circle is often composed of other substance abusers, making it hard for the individual to maintain relationships while becoming or remaining abstinent — the goal in treatment. A wide range of intervention may be needed, including a general assessment of the drug abuse, and evaluation of medical, social, and psychological problems. It is best to involve partner/family/friends to help the person gain new understanding of the problem and to make the general assessment complete. An explicit treatment plan should be worked out with the person (and partner/family/friends if appropriate) with concrete goals for which the person takes responsibility, which should include not only stopping substance use, but dealing with associated problems concerning health, personal relationships and work. Severe withdrawal symptoms may require hospitalization.

Associations & Agencies

81   Alcoholics Anonymous (AA): Worldwide
475 Riverside Drive
11th Floor
New York, NY 10115
212-870-3400
Fax: 212-870-3003
E-mail: cpc@aa.org
www.aa.org

Irene Kontje, CPC Coordinator

A fellowship of men and women who share their experience, strength and hope with each other that they may solve their common problem and help others to recover from alcoholism.

82   American Academy of Addiction Psychiatry (AAAP)
345 Blackstone Boulevard
1st Floor - Weld
Providence, RI 02906
401-524-3076
Fax: 401-272-0922
E-mail: info@aaap.org
www.aaap.org

John T. Pichot, Board Member

Professional membership organization with approximately 1,000 members in the United States and around the world. The membership consists of psychiatrists who work with addiction in their practices, faculty at various academic institutions.

83   American Council on Alcoholism
1000 E. Indian School Road
Phoenix, AZ 85014
800-527-5344
Fax: 602-264-7403
E-mail: info@aca-usa.org
www.aca-usa.org

Lloyd Vacovsky, Executive Director
Percy Menzies, Acting Chairman

ACA is dedicated to educating the public about the effects of alcohol, alcoholism, alcohol abuse & the need for prompt, effective, readily-available & affordable alcoholism treatment.

84 American Public Human Services Association

810 1st Street NE
Suite 500
Washington, DC 20002
202-682-0100
Fax: 202-289-6555
E-mail: jfriedman@aphsa.org
www.aphsa.org

Karl Kurtz, President
Jerry Friedman, Executive Director

Nonprofit, bipartisan organization of individuals and agencies concerned with human services. Members include all state and many territotiral human service agencies, more than 1,200 local agencies and thousands of individuals.

85 Career Assessment & Planning Services
Goodwill Industries-Suncoast

10596 Gandy Boulevard
PO Box 14456
St. Petersburg, FL 33702
727-523-1512
888-279-1988
Fax: 727-577-2749
E-mail: gw.marketing@goodwill-suncoast.com
www.goodwill-suncoast.org

R. Lee Waits, President/CEO
Deborah A Passerini, VP Operations

Provides a comprehensive assessment, which can predict current and future employment and potential adjustment factors for physically, emotionally, or developmentally disabled persons who may be unemployed or underemployed.

86 Center for Family Support (CFS)

333 7th Avenue
New York, NY 10001-5004
212-629-7939
Fax: 212-239-2211
www.cfsny.org

Steven Vernickofs, Executive Director
Melanie Singleton, Human Resources Director

Service agency devoted to the physical well-being and development of the retarded child and the sound mental health of the parents. Helps families with retarded children with all aspects of home care including counseling, referrals, home aide service and consultation. Offers intervention for parents at the birth of a retarded child with in home support, guidance and infant stimulation. Pioneered training of non-professional women as home aides to provide supportive services in homes.

87 Center for Mental Health Services Knowledge

PO Box 42557
Washington, DC 20015-4800
800-789-2647
Fax: 301-984-8796
E-mail: ken@mentalhealth.org
www.mentalhealth.org

A Kathryn Power, MEd, Director
Edward B Searle, Deputy Director

Information about resources, technical assistance, research, training, networks, and other federal clearing houses, and fact sheets and materials. Information specialists refer callers to mental health resources in their communities as well as state, federal and nonprofit contacts. Staff available Monday through Friday, 8:30 AM - 5:00 PM, EST, excluding federal holidays. After hours, callers may leave messages and an information specialist will return their call.

88 Grief Recovery After Substance Passing (GRASP)

C/O Patricia Wittberger
1088 Torrey Pines Road
Chula Vista, CA 91915
619-656-8414
Fax: 619-397-3493
E-mail: mom@jennysjourney.org
www.grasphelp.org

Support and advocacy group for parents who have suffered the death of a child due to substance abuse. Provides opportunity for parents to share theri grief and experiences without shame or recrimination. They will provide information and suggestions for those wanting to start a similar group elsewhere.

Year Founded: 2002

89 National Alliance on Mental Illness

2107 Wilson Boulevard
Suite 300
Arlington, VA 22201-3042
703-524-7600
800-950-6264
Fax: 703-524-9094
E-mail: info@nami.org
www.nami.org

Suzanne Vogel-Scibilia, President
Fredrick Sandoval, VP

Nation's leading self-help organization for all those affected by severe brain disorders. Mission is to bring consumers and families with similar experiences together to share information about services, care providers, and ways to cope with the challenges of depression, schizophrenia, bipolar disorder, and other serious mental illnesses. Organization advocates for improvement in the public mental health system, health insurance coverage, housing, employment, income supports and other issues affecting individuals living with mental illness.

Year Founded: 1979

90 National Association of Alcohol and Drug Abuse Counselors (NAADAC)

1001 N. Fairfax St.
Suite 201
Alexandria, VA 22314
703-741-7686
800-548-0497
Fax: 800-377-1136
E-mail: naadac@naadac.org
www.naadac.org

Patricia Greer, President
Cynthia Moreno Tuohy, Executive Director

The only professional membership organization that serves counselors who specialize in addiction treatment. With 14,000 members and 47 state affiliates representing more than 80,000 addiction counselors, it is the nation's largest network of alcoholism and drug abuse treatment professionals. Among the organization's national certification programs are the National Certified Addiction Counselor and the Masters Addiction Counselor designations.

91 National Association of State Alcohol and Drug Abuse Directors
1025 Connecticut Avenue NW
Suite 605
Washington, DC 20036
202-293-0090
Fax: 202-293-1250
E-mail: dcoffice@nasadad.org
www.nasadad.org

Lewis Gallant PhD, Executive Director
Alan Moghul, Prevention Director
Hollis McMullen, Director Finance

A private, nonprofit educational, scientific and informational organization that serves all state alcoholism and drug agency directors. NASADADs basic purpose is to foster and support the development of effective alcohol and other drug abuse prevention.
Year Founded: 1971

92 National Clearinghouse for Alcohol and
PO Box 2345
Rockville, MD 20847-2345
800-729-6686
Fax: 301-468-6433
www.health.org

Godfrey Jacobs, Deputy Director
John Noble, Project Director

One-stop resource for information about abuse prevention and addiction treatment.

93 National Clearinghouse for Alcohol and Drug
PO Box 2345
Rockville, MD 20847-2345
800-729-6686
Fax: 301-468-7394
www.ncadi.samhsa.gov/govpubs/ph317/

Godfrey Jacobs, Deputy Director
John Noble, Project Director

One-stop resource for information about substance abuse prevention and addiction treatment.

94 National Council for Community Behavioral Healthcare
12300 Twinbrook Parkway
Suite 320
Rockville, MD 20852
301-984-6200
Fax: 301-881-7159
E-mail: administration@thenationalcouncil.org
www.thenationalcouncil.org

Linda Rosenberg, President/CEO
Jeannie Campbell, Executive VP

Promotes professionalism among those working in healthcare management. Serves as a network for sharing information and fellowship among members. Provides technical assistance to members and functions as a liaison to related professional organizations.

95 National Council on Alcoholism and Drug Dependence
244 East 58th Street
4th Floor
New York, NY 10022-2001
212-269-7797
Fax: 212-269-7510
E-mail: officemanager@ncadd.org
www.ncadd.org

Anand Pandya, MD, President
Leah Brook, Affiliate Services

Fights the stigma and the disease of alcoholism and other drug addictions. Founded by Marty Mann, the first woman to find long-term sobriety in Alcoholics Anonymous, NCADD provides education, information, intervetion and treatment through offices in New York and Washington, and a nationwide network of Affiliates.
Year Founded: 1944

96 National Institute on Alcohol Abuse and Alcoholism
5635 Fishers Lane
MSC 9304
Bethesda, MD 20892-9304
301-443-3860
Fax: 301-443-8774
E-mail: niaaweb-r@exchange.nih.gov
www.niaaa.nih.gov

Ting-Kai Li, Director
Faye Calhoun, Deputy Director

Federal agency that supports research nationwide on alcohol abuse and alcoholism. Includes investigator-initiated research on homeless persons.

97 National Mental Health Association
2000 N. Beauregard Street
6th Floor
Alexandria, VA 22311
703-684-7722
800-969-6642
Fax: 703-684-5968
TTY: 800-433-5959
E-mail: infoctr@mentalhealthamerica.net
www.www.mentalhealthamerica.net

David Sheon, PhD., President/CEO
Danielle Fritze, Project Manager and Public Affai

NMHA is America's oldest and only nonprofit organization that addresses all the aspects of mental health and mental illness.

98 National Mental Health Consumer's
1211 Chestnut Street
Suite 1207
Philadelphia, PA 19107
215-751-1810
800-553-4539
Fax: 215-636-6312
E-mail: info@mhselfhelp.org
www.mhselfhelp.org

Christine Simiriglia, Executive Director
Jennifer Melinn, Info/Referral Dept.

Funded by the National Institute of Mental Health Community Support Program, the purpose of the Clearinghouse is to encourage the development and growth of consumer self-help groups.

99 National Mental Health Consumers' Self-Help Clearinghouse
1211 Chestnut Street
Suite 1207
Philadelphia, PA 19107
215-751-1810
800-553-4539
Fax: 215-636-6312
E-mail: info@mhselfhelp.org
www.mhselfhelp.org

Joseph Rogers, Executive Director

A national consumer technical assistance center that has played a major role in the development of the mental health consumer movement.

Year Founded: 1986

100 National Organization on Fetal Alcohol Syndrome
900 17th Street NW
Suite 910
Washington, DC 20006
202-785-4585
800-666-6327
Fax: 202-466-6456
E-mail: information@nofas.org
www.nofas.org

Tom Donaldson, President
Kathleen Tavenner Mitchell, Program Director/Spokesperson

Develops and implements innovative prevention and education strategies assessing fetal alcohol syndrome - the leading known preventable cause of mental retardation - including information, resource and referral clearinghouse.

101 SAMHSA's National Mental Health Information Center
US Department of Health and Human Services
PO Box 42557
Washington, DC 20015
240-221-4021
800-789-2647
Fax: 240-221-4295
TDD: 866-889-2647
www.mentalhealth.org

A Kathryn Power MEd, Director
Edward B Searle, Deputy Director

Provides information about mental health via a toll-free telephone number, this web site, and more than 600 publications. Developed for users of mental health services and their families, the general public, policy makers, providers, and the media.

102 Samhsa's National Clearinghouse For Alcohol And Drug Information
PO Box 2345
Rockville, MD 20847-2345
240-221-4019
800-729-6686
Fax: 240-221-4292
TDD: 800-487-4889
www.www.ncadi.samhsa.gov

One-stop resource for information about abuse prevention and addiction treatment.

103 Section for Psychiatric and Substance Abuse Services (SPSPAS)
1 N Franklin Street
Chicago, IL 60606-3421
312-422-3000
Fax: 312-422-4796
www.http://www.aha.org/aha/member-center/constituency-

Dick Davidson, President
Pamela Thompson, Executive Director

Institutional members of the American Hospital Association who provide psychiatric substance abuse, clinical psychology and other behavorial health services and assists the AHA in development and implementation of policies and programs.

104 Suncoast Residential Training Center/Developmental Services Program
Goodwill Industries-Suncoast
10596 Gandy Boulevard
PO Box 14456
St. Petersburg, FL 33702
727-523-1512
888-279-1988
Fax: 727-577-2749
E-mail: gw.marketin@goodwill-suncoast.org
www.goodwill-suncoast.org

R. Lee Waits, President/CEO
Deborah A Passerini, VP Operationse

A large group home which serves individuals diagnosed as mentally retarded with a secondary diagnosed of psychiatric difficulties as evidenced by problem behavior. Providing residential, behavioral and instructional support and services that will promote the development of adaptive, socially appropriate behavior. Each individual is assessed to determine, socialization, basic academics and recreation. The primary intervention strategy is applied behavior analysis. Professional consultants are utilized to address the medical, dental, psychiatric and pharmacological needs of each individual. One of the most popular features is the active community integration component of SRTC. Program customers attend an average of 15 monthly outings to various community events.

Books

105 Addiction Workbook: A Step by Step Guide to Quitting Alcohol and Drugs
New Harbinger Publications
5674 Shattuck Avenue
Oakland, CA 94609-1662
510-652-2002
800-748-6273
Fax: 510-652-5472
E-mail: customerservice@newharbinger.com
www.newharbinger.com

This comprehensive workbook explains the facts about addiction and provides simple, step by step directions for working through the stages of the quitting process. *$18.95*

160 pages ISBN 1-572240-43-1

106 Addiction: Why Can't They Just Stop?
Rodale Books
733 Third Avenue
15th Floor
New York, NY 10017-3204

212-697-2040
Fax: 212-682-2237
Susan Cheever, Author

Addiction offers a comprehensive and provocative look at the impact of chemical dependency on addicts, their loved ones, society, and the economy.

ISBN 1-594867-15-1

107 Alcohol & Other Drugs: Health Facts
ETR Associates
4 Carbonero Way
Scotts Way, CA 95066
831-438-4060
800-321-4407
Fax: 800-435-8433
E-mail: customerservice@etr.org
www.etr.org

Offers clear, concise background information on alcohol and other drugs, and provides assessment of the impact on youth. Also, discusses risk and protective factors, current trends, and prevention strategies. *$17.00*

108 Alcohol and the Community
Cambridge University Press
40 W 20th Street
New York, NY 10011-4221
212-924-3900
800-872-7423
Fax: 212-691-3239
E-mail: marketing@cup.org
www.cup.org

The authors challenge the current implicit models used in alcohol problem prevention and demonstrate an ecological perspective of the community as a complex adaptive system composed of interacting subsystems. This volume represents a new and sensible approach to the prevention of alcohol dependence and alcohol-related problems. *$110.00*

197 pages ISBN 0-521591-87-2

109 Alcoholism Sourcebook
Omnigraphics
PO Box 625
Holmes, PA 19043
800-234-1340
Fax: 800-875-1340
E-mail: info@omnigraphics.com
www.omnigraphics.com

Omnigraphics is the publisher of the Health Reference Series, a growing consumer health information resource with more than 100 volumes in print. Each title in the series features an easy to understand format, nontechnical language, comprehensive indexing, and resources for further information. Material in each book has been collected from a wide range of government agencies, professional associations, periodicals, and other sources. *$78.00*

613 pages ISBN 0-780803-25-6

110 American Psychiatric Association Practice Guideline for the Treatment of Patients With Substance Use Disorders
American Psychiatric Publishing
1000 Wilson Boulevard
Suite 1825
Arlington, VA 22209-3901

703-907-7322
800-368-5777
Fax: 703-907-1091
E-mail: appi@psych.org
www.appi.org

Offers guidance to psychiatrists caring for patients with substance use disorders. Includes treatment for alcohol, cocaine and opioids addiction. *$29.50*

126 pages ISBN 0-890423-03-2

111 Broken
Penguin
375 Hudson Street
New York, NY 10014
212-366-2372
Fax: 212-366-2933
www.www.penguin.com

William Cope Moyers, Author

Broken tells the story of what happened between then and now-from growing up the privileged son of Bill Moyers to his descent into alcholism and drug addiction, his numerous stabs at getting clean, his many relapses, and how he managed to survive.

ISBN 0-143112-45-7

112 Clinical Supervision in Alcohol and Drug Abuse Counseling
Jossey-Bass / Wiley & Sons
111 River Street
Hoboken, NJ 07030-5774
201-748-6000
Fax: 201-748-6088
E-mail: custserv@wiley.com
www.josseybass.com

This is the throughly revised edition of the groundbreaking, definitive text for supervisors in substance abuse counseling. *$25.95*

400 pages ISBN 0-787973-77-7

113 Concerned Intervention: When Your Loved One Won't Quit Alcohol or Drugs
New Harbinger Publications
5674 Shattuck Avenue
Oakland, CA 94609-1662
510-652-2002
800-748-6273
Fax: 510-652-5472
E-mail: customerservice@newharbinger.com
www.newharbinger.com

Practical guide to group intervention techniques with lessons from experiences of families seeking counseling and treatment. *$13.95*

208 pages ISBN 1-879237-36-9

114 Concise Guide to Treatment of Alcoholism and Addictions
American Psychiatric Publishing
1000 Wilson Boulevard
Suite 1825
Arlington, VA 22209-3901
703-907-7322
800-368-5777
Fax: 703-907-1091
E-mail: appi@psych.org
www.appi.org

Presents information on available treatment options for alcoholism and addictions, substance abuse in the workplace and laboratory testing. *$29.95*

172 pages ISBN 0-880483-26-1

115 Drug Abuse Sourcebook
Omnigraphics
615 Griswold
Detroit, MI 48226
800-234-1340
Fax: 800-875-1340
E-mail: info@omnigraphics.com
www.omnigraphics.com

Health information about illicit substance abuse and the misuse of prescription and over-the-counter medications, including depressants, hallucinogens, inhalants, marijuana, stimulants and anabolic steroids. *$78.00*

608 pages ISBN 0-780807-40-5

116 Dynamics of Addiction
Hazelden
15251 Pleasant Valley Road
PO Box 176
Center City, MN 55012-0176
651-213-2400
800-257-7810
Fax: 651-213-4411
E-mail: info@hazelden.org
www.hazelden.org

Pamphlet about addictions.

12 pages ISBN 0-935908-38-2

117 Eye Opener
Hazelden
15251 Pleasant Valley Road
PO Box 176
Center City, MN 55012-0176
651-213-4000
800-328-9000
Fax: 651-213-4590
www.hazelden.org

These daily meditations support core concepts of the AA program and help clients review key recovery ideas.
$12.00

381 pages ISBN 0-894860-23-2

118 Fetal Alcohol Syndrome & Fetal Alcohol Effect
Hazelden
15251 Pleasant Valley Road
PO Box 176
Center City, MN 55012-0176
651-213-4000
800-328-9000
Fax: 651-213-4590
E-mail: customersupport@hazelden.org
www.hazelden.org

If you're a chemical dependency counselor or work with women in pregnancy planning or self-care, this resource is filled with facts to help you better meet your clients needs.
$5.25

48 pages ISBN 0-894869-51-5

119 Getting Beyond Sobriety
Jossey-Bass / Wiley & Sons
111 River Street
Hoboken, NJ 07030-5774
201-748-5774
Fax: 201-748-6088
E-mail: custserv@wiley.com
www.wiley.com

This method will lead to a change in behavior within the individual, while developing and expanding connection with others. *$ 42.50*

198 pages Year Founded: 1997 ISBN 0-787908-40-1

120 Getting Hooked: Rationality and Addiction
Cambridge University Press
40 W 20th Street
New York, NY 10011-4221
212-924-3900
Fax: 212-691-3239
www.cambridge.org

The essays in this volume offer thorough and up-to-date discussion on the relationship between addiction and rationality. Includes contributions from philosophers, psychiatrists, neurobiologists, sociologists and economists. Offers the neurophysiology of addiction, examination of the Becker theory of rational addiction, an argument for a visceral theory of addiction, a discussion of compulsive gambling as a form of addiction, discussions of George Ainslie's theory of hyperbolic discounting, analyses of social causes and policy implications and an investigation into relapse. *$75.00*

296 pages Year Founded: 1999 ISBN 0-521640-08-3

121 Handbook of the Medical Consequences of Alcohol and Drug Abuse
Taylor & Francis
2 Park Square
Milton Park
Oxford, UK

Carlton Erickson, Author

Alcohol is one of the oldest and most widely used psychoactive drugs on earth.

122 Helping Women Recover: Special Edition for Use in the Criminal Justice System
Jossey-Bass / Wiley & Sons
111 River Street
Hoboken, NJ 07030-5774
201-748-6000
Fax: 201-748-6088
E-mail: custserv@wiley.com
www.wiley.com

Designed to meet the unique needs of substance-abusing women. Created for use with women's groups in a variety of correctional settings. Offers mental health professionals, corrections personnel, and program administrators the tools they need to implement this highly effective program.

384 pages ISBN 0-787946-10-5

123 Inside Recovery How the Twelve Step Program Can Work for You
The Rosen Publishing Group
29 E 21st Street
New York, NY 10010-6209

212-777-3017
800-237-9932
Fax: 888-436-4643
E-mail: info@rosenpublishing.com
www.rosenpublishing.com

A twelve step program to help with the recovery process.
$25.25

ISBN 0-823926-34-6

124 Inside a Support Group
Rosen Publishing Group
29 E 21st Street
New York, NY 10010-6209
212-777-3017
800-237-9932
Fax: 888-436-4643
E-mail: info@rosenpub.com
www.rosenpublishing.com

Lists support organizations for children of alcoholics. Explains what to expect at Alateen meetings and support groups for teenagers. *$25.25*

64 pages ISBN 0-823925-08-0

125 Kicking Addictive Habits Once & For All
Jossey-Bass / Wiley & Sons
111 River Street
Hoboken, NJ 07030
800-956-7739
Fax: 800-605-2665
E-mail: custserv@wiley.com
www.wiley.com

All aspects of changing bad habits and developing a balanced lifestyle are addressed in the book. *$22.50*

224 pages ISBN 0-787940-68-2

126 LSD: Still With Us After All These Years
Jossey-Bass / Wiley & Sons
111 River Street
Hoboken, NJ 07030
201-748-6000
Fax: 201-748-6088
E-mail: custserv@wiley.com
www.wiley.com

Facts about LSD. *$21.50*

176 pages ISBN 0-787943-79-7

127 Let's Talk Facts About Substance Abuse & Addiction
American Psychiatric Publishing
1000 Wilson Boulevard
Suite 1825
Arlington, VA 22209-3901
703-907-7322
800-368-5777
Fax: 703-907-1091
E-mail: appi@psych.org
www.appi.org

Straight talk about a difficult subject. *$26.95*

128 Living Skills Recovery Workbook
Elsevier Science
11830 Westline Industrial Drive
St. Louis, MO 63146
314-453-7010
800-545-2522

Fax: 314-453-7095
E-mail: custserv@elsevier.com
www.elsevier.com

Katie Hennessy, Medical Promotions Coordinator

Provides clinicians with the tools necessary to help patients with dual diagnoses acquire basic living skills. Focusing on stress management, time management, activities of daily living, and social skills training, each living skill is taught in relation to how it aids in recovery and relapse prevention for each patient's individual lifestyle and pattern of addiction. Book is now printed as ordered. *$39.95*

224 pages ISBN 0-750671-18-1

129 Living Sober I
Jossey-Bass / Wiley & Sons
111 River Street
Hoboken, NJ 07030
201-748-8677
Fax: 201-748-2665
www.wiley.com

Emphasizes the specific coping skills essential to a client's recovery. *$495.00*

87 pages Year Founded: 1999

130 Living Sober II
Jossey-Bass / Wiley & Sons
111 River Street
Hoboken, NJ 07030
201-748-6000
Fax: 201-748-6088
www.wiley.com

Emphasizes the specific coping skills essential to a client's recovery. *$395.00*

131 Meaning of Addiction
Jossey-Bass / Wiley & Sons
111 River Street
Hoboken, NJ 07030
201-748-6000
Fax: 201-748-6088
www.wiley.com

A controversial and persuasive analysis of addiction. *$30.50*

224 pages Year Founded: 1998 ISBN 0-787943-82-7

132 Medical Aspects of Chemical Dependency
Active Parenting Publishers
Hazelden
15251 Pleasant Valley Road
PO Box 176
Center City, MN 55012-0176
651-213-4000
800-328-9000
Fax: 651-213-4590
E-mail: info@hazelden.org
www.hazelden.org

This curriculum helps professionals educate clients in treatment and other settings about medical effects of chemical use and abuse. The program includes a video that explains body and brain changes that can occur when using alcohol or other drugs, a workbook that helps clients apply the information from the video to their own situations, a handbook that provides in-depth information on addiction, brain chemistry and the physiological effects of chemical dependency and a pamphlet that answers critical questions clients have about the medical effects of chemical dependency. Available to purchase separately. Program value packages available. *$244.70*

133 Mother's Survival Guide to Recovery: All About Alcohol, Drugs & Babies
New Harbinger Publications
5674 Shattuck Avenue
Oakland, CA 94609-1662
510-652-0215
800-748-6273
Fax: 510-652-5472
E-mail: customerservice@newharbinger.com
www.newharbinger.com

Offers a strong message of hope to help women cope with the challenges of recovering, deal with prenatal care and parenting issues, and take steps toward creating the healthy, happy families they want to have. A must read textbook for healthcare professionals and children's service workers. *$12.95*

138 pages ISBN 1-572240-49-0

134 Motivating Behavior Changes Among Illicit-Drug Abusers
American Psychological Association
750 First Street NE
Washington, DC 20002-4241
202-336-5500
800-374-2721
Fax: 202-216-7610
www.apa.org

Scientifically based method focused on the use of incentives to change behavior. Research in multiple applications of contingency management techniques. Test case of effective utilization of the method in treating illicit-drug abusers. *$39.95*

547 pages Year Founded: 1999 ISBN 1-557985-70-7

135 National Directory of Drug and Alcohol Abuse Treatment Programs
Substance Abuse & Mental Health Services Adminsitration
5600 Fishers Lane
Room 16-105, Office of Applied Studies
Rockville, MD 20857
301-443-6239
Fax: 301-443-9847
E-mail: findtreatment@samhsa.gov
www.findtreatment.samhsa.gov

Geraldine Scott Pinkney, Statistician

Directory of substance abuse treatment programs for use by persons seeking treatment and by professionals. Lists facility name, address, telephone number and services offered. Updated annually. Available in paperback. Searchable on-line version on web site.

596 pages 1 per year

136 New Treaments for Chemical Addictions
American Psychiatric Publishing
1000 Wilson Boulevard
Suite 1825
Arlington, VA 22209-3901
703-907-7322
800-368-5777
Fax: 703-907-1091

E-mail: appi@psych.org
www.appi.org

Katie Duffy, Marketing Assistant

Examines new approaches for an old problem. *$37.50*

248 pages ISBN 0-880488-38-7

137 Points for Parents Perplexed about Drugs
Hazelden
15251 Pleasant Valley Road
PO Box 176
Center City, MN 55012-0176
651-213-4000
800-257-7810
Fax: 651-213-4411
E-mail: info@hazelden.org
www.hazelden.org

Clear guidelines help teachers, parents, family members and others recognize, evaluate, and deal with adolescent drug abuse. Excellent support for family counseling programs. *$3.25*

16 pages Year Founded: 1996 ISBN 0-894861-40-9

138 Relapse Prevention for Addictive Behaviors: a Manual for Therapists
Blackwell Publishing
350 Main Street
Malden, MA 02148
781-388-8200
Fax: 781-388-8210
www.blackwellpublishing.com

Katie Duffy, Marketing Assistant

Applies cognitive-behavioral strategies and lifestyle procedures to treat people with addiction problems. *$43.95*

224 pages ISBN 0-632024-84-4

139 Rethinking Substance Abuse: What the Science Shows, and What We Should Do about It
The Guilford Press
72 Spring Street
New York, NY 10012
800-365-7006
Fax: 212-966-6708
E-mail: info@guilford.com
www.www.guilford.com

William R Miller, Author

Civilizations have long wrestled with problems linked to the use of alcohol and other psychoactive substances, and have made all manner of efforts to control.

ISBN 1-572302-31-3

140 Science of Prevention: Methodological Advances from Alcohol and Substance Research
American Psychological Association
750 First Street NE
Washington, DC 20002-4241
202-336-5500
800-374-2721
Fax: 202-216-7610
E-mail: executiveoffice@apa.org
www.apa.org

Carolyn Valliere, Marketing Specialist

This book explores ways for bringing greater methodological rigor to prevention research, gathering together the analyses and insights of prominent researchers who present examples of the problems and the solutions they have encountered in their own work. *$39.95*

458 pages Year Founded: 1997 ISBN 1-557984-39-5

141 Selfish Brain: Learning from Addiction
Hazelden
15251 Pleasant Valley Road
PO Box 176
Center City, MN 55012-0176
651-213-4000
800-328-9000
Fax: 651-213-4590
E-mail: customersupport@hazelden.org
www.hazelden.org

Helps clients or loved ones face addiction and recovery by exploring the biological, historical and cultural aspects of addiction and its destructiveness. *$18.95*

544 pages ISBN 1-568383-63-0

142 Seven Points of Alcoholics Anonymous
Hazelden
15251 Pleasant Valley Road
PO Box 176
Center City, MN 55012-0176
651-213-4000
800-328-9000
Fax: 651-213-4590
E-mail: customersupport.org
www.hazelden.org

The 7 points of Alcoholics Anonymous is the final work of Richmond Walker, author of the best-selling beloved book Twenty-Four Hours a Day. This book is the summation of Walker's knowledge on the practice and fundamentals of 12 Step recovery. Topics include an overview and history of A.A., the nature of alcoholism and recovery, the 12 Step way and fellowship, surrender, character defects, amends, living One Day at a Time, and sharing. *$9.95*

103 pages ISBN 0-934125-16-3

143 Sex, Drugs, Gambling and Chocolate: Workbook for Overcoming Addictions
Impact Publishers
PO Box 6016
Atascadero, CA 93423-6016
805-466-5917
800-246-7228
Fax: 805-466-5919
E-mail: info@impactpublishers.com
www.impactpublishers.com

There is an alternative to 12-step. You can reduce almost any type of addictive behavior from drinking to sex, eating, and the Internet. With this practical and effective workbook. Teaches general principles of addictive behavior change, so readers can apply them as often as they need. *$15.95*

240 pages ISBN 1-886230-55-2

144 Substance Abuse Treatment and the Stages of Change: Selecting and Planning Interventions (Guilford Substance Abuse Series)
The Guilford Press
72 Spring Street
New York, NY 10012
800-365-7006
Fax: 212-966-6708
E-mail: info@guilford.com
www.www.guilford.com

Gerard J Connors, Author

Alcohol and drug use is a common occurrence in today's society, with such use often associated with a variety of medical, psychological, and social problems.

ISBN 1-593850-97-2

145 Substance Abuse: Information for School Counselors, Social Workers, Therapists, and Counselors
Allyn & Bacon
230 Pearson Parkway
Lebanon, IN 46052
E-mail: pearsonstorecs@pearsoned.com
www.www.pearsonhighered.com

Gary L Fisher, Author

To provide counselors, social workers, and students with a detailed overview of the alcohol-and-other-drug field. The new edition provides updated coverage and clinical examples to reflect the rapid changes in this area.

ISBN 0-205591-76-0

146 Teach & Reach: Tobacco, Alcohol & Other Drug Prevention
ETR Associates
4 Carbonero Way
Scotts Valley, CA 95066
831-438-4060
800-321-4407
Fax: 800-435-8433
E-mail: customerservice@etr.org
www.etr.org

Helps to build commitment to stay tobacco, alcohol drug free. Also, looks to peer norms to support healthy, responsible choices, and enhances protective factors that prevent tobacco, alcohol and other drug use *$22.00*

147 Teen Guide to Staying Sober
Rosen Publishing
29 E 21st Street
New York, NY 10010-6209
212-777-3017
800-237-9932
Fax: 888-436-4643
E-mail: info@rosenpub.com
www.rosenpublishing.com

Helpful tips on how to keep teens from drinking. *$25.25*

64 pages ISBN 0-823927-65-2

148 The Science of Addiction: From Neurobiology to Treatment
W.W. Norton
500 Fifth Avenue
New York, NY 10110

212-354-5500
Fax: 212-869-0856
www.www.wwnorton.com
Carlton Erickson, Author

Indivdual chapters look at the general consequences of alcohol abuse, its neuropsychological consequences, effects on the brain, and effects of heavy prenatal alcohol exposure.

ISBN 0-393704-63-7

149 Treating Alcoholism
Jossey-Bass Publishers
10475 Crosspoint Blvd
Indianapolis, IN 46256
877-762-2974
Fax: 800-597-3299
www.josseybass.com

Presents a model of alcoholism treatment to help you guide alcoholics and their families on a path to long term recovery. *$40.00*

448 pages ISBN 0-787938-76-9

150 Twelve-Step Facilitation Handbook
Hazelden Publishing
15251 Pleasant Valley Road
PO Box 176
Center City, MN 55012-0176
651-213-4000
800-328-9000
Fax: 651-213-4590
E-mail: customersupport@hazelden.org
www.hazelden.com

This book provides clinicians with the tools they need to encourage chemically dependent clients to take advantage of the healing power of twelve-step programs. Learn how to integrate these time-tested principles into your practice. *$24.95*

214 pages Year Founded: 2003 ISBN 1-592850-96-0

151 Twenty-Four Hours a Day
Hazelden
15251 Pleasant Valley Road
PO Box 176
Center City, MN 55012-0176
651-213-4000
800-328-9000
Fax: 651-213-4590
E-mail: customersupport@hazelden.org
www.hazelden.org

Daily meditation in this classic book helps clients develop a solid foundation in a spiritual program, learn to relate the Twelve Steps to their everyday lives and accomplish their treatment and aftercare goals. Includes 366 daily meditations with special consideration and extra encouragement given during holidays. Helps clients find the power to stay sober each day and not to take that first drink. Hardcover - $12.95, Softcover - $10.95.

400 pages ISBN 0-894868-34-9

152 When Parents Have Problems: A Book for Teens and Older Children with an Abusive, Alcoholic, or Mentally Ill Parent
Charles C Thomas Publishers
PO Box 19265
Springfield, IL 62794-9265

217-789-8980
800-258-8980
Fax: 217-789-9130
www.ccthomas.com

This book is written with the idea that intelligent children can use sound ideas to improve thier lives, either on their own or with the help of adults. The author helps the reader be realistic about the sources of a problem, particularly if they are the result of a parents' difficulties. The text covers the kinds of problems that a parent's troubles can causes and offers ideas on how to deal constructively with the challenges. Available in paperback for $23.95. *$39.95*

94 pages Year Founded: 1995 ISBN 0-398059-89-6

153 Woman's Journal, Special Edition for Use in the Criminal Justice System
Jossey-Bass / Wiley & Sons
111 River Street
Hoboken, NJ 07030
201-748-6000
Fax: 201-748-6088
E-mail: customer@wiley.com
www.wiley.com

Designed to meet the unique needs of substance-abusing women. Created for use with women's groups in a variety of correctional settings. Offers mental health professionals, corrections personnel, and program administrators the tools they need to implement this highly effective program. *$23.50*

144 pages Year Founded: 1999 ISBN 0-787946-10-9

154 You Can Free Yourself From Alcohol & Drugs: Work a Program That Keeps You in Charge
New Harbinger Publications
5674 Shattuck Avenue
Oakland, CA 94609-1662
510-652-2002
800-748-6273
Fax: 510-652-5472
E-mail: customerservice@newharbinger.com
www.newharbinger.com

Reworking of the Twelve Steps approach into a program that helps addicts and alcoholics make needed changes in their lifestyle. *$13.95*

214 pages ISBN 1-572241-18-7

155 Your Brain on Drugs
Hazelden
15251 Pleasant Valley Road
PO Box 176
Center City, MN 55012-0176
651-213-4000
800-328-9000
Fax: 651-213-4590
E-mail: info@hazelden.org
www.hazelden.org

This pamphlet explains the effects of alcohol and other drugs on the brain through illustrations, activities and exercise that help to reinforce the easy-to-read text. *$4.00*

36 pages

Periodicals & Pamphlets

156 About Alcohol
ETR Associates
4 Carbonero Way
Scotts Valley, CA 95066
831-438-4060
800-321-4407
Fax: 800-435-8433
E-mail: customerservice@etr.org
www.etr.org

What it is, why it's dangerous, and its negative effects on the body and in prenatal development. Title #079.

157 About Crack Cocaine
ETR Associates
4 Carbonero Way
Scotts Valley, CA 95066
831-438-4060
800-321-4407
Fax: 800-435-8433
E-mail: customerservice@etr.org
www.etr.org

Describes what crack cocaine is and why it's dangerous and lists the effects on the body. *$16.00*

158 About Drug Addiction
ETR Associates
4 Carbonero Way
Scotts Valley, CA 95066
831-438-4060
800-321-4407
Fax: 800-435-8433
E-mail: customerservice@etr.org
www.etr.org

Includes answers to commonly asked questions about drug addiction, a 13'x 17' wall chart presents the stages of addiction and recovery, covers denial, withdrawal and relapse. *$18.00*

159 Alateen Talk
Al-Anon Family Group Headquarters
1600 Corporate Landing Parkway
Virginia Beach, VA 23454-5617
757-563-1600
888-425-2666
Fax: 757-563-1655
E-mail: wso@al-anon.org
www.al-anon.alateen.org

Newsletter with articles and drawings created by teenage and preteen Alateen members. Material relates to members' application of twelve step, and principles of Alateen program. Also includes articles by Alateen sponsors. *$7.50*

4 pages 4 per year ISSN 1054-1411

160 Alcohol ABC's
ETR Associates
4 Carbonero Way
Scotts Valley, CA 95066
831-438-4060
800-321-4407
Fax: 800-435-8433
E-mail: customerservice@etr.org
www.etr.org

Presents the consequenes of drinking and explains the difference between use and abuse in a straightforward, matter-of-fact way. Title #R712.

161 Alcohol Issues Insights
Beer Marketer's Insights
PO Box 264
W Nyack, NY 10994-0264
845-624-2337
Fax: 845-624-2340
E-mail: eric@beerinsights.com
www.beerinsights.com

Benjamin Steinman, Publisher

Newsletter that provides information on the use and misuses of alcohol. Covers such topics as misrepresentation in the media, minimum age requirements, advertising bans, deterrence of drunk driving, and the effects of tax increases on alcoholic beverage consumption. *$375.00*

4 pages 12 per year ISSN 1067-3105

162 Alcohol Self-Test
ETR Associates
4 Carbonero Way
Scotts Valley, CA 95066
831-438-4060
800-321-4407
Fax: 800-435-8433
E-mail: customerservice@etr.org
www.etr.org

Thought provoking questions include: What do I know about alcohol? How safely do I drink? When and why do I drink? Title #H259.

163 Alcohol: Incredible Facts
ETR Associates
4 Carbonero Way
Scotts Valley, CA 95066
831-438-4060
800-321-4407
Fax: 800-435-8433
E-mail: customerservice@etr.org
www.etr.org

Strange but true facts to trigger discussion about alcohol use, social consequences, and risks involved. Title #R719.

164 Alcoholism: A Merry-Go-Round Named Denial
Hazelden
15251 Pleasant Valley Road
PO Box 176
Center City, MN 55012-0176
651-213-4000
800-328-9000
Fax: 651-213-4590
E-mail: customersupport.org
www.hazelden.org

This pamphlet provides a clear description of alcoholism and defines the roles of the alcoholic and those affected by chemical dependency. *$2.95*

20 pages ISBN 0-894860-22-4

165 Alcoholism: A Treatable Disease
Hazelden
15251 Pleasant Valley Road
PO Box 176
Center City, MN 55012-0176

651-213-4000
800-328-9000
Fax: 651-213-4590
www.hazelden.org

A hard look at the disease of chemical dependence, the confusion and delusion that go with it, intervention and a hopeful conclusion - alcoholism is treatable. *$2.95*

18 pages ISBN 0-935908-37-4

166 American Journal on Addictions
American Academy of Addiction Psychiatry
7301 Mission Road
Suite 252
Prairie Village, KS 66208-3075
913-262-6161
Fax: 913-262-4311
E-mail: info@aaap.org
www.aaap.org

Jeanne G Trumble, Executive Director

Publishes overview articles, original, clinical, basic and research papers and updates.

ISSN 1055-0496

167 Binge Drinking: Am I At Risk?
ETR Associates
4 Carbonero Way
Scotts Valley, CA 95066
831-438-4060
800-321-4407
Fax: 800-435-8433
E-mail: customerservice@etr.org
www.etr.org

Easy-to-follow checklists help students decide if they have a problem with binge drinking, make a plan, and get help. Title #R018.

168 Chalice
Calix Society
2555 Hazelwood Avenue
Saint Paul, MN 55109-2030
651-773-3117
800-398-0524
Fax: 651-777-3069
www.calixsociety.org

Directed toward Catholic and non-Catholic alcoholics who are maintaining their sobriety through affiliation with and participation in Alcoholics Anonymous. Emphasizes the virtue of total abstinence, through contributed stories regarding spiritual and physical recovery. Recurring features include statistics, book announcements, and research. *$15.00*

4-6 pages 24 per year

169 Children and Youth Funding Report
CD Publications
8204 Fenton Street
Silver Spring, MD 20910-4509
301-588-6380
800-666-6380
Fax: 301-588-6385
E-mail: fsr@cdpublications.com
www.cdpublications.com

Mark Sherman, Editor

Helps social service professionals stay up-to-date on changing federal priorities and legislative developments in Wash-

ington, with insight from agency officials, Congressional staff, and advocates on what's likely to happen in the months ahead. Also provides updates on national and local news, with in-depth reports on welfare reform, the federal budget, and entitlement programs. Features program ideas from around the country, to help children and youth service providers learn about innovative new strategies they can implement in their communities. *$399.00*

18 pages 24 per year ISSN 1524-9484

170 Crossing the Thin Line: Between Social Drinking and Alcoholism
Hazelden
15251 Pleasant Valley Road
PO Box 176
Center City, MN 55012-0176
651-213-4000
800-328-9000
Fax: 651-213-4590
www.hazelden.org

This pamphlet explores the physical predisposition to alcoholism, as well as behavioral and emotional changes. *$2.50*

20 pages ISBN 0-894860-77-1

171 Designer Drugs
ETR Associates
4 Carbonero Way
Scotts Valley, CA 95066
831-438-4060
800-321-4407
Fax: 800-435-8433
E-mail: customerservice@etr.org
www.etr.org

Traces the evolution of designer drugs like China White and MDMA, explains how addiction works and suggests why designer drugs are so addictive. *$16.00*

172 Drinking Facts
ETR Associates
4 Carbonero Way
Scotts Valley, CA 95066
831-438-4060
800-321-4407
Fax: 800-435-8433
E-mail: customerservice@etr.org
www.etr.org

Addresses changing attitudes about drinking, and examines the basic facts of alcohol. Shows how to avoid risky situations, explains about the blood alcohol levels, and offers tips for curbing consumption. Title #R843

173 Drug ABC's
ETR Associates
4 Carbonero Way
Scotts Valley, CA 95066
831-438-4060
800-321-4407
Fax: 800-435-8433
E-mail: customerservice@etr.org
www.etr.org

26 good reasons to stay away from drugs, facts of different drugs, and motivation for being drug-free. *$16.00*

174 Drug Dependence, Alcohol Abuse and Alcoholism
Elsevier Publishing
11830 Westline Industrial Drive
St Louis, MO 63146
314-453-7010
800-542-2522
Fax: 314-453-7095
E-mail: usbkinfo@elsevier.com
www.elsevier.com

This journal aims to provide its readers with a swift, yet complete, current awareness service. This is achieved both by the scope and structure of the journal.

ISSN 0925-5958

175 Drug Facts Pamphlet
ETR Associates
4 Carbonero Way
Scotts Valley, CA 95066
831-438-4060
800-321-4407
Fax: 800-435-8433
E-mail: customerservice@etr.org
www.etr.org

Overview of 11 of the most commonly abused drugs includes: Description of drug, short-term effects and long-term effects. *$18.00*

176 Drug and Alcohol Dependence
Customer Support Services
PO Box 945
New York, NY 10159-0945
212-633-3730
800-654-2452
Fax: 212-633-3680
www.elsevier.com

International journal devoted to publishing original research, scholarly reviews, commentaries and policy analysis in the area of drug, alcohol and tobacco use and dependence. *$239.00*

15 per year ISSN 0376-8716

177 DrugLink
Facts and Comparisons
111 Westport Plaza
Suite 300
Saint Louis, MO 63146-3014
314-216-2100
800-223-0554
Fax: 314-878-5563
www.drugsfacts.com

DrugLink is an eight-page newsletter that provides abstracts of drug-related articles from various journals. DrugLink allows health care professionals to stay up-to-date on hot topics without having to subscribe to multiple publications. *$52.95*

8 pages ISBN 1-089559-0 -

178 Drugs: Talking With Your Teen
ETR Associates
4 Carbonero Way
Scotts Valley, CA 95066
831-438-4060
800-321-4407
Fax: 800-435-8433

E-mail: customerservice@etr.org
www.etr.org

Suggestions for effective communication include: avoid scare tatics, clarify family rules, other alternative for drug use. *$ 16.00*

179 Fetal Alcohol Syndrome & Fetal Alcohol Effect
Hazelden
15251 Pleasant Valley Road
PO Box 176
Center City, MN 55012-0176
651-213-4000
800-328-9000
Fax: 651-213-4590
www.hazelden.org

If you're a chemical dependency counselor or work with women in pregnancy planning or self-care, this resource is filled with facts to help you better meet your clients needs. *$5.95*

48 pages ISBN 0-894869-51-5

180 Five Smart Steps to Safer Drinking
ETR Associates
4 Carbonero Way
Scotts Valley, CA 95066
831-438-4060
800-321-4407
Fax: 800-435-8433
E-mail: customerservice@etr.org
www.etr.org

John Henry Ledwith, Sales

Steps to making healthy decisions about alcohol include: make choices, learn about alcohol, know your limits, have a plan, and watch for problems. Title # H252.

181 Getting Involved in AA
Hazelden
15251 Pleasant Valley Road
PO Box 176
Center City, MN 55012-0176
651-213-4000
800-328-9000
Fax: 651-213-4590
E-mail: customersupport@hazelden.org
www.hazelden.org

Twelve specific suggestions help clients through their early days in the AA fellowship. Topics include different types of meetings, expectations, common pitfalls, as well as do's and don'ts. *$2.95*

24 pages ISBN 0-894861-36-0

182 Getting Started in AA
Hazelden
15251 Pleasant Valley Road
PO Box 176
Center City, MN 55012-0176
651-213-4000
800-328-9000
Fax: 651-213-4590
www.hazelden.org

The principles and working of Alcoholics Anonymous provide an excellent resource for clients in early treatment and as a aftercare tool to provide ongoing support. *$10.95*

160 pages ISBN 1-568380-91-7

183 Getting What You Want From Drinking
ETR Associates
4 Carbonero Way
Scotts Valley, CA 95066
831-438-4060
800-321-4407
Fax: 800-435-8433
E-mail: customerservice@etr.org
www.etr.org

Practical ideas for drinking more safely, preventing hang-overs, weight gain, and injuries; blood alcohol chart shows the effect of alcohol on the mind and body. Title #H220.

184 Hazelden Voice
Hazelden Foundation
PO Box 11
Center City, MN 55012-0011
612-213-4000
800-257-7810
Fax: 651-213-4411
E-mail: info@hazelden.org
www.hazelden.org

Reports on Hazelden activities and programs, and discusses developments and issues in chemical dependency treatment and prevention. Carries notices of professional education opportunities, reviews of resources in the field, and a calendar of events.

185 I Can't Be an Alcoholic Because...
Hazelden
15251 Pleasant Valley Road
PO Box 176
Center City, MN 55012-0176
651-213-4000
800-328-9000
Fax: 651-213-4590
www.hazelden.org

This pamphlet describes fallacies and misconceptions about alcoholism and includes facts and figures about alcohol, its use, and its abuse. Available in Spanish. *$1.95*

9 pages ISBN 0-894861-58-1

186 ICPA Reporter
ICPADD
12501 Old Columbia Pike
Silver Spring, MD 20904-6601
301-680-6719
Fax: 301-680-6707
E-mail: The ICPA@hotmail.com
www.icpa-dd.org

Reports on activities of the Commission worldwide, which seeks to prevent alcoholism and drug dependency. Recurring features include a calendar of events and notices of publications available.

4 pages 4 per year

187 Journal of Substance Abuse Treatment
Elsevier Publishing
11830 Westline Industrial Drive
St Louis, MO 63146
314-453-7010
800-545-2522
Fax: 314-453-7095
E-mail: custserv@elsevier.com
www.elsevier.com

The Journal of Substance Abuse Treatment features original reviews, training and educational articles, special commentary, and especially research articles that are meaningful to the treatment of nicotine, alcohol, and other drugs of dependence.

ISSN 0740-5472

188 Marijuana ABC's
ETR Associates
4 Carbonero Way
Scotts Valley, CA 95066
831-438-4060
800-321-4407
Fax: 800-435-8433
E-mail: customerservice@etr.org
www.etr.org

Discusses the effects of marijuana, legal consequences, and strategies for saying no. *$16.00*

189 Motivational Interviewing: Preparing People to Change Addictive Behavior
Guilford Publications
72 Spring Street
New York, NY 10012-4019
212-431-9800
800-365-7006
Fax: 212-966-6708
E-mail: info@guilford.com
www.guilford.com

A nonauthoritarian approach to helping people free up their own motivations and resources, overcome ambivalence and help 'unstuck.' Presents a practical, research-tested approach to effecting change in persons with addictive behaviors. Paperback also available. *$42.00*

419 pages ISBN 1-572305-63-0

190 National Institute of Drug Abuse (NIDA)
6001 Executive Boulevard
Room 5213
Bethesda, MD 20892-9561
301-443-1124
Fax: 301-443-7397
E-mail: information@lists.nida.nih.gov
www.nida.nih.gov

Mora D Volkow, Director
Beverly Jackson, Public Information Director

Covers the areas of drug abuse treatment and prevention research, epidemiology, neuroscience and behavioral research, health services research and AIDS. Seeks to report on advances in the field, identify resources, promote an exchange of information, and improve communications among clinicians, researchers, administrators, and policymakers. Recurring features include synopses of research advances and projects, NIDA news, news of legislative and regulatory developments, and announcements.

191 Real World Drinking
ETR Associates
4 Carbonero Way
Scotts Valley, CA 95066
831-438-4060
800-321-4407
Fax: 800-435-8433
E-mail: customerservice@etr.org
www.etr.org

Credible young people talk about benefits of not drinking and risks of drinking. Title #R746.

192 Save Our Sons and Daughters Newsletter (SOSAD)
2441 W Grand Boulevard
Detroit, MI 48208
313-361-5200
E-mail: sosadb@aol.com

Serves as a forum for the organization, parents and supporters of children killed in street violence who began working together to create positive alternatives for young people. Provides commentaries, news of neighborhood coalitions, rallies, other social activities. Crisis Intervention and Violence Prevention News.

8 pages 12 per year

193 Teens and Drinking
ETR Associates
4 Carbonero Way
Scotts Valley, CA 95066
831-438-4060
800-321-4407
Fax: 800-435-8433
E-mail: customerservice@etr.org
www.etr.org

Includes common sense messages about drinking, binge drinking, and important things to know about drinking. Title #R717.

194 The Prevention Researcher
Integrated Research Services
66 Club Road
Suite 370
Eugene, OR 97401-2463
541-683-9278
800-929-2955
Fax: 541-683-2621
E-mail: info@tpronline.org
www.tpronline.org

Provides information on behavioral research to health and human services professionals, with a primary emphasis on adolescent substance abuse issues. *$20.00*

12-16 pages 4 per year ISSN 1086-4385

195 Understanding Dissociative Disorders and Addiction
Hazelden Publishing
15251 Pleasant Valley Road
Center City, MN 55012-0176
410-825-8888
800-328-9000
Fax: 651-213-4577
E-mail: customersupport@hazelden.org
www.hazelden.org

A Scott Winter, MD

This booklet discusses the origins and symptoms of dissociation, explains the links between dissociative disorder and chemical dependency. Addresses treatment options available to help in your recovery. The work book includes exercises and activities that help you acknowledge, accept and manage both your chemical dependency and your dissociative disorder. *$2.95*

ISBN 1-572850-14-6

196 When Someone You Care About Abuses Drugs and Alcohol: When to Act, What to Say
Hazelden
15251 Pleasant Valley Road
PO Box 176
Center City, MN 55012-0176
651-213-4000
800-328-9000
Fax: 651-213-4590
www.hazelden.org

This pamphlet shows family, friends, and co-workers how to confront someone who may be abusing alcohol or other drugs. *$2.50*

16 pages

197 Why Haven't I Been Able to Help?
Hazelden
15251 Pleasant Valley Road
PO Box 176
Center City, MN 55012-0176
651-213-4000
800-328-9000
Fax: 651-213-4590
E-mail: customersupport@hazelden.org
www.hazelden.org

Discusses how spouses of alcoholics are also trapped by deteriorating self-image, unconscious defense, destructive behavior, and offers change, especially through intervention. *$2.95*

12 pages ISBN 0-935908-40-4

Support Groups & Hot Lines

198 Adult Children of Alcoholics World Services Organization
PO Box 3216
Torrance, CA 90510
310-534-1815
E-mail: info@adultchildren.org
www.adultchildren.org

A 12-Step and 12-Tradition program for adults raised in an environment including alcohol or other dysfunctions.

199 Al-Anon Family Group National Referral Hotline
1600 Corporate Landing Parkway
Virginia Beach, VA 23454-5617
757-563-1600
Fax: 757-563-1655
E-mail: wso@al-anon.org
www.al-anon.alateen.org

Al - Anon's purpose is to help families and friends of alcoholics recover from the effects of living with the problem drinking of a relative or friend.

200 Alcoholics Anonymous (AA): World Services
PO Box 459
New York, NY 10163
212-870-3400
www.aa.org

For men and women who share the common problems of alcoholism.

201 Chemically Dependent Anonymous
PO Box 423
Severna Park, MD 21146
888-232-4673
E-mail: publicinfo@cdaweb.org
www.cdaweb.org

Twelve-step program for friends and relatives of chemically dependent people.

202 Cocaine Anonymous
3740 Overland Avenue
Suite C
Los Angeles, CA 90034
310-559-5833
Fax: 310-559-2554
E-mail: cawso@ca.org
www.www.ca.org

Fellowship of men and women who share their experience, stength and hope with each other in hope that they may solve their common problem and help others recover from their addiction.

203 Infoline
United Way of Connecticut
1344 Silas Deane Highway
Rocky Hill, CT 06067
800-203-1234
www.211infoline.org

Infoline is a free, confidential, help-by-telephone service for information, referral, and crisis intervention. Trained professionals help callers find information, discover options or deal with a crisis by locating hundreds of services in their area on many different issues, from substance abuse to elder needs to suicide to volunteering in your community. Infoline is certified by the American Association of Suicidology. Operates 24 hours a day, everyday. Multilingual caseworkers are available. For Child Care Infoline, call 1-800-505-1000.

204 Join Together Online
715 Albany Street
580-3rd Floor
Boston, MA 02118
617-437-1500
Fax: 617-437-9394
E-mail: info@jointogether.org
www.jointogether.org

A project of the Boston University School of Public Health, this association's mission is to help reduce substance abuse and gun violence.

205 MADD-Mothers Against Drunk Drivers
511 E John Carpenter Freeway
Suite 700
Irving, TX 75062
214-744-6233
800-438-6233
Fax: 972-869-2206
www.madd.org

Glynn Birch, National President

A crusade against alcohol consumption. Mission is to stop drunk driving, support the victims of the violent crime and prevent underage drinking.

206 Marijuana Anonymous
PO Box 2912
Van Nuys, CA 91404
800-766-6779
E-mail: office@marijuana-anonymous.org
www.marijuana-anonymous.org

Twelve-step program for marijuana addiction.

207 Nar-Anon Family Group
22527 Crenshaw Blvd
#200B
Torrance, CA 90505
310-534-8188
800-477-6291
Fax: 310-534-8688
E-mail: naranonWSO@hotmail.com
www.www.nar-anon.org

Twelve-step program for families and friends of addicts.

208 Narcotics Anonymous
PO Box 9999
Van Nuys, CA 91409
818-773-9999
Fax: 818-700-0700
www.na.org

For narcotic addicts: Peer support for recovered addicts.

209 Pathways to Promise
5400 Arsenal Street
Saint Louis, MO 63139
Fax: 314-877-6405
E-mail: pathways@mimh.edu
www.pathways2promise.org

Pathways to Promise is an interfaith technical assistance and resource center which offers liturgical and educational materials, program models, and networking information to promote a caring ministry with people with mental illness and their families.

210 Rational Recovery
PO Box 800
Lotus, CA 95651
530-621-2667
www.www.rational.org

Exclusive, worldwide source of counseling, guidance and direct instruction on self-recovery from addiction to alcohol and other drugs through planned, permanent abstinence.

211 SADD: Students Against Destructive Decisions
255 Main Street
Marlborough, MA 01752
877-723-3462
Fax: 508-481-5759
E-mail: webmaster@sadd.org
www.www.sadd.org

Peer leadership organization dedicated to preventing destructive decisions, particularly underage drinking, other drug use, impaired driving, teen violence and teen depression and suicide.

212 SMART-Self Management and Recovery Training
7537 Mentor Avenue
Suite 306
Mentor, OH 44060

440-951-5357
866-951-5357
Fax: 440-951-5358
E-mail: info@smartrecovery.org
www.smartrecovery.org

Free face-to-face and online mutual help groups. Helps people recover from all types of addictive behaviors. Also it is an alternative to AA-Alcoholics Anonymous and NA-Narcotics Anonymous.

Video & Audio

213 Alcohol and Sex: Prescription for Poor Decision Making
ETR Associates
4 Carbonero Way
Scotts Valley, CA 95066
831-438-4060
800-321-4407
Fax: 800-435-8433
E-mail: customerservice@etr.org
www.etr.org

Explains how alcohol use can interfere with healthy decisions about sex and intimacy, as well as describing the effects of alcohol on the brain. Also, includes information about the date rape drug, how alcohol affects relationships, and includes a Teacher Resource Book. *$139.95*

214 Alcohol: the Substance, the Addiction, the Solution
Hazelden
15251 Pleasant Valley Road
PO Box 176
Center City, MN 55012-0176
651-213-4000
800-328-9000
Fax: 651-213-4590
www.hazelden.org

Weaves dramatic personal stories of recovery from alcoholism with essential facts about alcohol itself. Emphasizes the impact of using and abusing alcohol in conjunction with other drugs. Educates about the dangers of this legally sanctioned drug, including the myth of safer versions such as wine and beer. *$225.00*

215 Binge Drinking
ETR Associates
4 Carbonero Way
Scotts Valley, CA 95066
831-438-4060
800-321-4407
Fax: 800-435-8433
E-mail: customerservice@etr.org
www.etr.org

Explains the physiological and psychological effects of alcohol, covers the warning signs for alcohol poisoning and procedures to take to save someone, and delivers a no-nonsense message about why binge drinking is dangerous. Describes the catastrophic realities that can result from party behavior, such as car crashes, falls, bad decisions and acquaintance rape. *$139.95*

216 Cocaine & Crack: Back from the Abyss
Hazelden
15251 Pleasant Valley Road
PO Box 176
Center City, MN 55012-0176
651-213-4000
800-257-7810
Fax: 651-213-4411
E-mail: info@hazelden.org
www.hazelden.org

Provides clients in correctional, educational, and treatment settings an understanding of the history, pharamacology, and medical impact of cocaine/crack use through personal stories of addiction and recovery. Reveals proven methods for overcoming addiction and discusses the best ways to maintain recovery. 46 minutes. *$225.00*

217 Cross Addiction: Back Door to Relapse
Hazelden
15251 Pleasant Valley Road
PO Box 176
Center City, MN 55012-0176
651-213-2121
800-328-9000
Fax: 651-213-4590
www.hazelden.org

Presents a overview of the nature of cross-addiction. What it looks like, how it happens and why the addict is so susceptible to it. Explains to clients understanding the impact of different drugs and multiple drugs on the mind and body. *$225.00*

218 Disease of Alcoholism Video
Hazelden
15251 Pleasant Valley Road
PO Box 176
Center City, MN 55012-0176
651-213-4000
800-328-9000
Fax: 651-213-4590
www.hazelden.org

This video is used daily in treatment, corporations, and schools. Dr. Ohlms discusses startling and convincing information on the genetic and physiological aspects of alcohol addiction. *$395.00*

219 Fetal Alcohol Syndrome & Fetal Alcohol Effect
Hazelden
15251 Pleasant Valley Road
PO Box 176
Center City, MN 55012-0176
651-213-4000
800-328-9000
Fax: 651-213-4590
www.hazelden.org

If you're a chemical dependency counselor or work with women in pregnancy planning or self-care, this resource is filled with facts to help you better meet your clients needs. *$225.00*

220 Fetal Alcohol Syndrome and Effect, Stories of Help and Hope
Hazelden
15251 Pleasant Valley Road
PO Box 176
Center City, MN 55012-0176

651-213-4000
800-328-9000
Fax: 651-213-4590
www.hazelden.org

Provides clients with a factual defintion of the medical diagonosis of fetal alcohol syndrome and its effects, including how children are diagnosed and the positive prognosis possible for these children. *$225.00*

221 Heroin: What Am I Going To Do?
Hazelden
15251 Pleasant Valley Road
PO Box 176
Center City, MN 55012-0176
651-213-4000
800-328-9000
Fax: 651-213-4590
E-mail: info@hazelden.org
www.hazelden.org

Shares powerful stories and keen insights from recovering heroin addicts and the rewards of clean living. Teaches clients how to use honesty, surrender and responsibility as the power tools for a successful recovery. Deglamorizes heroin use, with a portrait of drug's inevitable degration of the mind, body and spirit. 30 minutes. *$225.00*

222 I'll Quit Tomorrow
Hazelden
15251 Pleasant Valley Road
PO Box 176
Center City, MN 55012-0176
651-213-4000
800-328-9000
Fax: 651-213-4590
www.hazelden.org

Show clients the progressive nature of alcoholism through one of the most powerful films ever made about this disease. This three-part video series and facilitator's guide use a dramatic personal story to provide a clear and thorough introduction to the disease concept of alcoholism, enabling the intervention process, treatment and the hope of healing and recovery. *$300.00*

223 Marijuana: Escape to Nowhere
Hazelden
15251 Pleasant Valley Road
PO Box 176
Center City, MN 55012-0176
651-213-4000
800-328-9000
Fax: 651-213-4590
E-mail: info@hazelden.org
www.hazelden.org

Challenges myths about marijuana by clearly stating that marijuana is addictive and use results in physical, emotional and spiritual consequences. Explains to clients in simple language the pharmacology of today's more potent marijuana and shares the hope and healing of recovery. 30 minutes. *$225.00*

Year Founded: 1999

224 Medical Aspects of Chemical Dependency
Active Parenting Publishers
Hazelden
15251 Pleasant Valley Road
PO Box 176
Center City, MN 55012-0176
651-213-2121
800-328-9000
Fax: 651-213-4590
E-mail: info@hazelden.org
www.hazelden.org

This curriculum helps professionals educate clients in treatment and other settings about medical effects of chemical use and abuse. The program includes a video that explains body and brain changes that can occur when using alcohol or other drugs, a workbook that helps clients apply the information from the video to their own situations, a handbook that provides in-depth information on addiction, brain chemistry and the physiological effects of chemical dependency and a pamphlet that answers critical questions clients have about the medical effects of chemical dependency. Available to purchase separately. Program value packages available. *$225.00*

225 Methamphetamine: Decide to Live Prevention Video
Hazelden
15251 Pleasant Valley Road
PO Box 176
Center City, MN 55012-0176
651-213-4000
800-328-9000
Fax: 651-213-4590
E-mail: info@hazelden.org
www.hazelden.org

Methamphetamine: Decide to Live presents the latest information on the devastating consequences of meth addiction and the struggles and rewards of recovery. Facts, medical aspects, personal stories, and insights on the recovery process illuminate the path to healing. The video is divided into two parts and is 38 minutes long. *$225.00*

226 Prescription Drugs: Recovery from the Hidden Addiction
Hazelden
15251 Pleasant Valley Road
PO Box 176
Center City, MN 55012-0176
651-213-4000
800-328-9000
Fax: 651-213-4590
E-mail: info@hazelden.org
www.hazelden.org

Combines essential facts about prescription drugs with vivid personal stories of addiction and recovery. Classifies prescription medications and gives the corresponding street forms. Offers solutions to problems unique to presciption drugs, addresses the particular needs of older adults and elaborates on the dangers of cross-addiction. 31 minutes. *$225.00*

227 Reality Check: Marijuana Prevention Video
Hazelden
15251 Pleasant Valley Road
PO Box 176
Center City, MN 55012-0176

651-213-4000
800-328-9000
Fax: 651-213-4590
E-mail: info@hazelden.org
www.hazelden.org

This video creates a strong message for kids about the dangers of marijuana use. A combination of humor, animated graphics, testimonials and music deliver the facts on the pharmacology of marijuana and both it's short and long use consequences. Suitable for kids grades 7-12.
15 minute video. *$225.00*

228 SmokeFree TV: A Nicotine Prevention Video
Hazelden
15251 Pleasant Valley Road
PO Box 176
Center City, MN 55012-0176
651-213-4000
800-328-9000
Fax: 651-213-4590
E-mail: info@hazelden.org
www.hazelden.org

Key facts, consequences of use and refusal skills guide children in understanding why they should avoid nicotine. Animated graphics, stories, humor, and music appeal to young people. Pharmacology of nicotine, its consequences and ways to refuse it are also explored. 15 minute video.
$225.00

229 Straight Talk About Substance Use and Violence
ADD WareHouse
300 NW 70th Avenue
Suite 102
Plantation, FL 33317
954-792-8100
800-233-9273
Fax: 954-792-8545
E-mail: sales@addwarehouse.com
www.addwarehouse.com

Substance abuse and violence prevention begins with this three video program featuring the frank testimonials of 19 teens with significant chemical dependency issues who range in age from 13 to 22. In the starkest terms they discuss their most personal issues: substance abuse, sexual abuse, physical abuse, suicide attempts, violent acting out, depression, and abusive relationships. Includes 95 page discussion guide and three 30 minute videos. *$259.00*

230 What Should I Tell My Child About Drinking?
NADD-National Council on Alcoholism and Drug Dependence
22 Cortlandt Street
Suite 801
New York, NY 10007-3128
212-269-7797
800-622-2255
Fax: 212-269-7510
E-mail: national@ncadd.org
www.ncadd.org

A two-part video to help parents and other caregivers improvve their communications skills about alcohol. Includes brochures and a facilitators guide. Approximately 46 minutes. *$59.99*

Web Sites

231 www.Ncadi.Samhsa.Gov
National Clearinghouse for Alcohol & Drug Information

One-stop resource for information about abuse prevention and addiction treatment.

232 www.aa.org
AA-Alcoholics Anonymous

Group sharing their experience, strength and hope with each other to recover from alcoholism.

233 www.aca-usa.org
American Council on Alcoholism

Referrals to DWI classes and treatment centers.

234 www.addictionresourceguide.com
Addiction Resource Guide

Descriptions of inpatient, outpatient programs.

235 www.adultchildren.org
Adult Children of Alcoholics World Services Organization

12 step and 12 tradition program for adults raised in an environment including alcohol or other dysfunctions.

236 www.al-anon.alateen.org
Al-Anon/Alateen

Program for relatives and friends of persons with alcohol problems.

237 www.alcoholism.about.com/library
Alcohol and the Elderly

Links to other pages relevant to overuse of alcohol and drugs in the elderly.

238 www.cfsny.org
Center for Family Support

Providing care givers with all aspects of service needed.

239 www.doitnow.org/pages/pubhub.hmtl
The Do It Now Foundation

Copies of brochures on drugs, alcohol, smoking, drugs and kids, and street drugs.

240 www.jacsweb.org
Jewish Alcoholics Chemically Dependent Persons

Ten articles dealing with denial and ignorance.

241 www.jointogether.org
Join Together

Alcohol and substance abuse information, legislative alerts, new and updates.

242 www.madd.org
MADD-Mothers Against Drunk Driving

A crusade to stop alcohol consumption, and underage drinking.

243 www.mentalhealth.com
Internet Mental Health

On-line information and a virtual encyclopedia related to mental disorders, possible causes and treatments. News, articles, on-line diagnostic programs and related links. Designed to improve understanding, diagnosis and treatment of mental illness throughout the world. Awarded the Top Site Award and the NetPsych Cutting Edge Site Award.

244 **www.mentalhealth.samhsa.gov**
SAMHSA's National Mental Health Info Center

Information about resources, technical assistance, research, training, networks, and other federal clearing houses, and fact sheets and materials.

245 **www.mhselfhelp.org**
National Mental Health Consumers Self-Help Clearinghouse

Encourages the development and growth of consumer self-help groups.

246 **www.naadac.org**
National Association of Alcohol and Drug Abuse Counselors

Its mission is to lead, unify and empower global addiction focused professionals to achieve excellence through education, advocacy, knowledge, standards of practice, ethics, professional development and research. Advocates on behalf of addiction professionals and the people they serve. Establishes and promotes the highest possible standards of practice and qualifications for addiction professionals.

247 **www.nccbh.org**
National Council for Commuity Behavioral Healthcare

A network for sharing information and provding assistance among those working in the healthcare management field.

248 **www.niaaa.nih.gov**
National Institute on Alcohol Abuse & Alcoholism

Supports research nationwide on alcohol abuse and alcoholism.

249 **www.nida.nih.gov**
National Institute on Drug Abuse

Many publications useful for patients. Research Reports, summaries about chemicals and treatments.

250 **www.nida.nih.gov/drugpages**
Commonly Abused Drugs: Street Names for Drugs of Abuse

Current names, periods of detection, medical uses.

251 **www.nofas.org**
National Organization on Fetal Alcohol Syndrome

Develops and implements innovative prevention and education strategies assessing fetal alcohol syndrome.

252 **www.psychcentral.com**
Psych Central

Personalized one-stop index for psychology, support, and mental health issues, resources, and people on the Internet.

253 **www.sadd.org**
SADD-Students Against Destructive Decisions

Peer leadership organization dedicated to preventing destructive decisions.

254 **www.samhsa.gov**
Substance Abuse and Mental Health Services Administration

Provides links to government resources related to substance abuse and mental health.

255 **www.smartrecovery.org**
SMART: Self-Management and Recovery Training

Four-Point program includes maintaining motivation, coping with urges, managing feelings and behavior, balancing momentary/enduring satisfactions.

256 **www.soulselfhelp.on.ca/coda.html**
Souls Self Help Central

Discusses self-help, mental health, issues of co-dependency.

257 **www.unhooked.com**
LifeRing

Offers nonreligious approach with links to groups.

258 **www.well.com**
Web of Addictions

Links to fact sheets from trustworthy sources.

Anxiety Disorders

Introduction

It is perfectly normal to feel worried or nervous sometimes, especially if there is an obvious reason: a loved one is late coming home; you are about to have your yearly evaluation meeting at work; an important social event is looming. Even when you are nervous or anxious with good cause, you continue performing life's functions adequately. Indeed, some anxiety is not only normal, it is necessary, helping us to avoid trouble and danger - like preparing for a test in school, or making sure your child is safely buckled into a car. But if you can't rid yourself of your worry, you worry all the time, you worry about everything, if people close to you comment that you seem bothered and unlike yourself, or if your nervousness is affecting your relationships and your work, it is time to seek help. Sometimes a person who suffers from persistent anxiety turns to alcohol or other drugs in an effort to seek relief.

Different kinds of Anxiety Disorders have been identified. Several of the most prevalent are discussed in detail below. Treatment is tailored to the particular disorder and has become more effective as a result.

Repeated panic attacks, may be followed by continuous anxiety that another attack will occur, fear of terrible consequences (e.g. having a heart attack or going crazy), and behavior that is markedly changed because of the attacks. This behavior change may consist of agoraphobia. A panic attack is a period of intense fear in which four or more of the following symptoms escalate suddenly, reaching a peak within ten minutes, after which they diminish: Palpitations and pounding; rapid heartbeat; sweating; trembling or shaking; shortness of breath; feeling of choking; chest pain; nausea; feeling dizzy or faint; feelings of unreality or detachment; fear of losing control or going crazy; fear of dying; numbness or tingling; chills or hot flashes.

SYMPTOMS

Agoraphobia
• Usually involves fears connected with being outside the home and alone;
• Anxiety about being in places or situations from which it is difficult or embarrassing to escape (e.g., in the middle seat of a row in a theatre) or in which help may not be immediately available (as in an airplane);
• Such situations are avoided or endured with distress and fear of having a panic attack.

Social Anxiety Disorder
• Fear of being humiliated or embarrassed in a social situation with strangers or where other people are watching;
• Being in the situation causes intense anxiety, sometimes with panic attacks;
• Realizing that the fear is irrational;
• Unlike simple shyness, the fear leads to avoidance of important or uncomplicated social situations and interferes with the ability to function at work or with friends and family.

General Anxiety Disorder
• Excessive worry and anxiety on most days for at least six months about several events or activities such as work or school performance;
• Difficulty in controlling the worry;

• The anxiety is connected with at least three of the following: restlessness/feeling on edge; being easily tired; difficulty concentrating; irritability; muscle tension; difficulty falling/staying asleep or restless sleep;
• The anxiety or physical symptoms seriously affect the person's social life, work life, or other important areas.

Phobias
• Persistent, unreasonable, and exaggerated fear of the presence or anticipated presence of a particular object or situation (e.g., snake, flying in an airplane; blood);
• The presence of such an object or situation triggers immediate anxiety which may be a panic attack;
• Knowledge that the fear is exaggerated and unreasonable;
• The phobic situation is either avoided or experienced with extreme distress;
• The avoidance, fearful anticipation, and distress seriously affects the person's normal routine, work and social activities, and relationships.

ASSOCIATED FEATURES

Anxiety can be acute and intense such as the fear of imminent death in a panic attack or it can be experienced as a state of chronic nagging worry in Generalized Anxiety Disorder. Whatever its intensity or frequency, it persists over time. One of the hallmarks of Anxiety Disorders is that the person is unable to control the anxiety, even when he or she knows it is exaggerated and unreasonable. To other people, the person may seem edgy, irritable, fearful, or have unexpected outbursts of anger. For the anxious person, the problem takes up time and effort and becomes a major preoccupation. In addition to the psychological effects (and entangled with them) are the physical effects, that is, a frequent or constant state of physical arousal and tension. This can lead to gastrointestinal upset, headaches, and cardiovascular disease. Using alcohol or drugs to resolve the problem is ineffective and dangerous. Anxiety Disorders negatively affect all aspects of life-family, work, and friends.

PREVALENCE

Anxiety Disorders are the most common psychiatric disorders in the U.S. Anxiety Disorders are approximately twice as common in women as in men.

TREATMENT OPTIONS

It is very important to have a psychiatric evaluation so that a proper diagnosis can be made. (Some people can be adequately diagnosed by a primary care physician, nurse practitoner, or another mental health profesional. That is true of most of the disorders. In general, people should have a primary care evaluation as part of the diagnostic process for all disorders, so as to rule out a general medical condition that could be causing the signs and symptoms. For example, hyperthyroidism can cause anxiety problems; hypothyroidism can look like deperssion.) Self medication with alcohol, tranquilizers, or other drugs is dangerous and can lead to serious drug abuse. Many people who abuse drugs are suffering from an underlying Anxiety Disorder. Treatment will vary depending on which of the Anxiety Disorders is diagnosed. Medications, psychotherapy or both will be prescribed. Some psychotherapies which have proven helpful in certain cases are cognitive-behavioral therapies, including exposure therapy. Eye movement desensitization therapy is controversial. Benzodiazepines, or minor tranquillizers, can be useful for the acute treatment of anxiety symptoms; care must be taken, because these medications have addictive potential. Selective Serotonin Reuptake Inhibitors, or SSRIs, which were originally developed as Antidepressants, have proved to be effective in several Anxiety Disorders and are now the mainstays of treatment. Since new drugs are frequently introduced, and already approved medications given new therapeutic indications by the USDA, it is wise to consult an expert or recent expert reference before making a treatment decision.

Suddenly stopping an SSRI can cause rebound symptoms including sleeplessness, headaches, and irritability. Medications should be tapered under the care of a physician.

Associations & Agencies

260 Agoraphobics in Motion
1719 Crooks Road
Royal Oak, MI 48067-1306
248-547-0400
E-mail: anny@ameritech.net
www.aim-hq.org

AIM is a nationwide, nonprofit, support group organization, committed to the support and recovery of those suffering with anxiety disorders, and their families.

261 Anxiety Disorders Association of America
8730 Georgia Avenue
Suite 600
Silver Spring, MD 20910
240-485-1001
Fax: 240-485-1035
www.adaa.org

Alies Muskin, COO
J. Teichroew, Director, Media Relations and Co

A national non profit organization dedicated exclusively to promoting the prevention, treatment, and cure of anxiety disorders and improving the lives of all people touched by these disorders.

262 Anxiety and Phobia Treatment Center
White Plains Hospital Center
Davis Avenue at E Post Road
White Plains, NY 10601
914-681-1038
Fax: 914-681-2284
E-mail: jchessa@wphospital.org
www.phobia-anxiety.org

Fredrick J Neumen MD, Director
Judy Lake Chessa, Coordinator

Treatment groups for individuals suffering from phobias. Deals with fears through contextual therapy, a treatment and study of the phobia in the actual setting in which the phobic reactions occur.

263 Career Assessment & Planning Services
Goodwill Industries-Suncoast
10596 Gandy Boulevard
PO Box 14456
St. Petersburg, FL 33733
727-523-1512
888-279-1988
Fax: 727-563-9300
E-mail: gw.marketing@goodwill-suncoast.com
www.goodwill-suncoast.org

R Lee Waits, President/CEO
Deborah A Passerini, VP Operations

Provides a comprehensive assessment, which can predict current and future employment and potential adjustment factors for physically, emotionally, or developmentally disabled persons who may be unemployed or underemployed. Assessments evaluate interests, aptitudes, academic achievements, and physical abilities (including dexterity and coordination) through coordinated testing, interviewing and behavioral observations.

264 Center for Family Support (CFS)
333 7th Avenue
New York, NY 10001-5004
212-629-7939
Fax: 212-239-2211
www.cfsny.org

Steven Vernickofs, Executive Director

An agency that continues to develop new programs to serve families and individuals with their care needs. Offering services throughout the New York City Region including: New Jersey, Long Island and the Lower Hudson Valley.

265 Center for Mental Health Services Knowledge
PO Box 42557
Washington, DC 20015-4800
800-789-2647
Fax: 240-747-5484
E-mail: ken@mentalhealth.org
www.mentalhealth.org

A. Kathryn Power, Director
Edward B Searle, Deputy Director

Information about resources, technical assistance, research, training, networks, and other federal clearing houses, and fact sheets and materials. Information specialists refer callers to mental health resources in their communities as well as state, federal and nonprofit contacts. Staff available Monday through Friday, 8:30 AM-5:00 PM, EST, excluding federal holidays. After hours, callers may leave messages and an information specialist will return their call.

266 Freedom From Fear
308 Seaview Avenue
Staten Island, NY 10305
718-351-1717
Fax: 718-667-8893
E-mail: help@freedomfromfear.org
www.freedomfromfear.com

Jack D Maser PhD, Professor of Psychiatry

The mission of Freedom From Fear is to aid and counsel individuals and their families who suffer from anxiety and depressive illness.

267 International Critical Incident Stress Foundation
3290 Pine Orchard Lane
Suite 106
Ellicott City, MD 21042
410-750-9600
Fax: 410-750-9601
E-mail: info@icisf.org
www.icisf.org

Donald Howell, President/CEO
Stephanie Beam, General Information

A nonprofit, open membership foundation dedicated to the prevention and mitigation of disabling stress by education, training and support services for all emergency service professionals.

268 National Alliance on Mental Illness
2107 Wilson Boulevard
Suite 300
Arlington, VA 22201-3042
703-524-7600
800-950-6264
Fax: 703-524-9094
E-mail: helpline@nami.org
www.nami.org

Michael Fitzpatrick, Executive Director

Nation's leading self-help organization for all those affected by severe brain disorders. Mission is to bring consumers and families with similar experiences together to share information about services, care providers, and ways to cope with the challenges of schizophrenia, manic depression, and other serious mental illnesses.

269 National Anxiety Foundation
3135 Custer Drive
Lexington, KY 40517-4001
859-272-7166
www.lexington-on-line.com/naf.html

Stephanie Cox MD, President/Medical Director
Linda Vernon Blair, VP

To alleviate suffering and to save lives by educating the public about anxiety disorders.

270 National Association for the Dually Diagnose d (NADD)
132 Fair Street
Kingston, NY 12401-4802
845-334-4336
800-331-5362
Fax: 845-331-4569
E-mail: nadd@mhv.net
www.thenadd.org

Dr. Robert Fletcher, Founder/CEO

Nonprofit organization designed to promote interest of professional and parent development with resources for individuals who have the coexistence of mental illness and mental retardation. Provides conference, educational services and training materials to professionals, parents, concerned citizens and service organizations. Formerly known as the National Association for the Dually Diagnosed.

Year Founded: 1983

271 National Mental Health Consumer's
1211 Chestnut Street
Suite 1207
Philadelphia, PA 19107
215-751-1810
800-553-4539
Fax: 215-636-6312
E-mail: info@mhselfhelp.org
www.mhselfhelp.org

Christine Simiriglia, Executive Director
Jennifer Melinn, Information/Refferal Dept.

Funded by the National Institute of Mental Health Community Support Program, the purpose of the Clearinghouse is to encourage the development and growth of consumer self-help groups.

272 National Mental Health Consumers' Self-Help Clearinghouse
1211 Chestnut Street
Suite 1207
Philadelphia, PA 19107
215-751-1810
800-553-4539
Fax: 215-636-6312
E-mail: info@mhselfhelp.org
www.mhselfhelp.org

Joseph Rogers, Executive Director

A national consumer technical assistance center that has played a major role in the development of the mental health consumer movement.

Year Founded: 1986

273 SAMHSA's National Mental Health Information Center
US Department of Health and Human Services
PO Box 42557
Washington, DC 20015
240-221-4021
800-789-2647
Fax: 240-221-4295
TDD: 866-889-2647
www.www.mentalhealth.samhsa.gov

Provides information about mental health via a toll-free telephone number, this web site, and more than 600 publications. Developed for users of mental health services and their families, the general public, policy makers, providers, and the media.

274 Selective Mutism Foundation
PO Box 13133
Sissonville, WV 25360
305-748-7714
Fax: 305-748-7714
E-mail: sue@selectivemutismfoundation.org
www.selectivemutismfoundation.org

Sue Newman, Co-Founder/Director
Carolyn Miller, Co-Founder/Director

Promote awareness and understanding for individuals and families affected by selective mutism, an inherited anxiety disorder in which children with normal or deficient language skills are unable to speak in school or social situations.

275 Suncoast Residential Training Center/Developmental Services Program
Goodwill Industries-Suncoast
10596 Gandy Boulevard
St. Petersburg, FL 33733
727-523-1512
888-279-1988
Fax: 727-563-9300
E-mail: gw.marketing@goodwill-suncoast.com
www.goodwill-suncoast.org

R Lee Waits, President/CEO
Deborah A Passerini, VP Operations

A large group home which serves individuals diagnosed as mentally retarded with a secondary diagnosis of psychiatric difficulties as evidenced by problem behavior. Providing residential, behavioral and instructional support and services that will promote the development of adaptive, socially appropriate behavior. Each individual is assessed to determine, socialization, basic academics and recreation. The primary intervention strategy is applied behavior analysis. Professional consultants are utilized to address the medical, dental, psychiatric and pharmacological needs of each individual. One of the most popular features is the active community integration component of SRTC. Program customers attend an average of 15 monthly outings to various community events.

276 Territorial Apprehensiveness (TERRAP) Programs
14 Wood Lake Square
Houston, TX 77063
713-266-5111
800-274-6242
Fax: 337-474-2782
E-mail: terrap@cox.net
www.terraphouston.com

Shirley Riff, Director

Territorial Apprehensiveness was formed to disseminate information concerning the recognition, causes, and treatment of anxieties, fears and phobias especially agoraphobia.

Books

277 100 Q&A About Panic Disorder
Jones and Bartlett Publishers
40 Tall Pine Drive
Sudbury, MA 01776
978-443-5000
800-832-0034
Fax: 978-443-8000
E-mail: info@jbpub.com
www.www.jbpub.com

Carol Berman, Author
ISBN 0-763727-15-6

278 Acceptance and Commitment Therapy for Anxiet y Disorders
New Harbinger Publications
5674 Shattuck Avenue
Oakland, CA 94609-1662
510-652-2002
800-748-6273
Fax: 510-652-5472
E-mail: customerservice@newharbinger.com
www.newharbinger.com

The first step-by-step professional book that teaches how to apply and integrate acceptance and mindfulness for treatment with anxiety disorders. *$58.95*

304 pages ISBN 1-572244-27-5

279 An End to Panic: Breakthrough Techniques for Overcoming Panic Disorder
New Harbinger Publications
5674 Shattuck Avenue
Oakland, CA 94609-1662
510-652-2002
800-748-6273
Fax: 510-652-5472
E-mail: customerservice@newharbinger.com
www.newharbinger.com

A state of the art treatment program covers breathing retraining, taking charge of fear fueling thoughts, overcoming the fear of physical symptoms, coping with phobic situations, avoiding relapse, and living in the here and now. *$18.95*

230 pages ISBN 1-572241-13-6

280 Anxiety & Phobia Workbook
New Harbinger Publications
5674 Shattuck Avenue
Oakland, CA 94609-1662
510-652-2002
800-748-6273
Fax: 510-652-5472
E-mail: customerservice@newharbinger.com
www.newharbinger.com

This comprehensive guide is recommended to those struggling with anxiety disorders. Includes step by step instructions for the crucial cognitive - behavioral techniques that have given real help to hundreds of thousands of readers struggling with anxiety disorders. *$19.95*

448 pages ISBN 1-572240-03-2

281 Anxiety Cure: Eight Step-Program for Getting Well
John Wiley & Sons
605 3rd Avenue
New York, NY 10058-0180
212-850-6000
Fax: 212-850-6008
E-mail: info@wiley.com
www.wiley.com

Anxiety disorders are the most common type of emotional trouble and among the most treatable. Dupont provides a practical guide featuring a step-by-step program for curing the six kinds of anxiety. *$14.95*

256 pages ISBN 0-471247-01-4

282 Anxiety Disorders
Cambridge University Press
40 W 20th Street
New York, NY 10011-4211
212-924-3900
800-872-7423
Fax: 212-691-3239
E-mail: marketing@cup.org
www.cup.org

Stephen Bourne, Chief Press Executive / Director

This comprehensive text covers all the anxiety disorders found in the latest DSM and ICD classifications. Provides detailed information about seven principal disorders, including anxiety in the medically ill. For each disorder, the book covers diagnosis criteria, epidemiology, etiology and pathogenesis, clinical features, natural history and different diagnosis. Describes treatment approaches, both psychological and pharmacological. *$74.95*

354 pages

283 Anxiety and Its Disorders
Guilford Publications
72 Spring Street
New York, NY 10012
212-431-9800
800-365-7006
Fax: 212-966-6708

E-mail: info@guilford.com
www.guilford.com

Incorporating recent advances from cognitive science and neurobiology on the mechanisms of anxiety and using emotion theory as basic theoretical framework. Ties theory and research of emerging clinical knowledge to create a new model of anxiety with profound implications for treatment. *$75.00*

700 pages ISBN 1-572304-30-8

284 Anxiety, Phobias, and Panic
Grand Central Publishing
322 South Enterprise Blvd
Lebanon, IN 46052
800-759-0190
www.www.hachettebookgroupusa.com

Reneau Z Peurifoy, Author

Congratulations! You are about to start a journey along the path to freedom.

ISBN 0-446692-77-8

285 Anxiety, Phobias, and Panic: a Step-By-Step Program for Regaining Control of Your Life
Time Warner Books
3 Center Plaza
Boston, MA 02108
800-759-0190
Fax: 800-331-1664
E-mail: sales@aoltwbg.com
www.twbookmark.com

Helps you identify stress and reduce stress anxiety, recognize and change distorted mental habits, stop thinking and acting like a victim, eliminate the excessive need for approval, make anger your friend and ally, stand up for yourself and feel good about yourself, and conquer your fears and take charge of your life. *$11.00*

363 pages ISBN 0-446670-53-7

286 Beyond Anxiety and Phobia
New Harbinger Publications
5674 Shattuck Avenue
Oakland, CA 94609-1662
510-652-2002
800-748-6273
Fax: 510-652-5472
E-mail: customerservice@newharbinger.com
www.newharbinger.com

Helping people try to get beyond anxiety and their phobia. *$19.95*

264 pages ISBN 1-572242-29-9

287 Biology of Anxiety Disorders
American Psychiatric Publishing
1000 Wilson Boulevard
Suite 1825
Arlington, VA 22209-3901
703-907-7322
800-368-5777
Fax: 703-907-1091
E-mail: appi@psych.org
www.appi.org

Provides the most recent data on the neurobiology and pathophysiology af anxiety from a variety of perspectives. *$30.50*

280 pages Year Founded: 1993 ISBN 0-880484-76-4

288 Cognitive Therapy for Depression and Anxiety
American Psychiatric Publishing
1000 Wilson Boulevard
Suite 1825
Arlington, VA 22209-3901
703-907-7322
800-368-5777
Fax: 703-907-1091
E-mail: appi@psych.org
www.appi.org

Katie Duffy, Marketing Assistant

Detailed guide to using cognitive therapy in the treatment of patients suffering from depression and anxiety - two of the most prevalent disorders encountered in the community. *$44.95*

240 pages ISBN 0-632039-86-8

289 Comorbidity of Mood and Anxiety Disorders
American Psychiatric Publishing
1000 Wilson Boulevard
Suite 1825
Arlington, VA 22209-3901
703-907-7322
800-368-5777
Fax: 703-907-1091
E-mail: appi@psych.org
www.appi.org

Katie Duffy, Assistant Editor

Presents a systematic examination of the concurrence of different symptoms and syndromes in patients with anxiety or mood disorders. *$75.00*

868 pages ISBN 0-880483-24-5

290 Concise Guide to Anxiety Disorders
American Psychiatric Publishing
1000 Wilson Boulevard
Suite 1825
Arlington, VA 22209-3901
703-907-7322
800-368-5777
Fax: 703-907-1091
E-mail: appi@psych.org
www.appi.org

Robert S Pursell, Marketing

Concise Guide to Anxiety Disorders summarizes the latest research and translates it into practical treatment strategies for the best clinical outcomes. Designed for daily use in the clinical setting, it serves as an instant library of current information, quick to access and easy to understand. Every clinician who diagnoses and treats patients with anxiety disorders-including psychiatrists, residents and medical students, psychologists, and mental health professionals-will find this book invaluable for making informed treatment decisions. *$29.95*

272 pages Year Founded: 2003 ISBN 1-585620-80-7

291 Consumer's Guide to Psychiatric Drugs
New Harbinger Publications
5674 Shattuck Avenue
Oakland, CA 94609-1662
510-652-2002
800-748-6273
Fax: 510-652-5472

E-mail: customerservice@newharbinger.com
www.newharbinger.com

Helps consumers understand what treatment options are available and what side effects to expect. Covers possible interactions with other drugs, medical conditions and other concerns. Explains how each drug works, and offers detailed information about treatments for depression, bipolar disorder, anxiety and sleep disorders, as well as other conditions. *$16.95*

340 pages ISBN 1-572241-11-X

292   Coping with Anxiety
New Harbinger Publications
5674 Shattuck Avenue
Oakland, CA 94609-1662
510-652-2002
800-748-6273
Fax: 510-652-5472
E-mail: customerservice@newharbinger.com
www.newharbinger.com

Ten simple steps, proven to help relieve anxiety. *$ 10.95*

176 pages ISBN 1-572243-20-1

293   Coping with Social Anxiety: The Definitive G uide to Effective Treatment Options
Holt Paperbacks
175 Fifth Avenue
New York, NY 10010
646-307-5095
Fax: 212-633-0748
E-mail: publicity@hholt.com
www.henryholt.com

Eric Hollander, Author

An essential guide for the 5.3 million American sufferers of social anxiety from a leading psychiatrist and researcher.

ISBN 0-805075-82-8

294   Coping with Trauma: A Guide to Self Understanding
Anxiety Disorders Association of America
8730 Georgia Avenue
Suite 600
Silver Spring, MD 20910
301-231-9350
Fax: 301-231-7392
E-mail: AnxDis@adaa.org
www.adaa.org

Alies Muskin, COO
Michelle Alonso, Communications/Membership

Book will appeal to survivors of traumatic stress, as well as mental health professionals.

295   Don't Panic: Taking Control of Anxiety Attacks
Anxiety Disorders Association of America
8730 Georgia Avenue
Suite 600
Silver Spring, MD 20910
301-231-9350
Fax: 301-231-7392
E-mail: AnxDis@adaa.org
www.adaa.org

Alies Muskin, COO
Michelle Alonso, Communications/Marketing

Book on overcoming panic and anxiety.

296   Drug Therapy and Anxiety Disorders
Mason Crest Publishers
370 Reed Road
Suite 302
Broomall, PA 19008
610-543-6200
866-627-2665
Fax: 610-543-3878
E-mail: dtaylor@masoncrest.com
www.masoncrest.com

This volume provides readers with a clear introduction to anxiety disorders. Numerous case studies give insight into the world of mental disorders and helps readers understand the symptoms and treatments of this disorder, which includes: generalized anxiety disorder, social phobia, specific phobia, obsessive-compulsive disorder (covered more extensively in a separate column), post-traumatic stress disorder, and panic disorder.

ISBN 1-590845-61-7

297   Dying of Embarrassment: Help for Social Anxiety and Social Phobia
New Harbinger Publications
5674 Shattuck Avenue
Oakland, CA 94609-1662
510-652-2002
800-748-6273
Fax: 510-652-5472
E-mail: customerservice@newharbinger.com
www.newharbinger.com

Clear, supportive instructions for assessing your fears, improving or developing new social skills, and changing self defeating thinking patterns. *$13.95*

204 pages ISBN 1-879237-23-7

298   Encyclopedia of Phobias, Fears, and Anxieties
Facts on File
132 West 31st Street
17th Floor
New York, NY 10001-2006
800-322-8755
Fax: 800-678-3633
E-mail: custserv@factsonfile.com
www.factsonfile.com

Providing the basic information on common phobias and anxieties, some 2000 entries explain the nature of anxiety disorders, panic attacks, specific phobias, and obsessive-compulsive disorders. *$71.50*

576 pages Year Founded: 2000 ISBN 0-816039-89-5

299   Five Weeks to Healing Stress: the Wellness Option
New Harbinger Publications
5674 Shattuck Avenue
Oakland, CA 94609-1662
510-652-2002
800-748-6273
Fax: 510-652-5472
E-mail: customerservice@newharbinger.com
www.newharbinger.com

This workbook presents a quick and effective, body oriented program for regaining inner strength and calming stress. *$17.95*

216 pages ISBN 1-572240-55-5

300 Flying Without Fear
New Harbinger Publications
5674 Shattuck Avenue
Oakland, CA 94609-1662
510-652-2002
800-748-6273
Fax: 510-652-5472
E-mail: customerservice@newharbinger.com
www.newharbinger.com

Program to confront fears of flying and guides you through first takeoff and later flights. *$13.95*

176 pages ISBN 1-572240-42-3

301 Free from Fears: New Help for Anxiety, Panic and Agoraphobia
Anxiety Disorders Association of America
8730 Georgia Avenue
Suite 600
Silver Spring, MD 20910
301-231-9350
Fax: 301-231-7392
E-mail: AnxDis@adaa.org
www.adaa.org

Alies Muskin, COO
Michelle Alonso, Communications/Membership

Book shows you how to recognize the avoidance trap, combat fears, and modify your behavior for a lasting cure.

302 Freeing Your Child from Anxiety: Powerful, P ractical Solutions to Overcome Your Child's Fears, Worries, and Phobias
Broadway Books
1745 Broadway
New York, NY 10019
212-782-9000
E-mail: bwaypub@randomhouse.com
www.www.randomhouse.com

Tamar Chansky, Author
Phillip Stern, Author

"From the children: When I was little my mom worked the "graveyard shift" at the hospital

303 Healing Fear: New Approaches to Overcoming Anxiety
New Harbinger Publications
5674 Shattuck Avenue
Oakland, CA 94609-1662
510-652-2002
800-748-6273
Fax: 510-652-5472
E-mail: customerservice@newharbinger.com
www.newharbinger.com

Covers a wide range of healing strategies that help you learn how to relinquish control, discover a unique purpose that is bigger than your particular fears, and find ways to restructure your work and home environments to make them more congruent with the real you. *$ 16.95*

416 pages ISBN 1-572241-16-0

304 How to Help Your Loved One Recover from Agoraphobia
Anxiety Disorders Association of America
8730 Georgia Avenue
Suite 600
Silver Spring, MD 20910

301-231-9350
Fax: 301-231-7392
E-mail: AnxDis@adaa.org
www.adaa.org

Alies Muskin, COO
Michelle Alonso, Communications/Membership

Book is helpful for sufferer and family members to understand what a sufferer is going through.

305 Integrative Treatment of Anxiety Disorders
American Psychiatric Publishing
1000 Wilson Boulevard
Suite 1825
Arlington, VA 22209-3901
703-907-7322
800-368-5777
Fax: 703-907-1091
E-mail: appi@psych.org
www.appi.org

An overview of the spectrum of anxiety disorders, and reviews the treatment alternatives. *$67.00*

349 pages Year Founded: 1996 ISBN 0-880487-15-1

306 It's Not All In Your Head: Now Women Can Discover the Real Causes of their Most Misdiagnosed Health Problems
Anxiety Disorders Association of America
8730 Georgia Avenue
Suite 600
Silver Spring, MD 20910
301-231-9350
Fax: 301-231-7392
E-mail: AnxDis@adaa.org
www.adaa.org

Alies Muskin, COO
Michelle Alonso, Communications/Membership

This book will present you with information about when, how and from whom to seek treatment.

307 Managing Social Anxiety: A Cognitive-Behavio ral Therapy Approach Client Workbook (Treatments That Work)
Oxford University Press
2001 Evans Road
Carry, NC 27513
800-445-9714
Fax: 919-677-1303
E-mail: custserv.us@oup.com
www.www.oup.com/us

Debra A Hope, Author
Richard G Heimberg, Author

This is a client workbook for those in treatment or considering treatment for social anxiety.

ISBN 0-195183-82-7

308 Master Your Panic and Take Back Your Life
Anxiety Disorders Association of America
8730 Georgia Avenue
Suite 600
Silver Spring, MD 20910
301-231-9350
Fax: 301-231-7392
E-mail: AnxDis@adaa.org
www.adaa.org

Alies Muskin, COO
Michelle Alonso, Communications/Membership

This book will help those suffering from panic and agoraphobia.

309 **Master Your Panic and Take Back Your Life: Twelve Treatment Sessions to Overcome High Anxiety**
Impact Publishers
PO Box 6016
Atascadero, CA 93423-6016
805-466-5917
800-246-7228
Fax: 805-466-5919
E-mail: info@impactpublishers.com
www.impactpublishers.com

Practical, self empowering book on overcoming agoraphobia and debilitating panic attacks is now completely revised and expanded to include the latest information and research findings on relaxation, breathing, medication and other treatments. *$15.95*

304 pages Year Founded: 1998 ISBN 1-886230-08-0

310 **Mastery of Your Anxiety and Panic: Workbook**
Oxford University Press
2001 Evans Road
Cary, NC 27513
800-445-9714
Fax: 919-677-1303
E-mail: custserv.us@oup.com
www.www.oup.com/us

David H Barlow, Author

If you are prone to panic attacks and constantly worry about when the next attack may come, you may suffer from panic disorder and/or agoraphobia. Though panic disorder seems irrational and uncontrollable, it has been proven that a treatment like the one outlined in this book can help you take control of your life.

ISBN 0-195311-35-3

311 **My Quarter-Life Crisis: How an Anxiety Disorder Knocked Me Down, and How I Got Back Up**
Tucket Pub 01776

Lee Wellman, Author

ISBN 0-978751-57-4

312 **No More Butterflies: Overcoming Shyness, Stagefright, Interview Anxiety, and Fear of Public Speaking**
New Harbinger Publications
5674 Shattuck Avenue
Oakland, CA 94609-1662
510-652-2002
800-748-6273
Fax: 510-652-5472
E-mail: customerservice@newharbinger.com
www.newharbinger.com

Demonstrates how to pinpoint fears, refute fear - provoking thoughts, and exhibit confidence at interviews and auditions. *$13.95*

176 pages ISBN 1-572240-41-5

313 **Panic Disorder and Agoraphobia: A Guide**
Madison Institute of Medicine
7617 Mineral Point Road
Suite 300
Madison, WI 53717-1623
608-827-2470
Fax: 608-827-2479
E-mail: mim@miminc.org
www.miminc.org

Learn about the causes of panic disorder and agoraphobia and how patients can overcome these disabling disorders with medications and behavior therapy in this booklet written by leading experts on the subject. *$5.95*

69 pages

314 **Panic Disorder: Critical Analysis**
Guilford Publications
72 Spring Street
New York, NY 10012
212-431-9800
800-365-7006
Fax: 212-966-6708
E-mail: info@guilford.com
www.guilford.com

Provides a comprehensive, integrative exploration of panic disorder. Discusses the phenomenology of the disorder, with extensive reviews of the epidemiology, biological aspects and psychopharmacalogic treatments, followed by detailed explorations of psychological aspects, including predictability and controllability and psychological treatments including cognitive behavioral techniques. *$38.00*

276 pages ISBN 0-898622-63-8

315 **Pharmacotherapy for Mood, Anxiety and Cognit ive Disorders**
American Psychiatric Publishing
1000 Wilson Boulevard
Suite 1825
Arlington, VA 22209-3901
703-907-7322
800-368-5777
Fax: 703-907-1091
E-mail: appi@psych.org
www.appi.org

Takes a critical look at the different medications available for treating mood, anxiety and cognitive disorders. Also, it takes a look at their relevance to pathobiology and the underlying mechanisms, and the limitations. *$99.00*

832 pages Year Founded: 2000 ISBN 0-880488-85-9

316 **Phobias And How to Overcome Them: Understand ing and Beating Your Fears**
New Page Books
3 Tice Road
PO Box 687
Franklin Lakes, NJ 07417
201-848-0310
800-227-3371
www.www.newpagebooks.com

James Gardner, Author

Do you or does someone you care about suffer from phobias?

ISBN 1-564147-66-5

317 Relaxation & Stress Reduction Workbook
New Harbinger Publications
5674 Shattuck Avenue
Oakland, CA 94609-1662
510-652-2002
800-748-6273
Fax: 510-652-5472
E-mail: customerservice@newharbinger.com
www.newharbinger.com

Matthew McKay, Editor

Step by step instructions cover progressive muscle relaxation, meditation, autogenics, visualization, thought stopping, refuting irrational ideas, coping skills training, job stress management, and much more. *$17.95*

256 pages ISBN 1-879237-82-2

318 Shy Children, Phobic Adults: Nature and Treatment of Social Phobia
American Psychological Association
750 First Street, NE
Washington, DC 20002-4242
202-336-5500
800-374-2721
TTY: 202-336-6123
www.www.apa.org

Deborah C Beidel, Author

Medical University of South Charleston. Recent advances in the understanding of social phobia.

ISBN 1-557984-61-1

319 Social Anxiety Disorder: A Guide
Madison Institute of Medicine
7617 Mineral Point Road
Suite 300
Madison, WI 53717-1623
608-827-2470
Fax: 608-827-2479
E-mail: mim@miminc.org
www.miminc.org

Do you fear public speaking or do you avoid social situations because you worry you may do something embarrassing or humiliating? Learn how social anxiety disorder, also known as social phobia, is diagnosed and treated in this thorough publication written by leading experts on the subject. *$5.95*

61 pages

320 Social Phobia: From Shyness to Stage Fright
Anxiety Disorders Association of America
8730 Georgia Avenue
Suite 600
Silver Spring, MD 20910
301-231-9350
Fax: 301-231-7392
E-mail: AnxDis@adaa.org
www.adaa.org

Alies Muskin, COO
Michelle Alonso, Communications/Membership

Book on social phobia.

321 Stop Obsessing: How to Overcome Your Obsessions and Compulsions
Anxiety Disorders Association of America
8730 Georgia Avenue
Suite 600
Silver Spring, MD 20910
301-231-9350
Fax: 301-231-7392
E-mail: AnxDis@adaa.org
www.adaa.org

Alies Muskin, COO
Michelle Alonso, Communications/Membership

Book provides knowledgeable descriptions of the steps, the challenges, and the value of self - treatment.

322 Stress-Related Disorders Sourcebook
Omnigraphics
PO Box 625
Holmes, PA 19043
800-234-1340
Fax: 800-875-1340
E-mail: info@omnigraphics.com
www.omnigraphics.com

Omnigraphics is the publisher of the Health Reference Series, a growing consumer health information resource with more than 100 volumes in print. Each title in the series features an easy to understand format, nontechnical language, comprehensive indexing and resources for further information. Material in each book has been collected from a wide range of government agencies, professional associations, periodicals, and other sources. *$78.00*

600 pages ISBN 0-780805-60-7

323 Ten Simple Solutions To Panic
New Harbinger Publications
5674 Shattuck Avenue
Oakland, CA 94609-1662
510-652-2002
800-748-6273
Fax: 510-652-5472
E-mail: customerservice@newharbinger.com
www.newharbinger.com

Provides readers who have at one time or another experienced unexplainable, intense mental and physical attacks over time. *$11.95*

152 pages ISBN 1-572243-25-2

324 Textbook of Anxiety Disorders
American Psychiatric Publishing
1000 Wilson Boulevard
Suite 1825
Arlington, VA 22209-3901
703-907-732
800-368-5777
Fax: 703-907-1091
E-mail: appi@psych.org
www.appi.org

Katie Duffy, Marketing Assistant

US and international experts cover every major anxiety disorder, compare it with animal behavior and the similarities in the brain that exist, how disorders can relate to age specific groups, and covers the latest developments in understanding and treating these disorders. *$77.00*

544 pages ISBN 0-880488-29-8

325 The Agoraphobia Workbook
New Harbinger Publications
5674 Shattuck Avenue
Oakland, CA 94609-1662
510-652-2002
800-748-6273
Fax: 510-652-5472
E-mail: customerservice@newharbinger.com
www.newharbinger.com

Self-help resource to help readers overcome the disorder in all its forms *$19.95*

200 pages ISBN 1-572243-23-6

326 The American Psychiatric Publishing Textbook of Anxiety Disorders
American Psychiatric Publishing
1000 Wilson Boulevard
Suite 1825
Arlington, VA 22209-3901
703-907-7322
800-368-5777
Fax: 703-907-1091
E-mail: appi@psych.org
www.appi.org

Gives a detailed look at the history, classification, preclinical models, concepts and combined treatment of anxiety disorders. *$92.00*

536 pages Year Founded: 2002 ISBN 0-880488-29-8

327 The Anxiety & Phobia Workbook, Fourth Editio n
New Harbinger Publications
5674 Shattuck Avenue
Oakland, CA 94609-1662
510-652-2002
800-748-6273
Fax: 510-652-5472
E-mail: customerservice@newharbinger.com
www.newharbinger.com

Edmund J Bourne, Author

Research conducted by the National Institute of Mental Health has shown that anxiety disorders are the number one mental health problem among American women and.

ISBN 1-572244-13-5

328 The Anxiety Cure for Kids: A Guide for Paren ts
Wiley, John & Sons
111 River Street
Hoboken, NJ 07030-5774
201-748-6000
Fax: 201-748-6088
E-mail: info@wiley.com
www.www.wiley.com/wileyCDA

Elizabeth DuPont Spencer, Author
Robert L DuPont, Author

Welcome to an amazing world and to the upbeat story of a Dragon that is tamed by a Wizard.

329 Treatment Plans and Interventions for Depression and Anxiety Disorders
Guilford Publications
72 Spring Street
New York, NY 10012

212-431-9800
800-365-7006
Fax: 212-966-6708
E-mail: info@guilford.com
www.guilford.com

Provides information on treatments for seven frequently encountered disorders: major depression, generalized anxiety, panic, agoraphobia, PTSD, social phobia, specific phobia and OCD. Serving as ready to use treatment packages, chapters describe basic cognitive behavioral therapy techniques and how to tailor them to each disorder. Also featured are diagnostic decision trees, therapist forms for assessment and record keeping, client handouts and homework sheets. *$ 55.00*

320 pages ISBN 1-572305-14-2

330 Trichotillomania: A Guide
Madison Institute of Medicine
7617 Mineral Point Road
Suite 300
Madison, WI 53717-1623
608-827-2470
Fax: 608-827-2479
E-mail: mim@miminc.org
www.miminc.org

Learn more about compulsive hair pulling and its treatment with medications and behavior therapy in this informative guide. *$5.95*

49 pages

331 Triumph Over Fear: a Book of Help and Hope for People with Anxiety, Panic Attacks, and Phobias
Anxiety Disorders Association of America
8730 Georgia Avenue
Suite 600
Silver Spring, MD 20910
301-231-9350
Fax: 301-231-7392
E-mail: AnxDis@adaa.org
www.adaa.org

Alies Muskin, COO
Michelle Alonso, Communications/Marketing

Resource and guide for both lay and professional readers.

332 What to Do When You Worry Too Much: A Kid's Guide to Overcoming Anxiety
American Psychological Association
750 First Street, NE
Washington, DC 20002-4242
202-336-5500
800-374-2721
TTY: 202-336-6123
www.www.apa.org

Dawn Hubner, Author

Interactive self-help book designed to guide 6-12 year olds and thier parents through the techniques most often used in the treatments of generalized anxiety.

333 What to Do When You're Scared and Worried: A Guide for Kids
Free Spirit Publishing
217 Fifth Avenue North, Suite 200
Minneapolis, MN 55401-1299

800-735-7323
Fax: 866-419-5199
www.www.freespirit.com
James J Crist, Author

This book is all about fears and worries: things taht everyone deals with at some point in thier lives.

334 Worry Control Workbook
New Harbinger Publications
5674 Shattuck Avenue
Oakland, CA 94609-1662
510-652-2002
800-748-6273
Fax: 510-652-5472
E-mail: customerservice@newharbinger.com
www.newharbinger.com

Self help program that shares experiences of people who
have developed ways to overcome chronic worry. Step by
step format helps identify areas likely to reoccur and develop new skills. *$15.95*

266 pages ISBN 1-572241-20-9

Periodicals & Pamphlets

335 Anxiety Disorders
National Institute of Mental Health
6001 Executive Boulevard
Room 8184
Bethesda, MD 20892-9663
866-615-6464
Fax: 301-443-4279
TTY: 301-443-8431
E-mail: nimhinfo@nih.gov
www.nimh.nih.gov

This brochure helps to identify the symptoms of anxiety
disorders, explains the role of research in understanding the
causes of these conditions, describes effective treatments,
helps you learn how to obtain treatment and work with a
doctor or therapist, and suggests ways to make treatment
more effective.

336 Anxiety Disorders Fact Sheet
Center for Mental Health Services: Knowledge
Exchange Network
PO Box 42490
Washington, DC 20015
800-789-2647
Fax: 301-984-8796
TDD: 866-889-2647
E-mail: ken@mentalhealth.org
www.mentalhealth.org

This fact sheet presents basic information on the symptoms,
formal diagnosis, and treatment for generalized anxiety disorder, panic disorders, phobias, and post-traumatic stress
disorder.

3 pages

337 Facts About Anxiety Disorders
National Institute of Mental Health
6001 Executive Boulevard
Room 8184
Bethesda, MD 20892-9663
866-615-6464
Fax: 301-443-4279
TTY: 301-443-8431

E-mail: nimhinfo@nih.gov
www.nimh.nih.gov

Series of fact sheets that provide overviews and descriptions of generalized anxiety disorder, obsessive-compulsive
disorder, panic disorder, post-traumatic stress disorder, social phobia, and the Anxiety Disorders Education Program.

**338 Families Can Help Children Cope with Fear,
Anxiety**
Center for Mental Health Services: Knowledge
Exchange Network
PO Box 42490
Washington, DC 20015
800-789-2647
Fax: 301-984-8796
TDD: 866-889-2647
E-mail: ken@mentalhealth.org
www.mentalhealth.org

This fact sheet defines conduct disorder, identifies risk factors, discusses types of help available, and suggests what
parents or other caregivers to common signs of fear and
anxiety.

339 Five Smart Steps to Less Stress
ETR Associates
4 Carbonero Way
Scotts Valley, CA 95066-1200
831-438-4060
800-321-4407
Fax: 800-435-8433
E-mail: customerservice@etr.org
www.etr.org

Steps to managing stress include: know what stresses you,
manage your stress, take care of your body, take care of
your feelings, ask for help. *$16.00*

340 Five Ways to Stop Stress
ETR Associates
4 Carbonero Way
Scotts Valley, CA 95066
831-438-4060
800-321-4407
Fax: 800-435-8433
E-mail: customerservice@etr.org
www.etr.org

An easy to read pamphlet that discusses how to recognize
the signs of stress, explains the big and little changes that
can produce stress and the different causes of stress.
$16.00

341 Getting What You Want From Stress
ETR Associates
4 Carbonero Way
Scotts Valley, CA 95066-4200
831-438-4060
800-321-4407
Fax: 800-435-8433
E-mail: customerservice@etr.org
www.etr.org

Includes signs of stress, some stress can be healthy, and
when to change, when to adapt. *$16.00*

342 Journal of Anxiety Disorders
Elsevier Publishing
360 Park Avenue South
New York, NY 10010-1710

314-453-7010
800-325-4177
Fax: 314-453-7095
E-mail: custserv.ehs@elsevier.com
www.elsevier.com

Interdisciplinary journal that publishes research papers dealing with all aspects of anxiety disorders for all age groups (child, adolescent, adult and geriatrics).

8 per year Year Founded: 1987 ISSN 0887-6185

343 Let's Talk Facts About Panic Disorder
American Psychiatric Publishing
1000 Wilson Boulevard
Suite 1825
Arlington, VA 22209-3901
703-907-7322
800-368-5777
Fax: 703-907-1091
E-mail: appi@psych.org
www.appi.org

Contains an overview of the illness, its symptoms, and the illness's effect on family and friends. A biliography and list of resources make them ideal for libraries or patient education. *$29.95*

8 pages ISBN 0-890423-57-1

344 One Hundred One Stress Busters
ETR Associates
4 Carbonero Way
Scotts Valley, CA 95066
831-438-4060
800-321-4407
Fax: 800-435-8433
E-mail: customerservice@etr.org
www.etr.org

These 101 stress busters were written by students to help fellow students relieve stress: tell a joke, laugh out loud, beat a pillow to smitherines. *$16.00*

345 Panic Attacks
ETR Associates
4 Carbonero Way
Scotts Valley, CA 95066
831-438-4060
800-321-4407
Fax: 800-435-8433
E-mail: customerservice@etr.org
www.etr.org

Describes causes of panic attacks, including genetics, stress, and drug use; prevention and treatment, and how to stop a panic attack in its tracks. *$16.00*

346 Real Illness: Generalized Anxiety Disorder
National Institute of Mental Health
6001 Executive Boulevard
Room 8184
Bethesda, MD 20892-9663
866-615-6464
Fax: 301-443-4279
TTY: 301-443-8431
E-mail: nimhinfo@nih.gov
www.nimh.nih.gov

If you worry and feel tense a lot, even though others may assure you there are no real problems, you have a treatable disorder. Read this easy pamphlet to learn more.

9 pages

347 Real Illness: Panic Disorder
National Institute of Mental Health
6001 Executive Boulevard
Room 8184
Bethesda, MD 20892-9663
866-615-6464
Fax: 301-443-4279
TTY: 301-443-8431
E-mail: nimhinfo@nih.gov
www.nimh.nih.gov

Do you often have feelings of sudden fear that don't make sense? If so, you may have panic disorder. Read this pamplet of simple information about getting help.

9 pages

348 Real Illness: Social Phobia Disorder
National Institute of Mental Health
6001 Executive Boulevard
Room 8184
Bethesda, MD 20892-9663
866-615-6464
Fax: 301-443-4279
TTY: 301-443-8431
E-mail: nimhinfo@nih.gov
www.nimh.nih.gov

Are you terrified of talking in groups or even going to parties because you're afraid people will think badly of you? This simple pamphlet describes how to get help.

9 pages

349 Stress
ETR Associates
4 Carbonero Way
Scotts Valley, CA 95066
831-438-4060
800-321-4407
Fax: 800-435-8433
E-mail: customerservice@etr.org
www.etr.org

Includes common changes that cause stress, symptoms of stress, and effects on feelings, actions and physical health.

350 Stress Incredible Facts
ETR Associates
4 Carbonero Way
Scotts Valley, CA 95066
831-438-4060
800-321-4407
Fax: 800-435-8433
E-mail: customerservice@etr.org
www.etr.org

Strange-but-true facts to trigger discussion about how stress affects the body, how to use it and long-term risks. *$18.00*

351 Stress in Hard Times
ETR Associates
4 Carbonero Way
Scotts Valley, CA 95066
831-438-4060
800-321-4407
Fax: 800-435-8433
E-mail: customerservice@etr.org
www.etr.org

Discusses stress caused by troubling world events, describes short and long term symptoms, and suggests ways to cope. *$16.00*

352 Teen Stress!
ETR Associates
4 Carbonero Way
Scotts Valley, CA 95066
831-438-4060
800-321-4407
Fax: 800-435-8433
E-mail: customerservice@etr.org
www.etr.org

Explains what stress is, outlines the causes and effects and offers ideas for handling stress. *$16.00*

Support Groups & Hot Lines

353 Agoraphobics Building Independent Lives
3212 Cutshaw Ave
Richmond, VA 23230
804-257-5591
E-mail: mhav@mhav.org
www.www.mhav.org

Provides hope, support and advocacy for people suffering from debilitating phobias, panic attacks and/or agoraphobics by establishing self-help groups providing public education.

354 Pass-Group
6 Mahogany Drive
Williamsville, NY 14221
716-689-4399

Offers three-month telephone counseling program for panic attack suffers (agoraphobia). 'The Panic Attack Recovery Book' explains the cause and cure for panic attacks.

355 Phobics Anonymous
PO Box 1180
Palm Springs, CA 92263
760-322-2673

Twelve-step program for panic disorders and anxiety. Publications available.

356 Recovery
802 N Dearborn Street
Chicago, IL 60610-3364
312-337-5661
Fax: 312-337-5756
E-mail: inquiries@recovery-inc.com
www.recovery-inc.com

Kathy Garcia, Executive Director

Techniques for controlling behavior, changing attitudes for recovering mental patients. Systematic method of self-help offered.

Video & Audio

357 Anxiety Disorders
American Counseling Association
5999 Stevenson Avenue
Alexandria, VA 22304-3300
703-823-9800
800-347-6647
Fax: 800-473-2329

TDD: 703-823-6862
E-mail: webmaster@counseling.org
www.counseling.org

Increase your awareness of anxiety disorders, their symptoms, and effective treatments. Learn the effect these disorders can have on life and how treatment can change the quality of life for people presently suffering from these disorders. Includes 6 audiotapes and a study guide. *$140.00*

358 DSM-IV Anxiety Disorders New Diagnostic Issues
American Psychiatric Publishing
1000 Wilson Boulevard
Suite 1825
Arlington, VA 22209-3901
703-907-7322
800-368-5777
Fax: 703-907-1091
E-mail: appi@psych.org
www.appi.org

Series of three clinical programs that reveals additions and changes for mood, psychotic and anxiety disorders. Each video focuses on a different level of disorder as well as giving three 10 minute interviews. Approximately 60 minutes. *$57.00*

Year Founded: 1995 ISBN 0-880488-98-0

359 Driving Far from Home
New Harbinger Publications
5674 Shattuck Avenue
Oakland, CA 94609-1662
510-652-2002
800-748-6273
Fax: 510-652-5472
E-mail: customerservice@newharbinger.com
www.newharbinger.com

120 minute videotape that reduces fear associated with leaving the safety of your home base. *$11.95*

Year Founded: 1995 ISBN 1-572240-14-8

360 FAT City: How Difficult Can This Be?
ADD WareHouse
300 NW 70th Avenue
Suite 102
Plantation, FL 33317
954-792-8100
800-233-9273
Fax: 954-792-8545
E-mail: sales@addwarehouse.com
www.addwarehouse.com

Teachers and parents will understand the anxiety felt by students with learning disabilities after viewing this remarkable video. Presents a series of striking simulations to teachers, counselors and parents designed to emulate the daily experience of children with learning disabilities. Includes a discussion guide for group presentations. 70 minutes. *$58.00*

Web Sites

361 www.adaa.org
Anxiety Disorders Association of America
Dedicated to promoting the prevention, treatment and cure of anxiety disorders.

362 **www.aim-hq.org**
Agoraphobics in Motion

Nonprofit support group committed to the recovery of those suffering from anxiety disorders.

363 **www.algy.com/anxiety/files/barlow.html**
Causes of Anxiety and Panic Attacks

Overview by noted experts.

364 **www.apa.org**
Answers to Your Questions about Panic Disorder

Four-page overview American Psychological Association publication.

365 **www.cfsny.org**
Center for Family Support (CFS)

Devoted to the physical well-being and development of the retarded child and the sound mental health of the parents.

366 **www.cyberpsych.org**
CyberPsych

Hosts the American Psychoanalyists Foundation, American Association of Suicideology, Society for the Exploration of Psychotherapy Intergration, and Anxiety Disorders Association of America. Also subcategories of the anxiety disorders, as well as general information, including panic disorder, phobias, obsessive compulsive disorder (OCD), social phobia, generalized anxiety disorder, post traumatic stress disorder, and phobias of childhood. Book reviews and links to web pages sharing the topics.

367 **www.dstress.com/guided.htm**
Basic Guided Relaxation: Advanced Technique

Devoted to stress management for organizations and individuals, and information to enhance your levels of Health/Wellness and Productivity.

368 **www.factsforhealth.org**
Madison Institute of Medicine

Resource to help identify, understand and treat a number of medical conditions, including social anxiety disorder and posttraumatic stress disorder.

369 **www.freedomfromfear.org**
Freedom From Fear

Aid and counsel to individuals and their families who suffer from anxiety and depressive illness.

370 **www.goodwill-suncoast.org**
Career Assessment & Planning Services

A comprehensive assessment for the developmentally disabled persons who may be unemployed or underemployed.

371 **www.guidetopsychology.com**
A Guide To Psychology & Its Practice

Free information on various types of psychology.

372 **www.healthanxiety.org**
Anxiety and Phobia Treatment Center

Treatment groups for individuals suffering from phobias.

373 **www.healthyminds.org**
Anxiety Disorders

American Psychiatric Association publication diagnostic criteria and treatment.

374 **www.icisf.org**
International Critical Incident Stress Foundation

A nonprofit, open membership foundation dedicated to the prevention and mitigation of disabling stress by education, training and support services for all emergency service professionals. Continuing education and training in emergency mental health services for psychologists, psychiatrists, social workers and licensed professional counselors.

375 **www.intelihealth.com**
Mastering Your Stress Demons

376 **www.jobstresshelp.com**
Job Stress Help

377 **www.lexington-on-line.com**
Panic Disorder

Explains development and treatment of panic disorder.

378 **www.mentalhealth.Samhsa.Gov**
Center for Mental Health Services Knowledge Exchange Network

Information about resources, technical assistance, research, training, networks and other federal clearinghouses.

379 **www.nami.org**
National Alliance for the Mentally Ill

Self-help organization for those affected by brain disorder.

380 **www.npadnews.com**
National Panic/Anxiety Disorder Newsletter

This resource was founded by Phil Darren who collects and collates information of recovered anxiety disorder sufferers who want to distribute some of the lessons that they learned with a view to helping others.

381 **www.panicattacks.com.au**
Anxiety Panic Hub

Information, resources and support.

382 **www.panicdisorder.about.com**
Agoraphobia: For Friends/Family

383 **www.planetpsych.com**
Planetpsych.com

Learn about disorders, their treatments and other topics in psychology. Articles are listed under the related topic areas. Ask a therapist a question for free, or view the directory of professionals in your area. If you are a therapist sign up for the directory. Current features, self-help, interactive, and newsletter archives.

384 **www.psychcentral.com**
Psych Central

Personalized one-stop index for psychology, support, and mental health issues, resources, and people on the Internet.

385 **www.selectivemutismfoundation.org**
Selective Mutism Foundation

Promotes awareness and understanding for individuals and families affected by mutism.

386 **www.selfhelpmagazine.com/articles/stress**
Meditation, Guided Fantasies, and Other Stress Reducers

387 **www.terraphouston.com**
Territorial Apprehensiveness Programs (TERRAP)

Formed to disseminate information concerning the recognition, causes and treatment of anxieties, fears and phobias.

388 **www.thenadd.org**
NADD: National Association for the Dually Diagnosed

Promotes interest of professional and parent development with resources for individuals who have coexistence of mental illness and mental retardation.

ADHD

Introduction

Attention-Deficit/Hyperactivity Disorder (AD/HD) includes: (1) a pervasive pattern of inattention, (2) difficulty in controlling impulses including the impulse to be constantly on the move. Since many chilren are inattentive, impulsive, and rambunctious at times, it is important to note that the disgnosis in not made unless these behaviors are more severe than is typical for a person at a comparable developmental level. The symptoms must appear before age seven.

The problems of hyperactivity show themselves in constant movement, especially among younger children. Preschool children with hyperactivity cannot sit still, even for quiet activities that usually absorb children of the same age, are always on the move, run rather than walk, and jump on furniture. In older children the intensity of the hyperactivity is reduced but fidgeting, getting up during meals or homework, and excessive talking continue.

People with Attention-Deficit/Hyperactivity Disorder have great difficulty controlling all their impulses, not just the craving for movement and stimulation. They have little sense of time (five minutes seems like hours), and waiting for something is intolerable. Thus, they are impatient, interrupt, make comments out of turn, grab objects from others, clown around, and cause trouble at home, in school, work, and in social settings.

The consequences of ADHD can be severe. From a young age, people with Attention-Deficit/Hyperactivity Disorder tend to experience failure repeatedly, including rejection by peers, resulting in low self-esteem and sometimes more serious problems.

SYMPTOMS

Inattention, as compared with others at the same developmental level
• Often fails to attend to details, or makes careless mistakes in schoolwork, work or other activities;
• Often finds it difficult to maintain attention in tasks or play activities;
• Often does not seem to listen when spoken to;
• Often doesn't follow through on instructions and doesn't finish schoolwork, chores, or tasks;
• Often has difficulty organizing tasks or activities;
• Often avoids tasks that demand sustained mental effort, such as schoolwork or homework;
• Often loses things needed for tasks or activities, such as toys and school assignments;
• Often is easily distracted;
• Often is forgetful in daily activities.

Hyperactivity, as compared with others at the same developmental level
• Often fidgets with hands or feet, or squirms in chair;
• Often leaves seat in classroom or other situations where remaining seated is expected;
• Often runs or climbs about in situations in which it is inappropriate (among adolescents or adults, this may be a feeling of restlessness);
• Often has difficulty playing or handling leisure activities quietly;
• Often is on the go, moving excessively;

• Often talks excessively.

Impulsivity, as compared with others at the same developmental level
• Often blurts out answers before questions are finished;
• Often has difficulty waiting in turn;
• Often interrupts or intrudes on others' games, activities, or conversations.

Parts of this description may apply to all or most children at times, but behaving in this way nearly all the time wreaks havoc on the child and family. Three distinctions are made in the diagnosis:

Attention-Deficit/Hyperactivity Disorder, Combined Type if six or more items from List (1) and six or more from List (2) are applicable;

Attention-Deficit/Hyperactivity Disorder, Predominantly Inattentive Type if six or more items from List (1) only are applicable;

Attention-Deficit/Hyperactivity Disorder, Predominantly Hyperactive-Impulsive Type if six or more items from List (2) only are applicable.

ASSOCIATED FEATURES

Certain behaviors often go along with Attention-Deficity/Hyperactivity Disorder. The person is often frustrated and angry, exhibiting outbursts of temper and bossiness. To others, the lack of application and inability to finish tasks may look like laziness or irresponsibility. Other conditions may also be associated with the disorder, including Hyperthyroidism (an overactive thyroid). There may be a higher prevalence of anxiety, depression, and learning disorders among people with AD/HD.

PREVALENCE

AD/HD occurs in various cultures. It is much more frequent in males than females, with male to female ratios at 4:1 in the general population, and 9:1 in clinic populations. The prevalence among school-age children is from three percent to five percent.

There is emerging literature concerning adult AD/HD, and evidence that some adults can benefit from the same treatments used for children.

TREATMENT OPTIONS

A careful assessment and diagnosis by a professional familiar with AD/HD are essential, especially since some of the typical AD/HD behaviors may resemble those of other disorders. Family, school, and other possible problems must be taken into account and addressed. This is a lifelong disorder, though sometimes attenuated in adulthood.

The diagnosis is especially difficult to establish in young children, e.g., at the toddler and preschool level, because behavior that is typical at that age is similar to the symptoms of AD/HD. Children at that age may be extremely active but not develop the disorder. Current treatments can have a positive impact and, in some cases, transform behaviors so that a formerly chaotic life becomes one over which the person has much greater control and more frequent experience of success. Treatment should be based on an understanding that

Attention-Deficit/Hyperactivity Disorder is not intentional, and punishment is not a cure.

The AD/HD person has great need for external motivation, consistency, and structure. This should be provided by a professional who is familiar with the disorder. For a school-aged child, it is important to enlist the help of the school in designing a treatment plan which should include concrete steps aimed at developing specific compentencies (e.g., handling time, sequencing, problem-solving, and social interaction).

Medication is often prescribed but should not be the only treatment. Newer preparations of medicaions, such as Concerta, offer once or twice a day dosing, so that children do not need to take medication during the school day. Since this condition affects all members of the family, the family needs help in providing consistency and structure, and in changing the role of the AD/HD person as the family member who always gets into trouble.

Associations & Agencies

390 Attention Deficit Disorder Association
15000 Commerce Parkway
Suite C
Mount Laurel, NJ 08054
856-439-9099
Fax: 856-439-0525
E-mail: adda@ahint.com
www.add.org

Linda S Anderson M.A. & MCC, President
Evelyn Polk Green MS.Ed, VP

Provides children, adolescents and adults with ADD information, support groups, publications, videos, and referrals. Also, generates hope, awareness, empowerment and connections worldwide.

391 Center For Mental Health Services
PO Box 42557
Washington, DC 20015
240-221-4022
800-789-2647
Fax: 240-221-4295
TDD: 866-889-2647
www.www.mentalhealth.samhsa.gov

392 Center for Family Support (CFS)
333 7th Avenue
New York, NY 10001-5004
212-629-7939
Fax: 212-239-2211
www.cfsny.org

Steven Vernickofs, Executive Director

An agency that continues to develop new programs to serve families and individuals with their care needs. They offer services throughout the New York City region including: New Jersey, Long Island and the Lower Hudson Valley.

393 Center for Mental Health Services Knowledge
PO Box 42557
Washington, DC 20015-4800
800-789-2647
Fax: 240-747-5484
E-mail: ken@mentalhealth.org
www.mentalhealth.org

A. Kathryn Power, Director
Edward B Searle, Deputy Director

Information about resources, technical assistance, research, training, networks, and other federal clearing houses, and fact sheets and materials. Information specialists refer callers to mental health resources in their communities as well as state, federal and nonprofit contacts. Staff available Monday through Friday, 8:30 AM-5:00 PM, EST, excluding federal holidays. After hours, callers may leave messages and an information specialist will return their call.

394 Children and Adults with AD/HD (CHADD)
8181 Professional Place
Suite 150
Landover, MD 20785
301-306-7070
800-233-4050
Fax: 301-306-7090
www.chadd.org

Anne Teeter EdD, President
E Clarke Ross D.P.A, CEO

National nonprofit organization representing children and adults with attention deficit/hyperactivity disorder (AD/HD).

Year Founded: 1987

395 Learning Disabilities Association of America
4156 Library Road
Pittsburgh, PA 15234-1349
412-341-1515
Fax: 412-344-0224
E-mail: info@LDAamerica.org
www.ldanatl.org

Charlie Giglio, President
Connie Parr, VP

Educating individuals with learning disabilities and their parents about the nature of the disability and inform them of their rights, encourages research in neuro-physiological and psycological aspects of learning disabilities.

396 National Alliance on Mental Illness
2107 Wilson Boulevard
Suite 300
Arlington, VA 22201-3042
703-524-7600
800-950-6264
Fax: 703-524-9094
E-mail: helpline@nami.org
www.nami.org

Suzanne Vogel-Scibilia, President
Fredrick Sandoval, Vice President

Nation's leading self-help organization for all those affected by severe brain disorders. Mission is to bring consumers and families with similar experiences together to share information about services, care providers, and ways to cope with the challenges of schizophrenia, manic depression, and other serious mental illnesses.

Year Founded: 1979

397 National Association for the Dually Diagnosed (NADD)
132 Fair Street
Kingston, NY 12401-4802
845-334-4336
800-331-5362

Fax: 845-331-4569
E-mail: nadd@mhv.net
www.thenadd.org

Robert Fletcher DSW, Founder/CEO
Donna Nagy PhD, President

Nonprofit organization designed to promote interest of professional and parent development with resources for individuals who have the coexistence of mental illness and mental retardation. Provides conference, educational services and training materials to professionals, parents, concerned citizens and service organizations. Formerly known as the National Association for the Dually Diagnosed.

Year Founded: 1983

398 National Dissemination Center for Children with Disabilities (NICHCY)

PO Box 1492
Washington, DC 20013
202-884-8200
800-695-0285
Fax: 202-884-8441
TTY: 800-695-0285
E-mail: nichcy@aed.org
www.nichcy.org

Suzanne Ripley, Project Director
Lisa Kupper, Author/Editor

Provides support and services for children and youth with physical and mental disabilities, as well as education and training services for their families.

399 National Mental Health Consumer's

1211 Chestnut Street
Suite 1207
Philadelphia, PA 19107
215-751-1810
800-553-4539
Fax: 215-636-6312
E-mail: info@mhselfhelp.org
www.mhselfhelp.org

Christine Simiriglia, Executive Director
Jennifer Melinn, Information/Referral Dept.

Funded by the National Institute of Mental Health Community Support Program, the purpose of the Clearinghouse is to encourage the development and growth of consumer self-help groups.

400 National Mental Health Consumers' Self-Help Clearinghouse

1211 Chestnut Street
Suite 1207
Philadelphia, PA 19107
215-751-1810
800-553-4539
Fax: 215-636-6312
E-mail: info@mhselfhelp.org
www.mhselfhelp.org

Joseph Rogers, Executive Director

A national consumer technical assistance center that has played a major role in the development of the mental health consumer movement.

Year Founded: 1986

401 SAMHSA's National Mental Health Information Center
US Department of Health and Human Services

PO Box 42557
Washington, DC 20015-4800
240-221-4021
800-789-2647
Fax: 240-221-4295
TDD: 866-889-2647
www.mentalhealth.org

A Kathryn Power MEd, Director
Edward B Searle, Deputy Director

Provides information about mental health via a toll-free telephone number, this web site, and more than 600 publications. Developed for users of mental health services and their families, the general public, policy makers, providers, and the media.

Books

402 AD/HD Forms Book: Identification, Measurement, and Intervention
Research Press

Dept 24 W
PO Box 9177
Champaign, IL 61826
217-352-3273
800-519-2707
Fax: 217-352-1221
E-mail: rp@researchpress.com
www.researchpress.com

Russell Pense, VP Marketing

A collection of intervention procedures and over 30 reproducible forms and checklists for use with any AD/HD program for children or adolescents. Each item is prefaced by a brief description of its purpose and use. The AD/HD Forms Book helps educators, mental health professionals and parents translate their knowledge into action. *$ 25.95*
128 pages ISBN 0-878223-78-9

403 ADD & Learning Disabilities: Reality, Myths, & Controversial Treatments
Bantam Doubleday Dell Publishing

1745 Broadway
New York, NY 10019
212-782-9000
Fax: 212-782-9700

For parents of children with learning disabilities and attention deficit disorder - and for educational and medical professionals who encounter these children - two experts in the field have devised a handbook to help identify the very best treatments. *$10.36*
256 pages ISBN 0-385469-31-4

404 ADD & Romance
ADD WareHouse

300 NW 70th Avenue
Suite 102
Plantation, FL 33317
954-792-8100
800-233-9273
Fax: 954-792-8545
E-mail: sales@addwarehouse.com
www.addwarehouse.com

Romantic relationships are hard enough, but sustaining a stimulating and satisfying romantic relationship can be even more challenging if one partner has ADD. This book discusses how ADD can influence vital aspects of one's romantic life, such as intimacy and communication and provides effective techniques for communication, conflict resolution and ways to cope with ADD in a relationship. *$ 12.95*

230 pages

405 ADD Hyperactivity Handbook for Schools
ADD WareHouse
300 NW 70th Avenue
Suite 102
Plantation, FL 33317
954-792-8100
800-233-9273
Fax: 954-792-8545
E-mail: sales@addwarehouse.com
www.addwarehouse.com

A must read for anyone interested in learning evaluation methods for ADD and ways to effectively assist children with ADD in regular and special education. Contains an overview of the important facts about ADD and provides practical and proven techniques teachers can use in the classroom to help students and their families. *$29.00*

330 pages

406 ADD Kaleidoscope: The Many Facets of Adult Attention Deficit Disorder
Hope Press
PO Box 188
Duarte, CA 91009-0188
818-303-0644
800-321-4039
Fax: 818-358-3520
www.hopepress.com

A comprehensive presentation of all aspects of attention deficit disorder in adults. While often thought of as a childhood disorder, ADD symptoms usually continue into adulthood where they can cause a wide range of problems with personal interactions, work performance, attitude towards one's employer, and interactions with spouses and children. *$24.95*

ISBN 1-878267-03-5

407 ADD Success Stories: Guide to Fulfillment for Families with Attention Deficit Disorder
ADD WareHouse
300 NW 70th Avenue
Suite 102
Plantation, FL 33317
954-792-8100
800-233-9273
Fax: 954-792-8545
E-mail: sales@addwarehouse.com
www.addwarehouse.com

Real-life stories of people with ADD who achieved success in school, at work, in marriages and relationships. Thousands of interviews and histories as well as new research show children and adults from all walks of life how to reach the next-step, a fulfilling, successful life with ADD. Discover which occupations are best for people with ADD. *$12.00*

250 pages

408 ADD and Adolescence: Strategies for Success
CHADD
8181 Professional Place
Suite 150
Landover, MD 20785
301-306-7070
800-233-4050
Fax: 301-306-7090
www.chadd.org

A diversity of national experts present new information on the nature of ADD during adolescence; possible comorbid conditions that will be seen in many cases; strategies for parents and clinicians on the management of teens with ADD. Includes advice on school management, parent and teen counseling, and psychopharmacological treatment; and needed guidance for preparing the adolescent with ADD for college and the workplace. *$15.00*

136 pages

409 ADD in the Workplace: Choices, Changes and Challenges
ADD WareHouse
300 NW 70th Avenue
Suite 102
Plantation, FL 33317
954-792-8100
800-233-9273
Fax: 954-792-8545
E-mail: sales@addwarehouse.com
www.addwarehouse.com

It's one thing to deal with ADD in the doctor's office or at home, but quite another 'out there' in the workplace. This unique guide focuses on adults living with ADD, and illustrates various ways to initiate and maintain the best possible work situation. *$24.00*

248 pages

410 ADD/ADHD Checklist: an Easy Reference for Parents & Teachers
ADD WareHouse
300 NW 70th Avenue
Suite 102
Plantation, FL 33317
954-792-8100
800-233-9273
Fax: 954-792-8545
E-mail: sales@addwarehouse.com
www.addwarehouse.com

This resource for parents and teachers is packed with up-to-date facts, findings and proven strategies and techniques for understanding and helping children and adolescents with attention deficit problems and hyperactivity. *$12.00*

150 pages

411 ADHD Monitoring System
ADD WareHouse
300 NW 70th Avenue
Suite 102
Plantation, FL 33317
954-792-8100
800-233-9273
Fax: 954-792-8545
E-mail: sales@addwarehouse.com
www.addwarehouse.com

Provides a simple, cost effective way to carefully monitor how well a student with ADHD is doing at school. Parents and teachers will be able to easily track behavior, academic performance, quality of student classwork and homework. Contains monitoring forms along with instructions for use. *$8.95*

412 ADHD Parenting Handbook: Practical Advise fo r Parents
Taylor Trade Publishing
5360 Manhattan Circle #101
Boulder, CO 80303
303-543-7835
Fax: 303-543-0043
E-mail: rrinehart@rowman.com

Colleen Alexander-Roberts, Author

Practical advice for parents from parents, and proven techniques for raising hyperactive children without losing your temper.

413 ADHD Survival Guide for Parents and Teachers
Hope Press
PO Box 188
Duarte, CA 91009-0188
818-303-0644
800-321-4039
Fax: 818-358-3520
www.hopepress.com

Fills an important need expressed by parents, teachers, and other caretakers of ADHD children who have asked for clear, practical, and easily understood strategies to deal with ADHD children.

ISBN 1-878267-43-4

414 ADHD and Teens: Parent's Guide to Making it Through the Tough Years
ADD WareHouse
300 NW 70th Avenue
Suite 102
Plantation, FL 33317
954-792-8100
800-233-9273
Fax: 954-792-8545
E-mail: sales@addwarehouse.com
www.addwarehouse.com

Unlike the parents of elementary school children with ADHD, parents of ADHD teens must focus on gaining and keeping control of the situation because the risks are increased in severity and consequence. A manual of practical advice to help parents cope with the problems that can arise during these years. *$13.00*

208 pages

415 ADHD and the Nature of Self-Control
Guilford Publications
72 Spring Street
New York, NY 10012
212-431-9800
800-365-7006
Fax: 212-966-6708
E-mail: info@guilford.com
www.guilford.com

Provides a radical shift of perspective on ADHD, arguing that the disorder is a developmental problem of self control

and that an attention deficit is a secondary characteristic. Combines neuropsychological research and the theory on the executive functions, illustrating how normally functioning individuals are able to bring behavior under the control of time and orient their actions toward the future. *$46.00*

410 pages ISBN 1-572302-50-X

416 ADHD in the Young Child: Driven to Redirection
ADD WareHouse
300 NW 70th Avenue
Suite 102
Plantation, FL 33317
954-792-8100
800-233-9273
Fax: 954-792-8545
E-mail: sales@addwarehouse.com
www.addwarehouse.com

The authors sensitively and effectively describe what life is like living with a young child with ADHD. With the help of over 75 cartoon illustrations they provide practical solutions to common problems found at home, in school and elsewhere. *$18.95*

202 pages

417 ADHD: A Complete and Authoritative Guide
American Academy Of Pediatrics
141 Northwest Point Boulevard
Elk Grove Village, IL 60007-1098
847-434-4000
Fax: 847-434-8000
www.www.aap.org

Sherill Tippins, Author

Based on the American Academy of Pediatrics' own clinical practice guidelines for ADHD and written in clear, accessible language, ths book answers the common question: How is ADHD diagnosed? What are today's best treatment options? and Will my child outgrow ADHD?

418 Adventures in Fast Forward: Life, Love and Work for the ADD Adult
ADD WareHouse
300 NW 70th Avenue
Suite 102
Plantation, FL 33317
954-792-8100
800-233-9273
Fax: 954-792-8545
E-mail: sales@addwarehouse.com
www.addwarehouse.com

For all adults with ADD, this book is designed to be a practical guide for day-to-day life. No matter where you are in the scenario - curious about ADD, just diagnosed or experiencing particular problems, this book will give you effective strategies to help anticipate and negotiate the challenges that come with the condition. Filled with important tools and tactics for self-care and success. *$23.00*

210 pages

419 All About Attention Deficit Disorder: Revised Edition
ADD WareHouse
300 NW 70th Avenue
Suite 102
Plantation, FL 33317

954-792-8100
800-233-9273
Fax: 954-792-8545
E-mail: sales@addwarehouse.com
www.addwarehouse.com

A practical and comprehensive manual for parents and teachers interested in understanding the facts about ADD. Chapters on home management, the 1-2-3 Magic discipline method, facts about medication management and practical ideas for teachers to use in managing learning and classroom behavior. *$13.00*

165 pages

420   All Kinds of Minds
ADD WareHouse
300 NW 70th Avenue
Suite 102
Plantation, FL 33317
954-792-8100
800-233-9273
Fax: 954-792-8545
E-mail: sales@addwarehouse.com
www.addwarehouse.com

Primary and elementary students with learning disorders can now gain insight into the difficulties they face in school. This book helps all children understand and respect all kinds of minds and can encourage children with learning disorders to maintain their motivation and keep from developing behavior problems stemming from their learning disorders. *$31.00*

283 pages

421   Answers to Distraction
ADD WareHouse
300 NW 70th Avenue
Suite 102
Plantation, FL 33317
954-792-8100
800-233-9273
Fax: 954-792-8545
E-mail: sales@addwarehouse.com
www.addwarehouse.com

A user's guide to ADD presented in a question and answer format ideal for parents of children and adolescents with ADD, adults with ADD and teachers who work with students who have ADD. *$13.00*

334 pages

422   Attention Deficit Disorder and Learning Disabilities
Bantam Doubleday Dell Publishing
1745 Broadway
New York, NY 10019
212-782-9000
Fax: 212-782-9700

Discusses ADHD and learning disabilities as well as their effective treatments. Warns against nutritional and other alternative treatments. *$12.95*

256 pages ISBN 0-385469-31-4

423   Attention Deficit Hyperactivity Disorder in Children: A Medication Guide
Madison Institute of Medicine
7617 Mineral Point Road
Suite 300
Madison, WI 53717-1623
608-827-2470
Fax: 608-827-2479
E-mail: mim@miminc.org
www.miminc.org

Written for parents, this explains the various medications used commonly to treat ADHD/ADD. It includes a review of the symptoms of ADHD, medication therapy, commonly asked questions, and side effects of medications. *$5.95*

41 pages

424   Attention Deficits and Hyperactivity in Children: Developmental Clinical Psychology and Psychiatry
Sage Publications
2455 Teller Road
Thousand Oaks, CA 91320
805-499-9774
800-818-7243
Fax: 800-583-2665
E-mail: info@sagepub.com
www.sagepub.com

Provides background information and evaluates key debates and questions that remain unanswered about ADHD. Includes what tools can be used to gain optimal information about this disorder and which factors predict subsequent functioning in adolescence and adulthood. Advances, challenges and unresolved problems in diverse but relevant areas are analyzed and placed in context. Paperback also available. *$43.95*

161 pages Year Founded: 1993 ISBN 0-803951-96-5

425   Attention-Deficit Hyperactivity Disorder in Adults: A Guide
Madison Institute of Medicine
7617 Mineral Point Road
Suite 300
Madison, WI 53717-1623
608-827-2470
Fax: 608-827-2479
E-mail: mim@miminc.org
www.miminc.org

This guide provides an overview of adult ADHD and how it is treated with medications and other treatment approaches. *$5.95*

58 pages

426   Beyond Ritalin
ADD WareHouse
300 NW 70th Avenue
Suite 102
Plantation, FL 33317
954-792-8100
800-233-9273
Fax: 954-792-8545
E-mail: sales@addwarehouse.com
www.addwarehouse.com

Beyond Ritalin: Facts About Medication and Other Strategies for Helping Children, Adolescents and Adults with Attention Deficit Disorders. The authors respond to concerns all parents and individuals have about using medication to treat disorders such as ADHD, explain the importance of a treatment program for those with this condition and discuss fads and fallacies in current treatments. *$13.50*

254 pages

427 Birds-Eye View of Life with ADD and ADHD: Ad vice from Young Survivors, Second Edition
Cherish the Children
PO Box 189
Cedar Bluff, AL
Fax: 256-779-5203
E-mail: chirs@chrisdendy.com
www.www.chrisdendv.com

Chris A Zeigler Dendy, Author

428 Conduct Disorders in Children and Adolesents
American Psychiatric Publishing
1000 Wilson Boulevard
Suite 1825
Arlington, VA 22209-3901
703-907-7322
800-368-5777
Fax: 703-907-1091
E-mail: appi@psych.org
www.appi.org

Katie Duffy, Marketing Assistant

Examines the phenomenology, etiology, and diagnosis of conduct disorders, and describes therapeutic and preventive interventions. Includes the range of treatments now availaable, including individual, family, group, and behavior therapy; hospitalization; and residential treatment. *$52.00*

448 pages ISBN 0-880485-17-5

429 Consumer's Guide to Psychiatric Drugs
New Harbinger Publications
5674 Shattuck Avenue
Oakland, CA 94609-1662
510-652-2002
800-748-6273
Fax: 510-652-5472
E-mail: customerservice@newharbinger.com
www.newharbinger.com

Helps consumers understand what treatment options are available and what side effects to expect. Covers possible interactions with other drugs, medical conditions and other concerns. Explains how each drug works, and offers detailed information about treatments for depression, bipolar disorder, anxiety and sleep disorders, as well as other conditions. *$16.95*

340 pages ISBN 1-572241-11-X

430 Daredevils and Daydreamers: New Perspectives on Attention Deficit/Hyperactivity Disorder
ADD WareHouse
300 NW 70th Avenue
Suite 102
Plantation, FL 33317
954-792-8100
800-233-9273
Fax: 954-792-8545
E-mail: sales@addwarehouse.com
www.addwarehouse.com

Summarizes what has been learned about ADHD in the past ten years and explains how parents can use this knowledge to help their child. Explains how to obtain a good evaluation, how to spot coexisting problems like depression and learning disabilities, how to find the right professional to treat your child and answers many other questions about caring for a child with ADHD. *$11.00*

260 pages

431 Distant Drums, Different Drummers: A Guide for Young People with ADHD
ADD WareHouse
300 NW 70th Avenue
Suite 102
Plantation, FL 33317
954-792-8100
800-233-9273
Fax: 954-792-8545
E-mail: sales@addwarehouse.com
www.addwarehouse.com

Barbara Ingersoll PhD

This book presents a positive perspective of ADHD - one that stresses the value of individual differences. Written for children and adolescents struggling with ADHD, it offers young readers the opportunity to see themselves in a positive light and motivates them to face challenging problems. Ages 8-14. *$16.00*

48 pages

432 Don't Give Up Kid
ADD WareHouse
300 NW 70th Avenue
Suite 102
Plantation, FL 33317
954-792-8100
800-233-9273
Fax: 954-792-8545
E-mail: sales@addwarehouse.com
www.addwarehouse.com

Alex, the hero of this book, is one of two million children in the US who have learning disabilities. This book gives children with reading problems and learning disabilities a clear understanding of their difficulties and the necessary courage to learn to live with them. Ages 5-12. *$13.00*

433 Down and Dirty Guide to Adult Attention Deficit Disorder
ADD WareHouse
300 NW 70th Avenue
Suite 102
Plantation, FL 33317
954-792-8100
800-233-9273
Fax: 954-792-8545
E-mail: sales@addwarehouse.com
www.addwarehouse.com

A book about ADD that is immensely entertaining, informative and uncomplicated. Describes concepts essential to understanding how this disorder is best identified and treated. You'll find a refreshing absence of jargon and an abundance of common sense, practical advice and healthy skepticism. *$17.00*

194 pages

434 Driven to Distraction: Recognizing and Coping with Attention Deficit Disorder from Childhood through Adulthood
ADD WareHouse
300 NW 70th Avenue
Suite 102
Plantation, FL 33317
954-792-8100
800-233-9273
Fax: 954-792-8545
E-mail: sales@addwarehouse.com
www.addwarehouse.com

Edward M Hallowell MD
John J Ratey MD

Through vivid stories of the experiences of their patients (both adults and children), this books shows the varied forms ADD takes - from the hyperactive search for high stimulation to the floating inattention of daydreaming - and the transforming impact of precise diagnosis and treatment. The authors explain when and how medication can be helpful, and since both authors have ADD, their advice on effective behavior-modification techniques is enriched by their own experience. Also available on audiotape for $16.00. *$13.00*

319 pages

435 Drug Therapy and Childhood & Adolescent Diso rders
Mason Crest Publishers
370 Reed Road
Suite 302
Broomall, PA 19008
610-543-6200
866-627-2665
Fax: 610-543-3878
E-mail: dtaylor@masoncrest.com
www.masoncrest.com

This book provides readers with an easy-to-understand introduction to this topic. Numerous case sstudies and examples give insight in the four disorders first diagnosed in childhood and adolescence that can be treated with psychiatric drugs, and helps readers understand the symptoms and treatments of these disorders. The disorders included in this volume are: mental retardation, pervasive developmental disorders, attention-deficit and disruptive behavior disorders and tic disorders.

ISBN 1-590845-63-3

436 Eagle Eyes: A Child's View of Attention Deficit Disorder
ADD WareHouse
300 NW 70th Avenue
Suite 102
Plantation, FL 33317
954-792-8100
800-233-9273
Fax: 954-792-8545
E-mail: sales@addwarehouse.com
www.addwarehouse.com

Jeanne Gehret

This book helps readers of all ages understand ADD and gives practical suggestions for organization, social cues and self calming. Expressive illustrations enhance the book and encourage reluctant readers. Ages 5-12. *$13.00*

437 Eukee the Jumpy, Jumpy Elephant
ADD WareHouse
300 NW 70th Avenue
Suite 102
Plantation, FL 33317
954-792-8100
800-233-9273
Fax: 954-792-8545
E-mail: sales@addwarehouse.com
www.addwarehouse.com

Cliff Corman MD
Esther Trevino

A story about a bright young elephant who is not like all the other elephants. Eukee moves through the jungle like a tornado, unable to pay attention to the other elephants. He begins to feel sad, but gets help after a visit to the doctor who explains why Eukee is so jumpy and hyperactive. With love, support and help, Eukee learns ways to help himself and gain renewed self-esteem. Ideal for ages 3-8. *$15.00*

22 pages

438 Facing AD/HD: A Survival Guide for Parents
Research Press
Dept 24 W
PO Box 9177
Champaign, IL 61826
217-352-3273
800-519-2707
Fax: 217-352-1221
E-mail: rp@researchpress.com
www.researchpress.com

Russell Pense, VP Marketing

Provides parents with the skills they need to help minimize the everyday struggles and frustrations associated with AD/HD. The book addresses structure, routines, setting goals, using charts, persistency with consistency, teamwork, treatment options, medication and more. *$ 14.95*

232 pages ISBN 0-878223-81-9

439 First Star I See
ADD WareHouse
300 NW 70th Avenue
Suite 102
Plantation, FL 33317
954-792-8100
800-233-9273
Fax: 954-792-8545
E-mail: sales@addwarehouse.com
www.addwarehouse.com

Jaye Andras Caffrey

This entertaining and funny look at ADD without hyperactivity is a must-read for middle grade girls with ADD, their teachers and parents. *$11.00*

150 pages

440 Gene Bomb
Hope Press
PO Box 188
Duarte, CA 91009-0188
818-303-0644
800-321-4039
Fax: 818-358-3520
www.hopepress.com

Gene Bomb: Does Higher Education and Advanced Technology Accelerate the Selection of Genes for Learning Disorders, Addictive and Disruptive Behaviors? Explores the hypothesis that autism, learning disorders, alcoholism, drug abuse, depression, attention deficit disorder, and other disruptive behavioral disorders are increaseing in frequency because of an increasing selection, in the 20th century, for the genes associated with these conditions. *$29.95*

304 pages ISBN 1-878267-38-8

441 Give Your ADD Teen a Chance: A Guide for Parents of Teenagers with Attention Deficit Disorder
ADD WareHouse
300 NW 70th Avenue
Suite 102
Plantation, FL 33317
954-792-8100
800-233-9273
Fax: 954-792-8545
E-mail: sales@addwarehouse.com
www.addwarehouse.com

Lynn Weiss PhD

Parenting teenagers is never easy, especially if your teen suffers from ADD. This book provides parents with expert help by showing them how to determine which issues are caused by 'normal' teenager development and which are caused by ADD. *$15.00*

299 pages

442 Grandma's Pet Wildebeest Ate My Homework
ADD WareHouse
300 NW 70th Avenue
Suite 102
Plantation, FL 33317
954-792-8100
800-233-9273
Fax: 954-792-8545
E-mail: sales@addwarehouse.com
www.addwarehouse.com

Tom Quinn

Parents and teachers dealing with hyperactive or daydreaming kids will find this book outstanding. As an ADHD adult himself, Quinn draws upon his own experience, making use of straightforward, creative behavioral management techniques, along with a keen sense of humor. A highly informative and enlightened book. *$16.95*

272 pages

443 Healing ADD: Simple Exercises That Will Change Your Daily Life
ADD WareHouse
300 NW 70th Avenue
Suite 102
Plantation, FL 33317
954-792-8100
800-233-9273
Fax: 954-792-8545
E-mail: sales@addwarehouse.com
www.addwarehouse.com

Thom Hartmann

Presents simple methods involving visualization and positive thinking that can be readily picked up by adults and taught to children with ADD. *$10.00*

178 pages

444 Help 4 ADD@High School
ADD WareHouse
300 NW 70th Avenue
Suite 102
Plantation, FL 33317
954-792-8100
800-233-9273
Fax: 954-792-8545
E-mail: sales@addwarehouse.com
www.addwarehouse.com

This new book was written for teenagers with ADHD. Designed like a web site, it has short, easy-to-read information packed sections which tell you what you need to know about how to get your life together - for yourself, not for your parents or your teachers. Includes tips on studying, ways your high school can help you succeed, tips on getting along better at home, on dating, exercise and much more. *$19.95*

119 pages

445 HomeTOVA: Attention Screening Test
ADD WareHouse
300 NW 70th Avenue
Suite 102
Plantation, FL 33317
954-792-8100
800-233-9273
Fax: 954-792-8545
E-mail: sales@addwarehouse.com
www.addwarehouse.com

Screen yourself or your child (ages 4 to 80 plus) for attention problems. After a simple installation on your home computer (Windows 95/98 OS only), the Home TOVA program runs with use of a mouse. Takes 21.6 minutes and measures how fast, accurate and consistent a person is in responding to squares flashing on a screen. Each program is limited to two administrators. *$29.95*

446 How to Do Homework without Throwing Up
ADD WareHouse
300 NW 70th Avenue
Suite 102
Plantation, FL 33317
954-792-8100
800-233-9273
Fax: 954-792-8545
E-mail: sales@addwarehouse.com
www.addwarehouse.com

Cartoons and witty insights teach important truths about homework and strategies for getting it done. Learn how to make a homework schedule, when to do the hardest homework, where to do homework, the benefits of homework and more. Useful in motivating students with ADD. For ages 8-13. *$9.00*

67 pages

447 Hyperactive Child, Adolescent, and Adult
Oxford University Press
198 Madison Avenue
New York, NY 10016
212-726-6000
800-451-7556
Fax: 919-677-1303
www.oup-usa.org/orbs/

Discusses symptoms and treatment of ADD/ADHD in children and adults with practical suggestions for the management of children. *$27.00*

172 pages ISBN 0-195042-91-3

448 Hyperactive Children Grown Up: ADHD in Children, Adolescents, and Adults
Guilford Publications
72 Spring Street
New York, NY 10012
212-431-9800
800-365-7006
Fax: 212-966-6708
E-mail: info@guilford.com
www.guilford.com

Explores what happens to hyperactive children when they grow to adulthood. Based on the McGill prospective studies, which spans more than 30 years, the volume reports findings on the etiology, treatment and outcome of attention deficits and hyperactivity at all stages of development. Paperback also available. *$44.95*

473 pages ISBN 0-898620-39-2

449 I'm Somebody, Too!
ADD WareHouse
300 NW 70th Avenue
Suite 102
Plantation, FL 33317
954-792-8100
800-233-9273
Fax: 954-792-8545
E-mail: sales@addwarehouse.com
www.addwarehouse.com

Jeanne Gehret, Contact

Because it is written for an older, non-ADD audience, this book explains ADD in depth and explains methods to handle the feelings that often result from having a family member with ADD. For children ages 9 and older. *$13.00*

159 pages

450 Is Your Child Hyperactive? Inattentive? Impulsive? Distractible?
ADD WareHouse
300 NW 70th Avenue
Suite 102
Plantation, FL 33317
954-792-8100
800-233-9273
Fax: 954-792-8545
E-mail: sales@addwarehouse.com
www.addwarehouse.com

Written with compassion and hope, this parent guide prepares you for the process of determining if your child has ADD and guides you in your dealings with educators, doctors and other professionals. *$13.00*

235 pages

451 Learning to Slow Down and Pay Attention
ADD WareHouse
300 NW 70th Avenue
Suite 102
Plantation, FL 33317
954-792-8100
800-233-9273
Fax: 954-792-8545

E-mail: sales@addwarehouse.com
www.addwarehouse.com

Written for children to read, and illustrated with charming cartoons and activity pages, the book helps children identify problems and explains how their parents, teachers and doctors can help. For children 6-14. *$10.00*

70 pages

452 Living with Attention Deficit Disorder: a Workbook for Adults with ADD
New Harbinger Publications
5674 Shattuck Avenue
Oakland, CA 94609-1662
510-652-2002
800-748-6273
Fax: 510-652-5472
E-mail: customerservice@newharbinger.com
www.newharbinger.com

Includes strategies for handling common problems at work and school, dealing with intimate relationships, and finding support. *$17.95*

176 pages ISBN 1-572240-63-6

453 Medications for Attention Disorders and Related Medical Problems: Comprehensive Handbook
ADD WareHouse
300 NW 70th Avenue
Suite 102
Plantation, FL 33317
954-792-8100
800-233-9273
Fax: 954-792-8545
E-mail: sales@addwarehouse.com
www.addwarehouse.com

ADHD and ADD are medical conditions and often medical intervention is regarded by most experts as an essential component of the multimodal program for the treatment of these disorders. This text presents a comprehensive look at medications and their use in attention disorders. *$37.00*

420 pages

454 Meeting the ADD Challenge: A Practical Guide for Teachers
Research Press
Dept 24 W
PO Box 9177
Champaign, IL 61826
217-352-3273
800-519-2707
Fax: 217-352-1221
E-mail: rp@researchpress.com
www.researchpress.com

Dr Michael J Asher, Co-Author
Dr Steven B Gordon, Author
Dennis Wiziecki, Marketing

Information on the needs and treatment of children and adolescents with ADD. The book addresses the defining characteristics of ADD, common treatment approaches, myths about ADD, matching intervention to student, use of behavior rating scales and checklists, evaluating interventions, regular versus special class placement, helping students regulate their own behavior and more. Includes case examples. *$21.95*

196 pages ISBN 0-878223-45-2

455 **Misunderstood Child: Understanding and Coping with Your Child's Learning Disabilities**
ADD WareHouse
300 NW 70th Avenue
Suite 102
Plantation, FL 33317
954-792-8100
800-233-9273
Fax: 954-792-8545
E-mail: sales@addwarehouse.com
www.addwarehouse.com

In this revised and updated edition you will find promising treatment options for children, adolescents and adults with learning disabilities, discussion of ADHD, pros and cons of using medication, revision to federal and state laws covering discrimination and educational rights, new approaches for those of college age and older. *$15.00*

403 pages

456 **My Brother's a World Class Pain: a Sibling's Guide to ADHD**
ADD WareHouse
300 NW 70th Avenue
Suite 102
Plantation, FL 33317
954-792-8100
800-233-9273
Fax: 954-792-8545
E-mail: sales@addwarehouse.com
www.addwarehouse.com

While they frequently bear the brunt of the ADHD child's impulsiveness and distractibility, siblings usually are not afforded opportunities to understand the nature of the problem and to have their own feelings and thoughts addressed. This story shows brothers and sisters how they can play an important role in the family's quest for change. *$12.00*

34 pages

457 **Put Yourself in Their Shoes: Understanding Teenagers with Attention Deficit Hyperactivity Disorder**
ADD WareHouse
300 NW 70th Avenue
Suite 102
Plantation, FL 33317
954-792-8100
800-233-9273
Fax: 954-792-8545
E-mail: sales@addwarehouse.com
www.addwarehouse.com

Contains up-to-date information on how ADHD affects the lives of adolescents at home, in school, in the workplace and in social relationships. Chapters discuss how to get a good assessment, controversial treatments and medications for ADHD, building positive communication at home, problem-solving strategies to resolve family conflict, ADHD and the military, study strategies to improve learning, ADHD and delinquency, two hundred educational accommodations for ADHD teens and more. *$19.00*

249 pages

458 **RYAN: A Mother's Story of Her Hyperactive/Tourette Syndrome Child**
Hope Press
PO Box 188
Duarte, CA 91009-0188
818-303-0644
800-321-4039
Fax: 818-358-3520
www.hopepress.com

A moving and informative story of how a mother struggled with the many behavioral problems presented by her son with Tourette syndrome, ADHD and oppositional defiant disorder. *$9.95*

302 pages ISBN 1-878267-25-6

459 **Shelley, The Hyperative Turtle**
ADD WareHouse
300 NW 70th Avenue
Suite 102
Plantation, FL 33317
954-792-8100
800-233-9273
Fax: 954-792-8545
E-mail: sales@addwarehouse.com
www.addwarehouse.com

Deborah Moss

The story of a bright young turtle who's not like all the other turtles. Shelley moves like a rocket and is unable to sit still for even the shortest periods of time. Because he and the other turtles are unable to understand why he is so wiggly and squirmy, Shelley begins to feel naughty and out of place. But after a visit to the doctor, Shelley learns what 'hyperactive' means and that it is necessary to take special medicine to control that wiggly feeling. Ideal for ages 3-7. *$14.00*

24 pages

460 **Sometimes I Drive My Mom Crazy, But I Know She's Crazy About Me**
ADD WareHouse
300 NW 70th Avenue
Suite 102
Plantation, FL 33317
954-792-8100
800-233-9273
Fax: 954-792-8545
E-mail: sales@addwarehouse.com
www.addwarehouse.com

This warm and humorous story of a young boy with ADHD addresses the many difficult and frustrating issues kids like him confront every day - from sitting still in the classroom, to remaining calm, to feeling 'different' from other children. This book is an amusing look at how a youngster with ADHD can develop a sense of self-worth through better understanding of this disorder. Ages 6-12. *$16.00*

129 pages

461 **Stuck on Fast Forward: Youth with Attention Deficit/Hyperactivity Disorder**
Mason Crest Publishers
370 Reed Road
Suite 302
Broomall, PA 19008
610-543-6200
866-627-2665

Fax: 610-543-3878
E-mail: dtaylor@masoncrest.com
www.masoncrest.com

Provides a comprehensive, yet easy to understand, overview of attention deficit/hyperactivity disorder. ADHD is an increasingly common diagnosis for school-aged and pre-school children today, as parents, educators, and medical professionals struggle to deal with children who often don't sit still, don't pay attention, or act impulsively and even inappropriately. The debate over diagnosis and treatment of such symptoms is intense, and Stuck on Fast Forward explores all sides of the issue.

ISBN 1-590847-28-8

462 Succeeding in College with Attention Deficit Disorders: Issues and Strategies for Students, Counselors and Educators
ADD WareHouse
300 NW 70th Avenue
Suite 102
Plantation, FL 33317
954-792-8100
800-233-9273
Fax: 954-792-8545
E-mail: sales@addwarehouse.com
www.addwarehouse.com

Written for college students, their couselors and educators. Based on the real life experiances of adults who were interviewed as part of a research study, this book offers a vivid picture of how college students with ADD can cope and find success in school. *$18.00*

189 pages

463 Survival Guide for College Students with ADD or LD
ADD WareHouse
300 NW 70th Avenue
Suite 102
Plantation, FL 33317
954-792-8100
800-233-9273
Fax: 954-792-8545
E-mail: sales@addwarehouse.com
www.addwarehouse.com

A useful guide for high school or college students diagnosed with attention deficit disorder or learning disabilities. Provides the information needed to survive and thrive in a college setting. Full of practical suggestions and tips from an experienced specialist in the field and from college students who also suffer from these difficulties. *$10.00*

56 pages

464 Survival Strategies for Parenting Your ADD Child
Underwood Books
PO Box 1609
Grass Valley, CA 95945
Fax: 530-274-7179
E-mail: timunderwd@cs.com
www.underwoodbooks.com

Survival Strategies for Parenting Your ADD Child: Dealing with Obsessions, Compulsions, Depression, Explosive Behavior and Rage. Provides parents with methods which can heal the fractures and pain that occur in families with troubled children. *$12.95*

268 pages ISBN 1-887424-19-9

465 Taking Charge of ADHD: Complete, Authoritative Guide for Parents
ADD WareHouse
300 NW 70th Avenue
Suite 102
Plantation, FL 33317
954-792-8100
800-233-9273
Fax: 954-792-8545
E-mail: sales@addwarehouse.com
www.addwarehouse.com

Written for parents who are ready to take charge of their child's life. Strong on advocacy and parental empowerment, this book provides step-by-step methods for managing a child with ADHD in a variety of everyday situations, gives information on medications and discusses numerous techniques for enhancing a child's school performance.
$18.00

350 pages

466 Teenagers with ADD and ADHD, 2nd Edition: A Guide for Parents and Professionals
Woodbine House
6510 Bells Mill Road
Bethesda, MD 20817
301-897-3570
800-843-7323
www.www.woodbinehouse.com

Chris A Zeigler Dendy, Author

The newly updated and expanded guide to raising a teenager with an attention deficit disorder is more comprehensive than ever. Thousands more parents can rely on Dendy's compassionately presented expertise based on the latest research and decades of her experience as a parent, teacher, school psychologist, and mental health counselor.

467 Teenagers with ADD: A Parent's Guide
Woodbine House
6510 Bells Mill Road
Bethesda, MD 20817
301-897-3570
800-843-7323
Fax: 301-897-5838
E-mail: info@woodbinehouse.com
www.woodbinehouse.com

Double-column book full of information, suggestions and case studies. Lively, upbeat, comprehensive and well targeted to the problems parents face with ADD teenagers.
$18.95

370 pages ISBN 0-933149-69-7

468 Understanding Girls with Attention Deficit Hyperactivity Disorder
ADD WareHouse
300 NW 70th Avenue
Suite 102
Plantation, FL 33317
954-792-8100
800-233-9273
Fax: 954-792-8545
E-mail: sales@addwarehouse.com
www.addwarehouse.com

Symptoms of ADHD are often overlooked or misunderstood in girls who are often diagnosed much later, and their ADHD symptoms may go untreated. This groundbreaking book reveals how ADHD affects girls from preschool through high school years. Gender differences are discussed along with issues related to school success, medication treatment, family relationships and susceptibility to other disorders such as anxiety, depression and learning problems. *$19.95*

291 pages

469   Voices From Fatherhood: Fathers, Sons and ADHD
ADD WareHouse
300 NW 70th Avenue
Suite 102
Plantation, FL 33317
954-792-8100
800-233-9273
Fax: 954-792-8545
E-mail: sales@addwarehouse.com
www.addwarehouse.com

Patrick J Kilcatt PhD
Patricia O Quinn MD

Written to specifically help fathers navigate the complex world of parenting and ADHD, this book helps fathers enhance and deepen their relationships with their sons while providing them with strategies for guiding their sons. *$20.00*

184 pages

470   What Makes Ryan Tick?
Hope Press
PO Box 188
Duarte, CA 91009-0188
818-303-0644
800-321-4039
Fax: 818-358-3520
www.hopepress.com

What Makes Ryan Tick? A Family's Triumph over Tourette's Syndrome and Attention Deficit Hyperactivity Disorder. A moving and informative story how a mother struggled with the many behavioral problems presented by her son with Tourettes syndrome, ADHD and oppositional defiant disorder. *$15.95*

303 pages   ISBN 1-878267-35-3

471   Women with Attention Deficit Disorder
ADD WareHouse
300 NW 70th Avenue
Suite 102
Plantation, FL 33317
954-792-8100
800-233-9273
Fax: 954-792-8545
E-mail: sales@addwarehouse.com
www.addwarehouse.com

Combines real-life histories, treatment experiences and recent clinical research to highlight the special challenges facing women with Attention Deficit Disorder. After describing what to look for and what to look out for in treatment and counseling, this book outlines empowering steps that women living with ADD may use to change their lives. Also available on audiotape. 3 hours on 2 cassettes for $20.00. *$12.00*

288 pages

472   You Mean I'm Not Lazy, Stupid or Crazy?
ADD WareHouse
300 NW 70th Avenue
Suite 102
Plantation, FL 33317
954-792-8100
800-233-9273
Fax: 954-792-8545
E-mail: sales@addwarehouse.com
www.addwarehouse.com

Katie Kelly
Peggy Ramundo

This book is the first written by ADD adults for ADD adults. A comprehensive guide, it provides accurate information, practical how-to's and moral support. Readers will also get information on unique differences in ADD adults, the impact on their lives, treatment options available for adults, up-to-date research findings and much more. Also available on audiotape. *$14.00*

426 pages

Periodicals & Pamphlets

473   ADDitude Magazine
ADD Warehouse
300 NW 70th Avenue
Suite 102
Plantation, FL 33317
954-792-8100
800-233-9273
Fax: 954-792-8545
E-mail: sales@addwarehouse.com
www.addwarehouse.com

Provides valuable resource information for professionals-teachers, healthcare providers, employers and others-who interact with AD/HD people everyday. *$19.97*

474   ADHD Report
Guilford Publications
72 Spring Street
New York, NY 10012
212-431-9800
800-365-7006
Fax: 212-966-6708
E-mail: info@guilford.com
www.guilford.com

This accessible newsletter provides a single reliable guide to the latest developments, newest topics, and current trends in ADHD. An indispensibe resource, the ADHD Report examines the nature, definition, diagnosis, developmental course, outcomes and etiologies associated with ADHD, as well as changes occuring in the fields of education and clinical management. It includes handouts for clinicians and parents, as well as annotated research findings. *$79.00*

6 per year   ISSN 1065-8025

475   Learning Disabilities: A Multidisciplinary Journal
Learning Disabilities Association of America
4156 Library Road
Pittsburgh, PA 15234-1349

412-341-1515
Fax: 412-344-0224
www.ldaamercia.org

The most current research designed for professionals in the field of LD. *$60.00*

476 Treatment of Children with Mental Disorders
National Institute of Mental Health
6001 Executive Boulevard
Room 8184
Bethesda, MD 20892-9663
866-615-6464
Fax: 301-443-4279
TTY: 301-443-8431
E-mail: nimhinfo@nih.gov
www.nimh.nih.gov

A short booklet that contains questions and answers about therapy for children with mental disorders. Includes a chart of mental disorders and medications used.

Video & Audio

477 ADHD & LD: Powerful Teaching Strategies & Ac comodations
ADD Warehouse
300 NW 70the Avenue
Suite 102
Plantation, FL 33317
954-792-8100
800-233-9273
Fax: 954-792-8545
E-mail: sales@addwarehouse.com
www.addwarehouse.com

Provides instructional strategies for engaging attention and active participation, classroom management and behavioral interventions, gives academic strategies and accomodations, and collaborates teaming for success. 45 minutes. *$129.00*

Year Founded: 2003

478 ADHD-Inclusive Instruction & Collaborative Practices
ADD Warehouse
300 NW 70th Avenue
Suite 102
Plantation, FL 33317
954-792-8100
800-233-9273
Fax: 954-792-8545
E-mail: sales@addwarehouse.com
www.addwarehouses.com

Describes classroom modifications, teaching strategies, and interventions that can be used to maximize learning and ensure that all students achieve success. 38 minutes. *$99.00*

Year Founded: 1995 ISBN 1-887943-04-8

479 ADHD: What Can We Do?
ADD WareHouse
300 NW 70th Avenue
Suite 102
Plantation, FL 33317
954-792-8100
800-233-9273
Fax: 954-792-8545

E-mail: sales@addwarehouse.com
www.addwarehouse.com

Can serve as a companion to ADHD: What Do We Know?, this video focuses on the most effective ways to manage ADHD, both in the home and in the classroom. Scenes depict the use of behavior management at home and accommodations and interventions in the classroom which have proven to be effective in the treatment of ADHD. Thirty five minutes. *$95.00*

ISBN 0-898629-72-1

480 ADHD: What Do We Know?
ADD WareHouse
300 NW 70th Avenue
Suite 102
Plantation, FL 33317
954-792-8100
800-233-9273
Fax: 954-792-8545
E-mail: sales@addwarehouse.com
www.addwarehouse.com

This video provides an overview of the disorder and introduces the viewer to three young people who have ADHD. Discusses how ADHD affects the lives of the children and adults, causes of the disorder, associated problems, outcome in adulthood and provides vivid illustrations of how individuals with ADHD function at home, at school and on the job. Thirty five minutes. *$95.00*

ISBN 0-898629-71-3

481 Adults with Attention Deficit Disorder: ADD Isn't Just Kids Stuff
ADD WareHouse
300 NW 70th Avenue
Suite 102
Plantation, FL 33317
954-792-8100
800-233-9273
Fax: 954-792-8545
E-mail: sales@addwarehouse.com
www.addwarehouse.com

Explains this often misunderstood condition and the effects it has on one's work, home and social life. With the help of a panel of six adults, four ADD adults and two of their spouses, the book addresses the most common concerns of adults with ADD and provides information that will help families who are experiencing difficulties. 86 minutes. *$47.00*

482 Educating Inattentive Children
ADD WareHouse
300 NW 70th Avenue
Suite 102
Plantation, FL 33317
954-792-8100
800-233-9273
Fax: 954-792-8545
E-mail: sales@addwarehouse.com
www.addwarehouse.com

This two-hour video is ideal for in-service to regular and special educators concerning problems experienced by inattentive elementary and secondary students. Provides educators with information necessary to indentify and evaluate classroom problems caused by inattention and a well-defined set of practical guidelines to help educate children with ADD. *$49.00*

483 Medication for ADHD
ADD WareHouse
300 NW 70th Avenue
Suite 102
Plantation, FL 33317
954-792-8100
800-233-9273
Fax: 954-792-8545
E-mail: sales@addwarehouse.com
www.addwarehouse.com

This comprehensive DVD addresses the critical questions regarding the use of medication in the treatment of ADD or ADHD. Allows those involved with ADHD to make well-informed and constructive decisions that may deeply change someone's life. *$39.95*

ISBN 1-889140-18-X

484 New Look at ADHD: Inhibition, Time and Self Control
Guilford Publications
72 Spring Street
New York, NY 10012
212-431-9800
800-365-7006
Fax: 212-966-6708
E-mail: info@guilford.com
www.guilford.com

This video provides an accessible introduction to Russell A Barkley's influential theory of the nature and origins of ADHD. The program brings to life the conceptual framework delineated in Barkley's other books. Discusses concrete ways that our new understanding of the disorder might facilitate more effective clinical interventions. This lucid, state of the art program is ideal viewing for clinicians, students and inservice trainees, parents of children with ADHD and adults with the disorder. 30 minutes. *$95.00*

Year Founded: 2000 ISBN 1-572304-97-9

485 Outside In: A Look at Adults with Attention Deficit Disorder
ADD Warehouse
300 NW 70th Avenue
Suite 102
Plantation, FL 33317
954-792-8100
800-233-9273
Fax: 954-792-8545
E-mail: sales@addwarehouse.com
www.addwarehouse.com

Documentary film about adults with ADD and their journeys and the strategies they used to succeed. 29 minutes *$27.95*

486 Understanding and Treating the Hereditary Psychiatric Spectrum Disorders
Hope Press
PO Box 188
Duarte, CA 91009-0188
626-303-0644
800-321-4039
Fax: 626-358-3520
E-mail: dcomings@mail.earthlink.net
www.hopepress.com

Learn with 10 hours of audio tapes from a two day seminar given in May 1997 by David E Comings, MD. Tapes cover:

ADHD, Tourette Syndrome, Obsessive-Compulsive Disorder, Conduct Disorder, Oppositional Defiant Disorder, Autism and other Hereditary Psychiatric Spectrum Disorders. Eight audio tapes. *$75.00*

Year Founded: 1997

487 Understanding the Defiant Child
Guilford Publications
72 Spring Street
New York, NY 10012
212-431-9800
800-365-7006
Fax: 212-966-6708
E-mail: info@guilford.com
www.guilford.com

Presents information on Oppositional Defiant Disorder and Conduct Disorder with scenes of family interactions, showing the nature and causes of these disorders and what can and should be done about it. Thirty five minutes with a manual that contains more information. 30 minutes. *$95.00*

Year Founded: 1997 ISBN 1-572301-66-X

488 Why Won't My Child Pay Attention?
ADD WareHouse
300 NW 70th Avenue
Suite 102
Plantation, FL 33317
954-792-8100
800-233-9273
Fax: 954-792-8545
E-mail: sales@addwarehouse.com
www.addwarehouse.com

Provides an easy-to-follow explanation concerning the effect ADD has on children at school, home and in the community. Provides guidelines to help parents and professionals successfully and happily manage the problems these behaviors can cause. 76 minutes. *$38.00*

Web Sites

489 www.CHADD.org
Children/Adults with Attention Deficit/Hyperactivity Disorder

490 www.LD-ADD.com
Attention Deficit Disorder and Parenting Site

491 www.aap.org
American Academy of Pediatrics Practice Guidelines on ADHD

Site serves the purpose of giving the public guidelines for diagnosing and evaluating children with possible ADHD.

492 www.add.about.com
Attention Deficit Disorder

Hundreds of sites.

493 www.add.org
Attention Deficit Disorder Association

Provides information, resources and networking to adults with ADHD and to the professionals who work with them.

494 www.additudemag.com
Happy Healthy Lifestyle Magazine for People with ADD

495 www.addvance.com
Answers to Your Questions About ADD

provides answers to questions about ADD, ADHD for families and individuals at every stage of life from preschool through retirement years.

496 www.adhdnews.com/Advocate.htm
Advocating for Your Child

497 www.adhdnews.com/sped.htm
Special Education Rights and Responsibilities

Writing IEP's and TIEPS. Pursuing special education services.

498 www.babycenter.com/rcindex.html
BabyCenter

499 www.cfsny.org
Center for Family Support

Devoted to the physical well-being and development of the retarded child and the sound mental health of parents.

500 www.cyberpsych.org
CyberPsych

Hosts the American Psychoanalyists Foundation, American Association of Suicideology, Society for the Exploration of Psychotherapy Intergration, and Anxiety Disorders Association of America. Also subcategories of the anxiety disorders, as well as general information, including panic disorder, phobias, obsessive compulsive disorder (OCD), social phobia, generalized anxiety disorder, post traumatic stress disorder, and phobias of childhood. Book reviews and links to web pages sharing the topics.

501 www.nami.org
National Aliance for the Mentally Ill

Brings consumers and families with similar experiences together to share information about services, care providers and ways to cope with the challenges.

502 www.nichcy.org
National Information Center for Children and Youth with Disabilities

Excellent information in English and Spanish.

503 www.nimh.nih.gov/publicat/adhd.cfm
Attention Deficit Hyperactivity Disorder

Thirty page booklet.

504 www.oneaddplace.com
One ADD Place

505 www.planetpsych.com
Planetpsych.com

Learn about disorders, their treatments and other topics in psychology. Articles are listed under the related topic areas. Ask a therapist a question for free, or view the directory of professionals in your area. If you are a therapist sign up for the directory. Current features, self-help, interactive, and newsletter archives.

506 www.psychcentral.com
Psych Central

Personalized one-stop index for psychology, support, and mental health issues, resources, and people on the Internet.

507 www.thenadd.org
National Association for the Dually Diagnosed

Nonprofit organization to promote interests of professional and parent development with resources for individuals who have coexistence of mental illness and mental retardation.

Asperger's Syndrome

Introduction

Asperger's Syndrome (AS) is an Autism Spectrum Disorder (ASD), a distinct group of neurological conditions characterized by impairment in language and communication skills. It is also associated with repetitive or restrictive patterns of thought and behavior.

It is named for Austrian pediatrician Hans Asperger who, in 1944, observed four children who had normal intelligence, but lacked nonverbal communication skills; in addition they did not demonstrate empathy with their peers, and were physically clumsy. Dr. Asperger called the condition 'autistic psychopathy' and described it as a personality disorder marked by social isolation.

Twin and family studies have shown a genetic predisposition to AS and the other ADs, but a specific gene has not yet been identified. Some researchers have proposed that the disorder may stem from abnormalities during critical stages of fetal development, including defects in the genes that control and regulate normal brain growth and growth patterns.

There is no standardized screening tool available to diagnose Asperger's Syndrome. Most doctors rely on the presence of a core group of behaviorsto diagnose the syndrome.

SYMPTOMS

In contrast to Autism, Asperger's Disorder causes two types of symptoms: problems with social interactions and stereotyped, repetitive patterns of behavior. Individuals with Asperger's Syndrome have limited interests and are preoccupied with a particular subject to the exclusion of other activities. Some other characteristics are: Repetitive routines or rituals; Peculiarities in speech and language, such as speaking in an overly formal manner or in a monotone, or taking figures of speech literally; Socially and emotionally inappropriate behavior and the inability to interact successfully with peers; Problems with non-verbal communication, including the restricted use of gestures, limited or inappropriate facial expressions, or a peculiar, stiff gaze; Clumsy and uncoordinated motor movements.

ASSOCIATED FEATURES

The person with Asperger's may not develop age-appropriate relationships or attempt to share interests or pleasures with others. He or she may be unable to reciprocate others' feelings, have difficulty using gestures or facial expressions, be extremely preoccupied with a very narrow area of interest, insist upon very rigid routines, make repetitive movements, and focus on parts of objects rather than the objects as a whole. Asperger's Disorder does not interfere with the development of language or thinking. However, its symptoms interfere with the individual's social or occupational functioning.

PREVALENCE

The incidence of Asperger's Syndrome is estimated to be two out of every 10,000 children. Boys are three to four times more likely than girls to have the disorder. Although diagnosed mainly in children, it is being increasingly diagnosed in adults with other mental health conditions such as depression, obsessive-compulsive disorder, and attention-deficit hyperactivity disorder.

TREATMENT OPTIONS

Treatment for Asperger's Syndrome addresses the core symptoms of the disorder: poor communication skills; obsessive or repetitive routines; and physical clumsiness. No single treatment works best, but the program would include social skills training, cognitive behavioral therapy, medication, occupational/physical therapy, and parent training and support.

Associations & Agencies

509 Apserger Syndrome Education Network of America (ASPEN)
9 Aspen Circle
Edison, NJ 08820-2832
732-321-0880
E-mail: info@aspennj.org
www.aspennj.org

Lori Shery, President

A non-profit organization which provides families and individuals whose lives are affected by Autism Spectrum Disorders with education about the issues surrounding the disorders; support in knowing that they are not alone, and in helping individuals achieve their maximum potential; advocacy in areas of appropriate educational programs, medical research funding, adult issues and increased public awareness and understanding.

510 Asperger's Association of New England (AANE)
85 Main Street
Suit 101
Watertown, MA 02472
617-393-3824
Fax: 617-393-3827
E-mail: info@aane.org
www.aane.org

Dania Jekel, MSW, Executive Director
Hank Miller, President

Fosters awareness, respect, acceptance and support for individuals with AS and related conditions and their families. AANE offers a full array of educational events for people with an interest in Asperger's Syndrome.

511 Autism Network International
PO Box 35448
Syracuse, NY 13235-5448
E-mail: jisincla@syr.edu
www.www.ani.ac

Jim Sinclair

ANI is an organization run by autistic people, for autistic people. We offer education, peer advocacy, and peer support.

512 Autism Research Institute
4182 Adams Avenue
San Diego, CA 92116
619-281-7165
866-366-3361
Fax: 619-563-6840
www.autsimreseachinstitute.com

Stephen M. Edelson, PhD, Director

Provides information on Autism and Asperger's Syndrome.

513 Autism Society of America
7910 Woodmont Avenue
Suite 300
Bethesda, MD 20814-3067
301-657-0881
800-328-8476
Fax: 301-657-0869
www.autism-society.org

Lee Grossman, President/CEO

Provides information on Autism and Asperger's Syndrome.

**514 Autism Treatment Center of America: The Son
-Rise Program**
The Option Institute
2080 S Undermountain Road
Sheffield, MA 01257
413-229-2100
Fax: 413-229-3202
E-mail: info@optioninstitute.com
www.autismtreatmentcenter.org

Neil Kaufman, Co-Founder/Co-Creator

A powerful, effective and totally unique treatment for children and adults challenged by Autism, Autism Spectrum Disorders, Pervasive Development Disorders, Asperger's Syndrome, and other developmental difficulties.

**515 Families of Adults Afflicted with Asperger's
Syndrome (FAAAS)**
PO Box 514
Centerville, MA 02632
508-790-1930
E-mail: faaas@faaas.org
www.faaas.org

Tony Attwood, Professional Advisory
Jack Kelley, Events Coordinator

The goals of FAAAS are to help families experience validation in their lives and the lives of their loved ones, and to supply information and insight to the medical, psychological and neurological communities. FAAAS is a non-profit organization.

Year Founded: 1997

**516 More Advanced Persons with Autism and
Asperger's Syndrome (MAAP)**
PO Box 524
Crown Point, IN 46307
219-662-1311
Fax: 219-662-0638
E-mail: info@maapservices.org
www.maapservices.org

Susan J. Moreno, Editior

A non-profit organization dedicated to providing information and advice to families of individuals with Autism, Asperger's Syndrom and other Pervasive Development Disorders. Conference and newsletter.

517 National Institute of Mental Health
National Institutes of Health DHHS
6001 Executive Boulevard Room 8184
MSC 9663
Bethesda, MD 20892-9663
301-443-4513
Fax: 301-443-4279

TTY: 301-443-8431
E-mail: nimhinfo@nih.gov
www.nimh.nih.gov

Provides information and support on Autism and Asperger's Syndrome.

**518 National Institute of Neurological Disorders
and Stroke Brain Information Network
(BRAIN)**
PO Box 5801
Bethesda, MD 20824
301-496-5751
800-352-9424
TTY: 301-468-5981
www.ninds.nih.gov

**519 National Institute on Deafness and Other
Communication Disorders Information
Clearinghouse**
31 Center Drive
MSC 2320
Bethesda, MD 20892-2320
800-241-1044
TTY: 800-241-1055
E-mail: nidcinfo@nidcd.nih.gov
www.nidcd.nih.gov

Barry ACHE, Director
Kaylin ADIPIETRO, Director

Support and services for individuals with Autism and Asperger's Syndrome.

Books

**520 A Parent's Guide to Asperger Syndrome and
High-Functioning Autism**
Guilford Press
72 Spring Street
New York, NY 10012
212-431-9800
800-365-7006
Fax: 212-966-6708
E-mail: info@guilford.com
www.guilford.com

Sally Ozonoff
Geraldine Dawson
James McPartland

How to Meet the Challenges and Help Your Child Thrive. Covers definitions, diagnsosis, causes and treatments as well as living with AS-HFA, channeling a child's strengths, and dealing with home and social world and life as an adult. *$18.95*

278 pages Year Founded: 2002 ISBN 1-572305-31-2

Periodicals & Pamphlets

521 The Source Newsletter
MAAP
PO Box 524
Crown Point, IN 46307
219-662-1311
Fax: 219-662-0638
E-mail: chart@netnitco.net

Susan J Moreno, Editor

Newsletter from the Global Information and Support Network for More Advanced Persons with Austism and Asperger's Syndrome.

4 per year

Video & Audio

522 **Asperger Syndrome: Living Outside the Bell Curve**
Program Development Associates
PO Box 2038
Syracuse, NY 13220-2038
315-452-0643
Fax: 315-452-0710
E-mail: info@disabilitytraining.com
www.disabilitytraining.com

This video combines in-depth interviews with Dr. Tina Lyama on Asperger Syndrome symptoms, causes and treatments with the success story of 12-year old Andrew, who develops skills and behaviors for the classroom. VHS or DVD *$79.95*

523 **Asperger's Syndrome: A Video Guide for Parents and Professionals**
Program Development Associates
PO Box 2038
Syracuse, NY 13220-2038
315-452-0643
Fax: 315-452-0710
E-mail: info@disabilitytraining.com
www.disabilitytraining.com

Dr. Tony Attwood, a Clinical Psychologist with extensive experience in early diagnosis and severe behaviors, presents theory of mind in the Asperger's challenge. He draws from his work with both profoundly disabled and high-functioning individuals. VHS or DVD, 180 minutes. *$99.95*

524 **Asperger's Syndrome: An Interview with Lars Perner and Philip Brousseau**
Program Development Associates
PO Box 2038
Syracuse, NY 13220-2038
315-452-0643
Fax: 315-452-0710
E-mail: info@disabilitytraining.com
www.disabilitytraining.com

Personal interviews offer living proof that people with Asperger's Syndrome and high functioning autism live successful lives...with guidance, training and support. Dr. Lars Perner, Marketing Professor and Philip Brosseau present insight, recommendations and inspiration. Available in VHS or DVD. 36 minutes. *$79.95*

525 **Asperger's Syndrome: Autism and Obsessive Behavior**
Program Development Associates
PO Box 2038
Syracuse, NY 13220-2038
315-452-0643
Fax: 315-452-0710
E-mail: info@disabilitytraining.com
www.disabilitytraining.com

This profile of Asperger's symptoms, phobias and anxieties of sufferes, and family responses, traces the source of this mild form of autism to the frontal cortex of the brain. This

video offers coping strategies and helpful socialization behaviors. VHS or DVD, 30 minutes. *$129.95*

526 **Asperger's Unplugged, an Interview with Jerry Newport**
Program Development Associates
PO Box 2038
Syracuse, NY 13220-2038
315-452-0643
Fax: 315-452-0710
E-mail: info@disabilitytraining.com
www.disabilitytraining.com

Meet the man who answered a question in the film 'Rain Man' - How much is 4,343 x 1,234? - before the autistic savant character played by Dustin Hoffman answered it. Jerry Newport discovered Asperger's Syndrome while watching 'Rain Man' and has since become an engaging speaker and self-help organizer. This inspiring interview, available on VHS or DVD, supports teachers, staff developers and people with high functioning autism. 40 minutes. *$79.95*

527 **Dr. Tony Attwood: Asperger's Syndrome Volume 2 DVD**
Program Development Associates
PO Box 2038
Syracuse, NY 13220-2038
315-452-0643
Fax: 315-452-0710
E-mail: info@disabilitytraining.com
www.disabilitytraining.com

Following rave national reviews that autism expert Dr. Tony Attwood received for his Volume 1 introduction to Asperger's Syndrome, here's the new DVD of his latest conference presentations. Volume 2 leaps off the DVD screen with Dr. Attwood's interactive, in-depth, theory-of-mind approach to Asperger's. 180 minutes. *$109.95*

528 **Rylee's Gift - Asperger Syndrome**
Program Development Associates
PO Box 2038
Syracuse, NY 13220-2038
315-452-0643
Fax: 315-452-0710
E-mail: info@disabilitytraining.com
www.disabilitytraining.com

This video or DVD spotlights Rylee - through his mother, grandparents, doctor, teacher - and adults with Asperger's Syndrome. Balances views of difficult transitions and meltdown behaviors, with sensory therapy, socialization and the amazing capabilities of people with this syndrome/gift. 56 minutes. *$89.95*

529 **Struggling with Life: Asperger's Syndrome**
Program Development Associates
PO Box 2038
Syracuse, NY 13220-2038
315-452-0643
Fax: 315-452-0710
E-mail: info@disabilitytraining.com
www.disabilitytraining.com

ABC News correspondent Jay Schadler's report on the neurological disorder called Asperger's focuses on the telling line between intense interests and obsessions. The latter may be an early symptom of the syndrome. This closed caption video is grounded on studies by Fred Voklmar at Yale that explore compulsive fixations and unreadable facial expressions, both of which are typical of Asperger's and inhibit normal peer interactions among children. VHS or DVD. 14 minutes. *$ 69.95*

Web Sites

530 Social Skills Training for Children and Adolescents with Asperger Syndrome and Social-Communications Problems
Autism Asperger Publishing
www.amazon.com

User-friendly book that provides a wealth of ready-to-use activities.

531 The Asperger Parent: How to Raise a Child with Asperger Syndrome and Maintain Your Sense of Humor
Autism Asperger Publishing Company
www.amazon.com

Great advice for the parent of a child with Asperger's Syndrome.

532 www.aspergerinfo.com
Aspergers Resource Links

AspergerInfo.com offers a safe place to ask questions, share experiences, and discuss treatments relating to Asperger Syndrome.

533 www.aspergers.com
Aspergers Resource Links

Asperger's Disorder Homepage

534 www.aspergersyndrome.org
Aspergers Resource Links

Barbara Kirby, Founder

A collection of web resources on Asperger's Syndrome and related topics. Hosted by the University of Delaware.

535 www.aspiesforfreedom.com
Aspies for Freedom

Aspies for Freedom (AFF) is a web site with chat rooms, forums and information relating to Austism and Asperger's Syndrome.

536 www.wrongplanet.net
Wrong Planet

WrongPlanet.net is a web community designed for individuals with Asperger's Syndrome and other PDDs. They provide a forum where members can communicate with each other, may read or submit essays or how-to guides about various subjects, and a chatroom for communication with other Aspies.

Conferences & Meetings

537 Asperger Syndrome Education Network (ASPEN) Conference
9 Aspen Circle
Edison, NJ 08820
732-321-0880

Lori Shery, President

Annual conference.

538 MAAP Services
PO Box 524
Crown Point, IN 46307
219-662-1311
Fax: 219-662-0638
E-mail: chart@netnitco.net

MAAP Services Conference on Autism, Asperger Syndrome and Pervasive Development Disorders.

Autistic Disorder

Introduction

Autistic Disorder is a pervasive developmental disorder whose main symptoms are a marked lack of interest in connecting, interacting, or communicating with others. People with this disorder cannot share something of interest with other people, rarely make eye contact with others, avoid physical contact, show little facial expression, and do not make friends. Autistic Disorder is a profound, lifelong condition associated with wide ranging and severe disabilities, including behavior problems, such as hyperactivity, obsessive compulsive behavior, self injury, and tics. Although present before age three, the disorder may not be apparent until later, although parents often sense that there is something wrong because of their child's marked lack of interest in social interaction. Very young children with autism not only show no desire for affection and cuddling, but show actual aversion to it. There is no socially directed smiling or facial responsiveness, and no responsiveness to the voices of parents and siblings. As a result, parents may sometimes worry that their child is deaf. Later, the child may be more willing to interact socially, but the quality of interaction is unusual, usually inappropriately intrusive with little understanding of social rules and boundaries. The autistic child seems not to have the abilities and desires that would make it possible for him or her to become a social being. Instead, the child seems locked up in an alien interior world which is both incomprehensible and inaccessible to parents, siblings, and others.

SYMPTOMS

Impairment in the Quality of Social Interaction
• Gross lack of nonverbal behavior (e.g., eye contact, facial expression, body postures, and gestures), which gives meaning to social interaction and social behavior;
• Failure to make friends in age-appropriate ways;
• Lack of spontaneously seeking to share interests or achievements with others (e.g., not showing things to others, not pointing to, or bringing interesting objects to others);
• Lack of social or emotional give and take (e.g., not joining in social play or simple games with others);
• Notable lack of awareness of others. Oblivious of other children (including siblings), of their excitement, distress, or needs.

Marked Impairment in the Quality of Communication
• Delay in, or lack of, spoken language development. Those who speak cannot initiate or sustain comunication with others;
• Lack of spontaneous make-believe or imitative play common among young children;
• When speech does develop, it may be abnormal and monotonous;
• Repetitive use of language.

Restricted Repetitive Patterns or Behavior
• Restricted range of interests often fixed on one subject and its facts (e.g., baseball);
• A great deal of exact repetition in play, (e.g., lining up play objects in the same way again and again);
• Resistance and distress if anything in the environment is changed, (e.g., a chair moved to a different place);
• Insistence on following certain rules and routines (e.g., walking to school by the same route each day);
• Repeated body movements (e.g., body rocking, hand clapping);
• Persistent preoccupation with details or parts of objects (e.g., buttons).

ASSOCIATED FEATURES

Autism seems to bring with it an increased risk of other disorders. Seventy-five percent of autistic children have cognitive deficits, and twenty-five percent, have cognitive abilities at or above average. Twenty-five percent of individuals with autism also have seizure disorders. The development of intellectual skills is usually uneven. An autistic child may be able to read extremely early, but not be able to comprehend what he or she reads. Other symptoms include hyperactivity, short attention span, impulsivity, aggressiveness, and self injury, such as head banging, hair pulling, and arm biting (particularly in young children). There may be unusual responses to stimuli: less than normal sensitivity to pain but extreme sensitivity to sounds or to being touched. There may be abnormalities in emotional expression, giggling or weeping for no apparent reason, and little or no emotional reaction when one would be expected. Similar abnormal responses may be shown in relation to fear; an absence of fear in response to real danger, but great fearfulness in the presence of harmless objects.

In adolescence or adulthood, people with Autistic Disorder who have the capacity for insight may become depressed when they realize how seriously impaired they are.

Autistic Disorder sometimes follows medical and obstetrical problems, such as encephalitis, anoxia (absence of oxygen) during birth, and maternal rubella during pregnancy.

There is some evidence of genetic transmission.

The disorder is not caused by inappropriate parenting pr by routine immunizations.

Some new, intensive, multi-dimensional treatments are promising, but few people have access to them at this time.

PREVALENCE

By definition, Autistic Director is present before age three. There are two to five cases of the disorder per 10,000 births. Rates of autism are four to five times greater among males than females. Females with Autistic Disorder are more likely to be severely retarded than are males with Autistic Disorder. Follow-up studies suggest that only a small percentage of people with Autistic Disorder live independent adult lives. Even the highest functioning adults continue to have problems in social interaction and communication, together with greatly restricted interests and activities. The siblings of people with the disorder are at increased risk.

TREATMENT OPTIONS

It is difficult or unusual to be able to eradicate all the symptoms of Autistic Disorder, but there are many intervention and education programs which help to improve functioning. It is extremely important, however, that a proper assessment and diagnosis be made. Since the disturbance in behavior is so wide ranging, this can require an array of professional skills - psychological, langugage development, neuropsychological, and medical. Such a multiple assessment establishes the presence or absence of other disorders, the level of intellectual functioning, together with individual strengths and weaknesses, and the child's capacity for social and personal self-sufficiency. Since the symptoms of Autistic Disorder vary widely from individual to individual, a proper assessment becomes the foundation for designing and planning an individually tailored intervention program.

The autistic person may benefit from a combination of educational and behavioral interventions, which may reduce many of the behavioral disturbances, and improve the quality of life for the person and his or her family. In some cases, medication may also be prescribed. The diagnosis of Autistic Disorder can be a shattering experience for any family. The outcome of the diagnosis is open-ended and uncertain and includes a lifetime of care. Every member of the family is affected and it is vital to work with and support them.

Associations & Agencies

540 Asperger Syndrome Education Network (ASPEN)
9 Aspen Circle
Edison, NJ 08820
732-321-0880
E-mail: info@aspennj.org
www.aspennj.org
Lori Shery, President
Claudia Loomis, Executive VP

Regionally based nonprofit organization headquarted in New Jersey, with 12 local chapters, providing families and those individuals affected with Asperger Syndrome, PDD-NOS, High Function Autism and related disorders. Provides education about the issues surronding Asperger Syndrome and other related disorders. Support in knowing that they are not alone and in helping individuals with AS achieve their maximum potential. Advocacy in areas of appropriate educational programs and placement, medical research funding and increased public awareness and understanding.

541 Asperger's Association of New England
182 Main Street
Watertown, MA 02472
617-393-3824
Fax: 617-393-3827
E-mail: info@aane.org
www.aane.autistics.org
Dania Jekel MSW, Executive Director
Jamie Field MSW, Adult Services Coordinator

Mission is to foster awareness, respect, acceptance, and support for individuals with Aspergers Syndrome and related conditions and their families.

542 Autism Research Foundation
c/o Moss-Rosene Lab, W701
715 Albany Street
Boston, MA 02118
617-414-7012
Fax: 617-414-7207
E-mail: tarf@ladders.org
www.ladders.org
Claudia Persico, Project Manager/Coordinator

A nonprofit, tax-exempt organization dedicated to researching the neurological underpinnings of autism and other related developmental brain disorders. Seeking to rapidly expand and accelerate research into the pervasive developmental disorders.

543 Autism Research Institute
4182 Adams Avenue
San Diego, CA 92116
619-281-7165
Fax: 619-563-6840
www.autismresearchinstitute.com
Dr. Bernard Rimland, Director
Mark Rimland, Assistant Director

A nonprofit organization which was established in 1967. ARI is primarily devoted to conducting research on the causes of autism and on methods of preventing, diagnosing and treating autism and other severe behavioral disorders of childhood. We provide information based on research to parents and professionals throughout the world. Relies primarily on the generosity of donors for its support. Publishes a quarterly newsletter called the Autism Research Review International, that covers various issues in autism, including Asperger's.
Year Founded: 1967

544 Autism Services Center
929 4th Avenue
PO Box 507
Huntington, WV 25710-0507
304-525-8014
Fax: 304-525-8026
www.autismservicescenter.org
Ruth C Sullivan PhD, Executive Director

Service agency for individuals with autism and other developmental disabilities and their families. Makes available technical assistance in designing programs.
Year Founded: 1979

545 Autism Society of America
7910 Woodmont Avenue
Suite 300
Bethesda, MD 20814-3067
301-657-0881
800-328-8476
Fax: 301-657-0869
www.autism-society.org
Lee Grossman, President/CEo
Jennifer Lefever, Director Information/Referral

Promotes lifelong access and opportunities for persons within the autism spectrum and their families, to be fully included, participating members of their communities through advocacy, public awareness, education and research related to autism.
Year Founded: 1965

546 Autistic Services
4444 Bryant Stratton Way
Williamsville, NY 14221
716-631-5777
888-288-4764
Fax: 716-565-0671
E-mail: veronica@autisticservices.org
www.autisticservices.com
Thomas Mazur, President
Veronica Federiconi, Executive Director

Agency exclusively dedicated to serving the unique lifelong needs of individuals with autism. Also a regional resource for parents, school districts, physicians and other professionals.

547 Center for Family Support (CFS)
333 7th Avenue
New York, NY 10001-5004
212-629-7939
Fax: 212-239-2211
www.cfsny.org

Steven Vernickofs, Executive Director

An agency that continues to develop new programs to serve families and individuals with their care needs. They offer services throughout the New York City region including: New Jersey, Long Island and the Lower Hudson Valley.

548 Center for Mental Health Services Knowledge
PO Box 42557
Washington, DC 20015-4800
800-789-2647
Fax: 240-747-5484
E-mail: ken@mentalhealth.org
www.mentalhealth.org

Information about resources, technical assistance, research, training, networks, and other federal clearing houses, and fact sheets and materials. Information specialists refer callers to mental health resources in their communities as well as state, federal and nonprofit contacts. Staff available Monday through Friday, 8:30 AM - 5:00 PM, EST, excluding federal holidays. After hours, callers may leave messages and an information specialist will return their call.

549 Community Services for Autistic Adults and Children
8615 East Village Avenue
Montgomery Village, MD 20886
240-912-2220
Fax: 301-926-9384
TTY: 800-735-2258
E-mail: csaac@csaac.org
www.csaac.org

Ian Paregol, Executive Director
Marcee Smith, Ph.D., Assistant Executive Director of

Enables individuals to achieve to their highest potential and contribute as confident members in their community, instead of living in institutions.

Year Founded: 1979

550 Families for Early Autism Treatment
PO Box 255722
Sacramento, CA 95865-5722
916-491-1033
Fax: 916-581-5029
E-mail: feat@feat.org
www.feat.org

A nonprofit organization of parents and professionals, designed to help families with children who are diagnosed with autism or pervasive developmental disorder.

551 More Advanced Autistic People Services (MAAPS)
PO Box 524
Crown Point, IN 46308-0524
219-662-1311
Fax: 219-662-0638
E-mail: chart@netnitco.net
www.maapservices.org

Susan J Moreno, President
Mary Anne Neiner, Assistant

Provides information and advice to people with Asperger syndrome, Autism and other pervasive developmental disorders. Provides parents and professionals a way to network with others to learn more within the autism spectrum.

552 National Alliance on Mental Illness
2107 Wilson Boulevard
Suite 300
Arlington, VA 22201-3042
703-524-7600
800-950-6264
Fax: 703-524-9094
E-mail: helpline@nami.org
www.nami.org

Michael Fitzpatrick, Executive Director

Nation's leading self-help organization for all those affected by severe brain disorders. Mission is to bring consumers and families with similar experiences together to share information about services, care providers, and ways to cope with the challenges of schizophrenia, manic depression, and other serious mental illnesses.

Year Founded: 1979

553 National Association for the Dually Diagnosed (NADD)
132 Fair Street
Kingston, NY 12401-4802
845-334-4336
800-331-5362
Fax: 845-331-4569
E-mail: nadd@mhv.net
www.thenadd.org

Robert Fletcher DSW, Founder/CEO
Donna Nagy PhD, President

Nonprofit organization designed to promote interest of professional and parent development with resources for individuals who have the coexistence of mental illness and mental retardation. Provides conference, educational services and training materials to professionals, parents, concerned citizens and service organizations. Formerly known as the National Association for the Dually Diagnosed.

Year Founded: 1983

554 National Mental Health Consumer's
1211 Chestnut Street
Suite 1207
Philadelphia, PA 19107
215-751-1810
800-553-4539
Fax: 215-735-0275
E-mail: info@mhselfhelp.org
www.mhselfhelp.org

Christine Smiriglia, Executive Director
Jennifer Melinn, Information/Referral Dept.

Funded by the National Institute of Mental Health Community Support Program, the purpose of the Clearinghouse is to encourage the development and growth of consumer self-help groups.

555 National Mental Health Consumers' Self-Help Clearinghouse
1211 Chestnut Street
Suite 1207
Philadelphia, PA 19107
215-751-1810
800-553-4539
Fax: 215-636-6312
E-mail: info@mhselfhelp.org
www.mhselfhelp.org

Joseph Rogers, Executive Director

A national consumer technical assistance center that has played a major role in the development of the mental health consumer movement.
Year Founded: 1986

556 New England Center for Children
33 Turnpike Road
Southborough, MA 01772-2108
508-481-1015
Fax: 508-485-3421
E-mail: info@necc.org
www.necc.org

L Vincent Strally Jr, Founder/Executive Director
Katherine E Foster MEd, Associate Executive Director

Serving students between the ages of 3 and 22 diagnosed with autism, learning disabilities, language delays, mental retardation, behavior disorders and related disabilities; educational curriculum encompasses both the teaching of functional life skills.

557 SAMHSA's National Mental Health Information Center
US Department of Health and Human Services
PO Box 42557
Washington, DC 20015-4800
240-221-4021
800-789-2647
Fax: 240-221-4295
TDD: 866-889-2647
www.mentalhealth.org

A Kathryn Power MEd, Director
Edward B Searle, Deputy Director

Provides information about mental health via a toll-free telephone number, this web site, and more than 600 publications. Developed for users of mental health services and their families, the general public, policy makers, providers, and the media.

558 Samhsa's National Mental Health Information Center
PO Box 42557
Washington, DC 20015
240-221-4022
800-789-2647
Fax: 240-221-4295
TDD: 866-889-2647
www.www.mentalhealth.samhsa.gov

information about resources, technical assistance,research,training,networks,and other federal clearing housesand fact sheets and materials.information specialists refer callers to mental health resources in their communities.as well as state,federal and non-profit contacts. staff available Mon-Fri , 8:30am - 5:00 pm, EST, excluding federal holidays. after hours, callers may leave   messages and an information specialist will return their call.

559 Son-Rise Program at the Option Institute
Autism Treatment Center of America
2080 S Undermountain Road
Sheffield, MA 01257
413-229-2100
Fax: 413-229-3202
E-mail: info@optioninstitute.com
www.son-rise.org

Barry Neil Kaufman, Co-Founder
Samahria Lyte Kaufman, Co-Founder

Training center for autism professionals and parents of autistic children. Programs focuses on the design and implementation of home-based/child-centered alternatives. Offers publications and other resource materials to educate parents, sufferers and professionals.

Books

560 1001 Great Ideas for Teaching or Raising Children with Autism Spectrum Disorders
Future Horizons
721 West Abram Street
Arlington, TX 76013
212-572-2882
800-489-0727
Fax: 817-277-2270
www.www.futurehorizons-autism.com/index.htm

Veronica Zysk, Author
Ellen Notbohm, Author

In a snappy, can-do format, 1001 Great Ideas for Teaching and Raising Children with Autism Specturm Disorders offers page after page of try-it-now solutions that have worked for thousands of children grappling with social, sensory, behavioral, and self-care issues, plus many more.

561 A Book: A Collection of Writings from the Advocate
Autism Society of North Carolina Bookstore
505 Oberlin Road
Suite 230
Raleigh, NC 27605-1345
919-743-0204
800-442-2762
Fax: 919-743-0208
www.autismsociety-nc.org

A collection of articles and writings from the Advocate, the national newsletter of the Autism Society of America.
$12.00

562 Activities for Developing Pre-Skill Concepts in Children with Autism
Autism Society of North Carolina Bookstore
505 Oberlin Road
Suite 230
Raleigh, NC 27605-1345
919-743-0204
800-442-2762
Fax: 919-743-0208
www.autismsociety-nc.org

Chapters include auditory development, concept development, social development and visual-motor integration.
$34.00

563 Adults with Autism
Cambridge University Press
40 W 20th Street
New York, NY 10011-4221
212-924-3900
Fax: 212-691-3239
E-mail: marketing@cup.org
www.cambridge.org

Provides pratical help and guidance specifically for those caring for the growing recognized population of adults with autism. *$ 50.00*

312 pages Year Founded: 1996 ISBN 0-521456-83-5

564 Are You Alone on Purpose?
Autism Society of North Carolina Bookstore
505 Oberlin Road
Suite 230
Raleigh, NC 27605-1345
919-743-0204
800-442-2762
Fax: 919-743-0208
www.autismsociety-nc.org

This is the story of Alison, the twin sister of an autistic boy, who develops a friendship with a boy who has become paralyzed. Alison's feelings of isolation from her family and brother are discussed as she develops a true friendship. *$14.95*

565 Aspects of Autism: Biological Research
Autism Society of North Carolina Bookstore
505 Oberlin Road
Suite 230
Raleigh, NC 27605-1345
919-743-0204
800-442-2762
Fax: 919-743-0208
www.autismsociety-nc.org

Reviews the evidence for a physical cause of autism and the roles of genetics, magnesium and vitamin B6. *$15.00*

566 Asperger Syndrome
Guilford Publications
72 Spring Street
New York, NY 10012
212-431-9800
800-365-7006
Fax: 212-966-6708
E-mail: info@guilford.com
www.guilford.com

Brings together preeminent scholars and practitioners to offer a definitive statement of what is currently known about Asperger syndrome and to highlight promising leads in research and clinical practice. Sifts through the latest developments in theory and research, discussing key diagnostic and conceptual issues and reviewing what is known about behavioral features and neurobiology. The effects of Asperger syndrome on social development, learning and communication are examined. *$48.00*

484 pages ISBN 1-572305-34-7

567 Asperger Syndrome: A Practical Guide for Teachers
ADD WareHouse
300 NW 70th Avenue
Suite 102
Plantation, FL 33317
954-792-8100
800-233-9273
Fax: 954-792-8545
E-mail: sales@addwarehouse.com
www.addwarehouse.com

A clear and concise guide to effective classroom practice for teachers and support assistants working with children with Asperger Syndrome in school. The authors explain characteristics of children with Asperger Syndrome, discusses methods of assessment and offers practical strategies for effective classroom interventions. *$24.95*

90 pages

568 Asperger's Syndrome: A Guide for Parents and Professionals
ADD WareHouse
300 NW 70th Avenue
Suite 102
Plantation, FL 33317
954-792-8100
800-233-9273
Fax: 954-792-8545
E-mail: sales@addwarehouse.com
www.addwarehouse.com

Providing a description and analysis of the unusual characteristics of Asperger's syndrome, with strategies to reduce those that are most conspicuous or debilitating. This guide brings together the most relevant and useful information on all aspects of the syndrome, from language and social behavior to motor clumsiness. *$18.95*

223 pages

569 Aspergers Syndrome: A Guide for Educators and Parents, Second Edition
Pro-Ed Publications
8700 Shoal Creek Boulevard
Austin, TX 78757-6816
512-451-3246
800-897-3202
Fax: 800-397-7633
E-mail: info@proedinc.com
www.proedinc.com

Packed with the current knowledge of a syndrome only recently applied in this country to individuals with significant social and language peculiarities. Will assist special education professionals and parents in understanding the special needs of children with AS, as well as how to address them in the classroom. For families, it offers helpful planning strategies for post secondary schooling. *$28.00*

130 pages

570 Autism
Autism Society of North Carolina Bookstore
505 Oberlin Road
Suite 230
Raleigh, NC 27605-1345
919-743-0204
800-442-2762
Fax: 919-743-0208
www.autismsociety-nc.org

In a question-and-answer format, the authors respond to questions about autism asked by countless parents and family members of children and youths with autism. *$26.00*

571 Autism & Asperger Syndrome
Cambridge University Press
40 W 20th Street
New York, NY 10011-4211
212-924-3900
800-872-7423
Fax: 212-691-3239
www.cup.org

Six clinician-researchers present aspects of Asperger Syndrome, one form of autism. Research summaries are enlivened by case studies. *$24.00*

247 pages

572 Autism & Sensing: The Unlost Instinct
Jessica Kingsley Publishers
325 Chestnut Street
Philadelphia, PA 19106
215-625-8900
Fax: 215-625-2940
www.jkp.com

Available in paperback. *$26.95*

200 pages Year Founded: 1998 ISBN 1-853026-12-3

573 Autism Bibliography
TASH
29 W Susquehanna Avenue
Suite 210
Baltimore, MD 21204
410-828-8274
Fax: 410-828-6706
E-mail: info@tash.org
www.tash.org

Three hundred recent references to publications on autism along with brief abstracts. *$9.00*

574 Autism Spectrum
Autism Society of North Carolina Bookstore
505 Oberlin Road
Suite 230
Raleigh, NC 27605-1345
919-743-0204
800-442-2762
Fax: 919-743-0208
www.autismsociety-nc.org

An excellent publication for new parents and professionals. *$28.95*

575 Autism Spectrum Disorders: The Complete Guid's to Understanding Autism, Asperger's Syndrome, Pervasive Developmental Disorder, and Other ASDs
Penguin Group (USA)
375 Hudson Street
New York, NY 10014
212-366-2372
Fax: 212-366-2933
www.www.penguin.com

Chantal Sicile-Kira, Author
Temple Grandin, Author

Twelve years ago, we were in the local doctor's office in a small village in England, where we had just moved.

576 Autism Treatment Guide
Autism Society of North Carolina Bookstore
505 Oberlin Road
Suite 230
Raleigh, NC 27605-1345
919-743-0204
800-442-2762
Fax: 919-743-0208
www.autismsociety-nc.org

A comprehensive book covering treatments and methods used to help individuals with autism. *$12.75*

577 Autism and Pervasive Developmental Disorders
Cambridge University Press
40 W 20th Street
New York, NY 10011-4221
212-924-3900
Fax: 212-691-3239
E-mail: marketing@cup.org
www.cup.org

Featuring contributions from leading authorities in the clinical and social sciences, this volume reflects recent progress in the understanding of autism and related conditions, and offers an international perspective on the present state of the discipline. Chapters cover current approaches to definition and diagnosis; prevalence and planning for service delivery; cognitive, genetic and neurobiological features and pathophysiological mechanisms. *$75.00*

294 pages Year Founded: 1998 ISBN 0-521553-86-5

578 Autism: An Inside-Out Approach An Innovative Look at the Mechanics of Autism and its Developmental Cousins
Jessica Kingsley Publishers
325 Chestnut Street
Philadelphia, PA 19106
215-625-8900
Fax: 215-625-2940
www.jkp.com

Marisa Kitsock, Marketing Representative

Written by an autistic person for people with autism and related disorders, carers, and the professionals who work with them, is a practical handbook to understanding, living with and working with autism. *$23.95*

336 pages ISBN 1-853023-87-6

579 Autism: An Introduction to Psychological Theory
Harvard University Press
79 Garden Street
Cambridge, MA 02138
800-405-1619
Fax: 800-406-9145
E-mail: CONTACT_HUP@harvard.edu
www.hup.harvard.edu

Provides a concise overview of current psychological theory and research that synthesizes the established work on the biological foundations, cognitive characteristics, and behavioral manifestations of this disorder. *$32.00*

160 pages Year Founded: 1998 ISBN 0-674053-12-5

580 Autism: Explaining the Enigma
Autism Society of North Carolina Bookstore
505 Oberlin Road
Suite 230
Raleigh, NC 27605-1345
919-743-0204
800-442-2762
Fax: 919-743-0208
www.autismsociety-nc.org

Explains the nature of autism. *$27.95*

581 Autism: From Tragedy to Triumph
Branden Publishing Company
PO Box 812094
Wellesley, MA 02482
Fax: 781-790-1056
E-mail: branden@branden.com
www.branden.com

A new book that deals with the Lovaas method and includes a foreward by Dr. Ivar Lovaas. The book is broken down into two parts, the long road to diagnosis and then treatment. *$12.95*

Year Founded: 1998 ISBN 0-828319-65-0

582 Autism: Identification, Education and Treatment
Autism Society of North Carolina Bookstore
505 Oberlin Road
Suite 230
Raleigh, NC 27605-1345
919-743-0204
800-442-2762
Fax: 919-743-0208
www.autismsociety-nc.org

Chapters include medical treatments, early intervention and communication and development in autism. *$36.00*

583 Autism: Nature, Diagnosis and Treatment
Guilford Publications
72 Spring Street
Department 4E
New York, NY 10012-4019
212-431-9800
800-365-7006
Fax: 212-966-6708
E-mail: exam@guilford.com
www.guilford.com

Foremost experts explore new perspectives on the nature and treatment of autism. Covering theory, research and the development of hypotheses and models, this book provides a balance between depth and breadth by focusing on questions most central to the field. For each question, an expert examines theoretical issues as well as empirical findings to offer new directions and testable hypotheses for future research. *$52.00*

417 pages ISBN 0-898627-24-9

584 Autism: Strategies for Change
Groden Center
86 Mount Hope Avenue
Providence, RI 02906
401-274-6310
Fax: 401-421-3280
E-mail: grodencenter@grodencenter.org
www.grodencenter.org

Andrea Pingitore, Administrative Assistant

A comprehensive approach to the education and treatment of children with autism and related disorders. Clinicians, parents, and students of autism who are, or want to be advocates for change will find in this book a blueprint, and much detail, on how to bring change about. This applies at the level of program planning and management as well as of clinical or education practice. *$21.95*

585 Autistic Adults at Bittersweet Farms
Haworth Press
10 Alice Street
Binghamton, NY 13904-1580
607-722-5857
800-429-6784
Fax: 607-722-1424
E-mail: getinfo@haworthpressinc.com
www.haworthpress.com

A touching view of an inspirational residential care program for autistic adolescents and adults. *$17.95*

212 pages ISBN 1-560240-57-1

586 Avoiding Unfortunate Situations
Autism Society of North Carolina Bookstore
505 Oberlin Road
Suite 230
Raleigh, NC 27605-1345
919-743-0204
800-442-2762
Fax: 919-743-0208
www.autismsociety-nc.org

A collection of tips and information from and about people with autism and other developmental disabilities. *$5.00*

587 Beyond Gentle Teaching
Autism Society of North Carolina Bookstore
505 Oberlin Road
Suite 230
Raleigh, NC 27605-1345
919-743-0204
800-442-2762
Fax: 919-743-0208
www.autismsociety-nc.org

A nonaversive approach to helping those in need. *$35.00*

588 Biology of the Autistic Syndromes
Autism Society of North Carolina Bookstore
505 Oberlin Road
Suite 230
Raleigh, NC 27605-1345
919-743-0204
800-442-2762
Fax: 919-743-0208
www.autismsociety-nc.org

A revision of the original, classic text in the light of new developments and current knowledge. This book covers the epidemiological, genetic, biochemical, immunological and neuropsychological literature on autism. *$74.95*

589 Children with Autism: A Developmental Perspective
Harvard University Press
79 Garden Street
Cambridge, MA 02138
800-405-1619
Fax: 800-406-9145

E-mail: CONTACT_HUP@harvard.edu
www.hup.harvard.edu

Views autism through the lens of developmental psychpathology, a discipline grounded in the belief that studies of normal and abnormal development can inform and enhance one another.

590 Children with Autism: Parents' Guide
Woodbine House
6510 Bells Mill Road
Bethesda, MD 20817
301-897-3570
800-843-7323
Fax: 301-897-5838
E-mail: info@woodbinehouse.com
www.woodbinehouse.com

Recommended as the first book parents should read, this completely revised volume offers information and a complete introduction to autism, while easing the family's fears and concerns as they adjust and cope with their child's disorder. *$14.95*

456 pages ISBN 1-890627-04-6

591 Communication Unbound: How Facilitated Communication Is Challenging Views
Baker & Taylor International
2709 Water Ridge Parkway
Charlotte, NC 28217
704-357-3500
800-775-1800
www.btol.com

Addresses the ways in which we receive persons with autism in our society, our community and our lives. *$18.95*

240 pages

592 Diagnosis and Treatment of Autism
Autism Society of North Carolina Bookstore
505 Oberlin Road
Suite 230
Raleigh, NC 27605-1345
919-743-0204
800-442-2762
Fax: 919-743-0208
www.autismsociety-nc.org

Various chapters written by professionals working with autistic children and adults. *$110.00*

593 Facilitated Communication and Technology Guide
Autism Society of North Carolina Bookstore
505 Oberlin Road
Suite 230
Raleigh, NC 27605-1345
919-743-0204
800-442-2762
Fax: 919-743-0208
www.autismsociety-nc.org

Chapters include technology and facilitated communication, augmentative and alternative communication, spelling boards, speech synthesizers and software. *$20.00*

594 Fighting for Darla: Challenges for Family Care & Professional Responsibility
Baker & Taylor International
2709 Water Ridge Parkway
Charlotte, NC 28217
704-357-3500
800-775-1800
www.btol.com

Follows the story of Darla, a pregnant adolescent with autism. *$18.95*

176 pages ISBN 0-807733-56-3

595 Fragile Success - Ten Autistic Children, Childhood to Adulthood
Autism Society of North Carolina Bookstore
505 Oberlin Road
Suite 230
Raleigh, NC 27605-1345
919-743-0204
800-442-2762
Fax: 919-743-0208
www.autismsociety-nc.org

A book about the lives of autistic children, whom the author has followed from their early years at the Elizabeth Ives School in New Haven, CT, through to adulthood. *$24.95*

596 Getting Started with Facilitated Communication
Syracuse University, Facilitated Communication Institute
370 Huntington Hall
Syracuse, NY 13244-2340
315-443-9657
Fax: 315-443-2274
E-mail: fcstaff@sued.syr.edu
www.soeweb.syr.edu/thefci

Describes in detail how to help individuals with autism and/or severe communication difficulties get started with facilitated communication.

597 Handbook of Autism and Pervasive Developmental Disorders
ADD WareHouse
300 NW 70th Avenue
Suite 102
Plantation, FL 33317
954-792-8100
800-233-9273
Fax: 954-792-8545
E-mail: sales@addwarehouse.com
www.addwarehouse.com

A comprehensive view of all information presently available about autism and other pervasive developmental disorders, drawing on findings and clinical experience from a number of related disciplines psychiatry, psychology, neurobiology and pediatrics. *$95.00*

1092 pages

598 Helping People with Autism Manage Their Behavior
Autism Society of North Carolina Bookstore
505 Oberlin Road
Suite 230
Raleigh, NC 27605-1345

919-743-0204
800-442-2762
Fax: 919-743-0208
www.autismsociety-nc.org

Covers the broad topic of helping people with autism manage their behavior. *$7.00*

599 Hidden Child: The Linwood Method for Reaching the Autistic Child
Woodbine House
6510 Bells Mill Road
Bethesda, MD 20817
301-897-3570
800-843-7323
Fax: 301-897-5838
E-mail: info@woodbinehouse.com
www.woodbinehouse.com

Chronicle of the Linwood Children's Center's successful treatment program for autistic children. *$14.95*

286 pages ISBN 0-933149-06-9

600 How to Teach Autistic & Severely Handicapped Children
Autism Society of North Carolina Bookstore
505 Oberlin Road
Suite 230
Raleigh, NC 27605-1345
919-743-0204
800-442-2762
Fax: 919-743-0208
www.autismsociety-nc.org

Book provides procedures for effectively assessing and teaching autistic and other severely handicapped children. *$9.00*

601 I'm Not Autistic on the Typewriter
TASH
29 W Susquehanna Avenue
Suite 210
Baltimore, MD 21204
410-828-8274
Fax: 410-828-6706
E-mail: info@tash.org
www.tash.org

Donna Gilles, President
Nancy Weiss, Executive Director
Jorge Pineda, Treasurer
Barbara Ransom, Secretary

An introduction to the facilitated communication training method. *$25.00*

602 Inner Life of Children with Special Needs
Taylor & Francis
325 Chestnut Street
Philadelphia, PA 19106
215-625-8900
Fax: 215-625-2940
www.taylorandfrancis.com

603 Joey and Sam
Autism Society of North Carolina Bookstore
505 Oberlin Road
Suite 230
Raleigh, NC 27605-1345
919-743-0204
800-442-2762

Fax: 919-743-0208
www.autismsociety-nc.org

A beautifully illustrated storybook for children, focusing on a family with two sons, one of whom suffers from autism. *$16.95*

604 Keys to Parenting the Child with Autism
Autism Society of North Carolina Bookstore
505 Oberlin Road
Suite 230
Raleigh, NC 27605-1345
919-743-0204
800-442-2762
Fax: 919-743-0208
www.autismsociety-nc.org

This book explains what autism is and how it is diagnosed. *$7.95*

605 Kristy and the Secret of Susan
Autism Society of North Carolina Bookstore
505 Oberlin Road
Suite 230
Raleigh, NC 27605-1345
919-743-0204
800-442-2762
Fax: 919-743-0208
www.autismsociety-nc.org

This book discusses Kristy and her new baby-sitting charge, Susan. Susan can't speak but sings beautifully. Susan is autistic. *$ 3.50*

606 Learning and Cognition in Autism
Kluwer Academic/Plenum Publishers
233 Spring Street
New York, NY 10013
212-620-8000
Fax: 212-463-0742
www.kluweronline.com

Collection of papers written by experts in the field of autism. Describes the cognitive and educational characteristics of people with autism and explains intervention techniques and strategies. Topics include motivating communication in children with autism and a chapter by a high-functioning woman with autism who discusses special learning problems and unique learning strengths that characterize their development and offers specific suggestions for working with people like herself. *$59.00*

368 pages ISBN 0-306448-71-8

607 Let Community Employment Be the Goal For Individuals with Autism
Autism Society of North Carolina Bookstore
505 Oberlin Road
Suite 230
Raleigh, NC 27605-1345
919-743-0204
800-442-2762
Fax: 919-743-0208
www.autismsociety-nc.org

A guide designed for people who are responsible for preparing individuals with autism to enter the work force. *$7.00*

608 Let Me Hear Your Voice
Autism Society of North Carolina Bookstore
505 Oberlin Road
Suite 230
Raleigh, NC 27605-1345
919-743-0204
800-442-2762
Fax: 919-743-0208
www.autismsociety-nc.org

The Maruice family's second and third children were diagnosed with autism. This book recounts their experience with a home program using behavior therapy. *$13.95*

609 Letting Go
Autism Society of North Carolina Bookstore
505 Oberlin Road
Suite 230
Raleigh, NC 27605-1345
919-743-0204
800-442-2762
Fax: 919-743-0208
www.autismsociety-nc.org

A book of poems about a journey, an emotional road of placing a child in a residential group home for children with autism. *$7.50*

610 Management of Autistic Behavior
Pro-Ed Publications
8700 Shoal Creek Boulevard
Austin, TX 78757-6816
512-451-3246
800-897-3202
Fax: 800-397-7633
E-mail: info@proedinc.com
www.proedinc.com

Comprehensive and practical book that tells what works best with specific problems. *$41.00*

450 pages ISBN 0-890791-96-1

611 Mindblindness: An Essay on Autism and Theory of Mind
Autism Society of North Carolina Bookstore
505 Oberlin Road
Suite 230
Raleigh, NC 27605-1345
919-743-0204
800-442-2762
Fax: 919-743-0208
www.autismsociety-nc.org

Interpretations and research into the theory of mindblindness in children with autism. *$19.95*

300 pages ISBN 0-262023-84-9

612 Mixed Blessings
Autism Society of North Carolina Bookstore
505 Oberlin Road
Suite 230
Raleigh, NC 27605-1345
919-743-0204
800-442-2762
Fax: 919-743-0208
www.autismsociety-nc.org

A real-life family discusses the raising of their autistic son. *$19.95*

613 More Laughing and Loving with Autism
Autism Society of North Carolina Bookstore
505 Oberlin Road
Suite 230
Raleigh, NC 27605-1345
919-743-0204
800-442-2762
Fax: 919-743-0208
www.autismsociety-nc.org

A collection of warm and humorous parent stories about raising a child with autism. *$9.95*

614 Neurobiology of Autism 2nd Edition
Johns Hopkins University Press
2715 N Charles Street
Baltimore, MD 21218-4363
410-516-6900
800-537-5487
Fax: 410-516-6968
www.press.jhu.edu/index.html

This book discusses recent advances in scientific research that point to a neurobiological basis for autism and examines the clinical implications of this research. *$44.95*

272 pages Year Founded: 2005 ISBN 0-801856-80-9

615 News from the Border: a Mother's Memoir of Her Autistic Son
Houghton Mifflin Company
222 Berkeley Street
Boston, MA 02116
617-351-5000
Fax: 617-351-1107
www.hmco.com

A searingly honest account of the author's family experiences with autism. Raising an autistic child is the central, ongoing drama of her married life in this riveting account of acceptance and coping. *$22.95*

384 pages

616 Nobody Nowhere
Autism Society of North Carolina Bookstore
505 Oberlin Road
Suite 230
Raleigh, NC 27605-1345
919-743-0204
800-442-2762
Fax: 919-743-0208
www.autismsociety-nc.org

An autobiography giving readers a tour of the author's life with autism. *$14.00*

617 Parent Survival Manual
Autism Society of North Carolina Bookstore
505 Oberlin Road
Suite 230
Raleigh, NC 27605-1345
919-743-0204
800-442-2762
Fax: 919-743-0208
www.autismsociety-nc.org

Compiled from three hundred fifty anecdotes told by parents of autistic and developmentally disabled children. *$38.50*

618 Parent's Guide to Autism
Autism Society of North Carolina Bookstore
505 Oberlin Road
Suite 230
Raleigh, NC 27605-1345
919-743-0204
800-442-2762
Fax: 919-743-0208
www.autismsociety-nc.org

An essential handbook for anyone facing autism. *$14.00*

619 Please Don't Say Hello
Human Sciences Press
233 Spring Street
New York, NY 10013-1522
212-620-8000
Fax: 212-807-1047

Paul and his family moved into a new neighborhood. Paul's brother was autistic. The children thought that Eddie was retarded until they learned that there were skills that he could do better than they could. *$10.95*

47 pages ISBN 0-898851-99-8

620 Preschool Issues in Autism
Kluwer Academic/Plenum Publishers
233 Spring Street
New York, NY 10013
212-620-8000
Fax: 212-463-0742
www.kluweronline.com

Combines some of the most important theory and data related to the early identifiction and intervention in autism and related disorders. Addresses clinical aspects, parental concerns and legal issues. Helps professionals understand and implement state-of-the-art services for young children and their families. *$54.00*

294 pages ISBN 0-306444-40-2

621 Psychoeducational Profile
Autism Society of North Carolina Bookstore
505 Oberlin Road
Suite 230
Raleigh, NC 27605-1345
919-743-0204
800-442-2762
Fax: 919-743-0208
www.autismsociety-nc.org

The PEP-R is a revision of the popular instrument that has been used for over twenty years to assess skills and behavior of autistic and communication-handicapped children who function between the ages of 6 months and 7 years. *$74.00*

622 Reaching the Autistic Child: a Parent Training Program
Brookline Books/Lumen Editions
PO Box 97
Newton Upper Falls, MA 02464
800-666-2665
Fax: 617-558-8011
www.brooklinebooks.com

Detailed case studies of social and behavioral change in autistic children and their families show parents how to implement the principles for improved socialization and behavior. Revised and updated 1998. *$15.95*

ISBN 1-571290-56-7

623 Record Books for Individuals with Autism
Indiana Institute on Disability and Community
Indiana University
2853 E Tenth Street
Bloomington, IN 47408-2696
812-855-6508
800-280-7010
Fax: 812-855-9630
TTY: 812-855-9396
E-mail: uap@indiana.edu
www.iidc.indiana.edu

This book was developed with parent information about an autistic child so that it is organized, easily accessible and can be copied as needed. *$5.00*

37 pages

624 Russell Is Extra Special
Autism Society of North Carolina Bookstore
505 Oberlin Road
Suite 230
Raleigh, NC 27605-1345
919-743-0204
800-442-2762
Fax: 919-743-0208
www.autismsociety-nc.org

A sensitive portrayal of an autistic boy written by his father. *$8.95*

625 Schools for Children With Autism Spectrum Disorders
Resources for Children with Special Needs
116 E 16th Street
Fifth Floor
New York City, NY 10003
212-677-4650
Fax: 212-254-4070
E-mail: info@resourcesnyc.org
www.resourcesnyc.org

Karen Schlesinger, Director

A Directory of Educational Programs in NYC and The Lower Hudson Valley. Detailed descriptions of more than 300 public and private schools with programs for children with Autism and Autism Spectrum Disorders. In addition, a general introduction on autism, educational approaches, available resources, supplementary services, definitions, and other related services are included. *$20.00*

626 Sex Education: Issues for the Person with Autism
Indiana Institute on Disability and Community
Indiana University
2853 E Tenth Street
Bloomington, IN 47408-2696
812-855-6508
800-280-7010
Fax: 812-855-9630
TTY: 812-855-9396
E-mail: uap@indiana.edu
www.iidc.indiana.edu

Discusses issues of sexuality and provides some methods of instruction for persons with autism. *$3.00*

18 pages

627   Siblings of Children with Autism: A Guide for Families
Autism Society of North Carolina Bookstore
505 Oberlin Road
Suite 230
Raleigh, NC 27605-1345
919-743-0204
800-442-2762
Fax: 919-743-0208
www.autismsociety-nc.org

Offers information on the needs of a child with autism. *$16.95*

628   Somebody Somewhere
Autism Society of North Carolina Bookstore
505 Oberlin Road
Suite 230
Raleigh, NC 27605-1345
919-743-0204
800-442-2762
Fax: 919-743-0208
www.autismsociety-nc.org

Offers a revealing account of the author's battle with autism. *$15.00*

629   Soon Will Come the Light
Autism Society of North Carolina Bookstore
505 Oberlin Road
Suite 230
Raleigh, NC 27605-1345
919-743-0204
800-442-2762
Fax: 919-743-0208
www.autismsociety-nc.org

Offers new perspectives on the perplexing disability of autism. *$19.95*

630   Teaching Children with Autism: Strategies to Enhance Communication
Autism Society of North Carolina Bookstore
505 Oberlin Road
Suite 230
Raleigh, NC 27605-1345
919-743-0204
800-442-2762
Fax: 919-743-0208
www.autismsociety-nc.org

This valuable new book describes teaching strategies and instructional adaptations which promote communication and socialization in children with autism. *$34.95*

631   Teaching and Mainstreaming Autistic Children
Love Publishing Company
9101 E Kenyon Avenue
Suite 2200
Denver, CO 80237
303-221-7333
Fax: 303-221-7444
E-mail: lpc@lovepublishing.com
www.lovepublishing.com

Dr Knoblock advocates a highly organized, structured environment for autistic children, with teachers and parents working together. His premise is that the learning and social needs of autistic children must be analyzed and a daily program be designed with interventions that respond to this functional analysis of their behavior. *$39.95*

Year Founded: 1982 ISBN 0-891081-11-9

632   The Hidden Child: Youth with Autism
Mason Crest Publishers
370 Reed Road
Suite 302
Broomall, PA 19008
610-543-6200
866-627-2665
Fax: 610-543-3878
E-mail: dtaylor@masoncrest.com
www.masoncrest.com

Hope is the keyword for the autistic child's future. Through education, early intervention, and continued research, children with autism can live normal lives. Factual information about autism, the Autism Society of America, sibshops, and different educational treatments will expand the reader's knowledge of this condition. A fictional story told from a sibling's point of view helps the reader understand the effects autism has on individuals and family members.

ISBN 1-590847-38-9

633   Then Things Every Child with Autism Wishes You Knew
Future Horizons
721 West Abram Street
Arlington, TX 76013
212-572-2882
800-489-0727
Fax: 817-277-2270
www.www.futurehorizons-autism.com/index.htm

Ellen Notbohm, Author

Framed in both humor and compassion, the book defines the top ten characteristics that illuminate the minds and hearts of cildren with autism. Ellen's personal experiences.

634   Thinking In Pictures, Expanded Edition: My Life with Autism
Vintage
1745 Broadway 20th Floor
New York, NY 10019
212-572-2882
800-733-3000
Fax: 212-572-6043
www.www.randomhouse.com/vintage/index.html

Temple Grandin, Author

ISBN 0-307275-65-5

635   Ultimate Stranger: The Autistic Child
Autism Society of North Carolina Bookstore
505 Oberlin Road
Suite 230
Raleigh, NC 27605-1345
919-743-0204
800-442-2762
Fax: 919-743-0208
www.autismsociety-nc.org

Delacato's thesis is that autism is neuro-genic and not psycho-genic in origin. *$10.00*

636   Understanding Autism
Fanlight Productions
4196 Washington Street
Boston, MA 02130

617-469-4999
800-937-4113
Fax: 617-469-3379
E-mail: fanlight@fanlight.com
www.fanlight.com

Parents of children with autism discuss the nature and symptoms of this lifelong disability, and outline a treatment program based on behavior modification principles. *$195.00*

ISBN 1-572951-00-1

637 **Until Tomorrow: A Family Lives with Autism**
Autism Society of North Carolina Bookstore
505 Oberlin Road
Suite 230
Raleigh, NC 27605-1345
919-743-0204
800-442-2762
Fax: 919-743-0208
www.autismsociety-nc.org

The central theme of this book is an effort to show what it is like to live with a child who cannot communicate. *$10.00*

638 **When Snow Turns to Rain**
Woodbine House
6510 Bells Mill Road
Bethesda, MD 20817
301-897-3570
800-843-7323
Fax: 301-897-5838
E-mail: info@woodbinehouse.com
www.woodbinehouse.com

A gripping personal account of one family's experiences with autism. Chronicles a family's journey from parental bliss to devastation, as they learn that their son has autism. This book delves into diagnosis, treatments, and attitudes toward persons with autism. *$14.95*

250 pages ISBN 0-933149-63-8

639 **Winter's Flower**
Autism Society of North Carolina Bookstore
505 Oberlin Road
Suite 230
Raleigh, NC 27605-1345
919-743-0204
800-442-2762
Fax: 919-743-0208
www.autismsociety-nc.org

The story of Ranae Johnson's quest to rescue her son from a world of silence. A story of love, patience and dedication. *$12.95*

640 **Without Reason**
Autism Society of North Carolina Bookstore
505 Oberlin Road
Suite 230
Raleigh, NC 27605-1345
919-743-0204
800-442-2762
Fax: 919-743-0208
www.autismsociety-nc.org

A story of a family coping with two generations of autism. *$19.95*

Periodicals & Pamphlets

641 **Autism Newslink**
Autism Society Ontario
1179A King Street W
Suite 004
Toronto, ON
416-246-9592
Fax: 416-246-9417
E-mail: mail@autismsociety.on.ca
www.autismsociety.on.ca

Covers society activities and contains information on autism. Recurring features include news of research, a calendar of events, reports of meetings, and book reviews. *$25.00*

10 pages 4 per year

642 **Autism Research Review International**
Autism Research Institute
4182 Adams Avenue
San Diego, CA 92116-2536
619-281-7165
Fax: 619-563-6840
www.autisimresearchinstitute.com

Discusses current research and provides information about the causes, diagnosis, and treatment of autism and related disorders. *$18.00*

8 pages 4 per year   ISSN 0893-8474

643 **Autism Society News**
Utah Parent Center
2290 E 4500 S
Suite 110
Salt Lake City, UT 84117-4428
801-272-1051
800-468-1160
Fax: 801-272-8907
www.utahparentcenter.org

Presents news, research information, and legislative updates regarding autism. Recurring features include a calendar of events and columns titled Parent Meetings, What's On in the News, Research News, Parent Corner, Legislative Summary, and A Big Thank You!

8 pages

644 **Autism in Children and Adolescents**
Center for Mental Health Services: Knowledge Exchange Network
PO Box 42557
Washington, DC 20015
800-789-2647
Fax: 301-984-8796
TDD: 866-889-2647
E-mail: ken@mentalhealth.org
www.mentalhealth.org.samhsa.gov

This fact sheet defines autism, describes the signs and causes, discusses types of help available, and suggests what parents or other caregivers can do.

2 pages Year Founded: 1997

645 **Facts About Autism**
Indiana Institute on Disability and Community
Indiana University
2853 E Tenth Street
Bloomington, IN 47408-2696

812-855-6508
800-280-7010
Fax: 812-855-9630
TTY: 812-855-9396
E-mail: uap@indiana.edu
www.iidc.indiana.edu

Provides concise information describing autism, diagnosis, needs of the person with autism from diagnosis through adulthood. Information on the Autism Society of America chapters in Indiana are listed in the back, along with a description of the Indiana Resource Center for Autism and suggested books to look for in the local library. Also available in Spanish. *$1.00*

646   Journal of Autism and Developmental Disorders
Springer Science & Business Media
Heidelberger Plate 3
14197 Berlin
Germany,
www.springer.com

Features research and case studies involving the entire spectrum of interventions and advances in the diagnosis and classification of disorders. *$98.00*

6 per year   ISSN 0162-3257

647   MAAP
MAAP Services
PO Box 524
Crown Point, IN 46307
219-662-1311
Fax: 219-662-0638
E-mail: chart@netnitco.net
www.maapservices.org

This quarterly newsletter provides the opportunity for parents and professionals to network with families of more advanced individuals with Autism, Asperger's syndrome, and Pervasive developmental disorder. Helps you to learn about more advanced individuals within the autism spectrum. *$22.00*

4 per year

648   Sex Education: Issues for the Person with Autism
Autism Society of North Carolina Bookstore
505 Oberlin Road
Suite 230
Raleigh, NC 27605-1345
919-743-0204
800-442-2762
Fax: 919-743-0208
www.autismsociety-nc.org

Discusses issues of sexuality and provides methods of instruction for people with autism. *$4.00*

649   Treatment of Children with Mental Disorders
National Institute of Mental Health
6001 Executive Boulevard
Room 8184
Bethesda, MD 20892-9663
866-615-6464
Fax: 301-443-4279
TTY: 301-443-8431
E-mail: nimhinfo@nih.gov
www.nimh.nih.gov

A short booklet that contains questions and answers about therapy for children with mental disorders. Includes a chart of mental disorders and medications used.

Research Centers

650   Facilitated Learning at Syracuse University
Syracuse University, Facilitated Communication Institute
370 Huntington Hall
Syracuse, NY 13244-2340
315-443-9657
Fax: 315-443-9218
E-mail: fcstaff@syr.edu
www.www.thefci.syr.edu

College offering facilitated learning research into communication with persons who have autism or severe disabilities. Offers books, videos and public awareness on research projects.

651   TEACCH
CB# 6305
University of NC at Chapel Hill
Chapel Hill, NC 27599-6305
919-966-2174
Fax: 919-966-4127
E-mail: teacch@unc.edu
www.www.teacch.com

Lee Marcus, Clinical Director
Jean Justice, Office Manager

This organization is the division for the treatment and education of autistic and related communication handicapped children.

Support Groups & Hot Lines

652   Autism Services Center
929 4th Avenue
PO Box 507
Huntington, WV 25710-0507
304-525-8014
Fax: 304-525-8026
www.autismservicescenter.org

Ruth Sullivan, Executive Director

ASC is a nonprofit, licensed bahavioral health center providing services to individuals with developmental disabilities in a four-county area in West Virginia. We also have an outside hotline (9-5) (M-F), which provides information to parents and other individuals.
Year Founded: 1979

653   Autism Society of America
7910 Woodmont Avenue
Suite 300
Bethesda, MD 20814-3067
301-657-0881
800-328-8476
www.autism-society.org

Cathy Pratt, Chair, Board Of Directors
Lee Grossman, President/Ceo

The mission of the Autism Society of America is to promote lifelong access and opportunities for persons within the autism spectrum and their families, to be fully included, participating members of their communities through advocacy, public awareness, education, and research related to autism.

Year Founded: 1965

654   Autism Treatment Center of America Son-Rise Program
2080 S Undermountain Road
Sheffield, MA 01257
413-229-2100
Fax: 413-229-3202
E-mail: correspondence@option.org
www.son-rise.org

Barry Neil Kaufman, Co Founder/Creator

Teaches parents and professionals caring for children and adults challenged by Autism how to design and implement home-based/child-centered programs.

Video & Audio

655   ASD: Heads Up for the Low Down
Program Development Associates
PO Box 2038
Syracuse, NY 13220-2038
315-452-0643
800-543-2119
Fax: 315-452-0710
E-mail: info@disabilitytraining.com
www.disabilitytraining.com/autism

Covers diagnosis symptoms and interventions with ASD, including experts in cognitive development and clinical pediatrics, plus young Jack's images mixed with his dad's original music. 14 minutes. *$79.95*

Year Founded: 2005

656   Autism DVD Package
Program Development Associates
PO Box 2038
Syracuse, NY 13220-2038
315-452-0643
800-543-2119
Fax: 315-452-0710
E-mail: info@disabilitytraining.com
www.disabilitytraining.com/autism

Delivers a full range of autism issues and instructional technique. Includes diagnoses and strategies on Asperger Syndrome and Autism Spectrum Disorders, talks with parents and kids about autism, and helps educators work with low-functioning students one-on-one. 5 DVD Set. *$289.95*

657   Autism Spectrum Disorders and the SCERTS
Program Development Associates
PO Box 2038
Syracuse, NY 13220-2038
315-452-0643
800-543-2119
Fax: 315-452-0710
E-mail: info@disabilitytraining.com
www.disabilitytraining.com/autism

Early intervention for children with Autism Spectrum Disorders. Shows a model in action with higher-functioning children who require less support. 105 minutes between three tapes. *$279.00*

Year Founded: 2004

658   Autism in the Classroom
Program Development Associates
PO Box 2038
Syracuse, NY 13220-2038
315-452-0643
800-543-2119
Fax: 315-452-0710
E-mail: info@disabilitytraining.com
www.disabilitytraining.com/autism

Overviews symptoms, behaviors and treatments, and interviews children with autism, along with their parents and their teachers. 16 minutes. *$69.95*

Year Founded: 2004

659   Autism is a World
Program Development Associates
PO Box 2038
Syracuse, NY 13220-2038
315-452-0643
800-543-2119
Fax: 315-452-0710
E-mail: info@disabilitytraining.com
www.disabilitytraining.com/autism

Takes a look inside the life of a woman who lives with the disorder. She explains how she feels, how she relates to others, her obsession and why her behavior can be so very different. Gives teachers and professionals striving to understand Autism Spectrum Disorder a glimpse from the inside out of this developmental disability. 40 minutes & can also be ordered as a DVD with special features. *$99.95*

Year Founded: 2004

660   Autism: A Strange, Silent World
Filmakers Library
124 E 40th Street
New York, NY 10016
212-808-4980
Fax: 212-808-4983
E-mail: info@filmakers.com
www.filmakers.com

British educators and medical personnel offer insight into autism's characteristics and treatment approaches through the cameos of three children. 52 minutes. *$295.00*

661   Autism: A World Apart
Fanlight Productions
4196 Washington Street
Suite 2
Boston, MA 01231
617-469-4999
800-937-4113
Fax: 617-469-3379
E-mail: fanlight@fanlight.com
www.fanlight.com

Kelli English, Publicity Coordinator

In this documentary, three families show us what the textbooks and studies cannot; what it's like to live with autism day after day, raise and love children who may be withdrawn and violent and unable to make personal connections with their families. Video cassette. 29 minutes. *$199.00*

ISBN 1-572950-39-0

662   Autism: Being Friends
Indiana Institute on Disability and Community
Indiana University
2853 E Tenth Street
Bloomington, IN 47408-2696
812-855-6508
800-280-7010
Fax: 812-855-9630
TTY: 812-855-9396
E-mail: uap@indiana.edu
www.iidc.indiana.edu

This autism awareness videotape was produced specifically for use with young children. The program portrays the abilities of the child with autism and describes ways in which peers can help the child to be a part of the everyday world. *$10.00*

Year Founded: 1991

663   Avoiding The Turbulance: Guiding Families of Children Diagnosed with Autism
Program Development Associates
PO Box 2038
Syracuse, NY 13220-2038
315-452-0643
800-543-2119
Fax: 315-452-0710
E-mail: info@disabilitytraining.com
www.disabilitytraining.com/autism

Focuses primarily on the best strategies of early intervention. Good resources for primary care medical providers and agency professionals involved in early intervention autism programs. 12 minutes. *$79.95*

Year Founded: 2005

664   Breakthroughs: How to Reach Students with Autism
ADD WareHouse
300 NW 70th Avenue
Suite 102
Plantation, FL 33317
954-792-8100
800-233-9273
Fax: 954-792-8545
E-mail: sales@addwarehouse.com
www.addwarehouse.com

This video is designed for instructors of children with autism, K-12. The program provides a fully-loaded teacher's manual with reproducible lesson plans that will take you through an entire school year as well as an award-winning video that demonstrates the instructional and behavioral techniques recommended in the manual. Covers math, reading, fine motor, self-help, vocational, social and life skills. Features a veteran instructor who was named 'Teacher of the Year' by the Autism Society of America. *$89.00*

665   Children and Autism: Time is Brain
Program Development Associates
PO Box 2038
Syracuse, NY 13220-2038
315-452-0643
800-543-2119
Fax: 315-452-0710
E-mail: info@disabilitytraining.com
www.disabilitytraining.com/autism

Video features Applied Behavior Analysis (ABA) as an autism treatment technique by focusing on two families raising a child with autism. Gives documentation on their interaction with therapists and behavior analysts. 28 minutes. *$99.95*

Year Founded: 2004

666   Going to School with Facilitated Communication
Syracuse University, Facilitated Communication Institute
370 Huntington Hall
Syracuse, NY 13244-2340
315-443-9657
Fax: 315-443-2274
E-mail: fcstaff@sued.syr.edu
www.soeweb.syr.edu/thefci

A video in which students with autism and/or severe disabilities illustrate the use of facilitated communication focusing on basic principles fostering facilitated communication.

667   Health Care Desensitization
Indiana Institute on Disability and Community
Indiana University
2853 E Tenth Street
Bloomington, IN 47408-2696
812-855-6508
800-280-7010
Fax: 812-855-9630
TTY: 812-855-9396
E-mail: uap@indiana.edu
www.iidc.indiana.edu

Training videotape for teachers, parents, health professionals and group home staff showing how the desensitization procedure to medical, dental and optometric exams was applied to preschool and adolescent students with autism and thier successful cooperation with the subsequent health care. *$25.00*

Year Founded: 1989

668   I'm Not Autistic on the Typewriter
Syracuse University, Facilitated Communication Institute
370 Huntington Hall
Syracuse, NY 13244-2340
315-443-9657
Fax: 315-443-2274
E-mail: fcstaff@sued.syr.edu
www.soeweb.syr.edu/thefci

A video introducing facilitated communication, a method by which persons with autism express themselves.

669   Interview with Dr. Pauline Filipek
Program Development Associates
PO Box 2038
Syracuse, NY 13220-2038
315-452-0643
800-543-2119
Fax: 315-452-0710
E-mail: info@disabilitytraining.com
www.disabilitytraining.com/autism

An interview that presents early stage developmental autism, with diagnosis and age-level comparisons, research, interventions and myths and false and future treatments. 14 minutes. *$79.95*

Year Founded: 2005

670 Matthew: Guidance for Parents with Autistic Children
Program Development Associates
PO Box 2038
Syracuse, NY 13220-2038
315-452-0643
800-543-2119
Fax: 315-452-0710
E-mail: info@disabilitytraining.com
www.disabilitytraining.com/autism

A resource video guide for parents of autistic children. Shows parents where they should go, who to consult and what did or did not work for Matthew and his parents. 28 minutes. *$79.95*

Year Founded: 2004

671 Rising Above a Diagnosis of Autism
Program Development Associates
PO Box 2038
Syracuse, NY 13220-2038
315-452-0643
800-543-2119
Fax: 315-452-0710
E-mail: info@disabilitytraining.com
www.disabilitytraining.com/autism

Focuses primarily on the period when a child receives a diagnosis of Autism. Meet with others who are involved somehow with autistic children, and hear recommendations from professionals and meet children that have Autism, PDD, Asperger's Syndrome or any other forms of Austism Spectrum Disorder. 30 minutes. *$99.95*

Year Founded: 2005

672 Sense of Belonging: Including Students with Autism in Their School Community
Indiana Institute on Disability and Community
Indiana University
2853 E Tenth Street
Bloomington, IN 47408-2696
812-855-6508
800-280-7010
Fax: 812-855-9630
TTY: 812-855-9396
E-mail: uap@indiana.edu
www.iidc.indiana.edu

Highlights the efforts of two elementary and one middle school student with autism in general education settings. Illustrates the value of inclusion and importance it plays for the future of all students. Practical strategies for teaching students with autism are described. *$40.00*

Year Founded: 1997

673 Straight Talk About Autism with Parents and Kids
ADD WareHouse
300 NW 70th Avenue
Suite 102
Plantation, FL 33317
954-792-8100
800-233-9273
Fax: 954-792-8545
E-mail: sales@addwarehouse.com
www.addwarehouse.com

These revealing videos contain intimate interviews with parents of kids with autism and the young people themselves. Topics discussed include friends and social isolation, communication difficulties, hypersensitivities, teasing, splinter skills, parent support groups and more. One video focuses on childhood issues, while the second covers adolescent issues. Two 40 minute videos. *$99.00*

Web Sites

674 www.aane.org
Asperger's Association of New England
Working advocacy group of Massachusetts parents of adults and teens with AS who have come together with the goal of getting state funding for residential supports for adults with AS. At the present time no state agency will provide these needed supports. Interested parents and AS adults are welcome to join this working group.

675 www.ani.ac
Autism Network International
This organization is run by and for the autistic people. The best advocates for autistic people are autistic people themselves. Provides a forum for autistic people to share information, peer support, tips for coping and problem solving, as well as providing a social outlet for autistic people to explore and participate in autistic social experiences. In addition to promoting self advocacy for high-functioning autistic adults, ANI also works to improve the lives of autistic people who, whether they are too young or because they do not have the communication skills, are not able to advocate for themselves. Helps autistic people by providing information and referrals for parenting and teachers. Also strives to educate the public about autism.

676 www.aspennj.org
Asperger Syndrome Education Network (ASPEN)
Regionally-based non-profit organization headquarted in New Jersey, with 11 local chapters, providing families and those individuals affected with Asperger Syndrome, PDD-NOS, High Function Autism, and related disorders. Provides education about the issues surrounding Asperger Syndrome and other related disorders. Support in knowing that they are not alone and in helping individuals with AS achieve their maximum potential. Advocacy in areas of appropriate educational programs and placement, medical research funding, and increased public awareness and understanding.

677 www.autism-society.org
Autism Society of America
Promotes lifelong access and opportunities for persons within the autism spectrum and their families, to be fully included, participating members of their communities through advocacy, public awareness, education and research related to autism.

678 www.autism.org
Center for the Study of Autism (CSA)
Located in the Salem/Portland, Oregon area. Provides information about autism to parents and professionals, and conducts research on the efficacy of various therapeutic interventions. Much of our research is in collaboration with the Autism Research Institute in San Diego, California.

679 www.autismresearchinstitute.org
Autism Research Institute

Devoted to conducting research on the causes of autism and on the methods of preventing, diagnosing and treating autism and other severe behavioral disorders of childhood.

680 www.autismservicescenter.org
Autism Services Center

Makes available technical assistance in designing programs. Provides supervised apartments, group homes, respite services, independent living programs and job-coached employment.

681 www.autismspeaks.org
National Alliance for Autism Research (NAAR)

National nonprofit, tax-exempt organization dedicated to finding the causes, preventions, effective treatments and, ultimately, a cure for the autism spectrum disorders. NAAR's mission is to fund, promote and support biomedical research into autism. Aims to have an aggressive and far-reaching research program. Seeks to encourage scientists outside the field of autism to apply their insights and experience to autism. Publishes a newsletter that focuses on developments in autism research. Supports brain banks and tissue consortium development.

682 www.autisticservices.com
Autistic Services

Dedicated to serving the unique lifelong needs of autistic individuals.

683 www.cfsny.org
Center for Family Support (CFS)

Devoted to the physical well-being and development of the retarded child and the sound mental health of the parents.

684 www.csaac.org
Community Services for Autistic Adults & Children

Enables individuals to achieve their highest potential and contribute as confident members in their community, instead of living in institutions.

685 www.cyberpsych.org
CyberPsych

Hosts the American Psychoanalyists Foundation, American Association of Suicideology, Society for the Exploration of Psychotherapy Intergration, and Anxiety Disorders Association of America. Also subcategories of the anxiety disorders, as well as general information, including panic disorder, phobias, obsessive compulsive disorder (OCD), social phobia, generalized anxiety disorder, post traumatic stress disorder, and phobias of childhood. Book reviews and links to web pages sharing the topics.

686 www.feat.org
Families for Early Autism Treatment

A nonprofit organization of parents and professionals, designed to help families with children who are diagnosised with autism or pervasive developmental disorder. It offers a network of support for families. FEAT has a Lending Library, with information on autism and also offers Support Meetings on the third Wednesday of each month.

687 www.iidc.indiana.edu
Indiana Resource Center for Autism (IRCA)

Conducts outreach training and consultations, engage in research and develop and disseminate info on behalf of individuals across the autism spectrum.

688 www.ladders.org
The Autism Research Foundation

A nonprofit, tax-exempt organization dedicated to researching the neurological underpinnings of autism and other related developmental brain disorders. Seeking to rapidly expand and accelerate research into the pervasive developmental disorders. To do this, time and efforts goes into investigating the neuropathology of autism in their laboratories, collecting and redistributing brain tissue to promising research groups for use by projects approved by the Tissue Resource Committee, studies frozen autistic brain tissue collected by TARF. They believe that only aggressive scientific and medical research will reveal the cure for this lifelong disorder.

689 www.maapservices.org
MAAP Services

Provides information and advice to people with Asperger Syndrome, Autism and Pervasive Developmental Disorders. Provides parents and professionals a chance to network with others to learn more within the autism spectrum.

690 www.mentalhealth.Samhsa.Gov
Center for Mental Health Services Knowledge Exchange Network

Information about resources, technical assistance, research, training, networks and other federal clearinghouses and fact sheets and materials.

691 www.mhselfhelp.org
National Mental Health Consumer's Self-Help Clearinghouse

Encourages the development and growth of consumer self-help groups.

692 www.nami.org
National Alliance for the Mentally Ill

Mission is to bring consumers and families with similar experiences together to share information about services, care providers and ways to cope with the challenges.

693 www.necc.org
New England Center for Children

Serves students diagnosed with autism, learning disabilities, language delays, mental retardation, behavior disorders and related disabilities.

694 www.planetpsych.com
Planetpsych.com

Learn about disorders, their treatments and other topics in psychology. Articles are listed under the related topic areas. Ask a therapist a question for free, or view the directory of professionals in your area. If you are a therapist sign up for the directory. Current features, self-help, interactive, and newsletter archives.

695 www.resourcesnyc.org
Resources for Children with Special Needs

Gives a general introduction on autism, educational approaches, available resources, supplementary services, definitions and other related services are included.

696 www.son-rise.org
Son-Rise Autism Treatment Center of America

Training center for autism professionals and parents of autistic children. Programs focus on the design and implementation of home-based/child-centered alternatives.

697 www.thenadd.org
NADD-National Association for the Dually Diagnosed

Promotes the interest of professional and parent development with resources for individuals who have the coexistence of mental illness and mental retardation.

Directories & Databases

698 After School and More
Resources for Children with Special Needs
116 E 16th Street
5th Floor
New York, NY 10003
212-677-4650
Fax: 212-254-4070
E-mail: info@resourcesnyc.org
www.resourcesnyc.org

Second Edition: After School, Weekend and Holiday Programs for Children an Youth with Disabilities and Special Needs in the Metro New York Area. Information about suitable after school programs for parents and care givers of children with disabilities. Over 400 providers of after school, holiday, weekend and pre-and post-camp programs for children and youth from 6 to 21 with disabilities and special needs. Arts, crafts, dance and music to homework help, tutoring and sports. *$25.00*

240 pages

699 Camps 2008
Resources for Children with Special Needs
116 E 16th Street
5th Floor
New York, NY 10003
212-677-4550
Fax: 212-254-4070
E-mail: info@resourcesnyc.org
www.resourcesnyc.org

A Directory of Camps and Summer Programs for Children and Youth with Disabilities and Special Needs in the Metro New York Area. Our guide includes profiles of more than 300 day camps, recreation, tutoring, and travel programs, museums, nature experience and summer employment in New York City, sleep away programs in the northeast, and travel programs throughout the U.S. that serve both special and mainstream children. *$25.00*

1 per year ISBN 0-967836-57-3

700 Schools and Services for Children with Autism Spectrum Disorders
Resources For Children with Special Needs
116 E 16th Street
5th Floor
New York, NY 10003
212-677-4650
Fax: 212-254-4070
E-mail: info@resourcesnyc.org
www.www.resourcesnyc.org

A Directory of Educational Programs in NYC and the Lower Hudson Valley. Includes over 700 schools, organizations and programs that serve children and youth with autism spectrum disorders in NYC, Westchester, Orange, Rockland, Putnam, Dutchess, Ulster and Sullivan counties. Includes early intervention programs, camps, day care, respite, evaluations, recreation, parent support, mentoring, health services, tutoring, employment preparation, social skills training, housing options and more. *$40.00*

288 pages ISBN 0-967836-59-X

701 The Comprehensive Directory
Resources For Children with Special Needs
116 E 16th Street
5th Floor
New York, NY 10003
212-677-4650
Fax: 212-254-4070
E-mail: info@resourcesnyc.org
www.resourcesnyc.org

Programs and Services for Children with Disabilities and their Families in the Metro New York Area. Provides information about more than 5000 programs and services for children and youth with disabilities and special needs, and their families. Up-to-date information about agencies, schools, afterschool social, recreational and cultural programs, camps and summer programs, family support and respite services. *$55.00*

1096 pages ISBN 0-967836-51-4

702 Transition Matters-From School to Independence
Resources for Children with Special Needs
116 E 16th Street
5th Floor
New York, NY 10003
212-677-4650
Fax: 212-254-4070
E-mail: info@resourcesnyc.org
www.resourcesnyc.org

A Guide and Directory of Services for Youth with Disabilities and Special Needs in the Metro New York Area. Takes you through the systems involved and covers rights, entitlements, options and programs. Over 1000 organization descriptions cover college, specialized education, job training, supported work, independent living and more. *$35.00*

500 pages ISBN 0-967836-56-5

Bipolar Disorders

Introduction

Bipolar Disorder (Manic Depression) is the name for a group of severe mental illnesses characterized by alterations between depression and manic euphoria or irritability.

The two states are not independent of each other, but part of the same illness. Individuals in the manic phase of Bipolar Disorder may feel exuberant, invincible, or even immortal. They may be awake for days at a time, and be able to work tirelessly; they may rush from one idea to the next carried by a nearly uncontrollable burst of energy that leaves others bewildered and unable to keep up. (Some extraordinarily creative people, Vincent Van Gogh, for example, have had Bipolar Disorder. Whether or not the disorder makes a positive contribution to creativity is a controversial question.)

In the depressed phase which follows a manic high, the patient may be suicidal. The depressed phase of the illness mirrors a major depressive episode. There are three forms of Bipolar Disorders: Bipolar I Disorder, Bipolar II Disorder, and Cyclothymic Disorder. Bipolar II Disorder consists of repeated depressive episodes interspersed with hypomanic (not full blown mania) episodes. The individual with Cyclothymic Disorder has a history of at least two years of repeated episodes of elevated and depresed mood which don't meet all the criteria for mania or depression but which cause distress and/or decreased ability to function.

A number of researchers are closing in on genetic links to the illness. Like all mental disorders, however, the relationship between genetic physiologic, psychological, and environmental causes is complex. Lithium was the first medication found to be effective; several other medications are now available and effective. Many patients with Bipolar Disorders need a combination of medications to address both the manic and depressive aspects. While medication is quite effective, patients need psychotherapy as well, in order to address issues like compliance with medication, noting early signs of relapse, dealing with friends and family and environmental life stressors.

SYMPTOMS

A **manic episode** consists of the following:

• A distinct period of abnormally and persistently elevated, expansive, or irritable mood, lasting at least one week;
• Inflated self-esteem or grandiosity; decreased need for sleep;
• More talkative than usual;
• Flight of ideas (a succession of topics with little relationship to one another) or a subjective experience that thoughts are racing;
• Distractibility;
• Increase in goal-directed activity;
• Excessive involvement in activities that have a high potential for painful consequences;
• The mood disturbances are severe enough to cause impairment in social or occupational functioning;
• The symptoms are not due to the direct physiological effects of a substance.

The **depressive phase** of Bipolar Disorder consists of the following:

• Depressed mood most of the day, nearly every day, as indicated by either subjective report or observation;
• Markedly diminished interest or pleasure in almost all activities most of the day;
• Significant weight loss when not dieting, or weight gain, or decrease or increase in appetite nearly every day;
• Insomnia or hypersomnia nearly every night;
• Psychomotor agitation or retardation nearly every day;
• Fatigue or loss of energy nearly every day;
• Feelings of worthlessness or excessive or inappropriate guilt nearly every day.

ASSOCIATED FEATURES

Bipolar Disorder is a severe mental illness that can cause extreme disruption to individual lives and careers, and to whole families. While manic, patients may spend all of a family's money, borrow great sums, engage in indiscriminate sexual activity, and behave in other ways that leave lasting negative effects. Suicide is a risk factor in the illness, and an estimated ten percent to fifteen percent of individuals with Bipolar I Disorder commit suicide. Abuse of children, spouses or other family members, or other types of violence, may occur during the manic phase of the illness. Untreated mania, during which the individual gets no sleep, little or no nutrition, and expends great quantities of energy, can result in death as well.

It is important for patients with depression to be carefully screened for any manic or hypomanic symptoms so that Bipolar Disorder can be diagnosed and the appropriate treatment prescribed. Most people with Bipolar Disorder present, or are referred, for care while in the depressive state; it is essential to obtain a history of episodes of elevated mood in any depressed individual receiving an antidepressant for the first time. Antidepressant medication alone can precipitate a manic episode in an individual with Bipolar Disorder. The cycles of mood changes tend to become more frequent, shorter, and more intense as the patient gets older.

Disturbances in work, school or social functioning are common, resulting in frequent school truancy or failure, occupational failure, divorce, or episodic antisocial behavior. A variety of other mental disorders may accompany Bipolar Disorder; these include Anorexia Nervosa, Bulimia Nervosa, Attention Deficit/Hyperactivity Disorder, Panic Disorder, Social Phobia, and Substance-Abuse Related Disorder.

PREVALENCE

The prevalence of Bipolar I Disorder varies from 0.4 percent to 0.6 percent in the community. Community prevalence of Bipolar II Disorder is approximately 0.5 percent. The prevalence of Cyclothymic Disorder is estimated at 0.4 percent to one percent, and from three percent to five percent in clinics specializing in mood disorders.

TREATMENT OPTIONS

Lithium is the most commonly prescribed drug for Bipolar Disorder and is effective for stabilizing patients in the manic phase of the illness and preventing mood swings. However, compliance is a problem among patients both because of the nature of the condition (some patients may actually miss the high of their mood swings and other people often envy their enthusiasm, energy, and confidence) and because of the side effects associated with the drug. These include weight gain, excessive thirst, tremors and muscle weakness. Lithium is also very toxic in overdose. Blood levels of lithium must be measured daily or weekly to begin with, and in at least six-month intervals thereafter. The distruptive nature of the condition also necessitates the use of psychotherapy and family therapy to help patients rebuild relationships, to maintain compliance with treatment and a positive attitude toward living with chronic illness, and to restore confidence and self-esteem.

Anticonvulsants/mood stabilizers, such as Valproate, Carbamazepine, Lamotrigine, Gabapentin, and Topiramate have also become first-line treatments.

Education of the family is crucial for successful treatment, as is education of patients about the disorder and treatment.

Associations & Agencies

704   Bipolar Disorders Treatment Information Center
Madison Institute of Medicine
7617 Mineral Point Road
Suite 300
Madison, WI 53717
608-827-2470
Fax: 608-827-2479
E-mail: mim@miminc.org
www.miminc.org

Margaret Baudhuin, Coordinator
David Katzelnick, Founder

Provides information on mood stabilizers other than lithium for bipolar disorder. With more than 4,000 references on file, the Center collects and disseminates information about all medications and other forms of treatment of bipolar disorder, including divalproex sodium (valproate), carbamazepine, lamotrigine, gabapentin and topiramate.

705   Career Assessment & Planning Services
Goodwill Industries-Suncoast
10596 Gandy Boulevard
PO Box 14456
St. Petersburg, FL 33702
727-523-1512
888-279-1988
Fax: 727-563-9300
E-mail: gw.marketing@goodwill-suncoast.com
www.goodwill-suncoast.org

R Lee Waits, President/CEO
Deborah Passerini, VP Operations

Provides a comprehensive assessment, which can predict current and future employment and potential adjustment factors for physically, emotionally, or developmentally disabled persons who may be unemployed or underemployed. Assessments evaluate interests, aptitudes, academic achievements, and physical abilities (including dexterity and coordination) through coordinated testing, interviewing and behavioral observations.

706   Center for Family Support (CFS)
333 7th Avenue
New York, NY 10001-5004
212-629-7939
Fax: 212-239-2211
www.cfsny.org

Steven Vernickofs, Executive Director

An agency that continues to develop new programs to serve families and individuals with their care needs. Currently offering services throughout the New York City region including: New Jersey, Long Island and the Lower Hudson Valley.

707   Center for Mental Health Services Knowledge
PO Box 42557
Washington, DC 20015-4800
800-789-2647
Fax: 240-747-5484
E-mail: ken@mentalhealth.org
www.mentalhealth.org

Information about resources, technical assistance, research, training, networks, and other federal clearing houses, and fact sheets and materials. Information specialists refer callers to mental health resources in their communities as well as state, federal and nonprofit contacts. Staff available Monday through Friday, 8:30 AM - 5:00 PM, EST, excluding federal holidays. After hours, callers may leave messages and an information specialist will return their call.

708   Depression & BiPolar Support Alliance
730 N Franklin Street
Suite 501
Chicago, IL 60610-7224
312-642-0049
800-826-3632
Fax: 312-642-7243
E-mail: questions@dbsalliance.org
www.dbsalliance.org

Lydia Lewis, President
Susan Bergeson, VP

Educates patients, families, professionals, and the public concerning the nature of depressive and manic-depressive illnesses as treatable medical diseases, fosters self-help for patients and families, eliminates discrimination and stigma.

709   Lithium Information Center
Madison Institute of Medicine
7617 Mineral Point Road
Suite 300
Madison, WI 53717-1623
608-827-2470
Fax: 608-827-2479
E-mail: mim@miminc.org
www.miminc.org

Margaret Baudhuin, Coordinator
David Katzelnick, Founder

A resource for information on lithium treatment of bipolar disorders and on the other medical and biological applications of lithium. The Center currently has more than 32,000 references on file.

710   National Alliance on Mental Illness
2107 Wilson Boulevard
Suite 300
Arlington, VA 22201-3042
703-524-7600
800-950-6264
Fax: 703-524-9094
E-mail: helpline@nami.org
www.nami.org

Michael Fitzpatrick, Executive Director

Nation's leading self-help organization for all those affected by severe brain disorders. Mission is to bring consumers and families with similar experiences together to share information about services, care providers, and ways to cope with the challenges of schizophrenia, manic depression, and other serious mental illnesses.

711 National Assocaition for the Dually
132 Fair Street
Kingston, NY 12401-4802
845-334-4336
800-331-5362
Fax: 845-331-4569
E-mail: nadd@mhv.net
www.thenadd.org

Robert Fletcher DSW, Founder/CEO
Donna Nagy PhD, President

Nonprofit organization designed to promote interest of professional and parent development with resources for individuals who have the coexistence of mental illness and mental retardation. Provides conference, educational services and training materials to professionals, parents, concerned citizens and service organizations. Formerly known as the National Association for the Dually Diagnosed.

712 National Association for the Dually Diagnosed (NADD)
132 Fair Street
Kingston, NY 12401
845-334-4336
800-331-5362
Fax: 845-331-4569
E-mail: info@thenadd.org
www.thenadd.org

Robert J Fletcher, CEO

A not-for-profit membership association established for professionals, care providers and families to promote understanding of and services for individuals who have developmental disabilities and mental health needs.

Year Founded: 1983

713 National Mental Health Consumer's Self-Help
1211 Chestnut Street
Suite 1207
Philadelphia, PA 19107
215-751-1810
800-553-4539
Fax: 215-735-0275
E-mail: info@mhselfhelp.org
www.mhselfhelp.org

Christine Smiriglia, Executive Director
Jennifer Melinn, Information/Referral Dept.

Funded by the National Institute of Mental Health Community Support Program, the purpose of the Clearinghouse is to encourage the development and growth of consumer self-help groups.

714 National Mental Health Consumers' Self-Help Clearinghouse
1211 Chestnut Street
Suite 1207
Philadelphia, PA 19107
215-751-1810
800-553-4539
Fax: 215-636-6312
E-mail: info@mhselfhelp.org
www.mhselfhelp.org

Joseph Rogers, Executive Director

A national consumer technical assistance center that has played a major role in the development of the mental health consumer movement.

Year Founded: 1986

715 SAMHSA's National Mental Health Information Center
PO Box 42557
Washington, DC 20015-4800
240-221-4025
800-789-2647
Fax: 240-221-4295
TDD: 866-889-2647
TTY: 301-443-9006
www.mentalhealth.org

A Kathryn Power MEd, Director
Edward B Searle, Deputy Director

Provides information about mental health via a toll-free telephone number, this web site, and more than 600 publications. Developed for users of mental health services and their families, the general public, policy makers, providers, and the media.

716 Suncoast Residential Training Center/Developmental Services Program
Goodwill Industries-Suncoast
10596 Gandy Boulevard
PO Box 14456
St. Petersburg, FL 33702
727-523-1512
Fax: 727-577-2749
E-mail: gw.marketing@goodwill-suncoast.org
www.goodwill-suncoast.org

R Lee Waits, President/CEO
Deborah A Passerini, VPÆOperations

Large group home which serves individuals diagnosed as mentally retarded with a secondary diagnosed of psychiatric difficulties as evidenced by problem behavior. Providing residential, behavioral and instructional support and services that will promote the development of adaptive, socially appropriate behavior, each individual is assessed to determine socialization, basic academics and recreation. The primary intervention strategy is applied behavior analysis. Professional consultants are utilized to address the medical, dental, psychiatric and pharmacological needs of each individual. One of the most popular features is the active community integration component of SRTC. Program customers attend an average of 15 monthly outings to various community events.

Books

717 A Story of Bipolar Disorder (Manic- Depressive Illness) Does this Sound Like You?
National Institute of Mental Health
6001 Executive Boulevard
Room 8184
Bethesda, MD 20892-9663
866-615-6464
Fax: 301-443-4279
TTY: 301-443-8431
E-mail: nimhinfo@nih.gov
www.nimh.nih.gov

Feeling really down sometimes and really up other times? Are these mood changes causing problems at work, school, or home? If yes, you may have bipolar disorder, also called manic-depressive illness.

20 pages

718 Bipolar Disorder Survival Guide: What You and Your Family Need to Know
The Guilford Press
72 Spring Street
New York, NY 10012
800-365-7006
Fax: 212-129-6667
E-mail: info@guilford.com
www.www.guilford.com

Gives ideas to the person diagnosed with the disorder how to come to terms with the diagnosis. Also shows who you should confide in and how to recognize mood swings. *$19.95*

322 pages Year Founded: 2002 ISBN 1-572305-25-8

719 Bipolar Disorder for Dummies
John Wiley and Sons
10475 Crosspoint Blvd
Indianapolis, IN 46256
877-762-2974
Fax: 800-597-3299
www.wiley.com

Guide explains the brain chemistry behind the disease, and covers the latest medications and therapies. Sound advice and self-help techniques that everyone can use including children to ease and eliminate syptoms, function in a crisis, and plan ahead for manic or depressive episodes. *$19.99*

340 pages Year Founded: 2005 ISBN 0-764584-51-0

720 Bipolar Disorders: A Guide to Helping Children and Adolescents
ADD WareHouse
300 NW 70th Avenue
Suite 102
Plantation, FL 33317
954-792-8100
800-233-9273
Fax: 954-792-8545
E-mail: sales@addwarehouse.com
www.addwarehouse.com

Mitzi Waltz

A million children and adolescents in the US may have childhood-onset bipolar disorder-including a significant number with ADHD. This new book helps parents and professionals recognize, treat and cope with bipolar disorders. It covers diagnosis, family life, medications, talk therapies, school issues, and other interventions. *$24.95*

340 pages

721 Bipolar Disorders: Clinical Course and Outcome
American Psychiatric Publishing
1000 Wilson Boulevard
Suite 1825
Arlington, VA 22209-3901
703-907-7322
800-368-5777
Fax: 703-907-1091

E-mail: appi@psych.org
www.appi.org

Katie Duffy, Marketing Assistant

Provides a concise, up to date summary of affective relapse, comorbid psychopathalogy, functional disability, and psychosocial outcome in contemporary bipolar disorders. *$49.95*

312 pages ISBN 0-880487-68-2

722 Bipolar Puzzle Solution
National Alliance on Mental Illness
2107 Wilson Boulevard
Suite 300
Arlington, VA 22201-3042
703-524-7600
800-950-6264
Fax: 703-524-9094
TDD: 703-516-7227
www.nami.org

An informative book on bipolar illness in a 187 question-and-answer format. *$17.00*

723 Carbamazepine and Manic Depression: A Guide
Madison Institute of Medicine
7617 Mineral Point Road
Suite 300
Madison, WI 53717-1623
608-827-2470
Fax: 608-827-2479
E-mail: mim@miminc.org
www.miminc.org

A concise guide to the use of carbamazepine for the treatment of manic depression with information about dosing, monitoring and side effects. *$5.95*

32 pages

724 Consumer's Guide to Psychiatric Drugs
New Harbinger Publications
5674 Shattuck Avenue
Oakland, CA 94609-1662
510-652-2002
800-748-6273
Fax: 510-652-5472
E-mail: customerservice@newharbinger.com
www.newharbinger.com

Helps consumers understand what treatment options are available and what side effects to expect. Covers possible interactions with other drugs, medical conditions and other concerns. Explains how each drug works, and offers detailed information about treatments for depression, bipolar disorder, anxiety and sleep disorders, as well as other conditions. *$16.95*

340 pages ISBN 1-572241-11-X

725 Divalproex and Bipolar Disorder: A Guide
Madison Institute of Medicine
7617 Mineral Point Road
Suite 300
Madison, WI 53717-1623
608-827-2470
Fax: 608-827-2479
E-mail: mim@miminc.org
www.miminc.org

Written by leading experts on bipolar disorder (manic depression) and its treatment, this concise, up-to-date guide includes the most important information every patient taking divalproex (valproate) for bipolar disorder needs to know about this medication. *$5.95*

32 pages

726 Guildeline for Treatment of Patients with Bipolar Disorder
American Psychiatric Publishing
1000 Wilson Boulevard
Suite 1825
Arlington, VA 22209-3901
703-907-7322
800-368-5777
Fax: 703-907-1091
E-mail: appi@psych.org
www.appi.org

Katie Dufffy, Marketing Assistant

Provides guidance to psychiatrists who treat patients with bipolar I disorder. Summarizes the pharmacologic, somatic, and psychotherapeutic treatments used for patients. *$22.50*

96 pages ISBN 0-890423-02-4

727 Lithium and Manic Depression: A Guide
Madison Institute of Medicine
7617 Mineral Point Road
Suite 300
Madison, WI 53717-1623
608-827-2470
Fax: 608-827-2479
E-mail: mim@miminc.org
www.miminc.org

A concise, up-to-date guide written by a leading expert on manic depression (bipolar disorder) and its treatment. This publication includes the most important information every patient taking lithium needs to know about lithium dosing, monitoring and side effects. *$5.95*

31 pages

728 Living Without Depression & Manic Depression: a Workbook for Maintaining Mood Stability
New Harbinger Publications
5674 Shattuck Avenue
Oakland, CA 94609-1662
510-652-2002
800-748-6273
Fax: 510-652-5472
E-mail: customerservice@newharbinger.com
www.newharbinger.com

Outlines a program that helps people achieve breakthroughs in coping and healing. Contents include: self advocacy, building a network of support, wellness lifestyle, symptom prevention strategies, self-esteem, mood stability, a career that works, trauma resolution, dealing with sleep problems, diet, vitamin and herbal therapies, dealing with stigma, medication side effects, psychotherapy, and counseling alternatives. *$18.95*

263 pages ISBN 1-879237-74-1

729 Management of Bipolar Disorder: Pocketbook
American Psychiatric Publishing
1000 Wilson Boulevard
Suite 1825
Arlington, VA 22209-3901
703-907-7322
800-368-5777
Fax: 703-907-1091
E-mail: appi@psych.org
www.appi.org

Katie Duffy, Marketing Assistant

Contains the need for treatment, what defines bipolar disorders, spectrum of the disorder, getting the best out of treatment, treatment of mania and bipolar depression, preventing new episodes, special problems in treatment, mood stabilizers and case studies. *$ 14.95*

96 pages ISBN 1-853172-74-X

730 Mania: Clinical and Research Perspectives
American Psychiatric Publishing
1000 Wilson Boulevard
Suite 1825
Arlington, VA 22209-3901
703-907-7322
800-368-5777
Fax: 703-907-1091
E-mail: appi@psych.org
www.appi.org

Katie Duffy, Marketing Assistant

Diagnostic considerations, biological aspects, and treatment of mania. *$59.95*

478 pages ISBN 0-880487-28-3

731 Oxcarbazepine and Bipolar Disorder: A Guide
Madison Institute of Medicine
7617 Mineral Point Road
Suite 300
Madison, WI 53717-1623
608-827-2470
Fax: 608-827-2479
E-mail: mim@miminc.org
www.miminc.org

This 31 page booklet provides patients with the information they need to know about the use of oxcarbazepine in the treatment of bipolar disorder, including information about proper dosing, medication management, and possible side effects. *$5.95*

31 pages

732 Physician's Guide to Depression and Bipolar Disorders
McGraw-Hill Companies
PO Box 182604
Columbus, OH 43272
877-833-5524
Fax: 614-759-3749
E-mail: customer.service@mcgraw-hill.com
www.mcgraw-hill.com

Offers a clear definitive instruction on drug treatments for bipolar disorders with the exact dosages needed. Crucial to a diagnosis and treatment is the ability to identify a patients symptoms. *$59.00*

400 pages Year Founded: 2005 ISBN 0-071441-75-1

733 Taming Bipolar Disorders
Alpha
1101 Enterprise Drive
PO Box 255
Royersford, PA 19468-0255
800-992-9124
www.alphapub.com

Contains cutting-edge research and straightforward advice from the most respectable names on bipolar disorder, along with the most up-to-date information on mental health organizations, support and advocacy groups. *$17.95*

400 pages Year Founded: 2004 ISBN 1-592572-85-5

Periodicals & Pamphlets

734 Bipolar Disorder
National Institute of Mental Health
6001 Executive Boulevard
Room 8184
Bethesda, MD 20892-9663
866-615-6464
Fax: 301-443-4279
TTY: 301-443-8431
E-mail: nimhinfo@nih.gov
www.nimh.nih.gov

Bipolar disorder, also known as manic-depressive illness, is a brain disorder that causes unusual shifts in a person's mood, energy, and ability to function. Different from the normal ups and downs that everyone goes through, the symptoms of bipolar disorder are severe. They can result in damaged relationships, poor job or school performance, and even suicide. But there is good news: bipolar disorder can be treated, and people with this illness can lead full and productive lives.

24 pages

735 Child and Adolescent Bipolar Disorder: An Update from the National Institute of Mental Health
National Institute of Mental Health
6001 Executive Boulevard
Room 8184
Bethesda, MD 20892-9663
866-615-6464
Fax: 301-443-4279
TTY: 301-443-8431
E-mail: nimhinfo@nih.gov
www.nimh.nih.gov

Research findings, clinical experience, and family accounts provide substantial evidence that bipolar disorder, also called manic-depressive illness, can occur in children and adolescents. Bipolar disorder is difficult to recognize and diagnose in youth. Better understanding of the diagnosis and treatment is urgently needed. In pursuit of this goal, the NIMH is conducting and supporting research on child and adolescent bioplar disorder.

3 pages Year Founded: 2000

736 Coping With Unexpected Events: Depression & Trauma
Depression & BiPolar Support Alliance
730 N Franklin Street
Suite 501
Chicago, IL 60610-7204

312-642-0049
800-826-3632
Fax: 312-642-7243
E-mail: programs@dbsalliance.org
www.ndmda.org

How to cope with depression after trauma, helping others and preventing suicide.

737 Coping with Mood Changes Later in Life
Depression and Bipolar Support Alliance
730 N Franklin Street
Suite 501
Chicago, IL 60610-7224
312-642-0049
800-826-3632
Fax: 312-642-7243
www.dbsallince.org

A large print guide that discusses symptoms, causes and treatment options. Also contains resources that may be helpful to older adults.

14 pages Year Founded: 2003

738 DBSA Support Groups: An Important Step on the Road to Wellness
Depression and Bipolar Support Alliance
730 N Franklin Street
Suite 501
Chicago, IL 60610-7224
312-642-0049
800-826-3632
Fax: 312-642-7243
www.dbsalliance.org

Support groups for people with depression or bipolar disorder to discuss the experiences, and helpful treatments.

10 pages Year Founded: 2003

739 Finding Peacce of Mind: Treatment Strategies for Depression and Bipolar Disorder
Depression and Bipolar Support Alliance
730 N Franklin Street
Suite 501
Chicago, IL 60610-7224
312-642-0049
800-826-3632
Fax: 312-642-7243
www.dbsalliance.org

Helps to build a good, cooperative relationship with your doctor by explaining some of the treatments for mood disorders and how they work. Also includes a guide for medication that has been frequently prescribed and new treatments that are being investigated.

20 pages Year Founded: 2003

740 Getting Better Sleep: What You Need to Know
Depression and Bipolar Support Alliance
730 N Franklin Street
Suite 501
Chicago, IL 60610-7224
312-642-0049
800-826-3632
Fax: 312-642-7243
www.dbsalliance.org

Describes some causes of sleep loss, and how sleep loss relates to bipolar disorder and depression. Also provides information on how to get better sleep.

741 Introduction to Depression and Bipolar Disorder
Depression and Bipolar Support Alliance
730 N Franklin Street
Suite 501
Chicago, IL 60610-7224
312-642-0049
800-826-3632
Fax: 312-642-7243
www.dbsalliance.org

Quick and easy-to-read brochure describing syptoms and treatments for mood disorders.

742 McMan's Depression and Bipolar Weekly
McMan's Depression and Bipolar Web
PO Box 5093
Kendall Park, NJ 08824
E-mail: mcman@mcmanweb.com
www.mcmanweb.com

John McManamy, Editor/Publisher

Online newsletter devoted to the issues of bipolar and depression disorders. There is no charge, just for you to understand different things about the disorders.

743 Mood Disorders
Center for Mental Health Services: Knowledge Exchange Network
PO Box 42490
Washington, DC 20015
800-789-2647
Fax: 301-984-8796
TDD: 866-889-2647
E-mail: ken@mentalhealth.org
www.mentalhealth.org

This fact sheet provides basic information on the symptoms, formal diagnosis, and treatment for bipolar disorder.

3 pages

744 Myths and Facts about Depression and Bipolar Disorders
Depression and Bipolar Support Alliance
730 N Franklin Street
Suite 501
Chicago, IL 60610-7224
312-642-0049
800-826-3632
Fax: 312-642-7243
www.dbsalliance.org

Gives some myths about depression and bipolar disorder and the truths that combat them.

745 You've Just Been Diagnosed...What Now?
Depression and Bipolar Support Alliance
730 N Franklin Street
Suite 501
Chicago, IL 60610-7224
312-642-0049
800-826-3632
Fax: 312-642-7243
www.dbsalliance.org

Pamphlet to help you understand about the disorder you have just been diagnosed with. Tells you basic facts about mood disorders and will help you work towards a diagnosis.

19 pages Year Founded: 2002

Research Centers

746 Bipolar Clinic and Research Program
The Massachusetts General Hospital Bipolar Clinic & Research Program
50 Staniford Street
Suite 580
Boston, MA 02114
617-726-6188
Fax: 617-726-6768
www.manicdepressive.org

Gary S Sachs MD, Founder/Director

Dedicated to providing quality clinical care, conducting clinically informative research, and educating our colleagues, patients, as well as the community.

747 Bipolar Disorders Clinic
Standford School of Medicine
401 Quarry Road
Stanford, CA 94305-5723
650-724-4795
www.bipolar.stanford.edu

Terence A Ketter MD, Clinic Chief
Jenifer Culver PhD, Clinical Assistant Professor

Offers an on-going clinical treatment, manage clinical trials and neuroimaging studies, lecture and teach seminar courses at Stanford University and train residents in the School of Medicine.

748 Bipolar Research at University of Pennsylvan ia
University of Pennsylvania
Clinical Research Building Room 11
125 S 31st Street Suite 2200
Philadelphia, PA 19104
215-746-3657
E-mail: balthrop@mail.med.upenn.edu
www.bipolargenes.org/penn.html

A study that invites individuals age 16 or older to participate in a neurobiology and behavior study. The individuals have to have bipolar disorder or schizoaffective disorder.

749 Epidemiology-Genetics Program in Psychiatry
John Hopkins University School of Medicine
733 N Broadway
Suite G49
Baltimore, MD 21231-2125
410-955-3182
www.hopkinsmedicine.org

The research program is to help characterize the genetic (biochemical) developmental, and environmental components of bipolar disorder. The hope is that once scientists understand the biological causes of this disorder new medications and treatments can be developed.

750 UT Southwestern Medical Center
5323 Harry Hines Blvd
Dallas, TX 75390
214-648-3111
Fax: 214-648-8955
www.www.utsouthwestern.edu

Researching corticosteroid effects on the brain, dual-diagnosed patients, and depression in asthma patients.

751 Yale Mood Disorders Research Program
Department of Psychiatry
300 George Street
New Haven, CT 06511
203-785-2117
www.www.med.yale.edu

Brings together a multi-disciplinary group of scientists who use a wide variety of research methods in a highly collaborative research effort to study the genetic and environmental factors that contribute to mood disorders.

Video & Audio

752 Covert Modeling & Covert Reinforcement
New Harbinger Publications
5674 Shattuck Avenue
Oakland, CA 94609-1662
510-652-2002
800-748-6273
Fax: 510-652-5472
E-mail: customerservice@newharbinger.com
www.newharbinger.com

Based on the essential book of cognitive behavioral techniques for effecting change in your life, Thoughts & Feelings. Learn step-by-step protocols for controlling destructive behaviors such as anxiety, obsessional thinking, uncontrolled anger, and depression. *$ 11.95*

ISBN 0-934986-29-0

753 Dark Glasses and Kaleidoscopes: Living with Manic Depression
Depression and Bipolar Support Alliance
730 N Franklin Street
Suite 501
Chicago, IL 60610-7224
312-642-0049
800-826-3632
Fax: 312-642-7243
www.dbsalliance.org

Video featuring people who have bipolar disorder (manic depression) and doctors outlining syptoms and coping strategies. 33 minutes. *$5.00*

Year Founded: 1997

754 Families Coping with Mental Illness
Mental Illness Education Project
PO Box 470813
Brookline Village, MA 02247-0244
617-562-1111
800-343-5540
Fax: 617-779-0061
E-mail: info@miepvideos.org
www.miepvideos.org

Ten family members share their experiences of having a family member with schizophrenia or bipolar disorder. Designed to provide insights and support to other families, the tape also profoundly conveys to professionals the needs of families when mental illness strikes. In two versions: a 22-minute version ideal for short classes and workshops, and a richer 43-minute version with more examples and details. Discounted price for families/consumers. *$99.95*

755 The Bonnie Tapes Mental Illness in the Family; Recovering from Mental Illness; My Sister is Mentally Ill
The Mental Illness Education Project
PO Box 470813
Brookline Village, MA 02447
617-562-1111
E-mail: info@miepvideos.org
www.miepvideos.org

Talks with a young woman with schizophrenia, how it has affected her and her family. Also talks with mental health professionals to see how she is handling everything. Talks about what happens when mental illness enters a family, and how the person with the illness feels, and what are steps to get better. Each video is $99.95

Web Sites

756 www.bpso.org
BPSO-Bipolar Significant Others

Informational site intended to provide information and support to the spouses, families, friends and other loved ones of those who suffer from bi-polar.

757 www.bpso.org/nomania.htm
How to Avoid a Manic Episode

Provides different ways to avoid an episode, and factors what causes episodes.

758 www.cfsny.org
Center for Family Services

Devoted to the physical well-being and development of the reatrded child and the sound mental health of the parents.

759 www.cyberpsych.org
CyberPsych

Hosts the American Psychoanalyists Foundation, American Association of Suicideology, Society for the Exploration of Psychotherapy Intergration, and Anxiety Disorders Association of America. Also subcategories of the anxiety disorders, as well as general information, including panic disorder, phobias, obsessive compulsive disorder (OCD), social phobia, generalized anxiety disorder, post traumatic stress disorder, and phobias of childhood. Book reviews and links to web pages sharing the topics.

760 www.dbsalliance.org
Depression & Bi-Polar Support Alliance

Mental health news updates and local support group information.

761 www.geocities.com/enchantedforest/1068
Bipolar Kids Homepage

Set of links.

762 www.goodwill-suncoast.org
Suncoast Residential Training Center

Group home that serves individuals diagnosed as mentally retarded with a secondary diagnosis of psychiatric difficulties as evidenced by problem behavior.

763 **www.manicdepressive.org**
The Massachusetts General Hospital Bipolar Clinic/Research Program

Dedicated to providing quality clinical care, conducting clinically informative research, and educating colleagues, patients and the community.

764 **www.med.yale.edu**
Yale University School of Medicine

Research center dedicated to understanding the science of mood disorders.

765 **www.mentalhealth.Samhsa.Gov**
Center for Mental Health Services Knowledge Exchange Network

Information about resources, technical assistance, research, training, networks, and other federal clearinghouses, fact sheets and materials.

766 **www.mhselfhelp.org**
National Mental Health Consumer's Self-Help Clearinghouse

Encourages the development and growth of consumer self-help groups.

767 **www.miminc.org**
Bipolar Disorders Treatment Information Center

Provides information on mood stabilizers other than lithium for bipolar disorders.

768 **www.moodswing.org/bdfaq.html**
Bipolar Disorder Frequently Asked Questions

Excellent for those newly diagnosed. Gives information on symptoms, stories, causes and helpful treatments.

769 **www.nami.org**
National Alliance for the Mentally Ill

Mission is to bring consumers and families with similar experiences experiences together to share information about services, care providers and ways to cope with the challenges.

770 **www.planetpsych.com**
Planetpsych.com

Learn about disorders, their treatments and other topics in psychology. Articles are listed under the related topic areas. Ask a therapist a question for free, or view the directory of professionals in your area. If you are a therapist sign up for the directory. Current features, self-help, interactive, and newsletter archives.

771 **www.psychcentral.com**
Psych Central

Personalized one-stop index for psychology, support, and mental health issues, resources, and people on the Internet.

772 **www.thenadd.org**
NADD: National Association for the Dually Diagnosed

Promotes interest of professional and parent development with resources for individuals who have the coexistence of mental illness and mental retardation.

773 **www.utsouthwestern.edu**
UT Southwestern Medical Center

Research to find the corticosteroid effects on the human brain, dual-diagnosed patients, and depression in asthma patients.

Cognitive Disorders

Introduction

Cognitive disorders are a group of conditions characterized by impairments in the ability to think, reason, plan and organize. There are three types of cognitive disorders; delirium, dementia (of which Alzheimer's Disease is the most common) and amnestic disorder.

Delirium is a relatively short-term condition in which the level of conciousness waxes and wanes. It is common in patients after surgery or during illness, as with high fever. It resolves when the underlying problem resolves. There are three categories of causes of delirium: a general medical condition; substance-induced; and multiple causes. An amnestic disorder, in contrast to delirium or dementia, is a condition in which only memory is impaired; for instance the person is unable to recall important facts or events, making it difficult to function normally. Dementia is a chronic impairment of multiple cognitive functions. Persons with dementia may have severe memory loss and also be unable to plan or prepare for events or to care for themselves.

Dementia, Alzheimer's type, is a progressive disorder that slowly kills nerve cells in the brain. While definitive treatments are lacking, there is a prodigious amount of research on the condition, some of which suggests that a vaccine may eventually prevent the condition. Though such hopeful breakthroughs remain distant, there is much that families and patients can do when the condition is recognized and care and support are sought early in the disorder's progression. Since other, serious, treatable disorders can resemble Alzeimer's Disease, it is very important for individuals who are losing cognitive functions to be evaluated by a physician. Early detection of Alzheimer's Disease, with early treatment, may improve the chances for slowing the rate of decline.

Here we will describe only Alzheimer's dementia, the most prevalent Cognitive Disorder.

SYMPTOMS

- Langugage disorders;
- Impaired ability to carry out motor activities despite intact motor function;
- Failure to recognize or identify objects despite intact sensory perception;
- Disturbance in executive functioning (planning, organizing, sequencing, abstracting);
- The deficits cause impairment in social or occupational functioning and represent a decline from previous level of functioning;
- The course is gradual and continuous;
- The deficits are not due to central nervous system conditions such as Parkinson's Disease, other conditions known to cause dementia, and are not substance-induced;
- The deficits do not occur during the course of delirium and are not better accounted for by severe depression or schizophrenia.

ASSOCIATED FEATURES

Dementia, Alzheimer's type, generally begins gradually, not with deficits in cognition but with a marked change in personality. For instance, a person may suddenly become given to fits of anger for no apparent reason.

Soon, however, family and acquaintances may notice that the individual begins to mix up facts, or gets lost driving to a familiar place. In the early stages the afflicted individual may become aware of slipping cognitive functions, adding to confusion, fright and depression. After a period, lapses in memory grow more obvious; patients with Alzheimer's are apt to repeat themselves, and may forget the names of grandchildren or longtime friends. They may also be increasingly agitated and combative when family members or other caretakers try to correct them or help with accustomed tasks. The memory lapses in patients with Alzheimer's differ markedly from those in normal aging: a patient with Alzheimer's may often forget entire experiences and rarely remembers them later; the patient only grudgingly acknowledges lapses. In contrast, the individual with normal aging or depression is extremely concerned about, and may even exaggerate, the extent of memory loss. In Alzheimer's, skills deteriorate and a patient is increasingly unable to follow directions, or care for him/herself. Eventually the disease leads to death.

PREVALENCE

An estimated two percent to four percent of the population over age 65 has dementia, Alzheimer's type. Other types of dementia are believed to be much less common. Prevalance of the condition increases with age, particularly after age 75; in persons over 85, an estimated twenty percent have dementia, Alzheimer's type.

TREATMENT OPTIONS

There is no known cure or definitive treatment for dementia, Alzheimer's type. However, research has suggested avenues that involve drugs, such as THA, Donepezil, and Rivastigmine, for regulating acetylcholine, seratonin or norepinephrine in the brain. According to the American Psychiatric Association, some progress has been seen in slowing the death rate among nerve cells using a chemical known as Alcar (acetyl-l-carnitine). Psychiatrists treating patients with dementia, Alzheimer's type, may also be able to prescribe medications that can treat the depression and anxiety that accompanies the condition. And families are strongly encouraged to take advantage of adjunctive services including support groups, counseling and psychotherapy. There is a high incidence of depression among family members caring at home for persons with Alzheimer's Disease.

Associations & Agencies

775 Alzheimer's Association National Office
225 N Michigan Avenue
Suite 1000
Chicago, IL 60601-7633
312-335-8700
888-572-8566
Fax: 866-699-1246
TDD: 866-403-3073
E-mail: info@alz.org
www.alz.org

Harry John, President/CEO

Headquarters for the nation's leading organization for all those suffering with alzheimer's disease and their families and support network. Offers referrals, support groups, workshops, training seminars, publications.

776 Alzheimer's Disease Education and Referral Center
PO Box 8250
Silver Spring, MD 20907-8250
301-495-3311
800-438-4380
Fax: 301-495-3334
TTY: 800-222-4225
E-mail: adear@alzheimers.org
www.alzheimers.org

Alison Serey, Executive Director

The ADEAR Center provides information about Alzheimer's Disease and related disorders to health professionals, patients and their families, and the public.

777 American Health Assistance Foundation
22512 Gateway Center Drive
Clarksburg, MD 20871
301-948-3244
800-437-2423
Fax: 301-258-9454
E-mail: janthony@ahaf.org
www.ahaf.org

Brian K Regan, PhD, President
Jonathan Rise, Esq, VP
Gayle Handiboe, Manager Of Development

Provides information on treatment, symptoms risk factors and healthy exercises.

778 Center for Family Support (CFS)
333 7th Avenue
New York, NY 10001-5004
212-629-7939
Fax: 212-239-2211
www.cfsny.org

Steven Vernickofs, Executive Director
Melaine Singleton, Director Human Resources

Service agency devoted to the physical well-being and development of the retarded child and the sound mental health of the parents. Helps families with retarded children with all aspects of home care including counseling, referrals, home aide service and consultation. Offers intervention for parents at the birth of a retarded child with in-home support, guidance and infant stimulation. Pioneered training of nonprofessional women as home aides to provide supportive services in homes.

779 Center for Mental Health Services Knowledge
PO Box 42490
Washington, DC 20015-4800
800-789-2647
Fax: 301-984-8796
E-mail: ken@mentalhealth.org
www.mentalhealth.smahsa.gov

Information about resources, technical assistance, research, training, networks, and other federal clearing houses, and fact sheets and materials. Information specialists refer callers to mental health resources in their communities as well as state, federal and nonprofit contacts. Staff available Monday through Friday, 8:30 AM - 5:00 PM, EST, excluding federal holidays. After hours, callers may leave messages and an information specialist will return their call.

780 National Association Councils on Developmental Disabilities
225 Reinekers Lane
Suite 650-B
Alexandria, VA 22314
703-739-4400
Fax: 703-739-6030
E-mail: info@nacdd.org
www.nacdd.org

Karen Flippo, Executive Director
Anne Rohall, Director Government Relations
Phyllis Guinivan, Council Services Liason

Provide support and assistance to member Councils in order to promote a consumer and family centered system of services and support for individuals with developmental disabilities.

781 National Association for the Dually Diagnosed (NADD)
132 Fair Street
Kingston, NY 12401-4802
845-334-4336
800-331-5362
Fax: 845-331-4569
E-mail: nadd@mhv.net
www.thenadd.org

Dr. Robert Fletcher, Founder/CEO

Nonprofit organization designed to promote interest of professional and parent development with resources for individuals who have the coexistence of mental illness and mental retardation. Provides conference, educational services and training materials to professionals, parents, concerned citizens and service organizations. Formerly known as the National Association for the Dually Diagnosed.

Year Founded: 1983

782 National Family Caregivers Association
10400 Connecticut Avenue
Suite 500
Kensington, MD 20895-3944
301-942-6430
800-896-3650
Fax: 301-942-2302
E-mail: info@thefamilycaregiver.org
www.nfcacares.org

Suzanne Mintz, Co-Founder/President
Cindy Fowler, Co-Founder/Secretary

Acts as a support and an advocate for family caregivers.

783 National Institute of Neurological Disorders and Stroke
NIH Neurological Institute
PO Box 5801
Bethesda, MD 20824
301-496-5751
800-352-9424
Fax: 301-402-2186
TTY: 301-468-5981
E-mail: braininfo@ninds.nih.gov
www.ninds.nih.gov

Story C Landis, PhD, Director
Audrey S Penn, MD, Deputy Director

Federal agency that supports research nationwide on disorders of the brain and nervous system. Website has updated neuroscience news and articles.

784 National Mental Health Consumer's Self-Help
1211 Chestnut Street
Suite 1207
Philadelphia, PA 19107
215-751-1810
800-553-4539
Fax: 215-636-6312
E-mail: info@mhselfhelp.org
www.mhselfhelp.org

Joseph Rodgers, Founder/Executive Director
Christine Simiriglia, Director

Funded by the National Institute of Mental Health Community Support Program, the purpose of the Clearinghouse is to encourage the development and growth of consumer self-help groups.

785 National Mental Health Consumers' Self-Help Clearinghouse
1211 Chestnut Street
Suite 1207
Philadelphia, PA 19107
215-751-1810
800-553-4539
Fax: 215-636-6312
E-mail: info@mhselfhelp.org
www.mhselfhelp.org

Joseph Rogers, Executive Director

A national consumer technical assistance center that has played a major role in the development of the mental health consumer movement.

Year Founded: 1986

786 National Niemann-Pick Disease Foundation
401 Madison Avenue, Suite B
PO Box 49
Ft Atkinson, WI 53538
920-563-0930
877-287-3672
Fax: 920-563-0931
E-mail: nnpdf@idcnet.com
www.nnpdf.org

Barbara Wedehase, Executive Director
Nadine Hill,, Director of Family Services

Offers support and funding for individuals with cognitive disorders and their support network.

787 SAMHSA's National Mental Health Information Center
US Department of Health and Human Services
PO Box 42490
Washington, DC 20015-4800
240-221-4021
800-789-2647
Fax: 240-221-4295
TDD: 866-889-2647
www.mentalhealth.smahsa.gov

Provides information about mental health via a toll-free telephone number, this web site, and more than 600 publications. Developed for users of mental health services and their families, the general public, policy makers, providers, and the media.

Books

788 Agitation in Patients with Dementia: a Practical Guide to Diagnosis and Management
American Psychiatric Publishing
1000 Wilson Boulevard
Suite 1825
Arlington, VA 22209-3901
703-907-7322
800-368-5777
Fax: 703-907-1091
E-mail: appi@psych.org
www.appi.org

James Scully, MD, President
Donald P Hay, MD, Editor

Appealing to a wide audience of geriatric psychiatrists, primary care physicians and internists, general practitioners, nurses, social workers, psychologists, pharmacists and mental health care workers and practitioners in hospitals, nursing homes and clinics, this remarkable monograph offers practical direction on assessing and managing agitation in patients with dementia. *$57.00*

250 pages Year Founded: 2003 ISBN 0-880488-43-3

789 Alzheimer's Disease Sourcebook
Omnigraphics
PO Box 625
Holmes, PA 19043
800-234-1340
Fax: 800-875-1340
E-mail: info@omnigraphics.com
www.omnigraphics.com

Omnigraphics is the publisher of the Health Reference Series, a growing consumer health information resource with more than 100 volumes in print. Each title in the series features an easy to understand format, nontechnical language, comprehensive indexing and resources for further information. Material in each book has been collected from a wide range of government agencies, professional associations, periodicals, and other sources. *$78.00*

524 pages ISBN 0-780802-23-3

790 Alzheimer's Disease: Activity-Focused Care, Second Edition
Therapeutic Resources
PO Box 16814
Cleveland, OH 16814
440-331-7114
888-331-7114
Fax: 440-331-7118
E-mail: contactus@therapeuticresources.com
www.therapeuticresources.com

Katie Hennessy, LCSW, Medical Promotions Coordinator

Provides practical and innovative strategies for care of people with Alzheimer's disease, emphasizing the activities that make up daily living - dressing, toileting, eating, exercising, and communication. The text is written from the viewpoint that activity-focused care promotes the resident's cognitive, physical, psychosocial, and spiritual well-being.

436 pages ISBN 0-750699-08-6

791 American Psychiatric Association Practice Guideline for the Treatment of Patients with Delirium
American Psychiatric Publishing
1000 Wilson Boulevard
Suite 1825
Arlington, VA 22209-3901
703-907-7322
800-368-5777
Fax: 703-907-1091
E-mail: appi@psych.org
www.appi.org

James Scully, MD, President

Best practices examined from the group whose vision is a society that has available, accessible quality psychiatric diagnosis and treatment. *$30.95*

75 pages Year Founded: 1999 ISBN 0-890423-13-X

792 Behavioral Complications in Alzheimer's Disease
American Psychiatric Publishing
1000 Wilson Boulevard
Suite 1825
Arlington, VA 22209-3901
703-907-7322
800-368-5777
Fax: 703-907-1091
E-mail: appi@psych.org
www.appi.org

James Scully, MD, President
Brian A Lawlor, Editor

Practical management strategies for the identification, measurement and treatment of behavioral symptoms in patient with Alzheimer's disease. *$36.50*

272 pages Year Founded: 1995 ISBN 0-880484-77-2

793 Care That Works: A Relationship Approach to Persons With Dementia
Johns Hopkins University Press
2715 N Charles Street
Baltimore, MD 21218-4319
410-516-6936
800-537-5487
Fax: 410-516-6998
www.press.jhu.edu

William DeJohn, Marketing/Sales Manager
Jitka M Zagola, Author

Provides caregivers the information with which they can develop their own approaches, evaluate their effectiveness, and continue to grow in skill and insight. Real life strategies for a challenging task. *$58.00*

272 pages Year Founded: 1999 ISBN 0-801860-25-3

794 Dementia: A Clinical Approach
Elsevier Health Sciences
11830 Westline Industrial Drive
St. Louis, MO 63146
314-453-7010
800-568-5136
Fax: 314-453-7095
E-mail: orders@bhusa.com or custserv@bhusa.com
www.bh.com

Mario F Mendez, Author
Jeffrey L Cummings, Author

Third Edition, this is both a scholarly review of the dementias and a practical guide to their diagnosis and treatment. *$ 99.00*

654 pages Year Founded: 2003 ISBN 0-750674-70-9

795 Disorders of Brain and Mind: Volume 1
Cambridge University Press
40 W 20th Street
New York, NY 10011-4221
212-924-3900
Fax: 212-691-3239
E-mail: marketing@cup.org
www.cup.org

Maria A Ron, Editor
Anthony S David, Editor

Discusses various neuropsychiatry topics where the brain and mind come together. *$65.00*

388 pages Year Founded: 1999 ISBN 0-521778-51-4

796 Drug Therapy and Cognitive Disorders
Mason Crest Publishers
370 Reed Road
Suite 302
Broomall, PA 19008
610-543-6200
866-627-2665
Fax: 610-543-3878
E-mail: dtaylor@masoncrest.com
www.masoncrest.com

Alzheimer's disease is one of the most common cognitive disorder, one that affects millions of people. Patients, caregivers and loved ones all suffer as they experience the devastation of this often misunderstood disease. Researchers are working hard to find a cure for the symptoms of Alzheimer's and other cognitive disorders, and this book describes the most recent research. Coauthored by someone who has experienced the early stages of Alzheimer's firsthand, this volume will give readers a new understanding and appreciation of the treatment options for those who experience a cognitive disorder.

ISBN 1-590845-62-5

797 Progress in Alzheimer's Disease and Similar Conditions
American Psychiatric Publishing
1000 Wilson Boulevard
Suite 1825
Arlington, VA 22209-3901
703-907-7322
800-368-5777
Fax: 703-907-1091
E-mail: appi@psych.org
www.appi.org

James Scully, MD, President
Leonard L Heston, MD, Editor

Details advances in research on human genetics that is broadening our knowledge of Alzheimer's disease and other related afflictions. Describes disease mechanisms, including prisons, that provide insight into the role environment plays in the development of disease. Includes stories about the pain inflicted by this disease on the patients and their family and friends as well as current efforts in management and treatment. *$77.00*

318 pages Year Founded: 1997 ISBN 0-880487-60-7

798 Victims of Dementia: Service, Support, and Care
Haworth Press
10 Alice Street
Binghamton, NY 13904
607-722-5857
800-429-6784
Fax: 607-721-0012
E-mail: getinfo@haworthpressinc.com
www.haworthpress.com

Jackie Blakeslee, Advertising/Journal Liaison
William M Clemmer, PhD, Editor

Provides an in depth look at the concept, construction and operation of Wesley Hall, a special living area at the Chelsea United Methodist retirement home in Michigan. *$27.95*

155 pages Year Founded: 1993 ISSN 978156024-265-9

Periodicals & Pamphlets

799 Alzheimer's Disease Research and the American Health Assistance Foundation
American Health Assistance Foundation
22512 Gateway Center Drive
Clarksburg, MD 20871
301-948-3244
800-437-2423
Fax: 301-258-9454
E-mail: jwilson@ahaf.org
www.ahaf.org

Jarmal Wilson, LSWA, AFRP Manager

Provides information on treatment, medication, medical referrals.

Video & Audio

800 A Change of Character
Fanlight Productions
4196 Washington Street
Suite 2
Boston, MA 02131
617-469-4999
Fax: 617-439-3379
E-mail: fanlight@fanlight.com
www.fanlight.com

Truett Allen's personality changed drastically after a series of strokes resulted in damage to the frontal lobes of his brain. this captivating video features neuroscientist Dr. Elkhonon Goldberg, author of The Executive Brain, as well as neurologist and best-selling author Dr. Oliver Sacks.

Web Sites

801 www.Nia.Nih.Gov/Alzheimers
Alzheimer's Disease Education and Referral
Fax: 301-495-3334

A division of the National Institute on Aging of the National Institute of Health. Solid information and a list of federally funded centers for evaluation, referral, treatment.

802 www.aan.com
American Academy of Neurology

Provides information for both professionals and the public on neurology subjects, covering Alzheimer's and Parkin-

son's diseases to stroke and migraine, includes comprehensive fact sheets.

803 www.agelessdesign.com
Ageless Design

Information on age related diseases such as Alzheimer's disease.

804 www.ahaf.org/alzdis/about/adabout.htm
American Health Assistance Foundation

Alzheimer's resource for patients and caregivers.

805 www.alz.co.uk
Alzheimer's Disease International

Umbrella organization of associations that support people with dementia.

806 www.alzforum.org
Alzheimer Research Forum

Information in layman's terms, plus many references and resources listed.

807 www.alzheimersbooks.com/
Alzheimer's Disease Bookstore

808 www.alzheimersupport.Com
AlzheimerSupport.com

Information and products for people dealing with Alzheimer's Disease.

809 www.biostat.wustl.edu
Washington University - Saint Louis

Page on Alzheimer's information, from basic care to friends and family networking experiences for support.

810 www.cyberpsych.org
CyberPsych

Hosts the American Psychoanalyists Foundation, American Association of Suicideology, Society for the Exploration of Psychotherapy Intergration, and Anxiety Disorders Association of America. Also subcategories of the anxiety disorders, as well as general information, including panic disorder, phobias, obsessive compulsive disorder (OCD), social phobia, generalized anxiety disorder, post traumatic stress disorder, and phobias of childhood. Book reviews and links to web pages sharing the topics.

811 www.elderlyplace.com
Elderly Place

Includes Caregiver's Guide to Alzheimer's.

812 www.habitsmart.com/cogtitle.html
Cognitive Therapy Pages

Offers accessible explanations.

813 www.mayohealth.org/mayo/common/htm/
MayoClinic.com

Information for dealing with Alzheimer's Disease.

814 www.mentalhealth.com
Internet Mental Health

On-line information and a virtual encyclopedia related to mental disorders, possible causes and treatments. News, articles, on-line diagnostic programs and related links. Designed to improve understanding, diagnosis and treatment of mental illness throughout the world. Awarded the Top Site Award and the NetPsych Cutting Edge Site Award.

815 www.mentalhealth.smahsa.gov
SMAHSA'S National Mental Health Information Center

US Department of Health and Human Services website with current Alzheimer's information.

816 www.mindstreet.com/training.html
Cognitive Therapy: A Multimedia Learning Program

The basics of cognitive therapy are presented.

817 www.ninds.nih.gov
National Institute of Neurological Disorders & Stroke

Neuroscience updates and articles.

818 www.noah-health.org/en/bns/disorders/ alzheimer.html
Ask NOAH About: Aging and Alzheimer's Disease

Links to brochures on medical problems of the elderly.

819 www.ohioalzcenter.org/facts.html
University Memory and Aging Center

Alzheimer's disease fact page.

820 www.planetpsych.com
Planetpsych.com

Learn about disorders, their treatments and other topics in psychology. Articles are listed under the related topic areas. Ask a therapist a question for free, or view the directory of professionals in your area. If you are a therapist sign up for the directory. Current features, self-help, interactive, and newsletter archives.

821 www.psych.org/clin_res/pg_dementia.cfm
American Psychiatric Association

Practice guidelines for the treatment of patients with Alzheimer's.

822 www.psychcentral.com
Psych Central

Personalized one-stop index for psychology, support, and mental health issues, resources, and people on the Internet.

823 www.rcpsych.ac.uk/info/help/memory
Royal College of Psychiatrists

Memory and Dementia

824 www.zarcrom.com/users/alzheimers
Alzheimer's Outreach

Detailed and practical information.

825 www.zarcrom.com/users/yeartorem
Year to Remember

A memorial site covering many aspects of Alzheimer's disease.

Conduct Disorder

Introduction

Conduct disorder is the diagnosis of children who demonstrate a repetitive and persistent pattern of behavior in which societal norms and the basic rights of others are violated. These behaviors can include physical harm to people or animals, damage to property, deceitfulness or theft, and extreme violations of rules. It is important to note that troublesome behavior can also result from adverse circumstances; the circumstances need to be fully investigated, and attempts to rectify adversity made, before Conduct Disorder is diagnosed. The diagnosis can be divided into two types, depending on the age of diagnosis: childhood-onset type and adolescent-onset type.

SYMPTOMS

• Aggression to people and animals, including bullying, picking fights, using weapons, physical cruelty to people and animals, stealing or forcing someone into sexual activity;
• Destruction of property;
• Deceitfulness or theft, including breaking into someone's house, lying to obtain goods or favors, or shoplifting;
• Violations of rules, including staying out past curfews, running away from home, and truancy from school.

ASSOCIATED FEATURES

Conduct disorder is often associated with early onset of sexual activity, drinking and smoking. The disorder leads to school disruption, problems with the police, sexually transmitted diseases, unplanned pregnancy, and injury from accidents and fights. Suicide and suicidal attempts are more common among adolescents with Conduct Disorder, probably both because they have a history of abuse and neglect and because their behavior results in adverse consequences. Individuals with Conduct Disorder appear to have little remorse for their acts, though they may learn that expressing guilt can diminish punishment; and they often show little or no empathy for the feelings, wishes, and well-being of others.

PREVALENCE

Prevalence of Conduct Disorder appears to have increased in recent years. For males under 18 years of age, rates range from six percent to sixteen percent; for females, rates range from two percent to nine percent.

TREATMENT OPTIONS

Both psychotherapy and medication can be useful in treating Conduct Disorder. As with many mental disorders, family members are often affected and it is crucial that they are supported and involved in the treatment.

Associations & Agencies

827 **Association for Behavioral and Cognitive Therapies**
305 Seventh Avenue
16th Floor
New York, NY 10001-6008
212-647-1890
Fax: 212-647-1865
E-mail: mebrown@aabt.org
www.aabt.org
Mary Jane Eimer, Executive Director
Mary Ellen Brown, Administration/Convention
Lisa Yarde, Membership

Membership listing of mental health professionals focusing in behavior therapy.

828 **Career Assessment & Planning Services**
Goodwill Industries-Suncoast
10596 Gandy Boulevard
St. Petersburg, FL 33702
727-523-1512
Fax: 727-563-9300
www.goodwill-suncoast.org
R Lee Waits, President/CEO
Jay McCloe, Resource Development

Provides a comprehensive assessment, which can predict current and future employment and potential adjustment factors for physically, emotionally, or developmentally disabled persons who may be unemployed or underemployed. Assessments evaluate interests, aptitudes, academic achievements, and physical abilities (including dexterity and coordination) through coordinated testing, interviewing and behavioral observations.

829 **Center for Family Support (CFS)**
333 7th Avenue
New York, NY 10001-5004
212-629-7939
Fax: 212-239-2211
www.cfsny.org
Steven Vernickofs, Executive Director
Melanie Singleton, Director Human Resource

Service agency devoted to the physical well-being and development of the retarded child and the sound mental health of the parents. Helps families with retarded children with all aspects of home care including counseling, referrals, home aide service and consultation. Offers intervention for parents at the birth of a retarded child with in-home support, guidance and infant stimulation. Pioneered training of nonprofessional women as home aides to provide supportive services in homes.

830 **National Association for the Dually Diagnosed (NADD)**
132 Fair Street
Kingston, NY 12401-4802
845-334-4336
800-331-5362
Fax: 845-331-4569
E-mail: nadd@mhv.net
www.thenadd.org
Dr. Robert Fletcher, Founder/CEO

Nonprofit organization designed to promote interest of professional and parent development with resources for individuals who have the coexistence of mental illness and mental retardation. Provides conference, educational services and training materials to professionals, parents, concerned citizens and service organizations. Formerly known as the National Association for the Dually Diagnosed.

Year Founded: 1983

831 National Mental Health Consumer's Self-Help
1211 Chestnut Street
Suite 1207
Philadelphia, PA 19107
215-751-1810
800-553-4539
Fax: 215-636-6312
E-mail: info@mhselfhelp.org
www.mhselfhelp.org

Joseph Rogers, Founder/Executive Director
Christine Simiriglia, Director

Funded by the National Institute of Mental Health Community Support Program, the purpose of the Clearinghouse is to encourage the development and growth of consumer self-help groups.

832 National Mental Health Consumers' Self-Help Clearinghouse
1211 Chestnut Street
Suite 1207
Philadelphia, PA 19107
215-751-1810
800-553-4539
Fax: 215-636-6312
E-mail: info@mhselfhelp.org
www.mhselfhelp.org

Joseph Rogers, Executive Director

A national consumer technical assistance center that has played a major role in the development of the mental health consumer movement.

Year Founded: 1986

833 Suncoast Residential Training Center/Developmental Services Program
Goodwill Industries-Suncoast
10596 Gandy Boulevard
PO Box 14456
St. Petersburg, FL 33702
727-523-1512
Fax: 727-563-9300
www.goodwill-suncoast.org

R Lee Waites, President/CEO
Deborah A Passerini, VP Operations
Lee C Zen, Corp Secretary/VP/Board Liason

Large group home which serves individuals diagnosed as mentally retarded with a secondary diagnosis of psychiatric difficulties as evidenced by problem behavior. Providing residential, behavioral and instructional support and services that will promote the development of adaptive, socially appropriate behavior, each individual is assessed to determine, socialization, basic academics and recreation. The primary intervention strategy is applied behavior analysis. Professional consultants are utilized to address the medical, dental, psychiatric and pharmacological needs of each individual. One of the most popular features is the active community integration component of SRTC. Program customers attend an average of 15 monthly outings to various community events.

Books

834 Antisocial Behavior by Young People
Cambridge University Press
40 W 20th Street
New York, NY 10011-4221
212-924-3900
Fax: 212-691-3239
E-mail: marketing@cup.org
www.cup.org

Michael Rutter, MRC Child Psychiarty Unit
Ann Hagell
Henri Giller

Written by a child psychiatrist, a criminologist and a social psychologist, this book is a major international review of research evidence on anti-social behavior. Covers all aspects of the field, including descriptions of different types of delinquency and time trends, the state of knowledge on the individuals, social-psychological and cultural factors involved and recent advances in prevention and intervention. *$22.99*

490 pages Year Founded: 1998

835 Bad Men Do What Good Men Dream: a Forensic Psychiatrist Illuminates the Darker Side of Human Behavior
American Psychiatric Publishing
1000 Wilson Boulevard
Suite 1825
Arlington, VA 22209-3901
703-907-7322
800-368-5777
Fax: 703-907-1091
E-mail: appi@psych.org
www.appi.org

James Scully, MD, President
Robert I Simon, MD, Author

Provides insights into the minds of rapists, stalkers, serial killers, psychopaths, professional exploiters, and other individuals whose behavior both frightens and fascinates us. *$32.50*

376 pages Year Founded: 1996 ISBN 0-880489-95-2

836 Conduct Disorders in Childhood and Adolescence, Developmental Clinical Psychology and Psychiatry
Sage Publications
2455 Teller Road
Thousand Oaks, CA 91320
805-499-9774
800-818-7243
Fax: 800-583-2665
E-mail: info@sagepub.com
www.sagepub.com

Blaise Simqu, President/CEO
Alan E Kazdin, Author

Conduct disorder is a clinical problem among children and adolescents that includes aggressive acts, theft, vandalism, firesetting, running away, truancy, defying authority and other antisocial behaviors. This book describes the nature of conduct disorder and what is currently known from research and clinical work. Topics include psychiatric diagnosis, parent psychopathology and child-rearing processes. Paperback also available. *$51.95*

191 pages Year Founded: 1995 ISBN 0-803971-81-8

837 Creative Therapy 2: Working with Parents
Impact Publishers
PO Box 6016
Atascadero, CA 93423-6016

805-466-5917
800-246-7228
Fax: 805-466-5919
E-mail: info@impactpublishers.com
www.impactpublishers.com

Kate M Ollier, Psych, Author
Angela M Hobday, Sc, Author

Sequel and companion volume to the authors' highly successful Creative Therapy with Children and Adolesents. Creative Therapy 2 offers practicing therapists a wealth of resources for working with parents whose children are experiencing emotional and/or behavioral problems. The procedures and exercises are carefully crafted to provide help even when the parents have been less than understanding - or perhaps even abusive toward their children. Therapists will find dozens of creative ways to form good working relationships with parents, and to prepare them to help their children. *$21.95*

192 pages Year Founded: 2001 ISBN 1-886230-42-0

838   Difficult Child
Bantam Doubleday Dell Publishing
1745 Broadway
New York, NY 10019
212-782-9000
Fax: 212-782-9700
E-mail: books@randomhouse.com
www.randomhouse.com

Erik Engstrom, President/CEO
Stanley Turecki, Author

Help for parents dealing with behavioral problems. *$ 17.00*

320 pages Year Founded: 2000 ISBN 0-553380-36-2

839   Dysinhibition Syndrome How to Handle Anger and Rage in Your Child or Spouse
Hope Press
PO Box 188
Duarte, CA 91009-0188
818-303-0644
800-321-4039
Fax: 818-358-3520
www.hopepress.com

Rose Wood, Author

How to understand and handle rage and anger in your children or spouse. The book presents behavioral approaches that can be very effective and an understanding that can be family saving. *$24.95*

271 pages Year Founded: 1999 ISBN 1-878267-08-6

840   Helping Parents, Youth, and Teachers Understand Medications for Behavioral and Emotional Problems
American Psychiatric Publishing
1000 Wilson Boulevard
Suite 1825
Arlington, VA 20009-3901
703-907-7322
800-368-5777
Fax: 703-907-1091
E-mail: appi@psych.org
www.appi.org

James Scully, MD, President
Mina K Dulcan, MD, Editor
Claudia Lizarralde, MD, Editor

Resource Book of Medication Information Handouts, Second Edition. Valuable resource for anyone involved in evaluating psychiatric disturbances in children and adolescents. Provides a compilation of information sheets to help promote the dialogue between the patient's family, caregivers and the treating physician. *$62.00*

205 pages Year Founded: 2003 ISBN 1-585620-41-6

841   Preventing Antisocial Behavior Interventions from Birth through Adolescence
Guilford Publications
72 Spring Street
New York, NY 10012
212-431-9800
800-365-7006
Fax: 212-966-6708
E-mail: info@guilford.com
www.guilford.com

Robert Matloff, President
Joan McCord, Editor
Richard E Tremblay, Editor

Establishes the crucial link between theory, measurement, and intervention. Brings together a collection of studies that utilize experimental approaches for evaluating intervention programs for preventing deviant behavior. Demonstrates both the feasibility and necessity of independent evaluation. Also shows how the information obtained in such studies can be used to test and refine prevailing theories about human behavior in general and behavior changes in particular. *$55.00*

391 pages Year Founded: 1992 ISBN 0-898628-82-2

842   Skills Training for Children with Behavior Disorders
Courage to Change
PO Box 486
Wilkes-Barre, PA 18703-0486
800-440-4003
Fax: 800-772-6499
www.couragetochange.com

Michael L Bloomquist, Author

Written for both parents and therapists, this book provides backround, instructions, and many reproducible worksheets. Academic success, anger management, emotional well being and compliance/following rules are covered. *$36.00*

272 pages Year Founded: 1996 ISBN 1-572300-80-9

Periodicals & Pamphlets

843   Conduct Disorder in Children and Adolescents
SAMHSA'S National Mental Health Information Center
PO Box 42557
Washington, DC 20015
800-789-2647
Fax: 240-747-5470
TDD: 866-889-2647
E-mail: ken@mentalhealth.org
www.mentalhealth.samhsa.gov

A Kathryn Power, MEd, Director
Edward B Searle, Deputy Director

This fact sheet defines conduct disorder, identifies risk factors, discusses types of help available, and suggests what parents or other caregivers can do.

2 pages

844 Mental, Emotional, and Behavior Disorders in Children and Adolescents
SAMHSA'S National Mental Health Information Center
PO Box 42557
Washington, DC 20015
800-789-2647
Fax: 240-747-5470
TDD: 866-889-2647
E-mail: ken@mentalhealth.org
www.mentalhealth.samhsa.gov

A Kathryn Power, MEd, Director
Edward B Searle, Deputy Director

This fact sheet describes mental, emotional, and behavioral problems that can occur during childhood and adolescence and discusses related treatment, support services, and research.

4 pages

845 Treatment of Children with Mental Disorders
National Institute of Mental Health
6001 Executive Boulevard
Room 8184
Bethesda, MD 20892-9663
866-615-6464
Fax: 301-443-4279
TTY: 301-443-8431
E-mail: nimhinfo@nih.gov
www.nimh.nih.gov

Dr Thomas R Insel, Director
Ruth Dubois, Assistant Chief

A short booklet that contains questions and answers about therapy for children with mental disorders. Includes a chart of mental disorders and medications used.

Year Founded: 2004

Research Centers

846 Child & Family Center
Menninger Clinic
2801 Gessner Drive
Houston, TX 77080
713-275-5000
800-351-9058
Fax: 713-275-5107
E-mail: webmaster@menninger.edu
www.menninger.edu

The Center's goals: to further develop emerging understanding of the impact of childhood maltreatment and abuse; to chart primary prevention strategies that will foster healthy patterns of caregiving and attachment and reduce the prevalence of maltreatment and abuse; to develop secondary prevention strategies that will promote early detection of attachment-related problems and effective interventions to avert the development of chronic and severe disorders; and to develop more effective treatment approaches for those individuals whose early attachment problems have eventuated in severe psychopathology.

Video & Audio

847 Active Parenting Now
Active Parenting Publishers
1955 Vaughn Road NW
Suite 108
Kennesaw, GA 30144-7808
770-429-0565
800-825-0060
Fax: 770-429-0334
E-mail: cservice@activeparenting.com
www.activeparenting.com

Michael H Popkin, MD, Author

A complete video-based parenting education program curriculum. Helps parents of children ages two to twelve raise responsible, courageous children. Emphasizes nonviolent discipline, conflict resolution and improved communication. With Leader's Guide, videotapes, Parent's Guide and more. Also available in Spanish. *$ 349.00*

Year Founded: 2002 ISBN 1-880283-89-1

848 Understanding & Managing the Defiant Child
Courage to Change
PO Box 486
Wilkes-Barre, PA 18703-0486
800-440-4003
Fax: 800-772-6499
www.couragetochange.com

Russell A Barkley, PhD, Presenter

Understanding and Managing the Defiant Child provides a proven approach to behavior management. *$205.95*

849 Understanding and Treating the Hereditary Psychiatric Spectrum Disorders
Hope Press
PO Box 188
Duarte, CA 91009-0188
818-303-0644
800-321-4039
Fax: 818-358-3520
www.hopepress.com

David E Comings MD, Presenter

Learn with ten hours of audio tapes from a two day seminar given in May 1997 by David E Comings, MD. Tapes cover: ADHD, Tourette Syndrome, Obsessive-Compulsive Disorder, Conduct Disorder, Oppositional Defiant Disorder, Autism and other Hereditary Psychiatric Spectrum Disorders. Eight audio tapes. *$75.00*

Year Founded: 1997

Web Sites

850 www.cyberpsych.org
CyberPsych

Hosts the American Psychoanalyists Foundation, American Association of Suicideology, Society for the Exploration of Psychotherapy Intergration, and Anxiety Disorders Association of America. Also subcategories of the anxiety disorders, as well as general information, including panic disorder, phobias, obsessive compulsive disorder (OCD), social phobia, generalized anxiety disorder, post traumatic stress disorder, and phobias of childhood. Book reviews and links to web pages sharing the topics.

851 **www.planetpsych.com**
PlanetPsych.com

Learn about disorders, their treatments and other topics in psychology. Articles are listed under the related topic areas. Ask a therapist a question for free, or view the directory of professionals in your area. If you are a therapist sign up for the directory. Current features, self-help, interactive, and newsletter archives.

852 **www.psychcentral.com**
Psych Central

Personalized one-stop index for psychology, support, and mental health issues, resources, and people on the Internet.

Depression

Introduction

Feelings of sadness are common to everyone, and quite natural in reaction to unfortunate circumstances. The death of a loved one, the end of a relationship, or other traumatic life experiences are bound to bring on the blues. But when feelings of sadness and despair persist beyond a reasonable period, arise for no particular reason, or begin to affect a person's ability to function, help is needed. Depression is a diagnosis made by a psychiatrist or other mental health professional to describe serious and prolonged symptoms of sadness or despair. While it is quite common, it is also a disease that no one should take lightly; depression can be deadly. Many people who are deeply depressed think about or actually try to commit suicide; some commit suicide. Even a relatively mild depression, if untreated, can disrupt marriages and relationships or impede careers. Such depressions cost the U.S. economy billions of dollars a year in lost productivity.

After giving birth, women may suffer from a spectrum of psychiatric disorders related to the demands of new motherhood and the abrupt hormonal changes that occur after delivery. The most common postpartum condition is 'baby blues' which begins within a few days of birth and causes increased emotional sensitivity to events, sometimes demonstrated by happy or sad tears. Reassurance is the only treatment required and the condition goes away spontaneously.

More serious is Postpartum Depression which often begins before birth, during pregnancy. The symptoms are the same as those of depression at any other time, but the mother is preoccupied with concerns about whether she is a good mother. Unlike an average, tired new mother, the depressed woman cannot rest even when the baby is sleeping, loses her appetite and cannot enjoy her baby. She is often guilty and reluctant to tell her family about it because she knows she is supposed to appreciate her good fortune and be happy. Severe Postpartum Depression, or Postpartum Psychosis, that causes confusion, disorientation, delusions, and hallucinations, and can cause suicide or infanticide, is a serious medical condition demanding immediate professional attention. Fortunately, there is increasing awareness and understanding of postpartum depression among the general population.

SYMPTOMS

Depression is diagnosed when an individual experiences 1) persistent feelings of sadness or 2) loss of interest or pleasure in usual activities, in addition to five of the following symptoms for at least two weeks:
• Significant weight gain or loss unrelated to dieting;
• Inability to sleep or, conversely, sleeping too much;
• Restlessness and agitation;
• Fatigue or loss of energy;
• Feelings of worthlesness or guilt;
• Diminished ability to think or concentrate;
• Recurrent thoughts of death or suicide;
• Distress is not caused by a medication or the symptoms of a medical illness.

Postpartum Depression (in addition to symptoms above)
• Preoccupation with concerns of being a good mother;
• Inability to rest while the baby is sleeping;
• Inability to enjoy her baby accompanied with feeling of guilt.

ASSOCIATED FEATURES

Because Depression can range from moderate to severe, people who are depressed may exhibit a variety of behaviors. Often, people who are depressed are tearful, irritable, or brooding. Problems sleeping (either insomnia or sleeping too much) are common. People with Depression may worry unnecessarily about being sick or having a disease, or they may report physical symptoms such as headaches or other pains. Depression can seriously affect people's friendships and intimate relationships.

Depression can make people worry about having a disease, but this is not a central symptom. Depression very frequently coexists with anxiety disorder. There is a genetic predisposition in some people.

Abuse of alcohol, prescription drugs, or illegal drugs is also common among people who are depressed. The most serious risk associated with Depression is the risk of suicide: people who have tried to commit suicide in the past, or who have family members who have commited suicide are especially at risk. Individuals who have another mental disorder, such as Schizophrenia, in addition to Depression are also more likely to commit suicide.

PREVALENCE

Every year more than 17 million Americans suffer some type of depressive illness. Depression does not discriminate; anyone can have it. Children, adults and the elderly are susceptible. Nevertheless, studies do indicate that women are twice as likely to have Depression as men. Depression has significant adverse effects on children's functioning and development; among adolescents, suicide is believed to be the fifth leading cause of death. Depression is also common among the elderly, and can be treated as an illness distinct from the loneliness or sadness that may accompany old age.

Very mild depression after delivery, or baby blues, affects over half, perhaps up to 90% of postpartum women. Baby blues is actually not depression at all; rather it is a common condition characterized by sensitivity and emotionality, both happy and sad. Postpartum Depression affects approximately 10% of new mothers. Much postpartum depression is a continuation of depression that was already present during pregnancy. The use of antidepressant drugs both during and after pregnancy, for nursing mothers, can be discussed with a patient's psychiatrist. There is an increasing amount of literature on the safety of medications at those times. Untreated depression has adverse consequences for fetus, mother and baby. Women who have had depression following one birth have a 50% chance of becoming depressed after a second delivery, and those who have had Postpartum Depression twice have a 75% likelihood of beccoming depressed after having a third baby. Postpartum Psychosis, a rare permutation of postpartum conditions, affects fewer than 1% of women.

TREATMENT OPTIONS

Depression is a medical disease and does not respond to the usual ways we have of cheering up ourselves or others. In fact, attempts to cheer depressed inviduals may have the opposite and unfortunate consequence of making them feel worse, often because they are frustrated and feel guilty that others' well-meaning efforts do not help. If a person experiences the symptoms of Depression, he or she should seek treatment from a qualified professional. The vast majority of people with Depression get better when they are treated properly, and virtually everyone gets some relief from their symptoms.

A psychiatrist or other mental health professional should conduct a thorough evaluation, including an interview; a physical examination should be done by a primary care provider. On the basis of a complete evaluation, the appropriate treatment will be prescribed. Most likely, the treatment will be medication or psychotherapy, or both. Antidepressants usually take effect within three to six weeks after treatment has begun; usually the prescribing psychiatrist will recommend that patients continue to take medication at least nine months to a year after symptoms have improved. It is important to give medications long enough to work, and to increase dosages or change or add medications if depression does not resolve completely.

The natural course of depression is about nine months and then, even though patients may feel better on the medication, the depression is likely to come back if medication is discontinued too early. In addition, depression recurs later in about 50% of patients after one episode, and more frequently if there is a second or third episode, so that some patients choose to remain on medication indefinitely to decrease their risk of recurrence. Dysthymic disorder is more low-level and chronic, with depressed mood consistently for at least two years, than major depressive episodes which last about nine months. Dysthymia can be treated with medication and psychotherapy as well.

Psychotherapy, or talk therapy, may be used to help the patient improve the way he or she thinks about things and deals with specific life problems. Individual, family or couples therapy may be recommended, depending on the patient's life experiences. If the depression is not severe, treatment can take a few weeks; if the Depression has been a longstanding problem, it may take much longer, but in many cases, a patient will experience improvement in 10-15 sessions.

Treatment for Postpartum Depression is similar to treatment for depression in general. Possible risks of medications taken during pregnancy and breastfeeding have to be weighed against the risks of leaving the depression untreated. Women who discontinue antidepressant medication because they wish to become pregnant are at a very high risk of relapse.

Associations & Agencies

854 Center for Family Support (CFS)
333 7th Avenue
New York, NY 10001-5004
212-629-7939
Fax: 212-239-2211
www.cfsny.org
Steven Vernickofs, Executive Director

An agency that continues to develop new programs to serve families and individuals with their care needs. Currently offering services throughout the New York City region including: New Jersey, Long Island and the Lower Hudson Valley.

855 Depression & Bi-Polar Support Alliance
730 N Franklin Street
Suite 501
Chicago, IL 60610-7204
800-826-3632
Fax: 312-642-7243
www.dbsalliance.org
Lydia Lewis, President
Ingrid Deetz, Program Manager

Educates patients, families, professionals, and the public concerning the nature of depressive and manic-depressive illnesses as treatable medical diseases, fosters self-help for patients and families, works to eliminate discrimination and stigma, improves access to care, advocates for research toward the elimination of these illnesses.

856 Depression & Related Affective Disorders Association (DRADA)
8201 Greensboro Drive
Suite 300
McLean, VA 22102
703-610-9026
Fax: 410-614-3241
E-mail: drada@jhmi.edu
www.drada.org
Catherine Pollock, Executive Director
Elizabeth Boyce, Director Development

Non profit association whose mission is to alleviate the suffering arising from depression and manic depression by assisting self - help groups, providing education and information and lending support to research programs.

857 Depression After Delivery
91 E Somerset Street
Raritan, NJ 08869-2129
908-575-9121
800-944-4773
Fax: 908-541-9713
E-mail: dadorg@earthlink.net
www.depressionafterdelivery.com
Joyce A Venis, RNC, President
Donna Cangialosi, Office Manager

Twenty four information request line. Free information packet of referrals and volunteer contacts nationwide for women with postpartum disorders.

858 Depression and Bi-Polar Alliance
730 N Franklin Street
Suite 501
Chicago, IL 60610-7204
800-826-3632
Fax: 312-642-7243
www.ndmda.org
Lydia Lewis, Executive Director
Julie Bremer, External Relations Director

Previously called the National Depressive and Manic Depressive Association, the Depression and Bi-Polar Alliance publishes a variety of educational materials for adults and teens on mood disorders, all available free of charge or for a nominial fee. Because the Alliance focuses on the consumer living with a mood disorder, their publications are written in language free from medical and scientific jargon and everything they produce conveys a strong message of hope and optimism.

859   Emotions Anonymous International Service Center
PO Box 4245
Saint Paul, MN 55104-0245
651-647-9712
Fax: 651-647-1593
E-mail: info@EmotionsAnonymous.org
www.EmotionsAnonymous.org

Karen Mead, Executive Director

Fellowship of men and women who share their experience, strength and hope with each other, that they may solve their common problem and help others recover from emotional illness.

860   Freedom From Fear
308 Seaview Avenue
Staten Island, NY 10305
718-351-1717
Fax: 718-980-5022
E-mail: help@freedomfromfear.org
www.freedomfromfear.com

Mary Guardino, Founder/President

The mission of Freedom From Fear is to aid and counsel individuals and their families who suffer from anxiety and depressive illness.

861   Mental Health Research Association (NARSAD)
60 Cutter Mill Road
Suite 404
Great Neck, NY 11021-3104
516-829-0091
800-829-8289
Fax: 516-487-6930
E-mail: info@narsad.org
www.narsad.org

Constance Lieber, President
Steven G Doochin, Executive Director

The Mental Health Research Association is a nonprofit organization that raises funds for scientific research on severe mental illnesses. It is the largest donor-supported organization in the world dedicated to finding the causes, improved treatments and cures for psychiatric brain and behavior disorders.

862   NARSAD: The Mental Health Research Associati on
60 Cutter Mill Road
Suite 404
Great Neck, NY 11021
516-829-0091
800-829-8289
Fax: 516-487-6930
E-mail: info@narsad.org
www.narsad.org

Steven G Doochin, President
Louis Innamorato, CFO

Previously known as the National Alliance for Research on Schizophrenia and Depression, NARSAD is a private, not-for-profit public charity organized for the purpose of raising funds for scientific research into the causes, cures, treatments and prevention of severe psychiatric brain and behavior disorders, such as schizophrenia and depression.

863   National Alliance on Mental Illness
2107 Wilson Boulevard
Suite 300
Arlington, VA 22201-3042
703-524-7600
800-950-6264
Fax: 703-524-9094
E-mail: info@nami.org
www.nami.org

Suzanne Vogel-Scibilia, MD, President
Frederick R Sandoval, First VP

Nation's leading self-help organization for all those affected by severe brain disorders. Mission is to bring consumers and families with similar experiences together to share information about services, care providers, and ways to cope with the challenges of schizophrenia, manic depression, and other serious mental illnesses.

Year Founded: 1979

864   National Association for the Dually Diagnosed (NADD)
132 Fair Street
Kingston, NY 12401-4802
845-334-4336
800-331-5362
Fax: 845-331-4569
E-mail: nadd@mhv.net
www.thenadd.org

Dr Robert Fletcher, Executive Director

Nonprofit organization designed to promote interest of professional and parent development with resources for individuals who have the coexistence of mental illness and mental retardation. Provides conference, educational services and training materials to professionals, parents, concerned citizens and service organizations. Formerly known as the National Association for the Dually Diagnosed.

Year Founded: 1983

865   National Institute of Mental Health
6001 Executive Boulevard
Room 8184
Bethesda, MD 20892-9663
866-615-6464
Fax: 301-443-4279
TTY: 301-443-8431
E-mail: nimhinfo@nih.gov
www.nimh.nih.gov

Information and resources concerning depression, manic depression, bi-polar disorder and other mental health issues.

866   National Mental Health Consumer's Self-Help
1211 Chestnut Street
Suite 1207
Philadelphia, PA 19107
215-751-1810
800-553-4539
Fax: 215-636-6312
E-mail: info@mhselfhelp.org
www.mhselfhelp.org

Christine Simiriglia, Executive Director
Jennifer Melinn, Information/Referral Dept.

Funded by the National Institute of Mental Health Community Support Program, the purpose of the Clearinghouse is to encourage the development and growth of consumer self-help groups.

867 National Mental Health Consumers' Self-Help Clearinghouse
1211 Chestnut Street
Suite 1207
Philadelphia, PA 19107
215-751-1810
800-553-4539
Fax: 215-636-6312
E-mail: info@mhselfhelp.org
www.mhselfhelp.org

Joseph Rogers, Executive Director

A national consumer technical assistance center that has played a major role in the development of the mental health consumer movement.

Year Founded: 1986

868 Postpartum Support International
927 N Kellogg Avenue
Santa Barbara, CA 93111
805-967-7636
Fax: 805-967-0608
E-mail: psioffice@postpartum.net
www.postpartum.net

Jane Honikman, Founding Director
Shoshana Bennett, PhD, PSI President

Increases awareness of emotional changes in women while pregnant and after childbirth.

869 SAMHSA'S National Mental Health Information Center
US Department of Health and Human Services
PO Box 42557
Washington, DC 20015
800-789-2647
Fax: 240-747-5470
TDD: 866-889-2647
E-mail: ken@mentalhealth.org
www.mentalhealth.samhra.gov

A Kathryn Power, MEd, Director
Edward B Searle, Deputy Director

Information about resources, technical assistance, research, training, networks, and other federal clearing houses, and fact sheets and materials. Information specialists refer callers to mental health resources in their communities as well as state, federal and nonprofit contacts. Staff available Monday through Friday, 8:30 AM - 5:00 PM, EST, excluding federal holidays. After hours, callers may leave messages and an information specialist will return their call.

870 Suncoast Residential Training Center/Developmental Services Program
Goodwill Industries-Suncoast
10596 Gandy Boulevard
PO Box 14456
St. Petersburg, FL 33702
727-523-1512
Fax: 727-577-2749
E-mail: gw.marketing@goodwill-suncoast.org
www.goodwill-suncoast.org

R Lee Waits, President/CEO
Deborah A Passerini, VP Operations

A large group home which serves individuals diagnosed as mentally retarded with a secondary diagnosed of psychiatric difficulties as evidenced by problem behavior. Providing residential, behavioral and instructional support and services that will promote the development of adaptive, socially appropriate behavior, each individual is assessed to determine, socialization, basic academics and recreation. The primary intervention strategy is applied behavior analysis. Professional consultants are utilized to address the medical, dental, psychiatric and pharmacological needs of ech individual. One of the most popular features is the active community integration component of SRTC. Program customers attend an average of 15 monthly outings to various community events.

Books

871 Against Depression
Viking Adult
375 Hudson Street
New York, NY 10014
212-366-2372
Fax: 212-366-2933
www.us.penguingroup.com

Peter D Kramer, Author

872 Anxiety and Depression in Adults and Children, Banff International Behavioral Science Series
Sage Publications
2455 Teller Road
Thousand Oaks, CA 91320
805-499-9774
800-818-7243
Fax: 800-583-2665
E-mail: info@sagepub.com
www.sagepub.com

Collection of papers by well respected researchers in the field of anxiety and depression. Brings together desparate areas of research and integrates them in an informative and interesting way. Focuses on recent advances in treating anxiety and depression in adults and children. Topics include self-management therapy, assessing and treating sexually abused children and unipolar depression. Integrates empirical research with clinical applications. Paperback also available. *$46.95*

296 pages ISBN 0-803970-20-X

873 Breaking the Patterns of Depression
Random House
1745 Broadway
New York, NY 10019
212-782-9000
800-733-3000
Fax: 212-572-6066
www.randomhouse.com

Presents skills that enable readers to understand and ultimately avert depression's recurring cycles. Focusing on future prevention as well as initial treatment, the book includes over one hundred structured activities to help sufferers learn the skills necessary to become and remain depression-free. Translates the clinical literature on psychotherapy and antidepressant medication into understandable language. Defines what causes depression and clarifies what can be done about it. With this knowledge in hand, readers can control their depression, rather than having depression control them. *$13.95*

362 pages ISBN 0-385483-70-8

874 Broken Connection: On Death and the Continuity of Life
American Psychiatric Publishing
1000 Wilson Boulevard
Suite 1825
Arlington, VA 22209
703-907-7322
800-368-5777
Fax: 703-907-1091
E-mail: appi@psych.org
www.appi.org

Katie Duffy, Marketing Assistant

Exploration of the inescapable connections between death and life, the psychiatric disorders that arise from these connections, and the advent of the nuclear age which has jeopardized any attempts to ensure the perpetuation of the self beyond death. *$38.00*

474 pages ISBN 0-880488-74-3

875 Clinical Guide to Depression in Children and Adolescents
American Psychiatric Publishing
1000 Wilson Boulevard
Suite 1825
Arlington, VA 22209-3901
703-907-7322
800-368-5777
Fax: 703-907-1091
E-mail: appi@psych.org
www.appi.org

Katie Duffy, Marketing Assistant

Integrates advances in the recognition, diagnosis, management, and treatment of depressive disorders and bipolar disorders in infancy, childhood, and adolescence. *$39.50*

304 pages ISBN 0-880483-56-3

876 Depression & Anxiety Management
New Harbinger Publications
5674 Shattuck Avenue
Oakland, CA 94609-1662
510-652-2002
800-748-6273
Fax: 510-652-5472
E-mail: customerservice@newharbinger.com
www.newharbinger.com

John D Preston, Author

Offers step-by-step help for identifying the thoughts that make one anxious and depressed, confronting unrealistic and distorted thinking, and replacing negative mental patterns with healthy, realistic thinking. *$11.95*

ISBN 1-879237-46-6

877 Depression Workbook: a Guide for Living with Depression
New Harbinger Publications
5674 Shattuck Avenue
Oakland, CA 94609-1662
510-652-2002
800-748-6273
Fax: 510-652-5472
E-mail: customerservice@newharbinger.com
www.newharbinger.com

Mary Ellen Copeland, Author

Based on responses of participants sharing their insights, experiences, and strategies for living with extreme mood swings. *$ 19.95*

352 pages Year Founded: 1992 ISBN 1-572242-68-X

878 Depression and Its Treatment
Time Warner Books
3 Center Plaza
Boston, MA 02108
800-759-0190
Fax: 800-331-1664
E-mail: sales@aoltwbg.com
www.twbookmark.com

A layman's guide to help one understand and cope with America's number one mental health problem. *$19.95*

157 pages

879 Depression, the Mood Disease
Johns Hopkins University Press
2715 N Charles Street
Baltimore, MD 21218-4319
410-516-6900
800-537-5487
Fax: 410-516-6998

Explores the many faces of an illness that will affect as many as 36 million Americans at some point in their lives. Updated to reflect state-of-the-art treatment. *$12.76*

240 pages ISBN 0-801851-84-X

880 Diagnosis and Treatment of Depression in Lat e Life: Results of the NIH Consensus Development Conference
American Psychiatric Publishing
1000 Wilson Boulevard
Suite 1825
Arlington, VA 22209-3901
703-907-7322
800-368-5777
Fax: 703-907-1091
E-mail: appi@psych.org
www.appi.org

Katie Duffy, Marketing Assistant

Provides comprehensive studies in early life depression versus late life depression, the prevalence of depression in elderly people and the risk factors involved. *$21.95*

536 pages ISBN 0-880485-56-6

881 Drug Therapy and Postpartum Disorders
Mason Crest Publishers
370 Reed Road
Suite 302
Broomall, PA 19008
610-543-3878
866-627-2665
Fax: 610-543-3878
E-mail: dtaylor@masoncrest.com
www.masoncrest.com

Pregnancy, childbirth and early motherhood are supposed to be times filled with the joy and wonder of bringing a new life into the world. Unfortunately, many women find that the struggles of early motherhood are accompanied by multiple sorrows that clash with the sentimental ideal. New mothers may feel alone in their struggles, but depression after childbirth is far more common than most people realize.

This book provides information about the psychiatric conditions that can accompany new motherhood and the treatments that can help.

ISBN 1-590846-70-6

882 Encyclopedia of Depression
Facts on File
132 W 31st Street
17th Floor
New York, NY 10001
800-322-8755
Fax: 800-678-3633
E-mail: custserv@factsonfile.com
www.factsonfile.com

This volume defines and explains all terms and topics relating to depression. *$58.50*

170 pages

883 Growing Up Sad: Childhood Depression and Its Treatment
WW Norton & Company
500 5th Avenue
New York, NY 10100-0017
212-354-5500
800-233-4830
Fax: 212-869-0856
E-mail: npb@wwnorton.com
www.wwnorton.com/psych

The authors have updated their classic study, Why Isn't Johnny Crying? that looks at the symptoms and treatment of childhood - onset depression. The authors give an authoritative summary of research, counsel prompt diagnosis, and assert that the disorder is treatable. *$25.00*

216 pages ISBN 0-393317-88-9

884 Help Me, I'm Sad: Recognizing, Treating, and Preventing Childhood and Adolescent Depression
Penguin Putnam
375 Hudson Street
New York, NY 10014-3658
212-366-2000
800-227-9604
Fax: 201-896-8569
www.pengiunputnam.com

Especially helpful to parents and other caregivers in recognizing the warning signs of depression whatever the development stage. Offers case histories to illustrate what childhood-onset depression looks like at different ages. *$14.00*

200 pages

885 Helping Your Depressed Teenager: a Guide for Parents and Caregivers
John Wiley & Sons
1 Wiley Drive
Somerset, NJ 08873
732-469-4400
800-225-5945
Fax: 732-302-2300
E-mail: compbks@wiley.com
www.wiley.com

Gerald D Oster, Author
Sarah S Montgomery, Author

The authors, a psychologist and a social worker, contrast clinical depression with normal adolescent mood changes. They deal realistically with teenage suicide and urge prompt intervention. *$ 19.95*

208 pages Year Founded: 1994 ISBN 0-471621-84-6

886 Lonely, Sad, and Angry: a Parent's Guide to Depression in Children and Adolescents
ADD Warehouse
300 NW 70th Avenue
Suite 102
Plantation, FL 33317
954-792-8100
800-233-9273
Fax: 954-792-8545
www.addwarehouse.com

Covers the symptoms of depression, its diagnosis, causes, treatment (including medication), suicide, and management strategies at home and at school. For parents and teenagers. *$14.95*

225 pages

887 Management of Depression
American Psychiatric Publishing
1000 Wilson Boulevard
Suite 1825
Arlington, VA 22209-3901
703-907-7322
800-368-5777
Fax: 703-907-1091
E-mail: appi@psych.org
www.appi.org

Katie Duffy, Marketing Assistant

Comprehensive text covers all the important issues in the management of depression. *$39.95*

136 pages ISBN 1-853175-47-1

888 Manic-Depressive Illness: Bipolar Disorders and Recurrent Depression
Oxford Univeristy Press
2001 Evans Road
Cary, NC 27513
800-445-9714
Fax: 919-677-1303
E-mail: custserv.us@oup.com
www.www.oup.com/us/

Frederick K Goodwin, Author

The revolution in psychiatry that began in earnest in the 1960s led to dramatic advances in the understanding and treatment of manic-depressive illness.

889 Mayo Clinic on Depression
Mason Crest Publishers
370 Reed Road
Suite 302
Broomall, PA 19008
866-627-2665
Fax: 610-543-3878
www.www.masoncrest.com/index.php

Keith G Kramlinger, Author

890 Mood Apart
Basic Books
387 Park Avenue S
New York, NY 10016

212-340-8100
Fax: 212-340-8125
An overview of depression and manic depression and the available treatments for them. *$24.00*

363 pages

891   Mood Apart: Thinker's Guide to Emotion & It's Disorders
Harper Collins
10 E 53rd Street
New York, NY 10022
212-207-7000
Fax: 212-207-7145
E-mail: sales@harpercollins.com
www.harpercollins.com

Discussion of depression and mania includes symptoms, human costs, biological underpinnings, and therapies. Authoritatively written, it uses case histories, appendices, and historical references. *$15.00*

ISBN 0-060977-40-X

892   Natural History of Mania, Depression and Schizophrenia
American Psychiatric Publishing
1000 Wilson Boulevard
Suite 1825
Arlington, VA 22209-3901
703-907-7322
800-368-5777
Fax: 703-907-1091
E-mail: appi@psych.org
www.appi.org

Katie Duffy, Marketing Assistant

An unusual look at the course of mental illness, based on data from the Iowa 500 Research Project. *$42.50*

336 pages   ISBN 0-880487-26-7

893   Overcoming Depression
Harper Collins
10 E 53rd Street
New York, NY 10022
212-207-7000
Fax: 800-822-4090
www.harpercollins.com

Described as one of the most comprehensive books available for the layperson on depression. Covers the full range of mood disorders. *$15.00*

ISBN 0-060927-82-8

894   Pain Behind the Mask: Overcoming Masculine Depression
Haworth Press
10 Alice Street
Binghamton, NY 13904-1580
607-722-5857
800-429-6784
Fax: 607-721-0012
E-mail: getinfo@haworthpress.com
www.haworthpress.com

Jackie Blakeslee, Advertising/Journal Liason
John Lynch, PhD, Author
Christopher Kilmartin, PhD, Author

Presents a model of masculinity based on the premise that men express depression through behaviors that distort the feelings and human conflicts they experience. *$22.95*

210 pages   Year Founded: 1999 ISBN 0-789005-58-1

895   Pastoral Care of Depression
Haworth Press
10 Alice Street
Binghamton, NY 13904-1503
607-722-5857
800-429-6784
Fax: 800-895-0582
E-mail: getinfo@haworthpressinc.com
www.haworthpress.com

Binford W Gilbert, PhD, Author

Helps caregivers by overcoming the simplistic myths about depressive disorders and probing the real issues. *$17.95*

127 pages   Year Founded: 1997 ISBN 0-789002-65-5

896   Post-Natal Depression: Psychology, Science and the Transition to Motherhood
Routledge
2727 Palisade Avenue
Suite 4H
Bronx, NY 10463-1020
888-765-1209
Fax: 718-796-0971
E-mail: vd6@columbia.edu

$23.95

ISBN 0-415163-62-5

897   Postpartum Mood Disorders
American Psychiatric Publishing
1000 Wilson Boulevard
Suite 1825
Arlington, VA 22209-3901
703-907-7322
800-368-5777
Fax: 703-907-1091
E-mail: appi@psych.orgg
www.appi.org

Katie Duffy, Marketing Assistant

Provides thorough coverage of a highly prevalent, but often misunderstood subject. *$38.50*

280 pages   ISBN 0-880489-29-4

898   Practice Guideline for Major Depressive Disorders in Adults
American Psychiatric Publishing
1000 Wilson Boulevard
Suite 1825
Arlington, VA 22209-3901
703-907-7322
800-368-5777
Fax: 703-907-1091
E-mail: appi@psych.org
www.appi.org

Katie Duffy, Marketing Assistant

Summarizes the specific forms of somatic, psychotherapeutic, psychosocial, and educational treatments developed to deal with major depressive order and its various subtypes. *$22.50*

51 pages   ISBN 0-890423-01-6

899 Predictors of Treatment Response in Mood Disorders
American Psychiatric Publishing
1000 Wilson Boulevard
Suite 1825
Arlington, VA 22209-3901
703-907-7322
800-368-5777
Fax: 703-907-1091
E-mail: appi@psych.org
www.appi.org

Katie Duffy, Marketing Assistant

Helps clinicians and managed care administrators assign the correct somatic therapy. *$29.00*

224 pages ISBN 0-880484-94-2

900 Prozac Nation: Young & Depressed in America, a Memoir
Houghton Mifflin Company
222 Berkeley Street
Boston, MA 02116
617-351-5000
Fax: 617-351-1117
www.hmco.com

Struck with depression at 11, Wurtzel, now 27, chronicles her struggle with the illness. Witty, terrifying and sometimes funny, it tells the story of a young life almost destroyed by depression. *$19.95*

317 pages

901 Questions & Answers About Depression & Its Treatment
Charles Press Publishers
117 S 17th Street
Suite 310
Philadelphia, PA 19103
215-496-9616
Fax: 215-496-9637
E-mail: mailbox@charlespresspub.com
www.charlespresspub.com

All the questions you'd like to ask, with answers.

136 pages

902 Seasonal Affective Disorder and Beyond: Light Treatment for SAD and Non-SAD Conditions
American Psychiatric Publishing
1000 Wilson Boulevard
Suite 1825
Arlington, VA 22209-3901
703-907-7322
800-368-5777
Fax: 703-907-1091
E-mail: appi@psych.org
www.appi.org

Katie Duffy, Marketing Assistant

Summarizes issues around the therapeutic uses of light treatment. *$45.00*

320 pages ISBN 0-880488-67-0

903 Stories of Depression: Does this Sound Like You?
National Institute of Mental Health
6001 Executive Boulevard
Room 8184
Bethesda, MD 20892-9663
866-615-6464
Fax: 301-443-4279
TTY: 301-443-8431
E-mail: nimhinfo@nih.gov
www.nimh.nih.gov

Are you feeling really sad, tired, and worried most of the time? Are these feelings lasting more than a few days? If yes, you may have depression.

20 pages

904 The Cognitive Behavorial Workbook for Depression: A Step-by-Step Program
New Harbinger Publications
5674 Shattuck Avenue
Oakland, CA 94609
615-793-5000
Fax: 615-213-3040
E-mail: ii.info@ingrambook.com
www.www.newharbinger.com

William J Knaus, Author
Albert Ellis, Author

This type of cognitive behavioral therapy, called rational emotive behavior therapy (REBT) by Ellis, proved especially effective at relieving problems like anger, anxiety, and depression.

905 Treatment Plans and Interventions for Depression and Anxiety Disorders
Guilford Publications
72 Spring Street
New York, NY 10012
212-431-9800
800-365-7006
Fax: 212-966-6708
E-mail: info@guilford.com
www.guilford.com

Provides information on treatments for seven frequently encountered disorders: major depression, generalized anxiety, panic, agoraphobia, PTSD, social phobia, specific phobia and OCD. Serving as ready to use treatment packages, chapters describe basic cognitive behavioral therapy techniques and how to tailor them to each disorder. Also featured are diagnostic decision trees, therapist forms for assessment and record keeping, client handouts and homework sheets. *$ 49.50*

332 pages ISBN 1-572305-14-2

906 Treatment for Chronic Depression: Cognitive Behavioral Analysis System of Psychotherapy (CBASP)
Guilford Publications
72 Spring Street
New York, NY 10012
212-431-9800
800-365-7006
Fax: 212-966-6708
E-mail: info@guilford.com
www.guilford.com

This book describes CBASP, a research based psychotherapeutic approach designed to motivate chronically depressed patients to change and help them develop needed problem solving and relationship skills. Filled with illustrative case material that brings challenging clinical situations to life, this book now puts the power of CBASP in the hands of the clinician. Readers are provided with two essential assets: an innovative framework for understanding the patient's psychopathology and a disciplined plan for helping the individual overthrow depression. *$35.00*

326 pages ISBN 1-572305-27-4

907 When Nothing Matters Anymore: A Survival Guide for Depressed Teens
Free Spirit Publishing
217 5th Avenue N
Suite 200
Minneapolis, MN 55401-1299
612-338-2068
866-735-7323
Fax: 612-337-5050
E-mail: help4kids@freespirit.com
www.freespirit.com

Written for teens with depression and those who feel despondent, dejected or alone. This powerful book offers help, hope, and potentially lifesaving facts and advice. *$13.95*

176 pages Year Founded: 1998 ISBN 1-575420-36-8

908 Winter Blues
Guilford Publications
72 Spring Street
New York, NY 10012
212-431-9800
800-365-7006
Fax: 212-966-6708
E-mail: info@guilford.com
www.guilford.com

Complete information about Seasonal Affective Disorder and its treatment. *$14.95*

909 Yesterday's Tomorrow
Hazelden
15251 Pleasant Valley Road
Center City, MN 55012-9640
612-257-4010
800-822-0080
Fax: 612-257-4449
www.hazelden.org

Meditation book that shows why and how recovery works, from the author's own experiences. *$12.00*

432 pages ISBN 1-568381-60-3

910 You Can Beat Depression: Guide to Prevention and Recovery
Impact Publishers
PO Box 6016
Atascadero, CA 93423-6016
805-466-5917
800-246-7228
Fax: 805-466-5919
E-mail: info@impactpublishers.com
www.impactpublishers.com

Includes material on prevention of depression, prevention of relapse after treatment, brief therapy interventions, exer-

cise, other non medical approaches and the Prozac controversy. Helps readers recognize when and how to help themsevles, and when to turn to professional treatment. *$14.95*

176 pages ISBN 1-886230-40-4

Periodicals & Pamphlets

911 Depression
National Institute of Mental Health
6001 Executive Boulevard
Room 8184
Bethesda, MD 20892-9663
866-615-6464
Fax: 301-443-4279
TTY: 301-443-8431
E-mail: nimhinfo@nih.gov
www.nimh.nih.gov

This brochure gives descriptions of major depression, dysthymia and bipolar disorder (manic depression). It lists symptoms, gives possible causes, tells how depression is diagnosed and discusses available treatments. This brochure provides help and hope for the depressed person, family and friends.

23 pages

912 Depression in Children and Adolescents: A Fact Sheet for Physicians
National Institute of Mental Health
6001 Executive Boulevard
Room 8184
Bethesda, MD 20892-9663
866-615-6464
Fax: 301-443-4279
TTY: 301-443-8431
E-mail: nimhinfo@nih.gov
www.nimh.nih.gov

Discusses the scope of the problem and the screening tools used in evaluating children with depression.

8 pages

913 Depression: Help On the Way
ETR Associates
4 Carbonero Way
Scotts Valley, CA 95066
831-438-4060
800-321-4407
Fax: 800-435-8433
E-mail: customerservice@etr.org
www.etr.org

Includes symptoms of minor depression, major depression, and seasonal affective depression; treatment options and medication, and the importance of exercise and laughter. Sold in lots of 50.

914 Depression: What Every Woman Should Know
National Institute of Mental Health
6001 Executive Boulevard
Room 8184
Bethesda, MD 20892-9663
866-615-6464
Fax: 301-443-4279
TTY: 301-443-8431
E-mail: nimhinfo@nih.gov
www.nimh.nih.gov

This booklet discusses the symptoms of depression and some of the reasons that make women so vulnerable. It also discusses the types of therapy and where to go for help.

24 pages

915 Let's Talk About Depression
National Institute of Mental Health
6001 Executive Boulevard
Room 8184
Bethesda, MD 20892-9663
866-615-6464
Fax: 301-443-4279
TTY: 301-443-8431
E-mail: nimhinfo@nih.gov
www.nimh.nih.gov

Facts about depression, and ways to get help. Target audience is teenaged youth.

916 Major Depression in Children and Adolescents
SAMHSA's National Mental Health Information Center
PO Box 42557
Washington, DC 20015
800-789-2647
Fax: 240-747-5470
TDD: 866-889-2647
E-mail: ken@mentalhealth.org
www.mentalhealth.samhsa.gov

A Kathryn Power, MEd, Director
Edward B Searle, Deputy Director

This fact sheet defines depression and its signs, identifies types of help available, and suggests what parents or other caregivers can do.

2 pages

917 Men and Depression
National Institute of Mental Health
6001 Executive Boulevard
Room 8184
Bethesda, MD 20892-9663
866-615-6464
Fax: 301-443-4279
TTY: 301-443-8431
E-mail: nimhinfo@nih.gov
www.nimh.nih.gov

Have you known a man who is grumpy, irritable, and has no sense of humor? Maybe he drinks too much or abuses drugs. Maybe he physically or verbally abuses his wife and his kids. Maybe he works all the time, or compulsively seeks thrills in high-risk behavior. Or maybe he seems isolated, withdrawn, and no longer interested in the people or activities he used to enjoy. Perhaps this man is you. Talk to a healthcare provider about how you are feeling, and ask for help.

36 pages

918 New Message
Emotions Anonymous
PO Box 4245
Saint Paul, MN 55104-0245
651-647-9712
Fax: 651-647-1593
E-mail: info@EmotionsAnonymous.org
www.EmotionsAnonymous.org

Karen Mead, Executive Director

Features stories and articles of recovery, plus the latest news from EA International. *$8.00*

4 per year

919 Recovering Your Mental Health: a Self-Help Guide
SAMHSA'S National Mental Health Informantion Center
PO Box 42557
Washington, DC 20015
800-789-2647
Fax: 240-747-5470
TDD: 866-889-2647
E-mail: ken@mentalhealth.org
www.mentalhealth.samhsa.gov

A Kathryn Power, MEd, Director
Edward B Searle, Deputy Director

This booklet offers tips for understanding symptoms of depression and other conditions and getting help. Also details the advantages of counseling, medications available, options for professional help, relaxation techniques and paths to positive thinking.

32 pages

920 Storm In My Brain
Depression & Bi-Polar Support Alliance
730 N Franklin Street
Suite 501
Chicago, IL 60610-7204
800-826-3632
Fax: 312-642-7243
www.dbsalliance.org

Lydia Lewis, President
Ingrid Deetz, Program Director

Pamphlet free on the Internet or by mail. Discusses child or adolesent Bi-Polar symptoms.

921 What Do These Students Have in Common?
National Institute of Mental Health
6001 Executive Boulevard
Room 8184
Bethesda, MD 20892-9663
866-615-6464
Fax: 301-443-4279
TTY: 301-443-8431
E-mail: nimhinfo@nih.gov
www.nimh.nih.gov

Provides college sutdents with clear descriptions of the most prevalent forms of depression. Discusses symptoms, causes and treatment options. Includes information about suicide and resources for help that are available to most college students.

4 pages

922 What to do When a Friend is Depressed: Guide for Students
National Institute of Mental Health
6001 Executive Boulevard
Room 8184
Bethesda, MD 20892-9663
866-615-6464
Fax: 301-443-4279
TTY: 301-443-8431
E-mail: nimhinfo@nih.gov
www.nimh.nih.gov

This brochure offers information on depression and its symptoms and suggests things a young person can do to guide a depressed friend in finding help. Especially good for health fairs, health clinics and school health units.

3 pages

Research Centers

923 National Alliance for Research on Schizophrenia and Depression
60 Cutter Mill Road
Suite 404
Great Neck, NY 11021
800-829-8289
Fax: 516-487-6930
E-mail: info@narsad.org
www.narsad.org

Constance Lieber, President

NARSAD raises funds for research on schizophrenia, depression, and other serious brain disorders.

924 Sid W Richardson Institute for Preventive Medicine of the Methodist Hospital
6565 Fannin Street
Houston, TX 77030-2704
713-790-3311

Alan Herd MD, Director

925 University of Texas: Mental Health Clinical Research Center
5323 Harry Hines Boulevard
Dallas, TX 75235
214-648-3111
www.www.utsouthwestern.edu
Research activity of major and atypical depression.

926 Yale University: Depression Research Program
Yale University Department of Psychiatry
333 Cedar Street
New Haven, CT 06510
203-785-4680
www.info.med.yale.edu/ysm

Successfuly treating people with depression for over three decades. Operated jointly by the Connecticut Mental Health Center and the Yale University School of Medicine, Department of Psychiatry.

Support Groups & Hot Lines

927 Depressed Anonymous
PO Box 17414
Louisville, KY 40217
502-569-1989
E-mail: info@depressedanon.com
www.depressedanon.com

Individuals suffering from depression or anxiety. A self-help organization with meetings and sharing of experiences. Similar to the 12 step program, uses mutual aid as a theraputic healing force. Website offers information on how to form groups in your area.

928 Recovery
802 N Dearborn Street
Chicago, IL 60610
312-337-5661
Fax: 312-337-5756
E-mail: inquiries@recovery-inc.com
www.recovery-inc.com

Kathy Garcia, Executive Director

Techniques for controlling behavior, changing attitudes for recovering mental patients. Systematic method of self-help offered.

Video & Audio

929 Bundle of Blues
Fanlight Productions
4196 Washington Street
Suite 2
Boston, MA 02131
617-469-4999
Fax: 617-439-3379
E-mail: fanlight@fanlight.com
www.fanlight.com

The stories in this thoughtful documentary represent a range of experiences from minor postpartum depression through postpartum psychosis. It stresses that PDD can happen to any new mother, but that it can be managed.

930 Coping with Depression
New Harbinger Publications
5674 Shattuck Avenue
Oakland, CA 94609-1662
510-652-2002
800-748-6273
Fax: 510-652-5472
E-mail: customerservice@newharbinger.com
www.newharbinger.com

Mary Ellen Copeland, Author

60 minute videotape that offers a powerful message of hope for anyone struggling with depression. *$39.95*

Year Founded: 1994 ISBN 1-879237-62-8

931 Day for Night: Recognizing Teenage Depression
DRADA-Depression and Related Affective Disorders Association
2330 W Joppa Road
Suite 100
Lutherville, MD 21097
410-583-2919
Fax: 410-583-2964
E-mail: drada@jhmi.edu
www.drada.org

Catherine Pollock, Executive Director
Sallie Mink, Director Education

Award winning video that provides an in depth look at teenage depression and offers educational support and hope for those who suffer this treatable condition. *$22.50*

932 Depression and Manic Depression
Fanlight Productions
47 Halifax Street
Boston, MA 02131
617-524-0980
800-937-4113
Fax: 617-524-8838
E-mail: info@fanlight.com
www.fanlight.com

Explores the realities of depression and manic depression, as well as provides an overview of available treatments, and a listing of other resources. *$149.00*

933 **Living with Depression and Manic Depression**
New Harbinger Publications
5674 Shattuck Avenue
Oakland, CA 94609-1662
510-652-2002
800-748-6273
Fax: 510-652-5472
E-mail: customerservice@newharbinger.com
www.newharbinger.com

Mary Ellen Copeland, Author

Describes a program based on years of research and hundreds of interviews with depressed persons. Warm, helpful, and engaging, this tape validates the feelings of people with depression while it encourages positive change. *$11.95*

Year Founded: 1994 ISBN 1-879237-63-6

934 **Why Isn't My Child Happy? Video Guide About Childhood Depression**
ADD WareHouse
300 NW 70th Avenue
Suite 102
Plantation, FL 33317
954-792-8100
800-233-9273
Fax: 954-792-8545
E-mail: sales@addwarehouse.com
www.addwarehouse.com

The first of its kind, this new video deals with childhood depression. Informative and frank about this common problem, this book offers helpful guidance for parents and professionals trying to better understand childhood depression. 110 minutes. *$55.00*

935 **Women and Depression**
Fanlight Productions
47 Halifax Street
Boston, MA 02131
617-524-0980
800-937-4113
Fax: 617-524-8838
E-mail: info@fanlight.com
www.fanlight.com

Clinical depression affects 19 million Americans, about 10 million of these are women. 28 minute video features women who talk about their own depression, and how it is viewed and handled in the African American community, and a therapist who deals with her own depression. Treatments are explored and practical strategies are offered. *$129.00*

Year Founded: 2000

Web Sites

936 **www.Depressedteens.Com**
Depression and Related Affective Disorders Association: DRADA

Educational site dedicated to helping teens, parents and teachers understand symptoms of teenage depression. Provides resources for those ready to seek help.

937 **www.Ifred.Org**
National Foundation for Depressive Illness
Support, helplines, and advice.

938 **www.befrienders.org**
Samaritans International
Support, helplines, and advice.

939 **www.blarg.net/~charlatn/voices**
Voices of Depression
Compilation of writings by people suffering from depression.

940 **www.cyberpsych.org**
CyberPsych

Hosts the American Psychoanalyists Foundation, American Association of Suicideology, Society for the Exploration of Psychotherapy Intergration, and Anxiety Disorders Association of America. Also subcategories of the anxiety disorders, as well as general information, including panic disorder, phobias, obsessive compulsive disorder (OCD), social phobia, generalized anxiety disorder, post traumatic stress disorder, and phobias of childhood. Book reviews and links to web pages sharing the topics.

941 **www.emdr.com**
EMDR Institute

Discusses EMDR-Eye Movement Desensitization and Reprocessing-as an innovative clinical treatment for trauma, including sexual abuse, domestic violence, combat, crime, and those suffering from a number of other disorders including depressions, addictions, phobias and a variety of self-esteem issues.

942 **www.klis.com/chandler/pamphlet/dep/**
Jim Chandler MD
White paper on depression in children and adolesents.

943 **www.nimh.nih.gov/publicat/depressionmenu.cfm**
National Institute of Mental Health

National Institute of Mental Health offers brochures organized by topic. Depression discusses symptoms, diagnosis, and treatment options.

944 **www.nimh.nih.gov/publist/964033.htm**
National Institute of Mental Health

Discusses depression in older years, symptoms, treatment, going for help.

945 **www.planetpsych.com**
Planetpsych.com

Learn about disorders, their treatments and other topics in psychology. Articles are listed under the related topic areas. Ask a therapist a question for free, or view the directory of professionals in your area. If you are a therapist sign up for the directory. Current features, self-help, interactive, and newsletter archives.

946 **www.psychcentral.com**
Psych Central

Personalized one-stop index for psychology, support, and mental health issues, resources, and people on the Internet.

947 **www.psychologyinfo.com/depression**
Psychology Information On-line: Depression

Information on diagnosis, therapy, and medication.

948 **www.psycom.net/depression.central.html**
Dr. Ivan's Depression Central

Medication-oriented site. Clearinghouse on all types of depressive disorders.

949 **www.queendom.com/selfhelp/depression/depression.html**
Queendom

Articles, information on medication and support groups.

950 **www.shpm.com**
Self Help Magazine

Articles and discussion forums, resource links.

951 **www.wingofmadness.com**
Wing of Madness: A Depression Guide

Accurate information, advice, support, and personal experiences.

Dissociative Disorders

Introduction

Dissociative Disorders are a cluster of mental disorders, united by a profound change in consciousness or a disruption in continuity of consciousness. People with a Dissociative Disorder may abruptly take on different personalities, or undergo long periods in which they do not remember anything that happened; in some cases, individuals may embark on lengthy international travels, returning home with no recollection of where they have been or why they had gone.

Dissociative Disorders are uncommon, mysterious and somewhat controversial; reports of Dissociative Disorders have grown more frequent in recent years and a degree of debate surrounds the validity of these reports. Some professionals say the disorders are far more rare than is reported, and that many individuals diagnosed with a Dissociative Disorder, while they may indeed be mentally or emotionally disturbed, are highly suggestible, experiencing symptoms subtly suggested by others.

Dissociative Disorders are believed to be related in many cases to severe trauma, although the historical validity of these cases is difficult to determine. There are five types of Dissociative Disorders: Dissociative Amnesia; Dissociative Fugue; Dissociative Identity Disorder; Depersonalization Disorder; and Dissociative Disorder Not Otherwise Specified.

SYMPTOMS

Dissociative Amnesia
• One or more episodes of inability to recall important personal information, usually of a traumatic or stressful nature, that is too extensive to be explained by ordinary forgetfulness;
• The disturbance does not occur exclusively during the course of any other Dissociative Disorder and is not due to the direct physiological effects of a substance abuse or general medical condition;
• The symptoms cause clinically significant distress or impairment in social, occupational or other important areas of functioning.

Dissociative Fugue
• A sudden, unexpected travel away from home or work, with inability to recall one's past;
• Confusion about personal identity or assumption of a new identity;
• The disturbance does not occur exclusively during the course of any other Dissociative Disorder and is not due to the direct physiological effects of a substance or a general medical condition;
• The symptoms cause clinically significant distress or impairment in social, occupational, or other important areas of functioning.

Dissociative Identity Disorder
• The presence of two or more distinct identities or personality states that take control of the person's behavior;
• Inability to recall important personal information;
• The disturbance is not due to the direct physiological effects of a substance or a general medical condition.

Depersonalization Disorder
• Persistent or recurrent experiences of feeling detached from one's body and mental processes;
• During the depersonalization experience, reality testing remains intact;
• The depersonalization causes clinically significant distress or impairment in social, occupational, or other important areas of functioning;
• The depersonalization does not occur during the course of another Dissociative Disorder or as a direct physiological effect of a substance or general medical condition;
• Akin to depersonalization (feeling one is not real) is derealization, which is feeling that one's environment and/or perceptions are not real.

ASSOCIATED FEATURES

Patients with any of the Dissociative Disorders may be depressed, and may experience depersonalization, or a feeling of not being in their own body. They will often experience impairment in work or interpersonal relationships, and they may practice self-mutilation or have aggressive and suicidal impulses. They may also have symptoms typical of a Mood or Personality Disorder. Individuals with Dissociative Amnesia and Dissociative Identity Disorder (sometimes known as multiple personality disorder) often report severe physical and/or sexual abuse in childhood. Controversy surrounds the accuracy of these reports, in part because of the unreliability of some childhood memories. Individuals with Dissociative Identity Disorder may have symptoms typical of Post-Traumatic Stress Disorder, as well as Mood, Substance Abuse Related, Sexual, Eating or Sleep Disorders.

PREVALENCE

The prevalence of Dissociative Disorders in most cases is either unknown, difficult to ascertain, or subject to controversy. The recent rise in the US in reports of Dissociative Amnesia and Dissociative Identity Disorder related to traumatic childhood abuse has been very controversial. Some say these disorders are overreported, the result of suggestibility in individuals and the unreliability of childhood memories. Others say the disorders are underreported, given the propensity for children and adults to dismiss or forget abusive memories and the tendency of perpetrators to deny or obscure their abusive actions. For Dissociative Fugue, a prevalence rate of 0.2 percent of the population has been reported. Dissociative Identity Disorder tends to be far more common in females than in males: the disorder is diagnosed three to nine times more frequently in females than in males.

Associations & Agencies

953 Center for Family Support (CFS)
333 7th Avenue
New York, NY 10001-5004
212-629-7939
Fax: 212-239-2211
www.cfsny.org

Steven Vernickofs, Executive Director

An agency that continues to develop new programs to serve families and individuals with their care needs. Currently offering services throughout the New York City region including: New Jersey, Long Island and the Lower Hudson Valley.

954 International Society for the Study of Dissociation
60 Revere Drive
Suite 500
Northbrook, IL 60062
847-480-0899
Fax: 847-480-9282
E-mail: issd@issd.org
www.issd.org

Steven N. Gold PhD, President
Ruth Blizard PhD, Director

The society is a nonprofit professional association organized for the porpuses of: information sharing and international networking of clinicians and researchers; providing professional and public education; promoting research and theory about dissociation.

955 National Association for the Dually Diagnosed (NADD)
132 Fair Street
Kingston, NY 12401-4802
845-334-4336
800-331-5362
Fax: 845-331-4569
E-mail: nadd@mhv.net
www.thenadd.org

Dr. Robert Fletcher, Executive Director

Nonprofit organization designed to promote interest of professional and parent development with resources for individuals who have the coexistence of mental illness and mental retardation. Provides conference, educational services and training materials to professionals, parents, concerned citizens and service organizations. Formerly known as the National Association for the Dually Diagnosed.

Year Founded: 1983

956 National Mental Health Consumer's Self-Help
1211 Chestnut Street
Suite 1207
Philadelphia, PA 19107
215-751-1810
800-553-4539
Fax: 215-636-6312
E-mail: info@mhselfhelp.com
www.mhselfhelp.org

Christine Simiriglia, Executive Director
Jennifer Melinn, Information/Referral Dept.

Funded by the National Institute of Mental Health Community Support Program, the purpose of the Clearinghouse is to encourage the development and growth of consumer self-help groups.

957 National Mental Health Consumers' Self-Help Clearinghouse
1211 Chestnut Street
Suite 1207
Philadelphia, PA 19107
215-751-1810
800-553-4539
Fax: 215-636-6312
E-mail: info@mhselfhelp.org
www.mhselfhelp.org

Joseph Rogers, Executive Director

A national consumer technical assistance center that has played a major role in the development of the mental health consumer movement.

Year Founded: 1986

958 SAMHSA'S National Mental Health Information
PO Box 42557
Washington, DC 20015
800-789-2647
Fax: 240-747-5470
E-mail: ken@mentalhealth.org
www.mentalhealth.samhsa.gov

A Kathryn Power, MEd, Director
Edward B Searle, Deputy Director

Information about resources, technical assistance, research, training, networks, and other federal clearing houses, and fact sheets and materials. Information specialists refer callers to mental health resources in their communities as well as state, federal and nonprofit contacts. Staff available Monday through Friday, 8:30 AM 5:00 PM, EST, excluding federal holidays. After hours, callers may leave messages and an information specialist will return their call.

959 SAMHSA's National Mental Health Information Center
US Department of Health and Human Services
PO Box 42557
Washington, DC 20015
240-221-4021
800-789-2647
Fax: 240-221-4295
TDD: 866-889-2647
www.mentalhealth.samhsa.gov

A Kathryn Power, MEd, Director
Edward B Searle, Deputy Director

Provides information about mental health via a toll-free telephone number, this web site, and more than 600 publications. Developed for users of mental health services and their families, the general public, policy makers, providers, and the media.

Books

960 Amongst Ourselves: A Self-Help Guide to Living with Dissociative Identity Disorder
New Harbinger Publications
5674 Shattuck Avenue
Oakland, CA 94609-1662
510-652-2002
800-748-6273
Fax: 510-652-5472
E-mail: customerservice@newharbinger.com
www.newharbinger.com

Tracy Alderman, PhD, Author
Karen Marshall, LCSW, Author

First person perspective of Dissociative Identity Disorder and practical suggestions to come to terms with and improve their lives. *$19.95*

256 pages Year Founded: 1998 ISBN 1-562241-22-5

961 Dissociation
American Psychiatric Publishing
1000 Wilson Boulevard
Suite 1825
Arlington, VA 22209-3901
703-907-7322
800-368-5777
Fax: 703-907-1091
E-mail: appi@psych.org
www.appi.org

Katie Duffy, Marketing Assistant

Combines cultural anthropology, congitive psychology, neurophysiology, and the study of psychosomatic illness to present the latest information on the dissociative process. Designed for professionals in cross cultural psychiatry and the influence of the mind on the body. *$33.50*

227 pages ISBN 0-880485-57-4

962 Dissociation and the Dissociative Disorders: DSM-V and Beyond
Routledge
270 Madison Avenue
New York, NY 10016
212-216-7800
Fax: 212-563-2269
www.www.routledge.com

Dell O'Neil, Author

This book draws together and integrates the most recent scientific and conceptual foundations of dissociation and the dissociative disorders field.

963 Dissociative Child: Diagnosis, Treatment and Management
Sidran Institute
200 E Joppa Road
Suite 207
Baltimore, MD 21286
410-825-8888
888-825-8249
Fax: 410-337-0747
E-mail: sidran@sidran.org
www.sidran.org

Esther Giller, President/CEO
J G Goellner, Director Emertius
Stanley Platman, MD, Medical Advisor
Joyanna Silberg, Author

This second groundbreaking edition addresses all aspects of caring for the dissociative child and adolescents. Contributors include experienced and eminent practitioners in the field of childhood DID. The section on diagnosis offers comprehensive coverage of various aspects of diagnosis, including diagnosis taxonomy, differential diagnosis, interviewing, testing and the special problems of male children and adolescents with DID. The section on treatment covers factors associated with positive theraputic outcome, therapeutic phases, the five-domain crisis model, promoting intergration in dissociative children, art therapy and group therapy. Includes ways school personnel can act to help the dissociative child, multiculturalism and other important information. *$35.00*

400 pages

964 Drug Therapy and Dissociative Disorders
Mason Crest Publishers
370 Reed Road
Suite 302
Broomall, PA 19008
610-543-6200
866-627-2665
Fax: 610-543-3878
E-mail: dtaylor@masoncrest.com
www.masoncrest.com

Dissociative disorders are some of the most controversial disorders in psychiatry today. Despite newfound recognition and numerous diagnosis the very existence of these disorders is still hotly debated in some academic circles. these disorders make us question our assumptions about memory, self, and personality, and shed unique light on the mysterious complexities of the human mind. From amnesia to multiple personalities, dissociative disorders present treatment challenges to psychotherapy and psychopharmacology alike. Through stories of individuals' struggles with dissociative disorders, this book provides both historical overview of treatment and reviews the most up-to-date treatments available today.

ISBN 1-590845-64-1

965 Got Parts? An Insider's Guide to Managing Li fe Successfully with Dissociative Identity Disorder (New Horizons in Therapy)
Loving Healing Press
5145 Pontiac Trail
Ann Arbor, MI 48105
734-929-0881
Fax: 734-663-6861
E-mail: info@lovinghealing.com
www.www.lovinghealing.com

This book is directed towards people treating Dissociative Identity Disorder.

966 Handbook for the Assessment of Dissociation: a Clinical Guide
American Psychiatric Publishing
1000 Wilson Boulevard
Suite 1825
Arlington, VA 22209-3901
703-907-7322
800-368-5777
Fax: 703-907-1091
E-mail: appi@psych.org
www.appi.org

Katie Duffy, Marketing Assistant

Offers guidelines for the systematic assessment of dissociation and posttraumatic syndromes for clinicians and researchers. Provides a comprehensive overview of dissociative symptoms and disorders and an introduction to the use of the SCID-D, a diagnostic interview for the dissociative disorders. *$54.00*

433 pages ISBN 0-880486-82-1

967 Lost in the Mirror: An Inside Look at Borderline Personality Disorder
Sidran Institute
200 E Joppa Road
Suite 207
Baltimore, MD 21286
410-825-8888
888-825-8249

Fax: 410-337-0747
E-mail: sidran@sidran.org
www.sidran.org

Esther Giller, President/CEO
J G Goellner, Director Emertius
Stanley Platman, MD, Medical Advisor
Richard Moskovitz, MD, Author

Dr. Moskovitz considers BPD to be part of the dissociative continuum, as it has many causes, symptoms and behaviors in common with Dissociative Disorder. This book is intended for people diagnosed with BPD, their families and therapists. Outlines the features of BPD, including abuse histories, dissociation, mood swings, self harm, impulse control problems and many more. Includes an extensive resource section. *$13.95*

190 pages

968   Rebuilding Shattered Lives: Responsible Treatment of Complex Post-Traumatic and Dissociative Disorders
John Wiley & Sons
1 Wiley Drive
Somerset, NJ 08873
732-469-4400
800-225-5945
Fax: 732-302-2300
E-mail: compbks@wiley.com
www.wiley.com

James Chu, Author

Essential for anyone working in the field of trauma therapy. Part I discusses recent findings about child abuse, the changes in attitudes toward child abuse over the last two decades and the nature of traumatic memory. Part II is an overview of principles of trauma treatment, including symptom control, establishment of boundaries and therapist self-care. Part III covers special topics, such as dissociative identity disorder, controversies, hospitalization and acute care. *$ 73.95*

288 pages   Year Founded: 1998 ISBN 0-471247-32-4

969   Treatment of Multiple Personality Disorder
American Psychiatric Publishing
1000 Wilson Boulevard
Suite 1825
Arlington, VA 22209-3901
703-907-7322
800-368-5777
Fax: 703-907-1091
E-mail: appi@psych.org
www.appi.org

Katie Duffy, Marketing Assistant

Authorities in the Multiple Personality Disorder field merge clinical understanding and research into therapeutic approaches that can be employed in clinical practice. *$22.50*

258 pages   ISBN 0-880480-96-3

970   Understanding Dissociative Disorders and Addiction
Sidran Institute
200 E Joppa Road
Suite 207
Townson, MD 21286
410-825-8888
888-825-8249
Fax: 410-337-0747

E-mail: sidran@sidran.org
www.sidran.org

Esther Giller, President/CEO
J Gila Goellner, Director Emertius
Stanley Plantman, MD, Medical Advisor
A Scott Winter, MD, Author

This booklet discusses the origins and symptoms of dissociation, explains the links between dissociative disorder and chemical dependency. Addresses treatment options available to help in your recovery. The work book includes exercises and activities that help you acknowledge, accept and manage both your chemical dependency and your disociative disorder. *$7.20*

971   Understanding Dissociative Disorders: A Guid e for Family Physicians and Healthcare Workers
Crown House Publishing
6 Trowbridge Drive
Suite 5
Bethel, CT 06801
203-778-1300
Fax: 203-778-9100
www.www.crownhouse.co.uk

Marlene E Hunter, Author

This volume outlines common presentations in the family physicians' practice, and offers realistic, practical answers to a multitude of questions.

Video & Audio

972   Different From You
Fanlight Publications
4196 Washington Street
Suite 2
Boston, MA 02131
617-469-4999
Fax: 617-439-3379
E-mail: fanlight@fanlight.com
www.fanlight.com

As a result of the 'deinstituionalization' of mental patients, people with mental illnesses now make up a majority of the homeless in many areas. This video explores the problem through the work of a compassionate physician who cares for mentally ill people living on the streets and in inadequate 'board and care' facilities in Los Angeles.

Web Sites

973   www.cyberpsych.org
CyberPsych

Hosts the American Psychoanalyists Foundation, American Association of Suicideology, Society for the Exploration of Psychotherapy Intergration, and Anxiety Disorders Association of America. Also subcategories of the anxiety disorders, as well as general information, including panic disorder, phobias, obsessive compulsive disorder (OCD), social phobia, generalized anxiety disorder, post traumatic stress disorder, and phobias of childhood. Book reviews and links to web pages sharing the topics.

974   www.fmsf.com
False Memory Syndrome Facts

Access to literature.

975 **www.isst-D.Org**
International Society for the Study of Dissociation

A nonprofit, professional society that promotes research and training in the identification and treatment of dissociative disorders, provides professional and public education about dissociative states, and serves as a catalyst for international communication and cooperation among clinicians and researchers working in this field.

976 **www.planetpsych.com**
Planetpsych.com

Learn about disorders, their treatments and other topics in psychology. Articles are listed under the related topic areas. Ask a therapist a question for free, or view the directory of professionals in your area. If you are a therapist sign up for the directory. Current features, self-help, interactive, and newsletter archives.

977 **www.psychcentral.com**
Psych Central

Personalized one-stop index for psychology, support, and mental health issues, resources, and people on the Internet.

978 **www.sidran.org**
Trauma Resource Area

Resources and Articles on Dissociative Experiences Scale and Dissociative Identity Disorder, PsychTrauma Glossary and Traumatic Memories.

Eating Disorders

Introduction

Eating is integral to human health, and for many people food is a pleasure that can be enjoyed without too much thought. But an increasing number of people (mostly, but not exclusively, women) have eating disorders, which cause them to use food and dieting in ways that are extremely unhealthy, even life-threatening. The two principal eating disorders are Anorexia Nervosa and Bulimia Nervosa; though different in the symptoms they manifest, the two disorders are quite similar in their underlying pathology: an obsessive concern with food, body image, and body weight.

Many people believe that eating disorders are, in part, culturally determined: in the Western world, and particularly the US, a pervasive cultural preference for slimness causes many people to spend extraordinary amounts of time, money and energy dieting and exercise to stay slim. At the same time, people are flooded with media images of delicous foods, restaurant portions grow ever larger, and driving replaces walking for daily activities. Cultural preference is likely to exert pressure on people, especially young women, who may be genetically or psychologically predisposed to the illness. It is important to be wary of media, including the internet, which can expose young people to counterproductive influences. Overeating is another type of Eating Disorder, as it reflects the paradox that, as society values thinness more and more, more and more people are obese. Eating Disorders may do serious and lasting physical damage; because of this, treatment must first restore a patient to a safe and healthy body weight. Treatment of the disorder is a long-term process, involving psychotherapy, family interventions and, for depressed or obsessional patients, antidepressant medication. Fortunately, most people who are appropriately treated can and do recover.

SYMPTOMS

Anorexia Nervosa:
• Refusal to maintain body weight at or above eighty-five percent of a minimally normal weight for age and height;
• Intense fear of gaining weight or becoming fat, even though underweight;
• Disturbance in the way one's body weight or shape is experienced, undue influence of body weight or shape on self-evaluation, or denial of the seriousness of the current low body weight;
• In menstruating females, the absence of at least three consecutive menstrual cycles;
• Physical damage often occurs, such as imbalances in body chemicals, which if severe can cause cardiac arrest; purging often erodes tooth enamel, in which case a dentist might make the diagnosis. A gynecologist may also diagnose Anorexia Nervosa, as it is associated with amenorrhea and often results in infertility.

Bulimia Nervosa:
• Recurrent episodes of binge eating characterized by eating more food than most people would eat during a similar period of time and under similar circumstances;
• A sense of loss of control over eating;
• Recurrent inappropriate behavior in order to prevent weight gain, such as self-induced vomiting or misuse of laxatives, and excessive fasting or exercise;
• The binge-eating and inappropriate behaviors both occur, on average, at least twice a week for three months;
• Self-evaluation is unduly influenced by body shape and weight;
• The disturbance does not occur exclusively during episodes of Anorexia Nervosa.

ASSOCIATED FEATURES

Patients with Anorexia Nervosa may be severely depressed, and may experience insomnia, irritability, and diminished interest in sex. These features may be exacerbated if the patient is severely underweight. People with Eating Disorders also share many of the features of Obsessive Compulsive Disorder. For instance, someone with an Eating Disorder may have an excessive interest in food; they may hoard food, or spend unusual amounts of time reading and researching about foods, recipes and nutrition. People with Anorexia Nervosa may also exhibit a strong need to control their environment, and may be socially and emotionally withdrawn.

Individuals with Bulimia Nervosa are often within the normal weight range, but prior to the development of the disorder they may be overweight. Depression and other Mood Disorders are common among people with bulimia, and patients often ascribe their bulimia to the Mood Disorders. In other cases, however, it appears that the Mood Disorders precede the Eating Disorders. Substance abuse occurs in about one-third of individuals with bulimia.

Anxiety Disorders are common, and fear of social situations can be a precipitating factor in binging episodes.

PREVALENCE

Prevalence studies in females have found rates of 0.5 to one percent for Anorexia Nervosa. There is only limited data for the prevalence of Anorexia Nervosa in males. The prevalence of Bulimia Nervosa among adolescent females is approximately one to three percent. The rate of the disorder among males is approximately one-tenth of that in females.

TREATMENT OPTIONS

Medications, especially the newest SSRIs (Selective Serotonin Reuptake Inhibitors, which were originally developed as antidepressants), have been found to be very effective in the treatment of Eating Disorders. They can help restore and build self-esteem, and thereby help the patient maintain a positive attitude as well as a safe and healthy body image and body weight.

Because of the physical damage that an Eating Disorder can do to a patient, nutritional counseling and monitoring is often vital to restore and maintain proper body weight.

It is critical to recognize that Eating Disorders are, in addition to being life-threatening, extremely complex: simply restoring the patient to an acceptable body weight is not enough. Many patients have complex and conflicting psychological issues that trigger the compulsion to binge, or the morbid fear of gaining weight. These issues need to be addressed by psychotherapy. Forms of psychotherapy that may be useful in treating Eating Disorders include psychodynamic psychotherapy (in which longstanding and sometimes unconscious emotional issues related to the eating disorders are explored) and cognitive behavior therapy, which aims to identify the thought patterns that trigger the Eating Disorder and to establish healthy eating habits. Recent literature suggests that psychotherapeutic approaches are often more effective than medications in the treatment of Anorexia. Family involvement in treatment is critical, and peer pressure can be utilized to compel patients to maintain adequate nutrition. Eating Disorders are serious — untreated Anorexia can kill a patient — and treatment may be required over a course of many years.

Associations & Agencies

980 American Anorexia/Bulimia Association
435 East 61st Street
6th Floor
New York, NY 10021
212-501-8351
800-522-2230
Fax: 212-501-0342

Judith Robinson, RN, PhD, Executive Director

Organization dedicated to increasing the awareness of eating disorders and offering information on prevention and treatment.

981 Anorexia Bulimia Treatment and Education Center
615 S New Ballas Road
Saint Louis, MO 63141-8221
314-569-6565
Fax: 314-569-6910

Offers education on the prevention of eating disorders and information on various treatment options.

982 Anorexia Nervosa and Related Eating Disorders
PO Box 5102
Eugene, OR 97405-0102
541-344-1144
E-mail: jarinor@rio.com
www.anred.com

We are a nonprofit organization that provides information about anorexia nervosa, bulimia nervosa, binge eating diorder, and other less-well-known food and weight disorders.

983 Center for Family Support (CFS)
333 7th Avenue
New York, NY 10001-5004
212-629-7939
Fax: 212-239-2211
www.cfsny.org

Steven Vernickofs, Executive Director

An agency that continues to develop new programs to serve families and individuals with their care needs. Currently offering services throughout the New York City region including: New Jersey, Long Island and the Lower Hudson Valley.

984 Change for Good Coaching and Counseling
3801 Connecticut Avenue NW
Washington, DC 20008-4530
202-362-3009
Fax: 202-204-6100
E-mail: brockhansenlcsw@aol.com
www.change-for-good.org

Brock Hansen, LCSW, President

Coaching on learnable emotional skills to see goals clearly, harness resources and get moving toward a successful outcome.

985 Council on Size and Weight Discrimination (CSWD)
PO Box 305
Mount Marion, NY 12456-0305
845-679-1209
Fax: 845-679-1206
E-mail: info@cswd.org
www.cswd.org

Miriam Berg, President
Lynn McAfee, Director of Medical Advocacy
William J. Fabrey, Media Project
Nancy Summer, Fund Raising

The Council on Size and Weight Discrimination is a not-for-profit group which works to change people's attitudes about weight. They act as consumer advocates for larger people, especially in the areas of medical treatment, job discrimination, and media images.

986 International Association of Eating Disorders Professionals
PO Box 1295
Pekin, IL 61555-1295
309-346-3341
800-800-8126
Fax: 309-346-2874
E-mail: iaedpmembers@earthlink.net
www.iaedp.com

Bonnie Harken, Managing Director
Emmett R Bishop MD CEDS, President

Offers professional counseling and assistance to the medical community, courts, law enforcement officials, and social welfare agencies.

987 Largesse, The Network for Size Esteem
PO Box 9404
New Haven, CT 06534-0404
203-787-1624
Fax: 203-787-1624
E-mail: size_esteem@yahoo.com
www.eskimo.com/~largesse

Karen W Stimson, Director

An international clearinghouse for information on size diversity empowerment. Their mission is to create personal awareness and social change which promotes a positive image, health and equal rights for people of size.

988 National Alliance on Mental Illness
2107 Wilson Boulevard
Suite 300
Arlington, VA 22201-3042
703-524-7600
800-950-6264
Fax: 703-524-9094
E-mail: helpline@nami.org
www.nami.org

Suzanne Vogel-Scibilia, MD, President
Frederick R Sandoval, First VP

Nation's leading self-help organization for all those affected by severe brain disorders. Mission is to bring consumers and families with similar experiences together to share information about services, care providers, and ways to cope with the challenges of schizophrenia, manic depression, and other serious mental illnesses.

Year Founded: 1979

989 National Association for the Dually Diagnose d (NADD)
132 Fair Street
Kingston, NY 12401-4802
845-334-4336
800-331-5362
Fax: 845-331-4569
E-mail: nadd@mhv.net
www.thenadd.org

Robert Fletcher MD, Founder/CEO
Donna Nagy PhD, President

Nonprofit organization designed to promote interest of professional and parent development with resources for individuals who have the coexistence of mental illness and mental retardation. Provides conference, educational services and training materials to professionals, parents, concerned citizens and service organizations. Formerly known as the National Association for the Dually Diagnosed.

Year Founded: 1983

990 National Association of Anorexia Nervosa and Associated Disorders (ANAD)
PO Box 7
Highland Park, IL 60035-0007
847-831-3438
Fax: 847-433-4632
E-mail: anad20@aol.com
www.anad.org

Vivian Hanson Meehan, DSc, President

Sponsors national and local programs to prevent eating disorders and assist people with eating disorders and their families. Provides a national clearinghouse of information and is a grassroots association for laypeople and professionals.

991 National Association to Advance Fat Acceptance (NAAFA)
PO Box 22510
Oakland, CA 48750-9460
916-558-6880
Fax: 415-373-0483
E-mail: naafa@naafa.org
www.naafa.org

Carole Cullum, Co-Chairman
Kara Brewer Allen, Co-Chairman

Nonprofit organization dedicated to improving the quality of life for fat people. Opposes discrimination against fat people including discrimination in advertising, employment, fashion, medicine, insurance, social acceptance, the media, schooling and public accomodations. Monitors legislative activity and litigation affecting fat people. Publications: NAAFA Newsletter, bimonthly. Annual conference and symposium, always mid-August.

992 National Eating Disorders Association
603 Stewart Street
Suite 803
Seattle, WA 98101
206-382-3587
800-931-2237
Fax: 206-829-8501
E-mail: info@NationalEatingDisroders.org
www.NationalEatingDisorders.org

Pauline Powers, MD, President
Lynn S Grefe, MA, CEO

Offers a national information phone line, an international treatment referral directory, and a support group directory. The organization sponsors an annual conference and offers a speakers' bureau with a wide range of eating disorder.

993 National Institute of Mental Health Eating Disorders Program
Building 10 Room 35231
Bethesda, MD 20892-0001
301-443-4513
866-615-6464
Fax: 301-443-4279

Thomas R Insel MD, President

Mission is to reduce the burden of mental illness and behavior disorders through research on mind, brain and behavior. NIMH is committed to educating the public about mental disorders and has developed many booklets and fact sheets that provide the latest research-based information on these illnesses.

994 National Mental Health Consumer's Self-Help
1211 Chestnut Street
Suite 1207
Philadelphia, PA 19107
215-751-1810
800-553-4539
Fax: 215-636-6312
E-mail: info@mhselfhelp.org
www.mhselfhelp.org

Christine Simiriglia, Executive Director
Jennifer Melinn, Information/Referral Dept.

Funded by the National Institute of Mental Health Community Support Program, the purpose of the Clearinghouse is to encourage the development and growth of consumer self-help groups.

995 National Mental Health Consumers' Self-Help Clearinghouse
1211 Chestnut Street
Suite 1207
Philadelphia, PA 19107
215-751-1810
800-553-4539
Fax: 215-636-6312
E-mail: info@mhselfhelp.org
www.mhselfhelp.org

Joseph Rogers, Executive Director

A national consumer technical assistance center that has played a major role in the development of the mental health consumer movement.

Year Founded: 1986

996 O-Anon General Service Office (OGSO)
PO Box 1314
North Folk, CA 93643
597-877-3615
Fax: 559-877-3015
E-mail: oanon@netptc.net

Jack Finley, Chairman

For families and friends of compulsive overeaters. Provides support groups that offer opportunities for the sharing of experiences and viewpoints to offer comfort, hope and friendship.

997 SAMHSA's National Mental Health Information Center
US Department of Health and Human Services
PO Box 42557
Washington, DC 20015
800-789-2647
Fax: 240-747-5470
TDD: 866-889-2647
E-mail: ken@mentalhealth.org
www.mentalhealth.samhsa.gov

A Kathryn Power, MEd, Director
Edward B Searle, Deputy Director

Information about resources, technical assistance, research, training, networks, and other federal clearing houses, and fact sheets and materials. Information specialists refer callers to mental health resources in their communities as well as state, federal and nonprofit contacts. Staff available Monday through Friday, 8:30 AM - 5:00 PM, EST, excluding federal holidays. After hours, callers may leave messages and an information specialist will return their call.

998 TOPS Club
4575 S 5th Street
PO Box 07360
Milwaukee, WI 53207-0360
414-482-4620
800-932-8677
Fax: 414-482-3955
E-mail: topsinteractive@tops.org
www.tops.org

Betty Domenoe, President

TOPS is an international family of all ages, sizes, and shapes from all walk of life. Dedicated to helping each other Take Off and Keep Off Pounds Sensibly. We offer fellowship while you change to a healthier, new lifestyle andlearn to maintain it.

999 We Insist on Natural Shapes
PO Box 19938
Sacramento, CA 95819
800-600-9467
E-mail: winsnews@aol.com
www.winsnews.org

Kara Garner, Executive Director

A nonprofit organization educates about normal, healthy shapes.

Books

1000 Anorexia Nervosa & Recovery: a Hunger for Meaning
Haworth Press
10 Alice Street
Binghamton, NY 13904-1503
607-722-5857
800-429-6784
Fax: 607-721-0012
E-mail: getinfo@haworthpress.com
www.haworthpress.com

Jackie Blakeslee, Advertising/Journal Liason
Karen Way, MA, Author

Presents the most objective, complete, and compassionate picture of what anorexia nervosa is about. *$19.95*

142 pages Year Founded: 1993 ISBN 0-918393-95-7

1001 Assessment of Eating Disorders
The Guilford Press
72 Spring Street
New York, NY 10012
800-365-7006
Fax: 212-966-6708
E-mail: info@guilford.com
www.www.guilford.com

Robert Matloff, President
James E Mitchell, Author
Carol B Peterson, Author

Provides a clear framework and a range of up-to-date tools for assessing patients with eating disorders.

1002 Beyond Anorexia
Cambridge University Press
40 W 20th Street
New York, NY 10011-4211
212-924-3900
800-872-7423
Fax: 212-691-3239
E-mail: marketing@cup.org
www.cup.org

Beyond Anorexia is a sociological exploration of how people recover from what medicince lables 'eating disorders'. *$59.95*

248 pages

1003 Binge Eating: Nature, Assessment and Treatment
Guilford Publications
72 Spring Street
New York, NY 10012
212-431-9800
800-365-7006
Fax: 212-966-6708
E-mail: info@guilford.com
www.guilford.com

Informative and practical text brings together original and significant contributions from leading experts from a wide variety of fields. Detailed manual covers all those who binge eat, including those who are overweight. *$21.95*

419 pages ISBN 0-898628-58-X

1004 Body Image Workbook: An 8 Step Program for Learning to Like Your Looks
New Harbinger Publications
5674 Shattuck Avenue
Oakland, CA 94609-1662
510-652-2002
800-748-6273
Fax: 510-652-5472
E-mail: customerservice@newharbinger.com
www.newharbinger.com

Thomas F Cash, PhD, Author

Workbook offering a program to help transform your relationship with your body. *$19.95*

240 pages Year Founded: 1997 ISBN 1-572240-62-8

1005 Body Image, Eating Disorders, and Obesity in Youth
APA Books
750 First Street NE
Washington, DC 20090

202-336-5500
800-374-2721
Fax: 202-336-5500
TDD: 202-336-6123
E-mail: order@apa.org
www.apa.org/books

Provides for clinicians including research, assessment and treatment suggestions on body image disturbances and eating disorders in children and adolescents. *$49.95*

517 pages ISBN 1-557987-58-0

1006 Brief Therapy and Eating Disorders
Jossey-Bass Publishers
989 Market Street
San Francisco, CA 94103
415-433-1740
Fax: 415-433-0499
www.josseybass.com

Demonstrates how solution-focused brief therapy is one of the more efficient approaches in treating eating disorders. *$36.95*

284 pages ISBN 0-787900-53-2

1007 Bulimia
Jossey-Bass Publishers
989 Martket Street
San Francisco, CA 94103
415-433-1740
Fax: 415-433-0499
www.josseybass.com

A step-by-step guide to this complex disease. Filled with practical information and advice, this essential resource offers hope to millions of bulimics and their loved ones. *$17.95*

167 pages ISBN 0-787903-61-2

1008 Bulimia Nervosa
University of Minnesota Press
111 3rd Avenue S
Suite 290
Minneapolis, MN 55401
612-627-1970
Fax: 612-627-1980
E-mail: ump@tc.umn.edu
www.upress.umn.edu

James E Mitchell, MD, Author

A practical guide for health-care professionals to the diagnosis, treatment and management of bulimia by a leading expert in the field of eating disorders. Hardcover. *$27.95*

188 pages ISBN 0-816616-26-4

1009 Bulimia Nervosa & Binge Eating: A Guide To Recovery
New York University Press
838 Broadway
3rd Floor
New York, NY 10003
212-998-2575
Fax: 212-995-3833
www.nyupress.nyu.edu

A self-help book designed to guide bilimics and binge-eaters to recovery. *$35.00*

160 pages ISBN 0-814715-22-2

1010 Bulimia: a Guide to Recovery
Gurze Books
PO Box 2238
Carlsbad, CA 92018-2238
760-434-7533
800-756-7533
Fax: 760-434-5476
E-mail: gzcatl@aol.com
www.gurze.net

Lindsey Cohn, Co-Owner Gurze Books

Guidebook offers a complete understanding of bulimia and a plan for recovery. Includes a two-week program to stop binging, things-to-do instead of binging, a two-week guide for support groups, specific advice for loved ones, and Eating Without Fear - Hall's story of self-cure which has inspired thousands of other bulimics. *$14.95*

285 pages ISBN 0-936077-31-X

1011 Clinical Handbook of Eating Disorders: An In tegrated Approach (Medical Psychiatry, 26)
Informa Healthcare
52 Vanderbilt Avenue
New York, NY 10017
212-262-8230
Fax: 212-262-8234
E-mail: healthcare.enquiries@informa.com
www.www.informahealthcare.com

Timothy D Brewerton, Author

Reviews the most current research on the assessment, epidemiology, etiology, risk factors, neurodevelopment, course of illness, and various empirically-based evaluation and treatment approaches relating to eating disorders-studying disordered eating in atypical patient populations, such as men, infants, and the elderly and highlighting gender, cultural, and age-related differences that have appeared in the study of these conditions.

1012 Controlling Eating Disorders with Facts, Advice and Resources
Oryx Press
88 Post Road W
Westport, CT 06881
203-226-3571
Fax: 603-431-2214
E-mail: info@oryxpress.com
www.oryxpress.com

1013 Conversations with Anorexics: A Compassionate & Hopeful Journey
Jason Aronson
230 Livingston Street
Northvale, NJ 07647
800-782-0015
Fax: 201-767-1576
www.aronson.com

A compassionate and hopeful journey through the theraputic process.In this book Bruch presents some of her most challenging cases, offering deeply moving accounts of the course and cure. *$30.00*

238 pages ISBN 1-568212-61-5

1014 Coping with Eating Disorders
Rosen Publishing Group
29 E 21st Street
New York, NY 10010-6209

800-237-9932
Fax: 888-436-4643
E-mail: info@rosenpub.com
www.rosenpublishing.com

Offers practical suggestions on coping with eating disorders. *$16.95*

ISBN 0-823921-33-6

1015 Cult of Thinness
Oxford University Press
198 Madison Avenue
New York, NY 10016
212-726-6003
800-445-9714
Fax: 919-677-1303
TTY: 800-445-9714
E-mail: custserv.us@oup.com
www.us.oup.com

Sharlene Hesse-Biber, Author

Discusses eating patterns and disorders and their relationship to emotional states and self-esteem. *$15.95*

208 pages Year Founded: 1997 ISBN 0-195082-41-9

1016 Developmental Psychopathology of Eating Disorders: Implications for Research, Prevention and Treatment
Lawrence Erlbaum Associates
10 Industrial Avenue
Mahwah, NJ 07430-2262
201-825-3200
800-926-6577
Fax: 201-236-0072
E-mail: orders@erlbaum.com
www.erlbaum.com

This text provides backround material from developmental psychology and psychopathology - following the theory that eating problems and disorders are typically rooted in childhood. Applications are then outlined, including research, treatment, protective factors and primary prevention. *$79.95*

456 pages ISBN 0-805817-46-8

1017 Eating Disorders & Obesity: a Comprehensive Handbook
Guilford Publications
72 Spring Street
New York, NY 10012
212-431-9800
800-365-7006
Fax: 212-966-6708
E-mail: info@guilford.com
www.guilford.com

Presents and integrates virtually all that is currently known about eating disorders and obesity in one authorative, accessible and eminently practical volume. *$57.95*

583 pages ISBN 0-898628-50-4

1018 Eating Disorders Sourcebook
Omnigraphics
PO Box 625
Holmes, PA 19043
800-234-1340
Fax: 800-875-1340
E-mail: info@omnigraphics.com
www.omnigraphics.com

Dawn D Matthews, Editor

Omnigraphics is the publisher of the Health Reference Series, a growing consumer health information resource with more than 100 volumes in print. Each title in the series features an easy to understand format, nontechnical language, comprehensive indexing and resources for further information. Material in each book has been collected from a wide range of government agencies, professional associations, periodicals and other sources. *$78.00*

322 pages Year Founded: 2001 ISBN 0-780803-35-3

1019 Eating Disorders and Obesity, Second Edition : A Comprehensive Handbook
The Guilford Press
72 Spring Street
New York, NY 10012
800-365-7006
Fax: 212-966-6708
E-mail: info@guilford.com
www.www.guilford.com

Robert Matloff, President
Christopher Fairburn, Author

This unique handbook presents and integrates virtually all that is currently known about eating disorders and obesity in one authoritative, accessible, and eminently practical volume.

1020 Eating Disorders: Reference Sourcebook
Oryx Press
88 Post Road W
Westport, CT 06881
203-226-3571
Fax: 603-431-2214
E-mail: info@oryxpress.com
www.oryxpress.com

Listings of 200 centers and groups for care and treatment of eating disorders, such as anorexia nervosa, bulimia nervosa, and compulsive overeating. *$49.95*

1021 Eating Disorders: When Food Turns Against You
Franklin Watts
90 Old Sherman Turnpike
Danbury, CT 06816-0001
800-621-1115
Fax: 203-797-3657
www.grolier.com

$14.50

96 pages ISBN 0-531111-75-X

1022 Emotional Eating: A Practical Guide to Taking Control
Lexington Books
4501 Forbes Boulevard
Suite 200
Lanham, MD 20706
717-794-3800
800-426-6420
Fax: 717-794-3803
www.lexingtonbook.com

Using case histories he explores some of the causes of emotional eating (childhood programming, family life, sexual abuse) and the manifestos of emotional eating ("sneaky snaking",grazing, and binging). Of particular interest is the last chaper, which helps the reader determine whether or not it is a good or bad time to diet. While not a diet book or a 12-step primer, this is a tool for developing healthier ways of handling emotions and food. *$19.95*

200 pages ISBN 0-029002-15-X

1023 Encyclopedia of Obesity and Eating Disorders
Facts on File
11 Penn Plaza
New York, NY 10001-2006
212-290-8090
800-322-8755
Fax: 212-678-3633

From abdominoplasty to Zung Rating Scale, this volume defines and explains these disorders, along with medical and other problems associated with them. *$50.00*

272 pages

1024 Etiology and Treatment of Bulimia Nervosa
Jason Aronson
506 Clement Street
Dunmore, PA 18512-1523
415-387-2272
Fax: 415-387-2377
E-mail: info@greepapplebooks.com
www.aronson.com

$35.00

352 pages ISBN 1-568213-39-5

1025 Feminist Perspectives on Eating Disorders
Guilford Publications
72 Spring Street
New York, NY 10012
212-431-9800
800-365-7006
Fax: 212-966-6708
E-mail: info@guilford.com
www.guilford.com

Explores the relationship between the anguish of eating disorder sufferers and the problems of ordinary women. Examines the sociocultural pressure on women to conform to culturally ideal body types and how this affects individual self concept. Controversial topics include the relationship between sexual abuse and eating disorders, the use of medications and the role of hospitalization and 12-step programs. *$ 25.95*

465 pages ISBN 1-572301-82-1

1026 Food for Recovery: The Next Step
Crown Publishing Group
201 E 50th Street
New York, NY 10022-7703
212-572-6117
Fax: 212-572-6161
www.randomhouse.com

A very practicle guide on every aspect needed by the patient and counselor to utilize nutrition as a therapeutic tool. *$ 14.00*

ISBN 0-517586-94-0

1027 Golden Cage, The Enigma of Anorexia Nervosa
Random House
1745 Broadway 15-3
New York, NY 10019

212-782-9000
Fax: 212-572-6066
www.randomhouse.com

One of the world's leading authorities offers a vivid and moving account of the causes, effects and treatment of this devastating disease. *$9.00*

ISBN 0-394726-88-X

1028 Group Psychotherapy for Eating Disorders
American Psychiatric Publishing
1000 Wilson Boulevard
Suite 1825
Arlington, VA 22209-3901
703-907-7322
800-368-5777
Fax: 703-907-1091
E-mail: appi@psych.org
www.appi.org

Katie Duffy, Marketing Assistant

The first book to fully explore the use of group therapy in the treatment of eating disorders. *$46.00*

353 pages ISBN 0-880484-19-5

1029 Helping Athletes with Eating Disorders
Human Kinetics Publishers
PO Box 5076
Champaign, IL 61825-5076
800-747-4457
Fax: 217-351-1549
E-mail: orders@hkusa.com

Gives readers the information they need to identify and address major eating disorders such as: anorexia, bulimia nervosa, and eating disorders not otherwise specified. *$25.00*

208 pages ISBN 0-873223-83-7

1030 Hunger So Wide and Deep
University of Minnesota Press
111 3rd Avenue S
Suite 290
Minneapolis, MN 55401
612-627-1970
Fax: 612-627-1980
E-mail: um@tc.umn.edu
www.upress.um.edu

ISBN 0-816624-35-6

1031 Hungry Self; Women, Eating and Identity
Harper Collins
10 E 53rd Street
New York, NY 10022
212-207-7000
Fax: 212-207-6978
www.harpercollins.com

Answers the need for help among the five million American women who suffer from eating disorders. Paperback. *$13.00*

256 pages ISBN 0-060925-04-3

1032 Insights in the Dynamic Psychotherapy of Anorexia and Bulimia
Jason Aronson
506 Clemant Street
San Francisco, CA 94118

415-387-2272
Fax: 415-387-2377
www.greenapplebooks.com

The clinical insights that guide the dynamic psychotheray of anorexic and bulimic patients. *$45.00*

288 pages ISBN 0-876685-68-8

1033 Lifetime Weight Control
New Harbinger Publications
5674 Shattuck Avenue
Oakland, CA 94609-1662
510-652-2002
800-748-6273
Fax: 510-652-5472
E-mail: customerservice@newharbinger.com
www.newharbinger.com

Patrick Fanning, Author

Program of lifetime weight management in seven steps: 1. Eat spontaneously to settle into your 'setpoint' weight. 2. Accept yourself as okay, regardless of your weight. 3. Determine how and why you eat, learning all the reasons besides hunger. 4. Satisfy emotional needs directly, saving food for satisfying real hunger. 5. Improve nutrition. 6. Increase activity. 7. Stick to it. *$13.95*

208 pages Year Founded: 1990 ISBN 0-934986-83-5

1034 Making Peace with Food
Harper Collins
10 E 53rd Street
New York, NY 10022-5244
212-207-7000
800-242-7737
Fax: 212-207-7617
www.harpercollins.com

For millions of diet-conscious Americans, the scientifically proven, step-by-step guide to overcoming repeated weight loss and gain, binge eating, guilt and anxieties about food and body image. *$15.00*

224 pages ISBN 0-060963-28-X

1035 Obesity: Theory and Therapy
Raven Press
I 185 Avenue of the Americas
New York, NY 10036
212-930-9500
800-638-3030
Fax: 212-869-3495
www.lww.com

A classic reference for clinicians dealing with obesity, this volume provides the most up-to-date research, preclinical and clinical information.

500 pages ISBN 0-881678-84-8

1036 Overeaters Anonymous
Metro Intergroup of Overeaters Anonymous
350 Third Avenue
PO Box 759
New York, NY 10001
212-946-4599
E-mail: NYOAMentroOffice@yahoo.com

Personal stories demonstrating the struggles overcome and accomplishments made. *$7.50*

204 pages

1037 Psychobiology and Treatment of Anorexia Nervosa and Bulimia Nervosa
American Psychiatric Publishing
1000 Wilson Boulevard
Suite 1825
Arlington, VA 22209-3901
703-907-7322
800-368-5777
Fax: 703-907-1091
E-mail: appi@psych.org
www.appi.org

Katie Duffy, Marketing Assistant

Combines clinical research concerning these distinct disorders and provides an overview of the psychobiology and treatment. *$48.50*

356 pages ISBN 0-880485-06-X

1038 Psychodynamic Technique in the Treatment of the Eating Disorders
Jason Aronson
400 Keystone Industrial Park
Dunmore, PA 18512-1523
570-342-1320
800-782-0015
Fax: 201-767-1576
www.aronson.com

Provides a blueprint for the treatment of the eating disorders. *$50.00*

440 pages ISBN 0-876686-22-6

1039 Psychosomatic Families: Anorexia Nervosa in Context
Harvard University Press
79 Garden Street
Cambridge, MA 02138
800-405-1619
Fax: 800-406-9145
E-mail: contact_hup@harvard.edu
www.hup.harvard.edu

Hardcover. *$38.50*

351 pages ISBN 0-674722-20-5

1040 Self-Starvation
Jason Aronson
400 Keystone Industrial Park
Dunmore, PA 18512-1523
570-342-1320
800-782-0015
Fax: 201-767-1576
www.aronson.com

Argues that anorexia nervosa is a social disease reflecting unbearable conflicts within the family. *$30.00*

312 pages ISBN 1-568218-22-2

1041 Starving to Death in a Sea of Objects
Jason Aronson
400 Keystone Industrial Park
Dunmore, PA 18512-1523
570-342-1320
800-782-0015
Fax: 201-840-7242
www.aronson.com

Makes the central dilemma clear: how emancipation can come to mean security and pleasure for the anorexic. *$30.00*

464 pages ISBN 0-876684-35-5

1042 Surviving an Eating Disorder: Perspectives and Strategies
Harper Collins
10 E 53rd Street
New York, NY 10022-5244
212-207-7132
Fax: 212-207-7946
www.harpercollins.com

Addresses the cutting-edge advances made in the field of eating disorders, discusses how the changes in health care have affected treatment and provides additional strategies for dealing with anorexia, bulemia and binge eating disorder. It also includes updated readings and a list of support organizations. A terrrific resource for those suffering from eating disorders, their families and professionals. Paperback. *$ 13.00*

256 pages ISBN 0-060952-33-4

1043 Treating Eating Disorders
Jossey-Bass Publishers
10475 Crosspoint Boulevard
Indianapolis, IN 46256
877-762-2974
Fax: 800-597-3299
E-mail: consumers@wiley.com
www.josseybass.com

Details how some of the most eminent clinicians in the field combine and intergrate a wide variety of contemporary therapies — ranging from psychodynamic to systematic to cognitive behavioral—to successfully treat clients with anorexia nervosa, bulimia nervosa, and binge eating diorders. Filled with up to date information and important approaches to assessment and treatment, the book offers a hands-on approach that cogently illustrates both theory and technique. *$29.95*

416 pages ISBN 0-787903-30-2

1044 When Food Is Love
Geneen Roth and Associates
PO Box 2852
Santa Cruz, CA 95063
877-243-6336
Fax: 831-685-8602
E-mail: GeneenRoth@GeneenRoth.com
www.geneenroth.com

Lindsey Cohn, Bookseller

Shows how dieting and compulsive eating often become a subsititue for intimacy. Drawing on painful personal experiece as well as the candid stories of those she has helped in her seminars, Roth claims the crucial issues that surrounds compulsive eating: need for control, dependency on melodrama, desire for what is forbidden, and the belief that the wrong move can mean catastrophe. She shows why many people overeat in an attempt to satisfy their emotional hunger, and why weight loss frequently just uncovers a new set of problems. This book will help readers break destructive, self-perpetuating patterns and learn to satisfy all the hungers - physical and emotional - that makes us human. *$10.00*

205 pages

1045 American Anorexia/Bulimia Association News
425 East 61st Streett
6th Floor
New York, NY 10021
212-501-8351
Fax: 212-501-0342

Offers information on the latest treatments, medications, books, conferences, support groups, and workshops for persons with eating disorders.

1046 Anorexia: Am I at Risk?
ETR Associates
4 Carbonero Way
Scotts Valley, CA 95066
831-438-4060
800-321-4407
Fax: 800-435-8433
E-mail: customerservice@etr.org
www.etr.org

Offers a clear overview of anorexia; Lists symptoms; Explains helath problems.

1047 Body Image
ETR Associates
4 Carbonero Way
Scotts Valley, CA 95066
831-438-4060
800-321-4407
Fax: 800-435-8433
E-mail: customerservice@etr.org
www.etr.org

Discusses the difference between healthy and distorted body image; the link between poor body image and low self esteem; five point list to help people check out their own body image.

1048 Bulimia
ETR Associates
4 Carbonero Way
Scotts Valley, CA 95066
831-438-4060
800-321-4407
Fax: 800-435-8433
E-mail: customerservice@etr.org
www.etr.org

Includes warning signs that someone's bulimic, health consequesnces of bulimia, and how to help a friend.

1049 Eating Disorder Sourcebook
Gurze Books
PO Box 2238
Carlsbad, CA 92018-2238
760-434-7533
800-756-7533
Fax: 760-434-5476
E-mail: gzcatl@aol.com
www.bulimia.com

Leigh Cohn, Co-Owner

Includes 125 books and tapes on eating disorders and related subjects for both lay and professional audiences, basic facts about eating disorders, a list of national organizations and treatment facilities. Also publishes a bimonthly newsletter for clinicians and are executive editors of Eating Disorders the Journal of Treatment and Prevention.

28 pages 1 per year

1050 Eating Disorders
ETR Associates
4 Carbonero Way
Scotts Valley, CA 95066
831-438-4060
800-321-4407
Fax: 800-435-8433
E-mail: customerservice@etr.org
www.etr.org

Includes anorexia and bulimia, eating patterns versus eating disorders, treatment and getting help.

1051 Eating Disorders Factsheet
SAMHSA'S National Mental Health Information Center
PO Box 42557
Washington, DC 20015
800-789-2647
Fax: 240-747-5470
TDD: 866-889-2647
E-mail: ken@mentalhealth.org
www.mentalhealth.samhsa.gov

A Kathryn Power, MEd, Director
Edward B Searle, Deputy Director

This fact sheet provides basic information on the symptoms, medical complications, formal diagnosis, and treatment for anorexia nervousa and bulimia nervosa.

2 pages

1052 Eating Disorders: Facts About Eating Disorders and the Search for Solutions
National Institute of Mental Health
6001 Executive Boulevard
Room 8184
Bethesda, MD 20892-9663
301-443-4513
866-615-6464
Fax: 301-443-4279
TTY: 301-443-8431
E-mail: nimhinfo@nih.gov
www.nimh.nih.gov

Eating is controlled by many factors, including appetite, food availability, family, peer, and cultural practices, and attempts at voluntary control. Dieting to a body weight leaner than needed for health is highly promoted by current fashion trends, sales campaigns for special foods, and in some activities and professions. Eating disorders involve serious disturbances in eating behavior, such as extreme and unhealthy reduction of food intake or severe overeating, as well as feelings of distress or extreme concern about body shape or weight. There is help, and there is every hope for recovery.

8 pages

1053 Fats of Life
ETR Associates
4 Carbonero Way
Scotts Valley, CA 95066
831-438-4060
800-321-4407
Fax: 800-435-8433
E-mail: customerservice@etr.org
www.etr.org

Stresses that health, not body weight, is what's important; dispels myths about dieting; includes chart to help people determine their body mass index.

1054 Food and Feelings
ETR Associates
4 Carbonero Way
Scotts Valley, CA 95066
831-438-4060
800-321-4407
Fax: 800-435-8433
E-mail: customerservice@etr.org
www.etr.org

Helps students recognize eating disorders; emphasizes the seriousness of eating disorders; encourages the sufferers to seek treatment.

1055 Getting What You Want from Your Body Image
ETR Associates
4 Carbonero Way
Scotts Valley, CA 95066
831-438-4060
800-321-4407
Fax: 800-435-8433
E-mail: customerservice@etr.org
www.etr.org

Discusses topics such as the influence of the media, the truth about dieting, and body image survival tips.

1056 Restrictive Eating
ETR Associates
4 Carbonero Way
Scotts Valley, CA 95066
831-438-4060
800-321-4407
Fax: 800-435-8433
E-mail: customerservice@etr.org
www.etr.org

Discusses the spectrum of eating patterns, signs of restrictive eating and why it is a problem, how to help a friend, and where to go for help.

1057 Teen Image
ETR Associates
4 Carbonero Way
Scotts Valley, CA 95066
831-438-4060
800-321-4407
Fax: 800-435-8433
E-mail: customerservice@etr.org
www.etr.org

Dispels unrealistic media images; offers ways to boost body image and self esteem; includes tips to maintain a good body image.

1058 Working Together
National Association of Anorexia Nervosa and Associated Disorders
PO Box 7
Highland Park, IL 60035-0007
847-831-3438
Fax: 847-433-4632
E-mail: anad20@aol.com
www.anad.org

Dawn Ries, Administrator

Designed for individuals, families, group leaders and professionals concerned with eating disorders. Provides updates on treatments, resources, conferences, programs, articles by therapists, recovered victims, group members and leaders.

2 pages 4 per year

Research Centers

1059 Center for the Study of Adolescence
Michael Reese Hospital and Medical Center
2929 S. Ellis Avenue
Chicago, IL 60616
312-791-2000
E-mail: info@michaelreesehospital.com
www.michaelreesehospital.com

Enrique Beckmann, Chair/Ceo

1060 Center for the Study of Anorexia and Bulimia
1841 Broadway 4th Floor
New York, NY 10023
212-333-3444
Fax: 212-333-5444
E-mail: csab@icpnyc.orgg
www.www.csabnyc.org

Established as a division of the Institute for Contemporary Psychotherapy in 1979 and is the oldest non-profit eating disorders clinic in New York City. Using an eclectic approach, the professional staff and affiliates are on the cutting edge of treatment in their field. The treatment staff includes social workers, psychologists, registered nurses and nutritionists, all with special training in the treatment of eating disorders.

1061 Eating Disorders Research and Treatment Program
Michael Reese Hospital and Medical Center
2929 S Ellis Avenue
Chicago, IL 60616
312-791-2000
E-mail: info@michaelreesehospital.com
www.www.michaelreesehospital.com

Enrique Beckmann, Chair/Ceo

1062 Obesity Research Center
St. Luke's-Roosevelt Hospital
1090 Amsterdam Avenue 14th Floor
New York, NY 10025
212-523-4196
Fax: 212-523-3416
E-mail: dg108@columbia.edu
www.nyorc.org

Janine Pangburn, Research Project Manager
Tony Sikora, Administrative Assistant

Helps reduce the the incidence of obesity and related diseases through leadership in basic research, clinical research, epidemiology and public health, patient care, and public education.

1063 University of Pennsylvania Weight and Eating Disorders Program
3535 Market Street
Suite 3108
Philadelphia, PA 19104

215-898-7314
Fax: 215-898-2878
E-mail: cwilson@mail.med.upenn.edu
www.www.med.upenn.edu

Conducts a wide variety of studies on the causes and treatment of weight-related disorders.

Support Groups & Hot Lines

1064 Food Addicts Anonymous
4623 Forest Hill Boulevard
Suite 109-4
W Palm Beach, FL 33415-9120
561-967-3871
Fax: 561-967-9815
E-mail: info@foodaddictsanonymous.org
www.foodaddictsanonymous.org

The FAA program is based on the belief that food addiction is a bio-chemical disease. We share our experience, strength, and hope with others allows us to recover from this disease.

1065 MEDA
92 Pearl Street
Newton, MA 02458
617-558-1881
866-343-6332
E-mail: info@medainc.org
www.medainc.org

MEDA ia a nonprofit organization dedicated to the prevention and treatment of eating disorders and disordered eating. MEDA'S mission is to prevent the continuing spread of eating disorders through educational awareness and early detection. MEDA serves as a support network and resource for clients, loved ones, clinicians, educators and the general public.

1066 National Center for Overcoming Overeating
PO Box 1257
Old Chelsea Station
New York, NY 10113
212-875-0442
E-mail: webmaster@overcomingovereating.com
www.overcomingovereating.com

Is an educational and training organization working to end body hatred and dieting.

1067 Overeaters Anonymous
World Service Office PO Box 44020
Rio Rancho, NM 87124-4020
505-891-2664
Fax: 505-891-4320
E-mail: info@oa.org
www.overeatersanonymous.org

Twelve step program for compulsive eaters.

Video & Audio

1068 Eating Disorder Video
Active Parenting Publishers
1955 Vaughn Road NW
Suite 108
Kennesaw, GA 30144-7808
770-429-0565
800-825-0060

Fax: 770-429-0334
E-mail: cservice@activeparenting.com
www.activeparenting.com

Features compelling interviews with several young people who have suffered from anorexia nervosa, bulimia and compulsive eating. Discusses the treatments, causes and techniques for prevention with field experts. *$39.95*

ISSN Q6456

1069 Eating Disorders: When Food Hurts
Fanlight Productions
4196 Washington Street
Suite 2
Boston, MA 01231
617-469-4999
800-937-4113
Fax: 617-469-3379
E-mail: info@fanlight.com
www.fanlight.com

Ben Achtenberg, President
Nicole Johnson, Publicity Coordinator

People recovering from anorexia and bulimia, together with a therapist specializing in eating disorders, discuss their experiences of confronting these dangerous conditions. Encourages people with eating disorders to get help, as well as educating teachers, counselors, and others who work with young women. *$195.00*

Year Founded: 1996

Web Sites

1070 www.alt.support.eating.disord
Alternative Support for Eating Disorder

Information for anorexics, also a bulletin board.

1071 www.anred.com
Anorexia Nervosa and Related Eating Disorders

The factual materials are detailed and organized.

1072 www.closetoyou.org/eatingdisorders
Close to You

Information about eating disorders, anorexia, bulimia, binge eating disorder, and compulsive overeating.

1073 www.cyberpsych.org
CyberPsych

Hosts the American Psychoanalyists Foundation, American Association of Suicideology, Society for the Exploration of Psychotherapy Intergration, and Anxiety Disorders Association of America. Also subcategories of the anxiety disorders, as well as general information, including panic disorder, phobias, obsessive compulsive disorder (OCD), social phobia, generalized anxiety disorder, post traumatic stress disorder, and phobias of childhood. Book reviews and links to web pages sharing the topics.

1074 www.edap.org
Eating Disorders Awareness and Prevention

A source of educational brochures and curriculum materials.

1075 www.gurze.com
Gurze Bookstore

Hundreds of books on eating disorders.

1076 www.healthyplace.com/Communities/
Peace, Love, and Hope

Click on Body Views for information on body dysmorphic disorder.

1077 www.kidsource.com/nedo/
National Eating Disorders Organization

Educational materials on dynamics, causative factors and evaluating treatment options.

1078 www.mentalhelp.net
Anorexia Nervosa General Information

Introductory text on Anorexia Nervosa.

1079 www.mirror-mirror.org/eatdis.htm
Mirror, Mirror

Relapse prevention for eating disorders.

1080 www.planetpsych.com
Planetpsych.com

Learn about disorders, their treatments and other topics in psychology. Articles are listed under the related topic areas. Ask a therapist a question for free, or view the directory of professionals in your area. If you are a therapist sign up for the directory. Current features, self-help, interactive, and newsletter archives.

1081 www.psychcentral.com
Psych Central

Personalized one-stop index for psychology, support, and mental health issues, resources, and people on the Internet.

1082 www.something-fishy.com
Something Fishy Music and Publishing

Continuously educating the world on eating disorders to encourage every sufferer towards recovery.

Factitious Disorder

Introduction

Factitious Disorders are a group of disorders in which patients deliberately fake or cause mental or physical symptoms: scratching wounds open; contaminating wounds so that they become infected; or using non-prescribed medications. In contrast with Malingering, the behaviors of Factitious Disorders are used to become a patient, to obtain medical or mental health care, rather than to achieve some personal gain, such as being excused from military duty or from responsibility for criminal activity.

The drive for those with a Factitious Disorder to be seen as sick goes well beyond the normal need everyone has for attention and care; patients with this disorder are willing to risk life and limb, both from the symptoms they cause and from the invasive diagnostic tests and treatments undertaken in attempts to discover and remedy what is wrong.

Patients with Factitious Disorders produce or exaggerate the symptoms of a physical or mental illness using a variety of methods, such as contaminating urine samples with blood, improperly taking medications, injecting substances, and other similar behaviors. The following disorders are included among the most prevalent: Munchausen Syndrome: Patients whose symptoms are dramatized and exaggerated. Many patients with Munchausen will undergo unnecessary exploratory surgeries and other procedures in the attempt to diagnose their illness.

Munchausen Syndrome by Proxy: When are parent or caregiver falsify a child's medical history, tamper with laboratory tests or somehow injure or cause a child to become ill and require treatment.

SYMPTOMS

Data on all of these disorders is incomplete, because most patients flee when discovered or suspected, and do not submit to a psychiatric examination. Several psychiatric diagnoses, including personality disorders and psychotic disorders, have been associated with Factitious Disorders. Some of the signs of factitious disorders are: dramatic but inconsistent medical history; extensive knowledge of medicine and/or hospitals; negative test results followed by further symptom development; symptoms that occur only when the patient is not being observed; eagerness to undergo operations or other procedures.

Diagnosis is based on the individual being observed performing the behaviors that cause the signs and symptoms of a Factitious Disorder, or in possession of the tools to do so. In diagnosing Munchausen's Syndrome by Proxy, the diagnosis is often made either when the caregiver is removed from the situation and the child recovers, or when the caregiver is witnessed causing harm to the child.

PREVALENCE

Factitious Disorders are more commen in men than in women, except in Munchausen's by Proxy, which most often affects a female caregiver.

TREATMENT OPTIONS

Treatment of Factitious Disorders is difficult. It involves the patient admitting his or her true illness and medical professionals stopping unnecessary medical tests, treatments or procedures. Psychotherapy has been of limited benefit. Antidepressent and antipsychotic medications have been helpful in a few cases. Successful treatment for individuals with chronic symptoms is rare; however, dangerous, expensive, and unnecessary medical interventions can be discontinued.

Associations & Agencies

1084 Center for Family Support (CFS)
333 7th Avenue
New York, NY 10001-5004
212-629-7939
Fax: 212-239-2211
www.cfsny.org

Steven Vernickofs, Executive Director
Melanie Singleton, Director Human Resources

Service agency devoted to the physical well-being and development of the retarded child and the sound mental health of the parents. Helps families with retarded children with all aspects of home care including counseling, referrals, home aide service, consultation. Offers intervention for parents at the birth of a retarded child with in-home support, guidance and infant stimulation. Pioneered training of nonprofessional women as home aides to provide supportive services in homes.

1085 Center for Mental Health Services Knowledge
PO Box 42557
Washington, DC 20015-4800
800-789-2647
Fax: 240-747-5484
E-mail: ken@mentalhealth.org
www.mentalhealth.samhsa.gov

A Kathryn Power, MEd, Director
Edward B Searle, Deputy Director

Information about resources, technical assistance, research, training, networks, and other federal clearing homes, and fact sheets and materials. Information specialists refer callers to mental health resources in their communities as well as state, federal and non-profit contacts. Staff available Monday through Friday, 8:30 AM - 5:00 PM, EST, excluding federal holidays. After hours callers may leave messages and an information specialist will return their call.

1086 National Association for the Dually Diagnosed (NADD)
132 Fair Street
Kingston, NY 12401
845-334-4336
800-331-5362
Fax: 845-331-4569
E-mail: nadd@mhv.net
www.thenadd.org

Dr Robert Fletcher, Founder/CEO

Nonprofit organization designed to promote interest of professional and parent development with resources for individuals who have the coexistences of mental illness and mental retardation. Provides conferences, educational services and training materials to professionals, parents, concerned citizens and service organizations. Formerly known as the National Association for the Dually Diagnosed.

Year Founded: 1983

1087 National Mental Health Consumer's Self-Help
1211 Chestnut Street
Suite 1207
Philadelphia, PA 19107
215-751-1810
800-553-4539
Fax: 215-636-6312
E-mail: info@mhselfhelp.org
www.mhselfhelp.org

Joseph Rogers, Founder/Executive Director
Christine Simiriglia, Director

Funded by the National Institute of Mental Health Community Support Program, the purpose of the Clearinghouse, is to encourage the development and growth of consumer self-help groups.

1088 National Mental Health Consumers' Self-Help Clearinghouse
1211 Chestnut Street
Suite 1207
Philadelphia, PA 19107
215-751-1810
800-553-4539
Fax: 215-636-6312
E-mail: info@mhselfhelp.org
www.mhselfhelp.org

Joseph Rogers, Executive Director

A national consumer technical assistance center that has played a major role in the development of the mental health consumer movement.

Year Founded: 1986

1089 SAMHSA's National Mental Health Information Center
US Department of Health and Human Services
PO Box 42557
Washington, DC 20015-4800
240-221-4021
800-789-2647
Fax: 240-221-4295
TDD: 866-889-2647
www.mentalhealth.samhsa.gov

A Kathryn Power, MEd, Director
Edward B Searle, Deputy Director

Provides information about mental health via a toll-free telephone number, this web site, and more than 600 publications. Developed for users of mental health services and their families, the general public, policy makers, providers, and the media.

Books

1090 Disorders of Simulation: Malingering, Factitious Disorders, and Compensation Neurosis
Psychosocial Press
59 Boston Post Road
Madison, CT
203-245-4000
Fax: 203-245-0775

Grant L Hutchinson, Author

1091 Do No Harm?
Independent Publishing Group
814 N Franklin Street
Chicago, IL 60610

312-337-0747
Fax: 312-337-5985
E-mail: frontdesk@ipgbook.com
www.www.ipgbook.com

Craig McGill, Author

Munchausen Syndrome by Proxy is the syndrome that causes parents and care workers to harm their children to get attention. Many families are separated after its diagnosis. But has the fertile imagination of social workers and the public turned MSBP into the trendy disorder of our time? *$16.95*

240 pages ISBN 1-901250-48-2

1092 Munchausen by Proxy: Identification, Intervention, and Case Management
Routledge
270 Madison Avenue
New York, NY 10016
212-216-7800
Fax: 212-563-2269
www.www.routledge.com

Mary Sheridan, Author
Louisa Lasher, Author

This step-by-step guide will help you identify and manage cases of this unique form of child maltreatment.

1093 Munchausen's Syndrome by Proxy
World Scientific Publishing Company
27 Warren Street
Suite 401-402
Hackensack, NJ 07601
201-487-9655
800-227-7562
Fax: 201-487-9656
E-mail: wspc@wspc.com
www.worldscientific.com

This book reviews the current state of knowledge of Munchausen's Syndrome by Proxy, a type of child abuse which causes wide concern. Two main areas are covered: new directions in research, and treatment of the perpetrator in and outside the family. *$53.00*

ISBN 1-860941-34-6

1094 Playing Sick
Routledge Publishing
270 Madison Avenue
New York, NY 10016
212-216-7800
Fax: 212-563-2269
www.www.routledge-ny.com

Marc Feldman, Author

Taken from bizarre cases of real patients, the first book to chronicle the devastating impact of phony illnesses-factitious disorders and Munchausen syndrome-on patients and caregivers alike. *$ 27.50*

328 pages ISBN 0-415949-34-7

1095 Playing Sick?: Untangling the Web of Munchausen Syndrome, Munchausen by Proxy, Malingering, and Factitious Disorder
Routledge
270 Madison Avenue
New York, NY 10016

212-216-7800
Fax: 212-563-2269
www.www.routledge.com
Marc Feldman, Author

Based on years of research and clinical practice, this book provides the clues that can help practitioners and family members recognize these disorders, avoid invasive procedures, and sort out the motives that drive people to hurt themselves and deceive others.

Periodicals & Pamphlets

1096 Asher Meadow Newsletter
18209 Smoke House Court
Germantown, MD 20874
www.ashermeadow.com

Asher Meadow is a wholly-owned non-profit subsidiary of American Marvels, an Internet development company that provides a newsletter for survivors of MSBP.

Support Groups & Hot Lines

1097 Asher Meadow
18209 Smoke House Court
Germantown, MD 20874
www.ashermeadow.com

A wholly-owned non profit subsidiary of American Marvels, and Internet development company that provides resources and links related to Munchausen's Syndrome by Proxy.

Web Sites

1098 www.mbpexpert.com
MBP Expert Services

Expert services from Louisa J Lasher, MA, provides Munchausen by Proxy maltreatment training, case consultation, technical assistance, and expert witness services in an objective manner and in the best interest of the child or children involved.

1099 www.msbp.com
Mothers Against Munchausen Syndrome by Proxy Allegations

Begun in response to the fast growing number of false allegations of Munchausen Syndrome by Proxy.

1100 www.munchausen.com
Munchause Syndrome

Dr. Marc Feldman's Munchausen Syndrome, Malingering, Factitious Disorder, & Munchausen by Proxy page. Includes articles, related book list, personal stories and links.

Gender Identity Disorder

Introduction

With a wide scope of questions and confusion surrounding human sexuality and gender-explicit roles in the modern era, many children, adolescents and adults have been perplexed by the concepts of homosexuality and cross-gender identification. Homosexuality is a matter of sexual orientation: whether one is sexually attracted to men or women. The American Psychiatric Association ceased to classify homosexuality as an illness in 1973. Gender identity, in contrast, is a matter of what gender one feels oneself to be; people with Gender Identity Disorder feel that their psychological experience conflicts with the physical body with which they were born. Gender Identity Disorders can have serious social and occupational repercussions.

Diagnosis of Gender Identity Disorder requires two sets of criteria: (1) a heavy and persistent insistence that the individual is, or has a strong desire to be, of the opposite sex, and (2) a constant discomfort about his/her designated sex, a feeling of inappropriateness towards his/her biological designation. Typically, boys meeting critera for the disorder are predisposed to dressing as girls, drawing explicit pictures of females, playing with pre-designated feminine toys, fantasizing and role playing as females and interacting primarily with girls. Girls with the condition tend to participate in contact sports, have an aversion to wearing dresses, are often mistaken for boys due to attire and hair style, and may assert that they will develop in to men. For adolescents and adults, ostracism in school and the workplace is likely to occur, as is a profound inability to associate with others and poor relationships with family members and members of either sex.

SYMPTOMS

In boys
- A marked preoccupation with traditionally feminine activites;
- A preference for dressing as a girl;
- Attraction to stereotypical female games and toys;
- Portraying female characters in role playing;
- Assertion he is a girl;
- Insistence on sitting to urinate;
- Displaying disgust for his genitals, wishing to remove them.

In girls
- Aversion to traditional female attire;
- Shared interest in contact games;
- A preference for associating with boys;
- Refusing to urinate sitting down;
- Show little interest in playing with stereotypical female toys such as dolls;
- Assertion that she will grow a penis, not breasts;
- Identification with strong male figures.

In adolescents
- Ostracism in school and social situations;
- Social isolation, peer rejection and peer teasing;
- Significant cross-gender identification and mannerisms;
- Similar symptoms as children.

In adults
- Adoption of social roles, physical appearance, and mannerisms of opposite sex;
- Surgical and/or hormonal manipulation of biological state;
- Discomfort in being regarded by others, or functioning, as his/her designated sex;
- Cross-dressing;
- Transvestic Fetishism.

ASSOCIATED FEATURES

Those who have Gender Identity Disorder are at risk of mental and physical harm resulting, not from the condition itself, but from the reactions of other people to the condition. In children, a manifestation of Separation Anxiety Disorder, Generalized Anxiety Disorder and symptoms of Depression may result. For adolescents, depression and suicidal thoughts or ideas, as well as actual suicide attempts can result from prolonged feelings of ostracism by peers. Relationships with either one or both parents may weaken from resentment, lack of communication and misunderstanding; many with this disorder may drop out of or avoid school due to peer teasing. For many, lives are built around attempts to decrease gender distress. They are often preoccupied with appearance. In extreme cases, males with the disorder perform their own castration. Prostitution has been linked with the disorder because young people who are rejected by their families and ostracized by others may resort to prostitution as the only way to support themselves, a practice which increases the risk of acquiring sexually transmitted diseases. Some people with the disorder resort to substance abuse and other forms of abuse in an attempt to deal with the associated stress.

TREATMENT OPTIONS

Therapists who attempt to pathologize and 'cure' sexual orientation have been generally unsuccessful. So-called conversion therapy can cause more harm than good. In contrast, some people with Gender Identity Disorder decide to live as members of the opposite sex; some choose to undergo sex-change surgery. There is some controversy about the diagnosis; 'transsexual' groups protest that their condition, like homosexuality, should not be classified as a mental disease. Psychological assistance can help individuals to gain acceptance of themselves, and can teach methods of dealing with discrimination, prejudice and violence.

Associations & Agencies

1102 Center for Family Support (CFS)
333 7th Avenue
New York, NY 10001-5004
212-629-7939
Fax: 212-239-2211
www.cfsny.org

Steven Vernickofs, Executive Director

An agency that continues to develop new programs to serve families and individuals with their care needs. They currently offer services throughout the New York City region including: New Jersey, Long Island and the Lower Hudson Valley.

1103 Center for Mental Health Services Knowledge
PO Box 42557
Washington, DC 20015-4800
800-789-2647
Fax: 240-747-5470
www.mentalhealth.samhsa.gov/

Information about resources, technical assistance, research, training, networks, and other federal clearing houses, and fact sheets and materials. Information specialists refer callers to mental health resources in their communities as well as state, federal and nonprofit contacts. Staff available Monday through Friday, 8:30 AM - 5:00 PM, EST, excluding federal holidays. After hours, callers may leave messages and an information specialist will return their call.

1104 National Association for the Dually Diagnose d (NADD)

132 Fair Street
Kingston, NY 12401-4802
845-331-4336
800-331-5362
Fax: 845-331-4569
E-mail: info@thenadd.org
www.thenadd.org

Dr. Robert Fletcher, Executive Director

Nonprofit organization designed to promote interest of professional and parent development with resources for individuals who have the coexistence of mental illness and mental retardation. Provides conference, educational services and training materials to professionals, parents, concerned citizens and service organizations. Formerly known as the National Association for the Dually Diagnosed.

Year Founded: 1983

1105 National Gay and Lesbian Task Force

1325 Massachusetts Avenue NW
Suite 600
Washington, DC 20005
202-393-5177
Fax: 202-393-2241
E-mail: info@TheTaskForce.org
www.thetaskforce.org

Jeff B Soref, Chair
Sandi Greene, Director of Administration

Offers community support for gay and lesbian individuals.

Year Founded: 1973

1106 National Institute of Mental Health

6001 Executive Blvd
Room 8184, MSC 9663
Bethesda, MD 20892-9663
301-443-4513
Fax: 301-443-4279
TTY: 301-443-8431
E-mail: nimhinfo@nih.gov
www.nimh.nih.gov

Thomas R Insel MD, Director

The mission of the National Institute of Mental Health is to reduce the burden of mental illness and behavioral disorders through research on mind, brain, and behavior.

1107 National Mental Health Consumers' Self-Help Clearinghouse

1211 Chestnut Street
Suite 1207
Philadelphia, PA 19107
215-751-1810
800-553-4539
Fax: 215-636-6312
E-mail: info@mhselfhelp.org
www.mhselfhelp.org

A consumer-run national technical assistance center serving the mental health consumer movement. They connect individuals to self-help and advocacy resources, and offer expertise to self-help groups and other peer-run services for mental health consumers.

Year Founded: 1986

1108 Parents and Friends of Lesbians and Gays

1726 M Street NW
Suite 400
Washington, DC 20036
202-467-8180
Fax: 202-467-8194
E-mail: info@pflag.org
www.pflag.org

Jody Huckaby, Executive Director
Nina Sevilla, Executive Office Administrator

Organization of families and friends of lesbian and gay individuals, dedicated to offer support and understanding.

1109 Parents, Families and Friends of Lesbians and Gays

1726 M Street NW
Suite 400
Washington, DC 20036
202-467-8180
Fax: 202-467-8194
E-mail: info@pflag.org
www.pflag.org

Jody Huckaby, Executive Director

A national non-profit organization with over 200,000 members and supporters and over 500 affiliates in the United States.

1110 SAMHSA's National Mental Health Information Center
US Department of Health and Human Services

PO Box 42557
Washington, DC 20015-4800
240-221-4021
800-789-2647
Fax: 240-221-4295
TDD: 866-889-2647
www.mentalhealth.samhsa.gov

A Kathryn Power MEd, Director
Edward B Searle, Deputy Director

Provides information about mental health via a toll-free telephone number, this web site, and more than 600 publications. Developed for users of mental health services and their families, the general public, policy makers, providers, and the media.

Books

1111 Gender Identity Disorder: A Medical Dictiona ry, Bibliography, and Annotated Research Guide to Internet References
ICON Health Publications

7404 Trade Street
San Diego, CA 92121
Fax: 858-635-9414
www.www.icongrouponline.com/Health

This book was created for medical professionals, students, and members of the general public who want to conduct medical research using the most advanced tools available and spending the least amount of time doing so.

1112 Handbook of Sexual and Gender Identity Disorder
John Wiley & Sons
111 River Street
Hoboken, NJ 07030-5774
201-748-6000
Fax: 201-748-6088
E-mail: info@wiley.com
www.www.wiley.com

William J Pesce, President/CEO
David L Rowland, Author

The Handbook of Sexual and Gender Identity Disorders provides mental health professionals a comprehensive yet practical guide to the understanding, diagnosis, and treatment of a variety of sexual problems. *$95.00*

1113 Identity Without Selfhood
Cambridge University Press
32 Avenue of the Americas
New York, NY 10013-2743
212-924-3900
Fax: 212-691-3239
www.cambridge.org

Mariam Fraser, Author

Situated at the crossroads of feminism, queer theory, and poststructuralist debates around identity, this is a book that shows how key Western concepts such as individuality constrain attempts to deconstruct the self and prevent bisexuality being understood as an identity. *$99.00*

ISBN 0-521623-57-x

Web Sites

1114 www.cyberpsych.org
CyberPsych

Presents information about psychoanalysis, psychotherapy and special topics such as anxiety disorders, the problematic use of alcohol, homophobia, and the traumatic effects of racism.

1115 www.health.nih.gov
National Institutes of Health

Part of the U.S. Department of Health and Human Services that is the nation's medical research agency-making important medical discoveries that improve health and save lives.

1116 www.healthfinder.gov
Healthfinder

Developed by the U.S. Department of Health and Human Services, a key resource for finding the best government and nonprofit health and human services information on the internet.

1117 www.intelihealth.com
Aetna InteliHealth

Aetna InteliHealth's mission is to empower people with trusted solutions for healthier lives.

1118 www.kidspeace.org
KidsPeace

KidsPeace is a private charity dedicated to serving the behavioral and mental health needs of children, preadolescents and teens.

1119 www.mayohealth.com
Mayo Clinic Health Oasis

Their mission is to empower people to manage their health. They accomplish this by providing useful and up-to-date information and tools that reflect the expertise and standard of excellence of Mayo Clinic.

1120 www.nlm.nih.gov
National Library of Medicine

The National Library of Medicine (NLM), on the campus of the National Institutes of Health in Bethesda, Maryland, is the world's largest medical library. The Library collects materials and provides information and research services in all areas of biomedicine and health care

1121 www.planetpsych.com
Planet Psych

The online resource for mental health information

1122 www.psychcentral.com
Psych Central

The Internet's largest and oldest independent mental health social network created and run by mental health professionals to guarantee reliable, trusted information and support communities.

Impulse Control Disorders

Introduction

Everyone has experienced a situation in which they are tempted to do something that is not good for them but do it anyway. This kind of behavior only becomes a disorder when a person is repeatedly and persistently unable to resist a temptation which is always harmful to them or to others. Usually the person feels a rising tension before acting on the need, feels pleasure and relief when giving in to the impulse and, sometimes, feels remorse and guilt afterwards. Four different disorders are included in this category.

KLEPTOMANIA

Symptoms
• Recurrent failure to resist the impulse to steal objects; often they are objects the individual could have paid for or doesn't particularly want;
• Increased sense of tension immediately before the theft;
• Pleasure and relief during the stealing;
• The theft is not due to anger, delusions or hallucinations.
• Awareness that stealing is senseless and wrong;
• Feelings of depression and guilt after stealing.

Associated Features
Kleptomania should not be confused with thefts which are deliberate and for personal gain, or those that are sometimes done by adolescents on a dare or as a rite of passage. Kleptomania is strongly associated with Depression, Anxiety Disorders, and Eating Disorders.

Prevalence
Kleptomania appears to be very rare; fewer than five percent of shoplifters have the disorder. However, Kleptomania is usually kept secret by the person, so this estimate may be low. It is much more common among females than males and may continue in spite of convictions for shoplifting.

Treatment Options
Behavior therapy, which is psychotherapy focusing on changing the behavior, has had some success, as has anti-depressant medication. A combination of these is most likely to help the person curb the impulse to steal while treating some of the underlying problems.

PYROMANIA

Symptoms
• Purposefully setting fires more than once;
• Increased tension before the deed;
• Fascination with and curiosity about fire and its paraphernalia;
• Pleasure or relief when setting or watching fires;
• The fire is not set for financial gain, revenge, or political reasons.

Associated Features
Many with this disorder make complicated preparations for setting a fire, and seem not to care about the serious consequences. They may get pleasure from the destruction. Most juveniles who set fires also have symptoms of Attention-Deficit/Hyperactivity Disorder or Adjustment Disorder.

Prevalence
Over forty percent of people arrested for arson in the US are under 18, but among children, the disorder is rare. Fire setting occurs mostly among males, and is more common for males with alcohol problems, learning problems and poor social skills.

Treatment Options
There is no agreed-upon best treatment. Pyromania is difficult to treat because the person usually does not take responsibility for the fire setting, and is in denial. Psychotherapy focused on the individual and with the family have been helpful. There is some indication that antidepressants may be effective.

PATHOLOGICAL GAMBLING

Symptoms
Recurrent gambling;
Gambling distrupts family, personal and work activities;
Preoccupation with gambling, thinking about past plays, planning future gambling and how to get money for more gambling;
Seeks excitement more than money. Bets become bigger and risks greater to produce the needed excitement;
Gambling continues despite repeated efforts to stop with accompanying restlessness and irritability;
Person may gamble to escape depression, anxiety, guilt;
Chasing losses may become a pattern;
May lie to family, therapists, and others to conceal gambling;
May turn to criminal behavior (forgery, fraud, theft) to get money for gambling;
May lose job, relationships, career opportunities;
Bailout behavior, that is turning to family and others, when in desperate financial straits.

Associated Features
Compulsive gamblers are distorted in their thinking. They are superstitious, deny they have a problem, and may be overconfident. They believe that money is the cause of, and solution to, all their problems. They are often competitive and easily bored. They may be extravagantly generous and very concerned with other people's approval. Compulsive gamblers are prone to medical problems connected with stress, such as hypertension and migraine. They also have a higher rate of Attention-Deficit/Hyperactivity Disorder; up to seventy-five percent suffer from Major Depressive Disorder, one third from Bipolar Disorder, and more than fifty percent abuse alcohol. Twenty percent are reported to have attempted suicide.

Prevalence
Gambling takes different forms in different cultures, e.g. cock-fights, horse racing, the stock market. Both males and females can be compulsive gamblers. Men usually begin gambling in adolescence, women somewhat later. Women are more likely to use gambling as an escape from Depression. The prevalence of pathological gambling is high and rising, now including between one percent and three percent of the adult US population.
It is estimated that half of pathological gamblers are women, though women only make up from two percent to four percent of Gamblers Anonymous. Women may not go to treatment programs because of greater stigma attached to women gamblers.

Treatment Options
It is a difficult disorder to treat, but psychotherapy that concretely targets the behavior had limited success.

Gamblers Anonymous, a 12-step program, may enable some to stop gambling. Treatment of the underlying disorders and involving family members may be helpful. It is important to note that, as specified in the American Psychiatric Association's Diagnostic and Statistical Manual of Mental Disorders, a psychiatric diagnosis, includng this one, does not, and is not meant to, exonerate an individual from criminal behavior.

TRICHOTILLOMANIA

Symptoms
Repeated hair pulling so that hair loss is noticeable; Increasing tension just before the behavior or when trying to resist it; Pleasure or relief when pulling; Causes clear distress and problems in personal work, or social functioning.

Associated Features
Examining the hair root, pulling the hair between the teeth, or eating hairs (Trichophagia) may accompany Trichotillomania. Hair pulling is usually done in private or in the presence of close family members. Pain is not usually reported. The hair pulling is mostly denied and concealed by wigs, hairstyling and cosmetics. People with this disorder may also have Major Depressive Disorder, General Anxiety Disorder, Eating Disorder or Mental Retardation.

Prevalence
Among children, both males and females can have the disorder, but among adults, it is far more frequent in females. There are no recent prevalence figures for the general population, but in studies of college students, one percent to two percent have experienced Trichotillomania.

Treatment Options
There is no agreement about the cause of this disorder, making treatment more difficult. Professionals are often not consulted. Variable treatments that have been proposed include behavior therapy, hypnosis, and stress reduction. Medication has sometimes been helpful.

Associations & Agencies

1124 Career Assessment & Planning Services
Goodwill Industries-Suncoast
10596 Gandy Boulevard
PO Box 14456
St. Petersburg, FL 33733
727-523-1512
888-279-1988
Fax: 727-563-9300
E-mail: gw.marketing@goodwill-suncoast.com
www.goodwill-suncoast.org

R Lee Waits, President/CEO
Deborah Passerini, VP Operations

Provides a comprehensive assessment, which can predict current and future employment and potential adjustment factors for physically, emotionally or developmentally disabled persons who may be unemployed or underemployed. Assessments evaluate interests, aptitudes, academic achievements, and physical abilities (including dexterity and coordination) through coordinated testing, interviewing and behavioral observations.

1125 Center for Family Support (CFS)
333 7th Avenue
New York, NY 10001-5004
212-629-7939
Fax: 212-239-2211
www.cfsny.org

Steven Vernickofs, Executive Director

An agency that continues to develop new programs to serve families and individuals with their care needs. Offering services throughout the New York City region including: New Jersey, Long Island and the Lower Hudson Valley.

1126 Center for Mental Health Services Knowledge
PO Box 42557
Washington, DC 20015-4800
800-789-2647
Fax: 240-747-5484
E-mail: ken@mentalhealth.org
www.mentalhealth.samhsa.gov

A Kathryn Power, MEd, Director

Information about resources, technical assistance, research, training, networks, and other federal clearing houses, and fact sheets and materials. Information specialists refer callers to mental health resources in their communities as well as state, federal and nonprofit contacts. Staff available Monday through Friday, 8:30 AM - 5:00 PM, EST, excluding federal holidays. After hours, callers may leave messages and an information specialist will return their call.

1127 Mental Health Matters
PO Box 82149
Kenmore, WA 98028
425-402-6934
E-mail: info@mental-health-matters.com
www.mental-health-matters.com

Founded to supply information and resources to mental health consumers, professionals, students and supporters.

1128 National Association for the Dually Diagnose d (NADD)
132 Fair Street
Kingston, NY 12401-4802
845-334-4336
800-331-5362
Fax: 845-331-4569
E-mail: nadd@mhv.net
www.thenadd.org

Robert Fletcher DSW, Founder/CEO
Donna Nagy PhD, President

Nonprofit organization designed to promote interest of professional and parent development with resources for individuals who have the coexistence of mental illness and mental retardation. Provides conference, educational services and training materials to professionals, parents, concerned citizens and service organizations. Formerly known as the National Association for the Dually Diagnosed.

Year Founded: 1983

1129 National Mental Health Consumer's Self-Help
1211 Chestnut Street
Suite 1207
Philadelphia, PA 19107
215-751-1810
800-553-4539
Fax: 215-636-6312

E-mail: info@mhselfhelp.org
www.mhselfhelp.org

Christine Simiriglia, Executive Director
Jennifer Melinn, Information/Referral Dept.

Funded by the National Institute of Mental Health Community Support Program, the purpose of the Clearinghouse is to encourage the development and growth of consumer self-help groups.

1130 National Mental Health Consumers' Self-Help Clearinghouse
1211 Chestnut Street
Suite 1207
Philadelphia, PA 19107
215-751-1810
800-553-4539
Fax: 215-636-6312
E-mail: info@mhselfhelp.org
www.mhselfhelp.org

Joseph Rogers, Executive Director

A national consumer technical assistance center that has played a major role in the development of the mental health consumer movement.

Year Founded: 1986

1131 SAMHSA's National Mental Health Information Center
US Department of Health and Human Services
PO Box 42557
Washington, DC 20015-4800
240-221-4021
800-789-2647
Fax: 240-221-4295
TDD: 866-889-2647
www.mentalhealth.samhsa.gov

A Kathryn Power, MEd, Director
Edward B Searle, Deputy Director

Provides information about mental health via a toll-free telephone number, this web site, and more than 600 publications. Developed for users of mental health services and their families, the general public, policy makers, providers, and the media.

1132 Suncoast Residential Training Center/Developmental Services Program
Goodwill Industries-Suncoast
10596 Gandy Boulevard
St. Petersburg, FL 33733
727-523-1512
Fax: 727-563-9300
E-mail: gw.marketing@goodwill-suncoast.com
www.goodwill-suncoast.org

R Lee Waits, President/CEO
Deborah A Passerini, VP Operations

A large group home which serves individuals diagnosed as mentally retarded with a secondary diagnosed of psychiatric difficulties as evidenced by problem behavior. Providing residential, behavioral and instructional support and services that will promote the development of adaptive, socially appropriate behavior, each individual is assessed to determine, socialization, basic academics and recreation. The primary intervention strategy is applied behavior analysis. Professional consultants are utilized to address the medical, dental, psychiatric and pharmacological needs of each individual. One of the most popular features is the ac-

tive community integration component of SRTC. Program customers attend an average of 15 monthly outings to various community events.

1133 Trichotillomania Learning Center
207 McPherson Street
Suite H
Santa Cruz, CA 95060
831-457-1004
Fax: 831-426-4383
www.www.trich.org

Nancy Keuthen, PhD, Chairman
Christina Pearson, Executive Director

Works to improve the quality of life of children, adolescents and adults with trichotillomania and related body-focused repetitive disorders such as skin picking through information dissemination, education, outreach, alliance building, and support of research into the causes and treatment of these disorders.

Year Founded: 1991

Books

1134 Angry All the Time
New Harbinger Publications
5674 Shattuck Avenue
Oakland, CA 94609
800-748-6273
Fax: 510-652-5472
E-mail: customerservices@newharbinger.com
www.www.newharbinger.com

An emergency guide for people who have anger control problems. *$12.95*

136 pages

1135 Clinical Manual of Impulse-Control Disorders
American Psychiatric Publishing
1000 Wilson Boulevard
Suite 1825
Arlington, VA 22209-3901
703-907-7322
800-368-5777
Fax: 703-907-1091
E-mail: appi@psych.org
www.www.appi.org

Ron McMillen, CEO
John McDuffie, Editorial Director

Focuses on all of the different impulse-control disorders as a group.

1136 Drug Therapy and Impulse Control Disorders
Mason Crest Publishers
370 Reed Road
Suite 302
Broomall, PA 19008
866-627-2665
Fax: 610-543-3878
www.masoncrest.com

Autumn Libal, Author

The stories and information in this book will tell you more about impulse-control disorders, how they affect people's lives, and how they can be treated. *$24.95*

128 pages ISBN 1-590845-66-0

1137 Dysinhibition Syndrome How to Handle Anger and Rage in Your Child or Spouse
Hope Press
PO Box 188
Duarte, CA 91009-0188
818-303-0644
800-321-4039
Fax: 818-358-3520
www.hopepress.com

How to understand and handle rage and anger in your children or spouse. The book presents behavioral approaches that can be very effective and an understanding that can be family saving. *$24.95*

271 pages ISBN 1-878267-08-6

1138 Impulse Control Disorders: A Clinician's Gui de to Understanding and Treating Behavioral Addictions
W.W. Norton & Company
500 Fifth Avenue
New York, NY 10110
212-354-5500
Fax: 212-869-0856
www.www.wwnorton.com

Jon E Grant, Author

A comprehensive book on impulse control disorders topic for clinicians provides a screening instrument and a detailed method for assessing and treating them.

1139 Impulsivity and Compulsivity
American Psychiatric Publishing
1000 Wilson Boulevard
Suite 1825
Arlington, VA 22209-3901
703-907-7322
800-368-5777
Fax: 703-907-1091
E-mail: appi@psych.org
www.appi.org

Katie Duffy, Marketing Assistant

Leading researchers and clinicians share their expertise on the phenomenological, biological, psychodynamic, and treatment aspects of these disorders. *$40.00*

294 pages ISBN 0-880486-76-7

1140 One Hundred Four Activities That Build
Sunburst Media
2 Skyline Drive
Suite 101
Hawthorne, NY 10532
888-367-6368
Fax: 914-347-1805
E-mail: info@Childswork.com
www.Childswork.com

Full of interactive and fun games that can be used to encourage, modification of behavior, increase interaction with others, start discussions and build other life and social skills. *$23.95*

71 pages

1141 Out of Control: Gambling and Other Impulse-Control Disorders
Chelsea House Publications
132 West 31st Street
17th Floor
New York, NY 10001
800-322-8755
Fax: 800-678-3633
E-mail: custserv@factsonfile.com
www.chelseahouse.infobasepublishing.com

This Encyclopedia of Psychological Disorders provides information on the history, causes and effects of, and treatment and therapies for problems affecting the human mind. *$35.00*

95 pages Year Founded: 2000 ISBN 0-791053-13-X

1142 Pyromania, Kleptomania, and Other Impulse-Control Disorder
Enslow Publishers
40 Industrial Road
Box 398
Berkeley Heights, NJ 07922-0398
908-771-9400
800-398-2504
Fax: 908-771-0925
E-mail: customerservice@enslow.com
www.enslow.com

Julie Williams, Author

Describes the characterisitics of impulsive control disorders, from their early diagnoses and methods of treatment to today's available medications. *$26.60*

128 pages Year Founded: 2002 ISBN 0-766018-99-7

1143 Stop Me Because I Can't Stop Myself: Taking Control of Impulsive Behavior
McGraw-Hill Companies
1221 Avenue of the Americas
New York, NY 10020-1095
212-904-2000
www.www.mcgraw-hill.com

Harold McGraw, III, Chairman/President/CEO
Jon E Grant, Author

Offers the latest research and practical help for those who engage in all types of impulse-related behaviors.

1144 The Anger Control Workbook
New Harbinger Publications
5674 Shattuck Avenue
Oakland Ca, 94
800-748-6273
Fax: 800-652-1613
www.newharbinger.com

Step by step exercises that will aid readers in identifying, understanding, responding to, and ultimately coping with their hostile feelings. *$17.95*

160 pages Year Founded: 2000 ISBN 1-572242-20-5

1145 When Anger Hurts: Quieting The Storm Within
New Harbinger Publications
5674 Shattuck Avenue
Oakland, CA 94609
800-748-6273
Fax: 800-652-1613
www.newharbinger.com

Step by step guide to changing habitual anger-controlled thoughts while developing healthier, more effective ways of meeting your needs. *$16.95*

325 pages Year Founded: 2003 ISBN 1-572243-44-9

1146 Youth with Impulse-Control Disorders: On the Spur of the Moment (Helping Youth with Mental, Physical, & Social Disabilities)
Mason Crest Publishers
370 Reed Road
Suite 302
Broomall, PA 19008
866-621-2665
Fax: 610-543-3878
www.www.masoncrest.com

Kenneth McIntosh, Author
Phyllis Livingston, Author

Support Groups & Hot Lines

1147 Gam-Anon Family Groups
PO Box 157
Whitestone, NY 11357
718-352-1671
Fax: 718-746-2571
www.gam-anon.org

The self-help organization of Gam-Anon is a life saving instrument for the spouse, family or close friends of compulsive gamblers.

1148 Gamblers Anonymous
PO Box 17173
Los Angeles, CA 90017
213-386-8789
Fax: 213-386-0030
E-mail: isomain@gamblersanonymous.org
www.gamblersanonymous.org

Fellowship of men and women who share their experience, strength and hope with each other so that they may solve their common problem and help others recover from a gambling problem.

1149 Trichotillomania Learning Center
207 McPherson Street
Suite H
Santa Cruz, CA 95060-5863
831-457-1004
Fax: 831-426-4383
E-mail: info@trich.org
www.trich.org

Groups of individuals who get together and help one another understand about their disease. Also, they show each other different ways to prevent a attack from happening.

Video & Audio

1150 A Desperate Act
Trichotillomania Learning Center
303 Potrero Street
Suite 51
Santa Cruz, CA 95060
831-457-1004
Fax: 831-426-4383
E-mail: info@trich.org
www.trich.org

A performance artist with TTM discusses her experiences in front of a live audience. 60 minutes.

1151 Our Personal Stories
Trichotillomania Learning Center
303 Potrero Street
Suite 51
Santa Cruz, CA 95060
831-457-1004
Fax: 831-426-4383
E-mail: info@trich.org
www.trich.org

Documentary detailing 8 women's personal experiences with TTM. 90 minutes. *$28.00*

1152 Trichotillomania: Overview and Introduction to HRT
Trichotillomania Learning Center
303 Potrero Street
Suite 51
Santa Cruz, CA 95060
831-457-1004
Fax: 831-426-4383
E-mail: info@trich.org
www.trich.org

A lecture on behavior therapy and Habit reversal Training for TTM. 120 minutes. *$30.00*

Web Sites

1153 www.apa.org/pubinfo/anger.html
Controlling Anger-Before It Controls You

From the American Psychological Association.

1154 www.cfsny.org
Center for Family Support

A not-for-profit human service agency that provides individualized support services and programs for individuals living with developmental and related disabilities, and for the families that care for them at home.

1155 www.cyberpsych.org
CyberPsych

Presents information about psychoanalysis, psychotherapy and special topics such as anxiety disorders, the problematic use of alcohol, homophobia, and the traumatic effects of racism.

1156 www.goodwill-suncoast.org
Suncoast Residential Training Center

Serves individuals diagnosed as mentally retarded with a secondary diagnosis of pychiatric difficulties as evidenced by problem behavior.

1157 www.members.aol.com/AngriesOut
Get Your Angries Out

Guidelines for kids, teachers, and parents.

1158 www.mentalhealth.org
Center for Mental Health Services Knowledge Exchange Network

Information about resources, technical assistance, research, training, networks and other federal clearinghouses, fact sheets and materials.

1159 www.mentalhelp.net/psyhelp/chap7
Anger and Aggression

Therapeutic approaches.

1160 www.mhselfhelp.org
National Mental Health Consumer's Self-Help
Clearinghouse

A national consumer technical assistance center, has played a major role in the development of the mental health consumer movement

1161 www.psychcentral.com
Psych Central

Internet's largest and oldest independent mental health social network created and run by mental health professionals to guarantee reliable, trusted information and support communities to you.

1162 www.stopbitingnails.com
Stop Biting Nails

Online organization created for those who bite their nails. Created a product which is used to prevent nailbiting.

1163 www.thenadd.org
National Association for the Dually Diagnosed

A not-for-profit membership association established for professionals, care providers and families to promote understanding of and services for individuals who have developmental disabilities and mental health needs.

Obsessive Compulsive Disorder

Introduction

Obsessive Compulsive Disorder (OCD) is the diagnosis for individuals who have overwhelming obsessions and/or compulsions. Obsessions are repeated, intrusive, unwanted thoughts that cause distressing emotions such as anxiety or disgust. A person may worry constantly about infection and contamination, or fear that he will engage in embarrassing behavior in public. A compulsion, which often accompanies an obsession, is a ceaseless urge to do something to lessen the anxiety and discomfort caused by the obession, such as handwashing to prevent contamination. People who have obsessions and compulsions often engage in rituals (a highly systematized set of repetitious actions).

Obsessive Compulsive Disorder may be mild or severe: an indvidual may engage in a private ritual that is out of the ordinary, but which does not significantly impede the individual from doing other activites. In more severe cases, the rituals may consume an entire day making normal functioning impossible. Because obsessions and compulsions cause anxiety and make the individual feel powerless, even mild cases can cause significant distress.

A remarkable amount of research is being conducted on OCD, and several treatments (including medication and behavior therapy) are available. The vast majority of patients who are properly treated can live normal lives.

SYMPTOMS

Recurrent and persistent thoughts, impulses or images that are experienced as intrusive and inappropriate and that cause marked anxiety or distress:
• The thoughts or images are not simply excessive worries about real-life problems;
• Repetitive behaviors that the person feels driven to perform in response to an obsession, or according to rules that must be applied rigidly;
• The person recognizes that the obession or compulsions are unreasonable;
• The obsessions or compulsions cause marked distress, are time consuming, or significantly interfere with the person's normal routine, occupational or academic functioning, or usual social activities.

ASSOCIATED FEATURES

The most common obsessions in people with OCD are repeated thoughts about contamination, repeated doubts (for instance about whether one has hurt someone in a traffic accident or left a door unlocked or the stove on) and a need to have things in a particular order. Other common obsessions include concern about aggressive impulses, such as a fear that one will hurt one's child or shout obscenities in a public place. In contrast, individuals with social anxiety disorder worry that others will see them and find them ridiculous even in the normal course of activities, such as eating in a restaurant or making an announcement in a meeting. Also common in OCD are unreasonable fears about one's health, because of contamination or exposure to germs, with repeated visits to the doctor. In contrast, individuals with hypochondria are hypersensitive to a wide range of normal bodily functions and worry that they are symptoms of serious or fatal disease.

The individual with OCD knows that these concerns are un-

reasonable, but feels powerless to stop them. And the individual usually undertakes some kind of ritualistic action to quell the anxieties caused by his or her obsession.

Because of the distress caused by the condition, people with OCD will often avoid situations that trigger the obsession. For instance, a person with a fear of contamination and a compulsion to wash hands may avoid shaking hands with strangers or eating in public restaurants. Performing compulsions can become virtually a full-time task, severely disrupting relationships and impeding the individual's ability to participate in normal life.

PREVALENCE

Although OCD usually begins in adolescence or early adulthood, it may begin in childhood. Age at onset is earlier in males than in females: between the ages of six and 15 years for males and 20 and 29 for females. Symptoms of OCD in children are generally similar to those in adults. Washing, checking, and ordering rituals are particularly common in children. The disorder is equally common in men as in women. Although OCD was once thought to be relatively rare, recent studies have estimated that two and one-half percent of the population may have the disorder.

TREATMENT OPTIONS

Patients with OCD may benefit from behavioral therapy and/or a variety of medications. Currently, one of the most effective treatments is a kind of behavior therapy called exposure and response prevention. Using this therapy, a patient, with a therapist, is carefully exposed to situations that cause anxiety and provoke the obsessive compulsive behavior. Slowly, the patient learns to decrease and later stop the ritualistic behavior altogether. In behavior therapy, a patient must sometimes agree to abide by certain guidelines established by the therapist. For instance, a patient who is a compulsive handwasher might agree to spend no more than ten minutes a day washing. People who are compulsive checkers might agree to check door locks and gas stoves only once a day.
Medications often used for depression have been found to be successful for OCD; these drugs include fluoxetine, fluvoxamine, paroxeatine, sertraline, and clomipramine. In very severe cases, in which the OCD is disabling, brain surgery is an option.

Associations & Agencies

1165 Career Assessment & Planning Services
Goodwill Industries-Suncoast
10596 Gandy Boulevard
St. Petersburg, FL 33733
727-523-1512
Fax: 727-563-9300
E-mail: gw.marketing@goodwill-suncoast.com
www.goodwill-suncoast.org

R Lee Waits, President / CEO
Loreen M Spencer, Chairman

Provides diagnostic services aimed at determining the readiness of individuals for employment and training. In addition to making employment and training recommendations, Goodwill identifies community resources that could improve the quality of life for those who are unprepared for immmediate placement in employment.

1166 Center for Family Support (CFS)
333 7th Avenue
New York, NY 10001-5004
212-629-7939
Fax: 212-239-2211
www.cfsny.org

Steven Vernickofs, Executive Director

An agency that continues to develop new programs to serve families and individuals with their care needs. They currently offer services throughout the New York City region including: New Jersey, Long Island and the Lower Hudson Valley.

1167 National Association for the Dually Diagnose d (NADD)
132 Fair Street
Kingston, NY 12401-4802
845-334-4336
800-331-5362
Fax: 845-331-4569
E-mail: nadd@mhv.net
www.thenadd.org

Dr. Robert Fletcher, Executive Director

Nonprofit organization designed to promote interest of professional and parent development with resources for individuals who have the coexistence of mental illness and mental retardation. Provides conference, educational services and training materials to professionals, parents, concerned citizens and service organizations. Formerly known as the National Association for the Dually Diagnosed.

Year Founded: 1983

1168 National Mental Health Consumer's Self-Help
1211 Chestnut Street
Suite 1207
Philadelphia, PA 19107
215-751-1810
800-553-4539
Fax: 215-636-6312
E-mail: info@mhselfhelp.org
www.mhselfhelp.org

Christine Simiriglia, Executive Director
Jennifer Melinn, Information/Referral Dept.

Funded by the National Institute of Mental Health Community Support Program, the purpose of the Clearinghouse is to encourage the development and growth of consumer self-help groups.

1169 National Mental Health Consumers' Self-Help Clearinghouse
1211 Chestnut Street
Suite 1207
Philadelphia, PA 19107
215-751-1810
800-553-4539
Fax: 215-636-6312
E-mail: info@mhselfhelp.org
www.mhselfhelp.org

Joseph A Rogers, Executive Director

A national consumer technical assistance center that has played a major role in the development of the mental health consumer movement.

Year Founded: 1986

1170 Obsessive Compulsive Anonymous
PO Box 215
New Hyde Park, NY 11040
516-739-0662
E-mail: west24th@aol.com
www.www.hometown.aol.com/west24th

Jim Broatch, Executive Director

National, nonprofit, self help organization consisting of a fellowship of individuals dedicated to sharing their experience, strength and hope with one another to enable them to solve their common problems and help others recover from OCD.

1171 Obsessive Compulsive Foundation
112 Water St
Suite 501
Boston, MA 2109
617-973-5801
Fax: 617-973-5803
E-mail: info@ocfoundation.org
www.ocfoundation.org

Michael Brogioli, Executive Director
Joy Kant, President

For sufferers of obsessive-compulsive disorder and their families and friends. To educate the public and professional communities about OCD and related disorders; to provide assistance to individuals with OCD and related disorders, their family and friends, and to support research into the causes and effective treatments.

1172 Obsessive Compulsive Information Center
Madison Institute of Medicine
7617 Mineral Point Road
Suite 300
Madison, WI 53717-1623
608-827-2470
Fax: 608-827-2479
E-mail: mim@miminc.org
www.miminc.org

Provides information packets, booklets, patient guides, and telephone information services.

Year Founded: 1990

1173 SAMHSA'S National Mental Health Information
PO Box 42557
Washington, DC 20015
800-789-2647
Fax: 240-747-5470
E-mail: ken@mentalhealth.org
www.mentalhealth.samhsa.gov

A Kathryn Power, MEd, Director
Edward B Searle, Deputy Director

Information about resources, technical assistance, research, training, networks, and other federal clearing houses, and fact sheets and materials. Information specialists refer callers to mental health resources in their communities as well as state, federal and nonprofit contacts. Staff available Monday through Friday, 8:30 AM - 5:00 PM, EST, excluding federal holidays. After hours, callers may leave messages and an information specialist will return their call.

1174 SAMHSA's National Mental Health Information Center
US Department of Health and Human Services
PO Box 42557
Washington, DC 20015-4800
240-221-4021
800-789-2647
Fax: 240-221-4295
TDD: 866-889-2647
www.mentalhealth.samhsa.gov

A Kathryn Power, MEd, Director
Edward B Searle, Deputy Director

Provides information about mental health via a toll-free telephone number, this web site, and more than 600 publications. Developed for users of mental health services and their families, the general public, policy makers, providers, and the media.

Books

1175 Boy Who Couldn't Stop Washing
Penguin Group
375 Hudson Street
New York, NY 10014
212-366-2000
800-631-8571
Fax: 201-366-2679
E-mail: online@penguinputnam.com
www.penguinputnam.com

The Boy Who Wouldn't Stop Washing: Experience and Treatment of Obsessive-Compulsive Disorder. A comprehensive treatment of obsessive-compulsive disorder that summarizes evidence that the disorder is neurobiological. It also describes the effect of medication combined with behavioral therapy. *$6.99*

304 pages Year Founded: 1991 ISBN 0-451172-02-7

1176 Brain Lock: Free Yourself from Obsessive Compulsive Behavior
Harper Collins
10 E 53rd Street
New York, NY 10022-5244
212-207-7000
Fax: 800-822-4090
www.harpercollins.com

Brian Murray, Group President
Jeffrey M Schwartz, Author

A simple four-step method for overcoming OCD that is so effective, it's now used in academic treatment centers throughout the world. Proved by brain-imaging tests to actually alter the brain's chemistry, this method dosen't rely on psychopharmaceuticals but cognitive self-therapy and behavior modification to develop new patterns of response. Offers real-life stories of actual patients. Paperback. *$13.00*

256 pages Year Founded: 1997 ISBN 0-060987-11-1

1177 Childhood Obsessive Compulsive Disorder
Sage Publications
2455 Teller Road
Thousand Oaks, CA 91320
805-499-9774
800-818-7243
Fax: 800-583-2665

E-mail: info@sagepub.com
www.sagepub.com

Childhood Obsessive Compulsive Disorder: Developmental Clinical Psychology and Psychiatry. *$21.95*

ISBN 0-803959-22-2

1178 Drug Therapy and Obsessive-Compulsive Disord er
Mason Crest Publishers
370 Reed Road
Suite 302
Broomall, PA 19008
610-543-6200
866-627-2665
Fax: 610-543-3878
E-mail: dtaylor@masoncrest.com
www.masoncrest.com

This volume provides readers with a clear and understandable introduction to obsessive-compulsive disorder (OCD). Numerous case studies are included, which give insight into the world of those who experience this disorder; these anecdotes also help readers understand the symptoms and treatments of this disease. Famous historical figures who suffered from OCD, such as Samuel Johnson (1709-1784) and Howard Hughes (1905-1975) are mentioned as well.

ISBN 1-590845-69-2

1179 Freeing Your Child from Obsessive-Compulsive Disorder: A Powerful, Practical Program for Parents of Children and Adolescents
Crown Publishing Group
1745 Broadway
New York, NY 10019
212-782-9000
Fax: 212-940-7868
E-mail: crownpublicity@randomhouse.com
www.www.randomhouse.com/crown/

Tamar Chansky PhD, Author

It is morning, and here I sit in tears while my daughter Kathy struggles to get dressed for school.

1180 Funny, You Don't Look Crazy: Life With Obsessive Compulsive Disorder
Dilligaf Publishing
64 Court Street
Ellsworth, ME 04605
207-667-5031

An honest look at people who live with Obsessive Compulsive Disorder and those who love them.

128 pages Year Founded: 1994 ISBN 0-963907-00-X

1181 Getting Control: Overcoming Your Obsessions and Compulsions
Penguin Putnam
375 Hudson Street
New York, NY 10014-3658
212-366-2000
800-227-9604
Fax: 201-896-8569
www.penguinputnam.com

Lee Baer, Author

Updated guide to treating OCD based on clinically proven techniques of behavior therapy. Offers a step-by-step program including assessing symptoms, setting realistic goals and creating specific therapeutic exercises. *$13.95*

272 pages Year Founded: 2000 ISBN 0-452281-77-6

1182 Imp of the Mind: Exploring the Silent Epidemic of Obsessive Bad Thoughts
Penguin Putnam
375 Hudson Street
New York, NY 10014-3658
212-366-2000
800-227-9604
Fax: 201-896-8569
www.penguinputnam.com

Draws on new advances to explore the causes of obsessive thoughts, and the difference between harmless and dangerous bad thoughts. *$14.00*

176 pages Year Founded: 2002 ISBN 0-525945-62-8

1183 Let's Talk Facts About Obsessive Compulsive Disorder
American Psychiatric Publishing
1000 Wilson Boulevard
Suite 1825
Arlington, VA 22209-3901
703-907-7322
800-368-5777
Fax: 703-907-1091
E-mail: appi@psych.org
www.appi.org

Katie Duffy, Marketing Assistant
$12.50

8 pages ISBN 0-890423-58-X

1184 OCD Workbook: Your Guide to Breaking Free From Obsessive-Compulsive Disorder
New Harbinger Publications
5674 Shattuck Avenue
Oakland, CA 94609-1662
510-652-2002
800-748-6273
Fax: 510-652-5472
E-mail: customerservice@newharbinger.com
www.newharbinger.com

Bruce Hyman, MD, Author
Cherry Pedrick, RN, Author

Offers the latest information about the neurobiological causes of obsessive-compulsive disorder(OCD), new developments in medication and other treatment options for the disorder, and a new chapter outlining cutting-edge daily coping strategies for sufferers. *$19.95*

198 pages ISBN 1-572244-22-4

1185 OCD in Children and Adolescents: A Cognitive-Behavioral Treatment Manual
Guilford Publications
72 Spring Street
New York, NY 10012
212-431-9800
800-365-7006
Fax: 212-966-6708
E-mail: info@guilford.com
www.guilford.com

Written for clinicians, the book includes tips for parents, and treatment guidelines. The cognitive - behavioral ap-

proach to OCD has been problematic for many to understand because patients with symptoms of increased anxiety are told that their treatment initially involves further increases in their anxiety levels. The authors provide this in a modified and developmentally appropriate approach. *$32.00*

298 pages

1186 Obsessive-Compulsive Disorder Casebook
American Psychiatric Publishing
1000 Wilson Boulevard
Suite 1825
Arlington, VA 22209-3901
703-907-7322
800-368-5777
Fax: 703-907-1091
E-mail: appi@psych.org
www.appi.org

Katie Duffy, Marketing Assistant

Presents 60 case histories of OCD with a discussion by the author and editors regarding their opinion on each diagnosis. *$39.95*

336 pages ISBN 0-880487-29-1

1187 Obsessive-Compulsive Disorder Spectrum
American Psychiatric Publishing
1000 Wilson Boulevard
Suite 1825
Arlington, VA 22209-3901
703-907-7322
800-368-5777
Fax: 703-907-1091
E-mail: appi@psych.org
www.appi.org

Katie Duffy, Marketing Assistant

Comprehensive examination of OCD, related disorders and treatment regimens. *$68.50*

338 pages ISBN 0-880487-07-0

1188 Obsessive-Compulsive Disorder in Children and Adolescents: A Guide
Madison Institute of Medicine
7617 Mineral Point Road
Suite 300
Madison, WI 53717-1623
608-827-2470
Fax: 608-827-2479
E-mail: mim@miminc.org
www.miminc.org

The guide is a comprehensive introduction to obsessive-compulsive disorder for parents who are learning about the illness. Discusses treating symptoms by a combination of behavioral therapy and medication and describes various drugs that can be used with children and adolescents in terms of their effects on brain functioning, symptom control, and side-effects. The book is attuned to the difficulties families of OCD children face. *$5.95*

66 pages ISBN 1-890802-28-X

1189 Obsessive-Compulsive Disorder in Children and Adolescents
American Psychiatric Publishing
1000 Wilson Boulevard
Suite 1825
Arlington, VA 22209-3901

703-907-7322
800-368-5777
Fax: 703-907-1091
E-mail: appi@psych.org
www.appi.org

Katie Duffy, Marketing Assistant

Examines the early development of obsessive - compulsive disorder and describes effective treatments. *$47.50*

360 pages ISBN 0-880482-82-6

1190 Obsessive-Compulsive Disorder: Theory, Research and Treatment
Guilford Publications
72 Spring Street
New York, NY 10012
212-431-9800
800-365-7006
Fax: 212-966-6708
E-mail: info@guilford.com
www.guilford.com

Part I: Psychopathology and Theoretical Perspectives; Part II: Assessment and Treatment; Part III: Obsessive Compulsive Spectrum Disorders; Appendix: List of Resources. *$50.00*

478 pages ISBN 1-572303-35-2

1191 Obsessive-Compulsive Disorders: A Complete Guide to Getting Well and Staying Well
Oxford University Press
198 Madison Avenue
New York, NY 10016
212-726-6000
800-451-7556
Fax: 919-677-1303
www.oup-usa.org

ISBN 0-195140-92-3

1192 Obsessive-Compulsive Disorders: A Complete G uide to Getting Well and Staying Well
Oxford University Press
2001 Evans Road
Cary, NC 27513
800-445-9714
Fax: 919-677-1303
E-mail: custserv.us@oup.com
www.www.oup.com/us

Fred Penzel, Author

In defining obsessive-compulsive disorders (OCDs), our language creates problems, because it treats the terms "obsessive" and "compulsion" very loosely.

1193 Obsessive-Compulsive Disorders: Practical Management
Elsevier
11830 Westline Industrial Drive
Saint Louis, MO 63146
314-453-7010
800-460-3110
Fax: 314-453-7095
www.elsevier.com

Michael A Jenike, MD, Author
Lee Baer, PhD, Author
Wiliam F Minichiello, EdD, Author

Topics include the clinical picture, illnesses relation to obsessive-compulsive disorder, spectrum disorders, patient and clinical management and pathophysiology and assessment. *$73.00*

886 pages Year Founded: 1998 ISBN 0-815138-40-7

1194 Obsessive-Compulsive Disorders: The Latest Assessment and Treatment Strategies
Compact Clinicals
7205 N.W. Waukomis Drive
Kansas City, MI 64151
816-587-0044
800-408-8830
Fax: 816-587-7198
E-mail: customerservice@compactclinicals.com
www.www.compactclinicals.com

Gail Steketee, Author

Previously considered a rare mental condition, obsessive compulsive disorder (OCD) now appears to be a hidden epidemic with over 6.5 million sufferers.

1195 Obsessive-Compulsive Related Disorders
American Psychiatric Publishing
1000 Wilson Boulevard
Suite 1825
Arlington, VA 22209-3901
703-907-7322
800-368-5777
Fax: 703-907-1091
E-mail: appi@psych.org
www.appi.org

Katie Duffy, Marketing Assistant

Discusses the way compulsivity and impulsivity are understood, diagnosed and treated. *$22.50*

286 pages ISBN 0-880484-02-0

1196 Over and Over Again: Understanding Obsessive-Compulsive Disorder
Jossey-Bass/Wiley
111 River Street
Hoboken, NJ 07030-5774
201-748-6000
Fax: 201-748-6088
E-mail: custserv@wiley.com
www.wiley.com

This sensitive and insightful book, the result of the author's years of research and experimentation, is a much needed survival manual for OCD sufferers and the families and friends who share their pain. *$25.00*

240 pages Year Founded: 1997 ISBN 0-787908-76-2

1197 Phobic and Obsessive-Compulsive Disorders: Theory, Research, and Practice
Kluwer Academic/Plenum Publishers
233 Spring Street
New York, NY 10013
212-620-8000
Fax: 212-463-0742
www.kluweronline.com

$80.00

Year Founded: 1990 ISBN 0-306410-44-3

1198 Real Illness: Obsessive-Compulsive Disorder
National Institute of Mental Health
6001 Executive Boulevard
Room 8184
Bethesda, MD 20892-9663
866-615-6464
Fax: 301-443-4279
TTY: 301-443-8431
E-mail: nimhinfo@nih.gov
www.nimh.nih.gov

Do you have disturbing thoughts and behaviors you know don't make sense but that you can't seem to control? This easy brochure explains how to get help.

9 pages

1199 Rewind, Replay, Repeat: A Memoir of Obsessive-Compulsive Disorder
Hazelden Publishing & Educational Services
PO Box 176
Center City, MN 55012-0176
651-213-4200
800-257-7810
Fax: 651-213-4411
E-mail: info@hazelden.org
www.www.hazelden.org

Jeff Bell, Author

The revealing story of one man's struggle with obsessive-compulsive disorder (OCD) and his hard-won recovery.

1200 School Personnel
Obsessive-Compulsive Foundation
676 State Street
New Haven, CT 06535-9573
203-401-2070
Fax: 203-401-2076
E-mail: info@ocfoundation.org
www.ocfoundation.org

Gail B Adams, Author

School Personnel: A Critical Link in the Identification, Treatment and Management of OCD in Children and Adolescents. Recognizing OCD in the school setting, current treatments, the role of school personnel in identification, assessment, and educational interventions, are thoroughly covered in this brief, but informative booklet especially targeted to educators and guidance counselors. *$4.00*

19 pages Year Founded: 1995 ISBN B-0006QK-6V-6

1201 Tormenting Thoughts and Secret Rituals: The Hidden Epidemic of Obsessive-Compulsive Disorder
Random House
1745 Broadway
3rd Floor
New York, NY 10019
212-782-9000
Fax: 212-572-6066
www.randomhouse.com

Discusses the various forms Obsessive-Compulsive Disorder (OCD) takes and, using the most common focuses of obsession, presents detailed cases whose objects are filth, harm, lust, and blasphemy. He explains how the disorder is currently diagnosed and how it differs from addiction, worrying, and preoccupation. He summarizes the recent findings in the areas of brain biology, neuroimaging and

genetics that show OCD to be a distinct chemical disorder of the brain. *$14.95*

336 pages Year Founded: 1999 ISBN 0-440508-47-9

1202 When Once Is Not Enough: Help for Obsessive Compulsives
New Harbinger Publications
5674 Shattuck Avenue
Oakland, CA 94609-1662
510-652-2002
800-748-6273
Fax: 510-652-5472
E-mail: customerservice@newharbinger.com
www.newharbinger.com

Gail Steketee, PhD, Author
Kerrin White, MD, Author

How to recognize and confront fears, using simple rituals, positive coping strategies and handling complications. *$14.95*

229 pages Year Founded: 1990 ISBN 0-934986-87-8

1203 When Perfect Isn't Good Enough: Strategies for Coping with Perfectionism
New Harbinger Publications
5674 Shattuck Avenue
Oakland, CA 94609-1662
510-652-2002
800-748-6273
Fax: 510-652-5472
E-mail: customerservice@newharbinger.com
www.newharbinger.com

Martin Antony, Author
Richard P Swinson, Author

This step by step guide explores the nature of perfectionism and offers a series of exercises to help you challenge unrealistic expectations and work on the specific situations in your life where perfectionism is a problem. *$14.95*

272 pages ISBN 1-572241-24-1

Periodicals & Pamphlets

1204 OCD Newsletter
676 State Street
New Haven, CT 06511
203-401-2070
Fax: 203-401-2076
E-mail: info@ocfoundation.org
www.ocfoundation.org

For sufferers of obsessive-compulsive disorder and their families and friends.

8-12 pages Year Founded: 1986

Support Groups & Hot Lines

1205 Obsessive-Compulsive Anonymous
PO Box 215
New Hyde Park, NY 11040-0910
516-739-0662
Fax: 212-768-4679
www.hometown.aol.com/west24th

Is a fellowship of people who share their Experience, Strength, and Hope with each other that they may solve their common problem and help others to recover from OCD.

1206 Obsessive-Compulsive Foundation
676 State Street
New Haven, CT 06511
203-401-2070
Fax: 203-401-2076
E-mail: info@ocfoundation.org
www.ocfoundation.org

An international not-for-profit organization compsed of people with obsessive compulsive disorder and related disorders, their families, friends, professionals and other concerned indidividuals.

Video & Audio

1207 Hope & Solutions for Obsessive Compulsive Disorder: Part III
Awareness Foundation for OCD
3N374 Limberi Lane
Afocd c/o Gail Adams
Saint Charles, IL 60175-7655
630-513-9234
www.ocawareness.com

An educational psychologist offers educators effective classroom strategies that school personnel may implement with students who have obsessive compulsive disorder and addresses federal law as it pertains to students with disabilities. *$19.95*

1208 Hope and Solutions for OCD
ADD WareHouse
300 NW 70th Avenue
Suite 102
Plantation, FL 33317
954-792-8100
800-233-9273
Fax: 954-792-8545
E-mail: sales@addwarehouse.com
www.addwarehouse.com

Finally, a video series about obsessive compulsive disorder with some straight forward solutions and advice for individuals with OCD, their families, doctors, and school personnel. Viewers will learn what OCD is and how to treat it. Discusses how OCD can affect students in school and the impact on the family life. 85 minutes. *$89.95*

1209 Touching Tree
Obsessive-Compulsive Foundation
676 State Street
New Haven, CT 06511
203-401-2070
Fax: 203-401-2076
E-mail: info@ocfoundation.org
www.ocfoundation.org

This video will foster awareness of early onset obsessive-compulsive disorder (OCD) and demonstrate the symptoms and current therapies that are most successful. Typical ritualistic compulsions of children and adolescents such as touching, hand washing, counting, etc. are explained. *$49.95*

Year Founded: 1993

1210 Understanding and Treating the Hereditary Psychiatric Spectrum Disorders
Hope Press
PO Box 188
Duarte, CA 91009-0188

818-303-0644
800-321-4039
Fax: 818-358-3520
www.hopepress.com

David E Comings MD, Presenter

Learn with ten hours of audio tapes from a two day seminar given in May 1997 by David E Comings MD. Tapes cover: ADHD, Tourette Syndrome, Obsessive-Compulsive Disorder, Conduct Disorder, Oppositional Defiant Disorder, Autism and other Hereditary Psychiatric Spectrum Disorders. Eight audio tapes. *$75.00*

Year Founded: 1997

Web Sites

1211 www.cyberpsych.org
CyberPsych

Presents information about psychoanalysis, psychotherapy and special topics such as anxiety disorders, the problematic use of alcohol, homophobia, and the traumatic effects of racism.

1212 www.fairlite.com/ocd/
OCD Web Server

Abstracts found from the University of Kentucky's Medical Library. Information on medications taken directly from the manufacturers' brochures.

1213 www.interlog.com/~calex/ocd
Obsessive-Compulsive Disorder Web Sites

List of links.

1214 www.lexington-on-line.com/
Obsessive-Compulsive Disorder

A five page explanation.

1215 www.mayoclinic.com
Mayo Clinic

Provides information on obsessive-compulsive disorder.

1216 www.nimh.nih.gov/anxiety/anxiety/ocd
National Institute of Health

Information on anxiety disorders and OCD.

1217 www.nimh.nih.gov/publicat/ocdmenu.cfm
Obsessive-Compulsive Disorder

Introductory handout with treatment recommendations.

1218 www.nursece.com/OCD.htm
Obsessive Compulsive Disorder

Features and treatments.

1219 www.ocdhope.com/gdlines.htm
Guidelines for Families Coping with OCD

1220 www.ocfoundation.org
Obsessive-Compulsive Foundation

An international not-for-profit organization composed of people with obsessive compulsive disorder and related disorders, their families, friends, professionals and other concerned individuals.

1221 www.planetpsych.com
Planetpsych.com

Online source for mental health information.

1222 www.psychcentral.com
Psych Central

The Internet's largest and oldest independent mental health social network created and run by mental health professionals to guarantee reliable, trusted information and support communities to you.

Paraphilias (Perversions)

Introduction

Paraphilias are sexual disorders or perversions in which sexual intercourse is not the desired goal. Instead, the desire is to use non-human objects or non-sexual body parts for sexual activities sometimes involving the suffering of, or inflicting pain onto, non-consenting partners.

SYMPTOMS

• Recurrent, intense, sexually arousing fantasies, urges, or behavior involving the particular perversion for at least six months;
• The fantasies, urges, or behavior cause distress and/or disruption in the person's functioning in social, work, and interpersonal areas.
There are eight Paraphilias, described below, categorized as either victimless, or as victimizing someone who has not consented to the sexual activity, with relevant associated features.

Exhibitionism

The exposure of the genitals to a stranger or group of strangers. Sometimes the paraphiliac masturbates during exposure. The onset of this disorder usually occurs before age 18 and becomes less severe after age 40.

Fetishism

Using non-living objects, known as fetishes, for sexual gratification. Objects commonly used by men with the disorder include women's underwear, shoes, or other articles of women's clothing. The person often masturbates while holding, rubbing, or smelling the fetish object. This disorder usually begins in adolescence; it is chronic and often lifelong.

Frotteurism

Sexual arousal, and sometimes masturbation to orgasm, while rubbing against a non-consenting person. The behavior is usually planned to occur in a crowded place, such as on a bus, subway, or in a swimming pool, where detection is less likely. Frotteurism usually begins in adolescence, is most frequent between the ages of 15 and 25, then gradually declines.

Pedophilia

Sexual Activity with a prepubertal child, generally 13 years or younger. The pedophiliac, him or herself, must be at least 16 and at least five years older than his victim when the behavior occurs. Pedophiliacs are usually attracted to children in one particular age range.
The frequency of the behavior may be associated with the degree of stress in the person's life. It usually begins in adolescence and is chronic. Pedophiles may be married, but have a higher than average incidence of severe marital discord.

Sexual Masochism

Acts of being bound, beaten, humiliated, or made to suffer in some other way in order to become sexually aroused. The behaviors can be self-inflicted or performed with a partner, and include physical bondage, blindfolding and humiliation. Masochistic sexual fantasies are likely to have been present since childhood. The activities themselves begin at different times but are common by early adulthood; they are usually chronic. The severity of the behaviors may increase over time.

Sexual Sadism

Acts in which the person becomes sexually excited through the physical or psychological suffering of someone else. Some Sexual Sadists may conjure up the sadistic fantasies during sexual activity without acting on them. Others act on their sadistic urges with a consenting partner (who may be a Sexual Masochist), or act on their urges with a non-consenting partner. The behavior may involve forcing the other person to crawl, be caged or tortured. Sdistic sexual fantasies are likely to have been present in childhood. The onset of the behavior varies but most commonly occurs by early adulthood. The disorder is usually chronic. The severity of the sadistic acts tends to increase over time. When the disorder is severe or coupled with Antisocial Personality Disorder, the person is likely to seriously injure or kill his victim.

Transvestic Fetishism

consists of heterosexual males dressing in women's clothes and makeup then masturbating. When not cross dressed, the man looks like an ordinary masculine man. It is important to note that there is considerable controversy over this diagnosis; some people who cross dress seem to have little distress and function normally. This condition typically begins in childhood or adolescence. Often the cross dressing is not done publicly until adulthood.

Voyeurism

Peeping Tom disorder, involving the act of observing one or more unsuspecting persons (usually strangers) who are naked, in the process of undressing, or engaged in sexual activity, in order for the voyeur to become sexually excited. Sexual activity with the people being observed is not usually sought. The voyeur may masturbate during the observation or later. The onset of this disorder is usually before age 15. It tends to be chronic.

PREVALENCE

Paraphiliacs are almost exclusively male. Very few volunteer to disclose their activities or to seek treatment. It is estimated that most have deficits in interpersonal or sexual relationships. In one study, two thirds were diagnosed with Mood Disorders and fifty percent had alcohol or drug abuse problems.

Recent studies provide evidence that the great majority of Paraphiliacs are active in more than one form of sexually perverse behavior; less than ten percent have only one form; and thirty-eight percent engage in five or more different sexually deviant behaviors. In a survey of college students, it was found that young males often fantasize about forced sex, and almost half have engaged in some form of sexual misconduct or sexual behavior with someone younger than age 14.

At the same time, the incidence and prevalence of some sexual perversions are hard to estimate, or unknown, because they are rarely reported or the people involved do not come into contact with the authorities or the health care system.

TREATMENT OPTIONS

All the Paraphilias are difficult to treat. It is important for the professional making the diagnosis to take a very careful history, and to be sensitive to the presence of other, e.g., personality, disorders. Relapse is common.

Diagnostic techniques can be useful. Penile plethysmography measures the degree of penile erection while the individual is exposed to visual sexual stimuli. Some people are treated in a formal Sex Offenders Program, developed for individuals arrested for and convicted of paraphilias that are crimes. Sometimes treatment occurs within the context of individual therapy where trust can be established. Others have been treated by means of conditioning techniques, e.g., where a fetish object is paired with an aversive stimulus such as mild electric shock. Medication is also used. Pedophilia is sometimes treated through so-called chemocastration which, through the use of female hormones or other medications, diminishes sexual appetite.

Treatment can be difficult because it is associated with the risk of reporting and punishment; many individuals do not have any real interest in being treated. They may deliberately deceive the professional, or deny the problem. Sex offenders are also more likely to exaggerate treatment gains, resist treatment, or end treatment prematurely.

The fact that these conditions are classified as mental disorders does not relieve individuals who violate laws of criminal responsibility.

Associations & Agencies

1224 Center for Family Support (CFS)
333 7th Avenue
New York, NY 10001-5004
212-629-7939
Fax: 212-239-2211
www.cfsny.org

Steven Vernickofs, Executive Director

An agency that continues to develop new programs to serve families and individuals with their care needs. They currently offer services throughout the New York City region including: New Jersey, Long Island and the Lower Hudson Valley.

1225 National Association for the Dually Diagnose d (NADD)
132 Fair Street
Kingston, NY 12401-4802
845-334-4336
800-331-5362
Fax: 845-331-4569
E-mail: nadd@mhv.net
www.thenadd.org

Dr. Robert Fletcher, Executive Director

Nonprofit organization designed to promote interest of professional and parent development with resources for individuals who have the coexistence of mental illness and mental retardation. Provides conference, educational services and training materials to professionals, parents, concerned citizens and service organizations. Formerly known as the National Association for the Dually Diagnosed.

Year Founded: 1983

1226 National Mental Health Consumer's Self-Help
1211 Chestnut Street
Suite 1207
Philadelphia, PA 19107
215-751-1810
800-553-4539

Fax: 215-636-6312
E-mail: info@mhselfhelp.org
www.mhselfhelp.org

Christine Simiriglia, Executive Director
Jennifer Melinn, Information/Referral Dept.

Funded by the National Institute of Mental Health Community Support Program, the purpose of the Clearinghouse is to encourage the development and growth of consumer self-help groups.

1227 National Mental Health Consumers' Self-Help Clearinghouse
1211 Chestnut Street
Suite 1207
Philadelphia, PA 19107
215-751-1810
800-553-4539
Fax: 215-636-6312
E-mail: info@mhselfhelp.org
www.mhselfhelp.org

Joseph A Rogers, Executive Director

A national consumer technical assistance center that has played a major role in the development of the mental health consumer movement.

Year Founded: 1986

1228 SAMHSA'S National Mental Health Information
PO Box 42557
Washington, DC 20015
800-789-2647
Fax: 204-747-5470
E-mail: ken@mentalhealth.org
www.mentalhealth.samhsa.gov

A Kathryn Power, MEd, Director
Edward B Searle, Deputy Director

Information about resources, technical assistance, research, training, networks, and other federal clearing houses, and fact sheets and materials. Information specialists refer callers to mental health resources in their communities as well as state, federal and nonprofit contacts. Staff available Monday through Friday, 8:30 AM - 5:00 PM, EST, excluding federal holidays. After hours, callers may leave messages and an information specialist will return their call.

1229 SAMHSA's National Mental Health Information Center
US Department of Health and Human Services
PO Box 42557
Washington, DC 20015-4800
240-221-4021
800-789-2647
Fax: 240-221-4295
TDD: 866-889-2647
www.mentalhealth.samhsa.gov

A Kathryn Power, MEd, Director
Edward B Searle, Deputy Director

Provides information about mental health via a toll-free telephone number, this web site, and more than 600 publications. Developed for users of mental health services and their families, the general public, policy makers, providers, and the media.

Books

1230 Perversion (Ideas in Psychoanalysis)
National Book Network
4501 Forbes Boulevard
Suite 200
Lanham, MD 20706
301-459-3366
800-462-6420
Fax: 301-429-5746
www.www.nbnbooks.com

Jed Lyons, President
Claire Pajaczkowska, Author

Perversion's relationship to feelings of contempt, triumph, sexual excitement and to shame, revulsion and fear, necessarily make it a troubling concept.

1231 The World of Perversion: Psychoanalysis and the Impossible Absolute of Desire
State University of New York Press
194 Washington Avenue
Suite 305
Albany, NY 12210-2384
518-472-5000
Fax: 518-472-5038
E-mail: info@sunypress.edu
www.www.sunypress.edu

Gary Dunham, Executive Director
James Penney, Author

An original critique of queer theory, from a psychoanalysis perspective.

Web Sites

1232 www.mentalhealth.com
Internet Mental Health

Website offers psychiatric diagnosis in the hope of reaching the two-thirds of individuals with mental illness who do not seek treatment.

1233 www.planetpsych.com
Planetpsych.com

The online resource for mental health information.

1234 www.psychcentral.com
Psych Central

The Internet's largest and oldest independent mental health social network created and run by mental health professionals to guarantee reliable, trusted information and support communities to you.

Personality Disorders

Introduction

Personality is deeply rooted in our sense of ourselves and how others see us; it is formed from a complex interminling of genetic factors and life experience. Everyone has personality characteristics that are likable and unlikable, attractive and unattractive, to others. By adulthood, most of us have personality traits that are difficult to change. Sometimes, these deeply rooted personality traits can get in the way of our happiness, hinder relationships, and even cause harm to ourselves or others.

For example, a person may have a tendency to be deeply suspicious of other people with no good reason. Another person may assume a haughty, arrogant manner that is difficult to be around. Personality Disorders, by definition, do not cause symptoms, which are experiences that are troublesome to the individual. They consist of whole sets of distorted experiences of the outside world that pervade every or nearly every aspect of a person's life, causing traits and behaviors leading to interpersonal problems which only secondarily cause distress to the individual. The problem is blamed on other people. For example, people with dependent personality disorder feel that they need more care and protection than others, not that they are inordinately demanding of care and protection. People with narcissistic personality disorder feel that others do not respect them, not that they demand more attention and admiration than others; people with paranoid personality disorder feel that othersare out to trick and cheat them, not that they are inordinately suspicious; people with obsessive personality disorder feel that others are sloppy, not that they are overly preoccupied with order and tidiness.

A diagnosis of a Personality Disorder should be distinguished from labeling someone as a bad or disagreeable person and not be used to stigmitize people who are simply unpopular, rebellious or otherwise unorthodox. A personality disorder is not simply a personality style, but a condition that interferes with successful living. A Personality Disorder refers to an enduring pattern or experience and behavior that is inflexible, long lasting (often beginning in adolescence or early childhood) and which leads to distress and impairment. Ten distinct personality disorders have been identified:
- Paranoid Personality Disorder;
- Schiziod Personality Disorder;
- Schizotypal Personality Disorder;
- Antisocial Personality Disorder;
- Borderline Personality Disorder;
- Histrionic Personality Disorder;
- Narcissistic Personality Disorder;
- Avoidant Personality Disorder;
- Dependent Personality Disorder;
- Obsessive-Compulsive Personality Disorder.

SYMPTOMS

An enduring pattern of inner experience and behavior that deviates markedly from the expectations of the individual's culture:
- This pattern is manifested in two or more of the following areas: cognition, affectivity, interpersonal functioning, and impulse control;
- The enduring pattern is inflexible and pervasive across a broad range of personal and social situations;
- The enduring pattern leads to clinically significant distress or impairment in social, occupational, or other important areas of functioning;
- The pattern is stable and of long duration and its onset can be traced back at least to adolescence or early adulthood;
- The enduring pattern is not better accounted for as a manifestation or consequence of another mental disorder;
- The enduring pattern is not due to the direct physiological effects of a substance or a general medical condition.

TREATMENT OPTIONS

Most people who suffer from a Personality Disorder do not see themselves as having psychological problems, and therefore do not seek treatment. For those who do, the most effective treatment is long-term (at least one year) psychotherapy. People with Personality Disorders generally seek treatment only because they are distressed that others do not behave as patients think they should, or because the patients' behaviors cause them to have significant problems with employment and relationships. It is important for a patient to find a mental health professional with expert knowledge and experience in treating personality disorders. Some therapists specialize in treating Borderline Personality Disorder and use a treatment called Dialectal Behavioral Therapy. Antisocial Personality Disorder is notably difficult to treat, especially in extreme cases, when the affected individual lacks all concern for others.

Psychotherapy encourages patients to talk about their suspicions, doubts and other personality traits that have a negative impact on their lives, and therefore helps to improve social interactions.

Psychotherapeutic treatment should include attention to family members, stressing the importance of emotional support, reassurance, explanation of the disorder, and advice on how to manage and respond to the patient. Group therapy is helpful in many situations.

Antipsychotic medication can be useful in patients with certain Personality Disorders, specifically Schizotypal and Borderline Disorders.

Associations & Agencies

1236 Career Assessment & Planning Services
Goodwill Industries-Suncoast
10596 Gandy Boulevard
St. Petersburg, FL 33702
727-523-1512
888-279-1988
Fax: 727-563-9300
E-mail: gw.marketing@goodwill-suncoast.org
www.goodwill-suncoast.org

Chris Ward, Marketing Media Manager
R Lee Waits, President/CEO

Provides a comprehensive assessment, which can predict current and future employment and potential adjustment factors for physically, emotionally, or developmentally disabled persons who may be unemployed or underemployed. Assessments evaluate interests, aptitudes, academic achievements, and physical abilities (including dexterity and coordination) through coordinated testing, interviewing and behavioral observations.

1237 Center for Family Support (CFS)

333 7th Avenue
New York, NY 10001-5004
212-629-7939
Fax: 212-239-2211
www.cfsny.org

Steven Vernickofs, Executive Director

An agency that continues to develop new programs to serve families and individuals with their care needs. They currently offer services throughout the New York City region including: New Jersey, Long Island and the Lower Hudson Valley.

1238 National Alliance on Mental Illness

2107 Wilson Boulevard
Suite 300
Arlington, VA 22201-3042
703-524-7600
800-950-6264
Fax: 703-524-9094
E-mail: info@nami.org
www.nami.org

Suzanne Vogel-Scibilia, MD, President
Frederick Sandoval, First VP

Nation's leading self-help organization for all those affected by severe brain disorders. Mission is to bring consumers and families with similar experiences together to share information about services, care providers, and ways to cope with the challenges of schizophrenia, manic depression, and other serious mental illnesses.

Year Founded: 1979

1239 National Association for the Dually Diagnose d (NADD)

132 Fair Street
Kingston, NY 12401-4802
845-334-4336
800-331-5362
Fax: 845-331-4569
E-mail: nadd@mhv.net
www.thenadd.org

Dr. Robert Fletcher, Executive Director

Nonprofit organization designed to promote interest of professional and parent development with resources for individuals who have the coexistence of mental illness and mental retardation. Provides conference, educational services and training materials to professionals, parents, concerned citizens and service organizations. Formerly known as the National Association for the Dually Diagnosed.

Year Founded: 1983

1240 National Mental Health Consumer's Self-Help

1211 Chestnut Street
Suite 1207
Philadelphia, PA 19107
215-751-1810
800-553-4539
Fax: 215-636-6312
E-mail: info@mhselfhelp.org
www.mhselfhelp.org

Christine Simiriglia, Executive Director
Jennifer Melinn, Information/Referral Dept.

Funded by the National Institute of Mental Health Community Support Program, the purpose of the Clearinghouse is to encourage the development and growth of consumer self-help groups.

1241 National Mental Health Consumers' Self-Help Clearinghouse

1211 Chestnut Street
Suite 1207
Philadelphia, PA 19107
215-751-1810
800-553-4539
Fax: 215-636-6312
E-mail: info@mhselfhelp.org
www.mhselfhelp.org

Joseph A Rogers, Executive Director

A national consumer technical assistance center that has played a major role in the development of the mental health consumer movement.

Year Founded: 1986

1242 SAMHSA'S National Mental Health Information

PO Box 42557
Washington, DC 20015
800-789-2647
Fax: 240-747-5470
E-mail: ken@mentalhealth.org
www.mentalhealth.smahsa.gov

A Kathryn Power, MEd, Director
Edward B Searle, Deputy Director

Information about resources, technical assistance, research, training, networks, and other federal clearing houses, and fact sheets and materials. Information specialists refer callers to mental health resources in their communities as well as state, federal and nonprofit contacts. Staff available Monday through Friday, 8:30 AM - 5:00 PM, EST, excluding federal holidays. After hours, callers may leave messages and an information specialist will return their call.

1243 SAMHSA's National Mental Health Information Center
US Department of Health and Human Services

PO Box 42557
Washington, DC 20015-4800
240-221-4021
800-789-2647
Fax: 240-221-4295
TDD: 866-889-2647
www.mentalhealth.samhsa.gov

A Kathryn Power, MEd, Director
Edward B Searle, Deputy Director

Provides information about mental health via a toll-free telephone number, this web site, and more than 600 publications. Developed for users of mental health services and their families, the general public, policy makers, providers, and the media.

1244 Suncoast Residential Training Center/Developmental Services Program
Goodwill Industries-Suncoast

10596 Gandy Boulevard
PO Box 14456
St. Petersburg, FL 33702
727-523-1512
Fax: 727-563-9300

E-mail: gw.marketing@goodwill-suncoast.org
www.goodwill-suncoast.org
R Lee Waits, President/CEO
Deborah A Passerini, VPÆOperations

A large group home which serves individuals diagnosed as mentally retarded with a secondary diagnosed of psychiatric difficulties as evidenced by problem behavior. Providing residential, behavioral and instructional support and services that will promote the development of adaptive, socially appropriate behavior, each individual is assessed to determine, socialization, basic academics and recreation. The primary intervention strategy is applied behavior analysis. Professional consultants are utilized to address the medical, dental, psychiatric and pharmacological needs of ech individual. One of the most popular features is the active community integration component of SRTC. Program customers attend an average of 15 monthly outings to various community events.

Books

1245 Angry Heart: Overcoming Borderline and Addictive Disorders
New Harbinger Publications
5674 Shattuck Avenue
Oakland, CA 94609-1662
510-652-2002
800-748-6273
Fax: 510-652-5472
E-mail: customerservice@newharbinger.com
www.newharbinger.com

Joseph Santoro, PhD, Author
Ronald Cohen, PhD, Author

This self help guide uses a variety of exercises and step by step techniques to help individuals with borderline and addictive disorders come to terms with their destructive lifestyle and take steps to break out of its dysfunctional cycle of self defeating thoughts and behavior. *$15.95*

272 pages Year Founded: 1997 ISBN 1-572240-80-6

1246 Assess Dialogue Personality Disorders
Cambridge University Press
40 W 20th Street
New York, NY 10011-4221
212-924-3900
Fax: 212-691-3239
E-mail: information@cup.org
www.cup.org

Cambridge University Press is the printing and publishing house of the University of Cambridge. It is an integral part of the University and is devoted constitutionally to printing and publishing for 'the acquisition, advancement, conservation, and dissemination of knowledge in all subjects'. As such, it is a charitable, not-for-profit organization, free from tax worldwide.

1247 Biology of Personality Disorders, Review of Psychiatry
American Psychiatric Publishing
1000 Wilson Boulevard
Suite 1825
Arlington, VA 22209-3901
703-907-7322
800-368-5777
Fax: 703-907-1091

E-mail: appi@psych.org
www.appi.org
Katie Duffy, Marketing Assistant

Contents include neurotransmitter function in personality disorders, new biological research strategies for personality disorders, genetics and psychobiology of seven - factor model of personality, psychopharmacological management, and significance of biological research for a biopsychosocial model of personality disorders. *$25.00*

166 pages ISBN 0-880488-35-2

1248 Borderline Personality Disorder
American Psychiatric Publishing
1000 Wilson Boulevard
Suite 1825
Arlington, VA 22209-3901
703-907-7322
800-368-5777
Fax: 703-907-1091
E-mail: appi@psych.org
www.appi.org
Katie Duffy, Marketing Assistant

Guide to the diagnosis and treatment of borderline personality disorder. *$34.00*

256 pages ISBN 0-880486-89-9

1249 Borderline Personality Disorder: Multidimensional Approach
American Psychiatric Publishing
1000 Wilson Boulevard
Suite 1825
Arlington, VA 22209-3901
703-907-7322
800-368-5777
Fax: 703-907-1091
E-mail: appi@psych.org
www.appi.org
Katie Duffy, Marketing Assistant

Practical approach to the management of patients with BPD. *$33.00*

288 pages ISBN 0-880486-55-4

1250 Borderline Personality Disorder: A Patient's Guide to Taking Control
WW Norton & Company
500 5th Avenue
New York, NY 10110-0017
212-354-5500
800-233-4830
E-mail: npb@wwnorton.com
www.wwnorton.com/psych

The Patient's Guide is your clients' means to begin to take command of their lives by following the therapeutic course described in these books. Provides a step-by-step cognitive program wich in worksheets and exercises to facilitate your clients' personal process of self-examination and problem solving.

ISBN 0-393703-53-3

1251 Borderline Personality Disorder: Etiology and Treatment
American Psychiatric Publishing
1000 Wilson Boulevard
Suite 1825
Arlington, VA 22209-3901
703-907-7322
800-368-5777
Fax: 703-907-1091
E-mail: appi@psych.org
www.appi.org

Katie Duffy, Marketing Assistant

Provides empirical data as the basis for progress in understanding and treating the borderline patient. *$50.00*

420 pages ISBN 0-880484-08-X

1252 Borderline Personality Disorder: Tailoring the Psychotherapy to the Patient
American Psychiatric Publishing
1000 Wilson Boulevard
Suite 1825
Arlington, VA 22209-3901
703-907-7322
800-368-5777
Fax: 703-907-1091
E-mail: appi@psych.org
www.appi.org

Katie Duffy, Marketing Assistant

Emphasizes how the clinician should decide between the use of supportive as opposed to expressive techniques, depending upon the characteristics of the patient. *$34.00*

256 pages ISBN 0-880486-89-9

1253 Challenging Behavior
Cambridge University Press
40 W 20th Street
New York, NY 10011-4221
212-924-3900
Fax: 212-691-3239
E-mail: marketing@cup.org
www.cup.org

1254 Clinical Assessment and Management of Severe Personality Disorders
American Psychiatric Publishing
1000 Wilson Boulevard
Suite 1825
Arlington, VA 22209-3901
703-907-7322
800-368-5777
Fax: 703-907-1091
E-mail: appi@psych.org
www.appi.org

Katie Duffy, Marketing Assistant

Focuses on issues relevant to the clinician in private practice, including the diagnosis of a wide range of personality disorders and alternative management approaches. *$33.00*

260 pages ISBN 0-880484-88-8

1255 Cognitive Analytic Therapy & Borderline Personality Disorder: Model and the Method
John Wiley & Sons
1 Wiley Drive
Somerset, NJ 08873

732-469-4400
800-225-5945
Fax: 732-302-2300
E-mail: compbks@wiley.com
www.wiley.com

Anthony Ryle, Author

This book documents CAT's recent theoretical and practical developments is a must for anyone interested in CAT itself and in integrative approaches, for those interested in brief, psychodynamically informed therapy, or indeed for those interested in developments in psychology generally. *$70.00*

206 pages Year Founded: 1997 ISBN 0-471976-18-0

1256 Cognitive Therapy of Personality Disorders, Second Edition
The Guilford Press
72 Spring Street
New York, NY 10012
800-365-7006
Fax: 212-966-6708
E-mail: info@guilford.com
www.www.guilford.com

Robert Matloff, President
Aaron T Beck, Author

Presents a cognitive framework for understanding and treating personality disorders.

1257 Developmental Model of Borderline Personality Disorder: Understanding Variations in Course and Outcome
American Psychiatric Publishing
1000 Wilson Boulevard
Suite 1825
Arlington, VA 22209-3901
703-907-7322
800-368-5777
Fax: 703-907-1091
E-mail: appi@psych.org
www.appi.org

Landmark work on this difficult condition. Emphasizes a developmental approach to BPD based on treatment of inpatients at Chestnut Lodge in Rockville, Maryland, during the years through 1975. Using information gleaned from the original clinical notes and follow-up studies, the authors present four intriguing case studies to chart the etiology, long-term course, and clinical manifestations of BPD. *$34.95*

256 pages Year Founded: 2002 ISBN 0-880485-15-9

1258 Disordered Personalities
Rapid Psychler Press
3560 Pine Grove Avenue
Suite 374
Port Huron, MI 48060
519-667-2335
888-779-2453
Fax: 888-779-2457
E-mail: rapid@psychler.com
www.psychler.com

David Robinson, MD, Publisher

Provides a comprehensive, practical and entertaining overview of the DSM-IV personality disorders. The diagnostic, theoretical and therapeutic principles relevant to understanding character pathology are detailed in the introductory chapters. *$39.95*

428 pages Year Founded: 2005 ISBN 1-894328-09-4

1259 Disorders of Narcissism: Diagnostic, Clinical, and Empirical Implications
American Psychiatric Publishing
1000 Wilson Boulevard
Suite 1825
Arlington, VA 22209-3901
703-907-7322
800-368-5777
Fax: 703-907-1091
E-mail: appi@psych.org
www.appi.org

Katie Duffy, Marketing Assistant

Addresses important subjects at the forefront of the study of narcissism, including cognitive treatment, normal narcissism, pathological narcissism and suicide, and the connection between pathological narcissism, trauma, and alexithymia. *$42.50*

304 pages ISBN 0-880487-01-1

1260 Drug Therapy and Personality Disorders
Mason Crest Publishers
370 Reed Road
Suite 302
Broomall, PA 19008
610-543-6200
866-627-2665
Fax: 610-543-3878
E-mail: dtaylor@masoncrest.com
www.masoncrest.com

This volume in the series explains the origins, symptoms and treatments of those personality disorders that can benefit from the use of psychiatric medications, including avoidant, paranoid, schizoid, schizotypal, obsessive-compulsive and borderline personality disorders. Case studies and examples of individuals with personality disorders are included to help readers gain a more complete understanding of how these disorders affect actual people.

ISBN 1-590845-71-4

1261 Fatal Flaws: Navigating Destructive Relationships with People with Disorders
American Psychiatric Publishing
1000 Wilson Boulevard
Suite 1825
Arlington, VA 22209-3901
703-907-7322
800-368-5777
Fax: 703-907-1091
E-mail: appi@psych.org
www.www.appi.org

Ron McMillen, CEO
Stuart C Yudofsky, Author

Featuring case vignettes from nearly 30 years of Dr. Yudofsky's clinical practice and incorporating the knowledge of gifted clinicians, educators, and research scientists with whom he has collaborated throughout that time.

1262 Field Guide to Personality Disorders
Rapid Psychler Press
3560 Pine Grove Avenue
Suite 374
Port Huron, MI 48060
519-667-2335
888-779-2453
Fax: 888-779-2457
E-mail: rapid@psychler.com
www.psychler.com

David Robinson, MD, Publisher

Provides a practical, comprehensive and enjoyable introduction to the DSM-IV-TR personality disorders. Diagnostic, theoretical and therapeutic principles are covered in detail, providing a basis for understanding character pathology. *$19.95*

212 pages Year Founded: 2005 ISBN 1-894328-10-8

1263 Lost in the Mirror: An Inside Look at Borderline Personality Disorder
Sidran Institute
200 E Joppa Road
Suite 207
Baltimore, MD 21286
410-825-8888
888-825-8249
Fax: 410-337-0747
E-mail: sidran@sidran.org
www.sidran.org

Esther Giller, President/CEO
J G Goellner, Director Emertius
Stanley Platman, MD, Medical Advisor
Richard Moskovitz, MD, Author

Dr. Moskovitz considers BPD to be part of the dissociative continuum, as it has many causes, symptoms and behaviors in common with Dissociative Disorder. This book is intended for people diagnosed with BPD, their families and therapists. Outlines the features of BPD, including abuse histories, dissociation, mood swings, self harm, impulse control problems and many more. Includes an extensive resource section. *$13.95*

190 pages

1264 Management of Countertransference with Borderline Patients
American Psychiatric Publishing
1000 Wilson Boulevard
Suite 1825
Arlington, VA 22209-3901
703-907-7322
800-368-5777
Fax: 703-907-1091
E-mail: appi@psych.org
www.appi.org

Katie Duffy, Marketing Assistant

Open and detailed discussion of the emotional reactions that clinicians experience when treating borderline patients. *$34.50*

254 pages ISBN 0-880785-63-9

1265 Personality Disorders in Modern Life
John Wiley & Sons
111 River Street
Hoboken, NJ 07030-5774

201-748-6000
Fax: 201-748-6088
E-mail: info@wiley.com
www.www.wiley.com

William J Pesce, President/CEO

Exploring the continuum from normal personality tests to the diagnosis amd treatment of severe cases of personality disorders.

1266 Personality and Psychopathology
American Psychiatric Publishing
1000 Wilson Boulevard
Suite 1825
Arlington, VA 22093-901
703-907-7322
800-368-5777
Fax: 703-907-1091
E-mail: appi@psych.org
www.appi.org

Katie Duffy, Marketing Assistant

Compiles the most recent findings from more than 30 internationally recognized experts. Analyzes the association between personality and psychopathology from several interlocking perspective, descriptive, developmental, etiological, and therapeutic. *$58.50*

496 pages ISBN 0-880489-23-5

1267 Role of Sexual Abuse in the Etiology of Borderline Personality Disorder
American Psychiatric Publishing
1000 Wilson Boulevard
Suite 1825
Arlington, VA 22209-3901
703-907-7322
800-368-5777
Fax: 703-907-1091
E-mail: appi@psych.org
www.appi.org

James Scully, MD, President
Mary C Zanarini, EdD, Editor

Presenting the latest generation of research findings about the impact of traumatic abuse on the development of BPD. This book focuses on the theoretical basis of BPD, including topics such as childhood factors associated with the development, the relationship of child sexual abuse to dissociation and self-mutilation, severity of childhood abuse, borderline symptoms and family environment. Twenty six contributors cover every aspect of BPD as it relates to childhood sexual abuse. *$65.00*

264 pages Year Founded: 1996 ISBN 0-880484-96-9

1268 Stop Walking on Eggshells
New Harbinger Publications
5674 Shattuck Avenue
Oakland, CA 94609-1662
510-652-2002
800-748-6273
Fax: 510-652-5472
E-mail: customerservice@newharbinger.com
www.newharbinger.com

Randi Kreger, Author
Paul Mason, MS, Author

Stop Walking on Eggshells: Taking Back Your Life When Someone You Care About Has Borderline Personality Disorder. This guide for the family and friends of those who have BPD is designed to help them understand how the disorder affects their loved ones and recognize what they can do to establish personal limits and enforce boundaries, communicate more effectively, cope with self destructive behavior, and take care of themselves. *$15.95*

272 pages Year Founded: 1998 ISBN 1-572241-08-X

1269 Structured Interview for DSM-IV Personality (SIDP-IV)
American Psychiatric Publishing
1000 Wilson Boulevard
Suite 1825
Arlington, VA 22209-3901
703-907-7322
800-368-5777
Fax: 703-907-1091
E-mail: appi@psych.org
www.appi.org

Katie Duffy, Marketing Assistant

Semistructured interview uses nonperorative questions to examine behavior and personality traits from the patient's perspective. *$21.95*

48 pages ISBN 0-880489-37-5

1270 The Borderline Personality Disorder Survival Guide
New Harbinger Publications
5674 Shattuck Avenue
Oakland, CA 94609
800-748-6273
Fax: 510-652-5472
www.www.newharbinger.com

Matt McKay, Cofounder/Author/Publisher
Alex Chapman, Author
Kim Gratz, Author

The book is organized as a series of answers to questions common to borderline personality disorder sufferers. Later chapters cover several common treatment approaches to borderline personality disorder.

Support Groups & Hot Lines

1271 SAFE Alternatives
7115 W North Avenue
PMB 319
Oak Park, IL 60302
708-366-9066
800-366-8288
Fax: 708-366-9065
E-mail: info@selfinjury.com
www.selfinjury.com

Karen Conterio, CEO
Wendy Lader, PhD, President/Clinical Director
Michelle Seliner, MSW/LCSW, COO

A national organized treatment appraoch, professional network and educational resource base, which is committed to helping you and others achieve an end to self-injurious behavior.

Web Sites

1272 www.cyberpsych.org
CyberPsych

Presents information about psychoanalysis, psychotherapy and special topics such as anxiety disorders, the problematic use of alcohol, homophobia, and the traumatic effects of racism

1273 www.mentalhealth.com
Internet Mental Health

Offers online psychiatric diagnosis in the hope of reaching the two-thirds of individuals with mental illness who do not seek treatment.

1274 www.mhsanctuary.com/borderline
Borderline Personality Disorder Sanctuary

Borderline personality disorder education, communities, support, books, and resources.

1275 www.nimh.nih.gov/publicat/ocdmenu.cfm
Obsessive-Compulsive Disorder

Introductory handout with treatment recommendations.

1276 www.ocdhope.com/gdlines.htm
Guidelines for Families Coping with OCD

1277 www.planetpsych.com
Planetpsych.com

The online resource for mental health information.

1278 www.psychcentral.com
Psych Central

The Internet's largest and oldest independent mental health social network created and run by mental health professionals to guarantee reliable, trusted information and support communities to you.

Post Traumatic Stress Disorder

Introduction

Traumatic events can stay with us for a long time. Such events can range from the rare and horrific, such as severe torture, to more common events such as an automobile accident or a violent crime. Veterans of war often spend years reliving, or trying to forget, the experience of combat. Effects of some childhood experiences can last well into adulthood. When the after-effects of a traumatic event are so severe and so persistent that they cause serious distress or impair functioning, professional help is necessary. Post-Traumatic Stress Disorder, or PTSD, consists of the psychological and physiological symptoms that arise in some people from experiencing, witnessing or participating in a traumatic event.

SYMPTOMS

Exposure to a traumatic event in which the person experienced, witnessed, or was confronted by death or serious injury, or a threat to the physical integrity of self or others, and the person's response involved intense fear, helplessness, or horror, can result in three basic types of symptoms: re-experiencing, numbing, and/or increased emotional arousal. Re-experiencing includes:
• Recurrent and intrusive distressing recollections of the event, including images, thoughts or perceptions;
• Recurrent distressing flashbacks, nightmares and/or dreams of the event;
• Acting or feeling as if the traumatic event were recurring. Increased arousal includes:
• Intense psychological distress at exposure to internal or external cues that symbolize or resemble an aspect of the traumatic event;
• Increased physiological reactivity (fast heartbeat or breathing, gastrointestinal distress) on exposure to internal or external cues that symbolize or resemble an aspect of the traumatic event;
• Persistent avoidance of stimuli associated with the trauma. Numbing includes:
• Diminished general responsiveness;
• Desensitization of emotional reactiveness.

Duration of the disturbance is more than one month, and the disturbance causes clinically significant distress or impairment in social, occupational, or other important settings.

ASSOCIATED FEATURES

Response to traumatic events can vary from person to person. Some characteristics, however, are common among individuals with PTSD. They are irritable and jumpy; they anger easily, and may get into trouble with the law. If a person has survived a life-threatening event, there may be a profound sense of guilt, particularly if others did not survive the event. These guilt feelings may be exacerbated if the individual perceives that his or her survival occurred at the expense of others' safety.

People with PTSD often avoid situations that remind them of the traumatic event, disrupting normal life because, for example, they make major detours to work or do errands. They may also experience dissociative symptoms, meaning that in certain threatening situations they revert to a state that they will be unable to recall later. In other cases, a person with PTSD may complain of physical symptoms that have no discernible anatomic or physiological explanation, but which are manifestations of psychic distress; these are known as somatic complaints. Patients with PTSD may feel that the trauma they experienced damaged them permanently and irreparably, or give up on previously strongly-held beliefs, such as belief in God; in some cases people with PTSD undergo a profound change of personality. Patients with PTSD may also have any number of other distinctive mental illnesses at the same time: Depression, Obsessive-Compulsive Disorder, Social Phobia, or Substance-Abuse Related Disorders.

PREVALENCE

Anyone who experiences a traumatic event can have Post Traumatic Stress Disorder. PTSD was first diagnosed in war veterans, and many people associate it with soliders, but women and children are actually more vulnerable to PTSD than are men, and account for more than half the cases. Studies in the community reveal a prevalence ranging from one percent to fourteen percent. Men and women tend to suffer different kinds of trauma; women are more likely to experience sexual assault than men, and sexual assault is more likely to result in PTSD than some other types of trauma. Yet when men are sexually assaulted, they are even more likely to develop PTSD than women are. When the study population is made up of combat veterans who have experienced a traumatic event, or victims of criminal violence, the prevalence ranges from three percent to fifty-eight percent. Each traumatic event makes the individual more vulnerable when further such events occur.

TREATMENT OPTIONS

As with many psychiatric disorders, treatment often involves some combination of therapy and medicine. SSRIs (Selective Seratonin Reuptake Inhibitors) medications can be especially helpful; some have specific FDA indications for PTSD. Also useful in some situations are benzodiazepines, which are tranquillizers that can be used to block the symptoms of anxiety at the time they occur. Beta-blocker medications block the physical signs and symptoms of anxiety, such as fast heart rate. SSRIs, on the other hand, are used on an everyday basis to prevent and treat the disease, rather than just when symptoms occur. Eye Movement Desensitization treatment has been used to help patients with PTSD, though the results are controversial and not consistent.

Behavior therapy is a kind of psychotherapy that focuses on helping the patient recognize the thought processes that result in traumatic stress reactions. By working with a professional and learning methods for relaxing and countering the stress reactions, the individual can master the reactions triggered by the traumatic event, or reminders of it. Behavior therapy may involve exposing the patient in a safe and controlled environment to stimuli that prompt a stress reaction; through repeated exposures, the patient slowly is desensitized and in time will be able to experience the stimuli without having a stress reaction. Traditional psychodynamic psychotherapy may also be useful to help the patient examine unconscious psychological conflicts related to the traumatic event. It can also be useful to rebuild self-confidence and self-esteem. Participation in a support group, discovering that others have had similar experiences and learning how they are coping with them, can also be extremely beneficial to individuals with PTSD. Groups have formed around particular issues and particular traumatic experiences; for instance, there are support groups for survivors of rape, incest, or the sudden loss of a loved one. Support groups also exist for combat veterans and other trauma victims.

Associations & Agencies

1280 Association of Traumatic Stress Specialists
PO Box 246
Phillips, ME 04966
207-639-2433
800-991-2877
Fax: 207-639-2434
E-mail: admin@atss.info
www.ATSS-HQ.com

Elena Cherepanov, Director
Susy Sanders, Ph.D., CTS, President
James Mc Aninch, Treasurer

ATSS is an international multidisciplinary membership organization offering certification to qualified individuals who provide services, intervention and treatment in the field of traumatic stress.

1281 Career Assessment & Planning Services
Goodwill Industries-Suncoast
10596 Gandy Boulevard
PO Box 14456
St. Petersburg, FL 33702
727-523-1512
Fax: 727-577-2749
www.goodwill-suncoast.org

Jay McCloe, Director Resource Development

Provides a comprehensive assessment, which can predict current and future employment and potential adjustment factors for physically, emotionally, or developmentally disabled persons who may be unemployed or underemployed. Assessments evaluate interests, aptitudes, academic achievements, and physical abilities (including dexterity and coordination) through coordinated testing, interviewing and behavioral observations.

1282 Center for Family Support (CFS)
333 7th Avenue
New York, NY 10001-5004
212-629-7939
Fax: 212-239-2211
www.cfsny.org

Steven Vernickofs, Executive Director

An agency that continues to develop new programs to serve famililes and individuals with their care needs. They currently offer services throughout the New York City region including: New Jersey, Long Island and the Lower Hudson Valley.

1283 E-Productivity-Services.Net
13 NW Barry Road, PMB 214
Kansas City, MO 64155-2728
816-468-4945
Fax: 816-468-6656
E-mail: nld@espn.netg
www.espn.net

Nancy L Day, Certified Trauma Specialist

Services include professional skills training in trauma resolutions and personal growth; and individual sessions.

1284 International Society for Traumatic Stress Studies
60 Revere Drive
Suite 500
Northbrook, IL 60062
847-480-9028
Fax: 847-480-9282
E-mail: istss@istss.org
www.istss.org

Stuart Turner, President

Provides a forum for sharing research, clinical strategies, public policy concerns and theoretical formulation on trauma in the US and worldwide. Dedicated to discovery and dissemination of knowledge and to the stimulation of policy, program and services.

Year Founded: 1985

1285 National Alliance on Mental Illness
2107 Wilson Boulevard
Suite 300
Arlington, VA 22201-3042
703-524-7600
800-950-6264
Fax: 703-524-9094
E-mail: info@nami.org
www.nami.org

Suzanne Vogel-Scibilia, MD, President
Frederick R Sandoval, First VP

Nation's leading self-help organization for all those affected by severe brain disorders. Mission is to bring consumers and families with similar experiences together to share information about services, care providers, and ways to cope with the challenges of schizophrenia, manic depression, and other serious mental illnesses.

Year Founded: 1979

1286 National Association for the Dually Diagnose d (NADD)
132 Fair Street
Kingston, NY 12401-4802
845-334-4336
800-331-5362
Fax: 845-331-4569
E-mail: nadd@mhv.net
www.thenadd.org

Dr. Robert Fletcher, President/CEO

Nonprofit organization designed to promote interest of professional and parent development with resources for individuals who have the coexistence of mental illness and mental retardation. Provides conference, educational services and training materials to professionals, parents, concerned citizens and service organizations. Formerly known as the National Association for the Dually Diagnosed.

1287 National Mental Health Consumer's Self-Help
1211 Chestnut Street
Suite 1207
Philadelphia, PA 19107
215-751-1810
800-553-4539
Fax: 215-636-6312
E-mail: info@mhselfhelp.org
www.mhselfhelp.org

Christine Simiriglia, Executive Director
Jennifer Melinn, Information/Referral Dept.

Funded by the National Institute of Mental Health Community Support Program, the purpose of the Clearinghouse is to encourage the development and growth of consumer self-help groups.

1288 National Mental Health Consumers' Self-Help Clearinghouse
1211 Chestnut Street
Suite 1207
Philadelphia, PA 19107
215-751-1810
800-553-4539
Fax: 215-636-6312
E-mail: info@mhselfhelp.org
www.mhselfhelp.org

Joseph A Rogers, Executive Director

A national consumer technical assistance center that has played a major role in the development of the mental health consumer movement.

Year Founded: 1986

1289 SAMHSA'S National Mental Health Information Center
US Department of Health and Human Services
PO Box 42557
Washington, DC 20015
800-789-2647
Fax: 301-984-8796
TDD: 866-889-2647
E-mail: ken@mentalhealth.org
www.mentalhealth.samhsa.gov

A Kathryn Power, MEd, Director
Edward B Searle, Deputy Director

Information about resources, technical assistance, research, training, networks, and other federal clearing houses, and fact sheets and materials. Information specialists refer callers to mental health resources in their communities as well as state, federal and nonprofit contacts. Staff available Monday through Friday, 8:30 AM - 5:00 PM, EST, excluding federal holidays. After hours, callers may leave messages and an information specialist will return their call.

1290 Suncoast Residential Training Center/Developmental Services Program
Goodwill Industries-Suncoast
10596 Gandy Boulevard
PO Box 14456
St. Petersburg, FL 33702
727-523-1512
Fax: 727-577-2749
E-mail: gw.marketing@goodwill-suncoast.org
www.goodwill-suncoast.org

R Lee Waits, President/CEO
Deborah A Passerini, VP Operations

A large group home which serves individuals diagnosed as mentally retarded with a secondary diagnosed of psychiatric difficulties as evidenced by problem behavior. Providing residential, behavioral and instructional support and services that will promote the development of adaptive, socially appropriate behavior, each individual is assessed to determine, socialization, basic academics and recreation. The primary intervention strategy is applied behavior analysis. Professional consultants are utilized to address the medical, dental, psychiatric and pharmacological needs of ech individual. One of the most popular features is the ac-

tive community integration component of SRTC. Program customers attend an average of 15 monthly outings to various community events.

Books

1291 After the Crash: Assessment and Treatment of Motor Vehicle Accident Survivors
American Psychological Publishing
750 1st Street NE
Washington, DC 20002-4242
202-336-5500
800-374-2721
Fax: 202-216-7610
TDD: 202-336-6123
TTY: 202-336-6123
www.apa.org

Edward B Blanchard, PhD, Author
Edward J Hickling, PsyD, Author

In this timely second edition, written in a clear and lucid style and illustrated by a wealth of charts, guides, case studies, and clinical advice, the authors report on new, international research and provide updates on their own longstanding research protocols within the groundbreaking Alabny MVA Project. *$59.95*

475 pages Year Founded: 2003 ISBN 1-591470-70-6

1292 Aging and Post Traumatic Stress Disorder
American Psychiatric Publishing
1000 Wilson Boulevard
Suite 1825
Arlington, VA 22209-3901
703-907-7322
800-368-5777
Fax: 703-907-1091
E-mail: appi@psych.org
www.appi.org

Katie Duffy, Marketing Assistant

Provides both literature reviews and data about animal and clinical studies and training for important current concepts of aging, the stress response and the interaction between them. *$37.50*

268 pages ISBN 0-880485-13-2

1293 Children and Trauma: Guide for Parents and Professionals
John Wiley & Sons
1 Wiley Drive
Somerset, NJ 08873
732-469-4400
800-225-5945
Fax: 732-302-2300
E-mail: compbks@wiley.com
www.wiley.com

Cynthia Monahon, Author

Comprehensive guide to the emotional aftermath of children's crises. Discusses warning signs that a child may need professional help, and explores how parents and professionals can help children heal, reviving a sense of well being and safety. *$21.95*

240 pages Year Founded: 1997 ISBN 0-787910-71-6

1294 Coping with Post-Traumatic Stress Disorder
Rosen Publishing Group
29 E 21st Street
New York, NY 10010
800-237-9932
Fax: 888-436-4643
E-mail: info@rosenpub.com
www.rosenpublishing.com

$26.50

Year Founded: 2002 ISBN 0-823934-56-X

1295 Coping with Trauma: A Guide to Self Understanding
American Psychiatric Publishing
1000 Wilson Boulevard
Suite 1825
Arlington, VA 22209-3901
703-907-7322
800-368-5777
Fax: 703-907-1091
E-mail: appi@psych.org
www.appi.org

James Scully, MD, President

$16.00

385 pages ISBN 0-880489-96-0

1296 Effecive Treatments for PTSD: Practice Guide lines from the International Society for Traumatic Stress Studies
The Guilford Press
72 Spring Street
New York, NY 10012
800-365-7006
Fax: 212-966-6708
E-mail: info@guilford.com
www.www.guilford.com

Edna B Foa, Author

The treatment guidelines presented in this book were developed under the auspices of the PTSD Treatment Guidelines Task Force established by the Board of Directors.

ISBN 1-593850-14-X

1297 Effective Treatments for PTSD
Guilford Publications
72 Spring Street
New York, NY 10012
212-431-9800
800-365-7006
Fax: 212-966-6708
E-mail: info@guilford.com
www.guilford.com

Represents the collaborative work of experts across a range of theoretical orientations and professional backgrounds. Addresses general treatment considerations and methodological issues, reviews and evaluates the salient literature on treatment approaches for children, adolescents and adults. *$44.00*

379 pages ISBN 1-572305-84-3

1298 Handbook of PTSD: Science and Practice
The Guilford Press
72 Spring Street
New York, NY 10012

800-365-7006
Fax: 212-966-6708
E-mail: info@guilford.com
www.www.guilford.com

Matthew J Friedman, Author

Unparalleled in its breadth and depth, this state-of-the-art handbook reviews the latest scientific advances in understanding trauma and PTSD.

ISBN 1-593854-73-0

1299 Haunted by Combat: Understanding PTSD in War Veterans
Praeger Security International General Interest-Cloth
88 Post Road West
Westport, CT 06881
203-226-3571
www.www.greenwood.com

Daryl S Paulson, Author

Across history, the condition has been called soldier's heart, shell shock, or combat fatigue.

ISBN 0-275991-87-3

1300 I Can't Get Over It: Handbook for Trauma Survivors
New Harbinger Publications
2674 Shattuck Avenue
Oakland, CA 94609-1662
510-652-2002
800-748-6273
Fax: 510-652-5472
E-mail: customerservice@newharbinger.com
www.newharbinger.com

Aphrodite Matsakis, Author

Guides readers through the healing process of recovering from Post Traumatic Stress Disorder. From the emotional experience to the process of healing, this book is written for survivors of all types of trauma including war, sexual abuse, crime, family violence, rape and natural catastrophes. *$16.95*

416 pages Year Founded: 1996 ISBN 1-572240-58-X

1301 Managing Traumatic Stress Risk: A Proactive Approach
Charles C Thomas Publishers
PO Box 19265
Springfield, IL 62794-9265
217-789-8980
800-258-8980
Fax: 217-789-9130
www.ccthomas.com

This volume represents the first systematic review of critical incident and disaster hazards, the contextual factors that influence risk, and their implications for traumatic stress risk management. It provides the hazard assessment and risk analysis information which, combined with information on resilience, facilitates the systematic analysis of traumatic stress risk and proactive and methodical development of mitigation and risk reduction strategies. This book is also available in paperback for $41.95. *$61.95*

258 pages Year Founded: 2004 ISBN 0-398075-17-4

1302 Post-Traumatic Stress Disorder: Assessment, Differential Diagnosis, and Forensic Evaluation
Professional Resource Press
PO Box 15560
Sarasota, FL 34277-1560
941-343-9601
800-443-3364
Fax: 941-343-9201
E-mail: orders@prpress.com
www.prpress.com

Carroll L Meek, Editor
Debra Fink, Managing Editor

A concise yet thorough examination of PTSD. An excellent resource for psychologists, psychiatrists, and lawyers involved in litigation concerning PTSD. *$26.95*

264 pages Year Founded: 1990 ISBN 0-943158-35-4

1303 Posttraumatic Stress Disorder in Litigation: Guidelines for Forensic Assessment
American Psychiatric Publishing
1000 Wilson Boulevard
Suite 1825
Arlington, VA 22209-3901
703-907-7322
800-368-5777
Fax: 703-907-1091
E-mail: appi@psych.org
www.appi.org

This essential collection by 13 leading US experts sheds important new light on forensic guidelines for effective assessment and diagnosis and determination of disability, serving both plaintiffs and defendants in litigation involving PTSD claims. Mental health and legal professionals, third-party payers, and interested laypersons will welcome this balanced approach to a complex and difficult field. *$44.95*

272 pages Year Founded: 2003 ISBN 1-585620-66-1

1304 Posttraumatic Stress Disorder: A Guide
Madison Institute of Medicine
7617 Mineral Point Road
Suite 300
Madison, WI 53717-1623
608-827-2470
Fax: 608-827-2479
E-mail: mim@miminc.org
www.miminc.org

This informative guide provides a comprehensive overview of the causes and effective treatments of posttraumatic stress disorder (PTSD). *$5.95*

69 pages

1305 Psychological Trauma
American Psychiatric Publishing
1000 Wilson Boulevard
Suite 1825
Arlington, VA 22209-3901
703-907-7322
800-368-5777
Fax: 703-907-1091
E-mail: appi@psych.org
www.appi.org

Katie Duffy, Marketing Assistant

Epidemiology of trauma and post-traumatic stress disorder. Evaluation, neuroimaging, neuroendocrinology and pharmacology. *$29.00*

206 pages ISBN 0-880488-37-9

1306 Rebuilding Shattered Lives: Responsible Treatment of Complex Post-Traumatic and Dissociative Disorders
John Wiley & Sons
1 Wiley Drive
Somerset, NJ 08873
732-469-4400
800-225-5945
Fax: 732-302-2300
E-mail: compbks@wiley.com
www.wiley.com

James Chu, Author

Essential for anyone working in the field of trauma therapy. Part I discusses recent findings about child abuse, the changes in attitudes toward child abuse over the last two decades and the nature of traumatic memory. Part II is an overview of principles of trauma treatment, including symptom control, establishment of boundaries and therapist self - care. Part III covers special topics, such as dissociative identity disorder, controversies, hospitalization and acute care. *$73.95*

288 pages Year Founded: 1998 ISBN 0-471247-32-4

1307 Risk Factors for Posttraumatic Stress Disorder
American Psychiatric Publishing
1000 Wilson Boulevard
Suite 1825
Arlington, VA 22209-3901
703-907-7322
800-368-5777
Fax: 703-907-1091
E-mail: appi@psych.org
www.appi.org

Katie Duffy, Marketing Assistant

Strategies to study risk for the development of PTSD including epidemiological risk factors for trauma and PTSD, genetic risk factors for a twin study, family studies, parental PTSD as a risk factor, neurocognitive risk factors and risk factors for the acute biological and psychological response to trauma. *$42.50*

320 pages ISBN 0-880488-16-6

1308 Take Charge: Handling a Crisis and Moving Forward
American Institute for Preventive Medicine
30445 Northwestern Highway
Suite 350
Farmington Hills, MI 48334-3102
248-539-1800
Fax: 248-539-1808
E-mail: aipm@healthy.net
www.HealthyLife.com

Don R Powell, PhD, President/CEO
Sue Jackson, VP Marketing

Take Charge helps people effectively live their lives after September 11th. This full color booklet provides just the right amount of information to effectively address the many concerns people have today. It will help people to be prepared for any kind of disaster, be it a terrorist attack, fire or flood. *$4.25*

32 pages

**1309 Traumatic Stress: Effects of Overwhelming
Experience on Mind, Body and Society**
Guilford Publications
72 Spring Street
New York, NY 10012
212-431-9800
800-365-7006
Fax: 212-966-6708
E-mail: info@guilford.com
www.guilford.com

The current state of research and clinical knowledge on
traumatic stress and its treatment. Contributions from leading authorities summarize knowledge emerging. Addresses
the uncertainties and controversies that confront the field of
traumatic stress, including the complexity of posttraumatic
adaptations and the unproven effectiveness of some approaches to prevention and treatment. *$62.00*

596 pages ISBN 1-572300-88-4

**1310 Trust After Trauma: A Guide to Relationships
for Survivors and Those Who Love Them**
New Harbinger Publications
5674 Shattuck Avenue
Oakland, CA 94609-1662
510-652-2002
800-748-6273
Fax: 510-652-5472
E-mail: customerservice@newharbinger.com
www.newharbinger.com

Aphrodite Matsakis, Author

Survivors guided through process of strengthening existing
bonds, building new ones, and ending cycles of withdrawal
and isolation. *$17.95*

352 pages Year Founded: 1998 ISBN 1-572241-01-2

**1311 Understanding Post Traumatic Stress Disorder
and Addiction**
Sidran Institute
200 E Joppa Road
Suite 207
Baltimore, MD 21286
410-825-8888
888-825-8249
Fax: 410-337-0747
E-mail: sidran@sidran.org
www.sidran.org

Katie Evans, Author

This booklet discusses PTSD, how to recognize it and how
to begin a dual recovery program from chemical dependency and PTSD. The workbook includes information to enhance your understanding of PTSD, activities to help
identify the symptoms of dual disorders, a self evaulation of
your recovery process and ways to handle situations that
may trigger PTSD. *$7.20*

38 pages

**1312 Who Gets PTSD? Issues of Posttraumatic Stress
Vulnerability**
Charles C Thomas Publishers
PO Box 19265
Springfield, IL 62794-9265
217-789-8980
800-258-8980

Fax: 217-789-9130
www.ccthomas.com

This book draws from research and life experiences on
trauma vulnerability to better understand how mental health
professionals and those concerned with the psychological
well-being of others may disentangle the perplexing questions of who gets PTSD, why they do, and how we may
prevent or minimize this from happening. This is also available in paperback for $29.95. *$46.95*

216 pages Year Founded: 2006 ISBN 3-980761-89-

Periodicals & Pamphlets

1313 Anxiety Disorders
**SAMHSA'S National Mental Health Information
Center**
PO Box 42557
Washington, DC 20015
800-789-2647
Fax: 240-747-5470
TDD: 866-889-2647
E-mail: ken@mentalhealth.org
www.mentalhealth.samhsa.gov

A Kathryn Power, MEd, Director
Edward B Searle, Deputy Director

This fact sheet presents basic information on the symptoms,
formal diagnosis, and treatment for generalized anxiety disorder, panic disorders, phobias, and posttraumatic stress
disorder.

3 pages

**1314 Helping Children and Adolescents Cope with
Violence and Disasters**
National Institute of Mental Health
6001 Executive Boulevard
Room 8184
Bethesda, MD 20892-9663
866-615-6464
Fax: 301-443-4279
TTY: 301-443-8431
E-mail: nimhinfo@nih.gov
www.nimh.nih.gov

Fact sheets that discuss children and adolescents' reactions
to violence and disasters, emphasizing the wide range of responses and the role that parents, teachers and therapists
can play in the healing process.

**1315 Let's Talk Facts About Post-Traumatic Stress
Disorder**
American Psychiatric Publishing
1000 Wilson Boulevard
Suite 1825
Arlington, VA 22209-3901
703-907-7322
800-368-5777
Fax: 703-907-1091
E-mail: appi@psych.org
www.appi.org

Katie Duffy, Marketing Assistant

$12.50

8 pages ISBN 0-890423-63-6

1316 Real Illness: Post-Traumatic Stress Disorder
National Institute of Mental Health
6001 Executive Boulevard
Room 8184
Bethesda, MD 20892-9663
866-615-6464
Fax: 301-443-4279
TTY: 301-443-8431
E-mail: nimhinfo@nih.gov
www.nimh.nih.gov

Do you avoid reminders of a bad accident, war or another traumatic event? Do you have nightmares, fear, emotional numbness? Read this pamphlet of simple information about how to get help.

9 pages

Video & Audio

1317 Treating Trauma Disorders Effectively
Colin A Ross Institute for Psychological Trauma
1701 Gateway
Suite 349
Richardson, TX 75080
972-918-9588
Fax: 972-918-9069
E-mail: rossinst@rossinst.com
www.rossinst.com

Colin A Ross MD, President
Trie Kole

This video illustrates two fundamental treatment principles: attachment to the perpetrator and loss of control shift. For clinicians, the program provides immediately usable techniques for their practices; for the layperson it provides a clear explanation for two consequences of childhood trauma. *$85.00*

Web Sites

1318 www.apa.org/practice/traumaticstress.html
American Psychological Association

Provides tips for recovering from disasters and other traumatic events.

1319 www.bcm.tmc.edu/civitas/caregivers.htm
Caregivers Series

Sophisticated articles describing the effects of childhood trauma on brain development and relationships.

1320 www.cyberpsych.org
CyberPsych

Presents information about psychoanalysis, psychotherapy and special topics such as anxiety disorders, the problematic use of alcohol, homophobia, and the traumatic effects of racism.

1321 www.factsforhealth.org
Madison Institute of Medicine

Resource to help identify, understand and treat a number of medical conditions, including social anxiety disorder, posttraumatic stress disorder, alzheimer's disease, and premenstrual dysphoric disorder.

1322 www.icisf.org
International Critical Incident Stress Foundation

A nonprofit, open membership foundation dedicated to the prevention and mitigation of disabling stress by education, training and support services for all emergency service professionals.

1323 www.mentalhealth.com
Internet Mental Health

On-line information and a virtual encyclopedia related to mental disorders, possible causes and treatments. News, articles, on-line diagnostic programs and related links. Designed to improve understanding, diagnosis and treatment of mental illness throughout the world. Awarded the Top Site Award and the NetPsych Cutting Edge Site Award.

1324 www.ncptsd.org
National Center for PTSD

Aims to advance the clinical care and social welfare of U.S. Veterans through research, education and training on PTSD and stress-related disorders

1325 www.planetpsych.com
Planetpsych.com

Online resource for mental health information

1326 www.psychcentral.com
Psych Central

The Internet's largest and oldest independent mental health social network created and run by mental health professionals to guarantee reliable, trusted information and support communities to you

1327 www.ptsdalliance.org
Post Traumatic Stress Disorder Alliance

Website of the Post Traumatic Stress Disorder Alliance.

1328 www.sidran.org
Sidran Institute

Helps people understand, recover from, and treat traumatic stress (including PTSD), dissociative disorders, and co-occuring issues, such as addictions, self injury, and suicidality.

1329 www.sidran.org/trauma.html
Trauma Resource Area

Resources and Articles on Dissociative Experiences Scale and Dissociative Identity Disorder, PsychTrauma Glossary and Traumatic Memories.

1330 www.sni.net/trips/links.html
Post Traumatic Stress Resources

Links to major pages and metasites.

1331 www.trauma-pages.com
David Baldwin's Trauma Information Pages

Focus primarily on emotional trauma and traumatic stress, including PTSD (Post-traumatic Stress Disorder) and dissociation, whether following individual traumatic experience(s) or a large-scale disaster.

Psychosomatic (Somatizing) Disorders

Introduction

Officially known as Somatizing Disorders, the disorders in this category are characterized by multiple physical symptoms or the conviction that one is ill despite negative medical examinations and laboratory tests. Those who have a Somatizing Disorder persist in believing they are ill, or experience physical symptoms over long periods, and their beliefs negatively affect all areas of their functioning. Two main types of Somatizing Disorders are Hypochondriasis, which consists of being convinced that one is ill despite evidence to the contrary, and Somatization Disorder, consisting of experiencing physical symptoms without a discernible basis.

HYPOCHONDRIASIS

• Preoccupation with fears of having a serious illness based on a misinterpretation of bodily symptoms or sensations;
• The preoccupation persists in spite of medical reassurance;
• The preoccupation is a source of distress and difficulty in social, work, and other areas;
• The duration of the preoccupation is at least six months.

SOMATIZATION DISORDER

• A history of physical complaints beginning before age 30 and continuing over years, resulting in a search for treatment or clear difficulties in social, work, or interpersonal areas;
• Four pain symptoms related to at least four anatomical areas or functions;
• Two gastrointestinal problems other than pain, e.g, nausea, diarrhea;
• One sexual symptom other than pain, e.g., irregular menstruation, sexual disinterest, erectile dysfunction;
• One pseudoneurological symptom other than pain, e.g., weakness, double vision;
• Symptoms cannot be explained by a medical condition;
• When a medical condition exists, physical complaints and social difficulties are greater than normal.

ASSOCIATED FEATURES

The person with either of these Somatizing Disorders visits many doctors, but physical examinations and negative lab results neither reassure them nor resolve their symptoms. They often believe they are not getting proper respect or attention, and, indeed, they may be viewed in medical settings as troublesome, because their problems are 'all in their heads.' Persons with these disorders often suffer from anxiety and depression as well. Physical symptoms appearing after the somatization diagnosis is made, however, should not be dismissed completely out of hand. Sufferers can have general medical disorders at the same time as Somatizing Disorders.

The person may be treated by several doctors at once, which can lead to unwitting and possibly dangerous combinations of treatments. There may be suicide threats and attempts, and deteriorating personal relationships. Individuals with these disorders often have associated Personality Disorders, such as Histrionic, Borderline, or Antisocial Personality Disorder.

PREVALENCE

Hypochondriasis is equally common in both sexes. Its prevalence in the general population is not known. In general medical practice, four percent to nine percent of patients have the disorder. It is usually chronic.

Somatization Disorder was once thought to be mainly a disease of women, but occurs in both sexes. It is slightly less common among men in the general population of the US than in other countries, but not uncommon in general medical practice. It is more common among Puerto Rican and Greek men, which suggests that cultural factors influence the sex ratios.

TREATMENT OPTIONS

These disorders are chronic by definition, and are difficult to manage. Repeated reassurance is not successful. The aim is to limit the extent to which the physical concerns and symptoms preoccupy an individual's thoughts and activities, and drain family emotional and financial resources. Individuals suffering from these disorders often resist mental health referral because they interpret it, sometimes correctly, as an indication that their symptoms are not being taken seriously. Treatment, whether by the primary care or mental health professional or both, should focus on maintaining function despite the symptoms. It is important that the psychological management and treatment is coordinated with medical treatment if possible by one physician only; one person should oversee all the medical treatment, including the psychological, so that care does not become fragmented and/or repetitive as the patient sees many different clinicians. Some individuals with Hypochondriasis respond to treatment which combines medication with intensive behavioral and cognitive techniques to manage anxiety and modify beliefs about the origin and course of physical symptoms.

Associations & Agencies

1333 Career Assessment & Planning Services
Goodwill Industries-Suncoast
10596 Gandy Boulevard
St. Petersburg, FL 33733
727-523-1512
Fax: 727-563-9300
E-mail: gw.marketing@goodwill-suncoast.com
www.goodwill-suncoast.org

R Lee Waits, President/CEO
Loreen M Spencer, Chair Person

Provides a comprehensive assessment, which can predict current and future employment and potential adjustment factors for physically, emotionally, or developmentally disabled persons who may be unemployed or underemployed. Assessments evaluate interests, aptitudes, academic achievements, and physical abilities (including dexterity and coordination) through coordinated testing, interviewing and behavioral observations.

1334 Center for Family Support (CFS)
333 7th Avenue
New York, NY 10001-5004
212-629-7939
Fax: 212-239-2211
www.cfsny.org

Steven Vernickofs, Executive Director

An agency that continues to develop new programs to serve families and individuals with their care needs. They currently offer services throughout the New York City region including: New Jersey, Long Island and the Lower Hudson Valley.

1335 Center for Mental Health Services
SAMSHA
PO Box 42557
Washington, DC 20015
800-789-2647
Fax: 240-747-5484
TDD: 866-889-2647
TTY: 301-443-9006
E-mail: ken@Mentalhealth.org
www.mentalhealth.samhsa.gov

Kathryn A Power, MEd, Director
Edward B Searle, Deputy Director

CMHS leads federal efforts to treat mental illnesses by promoting mental health and by preventing the development or worsening of mental health when possible.

1336 Deborah MacWilliams
548 SW 13th Street
Suite B-3
Bend, OR 97702
541-617-0351
Fax: 541-617-0351

Deborah MacWilliams PhD PMHNP

Providing individual psychiatric evaluation, psychotherapy, and medical management for adults and teens. Specializing in thorough assessments and personalized treatment planning.

1337 Institute for Contemporary Psychotherapy
1841 Broadway
4th Floor
New York, NY 10023
212-333-3444
Fax: 212-333-5444
www.icpnyc.org

Ron Taffel PhD, Chairman
Fred Lipschitz, Treasurer/Founder
Mildred Schwartz, Founder

One of the oldest and largest not-for-profit mental health training and treatment facilities in New York City, dedicated to providing high quality therapy at low to moderate cost, offering post-graduate training for therapists, and educating the public about mental health issues.

Year Founded: 1971

1338 Institute for Contemproary Psychotherapy
1841 Broadway 60th Street Fourth Floor
New York, NY 10023-7603
212-333-3444
Fax: 212-333-5444
www.icpnyc.org

Ron Taffel, PhD, Chairman
Fred Lipschitz, Treasurer

ICP is dedicated to providing high quality therapy at low to moderate cost, offering post-graduate training for therapists and educatiing the public about mental health issues.

1339 National Association for the Dually Diagnose d (NADD)
132 Fair Street
Kingston, NY 12401-4802
845-334-4336
800-331-5362
Fax: 845-331-4569
E-mail: nadd@mhv.net
www.thenadd.org

Dr. Robert Fletcher, Executive Director

Nonprofit organization designed to promote interest of professional and parent development with resources for individuals who have the coexistence of mental illness and mental retardation. Provides conference, educational services and training materials to professionals, parents, concerned citizens and service organizations. Formerly known as the National Association for the Dually Diagnosed.

1340 National Mental Health Consumer's
1211 Chestnut Street
Suite 1207
Philadelphia, PA 19107
215-751-1810
800-553-4539
Fax: 215-636-6312
E-mail: info@mhselfhelp.org
www.mhselfhelp.org

Christine Simiriglia, Executive Director
Jennifer Melinn, Information/Referral Dept.

Funded by the National Institute of Mental Health Community Support Program, the purpose of the Clearinghouse is to encourage the development and growth of consumer self-help groups.

1341 National Mental Health Consumers' Self-Help Clearinghouse
1211 Chestnut Street
Suite 1207
Philadelphia, PA 19107
215-751-1810
800-553-4539
Fax: 215-636-6312
E-mail: info@mhselfhelp.org
www.mhselfhelp.org

Joseph Rogers, Executive Director

A national consumer technical assistance center that has played a major role in the development of the mental health consumer movement.

Year Founded: 1986

1342 SAMHSA'S National Mental Health Information Center
US Department of Health and Human Services
PO Box 42557
Washington, DC 20015
800-789-2647
Fax: 240-747-5470
TDD: 866-889-2647
E-mail: ken@mentalhealth.org
www.mentalhealth.smahsa.org

A Kathryn Power, MEd, Director
Edward B Searle, Deputy Director

Information about resources, technical assistance, research, training, networks, and other federal clearing houses, and fact sheets and materials. Information specialists refer callers to mental health resources in their communities as well as state, federal and nonprofit contacts. Staff available Monday through Friday, 8:30 AM - 5:00 PM, EST, excluding federal holidays. After hours, callers may leave messages and an information specialist will return their call.

Books

1343 Drug Therapy and Psychosomatic Disorders
Masn Crest Publishers
370 Reed Road
Suite 302
Broomall, PA 19008
610-543-6200
866-627-2665
Fax: 610-543-3878
E-mail: dtaylor@masoncrest.com
www.masoncrest.com

Psychosomatic disorders are complex psychiatric conditions involving the mysterious connection between the body and the brain. From unexplained pain to nonepileptic seizures, the physical symptoms that result from psychopharmacology alike. Through stories of individuals' struggles with psychosomatic disorders combined with easily explained scientific information, this book provides both a historical overview of treatment and reviews the most up-to-date treatments available today.

ISBN 1-590845-73-0

1344 Essentials of Psychosomatic Medicine
American Psychiatric Publishing
1000 Wilson Boulevard
Suite 1825
Arlington, VA 22209-3901
703-907-7322
800-368-5777
Fax: 703-907-1091
E-mail: appi@psych.org
www.www.appi.org

Ron McMillen, CEO
James L Levenson, Author

This book focuses on psychiatric care for medically ill patients.

1345 Hypochondria: Woeful Imaginings
University of California Press
2120 Berkeley Way
Berkeley, CA 94720-5804
501-642-4247
Fax: 510-643-7127
E-mail: askucp@ucpress.edu
www.ucpress.edu

Susan Baur illuminates the process by which hypochondriacs come to adopt and maintain illness as a way of life. *$25.00*

260 pages Year Founded: 1989 ISBN 0-520067-51-7

1346 Mind-Body Problems: Psychotherapy with Psychosomatic Disorders
Jason Aronson
230 Livingston Street
Northvale, NJ 07647
570-342-1320
800-782-0015

Fax: 201-767-1576
www.aronson.com

Shows us the causes and treatments of the major pychosomatic symptons. *$70.00*

376 pages ISBN 1-568216-54-8

1347 Phantom Illness: Recognizing, Understanding, and Overcoming Hypochondria
Houghton Mifflin Company
222 Berkeley Street
Boston, MA 02116
617-351-5000
E-mail: inquiries@hmco.com
www.hmco.com

Offers hope to those who suffer from the debilitating disorder of hypochondria. Carla Cantor's long, dark road to hypochondria began when she crashed a car, killing a friend of hers. She couldn't forgive herself, and a few years later began imagining that she was suffering from Lupus. Many years and two hospitalizations later, she wrote this book not only about her experiences, but about hypochondria in general, now more politely referred to as a 'somatoform disorder'. Paperback. *$15.00*

351 pages ISBN 0-395859-92-1

1348 Somatoform and Factitious Disorders (Review of Psychiatry)
American Psychiatric Publishing
1000 Wilson Boulevard
Suite 1825
Arlington, VA 22209-3901
703-907-7322
800-368-5777
Fax: 703-907-1091
E-mail: appi@psych.org
www.www.appi.org

Ron McMillen, CEO
Katharine A Phillips, Author

Offers clinicians a broad synthesis of the current knowledge about somatoform and factitious disorders.

1349 The Divided Mind: The Epidemic of Mindbody Disorders
HarperCollins Publishers
10 East 53rd Street
New York, NY 10022-3901
212-207-7000
www.www.harpercollins.com

John E Sarno, Author

Explores the chasm between the conscious and unconscious minds where psychosomatic ailments originate.

Video & Audio

1350 Effective Learning Systems
3451 Bonita Bay Boulevard
Suite 205
Bonita Springs, FL 34134
239-948-1660
800-966-5683
Fax: 239-948-1664
E-mail: info@efflearn.com
www.efflearn.com

Robert E Griswold, President
Deirdre M Griswold, VP

Audio tapes for stress management, deep relaxation, anger control, peace of mind, insomnia, weight and smoking, self-image and self-esteem, positive thinking, health and healing. Since 1972, Effective Learning Systems has helped millions of people take charge of their lives and make positive changes. Over 75 titles available, each with a money-back guarantee. Price range $12-$14.

Web Sites

1351 www.mentalhealth.com
Internet Mental Health

Offers online psychiatric diagnosis in the hope of reaching the two-thirds of individuals with mental illness who do not seek treatment.

1352 www.planetpsych.com
Planetpsych.com

Online resource for mental health information

1353 www.psychcentral.com
Psych Central

The Internet's largest and oldest independent mental health social network created and run by mental health professionals to guarantee reliable, trusted information and support communities to you.

1354 www.users.lanminds.com/~eds/
Trauma Treatment Manual

On-line treatment manual gives professionals an overview of trauma treatment from one psychologist's viewpoint, treatment guidelines and examples.

Schizophrenia

Introduction

Schizophrenia is a devastating disease of the brain that severely impairs an individual's ability to think, feel and function normally. Though not a common disorder, it is one of the most destructive, disrupting the lives of sufferers, as well as of family members and loved ones. Long misunderstood, people with Schizophrenia and their families have also borne a burden of stigma in addition to the burden of their illness.

Although family and other environmental stressors can play a role in precipitating or exacerbating episodes of illness, theories that the disease is caused by poor parenting have been discredited. Much has been learned about the disease in recent years and treatments have improved markedly.

Schizophrenia is a largely genetically determined disorder of the brain. One theory is that it is a disorder of information processing resulting from a defect in the prefrontal cortex of the brain. Because this system is defective, an individual with Schizophrenia is easily overwhelmed by the amount of information and stimuli coming from the environment. Schizophrenia causes hallucinations, which are sensory experiences in th absence of actual stimuli (hearing voices when no one is speaking), and delusions, which are bizarre beliefs (that the individual is God, that the television is conveying messages specifically aimed at the individual, that some power is removing the individual's thoughts from his or her mind). Speech may be tangential or confused. These arecalled 'positive symptoms.' The individual also loses some normal behaviors and experiences, engaging in little behavior or social interaction. These are called 'negative symptoms.' Schizophrenia is a chronic disease and, once diagnosed, a person often needs treatment the rest of his or her life. However, great strides have been made in treating the disease and many individuals with schizophrenia can hold jobs, marry, parent children, and have gratifying and productive lives.

SYMPTOMS

So-called 'Positive' symptoms (experiences not shared by people in society):
• Delusions or false and bizarre beliefs;
• Hallucinations;

Negative symptoms (the loss of normal behaviors):
• Withdrawing from social contact;
• Speaking less;
• Losing interest in things and the ability to enjoy them;
• Disorganized speech;
• Grossly disorganized or catatonic behavior (extremely agitated or zombie-like);
• The symptoms cause social and occupational dysfunction;
• Signs of the disturbance persist for at least six months;
• The symptoms must not be related to mood or depressive disorders, substance abuse or general medical conditions.

ASSOCIATED FEATURES

People with Schizophrenia, because their disease causes difficulty in perceiving their environment and responding to it normally, will often act strange, and have odd beliefs. They sometimes react to stimuli (voices or images originating inside their brains) as though they were originating in their environment; hallucinations and delusions can make a person's behavior appear bizarre to others. A person with the disease may act socially inappropriately for instance, by smiling, laughing or being silly for no reason. Anhedonia, the inability to enjoy pleasurable activities is common in Schizophrenia, as are sleep disturbances and abnormalities of psychomotor activity. The latter may take the form of pacing, rocking, or immobility. Negative symptoms can be more disabling than positive ones. Family members often become annoyed because they think the individual is just lazy. Schizophrenia takes many forms, and there are a number of subtypes of the illness, including paranoid schizophrenia.

Individuals with untreated Schizophrenia, under the influence of hallucinations and delusions, have a slightly greater propensity for violence than the general population, especially when there is co-existing alcohol or substance abuse, which is quite common. However, it is important to emphasize that this is not always the case; Schizophrenia is known as a heterogenous disease, meaning that the illness takes many forms, depending on a variety of individual characteristics and circumstances. Patients who receive appropriate treatment are not more violent than the general population.

The life expectancy of people with Schizophrenia is shorter then the general population for a variety of reasons: suicide is common among people with the disease and people with Schizophrenia often have both poor medical care and poor health.

PREVALENCE

The first episode of Schizophrenia usually occurs in teenage years, although some cases may occur in the late thirties or forties. Onset prior to puberty is rare, though cases as early as five year olds have been reported. Women have a later average of onset and a better prognosis. Estimates of the prevalence of Schizophrenia vary widely around the world, but probably about one percent of the world population has the disease.

TREATMENT OPTIONS

Medications can diminish or eliminate many of the positive symptoms of Schizophrenia. Older medications, such as Haldol, are effective and inexpensive, but cause more side effects than newer medications, such as Zyprexa and Geodon. Clozapine was the first and is still one of the most effective treatments, but it causes a low incidence of a life-threatening blood disorder; therefore people who take it must have blood tests at regular intervals. The newer medications are more effective in treating the negative, as well as the positive, symptoms.

Antipsychotic medications can have serious side effects, the most prominent being Tardive Dyskinesia, which consists of involuntary muscular movements. Often, patients report that antipsychotic medications make them feel foggy, or lethargic. The newer antipsychotic medications are less sedating and have a decreased risk of causing Tardive Dyskinesia, but are associated with significant weight gain and increased risk of diabetes. There is considerable public controversy as to whether the weight gain, and risk of diabetes associated with the newer medications, along with their cost, outweighs their advantages.

Having Schizophrenia interferes with taking care of oneself

and getting proper medical care in several ways; Schizophrenia often depletes financial resources so that patients cannot afford medication, nutrition, and medical care. Schizophrenia can also interfere with an individual's ability to understand signs and symptoms of medical disorders. Compliance with medication is often a problem, and failure to continue taking medication is a major cause of relapse. For this reason, treatment should include supportive therapy, in which a psychiatrist or other mental health professional provides counseling aimed at helping the patient maintain a positive and optimistic attitude focused on staying healthy. Other forms of therapy, such as social skills training, have also found some success and may be useful in helping a person with schizophrenia learn appropriate social and interpersonal behavior. It is important to note that psychotic illness does not necessarily affect all aspects of an individual's thinking. People with schizophrenia may have bizarre beliefs or behaviour in one sphere of life but be perfectly able to make decisions and function in other areas. In addition, it is crucial not to destroy an individual or family's hopes fo a normal life by communicating the message that schizophrenia is hopeless.

Paranoid schizophrenia is especially difficult to treat. Paranoia, the irrational conviction that other people, institutions (the FBI), or alien beings are atempting to harm the individual, prevents the individual from forming trusting relationships with care providers and adhering to effective treatment regimens. The individual with paranoid schizophrenia can appear convincingly lucid before a judge or general physician, in order to obtain release from care, while maintaining behaviors,

Associations & Agencies

1356 Career Assessment & Planning Services
Goodwill Industries-Suncoast
10596 Gandy Boulevard
St. Petersburg, FL 33733
727-523-1512
Fax: 727-563-9300
E-mail: gw.marketing@goodwill-suncoast.org
www.goodwill-suncoast.org

R Lee Waits, President/CEO
Loreen M Spencer, Chair Person

Provides a comprehensive assessment, which can predict current and future employment and potential adjustment factors for physically, emotionally, or developmentally disabled persons who may be unemployed or underemployed. Assessments evaluate interests, aptitudes, academic achievements, and physical abilities (including dexterity and coordination) through coordinated testing, interviewing and behavioral observations.

1357 Center for Family Support (CFS)
333 7th Avenue
New York, NY 10001-5004
212-629-7939
Fax: 212-239-2211
www.cfsny.org

Steven Vernickofs, Executive Director

An agency that continues to develop new programs to serve families and individuals with their care needs. They currently offer services throughout the New York City region including: New Jersey, Long Island and the Lower Hudson Valley.

1358 Center for Mental Health Services
SAMSHA
PO Box 42557
Washington, DC 20015
800-789-2647
Fax: 240-747-5484
TDD: 866-889-2647
TTY: 301-443-9006
E-mail: ken@mentalhealth.org
www.mentalhealth.samhsa.gov

A Kathryn Power, Director
Edward B Searle, Deputy Director

Develops national mental health policies, that promote Federal/State coordination and benefit from input from consumers, family members and providers. Ensures that high quality mental health services programs are implemented to benefit seriously mentally ill populations, disasters or those involved in the criminal justice system.

1359 NARSAD: The Mental Health Research Associati on
60 Cutter Mill Road
Suite 404
Great Neck, NY 11021
516-829-0091
800-829-8289
Fax: 516-487-6930
E-mail: info@narsad.org
www.narsad.org

Constance Lieber, President
Stephen Doochin, Executive Director

A nonprofit organization that raises funds for scientific research on severe mental illness. It is the largest donor-supported organization in the world dedicated to finding the causes, improved treatments and cures for psychiatric brain and behavior disorders.

1360 National Alliance for Research on Schizophrenia and Depression
60 Cutter Mill Road
Suite 404
Great Neck, NY 11021
516-829-0091
800-829-8289
Fax: 516-487-6930
E-mail: info@narsad.org
www.narsad.org

Constance E Lieber, President

NARSAD is a private, not-for-profit public charity 501 (C) (3) organized for the purpose of raising and distributing funds for scientific research into the causes, cures, treatments and prevention of severe psychiatric brain disorders, such as schizophrenia and depression.

1361 National Alliance on Mental Illness
2107 Wilson Boulevard
Suite 300
Arlington, VA 22201-3042
703-524-7600
800-950-6264
Fax: 703-524-9094
E-mail: info@nami.org
www.nami.org

Suzanne Vogel-Scibila, MD, President
Frederick R Sandoval, First VP

Nation's leading self-help organization for all those affected by severe brain disorders. Mission is to bring consumers and families with similar experiences together to share information about services, care providers, and ways to cope with the challenges of schizophrenia, manic depression, and other serious mental illnesses.

Year Founded: 1979

1362 National Association for The Dually Diagnose d (NADD)

132 Fair Street
Kingston, NY 12401-4802
845-334-4336
800-331-5362
Fax: 845-331-4569
E-mail: nadd@mhv.net
www.thenadd.org

Dr. Robert Fletcher, Executive Director

Nonprofit organization designed to promote interest of professional and parent development with resources for individuals who have the coexistence of mental illness and mental retardation. Provides conference, educational services and training materials to professionals, parents, concerned citizens and service organizations. Formerly known as the National Association for the Dually Diagnosed.

1363 National Mental Health Association

2001 N Beauregard Street
12th Floor
Alexandria, VA 22311
703-684-7722
800-969-6642
Fax: 703-684-5968
TTY: 800-433-5959
E-mail: infoctr@nmha.org
www.nmha.org

Mike Fienza, Executive Director
Chris Condayn, Communications

Dedicated to improving treatments, understanding and services for adults and children with mental health needs. Working to win political support for funding for school mental health programs. Provides information about a wide range of disorders.

1364 National Mental Health Consumer's Self-Help

1211 Chestnut Street
Suite 1207
Philadelphia, PA 19107
215-751-1810
800-553-4539
Fax: 215-735-0275
E-mail: info@mhselfhelp.org
www.mhselfhelp.org

Christine Simiriglia, Executive Director
Jennifer Melinn, Information/Referral Dept.

Funded by the National Institute of Mental Health Community Support Program, the purpose of the Clearinghouse is to encourage the development and growth of consumer self-help groups.

1365 National Mental Health Consumers' Self-Help Clearinghouse

1211 Chestnut Street
Suite 1207
Philadelphia, PA 19107

215-751-1810
800-553-4539
Fax: 215-636-6312
E-mail: info@mhselfhelp.org
www.mhselfhelp.org

Joseph Rogers, Executive Director

A national consumer technical assistance center that has played a major role in the development of the mental health consumer movement.

Year Founded: 1986

1366 SAMHSA'S National Mental Health Information Center
US Department of Health and Human Services

PO Box 42557
Washington, DC 20015
800-789-2647
Fax: 240-747-5470
TDD: 866-889-2647
E-mail: ken@mentalhealth.org
www.mentalhealth.samhsa.gov

A Kathryn Power, MEd, Director
Edward B Searle, Deputy Director

Information about resources, technical assistance, research, training, networks, and other federal clearing houses, and fact sheets and materials. Information specialists refer callers to mental health resources in their communities as well as state, federal and nonprofit contacts. Staff available Monday through Friday, 8:30 AM - 5:00 PM, EST, excluding federal holidays. After hours, callers may leave messages and an information specialist will return their call.

1367 Suncoast Residential Training Center/Developmental Services Program
Goodwill Industries-Suncoast

10596 Gandy Boulevard
St. Petersburg, FL 33733
727-523-1512
Fax: 727-563-9300
E-mail: gw.marketing@goodwill-suncoast.org
www.goodwill-suncoast.org

R Lee Waits, President/CEO
Deborah A Passerini, VP Operations

A large group home which serves individuals diagnosed as mentally retarded with a secondary diagnosed of psychiatric difficulties as evidenced by problem behavior. Providing residential, behavioral and instructional support and services that will promote the development of adaptive, socially appropriate behavior, each individual is assessed to determine, socialization, basic academics and recreation. The primary intervention strategy is applied behavior analysis. Professional consultants are utilized to address the medical, dental, psychiatric and pharmacological needs of ech individual. One of the most popular features is the active community integration component of SRTC. Program customers attend an average of 15 monthly outings to various community events.

Books

1368 Biology of Schizophrenia and Affective Disease
American Psychiatric Publishing

1000 Wilson Boulevard
Suite 1825
Arlington, VA 22209-3901

703-907-7322
800-368-5777
Fax: 703-907-1091
E-mail: appi@psych.org
www.appi.org

Katie Duffy, Marketing Assistant

Provides a state-of-the-art look at the biological basis of several mental illness from the perspective of the researchers making these discoveries. *$58.50*

464 pages ISBN 0-880487-46-1

1369 Breakthroughs in Antipsychotic Medications: A Guide for Consumers, Families, and Clinicians
National Alliance on Mental Illness
2107 Wilson Boulevard
Suite 300
Arlington, VA 22201-3042
703-524-7600
800-950-6264
Fax: 703-524-9094
TDD: 703-516-7227
E-mail: campaign@nami.org
www.nami.org

Helps consumers and their families weigh the pros and cons of switching from older antipsychotics to newer ones. Answers frequently asked questions about antipsychotics and guides readers through the process of switching. Includes fact sheets on the new medications and their side effects. *$22.95*

207 pages Year Founded: 1999 ISBN 0-393703-03-7

1370 Concept of Schizophrenia: Historical Perspectives
American Psychiatric Publishing
1000 Wilson Boulevard
Suite 1825
Arlington, VA 22209-3901
703-907-7322
800-368-5777
Fax: 703-907-1091
E-mail: appi@psych.org
www.appi.org

Katie Duffy, Marketing Assistant

$65.00

211 pages

1371 Contemporary Issues in the Treatment of Schizophrenia
American Psychiatric Publishing
1000 Wilson Boulevard
Suite 1825
Arlington, VA 22209-3901
703-907-7322
800-368-5777
Fax: 703-907-1091
E-mail: appi@psych.org
www.appi.org

Covers approaches to the patient by investigating biological, pharmacological and psychosocial treatments. *$99.95*

960 pages ISBN 0-880486-81-3

1372 Drug Therapy and Schizophrenia
Mason Crest Publishers
370 Reed Road
Suite 302
Broomall, PA 19008
610-543-6200
866-627-2665
Fax: 610-543-3878
E-mail: dtaylor@masoncrest.com
www.masoncrest.com

This volume provides a concise description of this disease, which is considered the most severe of the mental disorders. The book also includes a brief account of the disease in history, as well as explanations of how the brain operates and how psychiatric drugs work within the brain. Many case studies are presented to help readers better understand the nature of this difficult and potentially devastating mental disorder.

ISBN 1-590845-74-9

1373 Encyclopedia of Schizophrenia and the Psychotic Disorders
Facts on File
132 W 31st Street
17th Floor
New York, NY 10001-2006
800-322-8755
Fax: 800-678-3633
E-mail: custserv@factsonfile.com
www.factsonfile.com

Details recent theories and research findings on schizophrenia and psychotic disorders, together with a complete overview of the field's history. *$65.00*

368 pages Year Founded: 2000 ISBN 0-816040-70-2

1374 Family Care of Schizophrenia: a Problem-Solving Approach...
Guilford Publications
72 Spring Street
New York, NY 10012
212-431-9800
800-365-7006
Fax: 212-966-6708
E-mail: info@guilford.com
www.guilford.com

Falloon and his colleagues have developed a model for the broad-based community treatment of schizophrenia and other severe forms of mental illness that taps this underutilized potential. The goal of their program is not merely the reduction of stress that can trigger florid episodes, but also the restoration of the patient to a level of social functioning that permits employment and socialization with people outside the family. As the author demonstrates, families can, with proper guidance, be taught to modulate intrafamilial stress, whether it derives from family tensions or external life events. *$27.95*

451 pages ISBN 0-898629-23-3

1375 Family Work for Schizophrenia: a Practical Guide
American Psychiatric Publishing
1000 Wilson Boulevard
Suite 1825
Arlington, VA 22209-3901
703-907-7322
800-368-5777

Fax: 703-907-1091
E-mail: appi@psych.org
www.appi.org

Katie Duffy, Marketing Assistant

1376 First Episode Psychosis
American Psychiatric Publishing
1000 Wilson Boulevard
Suite 1825
Arlington, VA 22209-3901
703-907-7322
800-368-5777
Fax: 703-907-1091
E-mail: appi@psych.org
www.appi.org

Katie Duffy, Marketing Assistant

Professional discussion of early Psychosis presentation.
$39.95

160 pages ISBN 1-853174-35-1

1377 Group Therapy for Schizophrenic Patients
American Psychiatric Publishing
1000 Wilson Boulevard
Suite 1825
Arlington, VA 22209-3901
703-907-7322
800-368-5777
Fax: 703-907-1091
E-mail: appi@psych.org
www.appi.org

Katie Duffy, Marketing Assistant

Acquaints mental health practitioners with this cost-effective method of treatment. *$29.00*

192 pages ISBN 0-880481-72-2

1378 Guidelines for the Treatment of Patients with Schizophrenia
American Psychiatric Publishing
1000 Wilson Boulevard
Suite 1825
Arlington, VA 22209-3901
703-907-7322
800-368-5777
Fax: 703-907-1091
E-mail: appi@psych.org
www.appi.org

Katie Duffy, Marketing Assistant

Provides therapists with a set of patient care strategies that will aid their clinical decison making. Describes the best and most appropriate treatments available to patients.
$22.50

160 pages ISBN 0-890423-09-1

1379 How to Cope with Mental Illness In Your Family: A Guide for Siblings and Offspring
Health Source
1404 K Street, NW
Washington, DC 20005-2401
202-789-7303
800-713-7122
Fax: 202-789-7899
E-mail: healthsourcebooks@psych.org
www.healthsourcebooks.org

This book explores the nature of illnesses such as schizophrenia, major depression, while providing the tools to overcome the devasting effects of growing up or living in a family where they exist. Readers are led through the essential stages of recovery, from revisiting their childhood to revising their family legacy, and ultimately, to reclaiming their life. *$14.00*

240 pages ISBN 0-874779-23-5

1380 Innovative Approaches for Difficult to Treat Populations
American Psychiatric Publishing
1000 Wilson Boulevard
Suite 1825
Arlington, VA 22209-3901
703-907-7322
800-368-5777
Fax: 703-907-1091
E-mail: appi@psych.org
www.appi.org

Firsthand look at the future direction of clinical services. Focuses on services for individuals who use the highest proportion of mental health resources and for whom traditional services have not been effective. *$65.00*

512 pages ISBN 0-880486-80-5

1381 Me, Myself, and Them: A Firsthand Account of One Young Person's Experience with Schizophrenia (Adolescent Mental Health Initiative)
Oxford University Press
198 Madison Avenue
New York, NY 10016
212-726-6000
www.www.oup.com/us

Kurt Snyder, Author
Raquel E Gur, Author

Offers practical advice on topics of particular interest to young people, such as suggestions on managing the illness at home, school, and work, and in relationships with family and friends.

1382 Natural History of Mania, Depression and Schizophrenia
American Psychiatric Publishing
1000 Wilson Boulevard
Suite 1825
Arlington, VA 22209-3901
703-907-7322
800-368-5777
Fax: 703-907-1091
E-mail: appi@psych.org
www.appi.org

Katie Duffy, Yarketing Assistant

An unusual look at the course of mental illness, based on data from the Iowa 500 Research Project. *$42.50*

336 pages ISBN 0-880487-26-7

1383 New Pharmacotherapy of Schizophrenia
American Psychiatric Publishing
1000 Wilson Boulevard
Suite 1825
Arlington, VA 22209-3901
703-907-7322
800-368-5777

Fax: 703-907-1091
E-mail: appi@psych.org
www.appi.org

Discusses the new class of antipsychotic agents that promise superior efficacy and more favorable side-effects; offers an improved understanding of how to employ existing pharmachotherapeutic agents. *$32.50*

272 pages ISBN 0-880484-91-8

1384 Office Treatment of Schizophrenia
American Psychiatric Publishing
1000 Wilson Boulevard
Suite 1825
Arlington, VA 22209-3901
703-907-7322
800-368-5777
Fax: 703-907-1091
E-mail: appi@psych.org
www.appi.org

Katie Duffy, Marketing Director

Examines options in outpatient treatment of schizophrenic patients. *$31.00*

208 pages

1385 Practicing Psychiatry in the Community: a Manual
American Psychiatric Publishing
1000 Wilson Boulevard
Suite 1825
Arlington, VA 22209-3901
703-907-7322
800-368-5777
Fax: 703-907-1091
E-mail: appi@psych.org
www.appi.org

Katie Duffy, Marketing Assistant

Addressess the major issues currently facing community psychiatrists. *$67.50*

560 pages ISBN 0-880486-63-5

1386 Prenatal Exposures in Schizophrenia
American Psychiatric Publishing
1000 Wilson Boulevard
Suite 1825
Arlington, VA 22209-3901
703-907-7322
800-368-5777
Fax: 703-907-1091
E-mail: appi@psych.org
www.appi.org

Considers a range of epigenetic elements thought to interact with abnormal genes to produce the onset of illness. Attention to the evidence implicating obstetric complications, prenatal infection, autoimmunity and prenatal malnutrition in brain disorders. *$36.50*

352 pages ISBN 0-880484-99-3

1387 Psychiatric Rehabilitation of Chronic Mental Patients
American Psychiatric Publishing
1000 Wilson Boulevard
Suite 1825
Arlington, VA 22209-3901
703-907-7322
800-368-5777

Fax: 703-907-1091
E-mail: appi@psych.org
www.appi.org

Katie Duffy, Marketing Assistant

Provides highly detailed prescriptions for assessment and treatment techniques with case examples and learning exercises. *$28.00*

320 pages ISBN 0-880482-01-X

1388 Psychoses and Pervasive Development Disorders in Childhood and Adolescence
American Psychiatric Publishing
1000 Wilson Boulevard
Suite 1825
Arlington, VA 22209-3901
703-907-7322
800-368-5777
Fax: 703-907-1091
E-mail: appi@psych.org
www.appi.org

Katie Duffy, Marketing Assistant

Provides a concise summary of currently knowledge of psychoses and pervasive developmental disorders of childhood and adolescence. Discusses recent changes in aspects of diagnosis and definition of these disorders, advances in knowledge, and aspects of treatment. *$46.50*

368 pages ISBN 1-882103-01-7

1389 Return From Madness
Jason Aronson
200 Livingston Street
Northvale, NJ 07647
201-767-4093
800-782-1005
Fax: 201-767-1576
www.aronson.com

This book offers a new approach to helping people who have emerged from madness. *$50.00*

256 pages ISBN 1-568216-25-4

1390 Schizophrenia
American Psychiatric Publishing
1000 Wilson Boulevard
Suite 1825
Arlington, VA 22209-3901
703-907-7322
800-368-5777
Fax: 703-907-1091
E-mail: appi@psych.org
www.appi.org

Katie Duffy, Marketing Assistant

Ideas in treating the disease, and how many patients can lead productive lives without relapse. *$165.00*

760 pages ISBN 0-632032-76-6

1391 Schizophrenia Revealed: From Neurons to Social Interactions
W.W. Norton & Company
500 Fifth Avenue
New York, NY 10110
212-354-5500
Fax: 212-869-0856
www.www.wwnorton.com

Michael Foster Green, Author

1392 Schizophrenia Revealed: From Nuerons to Social Interactions
WW Norton & Company
500 5th Avenue
6th Floor
New York, NY 10110
212-354-5500
800-233-4830
Fax: 212-869-0856
E-mail: admalmud@wwnorton.com
www.wwnorton.com

John Darger, Contact
Michael F Gree, Author

Helps explain some of the former mysteries of Schizophrenia that are now possible to study through advances in neuroscience. *$ 19.95*

240 pages Year Founded: 2003 ISBN 0-393704-18-1

1393 Schizophrenia and Genetic Risks
National Alliance on Mental Illness
2107 Wilson Boulevard
Suite 300
Arlington, VA 22201
703-524-7600
800-950-6264
Fax: 703-524-9094
TDD: 703-516-7227
E-mail: info@nami.org
www.nami.org

Provides basic facts about schizophrenia and its familial distribution so consumers and mental health workers can become informed enough to initiate appropriate actions. Includes suggested resources.

1394 Schizophrenia and Manic Depressive Disorder
National Alliance for the Mentally Ill
2107 Wilson Boulevard
Suite 300
Arlington, VA 22201
703-524-7600
800-950-6264
Fax: 703-524-9094
TDD: 703-516-7227
E-mail: info@nami.org
www.nami.org

Explores the biological roots of mental illness with a primary focus on schizophrenia. *$27.00*

274 pages ISBN 0-465072-85-2

1395 Schizophrenia and Primitive Mental States
Jason Aronson Publishing
276 Livingston Street
Northvale, NJ 07647
570-342-1320
800-782-0015
Fax: 201-767-1576
www.aronson.com

In this volume, renowned therapist Peter Giovacchini shows readers how to do more for psychotic patients than rely on medication to reduce their florid symptoms. Instead, he demonstrates how schizophrenic patients can be offered true cure and the possibility of living a full and related life through intensive psychotherapeutic treatment. *$50.00*

288 pages ISBN 0-765700-27-1

1396 Schizophrenia in a Molecular Age
American Psychiatric Publishing
1000 Wilson Boulevard
Suite 1825
Arlington, VA 22209-3901
703-907-7322
800-368-5777
Fax: 703-907-1091
E-mail: appi@psych.org
www.appi.org

Katie Duffy, Marketing Assistant

Explores the multidimensional phenotype of schizophrenia, and use of molecular biology and anti-psychotic medications. Reviews the implications of early sensory procesing and subcortical involvement of cognitive dysfuntion in schizophrenia. Functional neuroimaging applied to the syndrome of schizophrenia. *$26.50*

224 pages ISBN 0-880489-61-8

1397 Schizophrenia: From Mind to Molecule
American Psychiatric Publishing
1000 Wilson Boulevard
Suite 1825
Arlington, VA 22209-3901
703-907-7322
800-368-5777
Fax: 703-907-1091
E-mail: appi@psych.org
www.appi.org

Katie Duffy, Marketing Assistant

Provides a thorough look at schizophrenia that includes neurobehavioral studies, traditional and emerging technologies, psychosocial and medical treatments, and future research opportunities. *$34.00*

278 pages ISBN 0-800489-50-2

1398 Schizophrenia: Straight Talk for Family and Friends
William Morrow & Company
10 East 53rd Street
New York, NY 10022
212-261-6500
Fax: 212-261-6549
www.williammorrow.com

Lists more than 150 local chapters of the National Alliance for the Mentally Ill. *$17.95*

Year Founded: 1985

1399 Stigma and Mental Illness
American Psychiatric Publishing
1000 Wilson Boulevard
Suite 1825
Arlington, VA 22209-3901
703-907-7322
800-368-5777
Fax: 703-907-1091
E-mail: appi@psych.org
www.appi.org

Katie Duffy, Marketing Assistant

Collection of firsthand accounts on how society has stigmatized mentally ill individuals, their families and their caregivers. *$36.00*

236 pages ISBN 0-880484-05-5

1400 Surviving Schizophrenia: A Manual for Families, Consumers and Providers
Harper Collins
10 E 53rd Street
New York, NY 10022-5244
212-207-7000
800-242-7737
Fax: 212-207-2271
www.harpercollins.com

Since its first publication nearly twenty years ago, this has become the standard reference book on this disease, helping thousands of patients, families and mental health professionals to better deal with the condition. Dr. Fuller Torrey explains the nature causes, symptoms, and treatment of this often misunderstood illness. This fully revised 4th edition of Surviving Schizophrenia is a must-have for the multitude of people affected both directly and indirectly by this serious, yet treatable, disorder. *$15.00*

544 pages ISBN 0-060959-19-3

1401 The Center Cannot Hold: My Journey Through M adness
Hyperion
77 West 66th Street
11th Floor
New York, NY 10023
212-633-4400
www.www.hyperionbooks.com

Elyn R Saks, Author

Demonstrates a novelist's skill of creating character, dialogue and suspense.

1402 The Complete Family Guide to Schizophrenia: Helping Your Loved One Get the Most Out of Life
The Guilford Press
72 Spring Street
New York, NY 10012
800-365-7006
Fax: 212-966-6708
E-mail: info@guilford.com
www.www.guilford.com

Robert Matloff, President
Kim T Mueser, Author
Susan Gingerich, Author

This book walks readers through a range of treatment and support options that can lead to a better life for the entire family. Individual chapters hightlight special issues for parents, siblings, and partners, while other sections provide tips for dealing with problems including cognitive difficulties, substance abuse, and psychosis.

1403 Treating Schizophrenia
Jossey-Bass / John Wiley & Sons
111 River Street
Hokoken, NJ 07030-5774
201-748-6000
Fax: 201-748-6088
E-mail: custserv@wiley.com
www.wiley.com

Using case studies from their own practices, the contributors describe how to conduct a successful assessment of schizophrenia. They then explore in detail the major treatment methods, including inpatient treatment, individual therapy, family therapy, group therapy, and the crucial role

of medication. Th authors also address the timely issue of treating schizophrenia in the era of managed care. *$ 121.60*

372 pages Year Founded: 1995

1404 Understanding Schizophrenia: Guide to the New Research on Causes & Treatment
Free Press
1120 Avenue of the Americas
New York, NY 10036-6700
800-456-6798
Fax: 800-943-9831
E-mail: consumer.customerservice@simonandschuster.com
www.simonsays.com

Two noted researchers provide an accessible, timely guide to schizophrenia, discussing the nature of the disease, recent advances in understanding brain structure and function, and the latest psychological and drug treatments. *$25.95*

283 pages Year Founded: 1994 ISBN 0-029172-47-0

1405 Water Balance in Schizophrenia
American Psychiatric Publishing
1000 Wilson Boulevard
Suite 1825
Arlington, VA 22209-3901
703-907-7322
800-368-5777
Fax: 703-907-1091
E-mail: appi@psych.org
www.appi.org

Katie Duffy, Marketing Assistant

Provides clinicians with a consolidated guide to polydipsia - hyponatramia, associated with schizophrenia. *$54.95*

304 pages ISBN 0-880484-85-3

Periodicals & Pamphlets

1406 Schizophrenia
National Institute of Mental Health
6001 Executive Boulevard
Room 8184
Bethesda, MD 20892-9663
866-615-6464
Fax: 301-443-4279
TTY: 301-443-8431
E-mail: nimhinfo@nih.gov
www.nimh.nih.gov

This booklet answers many common questions about schizophrenia, one of the most chronic, severe and disabling mental disorders. Current research-based information is provided for people with schizophrenia, their family members, friends and the general public about the symptoms and diagnosis of schizophrenia, possible causes, treatments and treatment resources.

28 pages Year Founded: 1999

1407 Schizophrenia Bulletin: Superintendent of Documents
Government Printing Office
732 N Capital Street NW
Washington, DC 20401
202-698-3277

ISBN 0-160105-89-7

1408 Schizophrenia Fact Sheet
SAMHSA'S National Mental Health Information Center
PO Box 42557
Washington, DC 20015
800-789-2647
Fax: 240-747-5470
TDD: 866-889-2647
E-mail: ken@mentalhealth.org
www.mentalhealth.samhsa.gov

A Kathryn Power, MEd, Director
Edward B Searle, Deputy Director

This fact sheet provides information on the symptoms, diagnosis, and treatment for schizophrenia.

2 pages

1409 Schizophrenia Research
11830 Westline Industrial Drive
St Louis, MO 63146
212-633-3730
800-545-2522
Fax: 800-535-9935
E-mail: usbkinfo@elsevier.com
www.elsevier.nl/locate/schres

A publication of new international research that contributes to the understanding of schizophrenia disorders. It is hoped that this journal will aid in bringing together previously separated biological, clinic and psychological research on this disorder, and stimulate the synthesis of these data into cohesive hypotheses.

ISSN 0920-9964

Research Centers

1410 NARSA: The Mental Health Research Associatio n
60 Cutter Mill Road
Suite 404
Great Neck, NY 11021
516-829-0091
800-829-8289
Fax: 516-487-6930
E-mail: info@narsad.org
www.narsad.org

Stephen G Doochin, Executive Vice President
Louis Innamorato, CFO

Previously known as the National Alliance for Research on Schizophrenia and Depression, NARSAD is a private, not-for-profit public charity organized for the purpose of raising funds for scientific research into the causes, cures, treatments and prevention of severe psychiatric brain and behavior disorders, such as schizophrenia and depression

1411 Schizophrenia Research Branch: Division of Clinical and Treatment Research
6001 Executive Boulevard
Room 18 MSC 9663
Bethesda, MD 20892-9663
301-443-4513
866-615-6464
Fax: 301-443-5158
TTY: 301-443-8431
E-mail: nimhinfo@nih.gov
www.nimh.nih.gov

Plans, supports, and conducts programs of research, research training, and resource development of schizophrenia and related disorders. Reviews and evaluates research developments in the field and recommends new program directors. Collaborates with organizations in and outside of the National Institute of Mental Health (NIMH) to stimulate work in the field through conferences and workshops.

1412 Schizophrenic Biologic Research Center
James J Peters VA Medical Center
130 W Kingsbridge Road
Bronx, NY 10468-3992
718-584-9000
Fax: 718-741-4269
www.va.gov/visns/visn03/bronxinfo.asp
Focuses on mental illness and schizophrenia.

Support Groups & Hot Lines

1413 Family-to-Family: National Alliance on Mental Illness
2107 Wilson Boulevard
Suite 300
Arlington, VA 22201-3042
703-524-7600
Fax: 703-524-9094
E-mail: info@nami.org
www.nami.org

Michael Fitzpatrick, Executive Director
Lynn Borton, COO

A free 12-week course for family caregivers of individuals with severe mental illnesses that discusses the clinical treatment of these illnesses and teaches the knowledge and skills that family members need to cope more effectively.

1414 Recovery
802 N Dearborn Street
Chicago, IL 60610-3364
312-337-5661
Fax: 312-337-5756
E-mail: inquiries@recovery-inc.com
www.recovery-inc.com

Kelly Garcia, Executive Director
Maurine Pyle, Assistant Director

Techniques for controlling behavior, changing attitudes for recovering mental patients. Systematic method of self-help offered.

1415 Schizophrenics Anonymous Forum
Mental Health Association in Michigan
30233 Southfield Road
Suite 220
Southfield, MI 48076
248-647-1711
Fax: 248-647-1732
E-mail: inquiries@nsfoundation.org
www.mha-mi.org

Elizabeth A Plant, Director

Self-help organization sponsored by American Schizophrenia Association. Groups are comprised of dignosed schizophrenics who meet to share experiences, strengths and hopes in an effort to help each other cope with common problems and recover from the disease, rehabilitation program follows the 12 principles of Alcoholics Anonymous.

Publications: Newsletter, semi-annual. Monthly support group meeting.

Video & Audio

1416 Bonnie Tapes
Mental Illness Education Project
PO Box 470813
Brookline Village, MA 02447-0813
617-562-1111
800-343-5540
Fax: 617-779-0061
E-mail: info@miepvideos.org
www.miepvideos.org

Christine Ledoux, Executive Director
Jack Churchill, President
Lucia Miller, Marketing Director

Bonnie's account of coping with schizophrenia will be a revelation to people whose view of mental illness has been shaped by the popular media. She and her family provide an intimate view of a frequently feared, often misrepresented, and much stigmatized illness-and the human side of learning to live with a psychiatric disability. Set of three tapes $143.88 or $59.95 per tape.

Year Founded: 1997

1417 Families Coping with Mental Illness
Mental Illness Education Project
PO Box 470813
Brookline Village, MA 02247-0244
617-562-1111
800-343-5540
Fax: 617-779-0061
E-mail: info@miepvideos.org
www.miepvideos.org

Christine Ledoux, Executive Director

10 family members share their experiences of having a family member with schizophrenia or bipolar disorder. Designed to provide insights and support to other families, the tape also profoundly conveys to professionals the needs of families when mental illness strikes. In two versions: a twenty two minute version ideal for short classes and workshops, and a richer forty three minute version with more examples and details. Discounted price for families/consumers. *$68.95*

Year Founded: 1997

Web Sites

1418 www.cyberpsych.org
CyberPsych

Presents information about psychoanalysis, psychotherapy and special topics such as anxiety disorders, the problematic use of alcohol, homophobia, and the traumatic effects of racism.

1419 www.health-center.com/mentalhealth/
schizophrenia/default.htm
Schizophrenia

Basic information for beginners.

1420 www.hopkinsmedicine.org/epigen
Epidemology-Genetics Program in Psychiatry

Learn more about research and how you can sign up for various studies.

1421 www.members.aol.com/leonardjk/USA.htm
Schizophrenia Support Organizations

1422 www.mentalhealth.com
Internet Mental Health

Offers online psychiatric diagnosis in the hope of reaching the two-thirds of individuals with mental illness who do not seek treatment.

1423 www.mentalhelp.net/guide/schizo.htm
Mentalhelp

Collection of articles and links.

1424 www.mgl.ca/~chovil
Experience of Schizophrenia

Home page containing a biography, advice, resources, and diagrams for teaching.

1425 www.mhsource.com/
advocacy/narsad/order.html
Schizophrenia

Brochures, books, and videos.

1426 www.mhsource.com/advocacy/
narsad/newsletter.html
Schizophrenia

Public service announcements.

1427 www.mhsource.com/advocacy/narsad
/narsadfaqs.html
Schizophrenia

Medical questions and answers.

1428 www.mhsource.com/advocacy/narsad/
studyops.html
Schizophrenia

Research studies.

1429 www.mhsource.com/narsad.html
National Alliance for Research on Schizophrenia and Depression

Raises funds for research on schizophrenia, depression and other mental illnesses. Affiliated with National Alliance for the Mentally Ill, National Depressive and Manic Depressive Association and National Mental Health Association.

1430 www.naminys.org
NAMI-New York State: National Alliance on Mental Illness

The purpose of the NAMI-New York State shall be to serve as an alliance of local mutual support, advocacy, self-help groups and individual members at-large dedicated to improving the quality of life for people with serious mental illness and to the eventual eradication of the severe effects of mental illnesses

1431 www.nimh.nih.gov/publicat/schizoph.htm
Schizophrenia

National Institute of Mental Health.

1432 **www.planetpsych.com**
Planetpsych.com

The online resource for mental health information.

1433 **www.psychcentral.com**
Psych Central

The Internet's largest and oldest independent mental health social network created and run by mental health professionals to guarantee reliable, trusted information and support communities to you.

1434 **www.recovery-inc.com**
Recovery

Describes the organizations approach.

1435 **www.schizophrenia.com**
Schizophrenia

A non-profit community providing in-depth information, support and education related to schizophrenia, a disorder of the brain and mind.

1436 **www.schizophrenia.com/discuss/**
Schizophrenia

On-line support for patients and families.

1437 **www.schizophrenia.com/newsletter**
Schizophrenia

Comprehensive psychoeducational site on schizophrenia.

1438 **www.schizophrenia.com/newsletter/buckets/**
success.html
Schizophrenia

Success stories including biographical accounts, links to stories of famous people who have schizophrenia, and personal web pages.

Sexual Disorders

Introduction

It is not possible to know what degree of sexual interest, desire, or activity is 'normal'; at best, we have averages, not indications of the optimal state. A Sexual Disorder is diagnosed when lack of desire or activity is repeated, persists over time and causes distress or interferes with the person's functioning in other important areas of life.

Sexual Disorders are divided into four groups: Disorders of Sexual Desire; Disorders of Sexual Arousal; Orgasmic Disorders; and Disorders involving Sexual Pain. It is essential to know whether the problem is lifelong or was precipitated by a recent event, and whether it occurs only with a particular partner or in a particular situation. It is also essential not to make assumptions about sexual activity based on age, socioeconomic status, or sexual orientation. The only way to know about an individual's sexual life is to ask.

SEXUAL DESIRE DISORDERS SYMPTOMS

Hypoactive Sexual Desire Disorder (HSDD)
• Persistent or repeated lack of sexual fantasies and desire for sexual activities;
• The lack of sexual fantasies and desire cause marked distress or interpersonal problems.

Sexual Aversion Disorder (SAD)
• Persistent or repeated extreme aversion to, and avoidance of, all or almost all genital sexual contact with a sexual partner;
• The aversion causes marked distress or interpersonal problems.

Associated Features
The person with a Sexual Desire Disorder commonly has a poor body image and avoids nudity. In HSDD, a person does not initiate sexual activity, or respond to the partner's initiation attempts. The disorder is often associated with the inability to achieve orgasm in women, and the inability to achieve an erection in men. It can also be associated with other psychiatric and medical problems, including a history of sexual trauma and abuse.

Prevalence
HADD is common in both men and women but twice as many women as men report it. It is estimated at twenty percent overall, and as high as sixty-five-percent among those seeking treatment for sexual disorders. The prevalence of SAD is unknown.

SEXUAL AROUSAL DISORDER SYMPTOMS

Female Sexual Arousal Disorder (FSAD)
• Persistent or repeated inability to attain or maintain adequate lubrication-swelling (sexual excitement) response throughout sexual activity;
• The disorder causes clear distress or interpersonal problems.

Male Erectile Disorder (MED)
• Persistent or repeated inability to maintain an adequate erection throughout sexual activity;
• The difficulty causes clear distress or interpersonal problems.

Associated Features
While both these disorders are common, men tend to be more upset by it than women. Contributing issues include performance anxiety (especially in men), fear of failure, inadequate stimulation, and relationship conflicts. Other problems are also associated with FSAD and MED, such as childhood sexual trauma, sexual identity concerns, religious orthodoxy, depression, lack of intimacy or trust, and power conflicts. MED is frequently associated with diabetes, peripheral nerve disorders, and hypertension, and is a side effect of a variety of medications; men with MED must be evaluated for these conditions. In addition, the medications used to treat MED are contraindicated in some medical conditions, such as heart conditions.

Prevalence
Prevalence information varies for FSAD. In one study, 13.6 percent of women overall reported a lack of lubrication during most or all sexual activity; twenty-three percent had such problems occasionally; and 4, 4.2 percent of post-menopausal women reported having lubrication problems. In a study of happily married couples, about one third of women complained of difficulty in achieving or maintaining sexual excitement.

Erectile difficulties in men are estimated to be very common, affecting 20-30 million men in the US. The frequency of erectile problems increases steeply with age. In one survey, fifty-two percent of men aged 40-70 reported erectile problems, with three times as many older men reporting difficulties. The disorder is common among married, single, heterosexual and homosexual men.

Treatment Options
In FSAD, a cognitive-behavioral psychotherapy is often recommended, including practical help such as the use of water-soluble lubricating products. Hormone treatment, such as testosterone-estrogen compounds, is sometimes helpful.

An array of treatments is available for Male Erectile Dysfunction, including prosthetic devices for physiological penile problems. In cases of hormonal problems, testosterone treatments have had some results. (However, the use of testosterone to treat sexual disorders in menopausal women is controversial and can have serious side effects.) Viagra is producing success for male erectile dysfunction, as are two newer medications for MED, vardenafil (Levitra) and tadalafil (Cialis).

When sexual problems are limited to a particular partner or situation, psychotherapy (individual or couple) is necessary to resolve the difficulty.

ORGASMIC DISORDER SYMPTOMS

Female and Male Orgasmic Disorders
Persistent or repeated delay in, or absence of, orgasm despite a normal sexual excitement phase;
The disorder causes clear distress of interpersonal problems.

Premature Ejaculation
Persistent or recurring ejaculation with minimal sexual stimulation before, upon, or shortly after penetration and earlier than desired;
The disorder causes clear distress of interpersonal problems.

Associated Features

When FOD or MOD occur only in certain situations, difficulty with desire and arousal are often also present.

All of these disorders are associated with poor body image, self-esteem or relationship problems. In FOD or MOD, medical or surgical conditions can also play a role, such as multiple sclerosis, spinal cord injury, surgical prostatectomy (males), and some medications. PE is likely to be very distruptive. Some males may have had the disorder all their lives, for others it may be situational. Few illnesses or drugs are associated with PE.

Prevalence

FOD is probably the most frequent sexual disorder among females. Among those who have sought sex therapy twenty-four percent to thirty-seven percent report the problem. In general population samples, 15.4 percent of premenopausal women report the disorder, and 34.7 percent of postmenopausal women do so. More single than married women report that they have never had an orgasm. There is no association between FOD and race, socioeconomic status, education, or religion. MOD is relatively rare; only three percent to eight percent of men seeking treatment report having the disorder, though there is a higher prevalence among homosexual males (ten percent to fifteen percent).

PE is very common: twenty-five percent to forty percent of adult males report having, or having had, this problem.

Treatment Options

Psychotherapeutic treatments are similar to those for Sexual Desire and Sexual Arousal Disorders. In both males and females with Orgasmic Disorders there may be a lack of desire, performance anxiety, and fear of impregnation or disease. Therapy should take into account contextual and historical information concerning the onset and course of the problem. Cognitive-behavioral methods to help change the assumptions and thinking of the person have sometimes been helpful.

SEXUAL PAIN DISORDER SYMPTOMS

Dyspareunia

Recurring or persistent pain with sexual intercourse in a male or female;
The disorder causes clear distress or interpersonal problems.

Vaginismus

Persistent or recurrent involunatry spasm of the vagina that interferes with sexual intercourse;
The disorder causes clear distress or interpersonal problems.

Associated Features

Both Dyspareunia and Vaginismus may be associated with lack of desire or arousal. Women with Vaginismus tend to avoid gynecological exams, and the disorder is most often associated with psychological and interpersonal issues. Various physical factors are associated with Dyspareunia, such as pelvic inflammatory disease, hymenal or childbirth-related scarring, and vulvar vestibulitis. Dyspareunia is not a clear symptom of any physical condition. In women it is often combined with Depression and interpersonal conflicts. Other associated psychosocial factors include religious orthodoxy, low self-esteem, poor body image, poor couple communication, and history of sexual trauma.

Prevalence

Dyspareunia is frequent in females but occurs infrequently in males. Vaginismus is seen quite often in sex therapy clinics - in fifteen percent to seventeen percent of women coming for treatment.

Treatment Options

Probably the most successful treatment for women with these disorders is the reinsertion of a graduated sequence of dilators in the vagina. The woman's sexual partner should be present, and a participant in this treatment. This treatment should be done in conjunction with relaxation training, sensate focusing exercises, (which help people focus on the pleasures of sex rather than the performance) and sex therapy.

General Treatment Options

The professional making the diagnosis of a Sexual Disorder should be trained and experienced in Sexual Disorders and sex therapy. It is important to know whether or not a medical or medication issue is present. However, many with these disorders do not seek treatment. Their lack of desire for sex is often combined with a lack of desire for sex therapy. Even with therapy, relapse is commonly reported. Treatments that have had some success are ones that challenge the cognitive assumptions and distortions of client(s), e.g., that sex should be perfect, that without intercourse and without both partners having an orgasm it isn't real sex. Therapy often also includes sensate focusing in which the person is encouraged and trained to give up the role of agitated spectator to love-making in favor of participating in it. A sexual history should be part of every mental health evaluation, and patients receiving psychotropic medications should be asked about sexual side effects. Having information about sexual function before medication is prescribed will prevent pre-existing sexual problems from being confused with any that may result from medication.

Associations & Agencies

1440 Center for Family Support (CFS)
333 7th Avenue
New York, NY 10001-5004
212-629-7939
Fax: 212-239-2211
www.cfsny.org

Steven Vernickofs, Executive Director

An agency that continutes to develop new programs to serve families and individuals with their care needs. They currently offer services throughout the New York City region including: New Jersey, Long Island and the Lower Hudson Valley.

1441 National Assocaition for the Dually Diagnose d (NADD)
132 Fair Street
Kingston, NY 12401-4802
845-334-4336
800-331-5362
Fax: 845-331-4569
E-mail: nadd@mhv.net
www.add.org

Dr. Robert Fletcher, Executive Director

Nonprofit organization designed to promote interest of professional and parent development with resources for individuals who have the coexistence of mental illness and mental retardation. Provides conference, educational services and training materials to professionals, parents, concerned citizens and service organizations. Formerly known as the National Association for the Dually Diagnosed.

Year Founded: 1983

1442 National Mental Health Consumer's Self-Help
1211 Chestnut Street
Suite 1207
Philadelphia, PA 19107
215-751-1810
800-553-4539
Fax: 215-636-6312
E-mail: info@mhselfhelp.org
www.mhselfhelp.org

Joseph Rodgers, Founder/Executive Director
Christine Simirglia, Director

Funded by the National Institute of Mental Health Community Support Program, the purpose of the Clearinghouse is to encourage the development and growth of consumer self-help groups.

1443 National Mental Health Consumers' Self-Help Clearinghouse
1211 Chestnut Street
Suite 1207
Philadelphia, PA 19107
215-751-1810
800-553-4539
Fax: 215-636-6312
E-mail: info@mhselfhelp.org
www.mhselfhelp.org

Joseph A Rogers, Executive Director

A national consumer technical assistance center that has played a major role in the development of the mental health consumer movement.

Year Founded: 1986

1444 SAMHSA'S National Mental Health Information Center
US Department of Health and Human Services
PO Box 42557
Washington, DC 20015
800-789-2647
Fax: 240-747-5470
TDD: 866-889-2647
E-mail: ken@mentalhealth.org
www.mentalhealth.samhsa.gov

A Kathryn Power, Director
Edward B Searle, Deputy Director

Information about resources, technical assistance, research, training, networks, and other federal clearing houses, and fact sheets and materials. Information specialists refer callers to mental health resources in their communities as well as state, federal and nonprofit contacts. Staff available Monday through Friday, 8:30 AM - 5:00 PM, EST, excluding federal holidays. After hours, callers may leave messages and an information specialist will return their call.

Books

1445 Back on Track: Boys Dealing with Sexual Abuse
200 E Joppa Road
Suite 207
Baltimore, MD 21286
410-825-8888
888-825-8249
Fax: 410-337-0747
E-mail: sidran@sidran.org
www.sidran.org

Leslie Bailey Wright
Mindy B Loiselle

Written for boys age ten and up, this wookbook addresses adolescent boys directly, answering commonly asked questions, offering concrete suggestions for getting help and dealing with unspoken concerns such as homosexuality. Contains descriptions of what therapy may be like and brief explanations of social services and courts, as well as sections on family and friends. Exercises and interesting graphics break up the text. The book's important message is TELL: Just keep telling until someone listens who STOPS the abuse. *$14.00*

144 pages

1446 Dangerous Sex Offenders: a Task Force Report of the American Psychiatric Association
American Psychiatric Publishing
1000 Wilson Boulevard
Suite 1825
Arlington, VA 22209-3901
703-907-7322
800-368-5777
Fax: 703-907-1091
E-mail: appi@psych.org
www.appi.org

Katie Duffy, Marketing Assistant

$40.95

224 pages ISBN 0-890422-80-X

1447 Handbook of Sexual and Gender Identity Disorder
John Wiley & Sons
111 River Street
Hoboken, NJ 07030-5774
201-748-6000
Fax: 201-748-6088
E-mail: info@wiley.com
www.www.wiley.com

William J Pesce, President/CEO
David L Rowland, Author

The Handbook of Sexual and Gender Identity Disorders provides mental health professionals a comprehensive yet practical guide to the understanding, diagnosis, and treatment of a variety of sexual problems. *$95.00*

1448 Interviewing the Sexually Abused Child
American Psychiatric Publishing
1000 Wilson Boulevard
Suite 1825
Arlington, VA 22209-3901
703-907-7322
800-368-5777
Fax: 703-907-1091

E-mail: appi@psych.org
www.appi.org

Katie Duffy, Marketing Assistant

Guide for mental health professionals who need to know if a child has been sexually abused. Presents guidelines on the structure of the interview and covers the use of free play, toys, and play materials by focusing on the investigate interview of the suspected victim. *$27.95*

80 pages ISBN 0-880486-12-0

1449 Masculinity and Sexuality: Selected Topics in the Psychology of Men
American Psychiatric Publishing
1000 Wilson Boulevard
Suite 1825
Arlington, VA 22209-3901
703-907-7322
800-368-5777
Fax: 703-907-1091
E-mail: appi@psych.org
www.appi.org

Katie Duffy, Marketing Assistant

$37.50

200 pages ISBN 0-880489-62-6

1450 Principles and Practice of Sex Therapy
The Guilford Press
72 Spring Street
New York, NY 10012
800-365-7006
Fax: 212-966-6708
E-mail: info@guilford.com
www.www.guilford.com

Robert Matloff, President
Sandra R Leiblum, Author

Provides a comprehensive guide to assessment and treatment of all of the major female and male sexual dysfunctions. *$95.00*

1451 Psychiatric Treatment of Victims and Survivors of Sexual Trauma: A Neuro-Bio-Psychological Approach
Charles C Thomas Publishers
PO Box 19265
Springfield, IL 62794-9265
217-789-8980
800-258-8980
Fax: 217-789-9130
www.ccthomas.com

This book originated on the basis of clinical observations and the authors believe that trauma is the region in which psych and soma meet each other and integrate, becoming a single entity. The authors attempt to integrate the psychosocial and bio-neuro-endcrine aspects of human experience, including trauma. Available in paperback for $33.95. *$53.95*

234 pages Year Founded: 2004 ISBN 0-398074-60-7

1452 Quickies: The Handbook of Brief Sex Therapy
W.W. Norton & Company
500 Fifth Avenue
New York, NY 10110

212-354-5500
Fax: 212-869-0856
www.www.wwnorton.com

Shelley K Green, Author
Douglas G Flemons, Author

All of the chapters present time-efficient, client-focused approaches supported by case examples, to working with clients with sexual problems.

ISBN 0-393705-27-7

1453 Sexual Aggression
American Psychiatric Publishing
1000 Wilson Boulevard
Suite 1825
Arlington, VA 22209-3901
703-907-7322
800-368-5777
Fax: 703-907-1091
E-mail: appi@psych.org
www.appi.org

Katie Duffy, Marketing Assistant

Appropriate diagnosis and treatment options are presented. *$64.00*

364 pages ISBN 0-880487-57-7

1454 Sexuality and People with Disabilities
Indiana Institute on Disability and Community
Indiana University
2853 E Tenth Street
Bloomington, IN 47408-2696
812-855-6508
800-280-7010
Fax: 812-855-9630
TTY: 812-855-9396
E-mail: uap@indiana.edu
www.iidc.indiana.edu

Sexuality information for people with disabilities is available but difficult to find. This publication discusses the importance of having sexuality information available and provides numerous sexuality-related resources. *$5.00*

16 pages

1455 Therapy for Adults Molested as Children: Beyond Survival
Springer Publishing Company
11 West 42nd Street
15th Floor
New York, NY 10036
877-687-7476
Fax: 212-941-7842
E-mail: contactus@springerpub.com
www.springerpub.com

Sheri W Sussman, SVP Editorial
John Briere, PhD, Author

Substantially expanded and revised, this new edition includes detailed information on how to treat sexual abuse survivors more effectively. Chapters cover topics such as client dissociation during therapy, the false/recovered memory controversy, gender differences in abuse treatment. The appendix analyzes the Trauma Symptom Inventory, a 100 item test of post traumatic stress and other psychological sequelae of traumatic events. *$39.95*

270 pages Year Founded: 1996 ISBN 0-826156-41-X

1456 Treating Intellectually Disabled Sex Offenders: A Model Residential Program
Safer Society Foundation
PO Box 340
Brandon, VT 05733-0340
802-247-3132
Fax: 802-247-4233
E-mail: gina@safersociety.org
www.safersociety.org

Gina Brown, Sales/Marketing Manager

Describes how the intensive residential specialized Social Skills Program at Oregon State Hospital combines the principles of respect, self-help, and experiential learning with traditional sex-offender treatment methods. *$24.00*

152 pages ISBN 1-884444-30-X

Periodicals & Pamphlets

1457 Family Violence & Sexual Assault Bulletin
Family Violence & Sexual Assault Institute
6160 Cornerstone Court E
San Diego, CA 92121
858-623-2777
Fax: 858-646-0761
www.fvsai.org

David Westgate, Director

Book club, research and quarterly newsletter. *$35.00*

60-70 pages

Web Sites

1458 www.cs.uu.nl/wais/html/na-bng/alt.support.abuse-partners.html

Partners of sexual abuse survivors.

1459 www.emdr.com
EMDR Institute

Eye Movement Desensitization and Reprocessing (EMDR) integrates elements of many effective psychotherapies in structured protocols that are designed to maximize treatment effects. These include psychodynamic, cognitive behavioral, interpersonal, experiential, and body-centered therapies.

1460 www.firelily.com/gender/sstgfaq
Support Transgendered

Transgendered and intersexed persons.

1461 www.mentalhealth.com
Internet Mental Health

Offers online psychiatric diagnosis in the hope of reaching the two-thirds of individuals with mental illness who do not seek treatment.

1462 www.planetpsych.com
Planetpsych.com

Online resource for mental health information.

1463 www.priory.com/sex.htm
Sexual Disorders

Diagnoses and treatments.

1464 www.psychcentral.com
Psych Central

The Internet's largest and oldest independent mental health social network created and run by mental health professionals to guarantee reliable, trusted information and support communities to you.

1465 www.shrinktank.com
Shrinktank

Psychology-related programs, shareware and freeware.

1466 www.xs4all.nl/~rosalind/cha-assr.html
Support and Information on Sex Reassignement

The purpose of this newsgroup is to provide a supportive and informative environment for people who are undergoing or who have undergone sex reassignment surgery (SRS) and for their relatives and significant others.

Sleep Disorders

Introduction

Sleep Disorders are a group of disorders characterized by extreme distruptions in normal sleeping patterns. These include Primary Insomnia, Primary Hypersomnia, Narcolepsy, Breathing-related Sleep Disorder, Circadian Rhythm Sleep Disorder, Substance Abuse Induced Sleep Disorder, Nightmare Disorder and Sleep Terror Disorder. Primary Insomnia consists of the inability to sleep, with excessive daytime sleepiness, for at least one month, as evidenced by either prolonged sleep episodes or daytime sleep episodes that occur almost daily. Narcolepsy is characterized by chronic, involuntary and irresistible sleep attacks; a person with the disorder can suddenly fall asleep at any time of the day and during nearly any activity, including driving a car.

Breathing-related Sleep Disorder is diagnosed when sleep is distrupted by an obstruction of the breathing apparatus. Circadian Rhythm Sleep Disorder is a disruption of normal sleep patterns leading to a mismatch between the schedule required by a person's environment and his or her sleeping patterns; i.e., the individual is irresistibly sleepy when he or she is required to be awake, and awake at those times that he or she should be sleeping. Nightmare Disorder is diagnosed when there is a repeated occurrence of frightening dreams that lead to waking. Sleep Terror Disorder is the repeated occurrence of sleep terrors, or abrupt awakenings from sleeping with a shriek or a cry.

SYMPTOMS

We will address here only the disorder with the greatest prevalence: Primary Insomnia. A diagnosis of Primary Insomnia is made if the following criteria are met:
• Difficulty initiating or maintaining sleep or nonrestorative sleep for at least one month;
• The impairment causes clinically significant distress or impairment in social, occupational or other important areas of functioning;
• The disturbance does not occur exclusively during the course of other sleep-related disorders;
• The disturbance is not due to another general medical or psychiatric disorder, or the direct physiological effects of a substance.

ASSOCIATED FEATURES

Individuals with primary insomnia have a history of light sleeping. Interpersonal or work-related problems typically arise because of lack of sleep. Accidents and injuries may result from lack of attentiveness during waking hours, and sleep inducing, tranquillizer, or other medications are liable to be misused or abused. Once general medical problems are ruled out, a careful sleep history will often reveal that the individual has poor sleep habits or is reacting to an adverse life situation. These problems can then be addressed with advice or psychotherapy.

PREVALENCE

Surveys indicate a one-year prevalence of insomnia complaints in thirty percent to forty percent of adults, though the percentage of those who would have a diagnosis of Primary Insomnia is unknown. In clinics specializing in Sleep Disorders, about fifteen percent to twenty-five percent of individuals with chronic insomnia are diagnosed with Primary Insomnia.

TREATMENT OPTIONS

Treatment for Sleep Disorders should combine an examination by a primary care physician to determine physical condition and sleeping habits, and a discussion with a somologist, a professional trained in Sleep Disorders, or other mental health professional to determine the individual's emotional state.

Referrals may be made to sleep clinics, which can be situated in hospitals, or sleep disorder centers, which could be part of hospitals, universities or psychiatric institutions. To determine the cause of sleep disturbances, an individual in a sleep clinic or sleep disorder center may undergo interviews, psychological tests and laboratory observation — sleeping in the sleep laboratory while various functions are monitored. Medications that may be part of treatment for Sleep Disorders include drugs known as Hypnotics, or sleeping pills, including temazepam, Ambien, Sonata, and Lunesta. Some medications are more helpful with falling, and others with staying, asleep; a new formulation of Ambien has been developed in an attempt to address both. Sleep medications can lose effectiveness if taken over extended periods; use should always be supervised by a physician. Many cases will resolve with improved sleep hygiene, and treatment of pain and other remediable causes. There is also a new drug, Provigil, which helps people with Narcoleopsy to stay awake.

Associations & Agencies

1468 American Academy of Sleep Medicine
One Westbrook Corporate Center
Suite 920
Westchester, IL 60154
708-492-0930
Fax: 708-492-0943
E-mail: inquiries@aasmnet.org
www.aasmnet.org

Jerome A Barrett, Executive Director
Jennifer Markkanen, Assistant Executive Director

National not-for-profit professional membership organization dedicated to the advancement of sleep medicine. The Academy's mission is to assure quality care for patients with sleep disorders, promote the advancement of sleep research and provide public and professional education. The AASM delivers programs, information and services to and through its members and advocates sleep medicine supportive policies in the medical community and the public sector.

Year Founded: 1975

1469 Center for Family Support (CFS)
333 7th Avenue
New York, NY 10001-5004
212-629-7939
Fax: 212-239-2211
www.cfsny.org

Steven Vernickofs, Executive Director

An agency that continues to develop new programs to serve families and individuals with their care needs. They currently offer services throughout the New York City region including: New Jersey, Long Island and the Lower Hudson Valley.

1470 National Alliance on Mental Illness
2107 Wilson Boulevard
Suite 300
Arlington, VA 22201-3042
703-524-7600
800-950-6264
Fax: 703-524-9094
E-mail: info@nami.org
www.nami.org

Suzanne Vogel-Scibilia, MD, President
Frederick R Sandoval, First VP

Nation's leading self-help organization for all those affected by severe brain disorders. Mission is to bring consumers and families with similar experiences together to share information about services, care providers, and ways to cope with the challenges of schizophrenia, manic depression, and other serious mental illnesses.

Year Founded: 1979

1471 National Association for the Dually Diagnose d (NADD)
132 Fair Street
Kingston, NY 12401-4802
845-334-4336
800-331-5362
Fax: 845-331-4569
E-mail: nadd@mhv.net
www.thenadd.org

Dr. Robert Fletcher, Executive Director

Nonprofit organization designed to promote interest of professional and parent development with resources for individuals who have the coexistence of mental illness and mental retardation. Provides conference, educational services and training materials to professionals, parents, concerned citizens and service organizations. Formerly known as the National Association for the Dually Diagnosed.

1472 National Mental Health Consumer's Self-Help
1211 Chestnut Street
Suite 1207
Philadelphia, PA 19107
215-751-1810
800-553-4539
Fax: 215-636-6312
E-mail: info@mhselfhelp.org
www.mhselfhelp.org

Joseph Rodgers, Founder/Executive Director
Christine Simiriglia, Director

Funded by the National Institute of Mental Health Community Support Program, the purpose of the Clearinghouse is to encourage the development and growth of consumer self-help groups.

1473 National Mental Health Consumers' Self-Help Clearinghouse
1211 Chestnut Street
Suite 1207
Philadelphia, PA 19107
215-751-1810
800-553-4539
Fax: 215-636-6312
E-mail: info@mhselfhelp.org
www.mhselfhelp.org

Joseph A Rogers, Executive Director

A national consumer technical assistance center that has played a major role in the development of the mental health consumer movement.

Year Founded: 1986

1474 SAMHSA'S National Mental Health Information Center
US Department of Health and Human Services
PO Box 42557
Washington, DC 20015
800-789-2647
Fax: 240-747-5470
TDD: 866-889-2647
E-mail: ken@mentalhealth.org
www.mentalhealth.samhsa.gov

A Kathryn Power, MEd, Director
Edward B Searle, Deputy Director

Information about resources, technical assistance, research, training, networks, and other federal clearing houses, and fact sheets and materials. Information specialists refer callers to mental health resources in their communities as well as state, federal and nonprofit contacts. Staff available Monday through Friday, 8:30 AM - 5:00 PM, EST, excluding federal holidays. After hours, callers may leave messages and an information specialist will return their call.

Books

1475 Concise Guide to Evaluation and Management of Sleep Disorders
American Psychiatric Publishing
1000 Wilson Boulevard
Suite 1825
Arlington, VA 22209-3901
703-907-7322
800-368-5777
Fax: 703-907-1091
E-mail: appi@psych.org
www.appi.org

Katie Duffy, Marketing Assistant

Overview of sleep disorders medicine, sleep physiology and pathology, insomnia complaints, excessive sleepiness disorders, parasomnias, medical and psychiatric disorders and sleep, medications with sedative-hypnotic properties, special problems and populations. *$29.95*

304 pages ISBN 0-880489-06-5

1476 Drug Therapy and Sleep Disorders
Mason Crest Publishers
370 Reed Road
Suite 302
Broomall, PA 19008
610-543-6200
866-627-2665
Fax: 610-543-3878
E-mail: dtaylor@masoncrest.com
www.masoncrest.com

What are sleep disorders? Which drugs do doctors prescribe to treat them? What risks and benefits are involved? This book answers these and other questions by examining various sleep disorders, their symptoms and causes, common treatments, the drugs used to treat them, and how sleep drugs affect the brain.

ISBN 1-590845-76-5

1477 Principles and Practice of Sleep Medicine
Elsevier/WB Saunders Company
Curtis Center, Suite 300E
170 S Independence Mall W
Philadelphia, PA 19106-3399
215-238-7800
800-523-1649
Fax: 800-238-7883
www.us.elsevierhealth.com

Covers the recent advances in basic sciences as well as sleep pathology in adults. Encompasses developments in this rapidly advancing field and also includes topics related to psychiatry, circadian rhythms, cardiovascualr diseases and sleep apnea diagnosis and treatment. Hardcover.
$159.00
1336 pages Year Founded: 2000 ISBN 0-721676-70-7

478 Sleep Disorders Sourcebook, Second Edition
Omnigraphics
PO Box 625
Holmes, PA 19043
800-234-1340
Fax: 800-875-1340
E-mail: info@omnigraphics.com
www.omnigraphics.com

Amy L Sutton, Editor

Omnigrahphics is the publisher of the Health Reference Series, a growing consumer health information resource with more than 100 volumes in print. Each title in the series features an easy to understand format, nontechnical language, comprehensive indexing and resources for further information. Material in each book has been collected from a wide range of government agencies, professional associations, periodicals and other sources. *$78.00*
567 pages Year Founded: 2005 ISBN 1-780807-43-X

Web Sites

1479 www.aasmnet.org
American Academy of Sleep Medicine

A professional society that is dedicated exclusively to the medical subspecialty of sleep medicine.

1480 www.cyberpsych.org
CyberPsych

Presents information about psychoanalysis, psychotherapy and special topics such as anxiety disorders, the problematic use of alcohol, homophobia, and the traumatic effects of racism.

1481 www.mentalhealth.com
Internet Mental Health

Offers on-line psychiatric diagnosis in the hope of reaching the two-thirds of individuals with mental illness who do not seek treatment.

1482 www.nhlbi.nih.gov/about/ncsdr
National Institute of Health National Center on Sleep Disorders

The Center seeks to fulfill its goal of improving the health of Americans by serving four key functions: research, training, technology transfer, and coordination.

1483 www.nlm.nih.gov/medlineplus/sleepdisorders. html
MEDLINEplus on Sleep Disorders

Compilation of links directs you to information on sleep disorders.

1484 www.planetpsych.com
Planetpsych.com

Online resource for mental health information.

1485 www.psychcentral.com
Psych Central

The Internet's largest and oldest independent mental health social network created and run by mental health professionals to guarantee reliable, trusted information and support communities to you.

1486 www.sleepdisorders.about.com
About.com on Sleep Disorders

Well-organized information including new developments and a chat room.

1487 www.sleepdisorders.com
SleepDisorders.com

Updated monthly and organized by sleep disorders with quality links.

1488 www.sleepfoundation.org
National Sleep Foundation

Dedicated to improving public health and safety by achieving understanding of sleep and sleep disorders, and by supporting sleep-related education, research, and advocacy.

1489 www.sleepnet.com
Sleepnet.com

Categorizes sleep disorders for research, forums are up-dated frequently and posts are thoughtful and insightful.

1490 www.talhost.net/sleep/links.htm
Sleep Disorder

For those who have sleep disorders and have a problem sleeping.

Suicide

Introduction

Suicide is an event, not a mental disorder, but it is the lethal consequence of some mental disorders. Suicide involves a complex interaction of psychological, neurological, medical, social, and family factors.

Most professionals distinguish at least two suicide groups: those who actually kill themselves, i.e., completed suicides; and those who attempt it, usually harming themselves, but survive. Those who succeed in killing themselves are nearly always suffering from one or more psychiatric disorders, most commonly depression, often along with alcohol or substance abuse. Some individuals plan suicide very carefully, taking steps to insure that they will not be discovered and rescued, and they use lethal means (shooting themselves, or jumping from high places). Some act impulsively, reacting to a life disappointment by jumping off a nearby bridge. Some suicide attempts or gestures use means that make discovery and rescue probable, and are not likely to be lethal (e.g. taking insufficient pills). Some people make repeated suicide attempts. Unfortunately, recurrent suicidal gestures cannot be dismissed; each unsuccessful attempt increases the likelihood of a completed suicide in the future.

ASSOCIATED FEATURES

Nine of 10 suicides are associated with some form of mental disorder, especially Depression, Schizophrenia, Alcohol Abuse, Bipolar Disorder, and Panic Disorder. In addition, Personality Disorders have been diagnosed in one-third to one-half of people who kill themselves. These suicides often occur in younger people who live in an environment where drug and alcohol abuse, as well as violence, are common. The most common personality disorders associated with suicide are Borderline Personality Disorder, Antisocial Personality Disorder, and Narcissistic Personality Disorder. Among people with Schizophrenia, especially those suffering from Paranoid Schizophrenia, suicide is the main reason for premature death; they have a lifetime risk of ten percent.

Drug and alcohol abuse is also a risk factor for suicide: among 113 young people who killed themselves in California, fifty-five percent had some kind of substance abuse problems, usually long standing and including several different drugs.

Some suicides result from insufficiently treated, severe, debilitating, or terminal physical illness. The pain, restricted function, and dread of dependence can all contribute to suicidal behavior, especially in illnesses such as Huntington's Disease, cancer, multiple sclerosis, spinal cord injuries, and AIDS. Some or many of these risk factors are present in most completed suicides. Depression and suicide are not inevitable for people with severe general medical illnesses or disabilities. The recognition and treatment of depression, when it occurs, can prevent many suicides.

PREVALENCE

Suicide is the ninth leading cause of death in the US and the third leading cause among 15-24 year-olds. It is estimated that over five million people have suicidal thoughts, though there are only 30,000 deaths from suicide each year. This may be a serious underestimate, however, since suicide is still stigmatized and often goes unreported. In the general population there are 11.2 reported suicides for every 100,000 people. The incidence among 5-14 year-olds is 0.7 percent per 100,000; even very young children can commit suicide. The rate among 15-19 year-olds, 13.2 percent per 100,000, has recently increased sharply. Boys are more likely to complete suicide than girls, largely because they use more lethal means, such as firearms. Compared to other countries, guns are particularly common in the US as a means of suicide. Children who kill themselves often have a history of antisocial behavior, and depression and suicide is more common in their families than in families in general.

More males than females commit suicide, both among adults and adolescents. Among adults, the most likely suicides are among men who are widowed, divorced, or single, who lack social support, who are unemployed, who have a diagnosis of mental disorder (especially Depression), who have a physical illness, a family history of suicide, who are in psychological turmoil, who have made previous suicide attempts, who use or abuse alcohol, and/or who have easy access to firearms. Among adolescents, the most likely suicides are married males (or unwed and pregnant females), who have suffered from parental absence or abuse, who have academic problems, affective disorders (especially Bioplar Disorder), who are substance abusers, suffer from Attention-Deficit/Hyperactivity Disorder or epilepsy, who have Conduct Disorder, problems with impulse control, a family history of suicide, and/or access to firearms. Keeping guns in the home is a suicide risk for both males and females.

Elderly people (those over age 65) are more likely than any other age group to commit suicide. While only twelve percent of the population is elderly, twenty percent of all those who kill themselves are elderly. As in other population groups, elderly men are more likely to kill themselves than elderly women but the difference between the sexes is much bigger in this age group than in other age groups. Among all ages, the rate of suicide for men is about 20 per 100,000 and for women five per 100,000. Among the elderly, the rate for men is about 42 per 100,000 and for women about six and one-half per 100,000. Thus the great overall gender differences become even bigger among the elderly and more so as the elderly get older. The highest rate of suicide is among white elderly men, probably because their economic and social status drops severely with age, because they usually do not have a good support system and because they are highly unlikely to ask for help.

Although all the factors discussed here are risk factors, it should be kept in mind that 99.9 percent of those at risk do not commit suicide.

TREATMENT OPTIONS

Considering the risk factors, a professional must first make a careful assessment, taking all the risk factors into account, including the availability of weapons, pills and other lethal means, as well as suicidal ideation and whether or not the person has conveyed the intention to commit suicide, and whether the method the patient plans to use is available (one can only jump off a bridge if there is a bridge, or drive into a wall if one has access to a vehicle). Every individual who feels that life is not worth living, or who is contemplating suicide, should be asked about guns in the home and should be encouraged to remove them.

Someone who has no thought of death or has thoughts of death that are not connected with suicide is at a lower risk than someone who is thinking of suicide. Among those who are thinking of it, those who have not worked out the means of committing suicide are at a lower risk than those who think of suicide and a specific method of carrying it out. Treatment is partly based on the level of intervention that is believed to be required. If the person is seriously depressed and is also anxious, tense, and angry, and in overwhelming psychological anguish, the risk is more acute. The first priority is to ensure the safety of the client. Sometimes hospitalization is necessary.

After safety is assured, treatment is aimed at the underlying disorder. It may include psychological support, medication and other therapies: group; art; dance/movement. Professional tretament may include psychological support, medication and other therapies: group; art; dance/movement. Professional treatment should involve working with the family if possible and other medical staff, e.g., a physician. Regular reassessments should take place.

In cases of Personality Disorders, there may be anger and aggression, and the suicidal thoughts and ideas may be chronic or repetitive. This is a particular strain on professionals, patients, and family. The patient, family, and clinician must work together to understand the chronicity of the condition, and the fact that suicide cannot always be prevented. It is essential to develop a working alliance between therapist and client, based on trust, mutual respect, and on the client's belief that the therapist genuinely cares about him/her, while at the same time setting limits on patient demands so that the clinician does not "burn out." Reassessments include getting information from other professionals involved in treating the person, including reassessment of medication with the prescribing physician, and from family members or others significant in the life of the client who should participate in planning and following up. Assessment must also include assessment of the client's ability to understand and participate in the treatment, information about his/her psychological state (hopeless, despairing, depressed) and cognitive competence.

Associations & Agencies

1492 American Association of Suicidology
5221 Wisconsin Avenue NW
Washington, DC 20015
202-237-2280
Fax: 202-237-2282
E-mail: info@suicidology.org
www.suicidology.org

James J Mazza, President
Alan Berman, PhD, Executive Director

A nonprofit organization devoted to understanding and preventing suicide. Promotes public awareness, research, public education, and training for professionals and volunteers.

Year Founded: 1968

1493 American Foundation for Suicide Prevention
120 Wall Street
22 Floor
New York, NY 10005-4023
212-363-3500
888-333-2377
Fax: 212-363-6237

E-mail: inquiry@afsp.org
www.afsp.org

Robert Gebbia, Executive Director
Herbert Hendin, MD, Medical Director

The American Foundation for Suicide Prevention (AFSP) is the only national not-for-profit exclusively dedicated to funding suicide prevention research, initiating treatment projects and offering educational programs and conferences.

1494 National Alliance on Mental Illness
2107 Wilson Boulevard
Suite 300
Arlington, VA 22201-3042
703-524-7600
800-950-6264
Fax: 703-524-9094
E-mail: info@nami.org
www.nami.org

Suzanne Vogel-Scibilia, MD, President
Frederick R Sandoval, First VP

Nation's leading self-help organization for all those affected by severe brain disorders. Mission is to bring consumers and families with similar experiences together to share information about services, care providers, and ways to cope with the challenges of schizophrenia, manic depression, and other serious mental illnesses.

Year Founded: 1979

1495 National Mental Health Consumer's Self-Help
1211 Chestnut Street
Suite 1207
Philadelphia, PA 19107
215-751-1810
800-553-4539
Fax: 215-636-6312
E-mail: info@mhselfhelp.org
www.mhselfhelp.org

Joseph Rodgers, Founder/Executive Director
Christine Simiriglia, Director

Funded by the National Institute of Mental Health Community Support Program, the purpose of the Clearinghouse is to encourage the development and growth of consumer self-help groups.

1496 National Mental Health Consumers' Self-Help Clearinghouse
1211 Chestnut Street
Suite 1207
Philadelphia, PA 19107
215-751-1810
800-553-4539
Fax: 215-636-6312
E-mail: info@mhselfhelp.org
www.mhselfhelp.org

Joseph Rogers, Executive Director

A national consumer technical assistance center that has played a major role in the development of the mental health consumer movement.

Year Founded: 1986

1497 SAMHSA'S National Mental Health Information Center
US Department of Health and Human Services
PO Box 42557
Washington, DC 20015
800-789-2647
Fax: 240-747-5470
TDD: 866-889-2647
E-mail: ken@mentalhealth.org
www.mentalhealth.samhsa.gov

A Kathryn Power, MEd, Director
Edward B Searle, Deputy Director

Information about resources, technical assistance, research, training, networks, and other federal clearing houses, and fact sheets and materials. Information specialists refer callers to mental health resources in their communities as well as state, federal and nonprofit contacts. Staff available Monday through Friday, 8:30 AM - 5:00 PM, EST, excluding federal holidays. After hours, callers may leave messages and an information specialist will return their call.

1498 Suicide Prevention Action Network USA (SPANUSA)
1025 Vermont Avenue NW
Suite 1066
Washington, DC 20005
202-449-3600
Fax: 202-449-3601
E-mail: info@spanusa.org
www.spanusa.org

Jerry Reed, Executive Director

SPAN USA is dedicated to preventing suicide through public education and awareness, community engagement, and federal, state and local grassroots advocacy. By empowering those who have been touched by suicide, SPAN USA seeks to advance the implementation of the National Strategy for Suicide Prevention.

Year Founded: 1996

Books

1499 Adolescent Suicide
American Psychiatric Publishing
1000 Wilson Boulevard
Suite 1825
Arlington, VA 22209-3901
703-907-7322
800-368-5777
Fax: 703-907-1091
E-mail: appi@psych.org
www.appi.org

Katie Duffy, Marketing Assistant

Presents techniques that allow psychiatrists and other professionals to respond to signs of distress with timely therapeutic intervention. *$38.95*

212 pages ISBN 0-873182-08-1

1500 Adolescent Suicide: A School-Based Approach to Assessment and Intervention
Research Press
Dept 24 W
PO Box 9177
Champaign, IL 61826
217-352-3273
800-519-2707

Fax: 217-352-1221
E-mail: rp@researchpress.com
www.researchpress.com

Dennis Wiziecki, Marketing
Dr William G Kirk, Author

Presents the information required to accurately identify potentially suicidal adolescents and provides the skills necessary for effective intervention. The book includes many case examples derived from information provided by parents, mental health professionals and educators, as well as adolescents who have considered suicide or survived suicide attempts. An essential resource for school counseling staff, psychologists, teachers and administrators. *$16.95*

190 pages ISBN 0-878223-36-3

1501 An Unquiet Mind: A Memoir of Moods and Madne ss
Knopf Publishing Group
1745 Broadway
New York, NY 10019
Fax: 212-940-7307
E-mail: knopfpublicity@randomhouse.com
www.www.randomhouse.com/knopf/

Kay Redfield Jamison, Author

Dr. Kay Redfield Jamison may be the foremost authority on manic-depressive illness. She is also one of its survivors. And it is this dual prespective—as healer and healed—that makes Jamison's memoir so lucid, learned, and profoundly affecting.

ISBN 0-961632-60-7

1502 Anatomy of Suicide: Silence of the Heart
Charles C Thomas Publisher
2600 S First Street
Springfield, IL 62704-4730
217-789-8980
800-258-8980
Fax: 217-789-9130
E-mail: books@ccthomas.com
www.ccthomas.com

The author explores the scope of this problem which involves clinical and ethical issues; the myth of depression; the path to suicide; unfinished business; staying alive; early warnings; first interventions; the self-contract; cases in point; and the future of suicide. Written for psychologists, counselors, and mental health professionals, this book is an excellent resource that will further our understanding of suicide and seek new ways for prevention. *$42.95*

170 pages Year Founded: 1998 ISSN 0-398-06803-8ISBN 0-398068-02-X

1503 Brilliant Madness: Living with Manic-Depressive Illness
Bantam Books
1745 Broadway
3rd Floor
New York, NY 10019
212-782-9000
Fax: 212-572-6066
E-mail: bdpublicity@randomhouse.com
www.www.randomhouse.com

Patty Duke, Author

1504 Exubernace: The Passion for Life
Knopf Publishing Group
1745 Broadway
New York, NY 10019
Fax: 212-940-7307
E-mail: knopfpublicity@randomhouse.com
www.www.randomhouse.com/knopf/

Kay Redfield Jamison, Author

1505 Harvard Medical School Guide to Suicide
Assessment and Intervention
Jossey-Bass / Wiley & Sons
111 River Street
Hoboken, NJ 07030-5774
201-748-6000
Fax: 201-748-6088
E-mail: consumers@wiley.com
www.wiley.com

Presents a multidimensional model of suicide assessment by offering clear techniques for intervention in both inpatient and outpatient settings. Also describes the use of psychopharmacology and prevention in the context of managed care. *$59.95*

736 pages Year Founded: 1998 ISBN 0-787943-03-7

1506 In the Wake of Suicide
Jossey-Bass / Wiley & Sons
111 River Street
Hoboken, NJ 07030-5774
201-748-6000
Fax: 201-748-6088
E-mail: consumers@wiley.com
www.wiley.com

Breathtaking stories of incredible power for anyone struggling to find the meaning in the suicide death of a loved one and for all readers seeking writing that moves and inspires. *$27.00*

256 pages Year Founded: 1998 ISBN 0-787940-52-6

1507 Left Alive: After a Suicide Death in the Family
Charles C Thomas Publisher
2600 S 1st Street
Springfield, IL 62704-4730
217-789-8980
800-258-8980
Fax: 217-789-9130
E-mail: books@ccthomas.com
www.ccthomas.com

$21.95

120 pages ISBN 0-398066-50-7

1508 Manic-Depressive Illness: Bipolar Disorders
and Recurrent Depression
Oxford University Press
2001 Evans Road
Cary, NC 27513
800-445-9714
Fax: 919-677-1303
E-mail: custserv.us@oup.com
www.www.oup.com/us

Frederick K Goodwin, Author

The revolution in psychiatry that began in earnest in the 1960s led to dramatic advances in the understanding and treamtent of manic-depressive illness. Hailed as the most outstanding book in the biomedical sciences when it was originally published in 1990.

1509 My Son...My Son: A Guide to Healing After De
ath, Loss, or Suicide
Bolton Press Atlanta
1090 Crest Brook Lane
Roswell, GA 30075-3403
770-645-1886
Fax: 770-649-0999
E-mail: contactus@boltonpress.com
www.www.boltonpress.com

Iris Bolton, Author

A moving story of love, loss and recovery that will grab your heart, nourish your soul and open your eyes. A must read for anyone who has experienced a great loss and is trying to find some path out of the darkness of their despair or to understand those that are.

ISBN 0-961632-60-7

1510 Night Falls Fast: Understanding Suicide
Vintage Books A Division Of Random House
1745 Broadway
20th Floor
New York, NY 10019
212-572-2882
800-733-3000
Fax: 212-572-6043
www.www.randomhouse.com/vintage/index.html

Kay Redfield Jamison, Author

ISBN 0-375701-47-8

1511 No Time to Say Goodbye: Surviving the Suicid
e of a Loved One
Broadway Books a Division of Random House
1745 Broadway
New York, NY 10019
212-782-9000
E-mail: bwaypub@randomhouse.com
www.www.randomhouse.com/broadway

Carla Fine, Author

1512 Suicidal Patient: Principles of Assesment,
Treatment, and Case Management
American Psychiatric Publishing
1000 Wilson Boulevard
Suite 1825
Arlington, VA 22209-3901
703-907-7322
800-368-5777
Fax: 703-907-1091
E-mail: appi@psych.org
www.appi.org

Katie Duffy, Marketing Assistant

Presents a clinical approach and valuable assessment strategies and techniques. Demonstrates an easy to use innovative clinical model with specific stages of treatment and associated interventions outlined for inpatient and outpatient settings. *$45.50*

282 pages ISBN 0-800485-54-X

1513 Suicide Over the Life Cycle
American Psychiatric Publishing
1000 Wilson Boulevard
Suite 1825
Arlington, VA 22209-3901
703-907-7322
800-368-5777
Fax: 703-907-1091
E-mail: appi@psych.org
www.appi.org

Katie Duffy, Marketing Assistant

Helps readers understand risk factors and treatment of suicidal patients. *$82.50*

836 pages ISBN 0-880483-07-5

1514 Touched with Fire: Manic-Depressive Illness and The Artistic Temperament
Free Press
40 Main Street
Suite 301
Florence, MA 01062
877-888-1533
Fax: 413-585-8904
www.www.freepress.net

Kay Redfield Jamison, Author

"We of the craft are all crazy." -remarked Lord Byron about himself and his fellow poets.

1515 Understanding and Preventing Suicide: New Perspectives
Charles C Thomas Publisher
2600 S 1st Street
Springfield, IL 62704-4730
217-789-8980
800-258-8980
Fax: 217-789-9130
E-mail: books@ccthomas.com
www.ccthomas.com

Seven perspectives for understanding and preventing suicidal behavior, illustrating their implications for prevention. This book discusses suicide from a crimnological perspective, and whether the theories in it have any applicability to suicidal behavior, both in furthering our understanding of suicide and in seeing new ways to prevent suicide. Armed with this information, we may move far toward understanding and preventing suicide in the twenty-first century. *$35.95*

137 pages Year Founded: 1990 ISSN 0-398-06235-8ISBN 0-398057-09-5

Periodicals & Pamphlets

1516 Suicide Talk: What To Do If You Hear It
ETR Associates
4 Carbonero Way
Scotts Valley, CA 95066
831-438-4060
800-321-4407
Fax: 800-435-8433
E-mail: customerservice@etr.org
www.etr.org

Includes suicide warning signs, how to help a friend, and ways to relieve stress. *$16.00*

1517 Suicide: Fast Fact 3
SAMHSA'S National Mental Health Information Center
PO Box 42557
Washington, DC 20015
800-789-2647
Fax: 240-747-5470
TDD: 866-889-2647
E-mail: ken@mentalhealth.org
www.mentalhealth.samhsa.org

A Kathryn Power MEd, Director
Edward B Searle, Deputy Director

This fact card provides statistics and a list of resources on suicide.

Year Founded: 2000

1518 Suicide: Who Is at Risk?
ETR Associates
4 Carbonero Way
Scotts Valley, CA 95066
831-438-4060
800-321-4407
Fax: 800-435-8433
E-mail: customerservice@etr.org
www.etr.org

Includes warning signs, symptoms, and what to do. *$ 16.00*

Support Groups & Hot Lines

1519 Friends for Survival
PO Box 214463
Sacramento, CA 95821
916-392-0664
www.friendsforsurvival.org

Marilyn Koenig, Director

An organization of people who have been affected by a death caused by suicide. Dedicated to providing a variety of peer support services that comfort those in grief, encourage healing and growth, foster the development of skills to cope with a loss and educate the entire community regarding the impact of suicide.

1520 NineLine
460 W 41st Street
New York, NY 10036
212-613-0300
800-999-9999
www.nineline.org

Bruce J Henry, Executive Director

Nationwide crisis/suicide hotline.

1521 Survivors of Loved Ones' Suicides (SOLOS)
PO Box 592
Dumfries, VA 22026-0592
E-mail: solos@1000deaths.com
www.1000deaths.com

Christine Smith, PhD, President

Provide help and support to Survivors of Loved Ones Suicides(SOLOS) through outreach, education and research.

Web Sites

1522 www.cyberpsych.org
CyberPsych

Presents information about psychoanalysis, psychotherapy and special topics such as anxiety disorders, the problematic use of alcohol, homophobia, and the traumatic effects of racism.

1523 www.lollie.com/about/suicide.html
Comprehensive Approach to Suicide Prevention

Readings for anyone contemplating suicide.

1524 www.members.aol.com/dswgriff/suicide.html
Now Is Not Forever: A Survival Guide

Print out a no-suicide contract, do problem solving, and other exercises.

1525 www.members.tripod.com/~suicideprevention/ index
Suicide Prevention Help

Coping with suicidal thoughts and friends.

1526 www.mentalhealth.com
Internet Mental Health

Offers online psychiatric diagnosis in the hope of reaching the two-thirds of individuals with mental illness who do not seek treatment.

1527 www.metanoia.org/suicide/
If You Are Thinking about Suicide...Read This First

Excellent suggestions, information and links for the suicidal.

1528 www.planetpsych.com
Planetpsych.com

Online resource for mental health information

1529 www.psychcentral.com
Psych Central

The Internet's largest and oldest independent mental health social network created and run by mental health professionals to guarantee reliable, trusted information and support to communities to you.

1530 www.psycom.net/depression.central.suicide. html
Suicide and Suicide Prevention

List of links to material on suicide.

1531 www.save.org
SA/VE - Suicide Awareness/Voices of Education

Prevents suicide through public awareness and education, reduce stigma, and serve as a resource for those touched by suicide.

1532 www.vcc.mit.edu/comm/samaritans/brochure. html
How to Help Someone You Care About

Guidelines for family.

1533 www.vvc.mit.edu/comm/samaritans/warning. html
Signs of Suicide Risk

Tic Disorders

Introduction

A tic is described as a sudden, rapid, recurrent, non-rhythmic motor movement or vocalization. Four disorders are associated with tics: Chronic Motor or Vocal Tick Disorder, Transient Tic Disorder, Tic Disorder Not Otherwise Specified, and Tourette's Syndrome. Tourette's Syndrome is the most extreme case, consisting of multiple motor tics and one or more vocal tics, and will be the focus of this chapter. The vocalizations of Tourette's Syndrome can consist of grunts, obscenities, or other words the individual otherwise would not make. They are disruptive and profoundly embarrassing.

SYMPTOMS

• Multiple motor, as well as one or more vocal tics have been present during the illness, not necessarily at the same time;
• The tics occur many times during a day (often in bouts) nearly every day or intermittently throughout for more than one year, and during this period there was never a tic-free period of more three consecutive months;
• The disturbance causes clear distress or difficulties in social, work, or other areas;
• The onset is before age 18;
• The involuntary movements or vocalizations are not due to the direct effects of a substance (e.g., stimulants) or a general medication condition.

ASSOCIATED FEATURES

Between ten percent and forty percent of people with Tourette's Syndrome also have echolalia (automatically repeating words spoken by others) or echopraxia (imitating someone else's movements). Fewer than ten percent have coprolalia (the involuntary uterance of obscenities). There seems to be a clear association between tic disorders, such as Tourette's Syndrome and Obsessive Compulsive Disorder (OCD). As many as twenty percent to thirty percent of people with OCD report having or having had tics, and between five percent and seven percent of those with OCD also have Tourette's Syndrome. In studies of patients with Tourette's Syndrome it was found that thirty-six percent to fifty-two percent also meet the criteria for OCD. This is evidence that Tourette's Syndrome and Obsessive Compulsive Disorder share a genetic basis or some underlying pathological/physiological disturbance. The genetic evidence is further strengthened by the concordance rate in twins (i.e., the likelihood that if one member of the pair has the disorder, the other will also develop it): in identical twins, who have the same genes, the concordance is fifty-three percent, whereas in fraternal twins, who are no more closely related than other siblings, it is eight percent.

Other conditions commonly associated with Tourette's Syndrome are hyperactivity, distractibility, impulsivity, difficulty in learning, emotional disturbances, and social problems. The disorder causes social uneasiness, shame, self-consciousness, and depression. The person may be rejected by others and may develop anxiety about the tics, negatively affecting social, school, and work functioning. In severe cases, the disorder may interfere with everyday activities like reading and writing.

PREVALENCE

Tourette's Syndrome is reported in a variety of ethnic and cultural groups. It is one and one-half to three times more common in males than females and about 10 times more prevalent in children and adolescents than in adults. Overall prevalence is estimated at between four and five people in 10,000.

While the age of onset can be as early as two years, it commonly begins during childhood or early adolescence. The median age for the development of tics is seven years. The disorder usually lasts for the life of the person, but there may be periods of remission of weeks, months, or years. The severity, frequency, and variability of the tics often diminish during adolescence and adulthood. In some cases, tics can disappear entirely by early adulthood.

TREATMENT OPTIONS

Many treatments have been tried. Haloperidol, an antipsychotic drug, is the most effective; it acts directly on the brain source of the tic, counteracting the overactivity, and can have a calming effect, but also can have unfortunate side effects. In very severe, disabling cases of OCD, brain surgery is an option. SSRIs (Selective Serotonin Reuptake Inhibitors) have also been effective in some cases of Tic Disorders. Symptoms of the disorder usually diminish with increasing age, and many people learn to live with them.

Associations & Agencies

1535 Center for Family Support (CFS)
333 7th Avenue
New York, NY 10001-5004
212-629-7939
Fax: 212-239-2211
www.cfsny.org

Steven Vernickofs, Executive Director

An agency that continues to develop new programs to serve families and individuals with their care needs. They currently offer services throughout the New York City region including: New Jersey, Long Island and the Lower Hudson Valley.

1536 National Alliance on Mental Illness
2107 Wilson Boulevard
Suite 300
Arlington, VA 22201-3042
703-524-7600
800-950-6264
Fax: 703-524-9094
E-mail: info@nami.org
www.nami.org

Joseph Rodgers, Founder/Executive Director
Christine Simirglia, Director

Nation's leading self-help organization for all those affected by severe brain disorders. Mission is to bring consumers and families with similar experiences together to share information about services, care providers, and ways to cope with the challenges of schizophrenia, manic depression, and other serious mental illnesses.

Year Founded: 1979

1537 National Association for the Dually Diagnose d (NADD)
132 Fair Street
Kingston, NY 12401-4802
845-334-4336
800-331-5362
Fax: 845-331-4569
E-mail: nadd@mhv.net
www.thenadd.org

Dr. Robert Fletcher, Executive Director

Nonprofit organization designed to promote interest of professional and parent development with resources for individuals who have the coexistence of mental illness and mental retardation. Provides conference, educational services and training materials to professionals, parents, concerned citizens and service organizations. Formerly known as the National Association for the Dually Diagnosed.

1538 National Mental Health Consumer's Self-Help
1211 Chestnut Street
Suite 1207
Philadelphia, PA 19107
215-751-1810
800-553-4539
Fax: 215-636-6312
E-mail: info@mhselfhelp.org
www.mhselfhelp.org

Christine Simiriglia, Executive Director
Jennifer Melinn, Information/Referral Dept.

Funded by the National Institute of Mental Health Community Support Program, the purpose of the Clearinghouse is to encourage the development and growth of consumer self-help groups.

1539 National Mental Health Consumers' Self-Help Clearinghouse
1211 Chestnut Street
Suite 1207
Philadelphia, PA 19107
215-751-1810
800-553-4539
Fax: 215-636-6312
E-mail: info@mhselfhelp.org
www.mhselfhelp.org

Joseph A Rogers, Executive Director

A national consumer technical assistance center that has played a major role in the development of the mental health consumer movement.

Year Founded: 1986

1540 SAMHSA'S National Mental Health Information Center
US Department of Health and Human Services
PO Box 42557
Washington, DC 20015
800-789-2647
Fax: 240-747-5470
TDD: 866-889-2647
E-mail: ken@mentalhealth.org
www.mentalhealth.samhsa.gov

A Kathryn Power, MEd, Director
Edward B Searle, Deputy Director

Information about resources, technical assistance, research, training, networks, and other federal clearing houses, and fact sheets and materials. Information specialists refer callers to mental health resources in their communities as well as state, federal and nonprofit contacts. Staff available Monday through Friday, 8:30 AM - 5:00 PM, EST, excluding federal holidays. After hours, callers may leave messages and an information specialist will return their call.

1541 Tourette Syndrome Association
42-40 Bell Boulevard
Suite 205
Bayside, NY 11361-2820
718-224-2999
888-486-8738
Fax: 718-279-9596
E-mail: ts@tsa-usa.org
www.tsa-usa.org

Tracy Flynn, Public Information

National, nonprofit voluntary health organization with 50 chapters in the US and over 45 contacts in other countries. Members include people with TS, their relatives and other interested, concerned supporters.

Year Founded: 1972

Books

1542 Adam and the Magic Marble
Hope Press
PO Box 188
Duarte, CA 91009-0188
800-321-4039
Fax: 818-358-3520
E-mail: dcomings@mail.earthlink.net
www.hopepress.com

Exciting reading for all ages, and a must for those who have been diagnosed with Tourette syndrome or other disabilities. An up-beat story of three heros, two with Tourette syndrome, one with cerebal palsy. Constantly taunted by bullies, the boys find a marble full of magic power, they aim a spell at the bullies and the adventure begins. *$6.95*

1543 Children with Tourette Syndrome: A Parent's Guide
ADD WareHouse
300 NW 70th Avenue
Suite 102
Plantation, FL 33317
954-792-8100
800-233-9273
Fax: 954-792-8545
E-mail: sales@addwarehouse.com
www.addwarehouse.com

The first guide written specifically for parents and other family members is a collaboration by a team of medical specialists, therapists, people with TS, and parents. It provides a complete introduction to TS and how it's diagnosed and treated. Also, chapters on family life, emotions, education and legal rights. *$17.00*

340 pages

1544 Children with Tourette Syndrome: A Parents' Guide
Woodbine House
6510 Bells Mill Road
Bethesda, MD 20817

800-843-7323
E-mail: info@woodbinehouse.com
www.www.woodbinehouse.com

Tracy Lynne Marsh, Author

Essays discuss the nature of Tourette Syndrome, how it is diagnosed and treated, daily life, family adjustments, and the educational needs of children with Tourette Syndrome.

ISBN 1-890627-36-4

1545 Don't Think About Monkeys: Extraordinary Stories Written by People with Tourette Syndrome
Hope Press
PO Box 188
Duarte, CA 91009-0188
800-321-4039
Fax: 626-358-3520
www.hopepress.com

Collection of fourteen stories written by teenager and adults with Tourette syndrome, describing how they have managed to cope and live with disorder. Especially inspiring to others with this and similar disorders. *$12.95*

200 pages ISBN 1-878267-33-7

1546 Echolalia: an Adult's Story of Tourette Syndrome
Hope Press
PO Box 188
Duarte, CA 91009-0188
818-303-0644
800-321-4039
Fax: 818-358-3520
www.hopepress.com

Adam Seligman, Author

Story of best selling writer Jackson Evans, who was diagnosed at age 35 as having Tourette syndrome and obsessive-compulsive disorder. At first he is grateful for the answers it brings him, but Jackson soon realizes that the real problems are just beginning. Story is told in a poetic style that captures the rhythms that smooth the Tourette. It ends with the ultimate truth, the answer isn't in being diagnosed, the answer is in living. *$11.95*

165 pages Year Founded: 1991 ISBN 1-878267-31-0

1547 Hi, I'm Adam: a Child's Story of Tourette Syndrome
Hope Press
PO Box 188
Duarte, CA 91009-0188
818-303-0644
800-321-4039
Fax: 818-358-3520
www.hopepress.com

Adam Buehrens, Author

Adam Buehrens is ten years old and has Tourette syndrome. Adam wrote and illustrated this book because he wants everyone to know he and other children with Tourette syndrome are not crazy. They just have a common neurological disorder. If you know a child that has tics, temper tantrums, unreasonable fears, or problems dealing with school, you will find this a reassuring story. *$4.95*

35 pages Year Founded: 1990 ISBN 1-878267-29-9

1548 I Can't Stop!: A Story About Tourette Syndrome
Albert Whitman & Company
6340 Oakton Street
Morton Grove, IL 60053-2723
847-581-0033
800-255-7675
Fax: 847-581-0039
E-mail: mail@awhitmanco.com
www.www.awhitmanco.com

Holly L Niner, Author

A picture book about tics (and TS, obviously) for kids. The kids portrayed in the book are in elementary school, and I'd say the text is good for grades 2-5, and easily read to kids somewhat younger.

ISBN 0-807536-20-2

1549 Mind of its Own, Tourette's Syndrome: Story and a Guide
Oxford University Press
198 Madison Avenue
New York, NY 10016
212-726-6000
800-451-7556
Fax: 919-677-1303
www.oup-usa.org/orbs/

Composed of two parts which interdigitate with each other. One part is an on-going story about Michael, a boy with TS, and his family and friends. Michael is a fictional composite character drawn from experience with many patients. Portrays a relatively mild case because the majority of the cases are mild. The second part consists of factual information which we have tried to present in a clear and readable manner. Includes illustration, some tables and other materials that may be of interest.

174 pages ISBN 0-195065-87-5

1550 RYAN: a Mother's Story of Her Hyperactive/Tourette Syndrome Child
Hope Press
PO Box 188
Duarte, CA 91009-0188
818-303-0644
800-321-4039
Fax: 818-358-3520
E-mail: dcomings@mail.earthlink.net
www.hopepress.com

A moving and informative story of how a mother struggled with the many behavioral problems presented by her son with Tourette syndrome, ADHD and oppositional defiant disorder. *$9.95*

302 pages ISBN 1-878267-25-6

1551 Raising Joshua
Hope Press
PO Box 188
Duarte, CA 91009-0188
818-303-0644
800-321-4039
Fax: 818-358-3520
E-mail: dcomings@mail.earthlink.net
www.hopepress.com

A mothers story of Josh, a boy with Tourette Syndrome and Attention Deficit Hyperactivity Disorder. *$14.95*

ISBN 0-965750-17-

1552 Tics and Tourette Syndrome: A Handbook for Parents and Professionals
Jessica Kingsley Publishers
116 Pentonville Road
London,
E-mail: post@jkp.com
www.www.jkp.com

Uttom Chowdhury, Author

This essential guide to tic disorders and Tourette Syndrome tackles problems faced both at home and at school, such as adjusting to the diagnosis, the effect on siblings and classroom difficulties.

ISBN 1-843102-03-X

1553 Tourette Syndrome
Dilligaf Publishing for Awareness Project
64 Court Street
Ellsworth, ME 04605
207-667-5031
E-mail: awareness@acadia.net

Includes an overview of the syndrome and tips of how to recognize traditional tics in the classroom; evaulation and referral are the basic components of this easy-to-read, basic book for the classroom teacher.

20 pages

1554 Tourette Syndrome and Human Behavior
Hope Press
PO Box 188
Duarte, CA 91009-0188
818-303-0644
800-321-4039
Fax: 818-358-3520
E-mail: dcomings@mail.earthlink.net
www.hopepress.com

How Tourette syndrome, a common hereditary disorder, provides insights into the cause and treatment of a wide range of human behavioral problems. It covers diagnosis, associated behaviors including ADHD, learning disorders, dyslexia, conduct disorder, obsessive-compulsive behaviors, alcoholism, drug abuse, obesity, depression, panic attacks, phobias, night terrors, bed wetting, sleep disturbances, lying, stealing, inappropiate sexual behavior, and others, brain structure and chemistry and implications for society. *$39.95*

850 pages ISBN 1-878267-28-0

1555 Tourette's Syndrome, Tics, Obsession, Compulsions: Developmental Psychopathology & Clinical Care
John Wiley & Sons
605 3rd Avenue
New York, NY 10058-0180
212-850-6000
Fax: 212-850-6008
E-mail: info@wiley.com
www.wiley.com

Once thought to be rare, Tourette's Syndeome is now seen as a relatively common childhood disorder either in its complete or partial incarnations. Drawing on the work of contributors hailing from the Yale Unversity Child Psychiatry Department, this edited volume explores the disorder from many perspectives, mapping out the diagnosis, genetics, phenomenology, natural history, and treatment of Tourette's Syndrome. *$189.00*

584 pages ISBN 0-471160-37-7

1556 Tourette's Syndrome: The Facts, Second Edition
Oxford University Press
198 Madison Avenue
New York, NY 10016
212-726-6000
800-451-7556
Fax: 919-677-1303
www.oup-usa.org

Mary M Robertson, Author

Explains the causes of the syndrome, how it is diagnosed, and the ways in which it can be treated. *$19.95*

110 pages Year Founded: 2005 ISBN 0-198523-98-X

1557 Tourette's Syndrome: Tics, Obsessions, Compulsions
ADD WareHouse
300 NW 70th Avenue
Suite 102
Plantation, FL 33317
954-792-8100
800-233-9273
Fax: 954-792-8545
E-mail: sales@addwarehouse.com
www.addwarehouse.com

Drawing on the work of contributors hailing from the prestigious Yale University Child Psychiatry Department, this edited volume explores the disorder from many perspectives, mapping out the diagnosis, genetics, phenomenology, natural history and treatment of Tourette's Syndrome. *$89.95*

584 pages

1558 Treating Tourette Syndrome and Tic Disorders : A Guide for Practitioners
The Guilford Press
72 Spring Street
New York, NY 10012
800-365-7006
Fax: 212-966-6708
E-mail: info@guilford.com
www.www.guilford.com

Peter Hollenbeck, Author

Grounded in a comprehensive model of Tourette syndrome (TS) and related disorders, this state-of-the-art volume provides a multidisciplinary framework for assessment and treatment.

ISBN 1-593854-80-3

1559 What Makes Ryan Tic?
Hope Press
PO Box 188
Duarte, CA 91009-0188
818-303-0644
800-321-4039
Fax: 818-358-3520
E-mail: dcomings@mail.earthlink.net
www.hopepress.com

What Makes Ryan Tic?: A Family's Triumph Over Tourette's Syndrome and Attention Deficit Hyperactivity Disorder. A moving and informative story of how a mother struggled with the many behavioral problems presented by her son with Tourette syndrome, ADHD and oppositional defiant disorder. *$15.95*

303 pages ISBN 1-878267-35-3

Support Groups & Hot Lines

1560 Tourette Syndrome Association
42-40 Bell Boulevard
Bayside, NY 11361-2820
718-224-2999
Fax: 718-224-9596
E-mail: ts@tsa-usa.org
www.tsa-usa.org

A national voluntary non-profit membership organization whose mission is to identify the cause of, find the cure for and control the effets of Tourette Syndrome.

Year Founded: 1972

Video & Audio

1561 After the Diagnosis...The Next Steps
Tourette Syndrome Association
42-40 Bell Boulevard
Suite 205
Bayside, NY 11361-2874
718-224-2999
888-486-8738
Fax: 718-279-9596
E-mail: ts@tsa-usa.org
www.tsa-usa.org

Judy Ungar, President
Gary Frank, EVP   ,
Mark Levine, VP Development
Richard Dreyfuss, Narrator

When the diagnosis is Tourette Syndrome, what do you do first? How do you sort out the complexities of the disorder? Whose advice do you follow? What steps do you take to lead a normal life? Six people with TS—as different as any six people can be—relate the sometimes difficult, but finally triumphant path each took to lead the rich, fulfilling life they now enjoy. Narrated by Academy Award-winning actor, Richard Dreyfuss, the stories are refreshing blends of poignancy, fact, and inspiration illustrating that a diagnosis of TS can be approached with confidence and hope. Includes comments by family and friends, teachers, counselors and leading medical authorities on Tourette Syndrome. A must-see for the newly diagnosed child, teen or adult. *$35.00*

1562 Clinical Counseling: Toward a Better Understanding of TS
Tourette Syndrome Association
42-40 Bell Boulevard
Suite 205
Bayside, NY 11361-2874
718-224-2999
888-486-8738
Fax: 718-279-9596
E-mail: ts@tsa-usa.org
www.tsa-usa.org

Judy Ungar, President
Gary Frank, EVP
Mark Levine, VP Development
Dylan McDermott, Narrator

Certain key issues often surface during the counseling sessions of people wwith TS and their families. These important areas of concern are explored for counselors, social workers, educators, psychologists and other allied professionals. Expert clinical practitioners offer invaluable insights for those working with people affected by Tourette Syndrome. *$30.00*

1563 Complexities of TS Treatment: Physician's Roundtable
Tourette Syndrome Association
42-40 Bell Boulevard
Suite 205
Bayside, NY 11361-2874
718-224-2999
888-486-8738
Fax: 718-279-9596
E-mail: ts@tsa-usa.org
www.tsa-usa.org

Judy Ungar, President
Gary Frank, EVP
Mark Levine, VP Development

Three of the most highly regarded experts in the diagnosis and treatment of Tourette Syndrome offer insight, advice and treatment strategies to fellow physicians and other healthcare professionals. *$30.00*

1564 Family Life with Tourette Syndrome... Personal Stories
Tourette Syndrome Association
42-40 Bell Boulevard
Suite 205
Bayside, NY 11361-2874
718-224-2999
888-486-8738
Fax: 718-279-9596
E-mail: ts@tsa-usa.org
www.tsa-usa.org

Judy Ungar, President
Gary Frank, EVP
Mark Levine, VP Development

In extended, in-depth interviews, all the people engagingly profiled in After the Diagnosis. The Next Steps, reveal the individual ways they developed to deal with TS. Each shows us that the key to leading a successful life in spite of having TS, is having a loving, supportive network of family and friends. Available in its entirety or as separate vignettes. *$50.00*

1565 Understanding and Treating the Hereditary Psychiatric Spectrum Disorders
Hope Press
PO Box 188
Duarte, CA 91009-0188
818-303-0644
800-321-4039
Fax: 818-358-3520
www.hopepress.com

David E Comings MD, Presenter

Learn with ten hours of audio tapes from a two day seminar given in May 1997 by David E Comings, MD. Tapes cover: ADHD, Tourette Syndrome, Obsessive-Compulsive Disorder, Conduct Disorder, Oppositional Defiant Disorder, Autism and other Hereditary Psychiatric Spectrum Disorders. Eight Audio tapes. *$75.00*

Year Founded: 1997

1566 www.mentalhealth.com
Internet Mental Health

Offers online psychiatric diagnosis in the hope of reaching the two-thirds of individuals with mental illness who do not seek treatment.

1567 www.planetpsych.com
Planetpsych.com

Online resource for mental health information.

1568 www.psychcentral.com
Psych Central

The Internet's largest and oldest independent mental health social network created and run by mental health professionals to guarantee reliable, trusted information and support communities to you.

1569 www.tourette-syndrome.com
Tourette Syndrome

Online community devoted to children and adults with Tourette Syndrome disorder and their families, friends, teachers, and medical professionals. Provides an interactive meeting place for those interested in Tourette Syndrome or people wanting to help others who have TS.

1570 www.tourettesyndrome.net
Tourette Syndrome Plus

Parent and teacher friendly site on Tourette Syndrome, Attention Deficit Disorder, Executive Dysfunction, Obsessive Compulsive Disorder, and related conditions.

1571 www.tsa-usa.com
Tourette Syndrome Association

Educational information for patients, caregivers and physicians.

1572 www.tsa-usa.org
Tourette Syndrome Association

Web site of the association dedicated to identifying the cause, finding the cure and controlling the effects of TS.

Pediatric & Adolescent Issues

Associations & Agencies

1573 American Academy of Child and Adolescent Psychiatry
3615 Wisconsin Avenue NW
Washington, DC 20016-3007
202-966-7300
800-333-7636
Fax: 202-966-2891
www.aacap.org

Virginia Anthony, Executive Director
Earl Magee, Administrator
William Bernet, Treasurer

Professional medical organization comprised of child and adolescent psychiatrist trained to promote healthy development and to evaluate, diagnose, and treat children and adolescents and their families who are affected by disorders of feeling, thinking, learning and behavior. Child and adolescent psychiatrists are physicians who are uniquely qualified to integrate knowledge about human behavior, social, and cultural perspectives with scientific, humanistic, and collaborative approaches to diagnosis, treatment and the promotion of mental health.

1574 American Academy of Pediatrics
141 NW Point Boulevard
Elk Grove Village, IL 60007
847-434-4000
Fax: 847-434-8000
E-mail: cme@aap.org
www.aap.org

Renée R. Jenkins, MD, President
Errol R. Alden, MD, Executive Director

Provides information on diagnosis and treatment of physical and mental pediatric conditions by offering programs, training, and resources.

1575 American Pediatrics Society
3400 Research Forest Drive
Suite B-7
The Woodlands, TX 77381
281-419-0052
Fax: 281-419-0082
E-mail: info@aps-spr.org
www.aps-spr.org

Debbie Anagnostelis, Executive Director
William W. Hay, Jr., M.D., President

Society of professionals working with pediatric health care issues; offers seminars and a variety of publications.

1576 Association for the Help of Retarded Children
83 Maiden Lane
New York, NY 10038
212-780-2500
Fax: 212-777-5893
E-mail: ahrcnyc@dti.net
www.ahrcnyc.org

Shirley Berenstein, Director
Jennifer Rossiter, Contact

Developmentally disabled children and adults, their families, and interested individuals. Provides support services, training programs, clinics, schools and residential facilities to the developmentally disabled.

1577 Center for Family Support (CFS)
333 7th Avenue
New York, NY 10001-5004
212-629-7939
Fax: 212-239-2211
www.cfsny.org

Steven Vernickofs, Executive Director

An agency that continues to develop new programs to serve families and individuals with their care needs. They currently offer services throughout the New York City Region including: New Jersey, Long Island and the Lower Hudson Valley.

1578 Federation for Children with Special Needs (FCSN)
1135 Tremont Street
Suite 420
Boston, MA 02120
617-236-7210
800-331-0688
Fax: 617-572-2094
E-mail: fcsninfo@fcsn.org
www.fcsn.org

Rich Robison, Executive Director

The federation provides information, support, and assistance to parents of children with disabilities, their professional partners and their communities.

1579 Federation of Families for Children's Mental Health
9605 Medical Center Drive
Suite 280
Rockville, MD 20850
240-403-1901
Fax: 240-403-1909
E-mail: ffcmh@ffcmh.org
www.ffcmh.org

Sandra Spencer, Executive Director
Arthur Penn, President

National family-run organization dedicated exclusively to children and adolescents with mental health needs and their families. Our voice speaks through our work in policy, training and technical assistance programs.

1580 Lifespire
350 Fifth Avenue
Suite 301
New York, NY 10118
212-741-0100
Fax: 212-242-0696
E-mail: info@lifespire.org
www.lifespire.org

Robert J. Krakow, Chairman

Professionals, parents, siblings, and others interested in mentally retarded and developmentally disabled adults.

1581 Mentally Ill Kids in Distress
755 E Willetta Street
Suite 128
Phoenix, AZ 85006
602-253-1240
800-356-4543
Fax: 602-523-1250
E-mail: Phoenix@MIKID.org
www.mikid.org

Mission is to provide support and assistance to families in Arizona with behaviorally challenged children, youth, and young adults.

1582 Michigan Association for Children's Mental Health
941 Abbott Road
Suite P
East Lansing, MI 48823-3104
517-336-7222
Fax: 517-336-8884
E-mail: acmhlori@acd.net
www.acmh-mi.org

Sara Way, Director

Promotes development of a system of care for families of children with emotional, behavioral or mental health disorders through community education and awareness, family support and involvement.

1583 National Child Support Network
PO Box 1018
Fayetteville, AR 72702-1018
800-729-5437
Fax: 479-582-2401
www.childsupport.org

A private bonded, licensed and insured child support collection agency.

1584 National Dissemination Center for Children with Disabilities
PO Box 1492
Washington, DC 20013
800-695-0285
Fax: 202-884-8441
E-mail: nichcy@aed.org
www.nichcy.org/

Suzanne Ripley, Project Director
Lisa Kupper, Author/Editor

Provides support and services for children and youth with physical and mental disabilities, as well as education and training services for their families.

1585 National Technical Assistance Center for Children's Mental Health
Georgetown University Child Development Center
Georgetown University Center for Child a
Box 571485
Washington, DC 20057
202-687-5000
Fax: 202-687-1954
TTY: 202-687-5503
E-mail: gucdc@georgetown.edu
www.http://gucchd.georgetown.edu/programs/ta_center

Integral part of the Georgetown University Center for Child and Human Development at the Georgetown University Medical Center. Nationally recognized for its work in assisting states and communities build systems of care for mental health concerns.

Year Founded: 1984

1586 Parents Helping Parents
3041 Olcott Street
Santa Clara, CA 9505
408-727-5775
Fax: 408-727-0182

E-mail: info@php.com
www.php.com

Mary Ellen Peterson, Executive Director

Nonprofit family resource center offering culturally sensitive information and peer counseling, provides a forum for parents and professionals to get information. PHP does not promote or recommend any treatment, therapy, institution or professional.

1587 Parents Information Network
1101 King Street
Suite 420
Alexandria, VA 22314
703-684-7710
Fax: 703-836-1040
E-mail: ffcmh@ffcmh.org
www.ffcmh.org/local.htm

Bridget Schneider, Facilitator

National parent run organization focused on the needs of children and youth with emotional, behavioral or mental disorders and their families.

1588 Pilot Parents: PP
Ollie Webb Center
1941 S 42nd Street
Suite 122
Omaha, NE 68105-2942
402-346-5220
Fax: 402-346-5253
E-mail: jvarner@olliewebb.org
www.olliebebb.org

Jennifer Varner, Coordinator

Parents, professionals and others concerned with providing emotional and peer support to new parents of children with special needs. Sponsors a parent-matching program which allows parents who have had sufficient experience and training.

1589 Research and Training Center for Children's Mental Health
University of South Florida
13303 Bruce B Downs Boulevard
Department of Child and Family
Tampa, FL 33612-3807
813-974-4661
Fax: 813-974-6257
www.rtckids.fmhi.usf.edu

Robert M Frieman PhD, Center Director
Albert Duchnowski, Deputy Director

State initiative for clinical studies of pediatric mental health issues.

1590 Research and Training Center on Family Support and Children's Mental Health
Portland State University/Regional Research Institute
PO Box 751
Portland State University
Portland, OR 97207-0751
503-725-4040
Fax: 503-725-4180
E-mail: rtcpubs@pdx.edu
www.rtc.pdx.edu

Nicole Ave, Public Information/Outreach
Janet Walker, Director of Research

Dedicated to promoting effective community based, culturally competent, family centered services for families and their children who are or may be affected by mental, emotional or behavioral disorders. This goal is accomplished through collaborative research partnerships with family members, service providers, policy makers, and other concerned persons. Major efforts in dissemination and training include: An annual conference, an award winning web site to share information about child and family mental services and policy issues which includes Focal Point, a national bulletin regarding family support and children's mental health.

1591 Resources for Children with Special Needs
116 E 16th Street
5th Floor
New York, NY 10003
212-677-4650
Fax: 212-254-4070
E-mail: info@resourcesnyc.org
www.resourcesnyc.org

Rachel Howard, Executive Director
Vicky Burton, Executive assitent

Information, referral, advocacy, training, publications for New York City parents of youth with disabilities or special needs and the professionals who work with them.

1592 United Families for Children's Mental Health
32 Norwich Avenue
Suite 103
Tampa, FL 33612
860-537-6125
86- 43- 078
Fax: 860-537-6130
E-mail: email@familiesunited.org
www.ctfamiliesunited.homestead.com

Jackie Hoope Hage, President
Cheryl Cole, VP

Run by and for caregivers of children with mental health issues. Children with emotional, behavioral, and mental health challenges can thrive at home, school, and in the community with appropriate, timely, and effective resources.

1593 Young Adult Institute and Workshop (YAI)
460 W 34th Street
New York, NY 10001-2382
212-273-6100
866- 49- 456
Fax: 212-268-1083
www.yai.org

Joel M Levy, CEO
Philip H. Levy, President/COO

Serves more than 15,000 people of all ages and levels of mental retardation, developmental and learning disabilities. Provides a full range of early intervention, preschool, family supports, employment training and placement, clinical and residential service.

1594 Youth Services International
6000 Cattleridge Drive
Suite 200
Sarasota, FL 34232
941-953-9199
Fax: 941-953-9198

E-mail: YSIWEB@youthservices.com
www.youthservices.com

Premier provider in the Youth Care Industry of educational and developmental services that change, dramatically, the thinking and behavior of troubled youth.

1595 Zero to Three
2000 M Street NW
Suite 200
Washington, DC 20036
202-638-1144
800-899-4301
Fax: 202-638-0851
E-mail: oto3@presswarehouse.com
www.zerotothree.org

Matthew E Melmed JD, Executive Director
Emily Fanichel, Associate Director

Professionals and researchers in the health care industry, policymakers and parents working to improve the healthy physical, cognitive and social development of infants, toddlers and their families. Sponsors training and technical assistance activities.

Books

1596 Aggression Replacement Training: A Comprehensive Intervention for Aggressive Youth
Research Press
Dept 24 W
PO Box 9177
Champaign, IL 61826
217-352-3273
800-519-2707
Fax: 217-352-1221
E-mail: rp@researchpress.com
www.researchpress.com

Russell Pense, VP Marketing

Aggression Replacement Training (ART) offers a comprehensive intervention program designed to teach adolescents to understand and replace aggression and antisocial behavior with positive alternatives. The book is designed to be user-friendly and teacher-oriented. It contains summaries of ART's outcome evaluations and it discusses recent applications in schools and other settings. *$24.95*

366 pages ISBN 0-878223-79-7

1597 Bibliotherapy Starter Set
Childs Work/Childs Play
135 Dupont Street
PO Box 760
Plainville, NY 11803-0760
800-962-1141
Fax: 800-262-1886
E-mail: info@Childswork.com
www.Childswork.com

Eight popular books for helping children ages four - twelve. Titles include Self Esteem, Divorce, ADHD, Feelings, and Anger. *$105.00*

1598 Book of Psychotherapeutic Homework
Childs Work/Childs Play
135 Dupont Street
PO Box 760
Plainville, NY 11803-0760

800-962-1141
Fax: 800-262-1886
E-mail: info@Childswork.com
www.Childswork.com

Lawrence E Shapiro, Author

More than 80 home activities to guarantee your therapy won't lose momentum. Appropriate for ages five - ten. *$20.95*

Year Founded: 2001 ISBN 1-882732-55-3

1599 Breaking the Silence: Teaching the Next Generation About Mental Illness
NAMI Queens/Nassau
1983 Marcus Avenue
Lake Success, NY 11042
516-326-0797
Fax: 576-437-5785
E-mail: btslessonplans@aol.com
www.btslessonplans.org

Amy Lax, Director PR/Educational Outreach
Janet Susin, Project Director
Lorraine Kaplan, Director Educational Training

Breaking the Silence (BTS) is an innovative teaching package which includes lesson plans, games and posters on serious mental illness for three grade levels: upper elementary, middle and high school. It is designed to fight stigma by putting a human face on mental illness, replacing fear and ridicule with compassion. BTS meets national health standards.

1600 CARE Child and Adolescent Risk Evaluation: A Measure of the Risk for Violent Behavior
Research Press
Dept 24 W
PO Box 9177
Champaign, IL 61826
217-352-3273
800-519-2707
Fax: 217-352-1221
E-mail: rp@researchpress.com
www.researchpress.com

Dennis Wiziecki, Marketing
Dr Kathryn Siefert, Author

The CARE was developed as a prevention tool to identify youth, as early as possible, who are at risk for committing acts of violence. Unlike other evaluation programs, CARE includes a case management planning form that provides the information needed to develop a risk management intervention plan. The CARE Kit includes 25 assessment forms, 25 case management planning forms and manual. *$75.00*

1601 Children and Trauma: Guide for Parents and Professionals
Courage to Change
375 Stewart Street
PO Box 486
Wilkes-Barres, PA 18703-0486
800-440-4003
Fax: 800-772-6499
www.couragetochange.com

Cynthia Monahon, Author

Comprehensive guide to the emotional aftermath of children's crises. Discusses warning signs that a child may need professional help, and explores how parents and professionals can help children heal, reviving a sense of well being and safety. *$19.95*

240 pages Year Founded: 1997 ISBN 0-787910-71-6

1602 Childs Work/Childs Play
135 Dupont Street
PO Box 760
Plainview, NY 11803-0760
800-962-1141
Fax: 800-262-1886
E-mail: info@Childswork.com
www.Childswork.com

Catalog of books, games, toys and workbooks relating to child development issues such as recognizing emotions, handling uncertainty, bullies, ADD, shyness, conflicts and other things that children may need some help navigating.

1603 Creative Therapy with Children and Adolescents
Impact Publishers
PO Box 6016
Atascadero, CA 93423-6016
805-466-5917
800-246-7228
Fax: 805-466-5919
E-mail: info@impactpublishers.com
www.impactpublishers.com

Over 100 activities to be used in working with children, adolescents and families. Encourages creativity in therapy and helps therapists facilitate change by gaining rapport with children and other clients who find it difficult to talk about feelings and experiences. *$21.95*

192 pages ISBN 1-886230-19-6

1604 Forms for Behavior Analysis with Children
Research Press
Dept 24 W
PO Box 9177
Champaign, IL 61826
217-352-3273
800-519-2707
Fax: 217-352-1221
E-mail: rp@researchpress.com
www.researchpress.com

Dr Joseph Cautela, Author
Dennis Wiziecki, Marketing

A unique collection of 42 reproducible assessment forms designed to aid counselors and therapists in making proper diagnoses and in developing treatment plans for children and adolescents. Different assessment formats are included, ranging from direct observations and interviews to informant ratings and self-reports. Certain forms are to be filled out by children and adolescents, while others are to be completed by parents, school personnel, significant others or the therapist. *$ 39.95*

208 pages ISBN 0-878222-67-7

1605 Forms-5 Book Set
Childs Work/Childs Play
135 Dupont Street
PO Box 760
Plainville, NY 11803-0760
800-962-1141
Fax: 800-262-1886
E-mail: info@Childswork.com
www.Childswork.com

Five-book pack with reproducible forms titled:
Oppositional Child, Children with OCD, Counseling
Children, ADHD Child and Socially Fearful Child.
$125.00

1606 Gangs in Schools: Signs, Symbols and Solutions
Research Press
Dept 24 W
PO Box 9177
Champaign, IL 61826
217-352-3273
800-519-2707
Fax: 217-352-1221
E-mail: rp@researchpress.com
www.researchpress.com

Russell Pense, VP Marketing

Written by noted authority Arnold Goldstein and gang expert Donald Kodluboy, this book is an essential resource for
educators and administrators who are concerned about gang
presence or the possibility of gang presence in their
schools. The book describes effective gang prevention and
intervention strategies. It includes a helpful checklist on
how to recognize early gang presence in schools. And it
presents a comprehensive plan for maximizing school
safety. *$19.95*

256 pages ISBN 0-878223-82-7

1607 Gender Respect Workbook
Childs Work/Childs Play
135 Dupont Street
PO Box 760
Plainville, NY 11803-0760
800-962-1141
Fax: 800-262-1886
E-mail: info@Childswork.com
www.Childswork.com

Over 100 activities appropriate for ages 8 and up, to help
teachers and counselors raise consciousness of sexisim and
sexist practices. *$20.95*

1608 I Wish Daddy Didn't Drink So Much
Childs Work/Childs Play
135 Dupont Street
PO Box 760
Plainville, NY 11803-0760
800-962-1141
Fax: 800-262-1886
E-mail: info@Childswork.com
www.Childswork.com

Judith Vigna, Author

Realistic and sensitive book about how a girl handles disappointment in her father's problems. Ages 6 - 12. *$6.95*

ISBN 0-807535-26-5

1609 Kid Power Tactics for Dealing with Depression
& Parent's Survival Guide to Childhood
Depression
Childs Work/Childs Play
135 Dupont Street
PO Box 760
Plainville, NY 11803-0760
800-962-1141
Fax: 800-262-1886
E-mail: info@Childswork.com
www.Childswork.com

Nicholas Dubuque, Author
Susan Dubuque, Author

Two-volume set was wriiten by a child who suffered from
depression and his mother. Plain language and a wealth of
information for children ages 8 and over, plus their parents
and teachers. *$12.95*

47 pages Year Founded: 1996 ISBN 1-882732-48-0

1610 My Body is Mine, My Feelings are Mine
Childs Work/Childs Play
135 Dupont Street
PO Box 760
Plainville, NY 11803-0760
800-962-1141
Fax: 800-262-1886
E-mail: info@Childswork.com
www.Childswork.com

Susan Hoke, Author
Bruce Van Patter, Illustrator
Charles Brenna, Designer

For ages 3 - 8. First part to be read to children, the second
part teaches adults how to educate children about body
safety. Sexual victimization can be prevented through explanation of how to identify inappropriate touching and
what to do about it. *$20.95*

78 pages Year Founded: 1995 ISBN 1-882732-24-3

1611 My Listening Friend: A Story About the
Benefits of Counseling
Childs Work/Childs Play
135 Dupont Street
PO Box 760
Plainview, NY 11803-0760
800-962-1141
Fax: 800-262-1886
E-mail: info@Childswork.com
www.Childswork.com

P J Michaels, Author
Anna Dewdney, Illustrator

For ages five - twelve, explores the feelings a child has the
first time they see a counselor. Written from the point of
view of the child. *$14.50*

57 pages Year Founded: 2001 ISBN 1-588150-43-7

1612 Saddest Time
Childs Work/Childs Play
135 Dupont Street
PO Box 760
Plainville, NY 11803-0760
800-962-1141
Fax: 800-262-1886
E-mail: info@Childswork.com
www.Childswork.com

Norma Simon, Author

Helps children ages 6 - 12 understand that death is sad and
sometimes tragic, but it is also part of life. *$13.95*

Year Founded: 1999 ISBN 0-613141-80-6

1613 Teen Relationship Workbook
Childs Work/Childs Play
135 Dupont Street
PO Box 760
Plainville, NY 11803-0760

516-349-5520
800-962-1141
Fax: 800-262-1886
E-mail: info@childswork.com
www.childswork.com

A reproducible workbook, this hands-on tool helps teens develop healthy relationships and prevent dating abuse and domestic violence. *$44.95*

135 pages

1614 Thirteen Steps to Help Families Stop Fightin Solve Problems Peacefully
Childs Work/Childs Play
135 Dupont Street
PO Box 760
Plainville, NY 11803-0760
800-962-1141
Fax: 800-262-1886
E-mail: info@Childswork.com
www.Childswork.com

Sharon Hernes Silverman, Author

Candid views on why families fight, and solutions to conflict. *$15.95*

Year Founded: 2001 ISBN 1-882732-77-4

1615 What Works When with Children and Adolescents: A Handbook of Individual Counseling Techniques
Research Press
Dept 24 W
PO Box 9177
Champaign, IL 61826
217-352-3273
800-519-2707
Fax: 217-352-1221
E-mail: rp@researchpress.com
www.researchpress.com

Dennis Wiziecki, Marketing
Dr Ann Vernon, Author

This practical handbook is designed for counselors, social workers and psychologists in schools and mental health settings. It offers over 100 creative activities and effective interventions for individual counseling with children and adolescents (ages 6-18). Dr. Vernon provides strategies for establishing a therapeutic relationship with students who are sometimes apprehensive or opposed to counseling. Several case studies are included to help illustrate the counseling techniques and interventions. The book also includes a chapter on working with parents and teachers. *$39.95*

344 pages ISBN 0-878224-38-6

Periodicals & Pamphlets

1616 Anxiety Disorders in Children and Adolescents
Center for Mental Health Services: Knowledge Exchange Network
PO Box 42557
Washington, DC 20015
800-789-2647
Fax: 240-747-5470
TDD: 866-889-2647
E-mail: ken@mentalhealth.org
www.mentalhealth.samhsa.gov/

This fact sheet defines anxiety disorders, identifies warning signs, discusses risk factors, describes types of help available, and suggests what parents or other caregivers can do.

3 pages

1617 Attention-Deficit/Hyperactivity Disorder in Children and Adolescents
Center for Mental Health Services: Knowledge Exchange Network
PO Box 42557
Washington, DC 20015
800-789-2647
Fax: 301-984-8796
TDD: 866-889-2647
E-mail: ken@mentalhealth.org
www.mentalhealth.samhsa.gov/publications/

This fact sheet defines attention-deficit/hyperactivity disorder, describes the warning signs, discusses types of help available, and suggests what parents or other caregivers can do.

3 pages Year Founded: 1997

1618 Autism Spectrum Disorders in Children and Adolescents
Center for Mental Health Services: Knowledge Exchange Network
PO Box 42490
Washington, DC 20015
800-789-2647
Fax: 301-984-8796
TDD: 866-889-2647
E-mail: ken@mentalhealth.org
www.mentalhealth.org

This fact sheet defines autism, describes the signs and causes, discusses types of help available, and suggests what parents or other caregivers can do.

2 pages

1619 Conduct Disorder in Children and Adolescents
Center for Mental Health Services: Knowledge Exchange Network
PO Box 42490
Washington, DC 20015
800-789-2647
Fax: 301-984-8796
TDD: 866-889-2647
E-mail: ken@mentalhealth.org
www.mentalhealth.org

This fact sheet defines conduct disorder, identifies risk factors, discusses types of help available, and suggests what parents or other caregivers can do.

2 pages

1620 Families Can Help Children Cope with Fear, Anxiety
Center for Mental Health Services: Knowledge Exchange Network
PO Box 42557
Washington, DC 20015
800-789-2647
Fax: 301-984-8796
TDD: 866-889-2647
E-mail: ken@mentalhealth.org
www.mentalhealth.org

This fact sheet defines conduct disorder, identifies risk factors, discusses types of help available, and suggests what parents or other caregivers to common signs of fear and anxiety.

1 pages Year Founded: 2002

1621 Helping Hand
Performance Resource Press
1270 Rankin Drive
Suite F
Troy, MI 48083-2843
248-588-7733
800-453-7733
Fax: 800-499-5718
www.prponline.com

Educates teachers and parents about child and adolescents behavioral health.

4 pages 9 per year

1622 Major Depression in Children and Adolescents
Center for Mental Health Services: Knowledge
Exchange Network
PO Box 42557
Washington, DC 20015
800-789-2647
Fax: 301-984-8796
TDD: 866-889-2647
E-mail: ken@mentalhealth.org
www.mentalhealth.org

This fact sheet defines depression and its signs, identifies types of help available, and suggests what parents or other caregivers can do.

2 pages Year Founded: 1997

1623 Mental, Emotional, and Behavior Disorders in
Children and Adolescents
Center for Mental Health Services: Knowledge
Exchange Network
PO Box 42557
Washington, DC 20015
800-789-2647
Fax: 301-984-8796
TDD: 866-889-2647
E-mail: ken@mentalhealth.org
www.mentalhealth.org

This fact sheet describes mental, emotional, and behavioral problems that can occur during childhood and adolescence and discusses related treatment, support services, and research.

4 pages Year Founded: 1996

Support Groups & Hot Lines

1624 Alateen and Al-Anon Family Groups
1600 Corporate Landing Parkway
Virginia Beach, VA 23454-5617
757-563-1600
888-425-2666
Fax: 757-563-1655
E-mail: wso@al-anon.org
www.al-anon.alateen.org/sitemap.html

Mary Ann Keller, Director Members Services

A fellowship of men, women, children and adult children affected by another persons drinking.

1625 Children and Adults with AD/HD (CHADD)
8181 Professional Place
Suite 150
Landover, MD 20785
301-306-7070
800-233-4050
Fax: 301-306-7090
www.chadd.org

Non-profit organization serving individuals with AD/HD and their families. Over 16,000 members in 200 local chapters throughout the United States. Chapters offer support for individuals, parents, teachers, professionals, and others.

1626 Covenant House Nineline
460 West 41st Street
New York, NY 10036
212-613-0300
800-999-9999
Fax: 212-989-9098
E-mail: info@covenanthouseny.org
www.covenanthouse.org/nineline/

Bruce Henry, Executive Director

Nationwide crisis/suicide hotline.

1627 Girls and Boys Town of New York
444 Park Avenue South
Suite 801
New York, NY 10016
212-725-4260
800-448-3000
Fax: 212-725-4385
E-mail: Hotline@girlsandboystown.org
www.girlsandboystown.org/aboutus/locations/newyork/

Anthony Dilauro, Site Director

Crisis intervention and referrals.

1628 Just Say No International
1777 North California Blvd.
Suite 210
Walnut Creek, CA 94596
510-939-6666
800-258-2766
E-mail: kci.org/meth_info/sites/drug_hotline.htm
www.justsayno.org/ and also

Provides numerous links to National Hotlines and Helplines in addition to Websites containing information on drug addiction/abuse, drug treatment/rehabilitation programs and centers, and also information on alcohol addiction/treatment and detox programs.

1629 Kidspeace National Centers
5300 Kidspeace Drive
Orefield, PA 18069
800-854-3123
Fax: 610-391-8280
E-mail: kpinfo@kidspeace.org.
www.kidspeace.org

C T O'Donnell II, President
Michael J Vogel, Chairman

KidsPeace is a private, not-for-profit charity dedicated to serving the critical behavioral and mental health needs of children, preadolescents and teens. Since 1882, KidsPeace has been helping kids develop the confidence and skills they need to overcome crisis. KidsPeace provides specialized residential treatment services and a comprehensive range of treatment programs and educational services to help families help kids anticipate and avoid crisis whenever possible.

1630 National Youth Crisis Hotline
5331 Mount Alifan Drive
San Diego, CA 92111-2622
800-448-4663
www.1800hithome.com/

Information and referral for runaways, and for youth and parents with problems.

1631 Rainbows
1111 Tower Road
Schaumburg, IL 60173
708-310-1880
Fax: 847-952-1774
E-mail: info@rainbows.org
www.www.rainbows.org/rainbows.html

Suzy Yehl Marta, Founder/President
Jessica Grata, Director of Administration

Peer support groups for adults and children who are grieving.

1632 SADD: Students Against Destructive Decisions
255 Main Street
Marlboro, MA 01752
508-481-3568
Fax: 508-481-5759
E-mail: info@sadd.org
www.sadd.org

Stephen Wallace, Chairman/CEO
Tiffany Corey, Student Leadership Council
Tinnelle Bombard, Marketing
Marlene Connelly, Family Focus Program

SADD's mission is to provide students with the best prevention and intervention tools possible to deal with the issues of underage drinking, other drug use, impaired driving and other destructive decisions, depression and suicide.

Video & Audio

1633 Aggression Replacement Training Video: A Comprehensive Intervention for Aggressive Youth
Research Press
Dept 24 W
PO Box 9177
Champaign, IL 61826
217-352-3273
800-519-2707
Fax: 217-352-1221
E-mail: rp@researchpress.com
www.researchpress.com

Dennis Wiziecki, Marketing

This staff training video illustrates the training procedures in the Aggression Replacement Training (ART) book.It features scenes of adolescents participating in group sessions for each of ART's three interventions: Prosocial Skills, Anger Control, and Moral Reasoning. A free copy of the book accompanies the video program. *$125.00*

1634 Are the Kids Alright?
Fanlight Productions
4196 Washington Street
Suite 2
Boston, MA 02131
617-469-4999
Fax: 617-439-3379
E-mail: fanlight@fanlight.com
www.fanlight.com

Filmed in courtrooms, correctional institutions, treatment centers, and family homes, this searing documentary documents the results of the tragic decline in mental health services for children and adolescents at risk.

1635 Children: Experts on Divorce
Courage to Change
375 Stewart Street
PO Box 486
Wilkes Barres, PA 18703-0486
800-440-4003
Fax: 800-772-6499
www.couragetochange.com/

Dede L Pitts, CEO

Children of divorced parents are interviewed about their feelings and views of how adults can relate to their children during and after a separation and divorce. The information on this video can help to prevent some of the long-term harm that they may feel. Ages of these children are four to fifteen. 38 minutes. *$34.95*

1636 Chill: Straight Talk About Stress
Childs Work/Childs Play
135 Dupont Street
PO Box 760
Plainview, NY 11803-0760
800-962-1141
Fax: 800-262-1886
E-mail: info@Childswork.com
www.Childswork.com

Encourages youth to recognize, analyze and handle the stresses in their lives. 22 minutes. *$96.95*

1637 Legacy of Childhood Trauma: Not Always Who They Seem
Research Press
Dept 24 W
PO Box 9177
Champaign, IL 61826
217-352-3273
800-519-2707
Fax: 217-352-1221
E-mail: rp@researchpress.com
www.researchpress.com

Russell Pense, VP Marketing

This powerful video focuses on the connection between so-called "delinquent youth" and the experience of childhood trauma such as emotional, sexual, or physical abuse. It inspires viewers to comprehend the emotional betrayal felt by abused children and encourages caregivers to identify strategies for healing and transformation. *$195.00*

1638 www.Al-Anon-Alateen.org
Al-Anon and Alateen

AA literature may serve as an introduction.

1639 www.CHADD.org
CHADD: Children/Adults with Attention Deficit/Hyperactivity Disorder

1640 www.abcparenting.com
ABCs of Parenting

1641 www.aboutteensnow.com/dramas
Teen Dramas

Realistic conflicts played out and discussed by a therapist.

1642 www.adhdnews.com.ssi.htm
Social Security

Applying for disability benefits for children with ADHD.

1643 www.adhdnews.com/Advocate.htm
Advocating for Your Child

1644 www.adhdnews.com/sped.htm
Special Education Rights and Responsibilities

Writing IEP's and TIEPS. Pursuing special education services.

1645 www.cfc-efc.ca/docs/00000095.htm
Helping Your Child Cope with Separation and Divorce

1646 www.couns.uiuc.edu
Self-Help Brochures

Address issues teens deal with.

1647 www.divorcedfather.com
Still a Dad

For divorced fathers.

1648 www.duanev/family/dads.html
So What are Dads Good For

1649 www.education.indiana.edu/cas/adol/adol.html
Adolescence Directory On-Line

A collection of documents on the growth and development of adolescents.

1650 www.ericps.crc.uiuc.edu/npin/index.html
NPIN: National Parent Information Network

Information on education.

1651 www.ericps.crc.uiuc.edu/npin/library/texts.html
NPIN Resources for Parents: Full Texts of Parenting-Related Material

1652 www.fathermag.com
Fathering Magazine

Hundreds of articles online.

1653 www.fathers.com
Fatherhood Project

1654 www.flyingsolo.com
Flying Solo

Site on single parenting.

1655 www.freedomvillageusa.com
Freedom Village USA

Faith-based home for troubled teens.

1656 www.fsbassociates.com/fsg/whydivorce.html
Breaking the News

Clear rules on how not to tell kids about divorce.

1657 www.geocities.com/enchantedforest/1068
Bipolar Kids Homepage

Set of links.

1658 www.home.clara.net/spig/guidline.htm
Guidelines for Separating Parents

1659 www.hometown.aol.com/DrgnKprl/BPCAT.html
Bipolar Children and Teens Homepage

1660 www.ianrpubs.unl.edu/family/nf223.htm
Supporting Stepfamilies: What Do the Children Feel

Deals with emotions of children in blended families.

1661 www.kidshealth.org/kid/feeling/index.html
Dealing with Feelings

Ten readings. Examples are: Why Am I So Sad; Are You Shy; Am I Too Fat or Too Thin; and A Kid's Guide to Divorce.

1662 www.kidsource.com/kidsource/pages/parenting
Parenting: General Parenting Articles

1663 www.klis.com/chandler/pamphlet/bipolar/bipolarpamphlet.html
Bipolar Affective Disorder in Children and Adolescents

An introduction for families.

1664 www.klis.com/chandler/pamphlet/bipolar/bipolarpamphlet.htm
Depression in Children and Adolescents

1665 www.klis.com/chandler/pamphlet/panic/
Panic Disorder, Separation, Anxiety Disorder, and Agoraphobia

1666 www.magicnet.net/~hedyyumi/child.html
Learning to Get Along for the Best Interest of the Child

1667 www.mentalhealth.org/publications/allpubs/
Attention-Deficit/Hyperactiviy Disorder in Children and Adolescents

Lists symptoms very fully.

1668 www.muextension.missouri.edu/xpor/hesguide/
Focus on Kids: The Effects of Divorce on Children

Discusses stresses on kids.

1669 www.naturalchild.com/home
Natural Child Project

Articles by experts.

1670 www.nichcy.org
National Information Center for Children and Youth with Disabilities

Excellent information in English and Spanish.

1671 www.nnfr.org/curriculum/topics/sep_div.html
Coping with Separation and Divorce: A Parenting Seminar

1672 www.nospank.org/toc.htm
Project NoSpank

Site for those against paddling in schools.

1673 www.npin.org/pnews/pnews997/
Temper Tantrums: What Causes Them and How Can You Respond?

Parents News publication.

1674 www.oznet.ksu.edu/library/famlf2/
Family Life Library

1675 www.parentcity.com/read/library
Parent City Library

Many articles on parenting.

1676 www.parenthoodweb.com
ParenthoodWeb

Focusing on early childhood.

1677 www.parenthoodweb.com/
Blended Families

Resolving conflicts.

1678 www.personal.psu.edu/faculty
Family Relations

Information parenting and family problems.

1679 www.positive-way.com/step.htm
Stepfamily Information

Introduction and tips for stepfathers, stepmothers and re-married parents.

1680 www.pta.org/commonsense
Common Sense: Strategies for Raising Alcoholic/Drug-/Free Children

Drug facts, warning signs, and guidence.

1681 www.stepfamily.org/tensteps.htm
Ten Steps for Steps

Guidelines for stepfamilies.

1682 www.stepfamilyinfo.org/sitemap.htm
Stepfamily Information

1683 www.teenwire.com/index.asp
Teenwire

Information on relationships and sexuality.

1684 www.todaysparent.com
Today's Parent Online

1685 www.users.aol.com:80/jimams/
Questions from Adolescents about ADD

Responses to children's questions.

1686 www.users.aol.com:80/jimams/answers1
Questions from Younger Children about ADD

Responses to children's questions.

1687 www.wholefamily.com/kidteencenter/
About Teens Now

Addresses important issues in teens lives.

1688 www.worldcollegehealth.org
World Health College

Dedicated to adolescent health issues including learning disabilities and grief. Written by experts.

1689 www2.mc.duke.edu/pcaad
Duke University's Program in Child and Adolescent Anxiety Disorder

Associations & Organizations

National

1690 AAMR: American Association on Mental Retardation
444 N Capitol Street NW
Suite 846
Washington, DC 20001-1512
800-424-3688
Fax: 202-387-2193
E-mail: dcroser@aaidd.org
www.www.aaidd.org

Paul Aitken, Director Finance/Administration
Doreen Croser, Executive Director
Bruce Appelgren, Director Publications

Promotes progressive policies, sound research, effective practices, and universal human rights for people with intellectual disabilities.

1691 Action Autonomie
#208 1260, rue Sainte-Catherine
Montreal, QC, ZZ
514-525-5060
Fax: 514-525-5580

Offers services for the protection and promotion of mental health rights.

1692 Advocates for Human Potential
323 Boston Post Road
Sudbury, MA 01776-3022
978-443-0055
Fax: 978-443-4722
E-mail: nshifman@ahpnet.com

Neal Shifman, President/CEO

Under contract with the Center for Mental Health Services (CMHS), Advocates for Human Potential (AHP) provides technical assistance to states and local providers regarding the Projects for Assistance in Transition from Homelessness (PATH) Program.

1693 Aleppos Foundation
39 Fairway E
Colts Neck, NJ 07722-1418
732-946-4489
Fax: 732-946-3344
E-mail: ilynch@monmouth.com
www.aleppos.org

Focuses on self-education: to learn about our inner and outer selves; to face up to our past; and to learn to communicate our true selves to others.

1694 Alliance of Genetic Support Groups
4301 Connecticut Avenue NW
Suite 404
Washington, DC 20008-2369
202-966-5557
800-336-4363
Fax: 202-966-8553
E-mail: info@geneticalliance.org
www.geneticalliance.org

A non-profit coalition of voluntary genetic support groups, consumers and professionals addressing the needs of individuals and families affected by genetic disorders from a national perspective. Specializes in linking people intrested in generic conditions with organization which can provide support and information.

1695 American Academy of Child and Adolescent Psychiatry
3615 Wisconsin Avenue NW
Washington, DC 20016-3007
202-966-7300
Fax: 202-966-2891
E-mail: communications@aacap.org
www.aacap.org

Robert Hendren, President
David Herzog, Secretary
William Bernet, Treasurer

Information is provided as a public service to aid in the understanding and treatment of the developmental, behavioral, and mental disorders which affect an estimated 7 to 12 million children and adolescents at any given time in the United States.

1696 American Academy of Pediatrics
141 NW Point Boulevard
Elk Grove Village, IL 60007
847-434-4000
Fax: 847-434-8000
E-mail: cme@aap.org
www.aap.org

Provides information on diagnosis and treatment of physical and mental pediatric conditions by offering programs, training, and resources.

1697 American Association for Geriatric Psychiatry
7910 Woodmont Avenue
Suite 1050
Bethesda, MD 20814-3004
301-654-7850
Fax: 301-654-4137
E-mail: main@aagponline.org
www.aagpgpa.org

Christine Devries, CEO/Executive Vice President
Annie Williams, Administrative Assistant

American Association for Geriatric Psychiatry (AAGP) is a national association representing and serving its members and the field of geriatric psychiatry. It is dedicated to promoting the mental health and well-being of older people and improving the care of those with late life mental disorders. AAGP enhances the knowledge base and standards of practice in geriatric psychiatry through education and research and by advocating for meeting the mental health needs of older Americans.

1698 American Association of Psychiatric Services for Children (AAPSC)
2345 Crystal Drive
Suite 250
Arlington, VA 22202
703-412-2400
Fax: 703-412-2401

Christine James-Brown, President/CEO

Fosters prevention and treatment of mental and emotional disorders of the child, adolescent and family and furthers the development and application of clinical knowledge. Researches and supports projects dealing with child and adolescent mental health. Sponsors educational programs and compiles statistics. Publications: AAPSC Membership Directory, annual. AAPSC Newsletter, bimonthly. Child Psychiatry and Human Development, quarterly. Annual conference and exhibit usually in February or March.

1699 American Holistic Health Association
PO Box 17400
Anaheim, CA 92817-7400
714-779-6152
E-mail: mail@ahha.org
www.ahha.org

Michael Morton, PhD., President
Suzan Walter, Secretary/Treasurer

Promotes holistic principles honoring the whole person and encouraging people to actively participate in their own health and healthcare.

1700 American Managed Behavioral Healthcare Association
1101 Pennsylvania Avenue NW
6th Floor
Washington, DC 20004
202-756-7726
Fax: 202-756-7308
E-mail: info@abhw.org
www.www.abhw.org

Pamela Greenberg, President/CEO

Represents and promotes the interests of specialty managed behavioral health care organizations.

1701 American Network of Community Options and Resources (ANCOR)
1101 King Street
Suite 380
Alexandria, VA 22314
703-532-7850
Fax: 703-535-7860
E-mail: ancor@ancor.org
www.ancor.org

Represents providers of care to persons with disabilities (including MR/NH). Promotes high standard of ethics. Conducts educational programs.

1702 American Pediatrics Society
3400 Research Forest Drive
Suite B-7
The Woodlands, TX 77381
281-419-0052
Fax: 281-419-0082
E-mail: info@aps-spr.org
www.aps-spr.org

Larry Shapiro, M.D., President
Elizabeth McAnarney, M.D., Vice President

Society of professionals working with pediatric health care issues; offers seminars and a variety of publications.

1703 American Psychiatric Association
1000 Wilston Boulevard
Suite 1825
Arlington, VA 22209-3901
703-907-7300
E-mail: apa@psych.org
www.psych.org

Carolyn Robinowitz, President

Medical specialty society recognized world-wide. Both U.S. and international member physicians work together to ensure humane care and effective treatment for all persons

with mental disorder, including mental retardation and substance-related disorders.

1704 American Psychological Association
750 1st Street NE
Washington, DC 20002-4242
202-336-5500
800-374-2721
Fax: 202-336-6063
TDD: 202-336-6123
TTY: 202-336-6123
www.apa.org

Largest scienctific and professional organziation representing psychology in the United States and is the world's largest association of psychologists. Works to advance psychology as a science, as a profession, and as a means of promoting human welfare.

1705 Association for the Care of Children's Health
19 Mantua Road
Mount Royal, NJ 08061-1006
609-224-1742
Fax: 609-224-1742

International, multidisciplinary membership organization of healthcare providers, parents, educators, researchers, chaplains, facility designers, social service professionals, corporations, institutions, and policy makers.

1706 Association for the Help of Retarded Children
200 Park Avenue S
Suite 1201
New York, NY 10003-1503
212-780-2500
Fax: 212-777-5893
E-mail: ahrcnyc@dti.net
www.ahrcnyc.org

Shirley Berenstein, Director

Offer disabled individuals day to day living that is as rich, absorbing and worthwhile as possible, with an emphasis on helping clients live up to their maximum potential in the community.

1707 Association of Mental Health Librarians (AMHL)
13301 Bruce B Downs Blvd
Tampa, FL 33612-3899
813-974-4471
Fax: 813-974-7242
E-mail: hanson@fmhi.usf.edu
www.fmhi.usf.edu/amhl

Ardis Hanson, President

An organization that is working in the field of mental health information delivery. Its members come from a variety of settings. AMHL provides opportunities for its members to enhance their professional skills; encourage research activities in mental health librarianship; and strengthens the role of the librarian within the mental health community.

1708 Bazelon Center for Mental Health Law
1101 15th Street NW
Suite 1212
Washington, DC 20005
202-467-5730
Fax: 202-223-0409

E-mail: webmaster@bazelon.org
www.bazelon.org

Robert Bernstein, Executive Director
Albert Archie, Operations Manager

National legal advocate for people with mental disabilities. Through precedent-setting litigation and in the public policy arena, the Bazelon Center works to advance and preserve the rights of people with mental illnesses and development disabilities.

1709 Best Buddies International (BBI)
100 SE 2nd Street
#1990
Miami, FL 33131
305-374-2233
800-892-8339
Fax: 305-374-5305
E-mail: LaverneLewis@BestBuddies.org
www.bestbuddies.org

Anthony Shriver, Founder
J.R. Fry, Director

A nonprofit organization dedicated to enhancing the lives of people with intellectual disabilities by providing opportunities for one-to-one friendships and integrated employment.

1710 Bethesda Lutheran Homes and Services
700 Hoffman Drive
Watertown, WI 53094
920-261-3050
800-369-4636
Fax: 920-261-8441

Matthew Becker

Provides religious education, habilitation services, therapeutic services, vocational training and residential care for persons with mental retardation. Paid summer co-op positions in nursing, social work, psychology, special education, recreation, Christian education. Provides free information and referral services nationwide for parents, pastors, teachers, and mental retardation professionals.

1711 Black Mental Health Alliance (BMHA)
733 W 40th Street
Suite 10
Baltimore, MD 21211-2107
410-338-2642
Fax: 410-338-1771

Seeks to increase clinicians, clergy, educators and social service professionals awareness of African-Americans mental health needs and concerns on issues including stress, violence, racism, substance abuse and parenting. Provides consultation, public information and resource referrals. Publications: Visions, quarterly. Annual meeting and dinner-dance. Annual Optimal Mental Health for African American Families Conference.

1712 Canadian Art Therapy Association
26 Earl Grey Road
Toronto ON, ZZ
416-461-9420
www.www.catainfo.ca

Nick Zwaagstra, President

To encourage and sponsor activities which enhance the progressive development of professional standards of art therapy, practice, training, research, publications & conferences.

1713 Canadian Federation of Mental Health Nurses
#104 1185 Eglinton Avenue E
Toronto ON, ZZ
416-426-7029
Fax: 416-426-7280
E-mail: info@cfmhn.ca
www.www.cfmhn.org

Sharyn Chapman, Treasurer/Membership

National voice for psychiatric and mental health nursing.

1714 Canadian Mental Health Association
#810 8 King Street E
Toronto ON, ZZ
416-484-7750
Fax: 416-484-4617
E-mail: info@cmha.ca
www.www.cmha.ca

Penelope Marrett, CEO

Promote mental health as well as support the resilience and recovery of people experiencing mental illness, through advocacy, education, research and service.

1715 Center for Attitudinal Healing (CAH)
33 Buchanan Drive
Sausalito, CA 94965-1650
415-331-6161
Fax: 415-331-4545
E-mail: home123@aol.com
www.attitudinalhealing.org

Don Gowewy, Executive Director

Nonsectarian organization established to supplement traditional health care by offering free attitudinal healing services for children and adults with life-threatening illnesses or other crisis. Offers support groups and arranges home and hospital visits for children, youth and adults. Publications: Advice to Doctors and Other Big People, book. Another Look at the Rainbow, book. Rainbow Connection, newsletter, three times a year. There is a Rainbow Behind Every Dark Cloud, book. Workshops, five times a year.

1716 Center for Family Support (CFS)
333 Seventh Avenue
9th Floor
New York, NY 10001-5004
212-629-7939
Fax: 212-239-2211
www.cfsny.org

Steven Vernickofs, Executive Director

A not-for-profit human service agency that provides individualized support services and programs for individuals living with developmental and related disabilities, and for the families that care for them at home.

1717 Center for Mental Health Services
SAMSHA
PO Box 42557
Washington, DC 20015
800-789-2647
Fax: 240-747-5484
TDD: 866-889-2647
TTY: 301-443-9006
www.mentalhealth.samhsa.org

Irene S Levine PhD, Deputy Director

Develops national mental health policies, that promote Federal/State coordination and benefit from input from consumers, family members and providers. Ensures that high quality mental health services programs are implemented to benefit seriously mentally ill populations, disasters or those involved in the criminal justice system.

1718 Center for the Study of Issues in Public Mental Health
Nathan S Kline Institute for Psychiatric Research
140 Old Orangeburg Road
Orangeburg, NY 10962-1157
845-398-6590
Fax: 845-398-6592
E-mail: siegel@nki.rfmh.org
www.csipmh.rfmh.org

Carole Siegel, PhD, Director
Kim Hopper, PhD, Co-Director
Dixianne Penney, Administrator Director

The Center is committed to developing and conducting research within the contents of a rigorous research program that is strongly influenced by the requirements of a public mental health system and, in turn, influences the development of policy and practice in this arena.

1719 Centre for Addiction & Mental Health
33 Russell Street
Toronto ON, ZZ
416-535-8501
800-463-6273
E-mail: public_affairs@camh.net
www.www.camh.net

Paul Beeston, Chair

Provide treatment for and research into substance abuse and mental health issues.

1720 Child & Parent Resource Institute
600 Sanatorium Road
London ON, ZZ
519-858-2774
Fax: 519-858-3913

Anne Stark, Administrator

Enhance the quality of life of children and youth with complex mental health or developmental challenges.

1721 Child Welfare League of America
2345 Crystal Drive
Suite 250
Arlington, VA 22202
703-412-2400
Fax: 703-412-2401
www.cwla.org

Christine James-Brown, President/CEO

Oldest and largest membership-based child welfare organization. Committed to engaging people everywhere in promoting the well-being of children, youth, and their families, and protecting every child from harm.

1722 Christian Horizons PO Box 3381 Grand Rapids, MI 49501
616-956-7063
Fax: 616-956-7063
E-mail: info@christianhorizonsinc.org
www.christianhorizonsinc.org

A Christian organization dedicated to enriching the lives of people with mental impairments. Provides day programs, camping ministries, and Bible studies. Assists churches in identifying persons with special needs and supports parents of those with special needs.

1723 Coalition of Voluntary Mental Health Agencies
90 Broad Street
8th Floor
New York, NY 10004
212-742-1600
Fax: 212-742-2080
E-mail: mailbox@cvmha.org
www.cvmha.org/

An umbrella advocacy organization of New York City's mental health community, representing over 100 non-profit community based mental health agencies that serve more than 500,000 clients in the five boroughs of New York City. Founded in 1972, the Coalition is entirely membership supported with limited foundation and government funding for special purpose advocacy and assistance projects.

1724 Community Access
666 Broadway
3rd Floor
New York, NY 10012-2317
212-780-1400
Fax: 212-780-1412
www.communityaccess.net

Donald Starcke, Director of Development

A nonprofit agency providing housing and advocacy for people with psychiatric disabilities. Provides 430 affordable housing units for people with psychiatric disabilities, families with disabilities, and low income people from local neighborhoods.

1725 Community Service Options
7575 S Kostner Avenueue
Chicago, IL 60652
773-884-1000
Fax: 773-838-9362
www.csol.org

Promotes access, 'choice' of service, options and independence to people with disabilities who reside in the City of Chicago, through the provision of information, education, planning and service coordination.

1726 Council for Learning Disabilities
PO Box 4014
Leesburg, VA 20177
571-258-1010
Fax: 571-258-1011
www.cldinternational.org

Kirsten McBride, Executive Secretary

Professional membership association for professionals working with individuals who have learning disabilities. Committed to enhancing the educational and life span development of the learning disabled. Sponsors conferences and publishes journals in the field of learning disabilities.

1727 Council on Quality and Leadership
100 W Road
Suite 406
Towson, MD 21204
410-583-0060
Fax: 410-583-0063

E-mail: info@thecouncil.org
www.thecouncil.org

James F Gardner PhD, President/CEO
Michael Chapman, VP

An international nonprofit organization dedicated to advancing the quality of services and supports to people with disabilities. This is accomplished through its accreditation services, training programs and research division. The Council is currently providing support to organizations and providers throughout the United States, Canada, England, Ireland and Australia.

1728 Eye Movement Desensitization and Reprocessing International Association (EMDRIA)
PO Box 141925
Austin, TX 78714-9125
512-451-5200
Fax: 512-451-5256
E-mail: info@emdria.org
www.emdria.org

Carol York, Executive Director
Rosalie Thomas, President

The primary objective of EMDRIA is to establish, maintain and promote the highest standards of excellence and integrity in Eye Movement Desensitization and Reprocessing practice, research and education.

1729 Families Anonymous
PO Box 3475
Culver City, CA 90231-3475
Fax: 310-815-9682
E-mail: famanon@familiesanonymous.org
www.familiesanonymous.org

For concerned relatives and friends of youth with drug abuse or related behavior problems.

1730 Family Advocacy & Support Association
PO Box 73367
Washington, DC 20056-3367
202-526-5436
Fax: 202-326-3039

Phyllis Morgan, President

Self-help, nonprofit, support, education and advocacy organization comprised of parents/family members and service providers dedicated to improving the quality of life for children and youth with emotional, behavioral and learning disabilities.

1731 Family Violence & Sexual Assault Institute
6160 Cornerstone Court E
San Diego, CA 92121
858-623-2777
Fax: 858-646-0761
www.fvsai.org

David Westgate, Director

Book club, research, and quarterly newsletter.

1732 Federation for Children with Special Needs (FCSN)
1135 Tremont Street
Suite 420
Boston, MA 02120
617-236-7210
800-331-0688

Fax: 617-572-2094
E-mail: fcsninfo@fcsn.org
www.fcsn.org

Rich Robison, Executive Director

The federation provides information, support, and assistance to parents of children with disabilities, their professional partners and their communities.

1733 Federation of Families for Children's Mental Health
1101 King Street
Suite 420
Alexandria, VA 22314
703-684-7710
Fax: 703-836-1040
E-mail: ffcmh@ffcmh.org
www.ffcmh.org

Barbara Huff, Executive Director

National family-run organization dedicated exclusively to children and adolescents with mental health needs and their families. Our voice speaks through our work in policy, training and technical assistance programs. Publishes a quarterly newsletter and sponsors an annual conference and exhibits.

1734 Healing for Survivors
PO Box 4698
Fresno, CA 93744-4698
559-442-3600
Fax: 559-442-3600
E-mail: hfshope@email.com
www.hfshope.org

Jan Kister, Director
Tammie Wineland, Administrative Assistant

Support center for adults who were physically, emotionally, or sexually abused as children. Provides weekly support groups, weekend workshops, individual counseling, partners groups and couples groups.

1735 Hincks-Dellcrest Centre
440 Jarvis Street
Toronto ON, ZZ
416-924-1164
Fax: 416-924-8208
E-mail: info@hincksdellcrest.org
www.www.hincksdellcrest.org

John F Spekkens, Executive Director

Provides mental health prevention and early intervention programs for infants, children and youth.

1736 Hong Fook Mental Health Association
1065 McNicoll Avenue
Scarborough ON, ZZ
416-493-4242
Fax: 416-493-2214
E-mail: info@hongfook.ca
www.www.hongfook.ca

Raymond CY Chung MSW RSW, Executive Director

To achieve optimal mental health status through activities of direct services, promotion and prevention.

1737 Human Services Research Institute
2336 Massachusetts Avenue
Cambridge, MA 02140

617-876-0426
Fax: 617-492-7401
E-mail: sjohniken@hsri.org
www.hsri.org

Sebrina Johniken, Office Manager

Assists state and federal government to enhance services and support people with mental illness and people with mental retardation.

1738 Information Centers for Lithium, Bipolar Disorders Treatment & Obsessive Compulsive Disorder
Madison Institute of Medicine
7617 Mineral Point Road
Suite 300
Madison, WI 53717-1623
608-827-2470
Fax: 608-827-2479
E-mail: mim@miminc.org
www.miminc.org

The Information Centers publish information booklets. Authored by experts on each disorder, these patient guides offer information about various psychiatric disorders and their treatments, and address the questions most frequently asked by patients and their families.

1739 Inner Peace Movement of Canada
#1106 100 Bronson Avenue
Ottawa ON, ZZ
613-238-7844
Fax: 613-238-7445

Rita Bunbury, Office Manager

Promote self-help techniques; to organize self-help programs for the public.

1740 Institute of Living Anxiety Disorders Center
Hartford Hospital
200 Retreat Avenue
Hartford, CT 06106
800-673-2411
Fax: 860-545-7068
www.instituteofliving.org/ADC

David Tolin, PhD, Director

Provides evaluation and treatment for individuals suffering from anxiety disorders as well as training and education for clinicians.

1741 International Photo Therapy Association
Photo Therapy Centre
#205 1300 Richards Street
Vancouver BC, ZZ
604-689-9709
Fax: 604-633-1505
E-mail: jweiser@phototherapy-centre.com
www.www.phototherapy-centre.com

Judy Weiser, Chair

Educate about therapeutic uses of still & video photography.

1742 International Society of Psychiatric-Mental Health Nurses
1211 Locust Street
Philadelphia, PA 19107-5409
215-545-2843
800-826-2950

Fax: 215-545-8107
E-mail: info@ispn-psych.org
www.ispn-psych.org

Lynette Jack PhD, RN, CARN, President
Geraldine S Pearson PhD, RN, CS, Secratary
Mary Jo Regan-Kubinski PhD, RN, Treasurer

To unite and enhance the presence and the voice of specialty psychiatric mental health nurses while influencing healthcare policy to promote equitable, evidence-based and effective treatment and care for individuals, families and communities.

1743 Judge Baker Children's Center
3 Blackfan Circle
Boston, MA 02115-5794
617-232-8390
Fax: 617-232-8399
E-mail: info@jbcc.harvard.edu
www.jbcc.harvard.edu

Stewart Hauser, MD, PhD, President
Kevin Lee Hepner, VP

A nonprofit organization dedicated to improving the lives of children whose emotional and behavioral problems threaten to limit their potential.

1744 Learning Disability Association of America
4156 Library Road
Pittsburgh, PA 15234-1349
412-341-1515
Fax: 412-344-0224
E-mail: info@ldaamerica.org
www.ldanatl.org

John E Muench, National Executive Director

Offers information and referral services to the learning disabled. Free pamphlets, fact sheets and bibliography regarding learning disabilities.

1745 Life Development Institute
18001 N 79th Avenue, Suite E71
Phoenix, AZ 85308
623-773-2774
Fax: 623-773-2788
E-mail: LDIinARIZ@aol.com
www.life-development-inst.org

Robert Crawford, President

Serves older adolescents and adults with learning disabilities and related disorders. Conducts programs to assist individuals to achieve careers/employment commensurate with capabilities and independent status.

1746 Lifespire
345 Hudson Street
3rd Floor
New York, NY 10014
212-741-0100
Fax: 212-463-9814
E-mail: info@lifespire.org
www.lifespire.com

Professionals, parents, siblings, and others interested in mentally retarded and developmentally disabled adults. Offers professionally supervised programs for mentally retarded and developmentally disabled adults including vocational rehabilitation, dual diagnosis programs, job placement, rehabilitation workshops, activities for daily living, day treatment, day training, supported work, and family support programs.

1747 Menninger Clinic
2801 Gessner
PO Box 809045
Houston, TX 77280-9045
713-275-5000
800-351-9058
Fax: 713-275-5107
www.menninger.edu

Dr. Herbert Spohn, Director

A national specialty psychiatric care facility offering diagnostic and treatment programs for adoloscents and adults.

1748 Mental Health and Aging Network (MHAN) of the American Society on Aging (ASA)
Ameican Society on Aging
833 Market Street
Suite 511
San Francisco, CA 94103
415-974-9600
800-537-9728
Fax: 415-974-0300
E-mail: info@asaging.org
www.asaging.org

Robert Stein, President/CEO
Robert Lowe, Director Of Operations

Dedicated to improving the supportive interventions for older adults with mental health problems and their caregivers by: Creating a cadre of professionals with expertise in geriatric mental health, Assuring that service professionals are multi capable, Improving the systems of care, Providing a voice for the underserved and Advocating for the services that advance quality of life for our clients.

1749 Mental Illness Education Project
PO Box 470813
Brookline Village, MA 02447-0813
617-562-1111
800-343-5540
Fax: 617-779-0061
E-mail: info@miepvideos.org
www.miepvideos.org

Christine Ledoux, Executive Director

Engaged in the production of video-based educational and support materials for the following specific populations: people with psychiatric disabilities; families, mental health professionals, special audiences, and the general public. The Project's videos are designed to be used in hospital, clinical and educational settings, and at home by individuals and families.

1750 Mentally Ill Kids in Distress
755 E Willetta Street
Phoenix, AZ 85006
602-253-1240
Fax: 602-523-1250
E-mail: mikidaz@qwest.net
www.mikid.org

Mission is to provide support and assistance to families in Arizona with behaviorally challenged children, youth, and young adults.

1751 Nathan S Kline Institute for Psychiatric Research
140 Old Orangeburg Road
Orangeburg, NY 10962
845-398-5500
Fax: 845-398-5510
E-mail: webmaster@nki.rfmh.org
www.rfmh.org/nki

Thomas O'Hara, Deputy Director Administration

Research programs in Alzheimers disease, analytical psychopharmacology, basic and clinical neuroimaging, cellular and molecular neurobiology, clinical trial data management, co-occuring disorders and many other mental health studies.

1752 National Alliance on Mental Illness
2107 Wilson Boulevard
Suite 300
Arlington, VA 22201-3042
703-524-7600
Fax: 703-524-9094
www.nami.org

Michael Fitzpatrick, Executive Director
Lynn Borton, COO

Dedicated to the eradication of mental illnesses and to the improvement of the quality of life of all whose lives are affected by these diseases.

Year Founded: 1979

1753 National Association for Rural Mental Health
3700 W Division Street
Suite 105
Saint Cloud, MN 56301-3728
320-202-1820
Fax: 320-202-1833
E-mail: NARMH@facts.ksu.edu
www.narmh.org

Rick Peterson, President
LuAnn Rice, Manager

Provides a forum for rural mental health professionals and advocates to identify problems, find solutions, and work cooperatively toward improving the delivery of rural mental health services, promote the unique needs and concerns of rural mental health policy and practice issues, sponsor an annual conference where rural mental health professionals benefit from the sharing of knowledge and resources. NARMH was founded to develop, enhance and support mental health services and providers in rural America.

Year Founded: 1977

1754 National Association for the Dually Diagnose d (NADD)
132 Fair Street
Kingston, NY 12401
845-334-4336
800-331-5362
Fax: 845-331-4569
E-mail: info@thenadd.org
www.thenadd.org

Robert J Fletcher, CEO

A not-for-profit membership association established for professionals, care providers and families to promote understanding of and services for individuals who have developmental disabilities and mental health needs.

Year Founded: 1983

1755 National Association of Protection and Advocacy Systems
900 2nd Street NE
Suite 211
Washington, DC 20002-3557
202-408-9514
Fax: 202-408-9520
TDD: 202-408-9521
E-mail: info@napas.org
www.protectionandadvocacy.com

Curtis L Decker, Executive Director

NAPAS was established under the Protection and Advocacy for Individuals with Mental Illness (PAIMI) Act. PAIMI programs protect and advocate for the legal rights of persons with mental illness. The programs investigate reports of abuse or neglect and provide technical assistance, information, and legal counseling. Publishes a free, quarterly newsletter, P&A News.

1756 National Association of State Mental Health Program Directors
66 Canal Center Plaza
Suite 302
Alexandria, VA 22314
703-739-9333
Fax: 703-548-9517
E-mail: roy.praschil@nasmhpd.org
www.nasmhpd.org

Robert W Glover PhD, Executive Director
Roy Praschil, Director Operations

Nonprofit membership organization that adovacates at the national level for the collective interests of state mental health agency commissioners and staff. Operates under a cooperative agreement with the National Governor's Association. NASMHPD is committed to working with other stakeholders to improve public mental health systems and the lives of persons with serious mental illnesses who access these and other systems. Its core services focus on legislative advocacy, technical assistance and information dissemination.

Year Founded: 1959

1757 National Association of Therapeutic Wilderness Camps
698 Dinner Bell-Ohiopyle Road
Ohiopyle, PA 15470
E-mail: info@natwc.org
www.natwc.org

Represents nearly fifty therapeutic wilderness camps located all over the US. We believe therapeutic wilderness camps represent the most effective method to help troubled young people change the way they deal with their parents, school, and other authorities.

1758 National Center for Learning Disabilities
381 Park Avenue S
Room 1401
New York, NY 10016
212-545-7510
888-575-7373
Fax: 212-545-9665
www.ncld.org

National, non profit organization dedicated to improving the lives of those affected by learning didabilities (LD).

Services include national information and referral, public outreach and communications, legislative advocacy and public policy. Its mission is to promote public awareness and understanding of learning disabilities and to provide national leadership on behalf of children and adults with LD so they may achieve thier potential and enjoy full participation in society. Our website offers a free monthly e mail newsletter, and much more information for contacts and referrals.

1759 National Center on Addiction and Substance Abuse at Columbia University
633 3rd Avenue
19th Floor
New York, NY 10017-6706
212-841-5200
Fax: 212-956-8020
E-mail: info@casacolumbia.org
www.casacolumbia.org

William H Foster PhD, COO
Richard Mulieri, Communications

Unique think/action tank that engages all disiplines to study every form of substance abuse as it affects our society.

1760 National Child Support Network
PO Box 1018
Fayetteville, AR 72702-1018
800-729-5437
Fax: 479-582-2401
www.childsupport.org

A private bonded, insured and licensed child support collection agency.

1761 National Council for Community Behavioral Healthcare
12300 Twinbrook Parkway
Suite 320
Rockville, MD 20852-1606
301-984-6200
Fax: 301-881-7159
E-mail: lindare@nccbh.org
www.nccbh.org

Linda Rosenberg, CEO
David Schuerholz, Marketing/Communications

Behavioral healthcare administrators. Publishes the Journal of Behavioral Health Sciences and Research, ABHM Leader. Annual training conferences. See web for additional information.

1762 National Empowerment Center
National Empowerment Center
599 Canal Street
Lawrence, MA 01840
978-685-1518
800-769-3728
Fax: 978-681-6426
www.power2u.org

Daniel B Fisher MD, PhD, Executive Director
Laurie Ahern, Educator

Technical assistance center, providing information and education to consumer/survivor/ex-patients, family members and professionals. Carries a message of recovery, empowerment, hope and healing to people who have been diagnosed with mental illness.

1763 National GAINS Center for People with Co-Occurring Disorders in the Justice System
345 Delaware Avenue
Delmar, NY 12054-1123
518-439-7415
800-311-4246
Fax: 518-439-7612
E-mail: sdavidson@prainc.com
www.gainsctr.com

Joseph J Cocozza PhD, Co-Director
Henry Steadman PhD, Co-Director
Susan Davidson, Division Manager

Center is a national focus for the collection and dissemination of information about effective, integrated mental health and substance abuse services for people with co-ocurring disorders who come in contact with the criminal justice system, including law enforcement, jails, prisons, and community corrections. The center is operated by Policy Research, Inc. of Delmar, NY and is supported by the National Institute of Corrections, the Center for Substance Abuse Treatment and the Center for Mental Health Services.

1764 National Institute of Drug Abuse (NIDA)
6001 Executive Boulevard
Room 5213
Bethesda, MD 20892-9561
301-443-1124
Fax: 301-443-7397
E-mail: information@lists.nida.nih.gov
www.nida.nih.gov

Beverly Jackson, Public Information

Covers the areas of drug abuse treatment and prevention research, epidemiology, neuroscience and behavioral research, health services research and AIDS. Seeks to report on advances in the field, identify resources, promote an exchange of information, and improve communications among clinicians, researchers, administrators, and policymakers. Recurring features include synopses of research advances and projects, NIDA news, news of legislative and regulatory developments, and announcements.

1765 National Institute of Mental Health Information Resources and Inquiries Branch
6001 Executive Boulevard
Room 8184
Bethesda, MD 20892-9663
866-615-6464
Fax: 301-443-4279
TTY: 301-443-8431
E-mail: nimhinfo@nih.gov
www.nimh.nih.gov

One of 27 components of the National Institutes of Health, the Federal government's principal biomedical and behavioral research agency.

1766 National Mental Health Association
2000 N Beauregard Street
6th Floor
Alexandria, VA 22311
703-684-7722
800-969-6642
Fax: 703-684-5968
TTY: 800-433-5959
www.nmha.org

David Shern, President/CEO
Kate Gaston, VP Afiliate Services

Dedicated to improving treatments, understanding and services for adults and children with mental health needs. Working to win political support for funding for school mental health programs. Provides information about a wide range of disorders, such as panic disorder, obsessive-compulsive disorder, post traumatic stress, generalized anxiety disorder and phobias. Also advocates for programs to diagnose and treat children in juvenille justice systems.

1767 National Mental Health Consumers' Self-Help Clearinghouse
1211 Chestnut Street
Suite 1207
Philadelphia, PA 19107
215-751-1810
800-553-4539
Fax: 215-636-6312
E-mail: info@mhselfhelp.org
www.mhselfhelp.org

Joseph Rogers, Executive Director

A national consumer technical assistance center that has played a major role in the development of the mental health consumer movement.

Year Founded: 1986

1768 National Network for Mental Health
#604 55 King Street
St. Catharine ON, ZZ
905-682-2423
888-406-4663
Fax: 905-682-7469
E-mail: info@nnmh.ca
www.www.nnmh.ca

Constance McKnight, Executive Director

Advocate, educate and provide expertise and resources for increased health and well-being of the Canadian mental health consumer.

1769 National Organization on Disability
910 16th Street NW
Suite 600
Washington, DC 20006
202-293-5960
Fax: 202-293-7999
TTY: 202-293-5968
E-mail: ability@nod.org
www.nod.org

Elizabeth A Davis, VP/Director
Charles Dey, VP/Director
Glynnis Breen, Development

Nonprofit organization dedicated to promoting the full and equal participation of America's 49 million women, men and children with disabilities in all aspects of life. Consisting of 4,500 members and 250 chapters, NOD produces educational materials including fact sheets, brochures, a directory and various booklets including From Barriers To Bridges and Loving Justice. Offers many groups, partnerships and programs all orientated around expanding, promoting and advocating for people affected with disabilities.

Year Founded: 1982

1770 National Rehabilitation Association
633 S Washington Street
Alexandria, VA 22314

703-836-0850
Fax: 703-836-0848
TDD: 703-836-0849
E-mail: info@nationalrehab.org
www.nationalrehab.org

Anne Marie Hohman, Executive Director
John D'Angelo, Director Operations

Concerned with the rights of people with disabilities, our mission is to provide advocacy, awareness and career advancement for professionals in the fields of rehabilitation. Our members include rehab counselors, physical, speech and occupational therapists, job trainers, consultants, independent living instructors and other professionals involved in the advocacy of programs and services for people with disabilities.

1771 National Resource Center on Homelessness & Mental Illness
345 Delaware Avenue
Delmar, NY 12054
518-439-7415
800-444-7415
Fax: 518-439-7612
E-mail: nrc@prainc.com
www.nrchmi.samhsa.gov

Francine Williams, Director
Deborah Dennis, VP/Project Director

Provides technical assistance and comprehensive information concerning the treatment, services and housing needs of persons who are homeless and who have serious mental illnesses. The Resource Center provides technical assistance to CHS grantees, provides or arranges technical assistance on the development of housing and services for special needs populations; maintains an extensive bibliographic database of published and unpublished materials, develops workshops and training institutes on the coordination of services and housing for homeless persons with mental illnesses, and responds to requests for information.

1772 National Self-Help Clearinghouse Graduate School and University Center
365 5th Avenue
Suite 3300
New York, NY 10016
212-817-1822
E-mail: info@selfhelpweb.org
www.selfhelpweb.org

Audrey Gardner, Co Director
Frank Riessman, Co Director

Facilitates access to self-help groups and increases the awareness of the importance of mutual support. The clearinghouse provides services by: assisting human service agencies on self-help principles, conducting training for self-help group leaders and group facilitators, researches the effectiveness of self-help and relationships with formal caregiving systems and provides media outreach.

Year Founded: 1976

1773 National Technical Assistance Center for Children's Mental Health
Georgetown University Child Development Center
3307 M Street NW
Washington, DC 20007
202-687-5000
Fax: 202-687-1954

TTY: 202-687-5503
E-mail: gucdc@georgetown.edu
www.dml.georgetown.edu/research/gucdc/cassp.html

Integral part of the Georgetown University Center for Child and Human Development at the Georgetown University Medical Center. Nationally recognized for its work in assisting states and communities build systems of care for mental health concerns.

Year Founded: 1984

1774 New Hope Foundation
PO Box 201
Kensington, MD 20895-0201
301-946-6395
Fax: 301-946-1402
E-mail: newhope@nhfi.org
www.newhopfoundationinc.org

Daphne Stegmaier, Volunteer

Nonprofit organization integrates the many techniques proven effective in dealing with serious mental problems. Presents an innovative, replicable program designed to maximize the ability of chronically ill mental patients to achieve stable, self supporting lives in the community.

1775 PRO Behavioral Health
7600 E Eastman Avenue
Denver, CO 80231
303-695-6007
888-687-6755
Fax: 303-695-0100
www.probh.com

Mari Teitelman LCSW, Business Development

PRO Behavioral Health is one of the nation's leading mental health and substance abuse managed care firms. Founded and directed by behavioral health clinicians and managers, PRO brings a clinically driven behavioral health service model to the market. Client organizations enjoy the benefits of PRO's client-specific customized programs, highly responsible customer service, behavioral health care coordinated with medical care, continuous quality improvement and reduced costs.

1776 Parents Helping Parents
3041 Olcott Street
Santa Clara, CA 95054
408-727-5775
Fax: 408-727-0182
E-mail: general@php.com
www.php.com

Lois Jones, Executive Director

Nonprofit family resource center offering culturally sensitive information, peer counseling and provides a forum for parents and professionals to get information. PHP does not promote or recommend any treatment, therapy, institution or professional.

1777 Parents Information Network
1101 King Street
Suite 420
Alexandria, VA 22314
703-684-7710
Fax: 703-836-1040
E-mail: ffcmh@ffcmh.org
www.ffcmh.org/local.htm

Bridget Schneider, Facilitator

National parent run organization focused on the needs of children and youth with emotional, behavioral or mental disorders and their families.

1778 Parents for Children's Mental Health
#309 40 St. Clair Avenue E
Toronto ON, ZZ
416-921-2109
Fax: 416-921-7600
E-mail: parents@parentsforchildrensmentalhealth.org
www.www.parentsforchildrensmentalhealth.org

Provide voice for children & their families who face the challenges of mental health problems in Ontario.

1779 Phoenix Care Systems, Inc: Willowglen Academy
1744 N Farwell Avenue
Milwaukee, WI 53202
414-225-4460
866-225-4459
Fax: 414-225-9403
E-mail: john.yopps@phoenixcaresystems.com
www.phoenixcaresystems.com

John A Yopps, Marketing/Development Director
Lin Daley, Exec Director-Wisconsin
Kathleen Tresemer, Exec Director-Illinois
Dwayne Mueller, Exec Director-Indiana

As a wholly owned subsidiary of Phoenix Care Systems, Inc, Willowglen Academy provides therapeutic residential treatment and educational services to children, adolescents and young adults with mental health, emotional, cognitive and developmental disabilities. Our accrediting bodies include COA, CARF and JCAHO.

1780 Professional Assistance Center for Education (PACE)
National-Louis University
2840 Sheridan Road
Evanston, IL 60201-1730
847-475-2670
Fax: 847-256-1057
E-mail: cburns@nl.edu
www.2.nl.edu/pace

Carol Burns, Director

Non-credit, non degree, two-year postsecondary program for students with learning disabilities. The program prepares young adults for careers as aides in preschools or human service agencies. In addition to professional preparation coursework, the curriculum also focuses on social skills and independent living skills. Students receive a certificate of completion at the conclusion of the program. College residential life is an integral part of the program. Transitional program where appropriate.

1781 Psychiatric Clinical Research Center
University of Illinois at Chicago
1740 W Taylor Street
Medical Center
Chicago, IL 60612-7232
312-996-0443
800-842-1002
www.uillinoismedcenter.org

Ramon Gomez, Director

The Center offers those whose quality of life is affected by severe mental disorders the opportunity to receive an accurate diagnosis and treatment for their condition using the latest methods of care. Those who participate in the clinical research give our staff the opportunity to learn more about these serious mental disorders.

1782 Reclamation
2502 Waterford Drive
San Antonio, TX 78217-5037
210-822-3569
www.community-2.webtv/stigmanet/

Don H Culwell, Director

Former mental patients and interested others. Seeks to eliminate the stigma of mental illness and reclaim members' dignity. Serves as a voice for mental health patients in consumer, social and political affairs. Helps members to live outside a hospital setting by providing assistance in the areas of resocialization, employment and housing. Monitors the media and encourages positive media coverage. Publications: Positive Visibility, quarterly newsletter. Annual Reclamation conference.

1783 Recovery
802 N Dearborn Street
Chicago, IL 60610-3364
312-337-5661
Fax: 312-337-5756
E-mail: inquiries@recovery-inc.com
www.recovery-inc.com

Kelly Garcia, Executive Director
Maurine Pyle

Recovery method is to help prevent relapses in former mental patients and to forestall chronicity in nervous patients. Recovery provides training in a systematic method of self-help aftercare for these patients, based on the system of self-help principles described in Low's book, Mental Health Through Will Training.

1784 Refuah
PO Box 1212
Randolph, MA 02368
781-961-2815
Fax: 781-986-5070
E-mail: nblrefuah@aol.com
www.refuahboston.org

Nancy Blake Lewis, Executive Director

Expanding network of concerned Jewish family members and friends with loved ones of any race or creed suffering from chronic mental illness.

1785 Research Center for Severe Mental Illnesses
11301 Wilshire Boulevard #116
W LA VA Medical Center, Building 208 R
Los Angeles, CA 90073-1003
310-477-7927
E-mail: rpl@ucla.edu
www.npi.ucla.edu/crc/products/products

Robert Paul Liberman MD, Director
Jim Mintz PhD, Associate Director

For more than 20 years the center has given priority to the design, validation and dissemination of the practical, user-friendly assesment, treatment and rehabilitation techniques for practitioners.

1786 Research and Training Center on Family Support and Children's Mental Health
Portland State University/Regional Research Institute
PO Box 751
Portland State University
Portland, OR 97207-0751
503-725-4040
Fax: 503-725-4180
E-mail: gordon@pdx.edu
www.rtc.pdx.edu

Lynwood Gordon, Public Information/Outreach
Janet Walker, Editor

Dedicated to promoting effective community based, culturally competent, family centered services for families and their children who are or may be affected by mental, emotional or behavioral disorders. This goal is accomplished through collaborative research partnerships with family members, service providers, policy makers, and other concerned persons. Major efforts in dissemination and training include: An annual conference, an award winning web site to share information about child and family mental services and policy issues which includes Focal Point, a national bulletin regarding family support and children's mental health.

1787 Resources for Children with Special Needs
116 E 16th Street
5th Floor
New York, NY 10003
212-677-4650
Fax: 212-254-4070
E-mail: info@resourcesnyc.org
www.resourcesnyc.org

Karen T Schlesinger, Executive Director
Dianne Littwin, Director Publications

Information, referral, advocacy, training, publications for New York City parents of youth with disabilities or special needs and the professionals who work with them.

1788 Sidran Traumatic Stress Institute
200 E Joppa Road
Suite 207
Towson, MD 21286
410-825-8888
888-825-8249
Fax: 410-337-0747
E-mail: sidran@sidran.org
www.sidran.org

Esther Giller, Executive Director

A nonprofit charitable organization devoted to education, advocacy and research to benefit people who are suffering from injuries of traumatic stress. Whether caused by family violence, crime, disaster, war or any other overwhelming experience, the disabling effects of trauma can be overcome with understanding, support and appropriate treatment. To support people with traumatic stress conditions and to educate mental health professionals and the public. Sidran has developed many service, training and bookshelf information sources.

1789 Systems Advocacy
National Mental Health Consumers' Self-Help Clearinghouse
1211 Chestnut Street
Suite 1000
Philadelphia, PA 19107-4103
215-751-1810
800-553-4539
Fax: 212-636-6312
E-mail: THEKEY@delphi.com
www.mhselfhelp.org

A consumer-run national technical assistance center serving the mental health consumer movement. Help connect individuals to self-help and advocacy resources, and we offer expertise to self-help groups and other peer-run services for mental health consumers.

1790 Thresholds Psychiatric Rehabilitation
4101 N Ravenswood Avenue
Chicago, IL 60613
773-880-6260
888-997-3422
Fax: 773-880-9050
E-mail: thresholds@thresholds.org
www.thresholds.org

Mary Jo Herseth, President
Tony M Zipple, CEO

Psychosocial rehabilitation agency serving persons with severe and persistent mental illness.

1791 United Families for Children's Mental Health
13301 Bruce B Downs Boulevard
FMHI Box 2, Room 2514
Tampa, FL 33612
813-974-7930
Fax: 813-974-7712
E-mail: ffcmh@earthlink.net

Carol Baier

Nonprofit family organization run by and for caregivers of children with mental health issues.

1792 Voice of the Retarded
5005 Newport Drive
Suite 108
Rolling Meadows, IL 60008-3837
847-253-6020
Fax: 847-253-6054
E-mail: vor@compuserve.com
www.vor.net

Tamie Hopp, Executive Director
Nancy Ward, President

VOR is a national advocacy organization. Its mission is to ensure quality care and choice in services and supports received by people with mental retardation. Through a weekly e-mail update, a quarterly newsletter and frequent action alerts, we empower our members and coordinate grass roots advocacy. Membership is $25 per year.

1793 Warren Grant Magnuson Clinical Center
9000 Rockville Pike
Building 10, Room 1C255
Bethesda, MD 20892-0001
301-496-2563
Fax: 301-402-2984
E-mail: occc@cc.nih.gov
www.cc.nih.gov

Established as the research hospital of the National Institutes of Health. Designed with patient care facilities close to research laboratories so new findings of basic and clinical scientists can be quickly applied to the treatment of patients. Upon referral by physicians, patients are admitted to NIH clinical studies.

Year Founded: 1953

1794 Windhorse Associates
211 North Street
Suite 1
Northampton, MA 01060
413-586-0207
Fax: 413-585-1521
www.windhorseassociates.org

Michael Herrick MA, Executive Director
Jeff Bliss CSW, Developmental Director
Sara Watters MA, Clinical Director

A therapeutic community approach to recovery for individuals struggling with psychiatric disturbances. Services are individually tailored in close communications with each client and family, and represent a wide range of intensity and structure. Clients may live alone or with a Windhorse housemate.

1795 Women's Counselling & Referral Education Cen tre
#303B 489 College Street
Toronto ON, ZZ
416-534-7501
Fax: 416-534-7501
E-mail: generalmail@wcrec.org

Coordinate and provide referrals to women seeking counselling and other resources.

1796 World Federation for Mental Health Secretariat
6564 Loisdale Court
Suite 301
Springfield, VA 22150
703-313-8680
Fax: 703-313-8683
E-mail: info@wfmh.com
www.wfmh.com

Preston Garrison, CEO

Education and advocacy organization. Our primary goal is to educate the public on mental health and to advocate for those who deal with mental health issues. Working to protect the human rights of those defined as mentally ill.

1797 Young Adult Institute and Workshop (YAI)
460 W 34th Street
New York, NY 10001-2382
212-273-6100
Fax: 212-268-1083
www.yai.org

Joel M Levy, Executive Director/CEO
Phil Levy, President/COO

Serves more than 15,000 people of all ages and levels of mental retardation, developmental and learning disabilities. Provides a full range of early intervention, preschool, family supports, employment training and placement, clinical and residential services, as well as recreation and camping services. YAI/National Intitute for People with Disabilities is also a professional organization, nationally renowned for its publications, conferences, training seminars, video training tapes and innovative television programs.

1798 Youth Services International
1819 Main Street
Suite 1000
Sarasota, FL 34236
941-953-9199
Fax: 941-953-9198
E-mail: YSIWEB@youthservices.com
www.youthservices.com

Premier provider in the youth care industry of educational and developmental services that change, dramatically, the thinking and behavior of troubled youth.

1799 Zero to Three
2000 M Street NW
Suite 200
Washington, DC 20036
202-638-1144
800-899-4301
Fax: 202-638-0851
E-mail: oto3@presswarehouse.com
www.zerotothree.org

Matthew E Melmed JD, Executive Director
Emily Fenichel, Associate Director

Professionals and researchers in the health care industry, policymakers and parents working to improve the healthy physical, cognitive and social development of infants, toddlers and their families. Sponsors training and technical assistance activities. Publications: Clinical Infant Reports, book series. Public Policy Pamphlets, 1 to 3 times per year. Zero to Three, 6 times per year, Annual National Training Institute conference and exhibits, usually in December.

Alabama

1800 Alabama Alliance for the Mentally Ill
6900 6th Avenue S
Suite B
Birmingham, AL 35212-1902
205-833-8336
800-626-4199
Fax: 205-833-8309
E-mail: alaami@aol.com

Ann Denbo, President

Advocacy, education and support for and about the Alabama mental health community.

1801 Birmingham Psychiatry
1 Independence Plaza
Homewood, AL
205-879-7953
Fax: 205-870-7987

1802 Horizons School
2111 University Boulevard
Birmingham, AL 35233
205-322-6606
800-822-6242
Fax: 205-322-6605
www.horizonsschool.org

Marie McElheny, Admissions Coordinator
Jade Carter, Director

College based, non degree program for students with specific learning disabilities and other mild learning problems. This specially-designed, two-year program prepares individuals for successful transitions to the community. Classes teach life skills, social skills and career training.

1803 Mental Health Board of North Central Alabama
4110 Highway 31 South
PO Box 2479
Decatur, AL 35603
256-355-5904
800-365-6008
Fax: 256-355-6092
E-mail: mentalhealth@mhcnca.org
www.mhcnca.org

1804 Mental Health Center of North Central Alabama
4110 Highway 31 S
Decatur, AL 35603
256-335-6091
800-337-3162
Fax: 256-355-6091
E-mail: mentalhealth@mhcna.org
www.mhcnca.org

We support all people with mental health disorders to achieve respect and dignity, to reach their full potential and to be free from stigma and prejudice.

1805 National Alliance on Mental Illness: Alabama
4122 Wall Street
Montgomery, AL 36106-2861
334-396-4797
800-626-4199
Fax: 334-396-4794
E-mail: terri@namialabama.org
www.namialabama.org

Greg Carlson, President
Terri Beasley, Executive Director

An organization comprised of local support and advocacy groups throughout the state dedicated to improving the quality of life for persons with a mental illness in Alabama.

Alaska

1806 Alaska Alliance for the Mentally Ill
144 W 15th Avenue
Suite B
Anchorage, AK 99501
907-277-1300
Fax: 907-277-1400
E-mail: info@nami-alaska.org
www.nami-alaska.org

Beth LaCross, Board President
Yvonne Evans, Support Group Facilitator

Mission is to bring consumers and families with similar experiences together to share information about services, care providers, and ways to cope with the challenges of schizophrenia, manic depression, and other serious mental illnesses.

1807 Mental Health Association in Alaska
4045 Lake Otis Parkway
Suite 209
Anchorage, AK 99508

907-563-0880
Fax: 907-563-0881
www.alaska.net/~mhaa/

1808 National Alliance on Mental Illness: Alaska
144 W 15th Avenue
Anchorage, AK 99501-5106
907-277-1300
800-478-4462
Fax: 907-277-1400
E-mail: info@nami-alaska.org
www.nami.org/sites/alaska

Jeanette Grasto, President

A nonprofit, support, education and advocacy organization of consumers, families and friends of people with severe brain disorders such as schizophrenia, schizoaffective disorder, bipolar disorder, major depressive disorder, obsessive-compulsive disorder, panic and anxiety disorders and attention deficit/hyperactivity disorder.

Arizona

1809 Arizona Alliance for the Mentally Ill
2210 N 7th Street
Phoenix, AZ 85006-1604
602-244-8166
800-626-5022
Fax: 602-244-9264
E-mail: azami@azami.org
www.az.nami.org

Sue Davis, Executive Director
Joan Abbot, Membership

Advocacy, education and support groups for families in Arizona who have loved ones dealing with mental health concerns.

1810 Community Partnership of Southern Arizona
4575 E Broadway
Tucson, AZ 85711
520-318-6900
Fax: 520-325-1441
E-mail: nogra@cpsa-rhba.org
www.cpsa-rhba.org

Neal Cash, CEO
Judy Johnson PhD, Deputy Director

Administrative organization responsible for the coordination of behavioral health treatment and preventitive services in southern and southeastern Arizona. We are a local community based nonprofit organization that is dedicated to ensuring the provision of accessible high quality and cost effective behavioral health services for adults and children.

1811 Devereux Arizona Treatment Network
11000 N Scottsdale Road
Suite 260
Scottsdale, AZ 85254-4581
480-998-2920
800-345-1292
Fax: 480-443-5587
www.devereux.org

Jim Cole, Executive Director

National non-profit treatment centers for emotional disorders.

1812 Mental Health Association of Arizona
6411 E Thomas Road
Scottsdale, AZ 85251-6005
480-994-4407
800-642-4407
Fax: 480-994-4744
www.mhaaz.com

Tiffany Bock, Executive Director
Julie Clark, Community Education

Allfiliate of the National Mental Health Association, we support all people with mental disorders to achieve respect and dignity, to reach their full potential and to be free from stigma and prejudice.

Year Founded: 1954

1813 National Alliance on Mental Illness: Arizona
2210 N 7th Street
Phoenix, AZ 85006-1604
602-244-8166
800-626-5022
Fax: 602-244-9264
E-mail: namiaz@namiaz.org
www.namiaz.org

Cheryl Fanning, President

The mission of NAMI Arizona shall be to serve as an alliance of local Arizona Affiliates of NAMI and their members and associate members who are dedicated to the eradication of mental illnesses and to the improvement of the quality of life of persons whose lives are affected by these diseases.

1814 Navajo Nation K'E Project
PO Box 3390
200 Parkway Administration Building 1
Window Rock, AZ 86515
928-871-7160
Fax: 928-871-7255

Janet Hillis

Children and families advocacy corporation.

1815 Navajo Nation K'E Project: Chinle
PO Box 3390
Chinle, AZ 86515
928-871-7160
Fax: 928-871-7255

Shirley Etsitty

Chinle children and families advocacy corporation.

1816 Navajo Nation K'E Project: Tuba City
PO Box 3390
200 Parkway Administration Building 1
Window Rock, AZ 86515
928-871-7160
Fax: 928-871-7255

Rueben McCabe

Childrens and families advocacy corporation.

1817 Navajo Nation K'E Project: Winslow
PO Box 3390
200 Parkway Administration Building 1
Window Rock, AZ 86515
928-871-7160
Fax: 928-871-7255

Jayne Clark

Children and families advocacy corporation.

Arkansas

1818 Arkansas Alliance for the Mentally Ill
4313 W Markham Street
Hendrix Hall, Room 203
Little Rock, AR 72205-4096
501-661-1548
800-844-0381
Fax: 501-664-0264
E-mail: tenewman@aol.com
www.nami.org

Laurie Flynn, Executive Director

Bringing consumers and families with similar experiences together to share information about services, care providers, and ways to cope with the challenges of schizophrenia, manic depression, and other serious mental illnesses.

1819 National Alliance on Mental Illness: Arkansa s
712 W 3rd Street
Suite 200
Little Rock, AR 72201-2222
501-661-1548
800-844-0381
Fax: 501-664-0264
E-mail: karnold@nami.org
www.ar.nami.org

Jerri Skaggs, President
Kim Arnold, Executive Director

A non-profit, grassroots organization dedicated to improving the lives of persons with severe mental illness, their families, and their communities. Formerly known as Arkansas Alliance for the Mentally Ill (AAMI), NAMI Arkansas operates a statewide organization and coordinates a network of affiliates, support groups and field services throughout the state.

California

1820 Assistance League of Southern California
1360 North Street
Andrews Plaza
Hollywood, CA 90028
323-469-1973
Fax: 323-469-3533
E-mail: email@assistanceleague.net
www.assistanceleague.net

Sandy Doerschlag, Chief Executive Director
Janet Harrison, Public Relations

Provides mental health services to children over 5 years of age, individuals and families. Parent education and domestic violence classes are available. Services in English, Spanish and Armenian.

Year Founded: 1919

1821 California Alliance for the Mentally Ill
National Alliance for the Mentally Ill
1111 Howe Avenue
Suite 475
Sacramento, CA 95825-8541
916-567-0163
Fax: 916-567-1757
E-mail: grace. mcandrews@namicalifornia.org
www.namicalifornia.org

Laurie Flynn, Executive Director

Nation's leading self-help organization for all those affected by severe brain disorders. Mission is to bring consumers and families with similar experiences together to share information about services, care providers, and ways to cope with the challenges of schizophrenia, manic depression, and other serious mental illnesses. The California office answers questions from hundreds of individuals and groups outside NAMI who turn to us for accurate information about mental illness, NAMI affiliates near them, and where to turn for help.

Year Founded: 1977

1822 California Association of Marriage and Family Therapists

7901 Raytheon Road
San Diego, CA 92111-1606
858-292-2638
Fax: 858-292-2666
www.camft.org

Mary Riemersma, Executive Director

Independent professional organization representing the interests of licensed marriage and family therapists. Dedicated to advancing the profession as an art and a science, to maintaining high standards of professional ethics, to upholding the qualifications for the profession and to expanding the recognition and awareness of the profession.

1823 California Association of Social Rehabilitation Agencies

815 Marina Vista, Suite D
PO Box 388
Martinez, CA 94553
925-229-2300
Fax: 925-229-9088
E-mail: casra@casra.org
www.casra.org

Betty Dahlquist, Executive Director
Peggy Harris, Executive Assistant
Dave Hosseini, Public Policy
Sheryle Stafford, Public Policy

Dedicated to improving services and social conditions for people with psychiatric disabilities by promoting their recovery, rehabilitation and rights. A diagnosis is not a destiny.

1824 California Health Information Association

1915 N Fine Avenue
Suite 104
Fresno, CA 93727-1510
559-251-5038
Fax: 559-251-5836
E-mail: info@californiahia.org
www.californiahia.org

LaVonne LaLamoreaux, Executive Director
Marilyn R Taylor, Operations Manager

Nonprofit association that provides leadership, education, resources and advocacy for California's health information management professionals. Contributes to the delivery of quality patient care through excellence in health information management practice.

1825 California Institute for Mental Health

2030 J Street
Sacramento, CA 95814-3904

916-556-3480
Fax: 916-446-4519
E-mail: sgoodwin@cimh.org
www.cimh.org

Sandra Naylor-Goodwin, Executive Director
Bill Carter, Deputy Director
Ed Diksa, Director Training

Promoting excellence in mental health services through training, technical assistances, research and policy development.

1826 California Psychiatric Association (CPA)

1400 K Street
Suite 302
Sacramento, CA 95814
916-442-5196
Fax: 916-442-6515
E-mail: calpsych@worldnet.att.net
www.calpsych.org

Barbara Gard, Executive Director
Randall Hagar, Director Government Relations

Represents psychiatrists and the interests of their patients as those interests are affected by state government. CPA is area six of the American Psychiatric Association, and is composed of members of APA's five district branches in California.

1827 California Psychological Association

1022 G Street
Sacramento, CA 95814-0817
916-325-9786
Fax: 916-325-9790
E-mail: calpsychlink@calpsychlink.org
www.calpsychlink.org

Claudia Foutz, Executive Director
Patricia VanWoerkom, Deputy Director
Annie Norris, Member Services

Nonprofit professional association for licensed psychologists and others affiliated with the delivery of psychological services. Sponsors many legislative proposals dealing with access to mental health care services, managed care, hospital practice, prescription privilege authority and other issues. Regularly provides free public service through programs such as the well respected disaster response service.

Year Founded: 1948

1828 Calnet

1916 Creston Road
Paso Robles, CA 93446-4465
805-239-3332
Fax: 805-239-4545
E-mail: blandis@calnetcare.com
www.calnetcare.com

Brent Lamb, President
Barbara Orlando, Marketing/Communications

Nonprofit membership association of mental health facilities networking mental health and chemical dependency treatment providers throughout the state of California.

1829 Community Resource Council

1945 Palo Verde Avenue
Suite 202
Long Beach, CA 90815-3445

562-430-3099
Fax: 562-749-3355

Barry Leedy, Executive Director

Agency provides groups and classes to all ages. Sliding fee scale.

1830 Five Acres: Boys and Girls Aid Society of Los Angeles County

760 W Mountain View Street
Altadena, CA 91001-4925
626-798-6793
Fax: 626-797-7722
TTY: 626-204-1375
E-mail: for5acres@earthlink.com
www.5acres.org

Robert A Ketch, Executive Director
Sandi Zaslow, Assistant Executive Director
Cathy Clement, Director Development

Works to: prevent child abuse and neglect, care for, treat and educate emotionally disturbed, abused and neglected children and their families in residential and outreach programs, advance the welfare of children and families in research, advocacy and collaboration, strive for the highest standards of excellence by professionals and volunteers, and provide research and educational resources to families, the community and professionals for the prevention and treatment of child abuse and neglect.

Year Founded: 1888

1831 Gold Coast Alliance for the Mentally Ill

520 N Main Street, Room 203
PO Box 1088
Angels Camp, CA 95222
209-736-4264
Fax: 209-736-4264
E-mail: gcami@goldrush.com
www.nami.org

Laurie Flynn, Executive Director

Local chapter of the national self-help organization (NAMI) for all those affected by severe brain disorders. Mission is to bring consumers and families with similar experiences together to share information about services, care providers, and ways to cope with the challenges of schizophrenia, manic depression, and other serious mental illnesses.

1832 Health Services Agency: Mental Health

1080 Emeline Avenue
Santa Cruz, CA 95060-1966
831-454-4000
Fax: 831-454-4770
TDD: 831-454-2123
E-mail: info@santacruzhealth.org
www.santacruzhealth.org

Rama Khalsa PhD, Health Services Administrator
David McNutt MD, County Health Officer

Exists to protect and improve the health of the people in Santa Cruz County. Provides programs in environmental health, public health, medical care, substance abuse prevention and treatment, and mental health. Clients are entitled to information on the costs of care and their options for getting health insurance coverage through a variety of programs.

1833 Langley Porter Psychiatric Institute at UCSF Parnassus Campus

University of California
401 Parnassus Avenue
San Francisco, CA 94143-9911
415-476-7000
www.psych.ucsf.edu

Samuel Barnodes MD, Director

Conducts clinical studies of psychiatric disorders.

1834 Nation Alliance on Mental Illness: Californi a

101 Hurley Way
Suite 195
Sacramento, CA 95825-3218
916-567-0163
Fax: 916-567-1757
E-mail: membership@namicalifornia.org
www.namicalifornia.org

Ralph Nelson, President
Grace McAndrews, Executive Director

An organization of families and individuals whose lives have been affected by serious mental illness. We advocate for lives of quality and respect, without discrimination and stigma, for all our constituents. We provide leadership in advocacy, legislation, policy development, education and support throughout California.

1835 National Association of Mental Illness: California

1111 Howe Avenue
Suite 475
Sacramento, CA 95825-8541
916-567-0163
Fax: 916-567-1757
E-mail: grace.mcandrews@namicalifornia.org
www.namicalifornia.org

Grace McAndrews, Executive Director

Provides support, information and education for families of seriously mentally ill individuals. NAMI California's efforts focus on support, referral, advocacy, research and education. Available are the Journal Magazine, videos, educational classes, and support groups.

1836 National Health Foundation

Hospital Association of Southern California
6633 Telephone Road
Suite 210
Ventura, CA 93003-5569
805-650-1243
Fax: 805-650-6456
E-mail: mclark@hasc.org
www.hasc.org

Monty Clark, Regional Vice President

Charitable affiliate whose mission is to improve and enhance the health of the underserved by developing and supporting inovative programs that can become independently viable, systemic solutions to gaps in healthcare access and delivery and have potential to be replicated nationally.

1837 Northern California Psychiatric Society

1631 Ocean Avenue
San Francisco, CA 94112-1796
415-334-2418
Fax: 415-239-2533

E-mail: info@ncps.org
www.ncps.org

Marvin Firestone, President
Byron Whittlin, VP
Janice Tagart, Executive Director

A district branch of the American Psychiatric Association. A nonprofit organization that tries to improve the treatment, rehabilitation, and care of the mentally ill, the developmentally disabled, and the emotionally disturbed.

1838 Orange County Psychiatric Society
300 S Flower Street
Orange, CA 92868-3417
949-978-3016
Fax: 949-978-6039

Works to improve public awareness of mental illness and increase financial support.

1839 UCLA Department of Psychiatry & Biobehavioral Sciences
C8-871 Neuropsychiatry Institute
Box 951759
Los Angeles, CA 90095-1759
310-825-0511
www.psychiatry.ucla.edu

Programs for clinical research treatment for adults and children suffering from psychiatric illness.

1840 United Advocates for Children of California
1401 El Camino Avenue
Suite 340
Sacramento, CA 95815
916-643-1530
Fax: 916-643-1592
TTY: 916-643-1532
E-mail: information@uacc4families.org
www.uacc4families.org

A nonprofit organization that works on behalf of children and youth with serious emotional disturbances and their families.

Colorado

1841 Adolescent and Family Institute of Colorado
10001 W 32nd Avenue
Wheat Ridge, CO 80033-5601
303-238-1231
Fax: 303-238-0500
www.aficonline.com

Eric Meyer, MD, Executive Director

A licensed and accredited adolescent psychiatric and substance abuse 24 hour facility.

1842 CHINS UP Youth and Family Services
25 Farragut Avenue
Colorado Springs, CO 80909-5601
719-475-0562
Fax: 719-634-0562
E-mail: shinsupinc@aol.com
www.chinsup.org

Gerard H Heneman, Executive Director

Chins Up is a nonprofit multi-service agency serving children and families in the child welfare and juvenile justice systems. Chins Up strives to heal the broken lives of children and families.

1843 Colorado Health Networks-Value Options
7150 Campus Drive
Suite 300
Colorado Springs, CO 80919
800-804-5040
Fax: 719-538-1433
www.valueoptions.com

CHN is comprised of partnerships between ValueOptions and seven community mental health centers.

1844 Craig Counseling & Biofeedback Services
611 Breeze Street
Craig, CO 81625-2503
970-824-7475
Fax: 970-824-7475
E-mail: drhadlee@hotmail.com

Frank Hadley MA, DAPA, Director
Bert Dech MD, Medical Director

Full-service mental health and biofeedback center with two male and one female therapist and a board certified adult, adolescent and child psychiatrist.

1845 Federation of Families for Children's Mental Health
Colorado Chapter
901 W 14th Avenue
Suite 1
Denver, CO 80204
303-572-0302
Fax: 303-572-0304
www.coloradofederation.org

To promote mental health for all children, youth and families.

1846 Mental Health Association of Colorado
6795 E Tennessee Avenue
Suite 425
Denver, CO 80224-1614
303-377-3040
800-456-3249
Fax: 303-377-4920
www.mhacolorado.org

Jeanne Mueller Rohner, Executive Director
Michelle Hoffer, Director Development
Kristen Gravatt, Director Community Relations

A nonprofit association providing leadership to address the full range of mental health issues in Colorado. The association is a catalyst for improving diagnosis, care and treatment for people of all ages with mental health problems.

1847 National Alliance on Mental Illness: Colorado o
1100 Fillmore Street
Suite 201
Denver, CO 80206-3334
303-321-3104
888-566-6261
Fax: 303-321-0912
E-mail: lberumen@nami.org
www.namicolorado.org

Dennis Hofts, President
Lacey Berumen, Executive Director

A statewide nonprofit organization whose mission is to give strength and hope to individuals with mental illness and their families.

Connecticut

1848 Connecticut Families United for Children's Mental Health
PO Box 151
New London, CT 06320
860-439-0710
866-439-0788
Fax: 860-439-0711
E-mail: ctfamiliesunited@sbcglobal.net
www.ctfamiliesunited.homestead.com

A nonprofit organization providing statewide emotional support, family and systems advocacy and information and referrals.

1849 Connecticut National Association of Mentally Ill
30 Jordan Lane
Wethersfield, CT 06109
860-882-0236
800-215-3021
Fax: 860-586-7477
www.namict.org

Marilyn Ricci, President
Debra Anderson, Executive Director

Dedicated to improving the lives of people with serious mental illnesses and their families.

1850 Family & Community Alliance Project
110 Washington Street
Hartford, CT 06106-4405
860-566-6810
Fax: 860-246-8778

Support group for families who have children with a mental illness.

1851 Mental Health Association: Connecticut
1480 Bedford Street
Stamford, CT 06905-5309
203-323-0124
Fax: 203-323-0383
www.mhct.org

To advocate and work for everyone's mental health.

1852 National Alliance on Mental Illness: Connecticut
241 Main Street
5th Floor
Hartford, CT 06106
860-882-0236
800-215-3021
Fax: 860-882-0240
E-mail: namicted@namict.org
www.namict.org

Allan Atherton, President
Kate Mattias, Executive Director

NAMI-CT is the only Connecticut organization affiliated with NAMI, the nation's leading grassroots family and consumer organization dedicated to improving the lives of people with serious mental illnesses and their families.

1853 Thames Valley Programs
1 Ohio Avenue
Norwich, CT 06360-1536

866-445-2616
Fax: 860-886-6567

Marek Kukulka, LMFT, Program Manager

The Thames Valley Programs offer a continuum of care services with the goal of stabilization for children and adolescents who suffer from a broad range of behavioral and emotional problems. Programs utilize a positive, goal oriented approach to treatment that emphasizes patients' strength and success in the effort to maintain recovery and desired outcomes. Individualized, highly structured treatment programs offered at Thames Valley include: Partial Hospital Program, Intensive Outpatient Program, and Extended Day Program.

1854 Women's Support Services
158 Gay Street
PO Box 341
Sharon, CT 06069
860-364-1080
Fax: 860-364-5767
E-mail: wssdv@snet.net

Judy Sheridan, Director

Support and advocacy for those affected by domestic violence and abuse as well as women in transition in the towns of Cannan, Cornwall, Kent, North Cannan, Salisbury, and Sharon, CT and nearby NY and MA.

Delaware

1855 Delaware Alliance for the Mentally Ill
2400 W 4th Street
Wilmington, DE 19805
302-427-0787
888-427-2643
Fax: 302-427-2075
E-mail: namide@namide.org
www.namide.org

John P Smoots, President
Richard Taylor, Vice President
Rita A Marocco, Executive Director

A statewide organization of families, mental health consumers, friends and professionals dedicated to improving the quality of life for those affected by life changing brain diseases such as schizophrenia, bipolar disorder and major depression.

1856 Delaware Guidance Services for Children and Youth
1156 Walker Road
Dover, DE 19904-6540
302-678-9316
Fax: 302-678-9317
www.delawareguidance.com

To provide quality mental health services for children, youth and their families.

1857 Mental Health Association of Delaware
100 W 10th Street
Wilmington, DE 19810
302-654-6833
Fax: 302-654-6838
www.mhinde.org

Marjorie Mudrick

To deliver mental health education, advocacy and support, and to collaborate to provide mental health leadership in Delaware

1858 National Alliance on Mental Illness: Delawar e
2400 W 4th Street
Wilmington, DE 19805-3306
302-427-0787
888-427-2643
Fax: 302-427-2075
E-mail: namide@namide.org
www.namide.org

Edward McNally, President
Rita Marocco, Executive Director

A statewide organization of families, mental health consumers, friends, and professionals dedicated to improving the quality of life for those affected by life-changing brain diseases such as schizophrenia, bipolar disorder, and major depression.

1859 National Association of Social Workers: Delaware Chapter
3301 Green Street
Claymont, DE 19703-2052
302-792-0356
Fax: 302-792-0678
E-mail: naswae@aol.com
www.naswdc.org

Works to enhance the professional growth and development of its members, to create and maintain professional standards, and to advance sound social policies.

District of Columbia

1860 DC Alliance for the Mentally Ill
422 8th Street SE
2nd Floor
Washington, DC 20003-2832
202-546-0646
Fax: 202-546-6817
E-mail: namidc@junc.com
www.nami.org/about/namidc

Adria A Green, President
Nancy Head, Executive Director

Nation's leading self-help organization for all those affected by severe brain disorders. Mission is to bring consumers and families with similar experiences together to share information about services, care providers, and ways to cope with the challenges of schizophrenia, manic depression, and other serious mental illnesses.

1861 Department of Health and Human Services/OAS
200 Independence Avenue SW
Washington, DC 20201
202-619-0257
877-696-6775
www.dhhs.gov

The DHHS is the United States government's principal agency for protecting the health of all Americans and providing essential human services, especially for those who are least able to help themselves.

1862 Family Advocacy & Support Association
1289 Brentwood Road NE
Washington, DC 20002

202-526-5436
Fax: 202-265-7877
www.mentalhealth.org

Comprehensive community mental health services program for children and their families.

1863 National Alliance on Mental Illness: Distric t of Columbia
422 8th Street SE
2nd Floor
Washington, DC 20003-2832
202-546-0646
Fax: 202-546-6817
E-mail: namidc@juno.com
www.nami.org/about.namidc

Adrian Green, President
Steven Newman, Executive Director

Established in 1978 as D.C. Threshold, NAMI-DC has been serving the families of persons with mental illness in the nation's capital for over a quarter century.

Florida

1864 Department of Human Services For Youth & Families
2929 NW 17th Avenue
Miami, FL 33125-1118
305-633-6481
Fax: 305-633-5632

1865 Family Network on Disabilities of Florida
2735 Whitney Road
Clearwater, FL 33760-1610
727-523-1130
800-825-5736
Fax: 727-523-8687
E-mail: fnd@fndfl.org
www.fndfl.org

Jan LaBelle, Executive Director
Laura Mataluni, Executive Assistant

A statewide network of families and individuals who may be at risk, have disabilities, or have special needs.

1866 Florida Alcohol and Drug Abuse Association
1030 E Lafayette Street
Suite 100
Tallahassee, FL 32301-4559
850-878-2196
Fax: 850-878-6584
E-mail: fadaa@fadaa.org
www.fadaa.org

John Daigle, Executive Director

Statewide membership organization that represents more than ninety community-based substance abuse treatment and prevention agencies throughout Florida. FADAA has provided advocacy for substance abuse programs and the clients they serve for the past twenty seven years, as well as quality training programs for substance abuse professionals and up-to-date information on substance abuse to the general public.

1867 Florida Federation of Families for Children' s Mental Health
734 Shadeville Highway
Crawfordville, FL 32327

850-926-3514
877-926-3514
Fax: 413-480-2947
E-mail: ejwells@sprynet.com
www.fifionline.org

Conni Wells

A nationally affiliated parent-run organization focused on the needs of children and youth with emotional, behavioral or mental disorders and their families.

1868 Florida Health Care Association

307 W Park Avenue
Tallahassee, FL 32301
850-224-3907
Fax: 850-681-2075
www.fhca.org

Kelley Rice-Schild, President

FHCA is dedicated to providing the highest quality care for elderly, chronically ill, and disabled individuals.

1869 Florida Health Information Management Association

7510 Ehrlich Road
Tampa, FL 33625
813-792-9550
Fax: 813-792-9442
E-mail: fhima@infionline.net
www.fhima.org

Holly Woemmel, MA RHIA, President
Anita Doupnik, RHIA, Director
Carolyn Glavan, MS RHIA, Executive Director

Fosters professional development for its members, promotes privacy and quality of health information through education, communication and advocacy.

1870 Florida National Alliance for the Mentally Ill

911 E Park Avenue
Tallahassee, FL 32301-2646
850-671-4445
Fax: 850-671-5272
E-mail: lynne@namifl.org
www.namifl.org

Lynn Montgomery, Executive Director

Nation's leading self-help organization for all those affected by severe brain disorders. Mission is to bring consumers and families with similar experiences together to share information about services, care providers, and ways to cope with the challenges of schizophrenia, manic depression, and other serious mental illnesses.

1871 Mental Health Association of West Florida

840 W Lakeview Avenue
Pensacola, FL 32501
850-438-9879
Fax: 850-438-5901

Offers special information and referrals for families of mental health.

1872 National Alliance on Mental Illness: Florida

1615 Village Square Boulevard
Suite 6
Tallahassee, FL 32309
850-671-4445
877-626-4352
Fax: 850-671-5272

E-mail: namifl@namifl.org
www.namifl.org

Linda McKinnon, President

Contains thirty-four affiliates in communities throughout Florida that provide education, advocacy, and support groups for people with mental illness and their loved ones.

1873 National Association of Social Workers Florida Chapter

1931 Dellwood Drive
Tallahassee, FL 32303
850-224-2400
800-352-6279
Fax: 850-561-6279
E-mail: naswfl@naswfl.org
www.naswfl.org

Jim Akin, Executive Director

NASW is a membership organization for professional social workers in Florida. NASWFL provides: continuing education, information center, advocacy for employment and legislation.

Georgia

1874 Georgia Association of Homes and Services for Children

34 Peachtree Street NW
Suite 710
Atlanta, GA 30303-2301
404-572-6170
Fax: 404-572-6171
E-mail: norman@gahsc.org
www.gahsc.org

GAHSC is an association that is dedicated to supporting those who care for children who are at risk of abuse and neglect. Member agencies of GAHSC include family foster care, community group homes, education programs and others.

1875 Georgia National Alliance for the Mentally Ill

3050 Presidential Drive
Suite 202
Atlanta, GA 30340-3916
770-234-0855
800-728-1052
Fax: 770-234-0237
E-mail: andymont@nami.org
www.nami.org or www.namigeorgia.org

Nora Haynes, President
Jean Dervan, Office Manager

NAMI is nonprofit, grassroots, self-help, support and advocacy organization of consumers, families and friends of people with severe mental illnesses such as schizophrenia, bipolar disorder, major despressive disorder, and other severe and persistent mental illnesses that affect the brain.

1876 Georgia Parent Support Network

1381 Metropolitan Parkway
Atlanta, GA 30310
404-758-4500
800-832-8645
Fax: 404-758-6833
E-mail: slsmith2@ix.netcom.com
www.gspn.org

Cynthia Wainscott, Chairperson
Kathy Dennis, Vice President
Linda Seay, Secretary/Treasurer

The Georgia Parent Support Network is dedicated to providing support, education and advocacy for children and youth with mental illness, emotional disturbances and behavioral difference and their families.

1877 Grady Health Systems: Central Fulton CMHC
80 Jesse Hill Jr Drive S.E.
Atlanta, GA 30303-3050
404-616-4307
Fax: 404-616-5998

Robert L Brown, FAIA Chairman
Clayton Sheptherd, Treasurer

Grady Health System improves the health of the community by providing quality, comprehensive health care in a compassionate, culturally competent, ethical and fiscally responsible manner. Grady maintains its commitment to the underserved of Fulton and DeKalb counties, while also providing care for residents of metro Atlanta and Georgia. Grady leads through its clinical exellence, innovative research and progressive medical education and training.

1878 National Alliance on Mental Illness: Georgia
3050 Presidential Drive
Suite 202
Atlanta, GA 30340-3916
770-234-0855
800-728-1052
Fax: 770-234-0237
E-mail: nami-ga@nami.org
www.namiga.org

Nora Hayes, President

The purpose of NAMI Georgia, Inc. is to relieve the suffering and improve the quality of life for mentally ill Georgians and their families.

Hawaii

1879 Hawaii Alliance for the Mentally Ill
770 Kapiolani Blvd
Suite 613
Honolulu, HI 96813-5240
808-591-1297
Fax: 808-591-2058
E-mail: MPoir14016@aol.com
www.nami.org

Laurie Flynn, Executive Director

Nation's leading self-help organization for all those affected by severe brain disorders. Mission is to bring consumers and families with similar experiences together to share information about services, care providers, and ways to cope with the challenges of schizophrenia, manic depression, and other serious mental illnesses.

1880 Hawaii Families As Allies
PO Box 700310
Kapolei, HI 96709-0310
808-487-8785
866-361-8825
Fax: 808-487-0514
www.mentalhealth.org

Sharon Nobriga, Co Executive Director

Parent Advocacy group for those with children who have mental disorders.

1881 NAMI Hawaii
85-175 Farrington Highway
Apt. A-418
Waianae, HI 96792-2171
808-524-5900
Fax: 808-585-9459
E-mail: nami-hi@hawaii.rr.com
www.nami.org

Mike Durant, President

NAMI is a support and advocacy organization. They sponsor local support groups and offer education and information about community services for people with mental illness and their families.

1882 National Alliance on Mental Illness: Hawaii
770 Kapiolani Boulevard
Suite 613
Honolulu, HI 96813-5212
808-591-1297
Fax: 808-591-2058
E-mail: namihawaii@hawaiiantel.net
www.namihawaii.org

Mike Durant, President
Marion Poirier, Executive Director

Idaho

1883 Idaho Alliance for the Mentally Ill
PO Box 68
Albion, ID 83311
208-673-6672
800-572-9940
Fax: 208-673-6685
www.nami.org

Laurie Flynn, Executive Director

NAMI Idaho is a non-profit, tax exempt family organization for people with brain disorders.

1884 National Alliance on Mental Illness: Idaho
PO Box 68
Albion, ID 83311-0068
208-673-6672
800-572-9940
Fax: 208-673-6685
E-mail: namiid@atcnet.net
www.nami.org/sites/namiidaho

Harry Holmberg, President
Lee Woodland, Executive Director

NAMI Idaho is a non-profit, tax-exempt family organization for people with brain disorders.

Illinois

1885 Allendale Association
PO Box 1088
Lake Villa, IL 60046-1088
847-356-2351
888-255-3631
Fax: 847-356-0289
www.allendale4kids.org

Mary Shahbazian, President
Ronald Howard, VP Reisdential Programs
Dr. Pat Taglione, VP Clinical/Community Services

The Allendale Association is a private, non-profit organization dedicated to the excellence and innovation in the care, education, treatment and advocacy for troubled children, youth and their families.

1886 Baby Fold

108 E Wilow Street
PO Box 327
Normal, IL 61761-0327
309-452-1170
Fax: 309-452-0115
E-mail: info@thebabyfold.org

The Baby Fold is a multi-service agency that provides Residential, Special Education, Child Welfare, and Family Support Services to children and families in central Illinois.

1887 Chaddock

205 S 24th Street
Quincy, IL 62301-4491
217-222-0034
888-242-3625
Fax: 217-222-3865
E-mail: dread@chaddock.org
www.chaddock.org

Debbie Reed, President

Chaddock's mission is to empower children and families to become capable, contributing members of their communities by providing quality programs and services in caring settings.

1888 Chicago Child Care Society

5467 S University Avenue
Chicago, IL 60615-5193
773-643-0452
Fax: 773-643-0620

Mrs. Hugo Sonnenschein, President
Robert L Rinder, Vice President
Mary O'Brian Pearlman, Vice President
Judith Lavender, Secretary

Chicago Child Care Society exists to protect vulnerable children and strengthen their families. We strive to be among the premier providers of high quality and effective child welfare services. We believe the quality of life for future generations depends upon the quality of care provided for children today. We believe children should be provided with services and opportunities that will enable them to reach their optimism physical, mental and social development. We believe all the children are entitled to the protection and nurturing care of adults, preferably within their birth families. However, if family can't fulfill these basic functions, we believe society, by either public or private means should provide the best alternative care.

1889 Children's Home Association of Illinois

2130 N Knoxville Avenue
Peoria, IL 61603-2460
309-685-1047
Fax: 309-687-7299
www.chail.org

James G , Sherman

Nonprofit, non-sectarian multiple program and social service organization. Giving children a childhood and future by protecting them, teaching them, healing them and by building strong communities and loving families.

1890 Coalition of Illinois Counselors Organization

PO Box 1086
Northbrook, IL 60065
847-205-4432
Fax: 847-205-4423

We collaberate with other mental health disciplines; human services organizations, industries and business as well as representatives of the government, to promote emotional health care interests. We are committed to upholding high standards for clients in Illinois.

1891 Family Service Association of Greater Elgin Area

22 S Spring Street
Elgin, IL 60120-6412
847-695-3680
Fax: 847-695-4552
E-mail: JZahm@fsaelgin.org
www.fsaelgin.org

Lisa A La Forge, Executive Director
Dr. Sandra Angelo, Dir. Consumer Credit Counseling
Jon A Zahm, Developmental/Community Rel.

A non-profit agancy, Family Service Association has served the Greater Elgin Area since 1931. Supported both publicly and privately, most of the funding is received from such local sources as United Ways, corporate and individual contributions and client fees.

1892 Human Resources Development Institute

222 S Jefferson Street
Chicago, IL 60661
312-441-9009
Fax: 312-441-9019
www.hrdi.org

Martina Jones, Executive Director
Kimberly Sutton PhD, Sr VP Clinical/Program Support

Community based behavioral health and human services organization. This nonprofit agency on the south side of Chicago, is concerned with mental health and substance abuse solutuions. Offering more than 40 programs at 20 sites.

Year Founded: 1974

1893 Illinois Alcoholism and Drug Dependency Association

937 S 2nd Street
Springfield, IL 62704-2701
217-528-7335
Fax: 217-528-7340
www.iadda.org

Angela M Bowman, CEO
Sara Moscato, Associate Director
Pel Thomas, Business Manage
May Jo Pevey, Prevention Coordinator

IADDA is a statewide organization established in 1967 respresenting more than 100 prevention and treatment agencies, as well as individuals who are interested in the substance abuse field. The Association advocates for sound public policy that will create healthier families and safer communites. IADDA members educate government officials in Springfield and Washington, and work to increase the public understanding of substance abuse and addiction.

1894 Illinois Alliance for the Mentally Ill
730 E Vine Street
Suite 209
Springfield, IL 62703-2553
217-522-1403
800-346-4572
Fax: 217-522-3598
E-mail: namiill@sbcglobal.net
www.il.namil.org

Tom Lambert, President

We are committed to a future where recovery is the expected outcome and when mental illness can be prevented or cured. We envision a nation where everyone with a mental illness will have access to early detection and the effective treatment and support essential to live, work, learn and participate fully in their community.

1895 Illinois Federation of Families for Children's Mental Health
PO Box 1357
Vienna, IL 62995
618-658-2059
800-871-8400
Fax: 618-658-2720
E-mail: iffcmh@msn.com
www.iffcmh.ner/contact.htm

Dian Ledbetter, Executive Director
Beth Berndt, Family Resource Director
Lejeune Burdine, Vienna Office Manager
Beverly Hartig, Austim Project Management

Goal is to create a statewide network for individuals and groups throughout Illinois so: Families are not alone in caring for their children with difficult behavior; Parents are better informed on social services, legal, educational and medica resources; research prevention, and early intervenion.

1896 Larkin Center
1212 Larkin Avenue
Elgin, IL 60123-6098
847-695-5656
Fax: 847-695-0897
www.larkincenter.org

Dennis L Graf MS, Executive Director
Richard Peterson MSW, Executive Director
Martine Lyle, Admissions And QA Director
Michelle Potter MS LCPC, Clinical Director

Our mission is achieved through the efforts of Larkins Center's team of skilled professionals in creative cooperation with the community.

1897 Little City Foundation (LCF)
1760 W Algonquin Road
Palatine, IL 60067-4799
847-358-5510
Fax: 847-358-3291
E-mail: people@littlecity.org
www.LittleCity.org

Alex Alexandrou, Pesident
Alex Gianaras, Vice President
Fred G Lebed, Secretary
Quentin Johnson, Treasurer

The mission of Little City Foundation is to provide state of the art services to help children and adults with mental retardation or other developmental emotional and behavioral challenges to lead meaningful, productive, and dignified lives.

1898 Metropolitan Family Services
14 E Jackson Boulevard
Chicago, IL 60604-2259
312-986-4340
Fax: 312-986-4187
E-mail: contactus@metrofamily.org
www.metrofamily.org

Richard L Jones PhD, President and CEO
Nancy Kim Philips, Chief Operating Officer
Denis Hurley, Chife Financial Offcer
Evelyn Engler, Vice President, Human ResourcesS

Our mission is to help Chicago - area families become strong, stable and self-sufficient.

1899 National Alliance on Mental Illness: Illinoi s
218 W Lawrence Avenue
Springfield, IL 32704-2612
217-522-1403
800-346-4572
Fax: 217-522-3598
E-mail: namiil@sbcglobal.net
www.il.nami.org

Carolyn Jakopin, President
Lora Thomas, Executive Director

A state-wide organization comprised of local Illinois Affiliates dedicated to the task of eradicating mental illness and improving the lives of persons with mental illness and their families.

Indiana

1900 Indiana Alliance for the Mentally Ill
PO Box 22697
Indianapolis, IN 46222-0697
317-925-9399
800-677-6442
Fax: 317-925-9398
www.nami.org

Laurie Flynn, Executive Director

NAMI Indiana is dedicated to improving the quality of life for those persons who are affected by mental illness.

1901 Indiana Resource Center for Autism (IRCA)
Indiana University
2853 E Tenth Street
Bloomington, IN 47408-2696
812-855-6508
800-280-7010
Fax: 812-855-9630
TTY: 812-855-9396
E-mail: uap@indiana.edu
www.iidc.indiana.edu/irca

Cathy Pratt PhD, Director
Scott Bellini PhD, Assistant Director

Conducts outreach training and consultations, engage in research, develop and disseminate information on behalf of individuals across the autism spectrum, Aspergers syndrome, and other pervasive developmental disorders. Provides communities, organizations, agencies and families with the knowledge and skills to support children and adults in typical early intervention, school, community work and home.

1902 Indiana University Psychiatric Management
PO Box 2087
Indianapolis, IN 46224-3784
317-278-9100
800-230-4876
Fax: 317-278-9142
E-mail: iupm@iupui.edu

IUPM is a managed mental health program development
within Indiana University which links quality mental health
and substance abuse providers in the community with a superior academic psychiatric program.

**1903 Mental Health Association in Marion County
Consumer Services**
2506 Willowbrook Parkway
Suite 100
Indianapolis, IN 46205-1542
317-251-0005
Fax: 317-254-2800
www.mcmha.org

Shary Johnson, President
Dan Collins, Vice President
Mike Simmons, Secretary
David Vonnegut-Gabovitch, Treasurer

The mission of the Association is to provide education, advocacy and service through programs designed to promote
health; positively affect public attiudes and perceptions of
mental illness through support and knowledge; and improve
care and treatment of persons with mental ilness.

1904 National Alliance on Mental Illness: Indiana
PO Box 22697
Indianapolis, IN 46222-0697
317-925-9399
Fax: 317-925-9398
E-mail: nami-in@nami.org
www.namiindiana.org

Teresa Hatten, President
Pamela McConey, Executive Director

Dedicated to improving the quality of life for those persons
who are affected by mental illness.

Iowa

1905 Iowa Alliance for the Mentally Ill
5911 Meredith Drive
Suite E
Des Moines, IA 50322-1903
515-254-0417
800-417-0417
Fax: 515-254-1103
E-mail: namiiowa@mchsi.com
www.nami.org

Bruce Sicleni, President
Margaret Stout, Executive Director

NAMI is dedicated to the education of mental illnesses and
to the improvement of the quality of life of all whose lives
are affected by these diseases.

**1906 Iowa Federation of Families for Children's
Mental Health**
112 S Williams
PO Box 362
Anamosa, IA 52205-7321
319-462-2187
888-400-6302

Fax: 319-462-6789
E-mail: help@iffcmh.org
www.ffcmh.org/local.htm

Lori Reynolds

Our mission is to link families to community, county and
state partners for needed support and services; and to promote system change that will enable families to live in a
safe, stable and respectful environment.

1907 National Alliance on Mental Illness: Iowa
5911 Meredith Drive
Suite E
Des Moines, IA 50322-1903
515-254-0417
800-417-0417
Fax: 515-254-1103
E-mail: namiiowa@mchsi.com
www.namiiowa.com

Bruce Sieleni, President
Margaret Stout, Executive Director

Mission is to raise public awareness and concern about
mental illness, to foster research, to improve treatment and
to upgrade the system of care for the people of Iowa.

**1908 University of Iowa, Mental Health: Clinical
Research Center**
University of Iowa Hospitals & Clinics
200 Hawkins Drive
Iowa City, IA 52242-1009
319-356-4720
877-575-2864
Fax: 319-356-2587

Dr. Nancy C Andreassen, Director

We seek to improve the precision with which specific disease categories are defined and to increase our understanding of their underlying mechanisms and causes. Our
primary emphasis is on schizophrenia spectrum disorders,
including schizophrenia, schizoaffective disorder,
schizophreniform disorder and schizotypal personality.

Kansas

1909 Kansas Schizophrenia Anonymous
112 SW 6th
PO Box 675
Topeka, KS 66601-0675
785-233-0755
800-539-2660
Fax: 785-233-4804
E-mail: namikansas@nami.org
www.namikansas.org

Laurie Flynn, Executive Director

Self-help organization for all those coping with the challenges of schizophrenia.

**1910 Keys for Networking: Kansas Parent Informati
on & Resource Center**
2311 West 33rd Street
Topeka, KS 66611
785-233-8732
800-499-8732
Fax: 785-235-6659
E-mail: jadams@keys.org
www.keys.org

A non-profit organization providing information, support, and training to families in Kansas whose children who have educational, emotional, and/or behavioral problems.

1911 National Alliance on Mental Illness: Kansas
PO Box 675
Topeka, KS 66601-0675
785-233-0755
800-539-2660
Fax: 785-233-4804
E-mail: namikansas@nami.org
www.namikansas.org

Rick e Cagan, Executive Director

Nation's leading self-help membership organization for all those affected by severe brain disorders. Mission is to provide peer support, education, advocacy and research on behalf of persons affected by serious mental illness and their family members.

Kentucky

1912 Children's Alliance
420 Capitol Avenue
Frankfort, KY 40601
502-875-3399
Fax: 502-223-4200
E-mail: melissa.lawson@childrensallianceky.org
www.childrensallianceky.org

Bart Baldwin, President
Melissa Lawson, Member Services
Nannette Lenington, Business Manager
David Graves, Chairman

Our mission is to shape public policy, inform constituencies and provide leadership in advocacy for Kentucky's children and families.

1913 FACES of the Blue Grass
570 E Main Street
Lexington, KY 40508-2342
606-254-3106
www.ffcmh.org/local.htm

Jim Powell

Support group for families who have children diagnosed with mental illness.

1914 KY-SPIN
10301-B Deering Road
Louisville, KY 40272
502-937-6894
800-525-7746
Fax: 502-937-6464
E-mail: spininc@aol.com
www.kyspin.com

Non-profit organization dedicated to promoting programs which will enable persons with disabilities and their families to enhance their quality of life.

1915 Kentucky Alliance for the Mentally Ill
10510 LeGrange Road
Building 103
Louisville, KY 40223-1228
502-245-5284
800-257-5081
Fax: 502-245-6390
E-mail: namiky@mindspring.com
www.nami.org

Harry Mills, Executive Director
Lois Anderson, President

Nation's leading self-help organization for all those affected by severe brain disorders. Mission is to bring consumers and families with similar experiences together to share information about services, care providers, and ways to cope with the challenges of schizophrenia, manic depression, and other serious mental illnesses.

1916 Kentucky IMPACT
275 E Main Street
Frankfort, KY 40621-0001
502-564-7610
Fax: 502-564-9010
E-mail: elizabeth.cloyd@uky.edu
www.ihdi.uky.edu/kydrm/contact_us.htm

Elizabeth Cloyd, Director

Kentucky IMPACT is a statewide program which coordinates services for children with severe emotional disabilities and their families.

1917 Kentucky Psychiatric Association
PO Box 198
Frankfort, KY 40602-0198
502-695-4843
877-597-7924
Fax: 502-695-4441
E-mail: waltonkpa@aol.com
www.kyppsych.org

Tom Brown, President
Theresa Walton, Executive Director

A non-profit association of medical doctors who have completed a psychiatry residency.

1918 National Alliance on Mental Illness: Kentuck y
10510 Lagrange Road
Building 103
Louisville, KY 40223-1277
502-245-5284
800-257-5081
Fax: 502-245-6390
E-mail: ccarrithers@bellsouth.net
www.ky.nami.org

Phillip Gunning, President
Carol Carrithers, Executive Director

NAMI Kentucky is a self-help organization that is part of a nation-wide network devoted to improving the lives of the seriously mentally ill and decreasing the prevailing stigma associated with mental illness.

1919 National Association of Social Workers: Kentucky Chapter
304 West Liberty Street
Suite 201
Louisville, KY 40202
800-526-8098
Fax: 502-589-3602
E-mail: naswky@aol.com
www.naswky.org

Professional membership organization, for state social workers.

1920 Project Vision
2210 Goldsmith Lane
Suite 118
Louisville, KY 40218-1038
502-456-0923
800-525-7746
Fax: 502-456-0893
www.ffcmh.org/local.htm

Laurie Cottrell

1921 SPOKES Federation of Families for Children's Mental Health
275 E Main Street
Frankfort, KY 40621-0001
502-564-7610
Fax: 502-564-9010
E-mail: danderson@mhrdmc.chr.state.ky.us
www.ffcmh.org/local.htm

Debbie Anderson

Non-profit organization focused on the need of children and youth with emotional, behavioral or mental disorders and their families.

1922 ValueOptions
4010 Dupont Circle
Suite 283
Louisville, KY 40207-4847
502-899-3999
Fax: 502-894-4445
www.valueoptions.com/

Founded in 1983, ValueOptions develops and implements managed behavioral health and Employee Assistance Program services for Fortune 500 companies, national and regional health plans, as well as federal, state and local governments.

Louisiana

1923 Louisiana Alliance for the Mentally Ill
PO Box 64585
Baton Rouge, LA 70896
504-343-6928
www.la.nami.org

Diane Pitts, President

Nation's leading self-help organization for all those affected by severe brain disorders. Mission is to bring consumers and families with similar experiences together to share information about services, care providers, and ways to cope with the challenges of schizophrenia, manic depression, and other serious mental illnesses.

1924 Louisiana Federation of Families for Children's Mental Health
200 Lafayette Street
Suite 420
Baton Rouge, LA 70801
225-346-4020
Fax: 225-346-0770
www.laffcmh.com

The purpose of the FFCMH is to serve the needs of children with serious emotional, behavioral and mental disorders and their families.

1925 National Alliance on Mental Illness: Louisia na
5700 Florida Boulevard
Suite 320
Baton Rouge, LA 70806
225-926-8770
866-851-6264
Fax: 225-926-8773
E-mail: namilouisiana@bellsouth.net
www.namilouisiana.org

Catherine Tridico, President
Jennifer Jantz, Executive Director

Maine

1926 Maine Alliance for the Mentally Ill
1 Bangor Street
Augusta, ME 04330
207-622-5767
800-464-5767
Fax: 207-621-8430
E-mail: NAMI-ME@nami.org
www.me.nami.org

David Sturtevant, Executive Director

Nation's leading self-help organization for all those affected by severe brain disorders. Mission is to bring consumers and families with similar experiences together to share information about services, care providers, and ways to cope with the challenges of schizophrenia, manic depression, and other serious mental illnesses.

1927 Maine Psychiatric Association
PO Box 190
Manchester, ME 04351-0190
207-622-7743
Fax: 207-622-3332
E-mail: weldridge@mainemed.com

Warene Chase Eldridge, Executive Secretary

To provide treatment for all persons with mental disorder, including mental retardation and substance-related disorders.

1928 National Alliance on Mental Illness: Maine
1 Bangor Street
Augusta, ME 04330-4701
207-622-5767
800-464-5767
Fax: 207-621-8430
E-mail: info@namimaine.org
www.namimaine.org

Julie O'Brien, President
Carol Carothers, Executive Director

Dedicated to improving the lives of all people affected by mental illness NAMI Maine provides services across the entire state of Maine

1929 United Families for Children's Mental Health
PO Box 2107
Augusta, ME 04338-2107
207-622-3309
Fax: 207-622-1661
www.ffcmh.org/local.htm

Pat Hunt

Non-profit organization providing statewide individual emotional suuport, information and referrals, help in locating services, news regarding children's mental health issues and current events, support groups, newsletter, family and professional collaborations, family and systems advocacy, family member participation in policy and system development.

Maryland

1930 Community Behavioral Health Association of Maryland: CBH
18 Egges Lane
Cantonsville, MD 21228-4511
410-788-1865
Fax: 410-788-1768
E-mail: mdcbh@aol.com
www.cbh.bluestep.net

Carol Veater, Administration

Professional association for Maryland's network of community behavioral health programs operating in the public and private sectors.

1931 Families Involved Together
2219 Maryland Avenue
Baltimore, MD 21218
410-235-5222
Fax: 410-235-4222
E-mail: diane@familiesinvolved.org

Diane Sakwa

Parents of children with special needs.

1932 Health Resources and Services Administration
Parklawn Building
5600 Fishers Lane
Rockville, MD 20857
301-594-4060
Fax: 301-594-4984
www.hrsa.gov

Elizabeth Duke PhD, Administrator
Stephen Smith, Senior Advisor

The Health Resources and Services Administration's mission is to improve and expand access to quality health care for all.

1933 Maryland Alliance for the Mentally Ill
711 W 40th Street
Suite 451
Baltimore, MD 21211
410-467-7100
800-467-0075
Fax: 410-467-7195
E-mail: amimd@aol.com
www.nami.org

Barbara Bellack, Executive Director

Nation's leading self-help organization for all those affected by severe brain disorders. Mission is to bring consumers and families with similar experiences together to share information about services, care providers, and ways to cope with the challenges of schizophrenia, manic depression, and other serious mental illnesses.

1934 Maryland Psychiatric Research Center
PO Box 21247
Baltimore, MD 21228-0747
410-402-7666
Fax: 410-402-7198
www.mprc.umaryland.edu

Dr. William Carpenter Jr, Director

To study the manifestations, causes, and innovative treatment of zchizophrenia.

1935 Mental Health Association of Maryland
711 W 40th Street
Suite 460
Baltimore, MD 21211-2110
410-235-1178
800-572-6426
Fax: 410-235-1180
E-mail: info@mhamd.org
www.mhamd.org

Christine McKee, Public Education Director
Diane Cabot, Regional Director
Linda Raines, Executive Director

The Mental Health Association of Maryland is dedicated to promoting mental health, preventing mental disorders and achieving victory over mental illness through advocacy, education, research and service.

1936 National Alliance on Mental Illness: Marylan d
804 Landmark Drive
Suite 122
Glen Burnie, MD 21061-4486
410-863-0470
800-467-0075
Fax: 410-863-0474
E-mail: namimd@nami.org
www.md.nami.org

Peggy Anderson, President
Lynn Albizo, Executive Director

Dedicated to the persons, families, and communities affected by mental illness.

1937 National Association of Social Workers: Maryland Chapter
5740 Executive Drive
Suite 208
Baltimore, MD 21228-1759
410-788-1066
800-867-6776
Fax: 410-747-0635
E-mail: nasw.md@verizon.net
www.nasw-md.org

The mission of the NASW-MD chapter is to support, promote and advocate for the social work profession and its clients, promote just and equitable social policies and for the health and welfare of the people of Maryland.

1938 National Federation of Families for Children 's Mental Health
9605 Medical Center Drive
Suite 280
Rockville, MD 20850
240-403-1901
Fax: 240-403-1909
E-mail: ffcmh@ffcmh.org
www.ffcmh.org/local.htm

Robert Dennis

Non-profit organization focused on the needs of children and youth, with emotional, behavioral or mental disorders and their families.

1939 Sheppard Pratt Health System
6501 N Charles Street
Baltimore, MD 21285
410-938-3000
888-938-4207
Fax: 410-938-3159
E-mail: info@sheppardpratt.org
www.sheppardpratt.org

Dr Steven S Sharfstein, President/CEO
Dr Robert Roca, VP & Medical Director

Private, nonprofit behavioral health system with inpatients, partial outpatient, residential, crisis, contract management.

1940 Survey & Analysis Branch
5600 Fishers Lane
Rockwall II Suite 15C
Rockville, MD 20857-0002
301-443-3343
Fax: 301-443-7926
www.samhsa.gov

Dr. Ronald Manderscheid, Branch Chief

Federally funded agency studying mental health issues.

Massachusetts

1941 Bridgewell
471 Broadway
Lynn, MA 01904
781-593-1088
Fax: 781-593-5731
E-mail: info@bridgewell.org
www.bridgewell.org

Robert Stearns, CEO

Private, non-profit corporation that provides residential, clinical, recreation, day and employment, work training, affordable housing, and multi-cultural and community education services for people with disabilities, their families, and advocates in Northeastern Massachusetts.

1942 Concord Family and Youth Services A Division of Justice Resource Institute
380 Massachusetts Avenue
Acton, MA 07120-3745
978-263-3006
Fax: 978-263-3088
www.jri.org

Gregory Canfield, Vice President

Concord Family and Youth Services, a division of the non-profit Justice Resource Institute, Inc., has been providing help to adolescents, young adults and families since 1814. Programs include a group home for boys, a therapeutic high school in Acton, two residential schools for girls, as well as, parenting and adoption support services through First Connections.

1943 Depressive and Manic-Depressive Association of Boston
115 Mill Street
PO Box 102
Belmont, MA 02478-0001
617-855-2795
Fax: 617-855-3666
E-mail: info@mddaboston.org
www.mddaboston.org/

MDDA-BOSTON is resource for people with affective disorders and their families and friends.

1944 Jewish Family and Children's Services
31 New Chardon Street
Boston, MA 02114-4701
617-227-6641
Fax: 617-227-3220

Jewish Family and Children's Services is here to help individuals and families of all ages through human service and health care programs that reflect Jewish values of social responsibility and concern for all members of the community.

1945 Massachusetts Alliance for the Mentally Ill
400 W Cummings Park
Suite 6650
Woburn, MA 01801-6528
781-938-4048
800-370-9085
Fax: 781-938-4069
E-mail: namimass@aol.com
www.namimass.org

Toby Fisher, Executive Director
Philip Hadley, President

Nation's leading self-help organization for all those affected by severe brain disorders. Mission is to bring consumers and families with similar experiences together to share information about services, care providers, and ways to cope with the challenges of schizophrenia, manic depression, and other serious mental illnesses.

1946 Massachusetts Behavioral Health Partnership
120 Front Street
Suite 315
Worcester, MA 01608
508-890-6400
Fax: 508-890-6410

The Massachusetts Behavioral Health Partnership manages the mental health and substance abuse services for MassHealth Members who select the Division's Primary Care Clinician Plan.

1947 Mental Health and Substance Abuse Corporations of Massachusetts
251 W Central Street
Natick, MA 01760
508-647-8385
Fax: 508-647-8311

To promote community-based mental health and substance abuse services as the most appropriate, clinically effective, and cost-sensitive method for providing care to individuals in need.

1948 National Alliance on Mental Illness: Massach usetts
400 West Cummings Park
Suite 6650
Woburn, MA 01801-6528
781-938-4048
800-370-9085
Fax: 781-938-4069
E-mail: namimass@aol.com
www.namimass.org

Phil Hadley, President
Toby Fisher, Executive Director

A nonprofit grassroots education and advocacy group dedicated to improving the quality of life for people affected by mental illness.

1949 Parent Professional Advocacy League
59 Temple Place
Suite 664
Boston, MA 02111
617-542-7860
800-537-0446
Fax: 617-542-7832
E-mail: info@ppal.net
www.http://ppal.net

Provides support, education, and advocacy around issues related to children's mental health

Michigan

1950 Ann Arbor Consultation Services Performance & Health Solutions
5331 Plymouth Road
Ann Arbor, MI 48105-9520
313-996-9111
Fax: 313-996-1950

Outpatient services for mental health and chemical dependency issues.

1951 Borgess Behavioral Medicine Services
1521 Gull Road
Kalamazoo, MI 49048
269-226-7000
Fax: 269-324-8665
www.borgess.com

Alan O Kogan MD, Medical Director
Denise Crawford MSW, Referal Development Division

Offers patients and families a wide array of services to address their mental health concerns.

1952 Boysville of Michigan
8759 Clinton Macon Road
Clinton, MI 49236-9572
517-423-7451
Fax: 517-423-5442
E-mail: djablons@boysville.org
www.boysville.org

David Jablonski, Director of Communications
Francis Boylan, President/CEO

Boysville of Michigan works with one thousand plus boys and girls and their families on a daily basis in both residential and community based programs throughout Michigan and northwestern Ohio.

1953 Justice in Mental Health Organizations
421 Seymour Avenue
Lansing, MI 48933-1116
517-371-2794
800-831-8035
Fax: 517-371-5770
E-mail: jimhojim@aol.com

Lisa Howell, Executive Director

The JMHO is a non-profit 501 (c) (3) organization in Lansing, Michigan. It is an advocacy group, as well as a mutual self-help organization that offers a network of support to thousands of individuals living in the community.

1954 Lapeer County Community Mental Health Center
1570 Suncrest Drive
Lapeer, MI 48446-1154
810-667-0500
Fax: 810-664-8728
E-mail: iccmhc@tir.com
www.countylapeer.org

Michael K Vizena, Executive Director
Lauren J Emmons, Associate Director

Comprehensive community mental health services to children and adults of all ages. Services are limited to Lapeer County residents. Most insurance plans are honored. A sliding fee schedule is applied for those without insurance benefits. The center is licensed by the state of Michigan and is fully accredited by JCAHO.

1955 Macomb County Community Mental Health
10 N Main
5th Floor
Mt Clemens, MI 48043
586-948-0222
Fax: 586-469-7674

Provides a wide variety of mental health treatment and support services to adults and children with mental illness, developmental disabilities, and substance abuse treatment needs.

1956 Manic Depressive and Depressive Association of Metropolitan Detroit
PO Box 32531
Detroit, MI 48232-0531
734-284-5563
www.mdda-metro-detroit.org

Educates patients, families, and professionals, and the public concerning the nature of depressive and manic-depressive illness as treatable medical diseases; to foster self-help for patients and families; to eliminate discrimination and stigma; to improve access to care; and to advocate for research toward the elimination of these illnesses.

1957 Metropolitan Area Chapter of Federation of Families for Children's Mental Health
5504 Kreger
Sterling Heights, MI 48310
810-978-1221
www.ffcmh.org/local.htm

Pat Boyer

Dedicated to children and adolescents with mental health needs and their families.

1958 Michigan Alliance for the Mentally Ill
921 N Washington Avenue
Lansing, MI 48906
517-485-4049
800-331-4264
Fax: 517-485-2333
E-mail: namimichigan@acd.net
www.mi.nami.org

Hubert Huebl, President

Nation's leading self-help organization for all those affected by severe brain disorders. Mission is to bring consumers and families with similar experiences together to share information about services, care providers, and ways to cope with the challenges of schizophrenia, manic depression, and other serious mental illnesses.

1959 Michigan Association for Children with Emotional Disorders: MACED
230233 Southfield Road
Suite 219
Southfield, MI 48076-0000
248-433-2200
Fax: 248-433-2299
E-mail: info@michkids.org
www.michkids.org

Samuel L Davis, Clinical Director

Ensures that children with serious emotional disorders receive appropriate mental health and educational services so that they reach their full potential. To provide support to families and to encourage community understanding of the need for specialized programs for their children.

1960 Michigan Association for Children's Mental Health
941 Abbott Road
Suite P
East Lansing, MI 48823-3104
517-336-7222
800-782-0883
Fax: 517-336-8884
E-mail: acmhlori@acd.net
www.ffcmh.org

Robin Laurain, Family Advocacy Consultant

Provides advocacy, resources and educational training to parents of emotionally impaired children.

1961 National Alliance on Mental Illness: Michiga n
921 N Washington Avenue
Lansing, MI 48906-5137
517-485-4049
800-331-4264
Fax: 517-485-2333
E-mail: namimichigan@acd.net
www.mi.nami.org

Hubert Huebl, President

To assist affiliates, provide support, promote education, pursue advocacy and encourage research on mental illness.

1962 Northpointe Behavioral Healthcare Systems
715 Pyle Drive
Kingsford, MI 49802-4456
906-774-9522
Fax: 906-774-1570
E-mail: info@nbhs.org
www.nbhs.org

Michigan Community Mental Health agency serving Dickinson, Menominee and Iron counties. Provides a full spectrum of managed behavioral healthcare services to the chronically mentally ill and developmentally disabled. A corporate services division provides employee assistance programs both in Michigan and outside the state.

1963 Southwest Counseling & Development Services
1700 Waterman Street
Detroit, MI 48209-3317

313-841-8905
Fax: 313-841-4470
www.comnet.org

John Van Camp, President/CEO
Graciela Villalobos, Program Director of Outpatient

A mental health agency working to promote community well being. The mission is to enhance the well being of individuals, families and the community by providing effective leadership and innovative, quality mental health services.

1964 Woodlands Behavioral Healthcare Network
960 M-60 East
Cassopolis, MI 49031
269-445-2451
Fax: 269-445-3216
www.woodlandsbhn.org

Provides community mental health services.

Minnesota

1965 Centre for Mental Health Solutions: Minnesota Bio Brain Association
2000 South Plymouth Road
Suite 220
Minnetonka, MN 55305
952-922-6916
877-853-6916
Fax: 952-922-3412
E-mail: info@mentalhealthsolutions.org
www.tcfmhs.org

Tamera Shumaker, Executive Director
Nicole Zivalich, CEO

Our goal and primary focus is to investigate the underlying core causes in the body's biochemistry that allows illness to present itself and to provide information and education about healthy lifestyles, exercise, nutritious foods, proper nutritional supplements, clean air and water, sunshine and right thinking and attitudes that will ultimately manifest into vibrant health.

1966 Minnesota Association for Children's Mental Health
165 Western Avenue
Suite 2
Saint Paul, MN 55102
651-644-7333
800-528-4511
Fax: 651-644-7391
E-mail: dsaxhaug@macmh.org
www.macmh.org

Deborah Saxhaug

The mission of the Minnesota Association for Children's Mental Health is to enhance the quality of life for children with emotional or behavioral disorders and their families.

1967 Minnesota Psychiatric Society
4707 Highway 61
#232
Saint Paul, MN 55110-3227
651-407-1873
Fax: 651-407-1754
www.mnpsychoc.org

Laura Vukelich, Executive Director

The Minnesota Psychiatric Society is a professional association of psychiatrists. Our vision is accessible, quality mental health care for the patients that we service.

1968 Minnesota Psychological Association
1711 W County Road B
Suite 310N
Roseville, MN 55113-4036
651-697-0440
Fax: 651-697-0439
www.mnpsych.org

Enhances public and psychological interests by promoting the science of psychology and its applications.

1969 NASW Minnesota Chapter
Iris Park Place, Suite 340
1885 University Avenue W
Saint Paul, MN 55104
651-293-1935
Fax: 651-293-0952
E-mail: email@naswmn.org
www.naswmn.org

To promote the profession of Social Work by establishing and maintaining professional standards and by advancing the authority and credibility of Social Work; to provide services to its members by supplying opportunities for professional development and leadership and by enhancing communication among its members; to advocate for clients by promoting political action and community education.

1970 National Alliance on Mental Illness: Minneso ta
800 Transfer Road
Suite 7A
Saint Paul, MN 55114-1414
651-645-2948
888-473-0237
Fax: 651-645-7379
E-mail: nami-mn@nami.org
www.namimn.org

David Hartford, President
Sue Abderholden, Executive Director

A non-profit organization dedicated to improving the lives of adults and children with mental illness and their families. NAMI-MN offers programs of education, support and advocacy, and supports research efforts.

1971 North American Training Institute: Division of the Minnesota Council on Compulsive Gambling
314 W Superior Street
Suite 702
Duluth, MN 55802-1805
218-722-1503
888-989-9234
Fax: 218-722-0346
E-mail: info@nati.org
www.nati.org

Elizabeth M George, Chief Executive Director

The NATI conducts web based clinical courses to provide specific knowledge and advanced training leading to national certification for professionals in the prevention, treatment, and rehabilitation of patholgical gamblers.

1972 Pacer Center
8161 Normandale Boulevard
Minneapolis, MN 55437

952-838-9000
800-537-2237
Fax: 952-838-0199
TTY: 952-838-0190
E-mail: pacer@pacer.org
www.pacer.org

To expand opportunities and anhance the quality of life of children and young adults with disabilities and their families, based on the concept of parents helping parents.

Mississippi

1973 Mississippi Alliance for the Mentally Ill
411 Briarwood Drive
Suite 401
Jackson, MI 39206
601-899-9058
800-357-0388
Fax: 601-956-6380
E-mail: namimiss1@aol.com
www.nami.org

Teri Brister, Executive Director
Annette Giessner, President

Nation's leading self-help organization for all those affected by severe brain disorders. Mission is to bring consumers and families with similar experiences together to share information about services, care providers, and ways to cope with the challenges of schizophrenia, manic depression, and other serious mental illnesses.

1974 Mississippi Families as Allies
5166 Keele Street
Suite B100
Jackson, MS 39206-4319
601-981-1618
800-833-9671
Fax: 601-981-1696
E-mail: msfam@netdoor.com
www.cecp.air.org

Tressa Eide, Family Support Coordinator

To provide information and emotional support to families, provide education and training for families and professionals and advocate for improvements in the System of Care for Mississippi's children.

1975 National Alliance on Mental Illness: Mississ ippi
411 Briarwood Drive
Suite 401
Jackson, MS 39206-3058
601-899-9058
803-570-3884
Fax: 601-956-6380
E-mail: namimiss1@aol.com
www.nami.org/sites/namimississippi

Anette Giessner, President
Shirley Montgomery, Executive Director

Missouri

1976 Depressive and Manic-Depressive Association of St. Louis
1905 S Grand Boulevard
Saint Louis, MO 63104-1542
314-776-3969
Fax: 314-776-7071

E-mail: dmdastl@aol.com
www.ndmda.org

A consumer drop-in center, friendship line, peer support and self-help group.

1977 Mental Health Association of Greater St. Louis
1905 S Grand Boulevard
Saint Louis, MO 63104-1542
314-773-1399
Fax: 314-773-5930
E-mail: mhagstleaol.com
www.mhagstl.org

The Mental Health Association (MHA) of Greater St. Louis serves St. Louis City and the counties of St. Louis, St. Charles, Lincoln, Warren, Franklin and Jefferson. Services include educational literature/reference library, referrals to mental health professionals and self-help groups, representative payee services, educational course (BRIDGES), speakers bureau and more.

1978 Missouri Alliance for the Mentally Ill
1001 SW Boulevard
Suite E
Jefferson City, MO 65109-2501
314-634-7727
800-374-2138
Fax: 573-761-5636
E-mail: mocami@aol.com

Steven R Wilhelm, President
Cindi Keele, Executive Director

The Missouri Coalition of Alliance for the Mentally Ill is a family organization for persons with brain disorders. It has 15 active chapters throughout Missouri.

1979 Missouri Institute of Mental Health
University of Missouri
5400 Arsenal Street
Saint Louis, MO 63139-1300
314-644-8787
Fax: 314-644-8834
www.mimh.edu

1980 Missouri Statewide Parent Advisory Network: MO-SPAN
440 A Rue Street Francois
Florissant, MO 63031
314-972-0600
Fax: 314-972-0606
www.mo.span.org

Donna Dittrich, Executive Director
Tina Var Vera, Administrative Assistant

The mission of MO-SPAN is to improve the lives of children and youth with serious emotional disorders and their families by supporting and mobilizing families through training, education, advocacy and systems change. MO-SPAN is a statewide, nonprofit organization which is directed by a Board of Directors, the majority of who are parents of children with severe emotional disabilities.

1981 National Alliance on Mental Illness: Missour i
1001 Southwest Boulevard
Suite E
Jefferson City, MO 65109-2501
573-634-7727
800-374-2138

Fax: 573-761-5636
E-mail: sonyabaumgartner@yahoo.com

Tim Harlan, President
Cindi Keele, Executive Director

Montana

1982 Family Support Network
3302 4th Avenue
Suite 103
Billings, MT 59104-1366
406-256-7783
Fax: 406-256-9879
www.ffcmh.org/local.htm

Barbara Sample, Executive Director

Dedicated to children and adolescents with mental health needs and their families.

1983 Mental Health Association of Montana
25 S Ewing
Suite 206
Helena, MT 59601
406-442-4276
Fax: 406-442-4986
E-mail: mmha@in-tch.com
www.mhamontana.org

Charles McCarthy, Executive Director
Betty DeYoung, Administrative Assistant

Providing public education and advocacy for mental health services in Montana for over fifty years. Provides a hot line, conferences, libraries and has five local affiliates. Over twelve hundred individual and organization memberships.

1984 Montana Alliance for the Mentally Ill
554 Toole Court
Helena, MT 59602-6946
406-443-7871
888-280-6264
Fax: 406-862-6357
E-mail: namimt@ixi.net
www.mt.nami.org

Gary Mihelish, President

1985 National Alliance on Mental Illness: Montana
Mihelish's Residence
554 Toole Court
Helena, MT 59602-6946
406-443-7871
888-280-6264
Fax: 406-862-6357
E-mail: namimt@ixi.net
www.namimt.org

Gary Mihelish, President

A self-help, support, education, and advocacy organization dedicated to improving the lives of all those affected by serious mental illness.

Nebraska

1986 Department of Health and Human Services Regulation and Licensure
Credentialing Division
301 Centennial Mall South 3rd Floor
Lincoln, NE 68509-5007

402-471-2155
Fax: 402-471-3577
E-mail: marie.mcclatchey@hhss.state.ne.us
www.hhs.state.ne.us/crl/crlindex.htm

Dick Nelson, Director
Helen Meeks, Division Administrator

The Credentialing Division's mission is to assure the public that health-related practices provided by individuals, facilities and programs are safe, of acceptable quality, and that the cost of expanded services is justified by the need.

1987 Mutual of Omaha's Health and Wellness Progra ms
Mutual of Omaha Plaza
Omaha, NE 68175-0001
402-342-7600
800-238-9354
Fax: 402-255-1600
E-mail: grouphealth@mutualofomaha.com.
www.mutualofomaha.com/products/index.html

Mutual of Omaha's Health and Wellness Programs provide assistance and professional support in a variety of areas including family concerns; depression/anxiety; gambling and other addictions; parenting issues; drug/alcohol abuse; grief issues and life changes.

1988 National Alliance on Mental Illness: Nebrask a
1941 S 42nd Street
Suite 517-Center Mall
Omaha, NE 68105-2986
402-345-8101
877-463-6264
Fax: 402-346-4070
E-mail: nami.nebraska@nami.org
www.nami.org/sites/ne

Ruth Few, President
Dan Jackson, Executive Director

Provides statewide support to families and friends of individuals with mental illness.

1989 National Association of Social Workers: Nebraska Chapter
PO Box 83732
Lincoln, NE 68501-3732
402-477-7344
877-816-6279
Fax: 402-476-6547
E-mail: naswne@assocoffice.net
www.naswne.org

June Remington, Executive Director

Nebraska chapter is an affiliate of the National Association of Social Workers with a membership of six hundred plus.

1990 Nebraska Alliance for the Mentally Ill
1941 S 42nd Street
Suite 517
Omaha, NE 68105
402-345-8101
877-463-6264
Fax: 402-346-4070
E-mail: cwuebben@nami.org
www.ne.nami.org

Colleen M Wuebben, Executive Director
Carole Denton, President

The office of NAMI Nebraska, a non-profit organization dedicated to providing support, education and advocacy to and for anyone whose life has been touched by a mental illness.

1991 Nebraska Family Support Network
3801 Harney Street
2nd Floor
Omaha, NE 68131
402-505-4608
800-245-6081
Fax: 402-444-7722

1992 Pilot Parents: PP
Ollie Webb Center
1941 S 42nd Street
Suite 122
Omaha, NE 68105-2942
402-346-5220
Fax: 402-346-5253
E-mail: jvarner@olliewebb.org
www.olliewebb.org

Jennifer Varner, Coordinator

Parents, professionals and others concerned with providing emotional and peer support to new parents of children with special needs. Sponsors a parent-matching program which allows parents who have had sufficient experience and training in the care of their own children to share their knowledge and expertise with parents of children recently diagnosed as disabled. Publications: The Gazette, newsletter, published 6 times a year. Also has chapters in Arizona and limited other states.

Nevada

1993 Carson City Alliance for the Mentally Ill Share & Care Group
PO Box 21477
Carson City, NV 89701-6122
775-882-9749
Fax: 775-665-1639
www.nami.org

Ruth Paxton

Part of the nation's leading self-help organization for all those affected by severe brain disorders. Mission is to bring consumers and families with similar experiences together to share information about services, care providers, and ways to cope with the challenges of schizophrenia, manic depression, and other serious mental illnesses.

1994 National Alliance on Mental Illness: Nevada
1170 Curti Drive
Reno, NV 89502
775-329-3260
775-688-3317
Fax: 775-329-1618
E-mail: joetyler@sdi.net
www.nami-nevada.org

Joe Tyler, President

1995 Nevada Alliance for the Mentally Ill
6150 Transverse Drive #104
Las Vegas, NV 89146
702-258-1618
Fax: 702-258-6931
www.nami-nevada.org

Rosetta Johnson, President

Organization composed of families, friends, and professionals who are dedicated to helping people with mental illness and their families in coping with the devastation of the illness.

1996 Nevada Principals' Executive Program
2355 Red Rock Street
Suite 106
Las Vegas, NV 89146
702-388-8899
800-216-5188
Fax: 702-388-2966
E-mail: pepinfo@nvpep.org
www.nvpep.org

Karen Taycher

To strengthen and renew the knowledge, skills, and beliefs of public school leaders so that they might help improve the conditions for teaching and learning in schools and school districts.

New Hampshire

1997 Monadnock Family Services
64 Main Street
Suite 301
Keene, NH 03431-3701
603-357-6878
Fax: 603-357-6896
E-mail: rboyd@mfs.org
www.mfs.org

Ken Jue, CEO
Gary Barnes, COO
Peter Skalahan, CFO

A nonprofit community mental health center serving the mental health needs of families, buisness and other public and private organizations with comprehensive continuum of education, prevention and treatment services.

1998 National Alliance on Mental Illness: New Hampshire
15 Green Street
Concord, NH 03301-4020
603-225-5359
800-242-6264
Fax: 603-228-8848
E-mail: info@naminh.org
www.naminh.org

Elizabeth Merry, President
Michael Cohen, Executive Director

A statewide education, support and advocacy organization working for a quality, comprehensive mental health service system.

1999 New Hampshire Alliance for the Mentally Ill
15 Green Street
Concord, NH 03301-4020
603-225-5359
800-242-6264
Fax: 603-228-8848
E-mail: naminh@naminh.org
www.naminh.org

Michael Cohen, Executive Director
Sam Adams, President

Nation's leading self-help organization for all those affected by severe brain disorders. Mission is to bring consumers and families with similar experiences together to share information about services, care providers, and ways to cope with the challenges of schizophrenia, manic depression, and other serious mental illnesses.

New Jersey

2000 Association for Advancement of Mental Health
819 Alexander Road
Princeton, NJ 08540-6303
609-452-2088
Fax: 609-452-0627
E-mail: info@aamh.org

Richard McDonnell, Executive Director
Bruce Moehler, Director of Development

A private, non-profit community-based mental health agency licensed by the NJ State Division of Mental Health and Hospitals, that provides comprehensive services to Mercer County individuals and their families whose lives are adversely affected by emotional distress, psychiatric illness and development disability. Fees are based on ability to pay.

2001 Association for Children of New Jersey
35 Halsey Street
2nd Floor
Newark, NJ 07102-3000
973-643-3876
Fax: 973-643-9153
www.acnj.org, www.kidlaw.org &
www.makekidscountnj.org

The organization primarily works through community education, research and public policy analysis to improve opportunities for all of New Jersey's children and their families.

2002 Eating Disorders Association of New Jersey
10 Station Place
Metuchen, NJ 08840
800-522-2230
Fax: 609-688-1544
E-mail: njaaba@aol.com
www.njaaba.org

Leigh Garfield, President

Self-help organization which offers information and referrals, and professionally-run support groups at 12 locations state-wide for people with eating disorders, their families, friends and interested professionals.

2003 Jewish Family Service of Atlantic County and Cape
3 S Weymouth Avenue
Ventnor City, NJ 08406-2948
609-822-1108
Fax: 609-882-1106
www.jfsatlantic.org

Multi-service familty counseling agency dedicated to promoting, strengthening and preserving individual, family, and community weel-being in a manner consistent with Jewish philosophy and values.

2004 Mental Health Association of New Jersey
1562 US Highway 130
North Brunswick, NJ 08902

732-940-0991
Fax: 732-940-0355
E-mail: naminj@optonline.net
www.naminj.org

Sylvia Axelrod, Executive Director
Mark Perrin, President

Nation's leading self-help organization for all those affected by severe brain disorders. Mission is to bring consumers and families with similar experiences together to share information about services, care providers, and ways to cope with the challenges of schizophrenia, manic depression, and other serious mental illnesses.

2005 National Alliance on Mental Illness: New Jersey

1562 US Highway 130
North Brunswick, NJ 08902-3004
732-940-0991
Fax: 732-940-0355
E-mail: info@naminj.org
www.naminj.org

Mark Perrin, President
Sylvia Axelrod, Executive Director

A statewide non profit organization dedicated to improving the lives of individuals and families who are affected by mental illness. Also provides education, support and systems advocacy to empower families and persons with mental illness.

2006 National Association for the Mentally Ill of New Jersey

1562 Route 130
N Brunswick, NJ 08902
732-940-0991
Fax: 732-940-0355
E-mail: naminj@optonline.net
www.naminj.org

Mark Perrin MD, President
Sylvia Axelrod, Executive Director

NAMI New Jersey is a statewide non profit organization dedicated to improving the lives of individuals and families who are affected by mental illness.

2007 New Jersey Association of Mental Health Agencies

The Neuman Building
3575 Quakerbridge Road, Suite 102
Mercerville, NJ 08619
609-838-5488
Fax: 609-838-5489
www.njamha.org

Debra L Wentz

To champion opportunities that advance its members' ability to deliver accessible, quality, efficient and effective integrated behavioral health care services to mental health consumers and their families.

2008 New Jersey Protection and Advocacy

210 S Broad Street
3rd Floor
Trenton, NJ 08608-2404
609-292-9742
800-922-7233
Fax: 609-777-0187
TTY: 609-633-7106

E-mail: advocate@njpanda.org
www.njpanda.org

Richard West, Secretary
Marilyn Goldstein, Vice-Chair

Legal and non legal advocacy, information and referral, technical assistance and training, outreach and education in support of the human, civil, and legal rights of people with disabilities in New Jersey.

2009 New Jersey Psychiatric Association

PO Box 8008
Bridgewater, NJ 08807-8008
908-685-0650
Fax: 908-725-8610
E-mail: psychnj@optonline.net

Carla A Ross, Executive Director

The New Jersey Psychiatric Association is a professional organization of about 900 physicians qualified by training and experience in the treatment of mental illness. NJPA is a District Branch of the American Psychiatric Association and is the official voice of organized psychiatry in New Jersey.

2010 New Jersey Support Groups
Anorexia/Bulimia Association of New Jersey

10 Station Place
Metuchen, NJ 08840
609-252-0202

Offers various support groups across the state for anorexics and bulimics.

New Mexico

2011 National Alliance on Mental Illness: New Mexico

6001 Marble NE, Suite 8
PO Box 3086
Alburquerque, NM 87190-3086
505-260-0154
Fax: 505-260-0342
E-mail: naminm@aol.com
www.nm.nami.org

Becky Beckett, President
Kim Ahlbom, Additional Contact

2012 Navajo Nation K'E Project-Shiprock

PO Box 1240
Shiprock, NM 87420-1240
505-368-4479
Fax: 505-368-5582

Evelyn Balwin

Provides community-based behavioral and/or mental health and related services to children and families with serious emotional difficulties.

2013 New Mexico Alliance for the Mentally Ill

6001 Marble NE Suite 8
PO Box 3086
Albuquerque, NM 87190-3086
505-260-0154
Fax: 505-260-0342
E-mail: naminm@aol.com
www.naminm.org

Elaine Jones, Executive Director
Elaine Miller, Administrator Assistant

Nation's leading self-help organization for all those affected by severe brain disorders. Mission is to bring consumers and families with similar experiences together to share information about services, care providers, and ways to cope with the challenges of schizophrenia, manic depression, and other serious mental illnesses.

New York

2014 Alliance for the Mentally Ill: Friends & Advocates of the Mentally Ill

255 W 98th Street
New York, NY 10018-6505
212-684-3264
Fax: 212-684-3364
E-mail: helpline@naminyc.org
www.nami-nyc-metro.org

Evelyn Roberts, Executive Director

The AMI/FAMI is an affiliate of the National Alliance for the Mentally Ill. Offers a wide range of support groups, educational lectures, a newsletter and public access cable television program, Resource Center, Help Line and advocacy efforts.

2015 Babylon Consultation Center

206 Deer Park Avenue
Babylon, NY 11702-1929
631-587-1924
Fax: 631-893-0618
www.kindesigns.com

Michael J Beck PhD, Founder
Dr Jacob Kesten PhD, Consulting Psychologist

The Babylon Consultation Center is a community based provider of a full gamut of mental health services for over 20 years, and consists of a multi-disciplinary group of professional independent contractors representing the fields of psychology, social work, marriage and family counseling, mediation also education and business consulting.

2016 Compeer

259 Monroe Avenue
Suite B1
Rochester, NY 14607-3632
585-546-8280
800-836-0475
Fax: 585-325-2558
E-mail: compeerp@rochester.rr.com
www.compeer.org

Bernice Skirboll, Executive Director
Andrea Miller, VP

National nonprofit organization which matches community volunteers in supportive friendship relationships with children and adults recieving mental health treatment.

2017 Eating Disorder Council of Long Island

50 Charles Lindbergh Boulevard
Suite 400
Uniondale, NY 11553
516-229-2393

The EDCLI is a non-profit organization devoted to prevention, education and support prevention of eating disorders, and support to sufferers of eating disorders, their families and their friends.

2018 Families Together in New York State

15 Elk Street
Albany, NY 12207
518-432-0333
888-326-8644
Fax: 518-434-6478
E-mail: info@ftnys.org
www.ftnys.org

Non-profit, parent-run organization that strives to establish a unified voice for children with emotional, behavioral, and social challenges.

2019 Finger Lakes Parent Network

25 W Steuben Street
Bath, NY 14810
585-928-9894
Fax: 585-928-9894

Patti DiNardo

Parent-governed, non-profit organization focused on the needs of children and youth with emotional, behavioral or mental disorders and their families.

2020 Healthcare Association of New York State

1 Empire Drive
Rensselaer, NY 12144
518-431-7600
Fax: 518-431-7915
E-mail: info@hanys.org
www.hanys.org

Cindy Levernois, Director Behavioral Health

Serves as the primary advocate for more than 550 non-profit and public hospitals, health systems, long-term care, home care, hospice, and other health care organizations throughout New York State.

2021 Mental Health Association in Albany County

260 S Pearl Street
Albany, NY 12202
518-447-4555
Fax: 518-447-4661

To ensure that persons with mental illness are provided a full range of services that promote stabilization, rehabilitation and recovery for the purpose of enhancing or improving their lives.

2022 Mental Health Association in Dutchess County

510 Haight Avenue
Poughkeepsie, NY 12603-2434
845-473-2500
Fax: 845-473-4870
E-mail: mhadc@hvc.rr.com
www.mhadc.com

The Mental Health Association in Dutchess County is a voluntary, not-for-profit dedicated to the promotion of mental health, the prevention of mental illness and the improved care and treatment of persons with mental illnesses.

2023 Metro Intergroup of Overeaters Anonymous

350 Third Avenue
PO Box 759
New York, NY 10010
212-946-4599
E-mail: NYOAMetroOffice@yahoo.com

Offers various support groups and meetings.

2024 National Alliance on Mental Illness: New Yor k
260 Washington Avenue
Albany, NY 12210-1312
518-462-2000
800-950-3228
Fax: 518-462-3811
E-mail: naminys@naminys.org
www.naminys.org

Sherry Grenz, President

The purpose shall be to serve as an alliance of local mutual support, advocacy, self-help groups and individual members at-large dedicated to improving the quality of life for people with serious mental illness and to the eventual eradication of the severe effects of mental illnesses.

2025 National Association of Social Workers New York State Chapter
188 Washington Avenue
Albany, NY 12210-2394
518-463-4741
Fax: 518-463-6446
E-mail: info@naswnys.com
www.naswnys.org

The National Association of Social Workers is the largest membership organization of professional social workers in the world, with more than 155,000 members. NASW works to enhance the professional growth and development of its members, to create and maintain professional standards, and to advance sound social policies.

2026 New York Association of Psychiatric Rehabilitation Services
1 Columbia Place
2nd Floor
Albany, NY 12207-1006
518-436-0008
Fax: 518-436-0044
E-mail: nyaprs@aol.com
www.nyaprs.org

Harvey Rosenthal, Executive Director
Kelly Adams, Administrative Coordinator

New York Association of Psychiatric Services (NYAPRS) is a statewide coalition of New Yorkers, who are in recovery from mental illness and the professionals who work alongside them in rehabilitation and peer support services located throughout New York State. NYAPRS' mission is to promote the partnership of consumers, providers and families seeking to increase opportunities for community integration and independence for persons who have experienced a mental illness.

2027 New York Business Group on Health
386 Park Avenue S
Suite 703
New York, NY 10016
212-252-7440
Fax: 212-252-7448
E-mail: nybgh@nybgh.org
www.nybgh.org

Laurel Pickering, Executive Director
Janaera J Gaston MPA, Programs Director

NYBGH is a not-for-profit coalition of 150 businesses and is the only organization in the New York Metropolitan area exclusively devoted to employer health benefit issues. The mission is to provide leadership and knowledge to employ-

ers to promote a value-based, market-driven healthcare system.

2028 New York City Depressive & Manic Depressive Group
100 LaSalle Street
Suite 5A
New York, NY 10027
917-445-2399
Fax: 646-349-1761
E-mail: nycdmdg@aol.com
www.columbia.edu/~jgg17/DMDA/PAGE_1.html

Support groups meets regularly at Mt. Siani Hospital. Web page has helpful information and links to mental health sites.

2029 New York State Alliance for the Mentally Ill
260 Washington Avenue
Albany, NY 12210-1336
518-462-2000
800-950-3228
Fax: 518-462-3811
E-mail: info@naminys.org
www.naminys.org

Sean C Moran, Program/Outreach Manager
J David Seay, Executive Director
Jeff Keller, Deputy Director

Organization comprised of families of individuals with mental illness. Members work to improve the quality of life for all people with mental illness and to eradicate the stigma associated with mental illness.

2030 Orange County Mental Health Association
20 Walker Street
Goshen, NY 10924
845-294-7411
Fax: 845-294-7348
www.mhaorangeny.com

Rosalyn Goldman

Promotes the positive mental health and emotional well-being of Orange County residents, working towards reducing the stigma of mental illness, developmental disabilities, and providing support to victims of sexual assault and other crimes.

2031 Parents United Network: Parsons Child Family Center
60 Academy Road
Albany, NY 12208
518-426-2600
Fax: 518-447-5234

Joan Valery

County wide peer support organization providing support and advocacy for the special needs of families caring for children suffering from emotional, social and behavioral disorders. Is a local chapter of the national organization Federation of Families united Network, and is affiliated with state chapter.

2032 Project LINK
Ibero-American Action League
817 E Main Street
Rochester, NY 14605-2722
585-256-8900
Fax: 585-256-0120

E-mail: eamarlin@iaal.org
www.iaal.org

Julio Vasquez, Executive Director

As well as our other activities in the Hispanic community, we continue to be committed to the betterment and quality of life of the mentally ill. We advocate for the severely and persistently mentally ill individual who is at risk of becoming involved or is involved with the criminal justice system. Project LINK operates in partnership with the University of Rochester, Strong-Memorial Department of Psychiatry, Action for a Better Community, Monroe County Mental Health Clinic for Socio-Legal Services, St. Mary's Hospital, the Urban League of Rochester and the Ibero-American Action League.

2033 State University of New York at Stony Brook Department of Psychiatry and Behavioral Science
101 Nicolls Road
Stony Brook, NY 11794-8101
631-444-2399
Fax: 631-444-7534
www.hsc.stonybrook.edu/som/psychiatry/

Mark J Sedler, MD/MPH, Director of Adult Psychiatry
Gabrielle Carlson, MD, Director of Child Psychiatry
Regina T Cline, JD, Administrator

2034 Westchester Alliance for the Mentally Ill
101 Executive Boulevard
Suite 2
Elmsford, NY 10523
914-592-5458
Fax: 914-592-5458
www.nami.org

Provides support and education for families who are feeling alone and in pain with a member of their family suffering from mental illness; no meeting fee.

2035 Westchester Task Force on Eating Disorders
3 Mount Joy Avenue
Scarsdale, NY 10583-2632
914-472-3701

Karen Cohen

A professionally-led support group for people with eating disorders including anorexia, bulimia and compulsive overeating; families and professionals interested in learning about the disorder are welcome to the meetings.

2036 Yeshiva University: Soundview-Throgs Neck Community Mental Health Center
2527 Glebe Avenue
Bronx, NY 10461-3109
718-904-4400
Fax: 718-931-7307

Dr. Itamar Salamon, Director

Mental health counseling for adults and children. Accepts Medicaid and private insurance. Sliding scale fee.

North Carolina

2037 Autism Society of North Carolina
505 Oberlin Road
Suite 230
Raleigh, NC 07605-1345

919-743-0204
E-mail: info@autismsociety-nc.org
www.autismsociety-nc.org

Jill Hinton Keel PhD, Executive Director
David Laxton, Director of Communications

Committed to providing support and promoting opportunities which enhance the lives of individuals within the autism spectrum and their families

2038 National Alliance on Mental Illness: North C arolina
309 W Millbrook Road
Suite 121
Raleigh, NC 27609-4394
919-788-0801
800-451-9682
Fax: 919-788-0906
E-mail: mail@naminc.org
www.naminc.org

Carol Matthieu, President
Debra Dihoff, Executive Director

The mission of NAMI North Carolina is to improve the quality of life for individuals and their families living with the debilitating effects of severe and persistent mental illness. We work to protect the dignity of people living with brain disorders through advocacy, education, and support.

2039 National Association of Social Workers: North Carolina Chapter
412 Morson Street
PO Box 27582
Raleigh, NC 27611-7582
919-828-9650
800-280-6207
Fax: 919-828-1341
E-mail: naswnc@naswnc.org
www.naswnc.org

Katherine Boyd, Executive Director

NASW is a membership organization that promotes, develops, and protects the practice of social work and social workers. NASW also seeks to enhance the effective functioning and well-being of individuals, families, and communities through its work and through advocacy.

2040 North Carolina Alliance for the Mentally Ill
309 W Millbrook Road
Suite 121
Raleigh, NC 27609
919-788-0801
800-451-9682
Fax: 919-788-0906
E-mail: mail@naminc.org
www.nami.nc.org

Gloria Harrison, Helpline Director

Nation's leading self-help organization for all those affected by severe brain disorders. Mission is to bring consumers and families with similar experiences together to share information about services, care providers, and ways to cope with the challenges of schizophrenia, manic depression, and other serious mental illnesses.

2041 North Carolina Mental Health Consumers Organization
PO Box 27042
Raleigh, NC 27611-7042

919-832-2286
800-326-3842
Fax: 919-828-6999

NC MHCO is a private non-profit organization not affilated with NAMI NC. This organization has been providing advocacy and support to adults with mental illness since 1989.

2042 Western North Carolina Families (CAN)
PO Box 665
Arden, NC 28704
828-277-7325
E-mail: wncfamilies@bellsouth.net

Ann May

Mutual support and community collaboration, provides resources, referrals, education, and advocacy for families who have children with challenging behaviors and serious emotional disorders.

North Dakota

2043 National Alliance on Mental Illness: North D akota
PO Box 3215
Minot, ND 58702-3215
701-852-8202
E-mail: naminwnd@min.midco.net

Janet Sabol, President

2044 National Association of Social Workers: North Dakota Chapter
PO Box 1775
Bismarck, ND 58502-1775
701-223-4161
Fax: 701-224-9824

Tom Tupa, Executive Director

NASW Dakotas, serves the critical and diverse needs of the entire social work profession.

2045 North Dakota Federation of Families for Children's Mental Health: Region II
PO Box 3061
Bismarck, ND 58502-3061
701-222-1223
Fax: 701-250-8835
E-mail: ndffrg19@idt.net

Valorie Keeney

To provide support and information to families of children and adolescents with serious emotional, behavioral, or mental disorders.

2046 North Dakota Alliance for the Mentally Ill
PO Box 3215
Minot, ND 58702-6016
701-852-8202
Fax: 701-725-4334
E-mail: jsabol@ndak.net
www.nami.org

Janet Sabol

Nation's leading self-help organization for all those affected by severe brain disorders. Mission is to bring consumers and families with similar experiences together to share information about services, care providers, and ways to cope with the challenges of schizophrenia, manic depression, and other serious mental illnesses.

2047 North Dakota Federation of Families for Children's Mental Health: Region V
214 2nd Avenue
W Fargo, ND 58078
701-235-9923
Fax: 701-235-9923

Pat Harles

To provide support and information to families fo children and adolescents with serious emotional, behavioral, or mental disorders.

2048 North Dakota Federation of Families for Children's Mental Health: Region VII
PO Box 3061
Bismarck, ND 58502-3061
701-222-1223
Fax: 701-250-8835
E-mail: ndffrg19@idt.net

Carlotta McCleary

To rpovide support and information to families of children and adolescents with serious emotional, behavioral, or mental disorders.

2049 North Dakota Federation of Families for Children's Mental Health
PO Box 3061
Bismarck, ND 58502-3061
701-222-1223
Fax: 701-250-8835
E-mail: ndffrg19@idt.net

Liz Sweet

To provide support and informatin to families of children and adolescents with serious emotional, behavioral, or mental disorders.

Ohio

2050 Concerned Advocates Serving Children & Families
9195 2nd Street
Canton, OH 44704-1132
330-454-7917
Fax: 330-455-2026

Connie Truman

Support group for families of children diagnosed with mental illness.

2051 Mental Health Association of Summit
405 Tallmadge Road
PO Box 639
Cuyahoga Falls, OH 44222
330-923-0688
Fax: 330-923-7573
E-mail: info@mhasc.net
www.mentalhealthassociationofsummitcounty.org

Rudy Libertini, Executive Director
Sandy Soful, Associate Director

The Mental Health Association of Summit is part of a network of professionals and volunteers committed to improving America's mental health seeking victory over mental illness. To help achieve this national goal we are working to improve mental health services, to initiate services where none exist and to monitor the use of mental health tax dollars in the community.

2052 Mount Carmel Behavioral Healthcare

1808 E Broad Street
Columbus, OH 43203-2003
614-251-8242
800-227-3256
Fax: 614-337-7027
E-mail: mcbhinfo@mchs.com
www.mcbh.com

Mark Ridenour, Executive Director
Marc Clemente MD, MBA, Medical Director

Mount Carmel Behavioral Healthcare is a behavioral healthcare management organization offering a cost-effective, comprehensive continuum of behavioral healthcare services.

2053 National Alliance on Mental Illness: Ohio

747 East Broad Street
Columbus, OH 43205
614-224-2700
800-686-2646
Fax: 614-224-5400
E-mail: amiohio@amiohio.org
www.namiohio.org

Harvey Snider, President
Jim Mauro, Executive Director

Mission is to improve the quality of life, ensure dignity and respect for persons with serious mental illness, and to support their families.

2054 National Association of Social Workers: Ohio Chapter

33 N Third Street
Suite 530
Columbus, OH 43215
614-461-4484
Fax: 614-461-9793
E-mail: ohnasw@ameritech.net
www.naswoh.org

Elaine C Schiwy, Executive Director
Sarah E Hamilton, Membership Coordinator

The mission of NASW is to strengthen, support, and unify the social work profession, to promote the development of social work standards and practice, and to advocate for social policies that advance social justice and diversity.

2055 Ohio Alliance for the Mentally Ill

747 E Broad Street
Columbus, OH 43205
614-224-2700
800-686-2646
Fax: 614-224-5400
E-mail: amiohio@amiohio.org
www.namiohio.org

Terry L Russell, Executive Director
Stacey Smith, Operations Director

Nation's leading self-help organization for all those affected by severe brain disorders. Mission is to bring consumers and families with similar experiences together to share information about services, care providers, and ways to cope with the challenges of schizophrenia, manic depression, and other serious mental illnesses.

2056 Ohio Association of Child Caring Agencies

400 E Town Street
Suite G-10
Columbus, OH 43215-4700
614-461-0014
Fax: 614-228-7004
E-mail: PWyman@oacca.org
www.oacca.org

Penny M Wyman, Executive Director
George E Biggs, Assistant Executive Director

The Ohio Association of Child Caring Agencies is to promote and strengthen a fully-integrated, private/public network of high-quality services for Ohio's children and their families through advocacy, education, and support of member agencies.

2057 Ohio Council of Behavioral Healthcare Providers

35 E Gay Street
Suite 401
Columbus, OH 43215-3138
614-228-0747
Fax: 614-228-0740
E-mail: staff@ohiocouncil-bhp.org
www.ohiocouncil-bhp.org

Pat Bridgman, Associate Director
Brenda Cornett, Membership Services

A trade association representing provider organizations throughout Ohio which provide behavioral healthcare services to their communities.

2058 Ohio Department of Mental Health

30 E Broad Street
Room 1180
Columbus, OH 43215-3414
614-466-2596
877-275-6364
Fax: 614-752-9453
TDD: 614-752-9696
TTY: 888-636-4889
www.mh.state.oh.us

State agency responsible for oversight and funding of public mental health programs and services.

2059 Planned Lifetime Assistance Network of Northeast Ohio

2490 Lee Boulevard
Suite 204
Cleveland Heights, OH 44118-1269
216-321-3611
Fax: 216-321-0021
E-mail: info@planNEohio.org
www.planneohio.org

Provides individualized home-based social services and advocacy to assist families who have a neurobiologically disabled family member to function at their maximum. LISW staff provides therapy and works with existing service providers to ensure quality of care. Offers a wide range of community-based, social, and recreational activities for its participants.

2060 Positive Education Program

3100 Euclid Avenue
Cleveland, OH 44115-2508
216-361-4400
Fax: 216-361-8600

E-mail: pepgen@pepcleve.org
www.pepcleve.org

Frank A Fecser Ph D, Executive Director
Tom Valore Ph D, Program Director

The Positive Education Program (PEP) is to help troubled and troubling children and their families build skills to grow and learn successfully.

2061 Six County
2845 Bell Street
Zanesville, OH 43701-1794
740-454-9766
Fax: 740-588-6452
E-mail: info@sixcounty.org
www.sixcounty.org

Helping community mental health needs in Coshocton, Guernsey, Morgan, Muskingum, Noble and Perry counties. In addition to the traditional treatment services, specialized services have been developed to reach people with ever changing needs. Employee assistance, sheltered employment, intensive outpatient, and residential services.

Oklahoma

2062 National Alliance on Mental Illness: Oklahom a
500 N Broadway Avenue
Suite 100
Oklahoma City, OK 73102-6200
405-230-1900
800-583-1264
Fax: 405-230-1903
E-mail: nami-ok@swbell.net
www.ok.nami.org

Wayne Merritt, President
Karina Forrest, Executive Director

2063 OK Parents as Partners
132 N.W. 13th Street
Oklahoma City, OK 73103
405-232-2796
866-492-5437
Fax: 405-232-2799
E-mail: parentsaspartners@coxinet.net
www.ffcmh-ok.org

Janice Garvin, President
Emma Mullendore, Vice President
Etka Ahluwalia, Phd., Oklahoma City Representative
George McCaffrey, Esq., Oklahoma City Representative

Oklahoma Federation of Families for Childrens' Mental Health dba Parents as Partners seeks to involve families in the decision making process; assist in meeting the needs of children with emotional, behavioral, mental health issues or disabilities; and improving the quality of mental health services the children receive in all settings: inpatient, outpatient, education, and within the juvenile justice system. Parents as Partners is a family run non-profit organization dedicated to providing support and advocacy for families of children and adolescents with emotional, behavioral, or mental health issues and/or disabilities.

2064 Oklahoma Alliance for the Mentally Ill
500 N Broadway Avenue
Suite 100
Oklamhoma City, OK 73102-6200
405-230-1900
800-583-1264

Fax: 405-230-1903
E-mail: nami-OK@swbell.net
www.ok.nami.org

Jeff Tallent, Executive Director
Hope Ingle, President

Nation's leading self-help organization for all those affected by severe brain disorders. Mission is to bring consumers and families with similar experiences together to share information about services, care providers, and ways to cope with the challenges of schizophrenia, manic depression, and other serious mental illnesses.

2065 Oklahoma Mental Health Consumer Council
3200 NW 48th
Suite 102
Oklahoma City, OK 73112
405-604-6975
888-424-1305
Fax: 405-605-8175
www.mentalhealth.samhsa.gov/

Kay Rote, Executive Director

OMHCC is the statewide advocacy organization of and for mental health consumers. Offers support groups, speakers' bureau and advocacy consultations on all issues affecting consumers.

2066 Oklahoma Psychiatric Physicians Association
PO Box 1328
Norman, OK 73070-1328
405-360-5066
Fax: 405-447-1053
E-mail: oklapsychiatry@yahoo.com
www.oklahomapsychiatry.org

District branch of the American Psychiatric Association, is a medical specialty society recognized world-wide. Psysicians specialize in the diagnosis and treatment of mental and emotional illnesses and substance abuse disorders.

Oregon

2067 National Alliance on Mental Illness: Oregon
3550 SE Woodward Street
Portland, OR 97202-1552
503-230-8099
800-343-6264
Fax: 503-230-2751
E-mail: namioregon@qwest.net
www.nami.org/sites/namioregon

Christopher Bouneff, President
David Delvallee, Executive Director

A statewide grassroots organization dedicated to improving the quality of life for individuals with mental illness and their families through support, education, and advocacy.

2068 Oregon Alliance for the Mentally Ill
2620 Greenway Drive NE
Suite 17
Salem, OR 97301-4538
503-370-7774
800-343-6264
Fax: 503-370-9452
E-mail: namior@comcast.net
www.namioregon.org

Monica Kosman, President
Stephen Loaiza, Executive Director

Dedicated to the eradication of mental illnesses and to the improvement of the quality of life of all whose lives are affected by these diseases. A self-help, support and advocacy organization of consumers, families, and friends of people with severe mental illnesses.

2069 Oregon Family Support Network
15544 S Clackamas River Drive
Oregon City, OR 97045
503-656-5440
Fax: 503-581-4841
E-mail: ofsn@open.org
www.ofsn.org

Maureen H Breckenridge, JD, Executive Director

Families throughout Oregon supporting other families who have children and adolescents with mental, emotional and behavioral disorders.

2070 Oregon Psychiatric Association
PO Box 2042
Salem, OR 97308-2042
503-370-7019
Fax: 503-587-8063
E-mail: assoc@wvi.com

John McCulley, Executive Secretary

To ensure human care and effective treatment for all persons with mental disorder, including mental retardation and substance-related disorders.

2071 People First of Oregon
PO Box 12642
Salem, OR 97309-0642
503-362-0336
Fax: 503-587-8459
E-mail: people1@open.org
www.open.org/people1

Develpmentally disabled people joining together to learn how to speak for themselves. Offers support, a united voice, advocacy to its members, information to communities, developing service projects to communities you live in, assistance in starting new People First groups, information to countries around the world, and participation on DD Council and A.R.C. Boards, Transit Boards.

Pennsylvania

2072 Health Federation of Philadelphia
1211 Chestnut Street
Suite 801
Philadelphia, PA 19107-4120
215-567-8001
Fax: 215-567-7743

Natalie Levkovich, Executive Director

A private, non-profit membership organization which provides shared services to a consortium of community and federally qualified health centers in Philadelphia.

2073 Mental Health Association of Southeastern Pennsylvania (MHASP)
1211 Chestnut Street
Philadelphia, PA 19107
215-751-1800
800-688-4226
Fax: 215-636-6300
E-mail: mha@mhasp.org
www.mhasp.org/

Joseph A Rogers, President/CEO
Jack Boyle, SVP/COO
Maryann E Ludwig, VP Finance/CFO
Stephen P Weinstein, Chairman

The Mental Health Association of Southeastern Pennsylvania (MHASP) is a nonprofit citizen's organization that develops, supports and promotes innovative education and advocacy programs. MHASP serves adults, children and family members through our programs and advocacy efforts. It is the mission of the Mental Health Association of Southeastern Pennsylvania to develop, maintain, and promote innovative education and advocacy programs and mental health services in the five counties we represent in a culturally competent manner, serving as a role model and technical assistance resource for state and national organizations and constituencies.

2074 National Alliance on Mental Illness: Pennsylvania
2149 North 2nd Street
Harrisburg, PA 17110-1005
717-238-1514
800-223-0500
Fax: 717-238-4390
E-mail: nami-pa@nami.org
www.namipa.nami.org

Jyoti Shah, President
James Jordan, Executive Director

A statewide non-profit organization dedicated to helping mental health consumers and their families rebuild their lives and conquer the challenges posed by severe and persistent mental illness.

2075 Parents Involved Network
1211 Chestnut Street
Philadelphia, PA 19107
215-751-1800
800-688-4226
E-mail: pin@pinofpa.org
www.pinofpa.org/

Janet Lonsdale, Director

Parents Involved Network of Pennsylvania is an organization that assists parents or caregivers of children and adolescents with emotional and behavioral disorders. PIN provides information, helps parents find services and will advocate on their behalf with any of the public systems that serve children.

2076 Pennsylvania Alliance for the Mentally Ill
2149 N 2nd Street
Harrisburg, PA 17110-1005
717-238-1514
800-223-0500
Fax: 717-238-4390
E-mail: nami-pa@nami.org
www.namipa.org

James W Jordan Jr, Executive Director
Carol Caruso, President

The largest statewide non-profit organization dedicated to helping mental health consumers and their families rebuild their lives and conquer the challenges posed by severe and persistent mental illness.

2077 Pennsylvania Chapter of the American Anorexia Bulimia Association
PO Box 1287
Langhorne, PA 19047
215-221-1864
Fax: 215-702-8944
www.aabaphila.org

The American Anorexia Bulimia Association of Philidelphia is a non-profit, providing services and programs for anyone interested in or affected by, Anorexia, Bulimia and/or related disorders.

2078 Pennsylvania Society for Services to Children
415 S 15th Street
Philadelphia, PA 19146-1637
215-875-3400
Fax: 215-875-3411
www.pssckids.org

Helen B Dennis, Executive Director
Carla Thompson Neal, Program Director

Philadelphia Society for Services to Children is a recognized leader in child abuse prevention in the Delaware Valley. Provides and advocate for services that will help each child to grow up in a safe, stable and supportive family environment.

2079 Southwestern Pennsylvania Alliance for the Mentally Ill
4721 McKnight Road
Suite 216
Pittsburgh, PA 15237-3415
412-366-3788
888-264-7972
Fax: 412-366-3935
E-mail: www.info@namiswpa.org
www.swpa.nami.org

NAMI Southwestern Pennsylvania is a non-profit organization that serves a ten-county region in Southwestern Pennsylvania. We address the increasing need for families and consumers to have a stronger voice in the mental health system.

2080 University of Pittsburgh Medical Center
200 Lothrop Street
Pittsburgh, PA 15213-2585
412-647-8762
800-533-8762
E-mail: upmcweb@upmc.edu
www.upmc.com

The University of Pittsburgh Medical Center is the leading health care system in western Pennsylvania and one of the largest nonprofit integrated health care systems in the United States.

Rhode Island

2081 East Bay Alliance for the Mentally Ill
St. Jean Baptiste
328 Main Street
Warren, RI 02885
401-245-2386
www.namiri.org/

Alice Tupaj, Executive Director

Nation's leading self-help organization for all those affected by severe brain disorders. Mission is to bring consumers and families with similar experiences together to share information about services, care providers, and ways to cope with the challenges of schizophrenia, manic depression, and other serious mental illnesses.

2082 Kent County Alliance for the Mentally Ill
Hillsgrove House
70 Minnesota Avenue
Warwick, RI 02818
401-821-5601
www.www.namiri.org

Shirley Lane, Executive Director

Nation's leading self-help organization for all those affected by severe brain disorders. Mission is to bring consumers and families with similar experiences together to share information about services, care providers, and ways to cope with the challenges of schizophrenia, manic depression, and other serious mental illnesses.

2083 National Alliance on Mental Illness: Rhode Island
154 Waterman Street
Suite 5B
Providence, RI 02906-3116
401-331-3060
800-749-3197
Fax: 401-274-3020
E-mail: chaznami@cox.net
www.namirhodeisland.org

Henry Saccoccia, President
Charles Gross, Executive Director

The mission of NAMI Rhode Island is to educate the public about mental illness; to offer resources and support to all whose lives are touched by mental illness; to advocate at every level to ensure the rights and dignity of those with mental illness; and to promote research in the science and treatment of mental illness.

2084 National Alliance on Mental Illness: Davis Park
VA Hospital
Room 384
Providence, RI 02908
401-568-7636
www.namiri.org

Gayle Frueh, Executive Director

NAMI Rhode Island (the National Alliance for the Mentally Ill of Rhode Island) was founded in 1983 by family members of people with serious mental illnesses. NAMI-RI is an independent organization which provides support to people with mental illness and their friends or family members, educates professionals and the public about mental illness, and advocates for improved services for all people with mental illness.

2085 National Alliance on Mental Illness: Rhode Island
82 Pitman Street
Providence, RI 02906
401-331-3060
Fax: 401-274-3020
E-mail: nicknami@aol.com
www.namiri.org/

Thomas Mack, President
Nicki Sahlin, Executive Director

NAMI Rhode Island (the National Alliance for the Mentally Ill of Rhode Island) was founded in 1983 by family members of people with serious mental illnesses. NAMI-RI is an independent organization which provides support to people with mental illness and their friends or family members, educates professionals and the public about mental illness, and advocates for improved services for all people with mental illness.

2086 New Avenues Alliance for the Mentally Ill

Johnston Mental Health Services
1516 Atwood Avenue
Johnston, RI 02919
401-952-5839
www.www.namiri.org

Gert Orenberg, Executive Director

Nation's leading self-help organization for all those affected by severe brain disorders. Mission is to bring consumers and families with similar experiences together to share information about services, care providers, and ways to cope with the challenges of schizophrenia, manic depression, and other serious mental illnesses.

2087 Newport County Alliance for the Mentally Ill

Channing Memorial
135 Pelham Street
Newport, RI 02840
401-331-3060
www.namiri.org

Mary Berry, Executive Director

Nation's leading self-help organization for all those affected by severe brain disorders. Mission is to bring consumers and families with similar experiences together to share information about services, care providers, and ways to cope with the challenges of schizophrenia, manic depression, and other serious mental illnesses.

2088 Northern Rhode Island Alliance for the Mentally Ill

Landmark Medical Center
Cass Avenue
Cumberland, RI 02864-6407
401-776-0865
www.namiri.org/

Stella Struzik, Executive Director

Nation's leading self-help organization for all those affected by severe brain disorders. Mission is to bring consumers and families with similar experiences together to share information about services, care providers, and ways to cope with the challenges of schizophrenia, manic depression, and other serious mental illnesses.

2089 Parent Support Network of Rhode Island

400 Warwick Avenue
Suite 12
Warwick, RI 02888
401-467-6855
800-483-8844
Fax: 401-467-6903
E-mail: psnofri@aol.com
www.mentalhealth.samhsa.gov/

Cathy Ciano, Executive Director

Organization of families supporting families with children and youth who are at risk for or have serious behavioral, emotional, and/or mental health challenges, having consideration for their backround and values. The goals of PSN are to: strengthen and preserve families; enable families in

advocacy; extend social networks, reduce family isolation and develop social policy systems of care. Parent Support Network accomplishes these goals through providing advocacy, education and training, promoting outreach and public awareness, facilitating social events for families, participating on committees responsible for developing, implementing and evaluating policies and systems of care.

2090 Siblings & Offspring Group Alliance for the Mentally Ill

1255 N Main Street
Providence, RI 02904
401-331-3060
www.namiri.org

Bill Emmet, Executive Director

Nation's leading self-help organization for all those affected by severe brain disorders. Mission is to bring consumers and families with similar experiences together to share information about services, care providers, and ways to cope with the challenges of schizophrenia, manic depression, and other serious mental illnesses.

2091 Spouses & Partners' Group Alliance for the Mentally Ill

Butler Hospital
345 Blackstone Boulevard
Providence, RI 02904
401-331-3060
www.namiri.org

Nicki Sahlin, Executive Director

Nation's leading self-help organization for all those affected by severe brain disorders. Mission is to bring consumers and families with similar experiences together to share information about services, care providers, and ways to cope with the challenges of schizophrenia, manic depression, and other serious mental illnesses.

2092 Washington County Alliance for the Mentally Ill

South Shore Mental Health
33 Cherry Lane
Wakefield, RI 02879
401-295-1956
www.namiri.org

Ginny Eastman, Executive Director

Nation's leading self-help organization for all those affected by severe brain disorders. Mission is to bring consumers and families with similar experiences together to share information about services, care providers, and ways to cope with the challenges of schizophrenia, manic depression, and other serious mental illnesses.

South Carolina

2093 Federation of Families of South Carolina

PO Box 1266
Columbia, SC 29202
803-779-0402
866-779-0402
Fax: 803-779-0017
www.ffcmh.org

Diane Revels-Flashnick, Executive Director

Nonprofit organization established to serve the families of children with any degree of emotional, behavioral or psychiatric disorder. The services and programs by the Federation are designed to meet the individual needs of families around the state. Through support networks, educational materials, publications, conferences, workshops and other activities, the Federation provides many avenues of support for families of children with emotional, behavioral or psychiatric disorders.

2094 National Alliance on Mental Illness: South Carolina
PO Box 1267
Columbia, SC 29202-1267
803-733-9592
800-788-5131
Fax: 803-733-9593
E-mail: namisc@namisc.org
www.namisc.org

John Balling, President
Bill Lindsey, Executive Director

2095 National Mental Health Association: Georgetown County
254 Yadkin Avenue
Georgetown, SC 29440
843-527-1435
Fax: 843-546-8101
www.nmha.org/affiliates/directory/index.cfm?doit=all

Everlena Lance, Executive Director

Advocates for people with mental illness including referrals to counseling and provides education about mental illness.

2096 South Carolina Alliance for the Mentally Ill
PO Box 1267
5000 Thurmond Mall Boulevard, Suite 338
Columbia, SC 29202-1267
803-733-9592
800-788-5131
Fax: 803-733-9593
E-mail: namiofsc@logicsouth.com
www.namisc.org

Ken Howell, President
David Almeida, Executive Director

Non-profit with 17 local groups throughout the state. Provide support, education and advocacy for families and friends of people with serious mental illness.

2097 South Carolina Alliance for the Mentally Ill
PO Box 2538
Columbia, SC 29202-2538
803-779-7849
800-788-5131
Fax: 803-733-9593
www.nami.org

Laurie Flynn, Executive Director

Nation's leading self-help organization for all those affected by severe brain disorders. Mission is to bring consumers and families with similar experiences together to share information about services, care providers, and ways to cope with the challenges of schizophrenia, manic depression, and other serious mental illnesses.

2098 South Carolina Family Support Network
PO Box 2538
Columbia, SC 29202-2538
803-779-7849
800-788-5131

Fax: 803-733-9593
www.ffcmh.org/local.htm

Diane Flashnick

Focused on the needs of children and youth with emotional, behavioral or mental disorders and their families.

South Dakota

2099 Brookings Alliance for the Mentally Ill
211 4th Street
PO Box 221
Brookings, SD 57006
605-692-8948
E-mail: zippy@brookings.net
www.nami.org/sites/NAMISouthDakota

Nancy Sonnenburg, Executive Director

Nation's leading self-help organization for all those affected by severe brain disorders. Mission is to bring consumers and families with similar experiences together to share information about services, care providers, and ways to cope with the challenges of schizophrenia, manic depression, and other serious mental illnesses.

2100 Huron Alliance for the Mentally Ill
79 Second Street SW
Huron, SD 57350-1204
605-353-6010
800-551-2531
Fax: 605-352-5573
E-mail: maskipper@ccs-sd.org
www.nami.org/sites/NAMISouthDakota

Marcia Skipper, Executive Director

Dedicated to the eradication of mental illness and the improvement of the quality of life of all whose lives are affected by these diseases.

2101 National Alliance on Mental Illness: South D akota
3920 S Western Avenue
PO Box 88808
Sioux Falls, SD 57109-8808
605-271-1871
800-551-2531
Fax: 605-271-1871
E-mail: namisd@midconetwork.com
www.nami.org/sites/namisouthdakota

Shelly Fuller, President
Phyllis Arends, Executive Director

To provide education and support for individuals and families impacted by brain-based disorders (mental illnesses), advocate for the development of a comprehensive system of services and lessen the stigma in the general public.

Tennessee

2102 Bridges: Building Recovery & Individual Dre ams & Goals Through Education & Support
480 Craighead Street
#200
Nashville, TN 37204
615-250-1176
800-539-0393
Fax: 615-383-1176
E-mail: bridges@tmhca-tn.org
www.3mhca-tn.org/About_Bridges.html

Irene Russell, Executive Director

Based on the belief that those with mental illness can and do recover a new and valued sense of self and purpose in accepting and overcoming the challenges of a disability that has affected every aspect of life: physical, intellectual, emotional, and spiritual.

2103 Memphis Business Group on Health

5050 Poplar Avenue
Suite 509
Memphis, TN 38157
901-767-9585
Fax: 901-767-6592
E-mail: information@memphisbusinessgroup.org
www.memphisbusinessgroup.org

To facilitate the purchase of efficient and effective health care services for the Memphis community.

2104 National Alliance on Mental Illness: Tenness ee

1101 Kermit Drive
Suite 608
Nashville, TN 37217-2126
615-361-6608
800-467-3589
Fax: 615-361-6698
E-mail: bstaceyscott@namitn.org
www.namitn.org

Elliot Garret, President
Sita Diehl, Executive Director

NAMI Tennessee is a grassroots, non-profit made up of families, consumers and professionals. We are dedicated to improving quality of life for people with mental illness and their families.

2105 Tennessee Alliance for the Mentally Ill

Cherry Cottage
5908 Lyons View Pike
Knoxville, TN 37919
423-602-7900
800-771-5491
www.namitn.org/

Sita Diehl, Executive Director

Nation's leading self-help organization for all those affected by severe brain disorders. Mission is to bring consumers and families with similar experiences together to share information about services, care providers, and ways to cope with the challenges of schizophrenia, manic depression, and other serious mental illnesses.

2106 Tennessee Association of Mental Health Organization

42 Rutledge Street
Nashville, TN 37210-2043
615-244-2220
800-568-2642
Fax: 615-254-8331
E-mail: tamho@tamho.org
www.tamho.org

Charles R Blackburn, Executive Director

State wide trade association representing primarily community mental health centers, community-owned corporations that have historically served the needs of the mentally ill and chemically dependent citizens of Tennessee regardless of their ability to pay.

2107 Tennessee Mental Health Consumers' Association

116 Dalton Street
Kingsport, TN 37665
800-459-2925
Fax: 423-245-6100
E-mail: tnmhca@aol.com

Irene Russell, Executive Director

Not-for-profit organization whose members are mental health consumers and other individuals and groups who support the mission of TMHCA.

2108 Tennessee Voices for Children

1315 8th Avenue S
Nashville, TN 37203
800-670-9882
Fax: 615-269-8914
E-mail: TVC@tnvoices.org
www.tnvoices.org/

Charlotte Bryson, Executive Director

Non-profit, non-partisan organization of families, professionals, business and community leaders, and government representatives committed to improving and expanding services related to the emotional and behavioral well-being of children.

2109 Vanderbilt University: John F Kennedy Center for Research on Human Development

PO Box 40
Peabody College
Nashville, TN 37203-5701
615-322-8240
Fax: 615-322-8236
TDD: 615-343-2958
E-mail: kc@vanderbilt.edu
www.kc.vanderbilt.edu

Pat Leavitt PhD, Center Acting Director
Jan Rosemergy PhD, Director Communications

Research and research training related to disorders of thinking, learning, perception, communication, mood and emotion caused by disruption of typical development. Available services include behavior analysis clinic, referrals, lectures and conferences, and a free quarterly newsletter.

Texas

2110 Children's Mental Health Partnership

1430 Collier Street
Austin, TX 78704
512-445-7780
Fax: 512-445-7701
www.mhatexas.org

A coalition of human services providers, parents, educators and juvenile court professionals who care about the special mental health needs of Austin area youth and families.

2111 Dallas Federation of Families for Children's Mental Health

2629 Sharpview Lane
Dallas, TX 75228-6047
214-320-1825
Fax: 214-320-3750
www.mentalhealth.samhsa.gov/databases/MHDR.asp?D1=
TX&T

Susan Rogers

The Dallas Federation is an advocacy service for families in need. They act as a liaison between professionals and families in need of specialized services for children with emotional/behavioral problems. They conduct trainings and workshops on national, state and local levels, regarding children's mental health.

2112 Depression and Bipolar Support Alliance of Houston and Harris County
10000 Memorial Drive
Suite 170
Houston, TX 77024-3486
713-528-1546
Fax: 713-812-1235
E-mail: info@dbsahouston.org
www.dbsahouston.org

Jennifer Urbach
Peggy Roe

Self-help, nonprofit organization for those who have been diagnosed or have symptoms of mood disorder. Families and friends of people with mood disorders are also involved. Provides personal support and direct services to its members, educates the public about the nature and management of these treatable disorders, and promotes related research.

2113 Fox Counseling Service
1900 Pease Street
Suite 310
Vernon, TX 76384-4625
940-553-3783
800-687-9439
Fax: 940-553-3783

Fred Fox, Sole Proprietor

Marital counseling using PREP, family counseling, ADHD diagnosis and management. Couseling for mental health issues, depression, anxiety, stress, etc.

2114 Jewish Family Service of Dallas
5402 Arapaho Road
Dallas, TX 75248
214-437-9950
Fax: 214-437-1988
E-mail: info@jfsdallas.org
www.jfsdallas.org

Michael Fleisher, Executive Director

2115 Jewish Family Service of San Antonio
12500 NW Military Hwy
#250
San Antonio, TX 78231-1871
210-302-6920
Fax: 210-349-6952
E-mail: johnsonb@jfs-sa.org

2116 Mental Health Association
670 N 7th Street
Beaumont, TX 77702-1741
409-833-9657
Fax: 409-833-3522
www.mhatexas.org/

Jayne Bordelon, Executive Director

Non-profit agency offering free information, referral services, educational programs, and advocay to all of Jefferson County.

2117 National Alliance on Mental Illness: Texas
Fountain Park Plaza III
2800 South IH35, Suite 140
Austin, TX 78704
512-693-2000
800-633-3760
Fax: 512-693-8000
E-mail: rpeyson@namitexas.org
www.namitexas.org

Lee Burns, President
Robin Peyson, Executive Director

The mission of NAMI Texas is to improve the lives of all persons affected by serious mental illness by providing support, education and advocacy through a grassroots network.

2118 Parent Connection
West Conroe Baptist Church
1855 Longmire Road
Conroe, TX 77304
936-760-1911
Fax: 936-760-1915
E-mail: wcbc@wcbc.us OR dany.daniel@wcbc.us
www.wcbc.us/wcb/ministries

Dany Daniel

For parents of teens which provides an opportunity for fellowship and a time of learning and sharing with other parents. Parents research and present information on relevant teen topics. There are small and large group discussions. Meets the first Sunday of the month at 5:00 p.m. in the new Student Ministry Building of the West Conroe Baptist Church.

2119 Texas Alliance for the Mentally Ill
Fountain Park Plaza III
2800 South IH35, Suite 140
Austin, TX 78704
512-693-2000
800-633-3760
Fax: 512-693-3760
E-mail: amidad@aol.com
www.namitexas.org

Joe Lovelace, Executive Director

Nation's leading self-help organization for all those affected by severe brain disorders. Mission is to bring consumers and families with similar experiences together to share information about services, care providers, and ways to cope with the challenges of schizophrenia, manic depression, and other serious mental illnesses.

2120 Texas Counseling Association
1204 San Antonio
Suite 201
Austin, TX 78701
512-472-3403
800-580-8144
Fax: 512-472-3756
E-mail: jan@txca.org
www.txca.org/tca/Default.asp

Jan Friese, Executive Director

The Texas Counseling Association is an association of professional counselors that provides leadership, service and advocacy and that promotes education and ethical standards.

2121 Texas Federation of Families for Children's Mental Health
7701 North Lama
Suite 518
Austin, TX 78752
512-407-8844
866-893-3264
Fax: 512-407-8266
E-mail: PattiDerr@txffcmh.org
www.ffcmh.org/

Patti Derr

The National family-run organization dedicated exclusively to helping children with mental health needs and their families achieve a better quality of life.

2122 Texas Psychological Association
1005 Congress Avenue
Suite 410
Austin, TX 78701
512-280-4099
888-872-3435
Fax: 512-476-7297
E-mail: itexaspsycholog@austin.rr.com
www.texaspsyc.org/

David White, Executive Director

2123 Texas Society of Psychiatric Physicians
401 W 15th Street
Suite 675
Austin, TX 78701
512-478-0605
Fax: 512-487-5223
E-mail: TxPsychiatry@aol.com
www.txpsych.org/

John R Bush, Executive Director

2124 University of Texas Southwestern Medical Center
5323 Harry Hines Boulevard
Dallas, TX 75390
214-648-3111
Fax: 214-648-8955
www.8.utsouthwestern.edu/

Kern Wildenthal, MD/Ph.D, President

Utah

2125 Allies for Youth & Families
2900 S State Street
Suite 301
Salt Lake City, UT 84115
801-467-1500
Fax: 801-467-0328
E-mail: wlolo@sisna.com
www.slsheriff.org/html/family_resources.html

Wilton Lolofie

2126 DMDA/DBSA: Uplift
444 W. Stonehedge Drive
Salt Lake City, UT 84107
801-264-8193
www.thewindsofchange.org/by_state.html

John W Kreipl

2127 Healthwise of Utah
2505 Parleys Way
Suite 30270
Salt Lake City, UT 84130-0270
801-333-2000
www.insurance.state.ut.us/Chpt30.html

2128 National Alliance on Mental Illness: Utah
450 2 900 E
Suite 160
Salt Lake City, UT 84102-2981
801-323-9900
Fax: 801-323-9799
E-mail: education@maniut.org
www.namiut.org

Alex Morrison, President
Sherri Wittwer, Executive Director

NAMI Utah's mission is to ensure the dignity and improve the lives of those who live with mental illness and their families through support, education and advocacy.

2129 Utah Parent Center
2290 E 4500 Street S
Suite 110
Salt Lake City, UT 84117-4428
801-272-1051
800-468-1160
Fax: 801-272-8907
E-mail: upcinfo@utahparentcenter.org
www.utahparentcenter.org

Helen Post, Executive Director
Jennie Gibson, Associate Director

The Utah Parent Center is a statewide nonprofit organization founded in 1984 to provide training, information, referral and assistance to parents of children and youth with all disabilities: physical, mental, learning and emotional. Staff at the center are primarily parents of children and youth with disabilities who carry out the philosophy of Parents Helping Parents.

2130 Utah Psychiatric Association
540 East 500 South
Salt Lake City, UT 84102
801-355-7477
Fax: 801-532-1550
E-mail: paige@utahmed.org
www.psych.org/dbs_state_soc/db_list/db_info_dyn.cfm

Paige De Mille, Executive Director

Vermont

2131 Fletcher Allen Health Care
111 Colchester Avenue
Burlington, VT 05401-1416
802-847-0000
800-358-1144
Fax: 802-656-2733
www.fahc.org/

Melinda L Estes, MD, President/CEO
Richarad Magnuson, CFO
Angeline Marano, COO
Theresa Alberghini Dipalma, VP/Government External Affairs

2132 National Alliance on Mental Illness: Vermont
132 South Main Street
Waterbury, VT 05676-1519
802-244-1396
800-639-6480
Fax: 802-244-1405
E-mail: namivt@verizon.net
www.namivt.org

Ann Moore, President
Larry Lewack, Executive Director

NAMI-Vermont is a statewide volunteer organization comprised of family members, friends, and individuals affected by mental illness. We have experienced the struggles and have joined together in membership to help ourselves and others by providing support, information, education and advocacy.

2133 Retreat Healthcare
Anna Marsh Lane
PO Box 803
Brattleboro, VT 05301-0803
802-257-7755
800-738-7328
Fax: 802-258-3791
TDD: 802-258-8770
www.retreathealthcare.org/

Richard T Palmisano, President/CEO
Gregory A Miller, VP Medical Affairs
Robert Soucy, COO
John E Blaha, VP/CFO

2134 Vermont Alliance for the Mentally Ill
132 South Main Street
Waterbury, VT 05676-1519
802-244-1396
800-639-6480
Fax: 802-244-1405
E-mail: namivt1@adelphia.net
www.www.namivt.org

Jerry Goessel, Executive Director

Nation's leading self-help organization for all those affected by severe brain disorders. Mission is to bring consumers and families with similar experiences together to share information about services, care providers, and ways to cope with the challenges of schizophrenia, manic depression, and other serious mental illnesses.

2135 Vermont Employers Health Alliance
104 Church Street
P O Box 987
Burlington, VT 05401-0987
802-865-0525
Fax: 805-862-5443

Jeanne Keller, MS/ARM, President

2136 Vermont Federation of Families for Children's Mental Health
28 Barre Street
PO Box 607
Montpelier, VT 05601-0607
802-223-4917
800-639-6071
Fax: 802-828-2159
E-mail: vffcmh@verizon.net
www.vffcmh.org

Kathy Holsopple, Executive Director

Virginia

2137 Anthem BC/BS of Virginia
2220/2221 Edward Holland Drive
Richmond, VA 23230-2518
804-354-2007
Fax: 804-354-2536

Clark Dumont, Anthem East Coast Media Contact

2138 First Hospital Corporation
240 Corporate Boulevard
Norfolk, VA 23502-4948
757-459-5100
866-867-2537
Fax: 757-459-5219

2139 Garnett Day Treatment Center
University of Virginia Health System/UVHS
1 Garnet Center Drive
Charlottesville, VA 22911-8572
434-977-3425
Fax: 434-977-8529
www.healthsystem.virginia.edu/internet/homehealth/

Byrd S Leavell Jr, MD, President UVHS

2140 NAMI
2107 Wilson Boulevard
Suite 300
Arlington, VA 22201-3042
703-524-7600
Fax: 703-524-9094
www.nami.org

Michael Fitzpatrick, Executive Director
Lynn Borton, COO

Dedicated to the eradication of mental illnesses and to the improvement of the quality of life of all whose lives are affected by these diseases.

2141 National Alliance on Mental Illness: Virgini a
PO Box 8260
Richmond, VA 23226-0260
804-285-8264
888-486-8264
Fax: 804-285-8464
E-mail: namiva@comcast.net
www.namivirginia.org

Bill Farrington, President
Mira Signer, Executive Director

Created in 1985 to provide support, education, and advocacy for consumers and families in Virginia affected by mental illness. It is our mission to improve the lives of all those who are affected by serious brain disorders and to fight the stigma that surrounds mental illness.

2142 Parent Resource Center
Division of Special Education And Student Services
Virginia Department of Education
P O Box 2120
Richmond, VA 23218-2120
804-371-7421
800-422-2083
Fax: 804-559-6835
E-mail: judy.hudgins@doe.virginia.gov
www.www.doe.virginia.gov/VDOE/sess

Judy Hudgins, Specialist

2143 Richmond Support Group
Warwick Medical & Professional Center
7149 Jahnke Road
Richmond, VA 23225
804-320-7881

Kenneth P Brooks, MD
Richard E Curtis, MD

2144 Virginia Beach Community Service Board
Pembroke 6
Suite 208
Virginia Beach, VA 23462
757-437-5770
Fax: 804-490-5736

Jerry W Brickeen, Media Contact

2145 Virginia Federation of Families
PO Box 26691
Richmond, VA 23261-6691
804-559-6833
800-447-0946
Fax: 804-559-6835
E-mail: pacct@infionline.net
www.pacct.net

Joyce B Kube, Executive Director
Randy Del Rossi, Family Support Coordinataor

Support and education for parents and family members of children and adolescents with mental, emotional and behavioral disorders.

2146 Virginia Federation of Families for Children's Mental Health
1101 King Street
Suite 420
Alexandria, VA 22314
703-684-7710
Fax: 703-836-1040
E-mail: ffcmh@ffcmh.org
www.ffcmh.org

Sandra Spencer, Executive Director
Gail Daniels, Coordinator Affiliate Relations
Marian Mealing, Administrative Assistant
Trina Osher, Coordinator Policy/Research

Family-run organization dedicated exclusively to children and adolescents with mental health needs and their families. Our work speaks through our work in policy, training and technical assistance programs. Publishes a quarterly newsletter and sponsors an annual conference and exhibits.

Washington

2147 Children's Alliance
2017 E Spruce
Seattle, WA 98122
206-324-0340
Fax: 206-325-6291
E-mail: seattle@childrensalliance.org
www.childrensalliance.org

Paola Maranan, Executive Director
Deborah Bowler, Administration
Ruth Schubert, Communications

Washington's statewide child advocacy organization. We champion public policies and practices that deliver the essentials that kids need to thrive — confidence, stability, health and safety.

2148 Common Voice for Pierce County Parents
801 141st Street E
Tacoma, WA 98445
253-537-2145
Fax: 253-537-2167
E-mail: margecritchlow@hotmail.com
www.mentalhealth.samhsa.gov/databases/MHDR.asp?D1=WA

Marge Critchlow

Family support group.

2149 Good Sam-W/Alliance for the Mentally Ill Family Support Group
325 Pioneer Avenue E
Puyallup, WA 98371
206-848-5571
Fax: 206-845-5355
www.nami.org

Gordon Bopp, Director Washington State Office

Nation's leading self-help organization for all those affected by severe brain disorders. Mission is to bring consumers and families with similar experiences together to share information about services, care providers, and ways to cope with the challenges of schizophrenia, manic depression, and other serious mental illnesses.

2150 Kitsap County Alliance for the Mentally Ill
Health Center
109 Austin Drive NE
Bremerton, WA 98310-0309
360-638-1960
E-mail: blackfish5@comcast.net
www.nami.org

Joyce Wilson
Myra Clodius

Nation's leading self-help organization for all those affected by severe brain disorders. Mission is to bring consumers and families with similar experiences together to share information about services, care providers, and ways to cope with the challenges of schizophrenia, manic depression, and other serious mental illnesses.

2151 Mental Health & Spirituality Support Group
Nami Eastside-Family Resource Center
16315 NE 87th Street
Suite B-11
Redmond, WA 98052
425-489-4084
E-mail: info@nami-eastside.org
www.nami-eastside.org/

John Radoslovich, Email: Johnrad14@Yahoo.Com
Kendra Perkins, Phone: 253-732-8010

Nation's leading self-help organization for all those affected by severe brain disorders. Mission is to bring consumers and families with similar experiences together to share information about services, care providers, and ways to cope with the challenges of schizophrenia, manic depression, and other serious mental illnesses.

2152 National Alliance on Mental Illness: Washington
500 108th Avenue NE
Suite 800
Bellevue, WA 98004-5580

425-990-6404
800-782-9264
E-mail: office@namigreaterseattle.org

Gordon Bopp, President

2153 North Sound Regional Support Network
117 North First Street
Suite 8
Mount Vernon, WA 98273-2858
360-416-7013
800-336-6164
Fax: 360-416-7017
TTY: 360-419-9008
E-mail: nsrsn@nsrsn.org
www.nsrsn.org

Charles Benjamin, Executive Director
Greg Long, Deputy Director

It is the purpose of the North Sound Regional Support Network (NSRSN) to ensure the provision of quality and integrated mental health services for the five counties (San Juan, Skagit, Snohomish, Island, and Whatcom) served by the NSRSN Prepaid Health Plan (PHP). We join together to enhance our community's mental health and support recovery for people with mental illness served in the North Sound region, through high quality culturally competent services.

2154 Nueva Esperanza Counseling Center
720 W Court Street
Suite 8
Pasco, WA 99301-4178
509-545-6506
Fax: 509-546-0520

2155 Pierce County Alliance for the Mentally Ill
304 7th Avenue NW
Puyallup, WA 98371
253-435-4518
www.nami.org

Eric Renz
Nola Renz

Nation's leading self-help organization for all those affected by severe brain disorders. Mission is to bring consumers and families with similar experiences together to share information about services, care providers, and ways to cope with the challenges of schizophrenia, manic depression, and other serious mental illnesses.

2156 Sharing & Caring for Consumers, Families Alliance for the Mentally Ill
NAMI-Eastside Family Resource Center
16315 NE 87th Street
Suite B-11
Redmond, WA 98052
425-885-6264
E-mail: info@nami-eastside.org
www.nami-eastside.org/

Susan Rynas
Bri Wiechmann

Nation's leading self-help organization for all those affected by severe brain disorders. Mission is to bring consumers and families with similar experiences together to share information about services, care providers, and ways to cope with the challenges of schizophrenia, manic depression, and other serious mental illnesses.

2157 South King County Alliance for the Mentally Ill
515 West Harrison Street
Suite 215
Kent, WA 98032
253-854-6264
E-mail: namisouthking@aol.com
www.nami.org/sites/NAMISouthKingCounty

Jim Adams
Sandy Klungness

Nation's leading self-help organization for all those affected by severe brain disorders. Mission is to bring consumers and families with similar experiences together to share information about services, care providers, and ways to cope with the challenges of schizophrenia, manic depression, and other serious mental illnesses.

2158 Spanish Support Group Alliance for the Mentally Ill
NAMI-Eastside
2601 Elliott Avenue
Suite 4143
Seattle, WA 98060
425-747-7892
E-mail: remmedicalraulmunoz@comcast.net
www.nami-eastside.org/

Gordon Bopp, NAMI-WA Contact Information

Nation's leading self-help organization for all those affected by severe brain disorders. Mission is to bring consumers and families with similar experiences together to share information about services, care providers, and ways to cope with the challenges of schizophrenia, manic depression, and other serious mental illnesses.

2159 Spokane Mental Health
107 South Division Street
Spokane, WA 99202-1586
509-838-4651
Fax: 509-458-7449
www.smhca.org/

Nancy Linerud, FCFH Supervisor
Jennifer Allen, UC Coordinator

Since 1970, Spokane Mental Health, a not-for-profit organization, has served children, families, adults and elders throughout Spokane County. Our professional staff provides quality treatment and rehabilitation for those with mental illness and co-occurring disorders. These services include crisis response services; individual, family and group therapy; case management and support; vocational rehabilitation; psychiatric and psychological services; medication management and consumer education. We tailor services to the unique needs and strengths of each person seeking care.

2160 Washington Advocates for the Mentally Ill
NAMI Eastside Family Resource Center
16315 NE 87th Street
Suite B-11
Redmond, WA 98052
425-885-6264
800-782-9264
E-mail: info@nami-eastside.org
www.nami-eastside.org/

Gordon Bopp, NAMI-WA Contact Information

Nation's leading self-help organization for all those affected by severe brain disorders. Mission is to bring consumers and families with similar experiences together to share information about services, care providers, and ways to cope with the challenges of schizophrenia, manic depression, and other serious mental illnesses.

2161 Washington Institute for Mental Illness Research and Training
Washington State University, Spokane
PO Box 1495
Spokane, WA 99210-1495
509-358-7514
Fax: 509-358-7619
www.spokane.wsu.edu/research&service/

Michael Hendrix, Director
Sandie Kruse, Training Coordinator

Governmental organization focusing on mental illness research.

2162 Washington State Psychological Association
711 North 35th Street
Suite 206
Seattle, WA 98103
206-547-4220
Fax: 206-547-6366
E-mail: wspa@wapsych.org
www.wapsych.org

Doug Wear, Ph.D, Executive Director
Wren St. Hilaire, Assistant Director

To support, promote and advance the science, education and practice of psychology in the public interest.

2163 Whidbey Island Alliance for the Mentally Ill
NAMI Whidbey Island Oak Harbor, WA
98277-8028
360-675-7358
Fax: 360-675-7358
E-mail: info@namiwi.org
www.nami.org OR namiwi.org

Margaret Houlihan

Nation's leading self-help organization for all those affected by severe brain disorders. Mission is to bring consumers and families with similar experiences together to share information about services, care providers, and ways to cope with the challenges of schizophrenia, manic depression, and other serious mental illnesses.

West Virginia

2164 CAMC Family Medicine Center of Charleston
1201 Washington Street East
Suite 108
Charleston, WV 25301
304-347-4600
Fax: 304-347-4621
www.hsc.wvu.edu/charleston/familymed/

Robert M D'Alessandri, MD, Vice President Health Sciences

2165 Mountain State Parents Children Adolescent Network
1201 Garfield Street
McMechen, WV 26040
304-233-5399
800-244-5385
Fax: 304-233-3847

E-mail: toothman@mspcan.org
www.mspcan.org

Teri Toothman, Executive Director
Susan Nally, CFO

Support, education and training for families who have a child with serious emotional disturbance.

2166 National Alliance on Mental Illness: West Virginia
PO Box 2706
Charleston, WV 25330-2706
304-342-0497
800-598-5653
Fax: 304-342-0499
E-mail: namiwv@aol.com
www.namiwv.org

Randal Johnson, President
Michael Ross, Executive Director

The voice for the families of those individuals with a serious mental illness.

2167 West Virginia Alliance for the Mentally Ill
PO Box 2706
Charleston, WV 25330-2706
304-342-0497
800-598-5653
Fax: 304-342-0499
E-mail: WVAMAIL@aol.com OR namiwv@aol.com
www.nami.org

Randal Johnson, President
Michael Ross, Executive Director

Nation's leading self-help organization for all those affected by severe brain disorders. Mission is to bring consumers and families with similar experiences together to share information about services, care providers, and ways to cope with the challenges of schizophrenia, manic depression, and other serious mental illnesses.

Wisconsin

2168 Charter BHS of Wisconsin/Brown Deer
4600 W Schroeder Drive
Brown Deer, WI 53223-1469
414-355-2273
Fax: 414-355-6726

2169 Child and Adolescent Psychopharmacology Information
Wisconsin Psychiatric Institute and Clinic
6001 Research Park Boulevard
#1568
Madison, WI 53719-1176
608-263-6171

2170 Families United of Milwaukee
2209 North Martin Luther King Drive
Suite 1
Milwaukee, WI 53212
414-265-2227
Fax: 414-265-2252
E-mail: families@ameritech.net
www.ffcmh.org/

Margaret Jefferson

2171 National Alliance on Mental Illness: Wiscons in
4233 West Beltline Highway
Madison, WI 53711-3814
608-268-6000
800-236-2988
Fax: 608-268-6004
E-mail: namiwisc@choiceonemail.com
www.namiwisconsin.org

Franklin Mixdorf, President
Cheryl Porior-Mayhew, Executive Director

The mission of NAMI Wisconsin is to improve the quality of life of people affected by mental illnesses and to promote recovery.

2172 Stoughton Family Counseling
1520 Vernon Street
Stoughton, WI 53589-2260
608-873-6422
Fax: 608-873-6014

2173 Wisconsin Alliance for the Mentally Ill
NAMI-Wisconsin
4233 West Beltline Highway
Madison, WI 53711-3814
608-268-6000
800-236-2988
Fax: 608-268-6004
E-mail: nami@namiwisconsin.org
www.namiwisconsin.org/

Nancy Phythyon, President
Donna Wren, Executive Director

Self-help organization for all those affected by severe brain disorders. Mission is to bring consumers and families with similar experiences together to share information about services, care providers, and ways to cope with the challanges of schizophrenia, manic depression, and other serious mental illnesses.

2174 Wisconsin Association of Family and Child Agency
131 W Wilson Street
Suite 901
Madison, WI 53703-3245
608-257-5939
Fax: 608-257-6067

2175 Wisconsin Family Ties
16 N Carroll Street
Suite 640
Madison, WI 53703-2726
608-267-6888
800-422-7145
Fax: 608-267-6801
E-mail: info@wifamilyties.org
www.wifamilyties.org

Hugh Davis, Executive Director
Joan Maynard, Information Referral Coordinator

Wyoming

2176 Central Wyoming Behavioral Health at Lander Valley
1320 Bishop Randall Drive
Lander, WY 82520-3939
307-332-5700
800-788-9446

Fax: 307-335-6465
www.landerhospital.com/patientservices.htm

Rebecca K Smith

2177 National Alliance on Mental Illness: Wyoming
133 W 6th Street
Casper, WY 82601-3124
307-234-0440
888-882-4968
Fax: 307-265-0968
E-mail: nami-wyo@qwest.net
www.nami.org/sites/namiwyoming

Theresa Bush, President
Anna Edwards, Executive Director

2178 Uplift
200 West 17th Street
Suite 664
Cheyenne, WY 82003-0664
307-778-8686
888-875-4383
Fax: 307-778-8681
E-mail: uplift@wyoming.com
www.upliftwy.org/

Ron Vigil, President
Peggy Nikkel, Executive Director
Jane Caton, Vice President

Wyoming Chapter of the Federation of Familes for Children's Mental Health. Providing support, education, advocacy, information and referral for parents and professionals focusing on emotional, behavioral and learning needs of children and youth.

2179 Wyoming Alliance for the Mentally Ill
NAMI Wyoming
133 W 6th Street
Casper, WY 82601-3124
307-234-0440
888-882-4968
Fax: 307-234-0440
E-mail: nami-wyo@qwest.net
www.nami.org/sites/namiwyoming

Theresa Bush, President

Nation's leading self-help organization for all those affected by severe brain disorders. Mission is to bring consumers and families with similar experiences together to share information about services, care providers, and ways to cope with the challenges of schizophrenia, manic depression, and other serious mental illnesses.

Government Agencies

Federal

2180 Administration for Children and Families
370 L'Enfant Promenade SW
Washington, DC 20201
202-401-4802
Fax: 202-401-5706
www.acf.hhs.gov/index.html

Kenneth Wolfe, Acting Director
Joan E Ohl, Commissioner

Responsible for federal programs that promotes the economic and social well-being of families, children, individuals, and communities.

2181 Administration for Children, Youth and Families
US Department of Health & Human Services
370 L'Enfant Promenade SW
Washington, DC 20201
202-401-4802
Fax: 202-401-5706
www.acf.hhs.gov/programs/acyf/acyf.htm

Kenneth Wolfe, Acting Director
Joan E Ohl, Commissioner

Advises Health and Human Services department on plans and programs related to early childhood development; operates the Head Start day care and other related child service programs; provides leadership, advice, and services that affect the general well-being of children and youths.

2182 Administration on Aging
1 Massachusetts Avenue
Suites 4100 & 5100
Washington, DC 20201
202-619-0724
E-mail: aoainfo@aoahhs.gov
www.www.aoa.gov

One of the nation's largest providers of home and community-based care for older persons and their caregivers. The mission is to promote the dignity and independence of older people, and help society prepare for an aging population.

2183 Administration on Developmental Disabilities
US Department of Health & Human Services
370 L'Enfant Promenade SW
Washington, DC 20201
202-690-6590
Fax: 202-690-6904
www.acf.hhs.gov/programs/add

Joan Ohl, Commissioner
Kenneth Wolfe, Acting Director

Develops and administers programs protecting rights and promoting independence, productivity and inclusion; funds state grants, protection and advocacy programs, University Affiliated Programs and other national projects.

2184 Agency for Healthcare Research and Quality: Office of Communications and Knowledge Transfer
540 Gaither Road
Suite 2000
Rockville, MD 20850

301-427-1364
www.ahrq.org

Provides policymakers and other health care leaders with information needed to make critical health care decisions.

2185 Association of Maternal and Child Health Programs (AMCHP)
1220 19th Street NW
Suite 801
Washington, DC 20036
202-775-0436
Fax: 202-775-0061
E-mail: lramo@amchp.org
www.amchp.org

Lauren Raskin-Ramos, Director Of Programs
Michael Fraser, CEO

National non-profit organization representing state public health workers. Provides leadership to assure the health and well-being of women of reproductive age, children, youth, including those with special health care needs and their families.

2186 Center for Mental Health Services Homeless Programs Branch
Substance Abuse and Mental Health Services Administration
1 Choke Cherry Road
Rockville, MD 20857
240-276-1310
Fax: 240-276-1320
www.samhsa.gov

Federal agency concerned with the prevention and treatment of mental illness and the promotion of mental health. Homeless Programs Branch administers a variety of programs and activities. Provides professional leadership for collaborative intergovernmental initiatives designed to assist persons with mental illnesses who are homeless. Also supports a contract for the National Resource Center on Homelessness and Mental Illness.

2187 Center for Substance Abuse Treatment
Substance Abuse Mental Health Services Administration
1 Choke Cherry Road
Rockville, MD 20857
240-276-1660
Fax: 240-276-1670
www.samhsa.gov

2188 Centers for Disease Control & Prevention
1600 Clifton Road
Atlanta, GA 30333
404-498-1515
800-311-3435
www.cdc.gov/

Protecting the health and safety of people — at home and abroad, providing credible information to enhance health decisions, and promoting health through strong partnership. Serves as the national focus for developing and applying disease prevention and control, environmental health, and health promotion in education activities designed to improve the health of the people of the United States.

2189 Centers for Medicare & Medicaid Services: Health Policy
7500 Security Blvd
Baltimore, MD 21244
410-786-3000
www.cms.hhs.gov/

2190 Committee for Truth in Psychiatry: CTIP
PO Box 1214
New York, NY 10003
212-665-6587
E-mail: ctip@erols.com
www.harborside.com/~equinox/ect.htm

Linda Andre, Director

Former psychiatric patients who have had electroconvulsive therapy (ECT's), working toward informed consent to shock treatment. Works to retain ECT's current FDA classification as a high-risk procedure. Publications: Synopsis of the Conflict Over ECT at the FDA, pamphlet. FDA's Regulatory Proceedings Concerning ECT, pamphlet. Shockwaves, quarterly. Future patients should be informed before they give their consent to such treatment.

2191 DC Department of Mental Health
64 New York Avenue, NE
4th Floor
Washington, DC 20002
202-673-7440
888-793-4357
www.dmh.dc.gov

The goal of the Department of Mental Health is to develop, support, and oversee a comprehensive, community-based, consumer-driven, culturally competent, quality mental health system. This system should be responsive and accessible to children, youths, adults, and their families. It should leverage continuous positive change through its ability to learn and to partner. It should also ensure that mental health providers are accountable to consumers and offer services that promote recovery from mental illness.

2192 Equal Employment Opportunity Commission
1801 L Street NW
Washington, DC 20507
202-663-4900
800-669-4000
TTY: 800-669-6820
E-mail: info@eeoc.gov
www.www.eeoc.gov

To eradicate employment discrimination at workplace.

2193 Health Care For All(HCFA)
30 Winter Street
10th Floor
Boston, MA 02108
617-350-7279
Fax: 617-451-5838
TTY: 617-350-0974
E-mail: mcdonough@hcfama.org
www.www.hcfama.org

John E McDonough, Executive Director
Lynn Wickwire, Director Communication/Develop.

2194 Health Systems and Financing Group
Health Resources and Services Administration
5600 Fishers Lane
Rockville, MD 20857
301-443-2194
www.www.hrsa.gov

Elizabeth Duke, Administrator
Dennis Williams, Deputy Administrator

2195 Health and Human Services Office of Assistant Secretary for Planning & Evaluation
200 Independence Avenue SW
Washington, DC 20201
202-619-0257
877-696-6775
www.wwww.aspe.hhs.gov

2196 Information Resources and Inquiries Branch
National Institute of Mental Health
6001 Executive Boulevard
Room 8184
Bethesda, MD 20892-9663
301-443-4513
866-615-6464
Fax: 301-443-4279
TTY: 301-443-8431
E-mail: nimhinfo@nih.gov
www.nimh.nih.gov

A component of the National Institute of Health, the NIMH conducts and supports research that seeks to understand, treat and prevent mental illness. The Institute's Information Resources and Inquiries Branch (IRIB) responds to information requests from the lay public, clinicians and the scientific community with a variety of publications on subjects such as basic behavioral research, neuroscience of mental health, rural mental, children's mental disorders, schizophrenia, paranoia, depression, bipolar disorder, learning disabilities, Alzheimer's disease, panic, obsessive compulsive and other anxiety disorders. A publication list is available upon request.

2197 National Institutes of Mental Health Division of Intramural Research Programs (DIRP)
10 Center Drive
Room 4N222 MSC 1381
Bethesda, MD 20892-1381
301-496-4183
Fax: 301-480-8348
www.intramural.nimh.nih.gov/

Maxine Steyer, Contact

The Division of Intramural Research Programs (DIRP) at the National Institute of Mental Health (NIMH) is the internal research division of the NIMH. NIMH DIRP scientists conduct research ranging from studies into mechanisms of normal brain function, conducted at the behavioral, systems, cellular, and molecular levels, to clinical investigations into the diagnosis, treatment and prevention of mental illness. Major disease entities studied throughout the lifespan include mood disorders and anxiety, schizophrenia, obsessive-compulsive disorder, attention deficit hyperactivity disorder, and pediatric autoimmune neuropsychiatric disorders.

2198 National Center for HIV, STD and TB Prevention
Centers For Disease Control and Prevention
1600 Clifton Road
NE Mailstop E-10
Atlanta, GA 30333
800-232-4636
TTY: 888-232-6348
E-mail: cdcinfo@cdc.gov
www.www.cdc.gov/nchstp/tb/default.htm

2199 National Clearinghouse for Drug & Alcohol
PO Box 2345
Rockville, MD 20847
800-729-6686
TDD: 800-487-4889
www.www.ncadi.samhsa.gov

2200 National Institute of Alcohol Abuse and Alcoholism: Treatment Research Branch
5635 Fishers Lane
MSC 9304
Bethesda, MD 20892-9304
301-443-3860
E-mail: niaaaweb-r@exchange.nih.gov
www.niaaa.nih.gov/

NIAAA provides leadership in the national effort to reduce alcohol-related problems by conducting and supporting research in a wide range of scientific areas including genetics, neuroscience, epidemiology, health risks and benefits of alcohol consumption, prevention, and treatment.

2201 National Institute of Alcohol Abuse and Alcoholism: Homeless Demonstration and Evaluation Branch
5600 Fishers Lane
Msc 9304
Rockville, MD 20892
301-443-3860
E-mail: niaaaweb-r@exchange.nih.gov
www.niaaa.nih.gov/

NIAAA provides leadership in the national effort to reduce alcohol-related problems by conducting and supporting research in a wide range of scientific areas including genetics, neuroscience, epidemiology, health risks and benefits of alcohol consumption, prevention, and treatment.

2202 National Institute of Alcohol Abuse and Alcoholism: Office of Policy Analysis
The Alcohol Policy Information System (APIS)
5600 Fishers Lane
Room 16-95
Rockville, MD 20857-0002
301-443-3864
E-mail: niaaaweb-r@exchange.nih.gov

The Alcohol Policy Information System (APIS) is an online resource that provides detailed information on a wide variety of alcohol-related policies in the United States at both State and Federal levels. It features compilations and analyses of alcohol-related statutes and regulations. Designed primarily as a tool for researchers, APIS simplifies the process of ascertaining the state of the law for studies on the effects and effectiveness of alcohol-related policies.

2203 National Institute of Drug Abuse: NIDA
6001 Executive Boulevard
Room 5213
Bethesda, MD 20892-9561
301-443-1124
E-mail: information@nida.nih.gov
www.nida.nih.gov

Covers the areas of drug abuse treatment and prevention research, epidemiology, neuroscience and behavioral research, health services research and AIDS. Seeks to report on advances in the field, identify resources, promote an exchange of information, and improve communications among clinicians, researchers, administrators, and policymakers. Recurring features include synopses of research advances and projects, NIDA news, news of legislative and regulatory developments, and announcements.

2204 National Institute of Mental Health: Schizophrenia Research Branch
6001 Executive Boulevard
Room 8184, MSC 9663
Bethesda, MD 20892-9663
301-443-4513
E-mail: nimhinfo@nih.gov
www.www.nimh.nih.gov

Information available includes a detailed booklet that provides an overview of schizophrenia and also describes symptoms, causes, and treatments, with information on getting help and coping.

2205 National Institute of Mental Health: Mental Disorders of the Aging
National Institutes of Health
6001 Executive Boulevard
Room 8184, MSC 9663
Bethesda, MD 20892-9663
301-443-4513
E-mail: nimhinfo@nih.gov
www.nimh.nih.gov/

The Aging Research Consortium was established in January 2002 by NIMH. Its mission is to: Stimulate research on mental health and mental illness to benefit older adults; Maintain an infrastructure to better coordinate aging research throughout the Institute; Provide a linkage to the Institute for researchers, advocates, and the public and advance research training for the study of late life mental disorders.

2206 National Institute of Mental Health: Office of Science Policy, Planning, and Communications
National Institutes of Health
6001 Executive Boulevard
Room 8208 MSC 9667
Bethesda, MD 20892-9667
301-443-4335
E-mail: nimhinfo@nih.gov
www.nimh.nih.gov

Plans and directs a comprehensive strategic agenda for national mental health policy, including science program planning and related policy evaluation, research training and coordination, and technology and information transfer. OSPPC plans and implements portfolio analysis, scientific disease coding, and program evaluations for developing and assessing NIMH strategic plans and portfolio management. OSPPC also creates and implements the Institute's communication efforts, including information dissemination, media relations activities, and internal communications. The Office proposes and guides science education activities concerned with informing the scientific community and public about mental health issues.

2207 National Institute on Drug Abuse: Office of Science Policy and Communications

6001 Executive Boulevard
Room 5153, MSC 9589
Bethesda, MD 20892-9589
301-443-6504
www.nida.nih.gov/

The Office of Science Policy and Communications (OSPC) carries out a wide variety of functions in support of the Director, NIDA, and on behalf of the Institute. We're made up of the Office of the Director and the International Program Office, and two branches, the Science Policy Branch and the Public Information and Liaison Branch.

2208 National Institute on Drug Abuse: Division of Clinical Neurosciences and Behavioral Research

6001 Executive Boulevard
Room 4123, MSC 9551
Bethesda, MD 20892-9551
301-443-4877
E-mail: sgrant@nida.nih.gov
www.nida.nih.gov

Steven Grant Ph.D, Chief

The Clinical Neuroscience Branch (CNB) advances a clinical research and research training program focused on understanding the neurobiological substrates of drug abuse and addiction processes and on characterizing how abused drugs affect the structure, function, development, and maturation of the human central nervous system. Another major emphasis of this program is on etiological studies examining individual differences in neurobiological, genetic, and neurobehavioral factors that underlie increased risk and/or resilience to drug abuse, addiction, and drug-related disorders, as well as on the neurobiological/neurobehavioral factors involved in the transition from drug use to addiction.

2209 National Institutes of Health: National Center for Research Resources (NCCR) 6701 Democracy Boulevard, MSC 4874 Baltimore, MD 20892

301-435-0888
Fax: 301-480-3558
E-mail: info@ncrr.nih.gov
www.ncrr.nih.gov/

The National Center for Research Resources (NCRR), a component of the National Institutes of Health that supports primary research to create and develop critical resources, models, and technologies. NCRR funding also provides biomedical researchers with access to diverse instrumentation, technologies, basic and clinical research facilities, animal models, genetic stocks, biomaterials, and more. These resources enable scientific advances in biomedicine that lead to the development of lifesaving drugs, devices, and therapies.

2210 National Institutes of Mental Health: Office on AIDS

National Institutes of Health
6001 Executive Boulevard
Room 6225, MSC 9621
Bethesda, MD 20892-9621

301-443-6100
www.nimh.nih.gov/oa/

(1) Plans, directs, coordinates, and supports biomedical and behavioral research designed to develop a better understanding of the biological and behavioral causes of HIV (AIDS virus) infection and more effective mechanisms for the diagnosis, treatment, and prevention of AIDS; (2) analyzes and evaluates National needs and research opportunities to identify areas warranting either increased or decreased program emphasis; and (3) consults and cooperates with voluntary and professional health organizations, as well as other NIH components and Federal agencies, to identify and meet AIDS-related needs.

2211 National Library of Medicine

National Instiues of Health
8600 Rockville Pike
Bethesda, MD 20894
301-594-5983
Fax: 301-496-2809
E-mail: custserv@nlm.nih.gov/
www.nlm.nih.gov/

Donald A B Lindberg MD, Director

The National Library of Medicine (NLM), on the campus of the National Institutes of Health in Bethesda, Maryland, is the world's largest medical library. The Library collects materials and provides information and research services in all areas of biomedicine and health care.

2212 Office of Applied Studies, SA & Mental Health Services

1 Choke Cherry Road
Rockville, MD 20857
240-276-2000
Fax: 240-276-2010
www.oas.samhsa.gov/

The Office of Applied Studies provides the latest national data on alchohol, tobacco, marijuana and other drug abuse in addition to drug related emergency department epidosdes, medical examiner cases and the nation's substance abuse treatment system.

2213 Office of Disease Prevention & Health Promotion

US Department of Health and Human Services
1101 Wootton Parkway, Suite Ll100
Rockville, MD 20852
240-453-8280
Fax: 240-453-8282
www.odphp.osophs.dhhs.gov/

CPT Penelope Royall PT/MSW, Director

The Office of Disease Prevention and Health Promotion, Office of Public Health and Science, Office of the Secretary, U.S. Department of Health and Human Services, works to strengthen the disease prevention and health promotion priorities of the Department within the collaborative framework of the HHS agencies.

2214 Office of National Drug Control Policy

Drug Policy Information Clearinghouse
PO Box 6000
Rockville, MD 20849-6000
800-666-3332
Fax: 301-519-5212
www.whitehousedrugpolicy.gov/

The goal of the Department of Mental Health is to develop, support, and oversee a comprehensive, community-based, consumer-driven, culturally competent, quality mental health system. This system should be responsive and accessible to children, youths, adults, and their families. It should leverage continuous positive change through its ability to learn and to partner. It should also ensure that mental health providers are accountable to consumers and offer services that promote recovery from mental illness.

2215 Office of Program and Policy Development
National Association of Community Health Centers
7200 Wisconcin Ave
Suite 210
Bethesda, MD 20814
301-347-0400
www.nachc.com/hco/hcops.asp

2216 Office of Science Policy OD/NIH
1 Center Drive
Building 1, Room 218
Bethesda, MD 20892
301-496-1454
Fax: 301-402-0280
www.www.ospp.od.nih.gov

Advises the NIH Director on science policy issues affecting the medical research community; Participates in the development of new policy and program initiatives; Monitors and coordinates agency planning and evaluation activities; Plans and implements a comprehensive science education program and Develops and implements NIH policies and procedures for the safe conduct of recombinant DNA and other biotechnology activities.

2217 President's Committee on Mental Retardation
US DHHS, Administration for Children & Families, PCMR
370 L'Enfatne Promenade SW
Washington, DC 20447
202-619-0634
www.acf.dhhs.gov/programs/pcmr

Wade F Horn PhD, Author
Curtis L Coy, Deputy Assistant Secretary

The PCMR acts in an advisory capacity to the President and the Secretary of Health and Human Services on matters relating to programs and services for persons with mental retardation. It has adopted several national goals in order to better recognize and uphold the right of all people with mental retardation to enjoy a quality of life that promotes independence, self-determination and participation as productive members of society.

2218 Presidential Commission on Employment of the Disabled
Frances Perkins Building
200 Constitution Avenue, NW
Washington, DC 20210
866-633-7365
Fax: 202-693-7888
TTY: 877-889-5627
www.www.dol.gov/odep

The Office of Disability Employment Policy (ODEP) was authorized by Congress in the Department of Labor's FY 2001 appropriation. Recognizing the need for a national policy to ensure that people with disabilities are fully integrated into the 21 st Century workforce, the Secretary of Labor Elaine L. Chao delegated authority and assigned responsibility to the Assistant Secretary for Disability Employment Policy. ODEP is a sub-cabinet level policy agency in the Department of Labor.

2219 Protection and Advocacy Program for the Mentally Ill
US Department of Health and Human Services
1 Choke Cherry Road
Rockville, MD 20857
240-276-1310
Fax: 240-276-1320
www.samhsa.gov/index.aspx

Federal formula grant program to protect and advocate the rights of people with mental illnesses who are in residential facilities and to investigate abuse and neglect in such facilities.

2220 Public Health Foundation
1300 L Street NW
Suite 800
Washington, DC 20005
202-218-4400
Fax: 202-218-4409
E-mail: info@phf.org
www.www.phf.org

Ricardo Martinez MD, President/CEO/Chairman

A high-performing public health system that protects and promotes health in every community by improving public health infrastructure and performance through innovative solutions and measurable results.

2221 Substance Abuse & Mental Health Services Adminstration (SAMHSA)
1 Choke Cherry Road
Rockville, MD 20857
240-276-1017
Fax: 240-276-1050
www.samhsa.gov/

Ronald Manderscheid, Director

Agency within the United States Department of health and human services that works to improve the quality and availability of substance abuse prevention, addiction treatment and mental health services.

2222 Substance Abuse and Mental Health Services Administration: Center for Mental Health Services
SAMHSA
PO Box 42557
Washington, DC 20015
240-221-4022
800-789-2647
Fax: 240-221-4021
TDD: 866-889-2647
www.www.mentalhealth.samhsa.gov

2223 US Department of Health & Human Services: Indian Health Service
801 Thompson Avenue, Suite 400
Rockville, MD 20852-1627
301-443-3024
E-mail: webmaster@ihs.gov
www.www.ihs.gov

The mission of Indian Health Service is to raise the physical, mental, social, and spiritual health of American Indians and Alaska Natives to the highest level; to assure that comprehensive, culturally acceptable personal and public health services are available and accessible to American Indian and Alaska Native people; and to uphold the Federal Government's obligation to promote healthy American Indian and Alaska Native people, communities, and cultures and to honor and protect the inherent sovereign rights of Tribes.

2224 US Department of Health and Human Services Planning and Evaluation
200 Independence Ave SW
Washington, DC 20201
202-619-0257
877-696-6775
www.www.hhs.gov

Mike Leavitt, Secretary

Responsible for policy development and for major activities in policy coordination, legislation development, strategic planning, policy research, evaluation, and economic analysis.

2225 US Department of Health and Human Services Bureau of Primary Health
Health Resources and Services Administration
5600 Fishers Lane
Rockville, MD 20857
301-594-4491
Fax: 301-594-0089
www.bphc.hrsa.gov/

Elizabeth Duke, Administrator

HRSA directs programs that improve the Nation's health by expanding access to comprehensive, quality health care for all Americans. HRSA works to improve and extend life for people living with HIV/AIDS, provide primary health care to medically underserved people, serve women and children through state programs, and train a health workforce that is both diverse and motivated to work in underserved communities.

2226 US Department of Health and Human Services: Office of Women's Health
200 Independence Avenue SW
Washington, DC 20201
202-690-7650
www.4woman.gov/owh/index.htm

Wanda Jones, Deputy Assistant Secretary

The Office on Women's Health (OWH) was established in 1991 within the U.S. Department of Health and Human Services. OWH coordinates the efforts of all the HHS agencies and offices involved in women's health. OWH works to improve the health and well-being of women and girls in the United States through its innovative programs, by educating health professionals, and motivating behavior change in consumers through the dissemination of health information.

2227 US Veterans Administration: Mental Health and Behavioral Sciences Services
810 Vermont Avenue NW
Room 900
Washington, DC 20410-0001
202-273-5400
www.va.gov/directory/guide/facility

Jonathan B Perlin MD/Ph.D, Secretary for Health
Michal J Kussman MD, Deputy Secretary for Health

The mission of the Veterans Healthcare System is to serve the needs of America's veterans by providing primary care, specialized care, and related medical and social support services. To accomplish this mission, VHA needs to be a comprehensive, integrated healthcare system that provides excellence in health care value, excellence in service as defined by its customers, and excellence in education and research, and needs to be an organization characterized by exceptional accountability and by being an employer of choice.

2228 California Department of Alcohol and Drug Programs
1700 K Street
Sacramento, CA 95811
916-327-3728
800-879-2772
www.adp.cahwnet.gov/

Renee Zito, Director

The California Department of Alcohol and Drug Program's mission is to lead California's strategy to reduce alcohol and other drug problems by developing, administering, and supporting prevention and treatment programs.

2229 Monatana Department of Human & Community Services
111 N Jackson Street
Helena, MT 59620
406-444-1788
www.dphhs.mt.gov/

The mission of the Montana Department of Human & Community Services is to promote job preparation and work as a means to help needy families become self-sufficient.

2230 Rhode Island Council on Alcoholism and Other Drug Dependence
500 Prospect Street
Pawtucket, RI 02860
401-725-0410
Fax: 401-725-0768
E-mail: info@ricaodd.org
www.ricaodd.org/

John Almeida, President

The Rhode Island Council on Alcoholism and Other Drug Dependence is a private, non-profit corporation whose mission is to help individuals, youth and families who are troubled with alcohol, tobacco and other drug dependence.

Alabama

2231 Alabama Department of Human Resources
Center For Communications
Gordon Persons Building, Suite 2104
50 North Ripley Street
Montgomery, AL 36130
334-242-1310
Fax: 334-353-1115
www.dhr.state.al.us/Index.asp

Member of the National Leadership Council. The mission of the Alabama Department of Human Resources is to partner with communities to promote family stability and provide for the safety and self-sufficiency of vulnerable Alabamians.

2232 Alabama Department of Mental Health and Mental Retardation
100 North Union Street
PO Box 301410
Montgomery, AL 36130-1410
334-242-3454
800-367-0955
Fax: 334-242-0725
E-mail: dmhmr@mh.alabama.gov
www.www.mh.alabama.gov

John Houston, Commissioner
Beth Sievers, Administrative Assistant

State agency charged with providing services to citizens with mental illness, mental retardation and substance abuse disorders.

2233 Alabama Department of Public Health
201 Monroe Street
Montgomery, AL 36104
334-206-5300
www.adph.org

Provides public health related information about the State of Alabama.

2234 Alabama Disabilities Advocacy Program
PO Box 870395
Tuscaloosa, AL 35487-0395
205-348-4928
800-826-1675
Fax: 205-348-3909
E-mail: adap@adap.ua.edu
www.adap.net/

Ellen Gillespie, Director

Federally mandated, statewide, Protection and Advocacy system serving eligible individuals with disabilities in Alabama. ADAP's five programs are: Protection and Advocacy for Persons with Developmental Disabilities, Protection and Advocacy for Individuals with Mental Illness, Protection and Advocacy of Individual Rights, Protection and Advocacy for Assistive Technology and Protection and Advocacy for Beneficiaries of Social Security.

Alaska

2235 Alaska Council on Emergency Medical Services
20321 Middle Road
Eagle River, AK 99577
907-465-3028
E-mail: shelley.owens@alaska.gov
www.chems.alaska.gov/ems/acems.htm

Shelley K Owens, Public Health Specialist

The mission of the Emergency Medical Services program in Alaska is to reduce both the human suffering and economic loss to society resulting from premature death and disability due to injuries and sudden illness.

2236 Alaska Department of Health & Social Services
350 Main Street, Room 404
PO Box 110601
Juneau, AK 99811-0601
907-465-3030
Fax: 907-465-3068

TDD: 907-586-4265
TTY: 907-586-4265
E-mail: karleen.jackson@alaska.gov
www.hss.state.ak.us/default.cfm

Karleen Jackson, Commissioner
Bill Hogan, Deputy Commissioner

The mission of the Alaska Department of Health and Social Services is to promote and protect the health and well being of Alaskans.

2237 Alaska Division of Mental Health and Developmental Disabilities
PO Box 110620
Juneau, AK 99811
907-465-3370
Fax: 907-465-5864
E-mail: stacy.toner@alaska.gov
www.hss.state.ak.us/dbh/resources/contacts/default.htm

Stacy Toner, Deputy Director

The mission of the Division of Behavioral Health is to manage an integrated and comprehensive behavioral health system based on sound policy, effective practices and partnerships.

2238 Alaska Health and Social Services Division of Behavioral Health
3601 C Street,
Suite 934
Anchorage, AK 99503
907-269-3410
Fax: 907-269-3786
E-mail: melissa.stone@alaska.gov
www.hss.state.ak.us/dbh/dir/default.htm

Melissa Witzler Stone, Director

The mission of the Division of Behavioral Health is to manage an integrated and comprehensive behavioral health system based on sound policy, effective practices and partnerships.

2239 Alaska Mental Health Board
431 N Franklin Street
Suite 200
Juneau, AK 99801
907-465-8920
Fax: 907-465-4410
E-mail: kathryn.craft@alaska.gov
www.http://hss.state.ak.us/amhb

Kathryn Craft, Executive Director

Planning and advocacy body for public mental health services. The board works to ensure that Alaska's mental health program is integrated and comprehensive. It recommends operating and capital budgets for the program. The Governor appoints twelve - sixteen members to the board. At least half the members must be consumers of mental health services or family members. Two members are mental health service providers and one an attorney.

2240 Mental Health Association in Alaska
4045 Lake Otis Parkway
Suite 209
Anchorage, AK 99508
907-563-0880
Fax: 907-563-0881
E-mail: mhaa2@pobox.alaska.net
www.alaska.net/~mhaa/

The Mental Health Association in Alaska (MHAA) is a Division of the National Mental Health Association and is dedicated to the promotion of good mental health, the prevention of mental illness and ongoing improvement in the care and treatment of the mentally ill through advocacy, education, referral, research, legislative input and the monitoring of existing programs.

Arizona

2241 Arizona Department of Health Services
150 North 18th Avenue
Phoenix, AZ 85007
602-542-1000
Fax: 602-154-0883
www.azdhs.gov/

Provides news and information about public health services and facilities.

2242 Arizona Department of Health Services: Behavioral Services
150 N. 18th Avenue
#200
Phoenix, AZ 85007
602-364-4558
Fax: 602-364-4570
www.azdhs.gov/bhs/

Administers Arizona's publicly funded behavioral health service system for individuals, families and communities.

2243 Arizona Department of Health Services: Child Fatality Review
Office of Women's and Children's Health
150 North 18th Avenue
Suite 320
Phoenix, AZ 85007
602-364-1463
Fax: 602-364-1496
E-mail: smithja@azdhs.gov
www.azdhs.gov/phs/owch/cfr.htm

Jamie Smith, Program Manager

The Child Fatality Review Program consists of locally developed multidisciplinary teams in counties throughout the state. These local teams conduct a detailed review of the circumstances surrounding the deaths of all children less than 18 years of age who resided in their county. During each review, teams complete a standardized data form and develop recommendations for reducing preventable childhood deaths.

2244 Arizona Department of Health: Substance Abuse
150 N 18th Avenue
#200
Phoenix, AZ 85007
602-542-1001
3 - -
Fax: 602-364-4570
TDD: 602-364-4558
E-mail: webmaster@azdhs.gov
www.azdhs.gov/bhs/bsagmh.htm

Crysty Dye, Bureau Chief

The Bureau of Substance Abuse Treatment and Prevention Services is responsible for the design, development and provision of technical assistance on substance abuse and

general mental health services to the Regional Behavioral Health Authorities (RBHAs) and provider community.

2245 Northern Arizona Regional Behavioral Health Authority
1300 South Yale Street
Flagstaff, AZ 86001
928-774-7128
www.narbha.org/

The Northern Arizona Regional Behavioral Health Authority's (NARBHA) mission is to improve the quality of life for individuals and families across northern Arizona who are eligible for state and federally funded behavioral health services.

Arkansas

2246 Arkansas Department Health & Human Services
Donaghey Plaza West
7th and Main Streets
Little Rock, AR 72203-1437
501-682-1001
Fax: 501-682-6836
TDD: 501-682-8933
www.arkansas.gov/dhhs/homepage.html

John Selig, Executive Director

The Arkansas Department of Health and Human Services provides Medicaid, mental health and substance abuse resources.

2247 Arkansas Division of Children & Family Service
700 Main Street
P O Box 1437 Slot S 560
Little Rock, AR 72203-1437
501-682-8770
Fax: 501-682-6968
TDD: 501-682-1442
www.arkansas.gov/dhhs/sgChildren.html

The Arkansas Division of Children's Services is a member of the National Leadership Council and provides information and resources on adoption, daycare and child abuse prevention.

2248 Arkansas Division on Youth Services
PO Box 1437
Slot 450
Little Rock, AR 72203-1437
502-682-8654
Fax: 501-682-1339
www.arkansas.gov/dhhs/dys/

The Division of Youth Services (DYS) provides in a manner consistent with public safety, a system of high quality programs to address the needs of the juveniles who come in contact with, or are at risk of coming into contact with the juvenile justice system.

2249 Arkansas State Mental Hospital
4313 West Markham
Little Rock, AR 72205
501-686-9000
Fax: 501-686-9464
E-mail: sheila.duncan@mail.state.ar.us
www.arkansas.gov/dhhs/dmhs/ar_state_hospital.htm

Albert Kittrell MD, Medical Director
Charles Smith, Administrator

The Arkansas State Hospital (ASH) is a 202-bed psychiatric inpatient facility licensed by the Arkansas Department of Health and the Centers for Medicare and Medicaid Services, and accredited by the Joint Commission on Accreditation of Healthcare Organizations (JCAHO). The hospital includes 90 beds for acute psychiatric admission; a 60-bed forensic treatment services program which offers assistance to circuit courts throughout the state; a 16-bed adolescent treatment program for youth 13-18; and a 16-bed program for juvenile sex offenders. The Arkansas State Hospital has been providing quality psychiatric care to the citizens of Arkansas since 1873.

2250 Mental Health Council of Arkansas

501 Woodlane Drive
Suite 104
Little Rock, AR 72201
501-372-7062
Fax: 501-372-8039
E-mail: mhca@mhca.org
www.mhca.org/

Kenny Whitlock, Executive Vice President
Tonia Ward, Administrative Assistant

The Mental Health Council of Arkansas is a non-profit organization governed by a board of directors with a representative from each of the 13 participating community mental health centers and their affiliates. The MHCA assists its members to achieve the goal of community based treatment which focuses on the whole person with emphasis on physical, mental and emotional wellness and promotes the comprehensive diagnostic, treatment, and wrap around services provided by the private non-profit community mental health centers of Arkansas. The MHCA is dedicated to improving the overall health and well-being of the citizens and communities of Arkansas.

California

2251 California Department of Alcohol and Drug Programs: Resource Center

1700 K Street
Sacramento, CA 95811
916-327-3728
800-444-3066
www.adp.cahwnet.gov

Renee Zito, Director

The Resource Center at the California Department of Alcohol and Drug Programs maintains a comprehensive collection of alcohol, tobacco, and other drug prevention and treatment information. This information is provided to all California residents at no cost through a Clearinghouse, a full-service Library, Internet communication links, and a telephone information and referral system. These services can be accessed by letter, fax, Internet, e-mail, telephone, or in person during the business hours of 8:00 a.m. to 4:30 p.m., Monday through Friday, excluding state holidays.

2252 California Department of Corrections and Rehabilitation

1515 S Street
Suite 502
Sacramento, CA 95814-7243
916-323-6001
www.www.cdcr.ca.gov

Our mission is founded on delivering a balance of quality and cost-effective health care in a safe, secure correctional setting.

2253 California Department of Education: Healthy Kids, Healthy California

PO Box 944272
Sacramento, CA 94244
510-670-4583
888-318-8188
Fax: 510-670-4582
www.californiahealthykids.org

The California Healthy Kids Resource Center was established to assist schools in promoting health literacy. Health literacy is the capacity of an individual to obtain, interpret, and understand basic health information and services and the competence to use such information and services in ways that are health enhancing.

2254 California Department of Health Services: Medicaid

714 P Street
Room 1253
Sacramento, CA 95814-6401
916-552-9100
www.cms.hhs.gov/medicaid/stateplans/toc.asp?state=CA

The mission of the California Department of Health Services is to protect and improve the health of all Californians. Website constains resources and links for detailed information on Medicaid.

2255 California Department of Health Services: Medi-Cal Drug Discount

714 P Street
Room 213
Sacramento, CA 95814-6401
916-654-0532
E-mail: mcreform@dhs.ca.gov. OR
MCRedesign@dhs.ca.gov
www.medi-calredesign.org/

Sandra Shewry, Director

The Department of Health Services Medi-Cal Redesign Website provides relevant information on the Medi-Cal Drug Program, the information of which will be updated periodically.

2256 California Department of Mental Health

1600 9th Street
Room 151
Sacramento, CA 95814
916-654-3890
800-896-4042
Fax: 916-654-3198
TTY: 800-896-2512
E-mail: dmh.dmh.ca.gov
www.dmh.ca.gov

2257 California Hispanic Commission on Alcohol Drug Abuse

2101 Capitol Avenue
Sacramento, CA 95816
916-443-5473
Fax: 916-443-1732
www.chcada.org

Services can consist of developing Latino-based agencies, program management, consultation related to proposal development, Board of Directors training, program planning, and information dissemination. Populations or groups served include Latino alcohol and drug service agencies, groups and/or individuals planning to initiate services to Latinos, other AOD agencies with a commitment to serve the Latino community, and County Alcohol and Drug Program offices.

2258 California Institute for Mental Health
2125 19th Street
2nd Floor
Sacramento, CA 95818
916-556-3480
Fax: 916-446-4519
E-mail: sgoodwin@cimh.org
www.cimh.org

Sandra Naylor-Goodwin, Executive Director
Bill Carter, Deputy Director

Promoting excellence in mental health services through training, technical asistances, research and policy development.

2259 California Mental Health Directors Association
2125 19th Street
Sacramento, CA 95818
916-556-3477
Fax: 916-446-4519
E-mail: pryan@cmhda.org
www.cmhda.org

Patricia Ryan, Executive Director

The mission of the Association is to provide leadership, advocacy, expertise and support to California's county and city mental health programs (and their system partners) that will assist them in serving persons with serious mental illness and serious emotional disturbance. Our goal is to assist in building a public mental health system that ensures the accessibility of quality, cost-effective mental health care that is consumer-and family-driven, resiliency-based and culturally competent.

2260 California Women's Commission on Addictions
14622 Victory Boulevard
Van Nuys, CA 91411-1621
818-376-0470
Fax: 818-376-1307

Colorado

2261 Colorado Department of Health Care Policy and Financing
1570 Grant Street
Denver, CO 80203
303-866-3513
800-221-3943
E-mail: diane.rodriguez.state.co.us
www.www.chcpf.state.co.us

Joan Henneberry, Executive Director

The Department of Health Care Policy and Financing manages the Colorado Medicaid Community Mental Health Services program. the program provides mental health care to medicaid clients in Colorado, through Behavioral Health Organization contracts.

2262 Colorado Department of Human Services (CDHS)
1575 Sherman Street
Denver, CO 80203
303-866-5700
Fax: 303-866-4047
www.cdhs.state.co.us/

Karen Beye, Executive Director

CDHS oversees the state's 64 county departments of social/human services, the state's public mental health system, Colorado's system of services for people with developmental disabilities, the state's juvenile corrections system and all state and veterans' nursing homes, through more than 5,000 employees and thousands of community-based service providers. Colorado is a state-supervised, county-administered system for the traditional social services, including programs such as public assistance and child welfare services.

2263 Colorado Department of Human Services: Alcohol and Drug Abuse Division
4055 S. Lowell Blvd.
Denver, CO 80236
303-866-7480
Fax: 303-866-7481
www.cdhs.state.co.us

Roxy Huber, Executive Director

The Alcohol and Drug Abuse Division (ADAD) of the Colorado Department of Human Services was established by state law in 1971 to: promote healthy, drug-free lifestyles; reduce alcohol and other drug abuse and to reduce abuse-associated illnesses and deaths.

2264 Colorado Division of Mental Health
Colorado Department of Human Services
3824 West Princeton Circle
Denver, CO 80236
303-866-7400
Fax: 303-866-7428
www.cdhs.state.co.us/dmh

The Division of Mental Health administers non-Medicaid community mental health services for people with serious emotional disturbance or serious mental illness of all ages, through contracts with six specialty clinics and seventeen private, nonprofit community mental health centers. The Division of Mental Health strives to ensure high quality, accessible mental health services for Colorado residents, by reviewing community mental health programs; adopting standards, rules and regulations; providing training and technical assistance; and responding to complaints from non-Medicaid consumers.

2265 Colorado Medical Assistance Program Information Center
Department of Health Care Policy and Financing
1570 Grant Street
Denver, CO 80203
303-866-3513
www.chcpf.state.co.us/

Provides numerous resources for policymakers, health care consumers, providers, and all citizens of Colorado.

2266 Colorado Traumatic Brain Injury Trust Fund Program
1575 Sherman Street
4th Floor
Denver, CO 80203
303-866-4085
Fax: 303-866-4905
www.cdhs.state.co.us

The TBI Trust Fund will strive to support all people in Colorado with traumatic brain injury through services, research and education.

2267 Denver County Department of Social Services
1200 Federal Boulevard
Denver, CO 80204-3221
720-944-3666
Fax: 720-944-3019
E-mail: codhs.fcs-sls@acs-inc.com
www.www.cdhs.state.co.us/servicebycounty.htm

Roxanne White, Manager

The vision of the Denver Department of Human Services is to help those in need and protect those in harm's way. The mission is to provide and coordinate services with courtesy and respect for each other and for the well being and protection of residents in the Denver community. These services are provided through partnerships that help families and individuals move toward independence, maintain pride and dignity and realize their potential.

2268 El Paso County Human Services
105 North Spruce Street
Colorado Springs, CO 80905
719-636-0000
www.dhs.elpasoco.com

The mission of the El Paso County Department of Human Services is to strengthen families, assure safety, promote self-sufficiency, eliminate poverty, and improve the quality of life in our community.

Connecticut

2269 Connecticut Department of Mental Health and Addiction Services
410 Capitol Avenue
P O Box 341431
Hartford, CT 06134
860-418-7000
800-446-7348
TDD: 860-418-6707
www.dmhas.state.ct.us/

The mission of the Department of Mental Health and Addiction Services is to improve the quality of life of the people of Connecticut by providing an integrated network of comprehensive, effective and efficient mental health and addiction services that foster self-sufficiency, dignity and respect.

2270 Connecticut Department of Children and Families
505 Hudson Street
Hartford, CT 06106
860-550-6301
866-637-4737
www.state.ct.us/dcf/

The mission of the Department of Children and Families is to protect children, improve child and family well-being

and support and preserve families. These efforts are accomplished by respecting and working within individual cultures and communities in Connecticut, and in partnership with others. Member of the National Leadership Council

Delaware

2271 Delaware Department of Health & Social Services
1901 North Dupont Highway
Main Building
New Castle, DE 19720
302-255-9040
Fax: 302-255-4429
www.dhss.delaware.gov/dhss/

Vincent P Meconi, Secretary

The mission of the Delaware Department of Health and Social Services is to improve the quality of life for Delaware's citizens by promoting health and well-being, fostering self-sufficiency, and protecting vulnerable populations.

2272 Delaware Division of Child Mental Health Services
1825 Faulkland Road
Wilmington, DE 19805
302-633-2600
Fax: 302-633-5118
E-mail: cmh.dscyf@state.de.us
www.state.de.us/kids/cmhs/cmhs.shtml

The Division of Child Mental Health Services (DCMHS) is part of the Delaware Department of Services for Children, Youth and Their Families. Its primary responsibility is to provide and manage a range of services for children who have experienced abandonment, abuse, adjudication, mental illness, neglect, or substance abuse. Its services include prevention, early intervention, assessment, treatment, permanency, and after care.

2273 Delaware Division of Family Services
1825 Faulkland Road
Wilmington, DE 19805
302-663-2665
E-mail: info.dscyf@state.de.us
www.state.de.us/kids/fs/fs.shtml

The Division of Family Services is mandated by law to investigate complaints about child abuse and neglect. Since 1875, state agencies have been balancing the children's right of safety and the parent's right to choose what is good for the family. The Adoption and Safe Families Act of 1997 clearly puts the focus on the protection, safety and permanency plan of children as the first priority. Services provided are child oriented and family focused.

District of Columbia

2274 California Department of Health and Human Services
200 Independence Avenue SW
Washington, DC 20201
202-619-0257
877-696-6775
www.www.hhs.gov

2275 DC Commission on Mental Health Services
64 New York Avenue, NE
4th Floor
Washington, DC 20002
202-673-7440
888-793-4357
www.dmh.dc.gov/dmh/site/default.asp

Regulates the District's mental health system for adults, children and youth, and their families, and provides mental health services directly through the Community Service Agency (for community-based consumers of mental health services) and St. Elizabeths Hospital.

2276 DC Department of Human Services
801 East Building
2700 Martin Luther King Jr Avenue SE
Washington, DC 20032
202-279-6002
Fax: 202-279-6014

2277 Health & Medicine Counsel of Washington
DDNC Digestive Disease National Coalition
507 Capital Court NE
Suite 200
Washington, DC 20002
202-544-7497
Fax: 202-546-7105
www.ddnc.org

Peter Banks, President
Linda Aukett, Chair

The Digestive Disease National Coalition (DDNC) is an advocacy organization comprised of the major national voluntary and professional societies concerned with digestive diseases. The DDNC focuses on improving public policy related to digestive diseases and increasing public awareness with respect to the many diseases of the digestive system. The DDNC was founded in 1978 and is based in Washington D.C.

Florida

2278 Florida Department Health and Human
Services: Substance Abuse Program
Department of Children and Families
1317 Winewood Boulevard
Building 1 Suite 207
Tallahassee, FL 32399-6570
850-487-2920
www.dcf.state.fl.us/mentalhealth/sa/

The Substance Abuse Program Office is dedicated to the development of a comprehensive system of prevention, emergency/detoxification, and treatment services for individuals and families at risk of or affected by substance abuse; to promote their safety, well-being, and self-sufficiency.

2279 Florida Department of Children and Families
1317 Winewood Boulevard
Building 1, Room 202
Tallahassee, FL 32399-0700
850-487-1111
Fax: 850-922-2993
www.state.fl.us/cf_web/

Robert Butterworth, Secretary

Provides rules, regulations, monitoring of fifteen district mental health program offices and mental health providers throughout the state.

2280 Florida Department of Health and Human
Services
2585 Merchants Row Boulevard
Tallahassee, FL 32399-6570
850-245-4444
www.doh.state.fl.us

The mission of the Florida Department of Health and Human Services is to promote and protect the health and safety of all people in Florida through the delivery of quality public health services and the promotion of health care standards.

2281 Florida Department of Mental Health and
Rehabilitative Services
Department of Children and Families
1317 Winewood Boulevard
Building 6
Tallahassee, FL 32399-0700
850-413-0935
www.dcf.state.fl.us/mentalhealth/

The Mental Health Program Office is committed to focusing its resources to meet the needs of people who cannot otherwise access mental health care.

2282 Florida Medicaid State Plan
2727 Mahan Drive
Tallahassee, FL 32308
888-419-3456
www.ahca.myflorida.com

Provides information about the Medicare plans, benefits and how to enroll in them. Medicaid is the state and federal partnership that provides health coverage for selected categories of people with low incomes. Its purpose is to improve the health of people who might otherwise go without medical care for themselves and their children. Florida implemented the Medicaid program on January 1, 1970, to provide medical services to indigent people. Over the years, the Florida Legislature has authorized Medicaid reimbursement for additional services. A major expansion occurred in 1989, when the United States Congress mandated that states provide all Medicaid services allowable under the Social Security Act to children under the age of 21.

Georgia

2283 Georgia Department of Human Resources
2 Peachtree Street NW
Suite 3-130
Atlanta, GA 30303
404-818-6600
866-351-0001
www.dhr.georgia.gov

Provides programs that control the spread of disease, enable older people to live at home longer, prevent children from developing lifelong disabilities, train single parents to find and hold jobs, and help people with mental or physical disabilities live and work in their communities.

2284 Georgia Department of Human Resources:
Division of Public Health
Two Peachtree Street, NW
Atlanta, GA 30303-3186

404-657-2700
E-mail: gdphinfo@dhr.state.ga.us
www.health.state.ga.us/

Our mission is to promote and protect the health of people in Georgia wherever they live, work, and play. We unite with individuals, families, and communities to improve their health and enhance their quality of life.

2285 Georgia Division of Mental Health Developmental Disabilities and Addictive Diseases (MHDDAD)
2 Peachtree Street NW
Atlanta, GA 30303
404-818-6600
www.mhddad.dhr.georgia.gov

Provides treatment and support services to people with mental illnesses and addictive diseases, and support to people with mental retardation and related developmental disabilities. MHDDAD serves people of all ages with the most severe and likely to be long-term conditions. The division also funds evidenced-based prevention services aimed at reducing substance abuse and related problems.

Hawaii

2286 Hawaii Department of Adult Mental Health
1250 Punchbowl #256
Honolulu, HI 96813
808-586-4686
Fax: 808-586-4745
www.amhd.org/

The mission of the Hawaii Department of Adult Mental Health is to provide a comprehensive, integrated mental health system supporting the recovery of adults with severe mental illness. The Adult Mental Health Division seeks to improve the mental health of Hawai'i's people by reducing the prevalence of emotional disorders, and mental illness. Services include mental health education, treatment and rehabilitation through community-based mental health centers, and an in-patient state hospital facility for the mentally-ill, including those referred through courts and the criminal justice system.

2287 Hawaii Department of Health
1250 Punchbowl Street
Honolulu, HI 96813
808-586-4416
www.hawaii.gov/health

Michelle R Hill, Director Behavioral Health

Idaho

2288 Department of Health and Welfare: Medicaid Division
450 West State Street
Boise, ID 83720-0036
208-334-5500
Fax: 208-364-1846
E-mail: APSPortal@idhw.state.id.us
www.healthandwelfare.idaho.gov/

Karl Kurtz, Director

Our mission is to promote and protect the health and safety of all Idahoans. From birth throughout life, we can help enrich and protect the lives of the people of our state.

2289 Department of Health and Welfare: Community Rehab
PO Box 83720
Boise, ID 83702-0036
208-332-6910
www.healthandwelfare.idaho.gov/

Our mission is to promote and protect the health and safety of all Idahoans. From birth throughout life, we can help enrich and protect the lives of the people of our state.

2290 Idaho Bureau of Maternal and Child Health
PO Box 83720
Boise, ID 83720-3720
208-332-6910
www.healthandwelfare.idaho.gov/

Our mission is to promote and protect the health and safety of all Idahoans. From birth throughout life, we can help enrich and protect the lives of the people of our state.

2291 Idaho Bureau of Mental Health and Substance Abuse, Division of Family & Community Service
PO Box 83720
Boise, ID 83720-0001
208-332-6910
www.healthandwelfare.idaho.gov/

Our mission is to promote and protect the health and safety of all Idahoans. From birth throughout life, we can help enrich and protect the lives of the people of our state.

2292 Idaho Department of Health & Welfare
PO Box 83720
Boise, ID 83720-0036
208-332-6910
www.healthandwelfare.idaho.gov/DesktopDefault.aspx

Our mission is to promote and protect the health and safety of all Idahoans. From birth throughout life, we can help enrich and protect the lives of the people of our state.

2293 Idaho Department of Health and Welfare: Family and Child Services
PO Box 83720
Boise, ID 83720-0036
203-332-6910
www.healthandwelfare.idaho.gov/

Our mission is to promote and protect the health and safety of all Idahoans. From birth throughout life, we can help enrich and protect the lives of the people of our state.

2294 Idaho Mental Health Center
PO Box 83720
Boise, ID 83720-0036
208-332-6910
www.www.healthandwelfare.idaho.gov/

The Idaho Department of Health and Welfare's programs and services are designed to help people live healthy and be productive, strengthening individuals, families and communities. From birth throughout life, we help people improve their lives.

Illinois

2295 Illinois Alcoholism and Drug Dependency Association
937 S 2nd Street
Springfield, IL 62704

217-528-7335
Fax: 217-528-7340
www.iadda.org

2296 Illinois Department of Alcoholism and Substance Abuse
100 W Randolph Street
Suite 5-600
Chicago, IL 60601
312-814-2300
Fax: 312-814-3838
E-mail: dhsa48@dhs.state.il.us
www.www.alcoholfreechildren.org

DASA consists of three operational Bureau's designed to reflect our mission and planning goals and objectives. Primary responsibilities are to develop, maintain, monitor and evaluate a statewide treatment delivery system designed to provide screening, assessment, customer-treatment matching, referral, intervention, treatment and continuing care services for indigents alcohol and drug abuse and dependency problems. These services are provided by numerous community-based substance abuse treatment organizations contracted by DASA according to the needs of various communities and populations.

2297 Illinois Department of Children and Family Services
100 W Randolph Street
Suite 6-200
Chicago, IL 60601
312-814-6800
TDD: 312-814-8783
www.state.il.us/dcfs/about/ab_about.shtml

Erwin McEwen, Acting Director

The Illinois Department of Children and Family Services provides child welfare services in Illinois. It is also the nation's largest state child welfare agency to earn accreditation from the Council on Accreditation for Children and Family Services (COA). The Department's organization includes the Divisions of Child Protection, Placement Permanency, Field Operations, Guardian & Advocacy, Clinical Practice & Professional Development, Service Intervention, Budget & Finance, Planning & Performance Management, and Communications.

2298 Illinois Department of Health and Human Services
401 South Clinton Street
Chicago, IL 60607
800-843-6154
TTY: 312-793-2354
www.dhs.state.il.us/

DHS serves Illinois citizens through seven main programs: Welfare programs, including temporary assistance for needy families, Food Stamps, and child care; Alcoholism and substance abuse treatment and prevention services; Developmental disabilities; Health services for pregnant women and mothers, infants, children, and adolescents; Prevention services for domestic violence and at-risk youth; Mental health and Rehabilitation services.

2299 Illinois Department of Human Services: Office of Mental Health
160 N LaSalle
10th Floor
Chicago, IL 60601

312-814-4964

Carol L Adams, Director

Works to improve the lives of persons with mental illness by integrating state operated services, community based programs, and other support services to create an effective and responsive treatment and care network. Management office which plans, organizes, and controls the activities of the organization, but does not offer services to the public.

2300 Illinois Department of Mental Health and Drug Dependence
Dhs-Division of Alcoholism and Substance Abuse
100 West Randolph Street
Suite 5-600
Chicago, IL 60652
800-843-6154
www.dhs.state.il.us/oasa/

Carol L Adams, Director

Primary responsibilities are to develop, maintain, monitor and evaluate a statewide treatment delivery system designed to provide screening, assessment, customer-treatment matching, referral, intervention, treatment and continuing care services for indigents alcohol and drug abuse and dependency problems. These services are provided by numerous community-based substance abuse treatment organizations contracted by DASA according to the needs of various communities and populations.

2301 Illinois Department of Mental Health and Developmental Disabilities
100 South Grand Avenue
2nd Floor
Springfield, IL 62765
217-524-7065
www.dhs.state.il.us/mhdd/dd/

Our mission is to provide a full array of quality, outcome-based, person- and community-centered services and supports for individuals with developmental disabilities and their families in Illinois.

2302 Illinois Department of Public Aid
201 S Grand Avenue E
Springfield, IL 62763
217-782-1200
Fax: 217-782-5672
www.hfs.illinois.gov/

The Illinois Department of Healthcare and Family Services, formerly the Department of Public Aid, is the state agency dedicated to improving the lives of Illinois' families through health care coverage, child support enforcement and energy assistance.

2303 Illinois Department of Public Health: Division of Food, Drugs and Dairies/FDD
535 W Jefferson Street
Springfield, IL 62761
217-782-4977
Fax: 217-782-3987
TTY: 800-547-0466
www.idph.state.il.us/

Damon Arnold, Director

The mission of the Illinois Department of Public Health is to promote the health of the people of Illinois through the prevention and control of disease and injury.

2304 Mental Health Association in Illinois
70 E Lake Street
Suite 900
Chicago, IL 60601
312-368-9070
www.www.mhai.org

Carol Wozniewski, Executive Director
Jennifer Okonma, Director Development

Works to promote mental health, prevent mental illnesses, and improve the care and treatment of persons suffering from mental and emotional problems. An affiliate of the National Mental Health Association, MHAI is Illinois' only statewide, non-profit, non-governmental advocacy organization concerned with the entire spectrum of mental and emotional disorders.

Year Founded: 1909

Indiana

2305 Indiana Department of Public Welfare Division of Family Independence: Food Stamps/Medicaid/Training
Family and Social Services Administration
402 W Washington Street
PO Box 7083
Indianapolis, IN 46207-7083
317-232-4946
Fax: 317-233-4693
www.www.in.gov/fssa

The mission of the Division of Family Independence is to strengthenfamilies and children through temporary assistance to needy families, food stamps, housing, child care, foster care, adoption, energy assistance, homeless services, and job programs.

2306 Indiana Family & Social Services Administration
402 W Washington Street
PO Box 7083
Indianapolis, IN 46207-7083
317-233-4454
Fax: 317-233-4693
www.in.gov/fssa/2474.htm

Ferzelle Jones, Administrative Assistant

The mission of the Indiana Department of Family and Social Services is to strengthen families and children through temporary assistance to needy families, food stamps, housing, child care, foster care, adoption, energy assistance, homeless services, and job programs.

2307 Indiana Family And Social Services Administration
402 W Washington Street
PO Box 7083
Indianapolis, IN 46207-7083
317-233-4454
Fax: 317-233-4693
www.in.gov/fssa//2474.htm

Ferzelle Jones, Administrative Assistant

The mission of the Indiana Bureau of Family Protection is to strengthen families and children through temporary assistance to needy families, food stamps, housing, child care, foster care, adoption, energy assistance, homeless services, and job programs.

2308 Indiana Family and Social Services Administration: Division of Mental Health
402 W Washington Street
Suite W-353
Indianapolis, IN 46204-2739
317-233-4319
Fax: 317-233-3472
www.in.gov/fssa/

The mission of the Indiana Family and Social Services Administration Division of Mental Health is to strengthening families and children through temporary assistance to needy families, food stamps, housing, child care, foster care, adoption, energy assistance, homeless services, and job programs.

2309 Office of Medicaid Policy & Planning (OMPP)
Indiana Family and Social Services Administration
402 W Washington Street
PO Box 7083
Indianapolis, IN 46207-7083
317-233-4454
Fax: 317-233-4693
www.in.gov/fssa/servicedisabl/medicaid/index.html

The Office of Medicaid Policy and Planning (OMPP) finances basic, cost-effective medical services for low-income residents of the State of Indiana.

2310 The Indiana Consortium for Mental Health Services Research (ICMHSR)
Institute for Social Research Indiana University
1022 East Third Street
Bloomington, IN 47405
812-855-3841
Fax: 812-856-5713
E-mail: acapshew@indiana.edu
www.indiana.edu/~icmhsr/

Bernice A Pescosolido Ph.D, Program Director

The Indiana Consortium for Mental Health Services Research (ICMHSR) focuses on developing high quality scholarly and applied research projects on mental health and related services for people with severe mental disorders. A major commitment of the ICMHSR is to use research to foster public awareness and improve public policy and decision-making regarding these devastating illnesses.

Iowa

2311 Iowa Department Human Services
1305 East Walnut
Des Moines, IA 50319
515-281-5454
Fax: 515-281-4980
E-mail: fdhs@dhs.state.ia.us
www.dhs.state.ia.us

Kevin W Concannon, Director

The Mission of the Iowa Department of Human Services is to help individuals and families achieve safe, stable, self-sufficient, and healthy lives, thereby contributing to the economic growth of the state. We do this by keeping a customer focus, striving for excellence, sound stewardship of state resources, maximizing the use of federal funding and leveraging opportunities, and by working with our public and private partners to achieve results.

2312 Iowa Department of Public Health
321 E 12th Street
Des Moines, IA 50319-0075
515-281-7689
www.idph.state.ia.us

Thomas Newton, Director

Under the direction of the director, the Iowa Department of Public Health exercises general supervision of the state's public health; promotes public hygiene and sanitation; does health promotion activities, prepares for and responds to bioemergency situations; and, unless otherwise provided, enforces laws on public health.

2313 Iowa Department of Public Health: Division of Substance Abuse
321 12th Street
Des Moines, IA 50319
515-242-6514
www.idph.state.ia.us/bh

G. Dean Austin, Bureau Chief

The Office of Substance Abuse Prevention/Staff of the Office of Substance Abuse Prevention provides the following services: technical assistance to individuals, groups, and contracted agencies and organizations; Coordinate and collaborate with multiple state agencies and organizations for assessment, planning, and implementation of statewide prevention initiatives; and Coordinate, train, and monitor funding to local community-based organizations for alcohol, tobacco, and other drug prevention services.

2314 Iowa Division of Mental Health & Developmental Disabilities: Department of Human Services
1305 E Walnut Street
Des Moines, IA 50319
515-281-5454
Fax: 515-281-4980
E-mail: fdhs@dhs.state.ia.us
www.dhs.state.ia.us

Kevin W Concannon, Director

The Division of Mental Health and Developmental Disabilities (MH/DD) is the agency designated as the state mental health authority by the Governor of Iowa. The Division: provides program support services for persons with mental illness, mental retardation and developmental disabilities; plans for state services; works with counties in the development and implementation of their services plans; develops policy for the state mental health institutes and the state resource centers for persons with developmental disabilities; provides consultation and technical assistance; and, provides accreditation for providers of MH/DD services.

Kansas

2315 Comcare of Sedgwick County
635 North Main Street
Wichita, KS 67203
316-660-7600
Fax: 316-383-7925
TTY: 316-267-0267
E-mail: mjarnold@sedgwick.gov
www.sedgwickcounty.org/comcare/

Mark J Arnold, Human Resources

COMCARE of Sedgwick County helps people with Mental Health and Substance Abuse needs to improve the quality of their lives

2316 Division of Health Care Policy
Kansas Department of Social and Rehabilitation Services
915 SW Harrison Street
Topeka, KS 66612
785-296-3959
Fax: 785-296-2173
www.srskansas.org

The Substance Abuse Treatment and Recovery Unit licenses all substance abuse treatment facilities in Kansas, oversees the credentialing of substance abuse counselors, and provides substance abuse treatment to low-income Kansans through a statewide network of funded providers.

2317 Kansas Council on Developmental Disabilities
Kansas Department of Social and Rehabilitation Services
Docking State Office Building
Room 141
Topeka, KS 66612
785-296-2608
Fax: 785-296-2861
www.www.kcdd.org

Donna Beauchamp, Council Chair

2318 Kansas Department of Mental Health and Retardation and Social Services
915 SW Harrison
Dsob 9th Floor
Topeka, KS 66612
785-296-3773
www.srskansas.org/hcp/

Ray Dalton, Deputy Secretary

The mission of the department of Mental Health in the Division of Health Care Policy is to provide individuals and families who experience mental illness alone or in combination with substance abuse problems, the support they need in order to achieve their personal goals.

Kentucky

2319 Kentucky Cabinet for Health and Human Services
275 East Main Street
1e-B
Frankfort, KY 40621
502-564-5497
Fax: 502-564-9523
E-mail: nancy.ovesen@ky.gov
www.chfs.ky.gov/

The goal of the Cabinet for Health and Family Services is to provide the finest health care possible for people in our state facilities; To provide the best preventative services through our public health programs; To provide the most outstanding service for our families and children; To protect and prevent the abuse of children, elders and people with disabilities and To build quality programs across-the-board; and by doing all of these things.

2320 Kentucky Department for Human Support Services
Kentucky Department for Health and Family Services
275 East Main Street
Mail Stop 3W-E
Frankfort, KY 40621
502-564-5343
Fax: 502-564-7478
www.chfs.ky.gov/dhss/default.htm

Sam Rodgers, Info Technology Client Manager

Consists of four divisions and one commission, all of which provide vital programs and services to Kentucky families. Divisions include Family Resource and Youth Services Centers, Aging Services, Women's Mental and Physical Health, and Child Abuse and Domestic Violence Services. This department also oversees the Kentucky Commission on Community Volunteerism and Service.

2321 Kentucky Department for Medicaid Services
Kentucky Cabinet for Health and Family Services
275 East Main Street
5w-A
Frankfort, KY 40621
502-564-2888
Fax: 502-564-3866
www.chfs.ky.gov

Steve D Davis, Deputy Inspector General

Owing to the unbridled spirit of our workforce, the mission of Kentucky Medicaid is to provide innovative opportunities to our members that will promote healthy lifestyles, personal accountability and responsible program governance for a healthier Kentucky.

2322 Kentucky Department of Mental Health and Mental Retardation
C/O The Commissioner's Office
100 Fair Oaks Lane 4E-B
Frankfort, KY 40621
502-564-4527
Fax: 502-564-5478
TTY: 502-564-5777
www.chfs.ky.gov/mhmr/

Dr. John M Burt, Commissioner Mental Health Dept

Our mission is to provide leadership, in partnership with others, to prevent disability, build resilience in individuals and their communities, and facilitate recovery for people whose lives have been affected by mental illness, mental retardation or other developmental disability, substance abuse or an acquired brain injury.

2323 Kentucky Justice Cabinet: Department of Juvenile Justice
1025 Capital Center Drive
Frankfort, KY 40601
502-573-2738
www.djj.ky.gov/

J. Ronald Haws, Commissioner

The Kentucky Department of Juvenile Justice's mission is to improve public safety by providing balanced and comprehensive services that hold youth accountable, and to provide the opportunity for youth to develop into productive, responsible citizens.

Louisiana

2324 Louisiana Commission on Law Enforcement and Administration (LCLE)
1885 Wooddale Boulevard
Room 1230
Baton Rouge, LA 70806-1511
225-925-4418
www.cole.state.la.us/

Judy A Dupuy, Executive Director

Lastest news and information on LCLE programs, resources, job openings, and general agency information on a monthly basis and for an in-depth review of our criminal justice programs.

2325 Louisiana Department of Health and Hospitals: Office of Mental Health
Bienville Building
628 N 4th Street
Baton Rouge, LA 70802
255-342-2540
Fax: 255-342-5066
www.dhh.state.la.us/offices/?ID=62

The Mission of the Office of Mental Health (OMH) is to perform the functions of the state which provide or lead to treatment, rehabilitation and follow-up care for individuals in Louisiana with mental and emotional disorders. OMH administers and/or monitors community-based services, public or private, to assure active quality care in the most cost-effective manner in the least restrictive environment for all persons with mental and emotional disorders.

2326 Louisiana Department of Health and Hospitals: Louisiana Office for Addictive Disorders
628 N 4th Street
PO Box 2790
Baton Rouge, LA 70821-2790
225-342-6717
Fax: 255-342-3875
www.dhh.louisiana.gov/offices/?ID=23

Michael Duffy, Assistant Secretary

It is the philosophy of this agency that treatment and prevention services should be of high quality and easily accessible to all citizens of the state. The Office for Addictive Disorders offers comprehensive treatment and prevention services through ten Regional/District Offices throughout the state.

Maine

2327 Maine Department Health and Human Services Children's Behavioral Health Services
11 State House Station
Augusta, ME 04333
207-287-5060
888-568-1112
TTY: 207-606-0215
www.www.maine.gov/dhhs/ocfs/cbhs/overview.html

Children's Behavioral Health Services (CBHS), a branch of the Department of Health and Human Services (DHHS) has a long tradition of advocacy for children with special needs. Once known as the Bureau of Children's with Special Needs (BCSN), this part of the Department became known as Children's Services in 1995. In a continuing effort to meet the diverse and growing needs of Maine families,

Children's Behavioral Health Services (CBHS) is going through a further transition. Most services formerly provided directly through the Department are now delivered through contracted community agencies.

2328 Maine Department of Behavioral and Developmental Services

Marguardt Building, 3rd Floor
159 State House Station
Augusta, ME 04333-0159
207-287-6415
Fax: 207-287-8910

Provides community services to individuals with mental illnesses, mental retardation, substance abuse issues and children with special needs. Provides psychiatric inpatient services at two mental health facilities.

2329 Maine Office of Substance Abuse: Information and Resource Center

11 State House Station
Augusta, ME 04333-0011
207-287-2595
800-499-0027
Fax: 207-287-8910
TTY: 800-606-0215
E-mail: osa.ircosa@maine.gov
www.maine.gov/bds/osa

Provides Maine's citizens with alcohol, tobacco and other drug information, resources and research for prevention, education and treatment.

Maryland

2330 Centers for Medicare & Medicaid Services/CMS: Office of Research, Statisctics, Data and Systems

7500 Security Boulevard
Baltimore, MD 21244
410-786-3000
www.cms.hhs.gov/home/rsds.asp

Information on CMS research, statistics, data & systems.

2331 Centers for Medicare & Medicaid Services

7500 Security Boulevard
Baltimore, MD 21244
410-786-3000
www.cms.hhs.gov

Information about the Centers for Medicare & Medicaid Services (CMS).

2332 Centers for Medicare & Medicaid Services: Office of Policy

7500 Security Boulevard
Baltimore, MD 21244
202-786-3000
www.cms.hhs.gov/

The OP assists the CMS Policy Council with immediate/rapid response on timely issues and transforms concepts into institutionalized processes.

2333 Centers for Medicare and Medicaid Services: Office of Financial Management/OFM

7500 Security Boulevard
Baltimore, MD 21244
410-786-3000
www.cms.hhs.gov/

OFM has overall reponsibility for the fiscal integrity of CMS' programs.

2334 Maryland Alcohol and Drug Abuse Administration

55 Wade Avenue
Baltimore, MD 21228
410-402-8600
Fax: 410-402-8601
www.maryland-adaa.org/ka/index.cfm

Peter F Luongo Ph.D, Director

The Alcohol and Drug Abuse Administration (ADAA) is the single state agency responsible for the provision, coordination, and regulation of the statewide network of substance abuse prevention, intervention and treatment services. It serves as the initial point of contact for technical assistance and regulatory interpretation for all Maryland Department of Health and Mental Hygiene (DHMH) prevention and certified treatment programs.

2335 Maryland Department of Health and Mental Hygiene

201 West Preston Street
Baltimore, MD 21201
410-767-6500
877-463-3464
E-mail: webadministrator@dhmh.state.md.us
www.dhmh.state.md.us/health/

Provides information on a variety of services including mental health and substance abuse, health plans and providers, nutrition and maternal care, environmental health and developmental disabilities.

2336 Maryland Department of Human Resources

311 West Saratoga Street
Baltimore, MD 21201
800-332-6347
TTY: 800-925-4434
E-mail: dhrhelp@dhr.state.md.us
www.dhr.state.md.us/help.htm

The mission of the Maryland Department of Human Resources is to assist people in economic need, provide prevention services, and protect vulnerable children and adults.

2337 Maryland Division of Mental Health

2301 Argonne Drive
Baltimore, MD 21218-1628
410-767-6860
Fax: 410-333-7482

Massachusetts

2338 Massachusetts Department of Mental Health

1 Ashburton Place
11th Floor
Boston, MA 02108
617-573-1600
www.mass.gov/dmh/

Judy Ann Bigby, Secretary

The Massachusetts Department of Mental Health provides clinical, rehabilitative and supportive services for adults with serious mental illness, and children and adolescents with serious mental illness or serious emotional disturbance.

2339 Massachusetts Department of Public Health

250 Washington Street
Boston, MA 02108-4619
617-624-6000
TTY: 617-624-6001
www.mass.gov/dph/

John Auerbach, Commissioner

Our mission, to serve all the people in the Commonwealth, particularly the under served, and to promote healthy people, healthy families, healthy communities and healthy environments through compassionate care, education and prevention. Your health is our concern.

2340 Massachusetts Department of Public Health: Bureau of Substance Abuse Services

250 Washington Street
Boston, MA 02108-4609
800-327-5050
TTY: 617-536-5872
www.mass.gov/dph/bsas/bsas.htm

The Bureau of Substance Abuse Services oversees the substance abuse prevention and treatment services in the Commonwealth. Responsibilities include: licensing programs and counselors; funding and monitoring prevention and treatment services; providing access to treatment for the indigent and uninsured; developing and implementing policies and programs; and, tracking substance abuse trends in the state.

2341 Massachusetts Department of Social Services

24 Farnsworth Street
Boston, MA 02210
617-748-2000
www.mass.gov/

Angelo McClain, Commissioner

The mission of the Massachusetts Department of Social Services is to ensure the safety of children in a manner that holds the best hope of nuturing a sustained, resilent network of relationships to support the child's growth and development into adulthood.

2342 Massachusetts Department of Transitional Assistance
Massachusetts Department of Health and Human Services

600 Washington Street
Boston, MA 02111
617-348-8500
www.mass.gov/dta/

The mission of the Department of Transitional Assistance is to serve the Commonwealth's most vulnerable families and individuals with dignity and respect, ensuring those eligible for our services have access to those services in an accurate, timely and culturally sensitive manner and in a way that promotes client's independence and long term self-sufficiency.

2343 Massachusetts Division of Medical Assistance
MassHealth Program

1 Ashburton Place
11th Floor
Boston, MA 02108
617-573-1600
www.mass/gov/dma/

Judy Ann Bigby, Secretary

The mission of the MassHealth program is to help the financially needy obtain high-quality health care that is affordable, promotes independence, and provides customer satisfacation.

2344 Massachusetts Executive Office of Public Safety

1 Ashburton Place
Suite 2133
Boston, MA 02108
617-727-7775
Fax: 617-727-4764
E-mail: eopsinfo@state.ma.us
www.www.mass.gov

Plans and manages public safety efforts by supporting, supervising and providing planning and guidance to a variety of state agencies.

Michigan

2345 Michigan Department of Community Health
Department of Mental Health

Capitol View Building
201 Townsend Street
Lansing, MI 48913
517-373-3740
E-mail: mccurtisj@michigan.gov
www.michigan.gov/mdch/

Janet Olszewski, Director
James McCurtis, Public Information Officer

Provides information on drug control and substance abuse treatment policies.

2346 Michigan Department of Human Services

235 S Grand Ave
PO Box 30037
Lansing, MI 48909
517-373-2305
Fax: 517-335-6101
TTY: 517-373-8071
www.michigan.gov/dhs/

The Department of Human Services (DHS) is Michigan's public assistance, child and family welfare agency. DHS directs the operations of public assistance and service programs through a network of over 100 county department of human service offices around the state.

2347 Michigan State Representative: Co-Chair
Public Health

S0688 House Office Building
P O Box 30014
Lansing, MI 48909-7514
517-373-1705
Fax: 517-373-5968
E-mail: shanellejackson@house.mi.gov
www.house.michigan.gov/rep.asp?DIST=009

Shanelle Jackson

2348 National Council on Alcoholism and Drug Dependence: Greater Detriot Area

4777 East Outer Drive
Detroit, MI 48234
313-369-5400
Fax: 313-369-5415
E-mail: info@ncadd-detroit.org
www.ncadd-detroit.org/

The National Council on Alcoholism and Drug Dependence-Greater Detroit Area is a voluntary, non-profit agency committed to improving health through providing substance abuse prevention, education, training, treatment and advocacy for the metropolitan Detroit area.

Minnesota

2349 Department of Human Services: Chemical Health Division
PO Box 64977
Saint Paul, MN 55164
651-431-2460
Fax: 651-431-7449
www.dhs.state.mn.us

The Chemical Health Division is the state alcohol and drug authority responsible for defining a statewide response to drug and alcohol abuse. This includes providing basic information on chemical health. It also includes planning a broad-based community service system, evaluating the effectiveness of various chemical dependency services, and funding innovative programs to promote reduction of alcohol and other drug problems and their effects on individuals, families and society

2350 Minnesota Department of Human Services
444 Lafayette Road
Saint Paul, MN 55155
651-431-3515
Fax: 651-431-7476
www.dhs.state.mn.us/

The Minnesota Department of Human Services helps people meet their basic needs by providing or administering health care coverage, economic assistance, and a variety of services for children, people with disabilities and older Minnesotans.

2351 Minnesota Youth Services Bureau
244 North Lake Street
Forest Lake, MN 55025
651-464-3685
Fax: 651-464-3687
E-mail: Jeanne.Walz@ysblakesarea.org
www.ysblakesarea.org

Jeanne Walz, Executive Director

Youth Service Bureau (YSB) was founded in 1976 by a group of concerned citizens, teachers, law enforcement, civic and community leaders in response to the changing needs of youth in our community. Programs and services reflect our commitment to prevention and intervention in problems affecting youth, which could result in youth entering the criminal justice system

Mississippi

2352 Mississippi Alcohol Safety Education Program
103 Mississippi Research Park
PO Box 5287
Mississippi State, MS 39762
662-325-3423
Fax: 662-325-9439
www.ssrc.misstate.edu/

MASEP is the statewide program for first-time offenders convicted of driving under the influence of alcohol or another substance which has impaired one's ability to operate a motor vehicle.

2353 Mississippi Department Mental Health Mental Retardation Services
1101 Robert E Lee Building
239 N. Lamar Street
Jackson, MS 39201
601-359-1288
877-210-8513
Fax: 601-359-6295
TDD: 601-359-6230
www.dmh.state.ms.us

Has the primary responsibility for the development and implementation of services to meet the needs of individuals with mental retardation/developmental disabilities. This public service delivery system is comprised of five state-operated comprehensive regional centers for individuals with mental retardation/developmental disabilities, a state-operated facility for youth who require specialized treatment and have mental retardation/developmental disabilities, 15 regional community mental health/mental retardation centers, and other nonprofit community agencies/organizations that provide community services.

2354 Mississippi Department of Human Services
750 North State Street
Jackson, MS 39202
601-359-4500
800-345-6347
www.www.mdhs.state.ms.us

Donald Taylor, Executive Director

The mission of the Department of Human Services is to provide services for people in need by optimizing all available resources to sustain the family unit and to encourage traditional family values thereby promoting self-sufficiency and personal responsibility for all Mississippians.

2355 Mississippi Department of Mental Health: Division of Alcohol and Drug Abuse
239 N Lamar Street
1101 Robert F Lee Building
Jackson, MS 39201
601-359-1288
Fax: 601-359-6295
TDD: 601-359-6230
www.dmh.state.ms.us
Edwin Legrand, Executive Director

The Division of Alcohol and Drug Abuse Services is responsible for establishing, maintaining, monitoring and evaluating a statewide system of alcohol and drug abuse services, including prevention, treatment and rehabilitation. The division has designed a system of services for alcohol and drug abuse prevention and treatment reflecting its philosophy that alcohol and drug abuse is a treatable and preventable illness.

2356 Mississippi Department of Mental Health: Division of Medicaid
Sillers Building 550 High Street
Suite 1000
Jackson, MS 39201-1399
601-359-6050
www.dom.state.ms.us/

Robert L Robinson, Executive Director

Medicaid is a national health care program. It helps pay for medical services for low-income people. For those eligible for full Medicaid services, Medicaid is paid to providers of health care. Providers are doctors, hospitals and pharmacists who take Medicaid. We strive to provide financial assistance for the provision of quality health services to our beneficiaries with professionalism, integrity, compassion and commitment. We are advocates for, and accountable to the people we serve.

2357 Mississippi Department of Rehabilitation Services: Office of Vocational Rehabilitation (OVR)
1281 Highway 51
PO Box 1698
Madison, MS 39110
601-853-5100
800-443-1000
www.mdrs.state.ms.us

Dr Norman Miller, Deputy Director

The Office of Vocational Rehabilitation (OVR) provides services designed to improve economic opportunities for individuals with physical and mental disabilities through employment. Work related services are individualized and may include but are not limited to: counseling, job development, job training, job placement, supported employment, transition services and employability skills training program. OVR has a network of 17 community rehabilitation centers (Allied Enterprises) located throughout the state, which provide vocational assessment, job training and actual work experience for individuals with disabilities. Thousands of Mississippians are successfully employed each year through the teamwork at OVR.

Missouri

2358 Missouri Department Health & Senior Services
PO Box 570
Jefferson City, MO 65102
573-751-6400
Fax: 573-751-6401
E-mail: info@dhss.mo.gov
www.dhss.mo.gov/

The Missouri Department of Health and Senior Services provides information on a variety of topics including senior services and health, current news and public notices, laws and regulations, and statistical reports.

2359 Missouri Department of Mental Health
1706 E Elm Street
P O Box 687
Jefferson City, MO 65102
573-751-4122
800-364-9687
Fax: 573-751-8224
TTY: 573-526-1201
E-mail: dmhmail@dmh.mo.gov
www.dmh.missouri.gov/

State law provides three principal missions for the department: (1) the prevention of mental disorders, developmental disabilities, substance abuse, and compulsive gambling; (2) the treatment, habilitation, and rehabilitation of Missourians who have those conditions; and (3) the improvement of public understanding and attitudes about mental disorders, developmental disabilities, substance abuse, and compulsive gambling.

2360 Missouri Department of Public Safety
301 W. High Street
Hst Building, Rm. 870, PO Box 749
Jefferson City, MO 65102

573-751-4905
Fax: 573-751-5399
E-mail: dpsinfo@dps.mo.gov
www.dps.mo.gov

Mark James, Director

The Office of the Director is the Department of Public Safety's central administrative unit. Our office administers federal and state funds in grants for juvenile justice, victims' assistance, law enforcement, and narcotics control. Other programs in the Director's Office provide support services and resources to assist local law enforcement agencies and to promote crime prevention.

2361 Missouri Department of Social Services
221 West High Street
P O Box 1527
Jefferson City, MO 65102-1527
573-751-4815
Fax: 573-751-3203
TDD: 800-735-2966
www.dss.mo.gov/

Deborah Scott, Director

A true measure of a society is the extent of its concern for those less fortunate-its intent of keeping families together, preventing abuse and neglect, and encouraging self-sufficiency and independence. In Missouri, programs dealing with these concerns are administered by the state Department of Social Services.

2362 Missouri Department of Social Services: Medical Services Division
615 Howerton Court
P O Box 6500
Jefferson City, MO 65102-6500
573-751-3425
Fax: 573-751-6564
www.dss.mo.gov/mhd/

The purpose of the Division of Medical Services is to purchase and monitor health care services for low income and vulnerable citizens of the State of Missouri. The agency assures quality health care through development of service delivery systems, standards setting and enforcement, and education of providers and recipients. We are fiscally accountable for maximum and appropriate utilization of resources

2363 Missouri Division of Alcohol and Drug Abuse
P O Box 687
1706 E Elm Street
Jefferson City, MO 65101
573-751-4942
E-mail: adamail@dmh.mo.gov
www.dmh.missouri.gov/ada/adaindex.htm

The Division provides funding for prevention, outpatient, residential, and detoxification services to community-based programs that work with communities to develop and implement comprehensive coordinated plans. The Division provides technical assistance to these agencies and operates a certification program that sets standards for treatment programs, qualified professionals, and alcohol and drug related educational programs.

2364 Missouri Division of Comprehensive Psychiatric Service
PO Box 687
1706 E Elm Street
Jefferson City, MO 65102
573-751-8017
E-mail: cpsmail@dmh.mo.gov
www.dmh.missouri.gov/cps/cpsindex.htm

The division is committed to serving four target populations: persons with serious and persistent mental illness (SMI); persons suffering from acute psychiatric conditions; children and youth with serious emotional disturbances (SED) and forensic clients. In addition, CPS has identified four priority groups within the target populations: (1) individuals in crisis, (2) people who are homeless, (3) those recently discharged from inpatient care and (4) substantial users of public funds. These target populations currently constitute the majority of clientele whom the Division serves both in inpatient and ambulatory settings.

2365 Missouri Division of Mental Retardation and Developmental Disabilities
1706 E Elm Street
PO Box 687
Jefferson City, MO 65101
573-751-8676
E-mail: mrddmail@dmh.mo.gov
www.dmh.missouri.gov/mrdd/mrddindex.htm

The Division of Mental Retardation and Developmental Disabilities (MRDD), established in 1974, serves a population that has developmental disabilities such as mental retardation, cerebral palsy, head injuries, autism, epilepsy, and certain learning disabilities. Such conditions must have occurred before age 22, with the expectation that they will continue. To be eligible for services from the Division, persons with these disabilities must be substantially limited in their ability to function independently.

Montana

2366 Montana Department of Health and Human Services: Child & Family Services Division
Cogswell Building
1400 Broadway
Helena, MT 59604
406-444-5900
www.dphhs.mt.gov/

The Child and Family Services Division (CFSD) is a part of the Montana Department of Public Health and Human Services. Its mission is to keep Montana's children safe and families strong. The division provides state and federally mandated protective services to children who are abused, neglected, or abandoned. This includes receiving and investigating reports of child abuse and neglect, working to prevent domestic violence, helping families to stay together or reunite, and finding placements in foster or adoptive homes.

2367 Montana Department of Public Health & Human Services: Addictive and Mental Disorders
555 Fuller Avenue
Helena, MT 59620
406-444-3964
www.dphhs.mt.gov/

The mission of the Addictive and Mental Disorders Division (AMDD) of the Montana Department of Public Health and Human Services is to implement and improve an appropriate statewide system of prevention, treatment, care, and rehabilitation for Montanans with mental disorders or addictions to drugs or alcohol.

2368 Montana Department of Public Health and Human Services: Montana Vocational Rehabilitation Programs
Disability Services Division
111 Sanders Street
Helena, MT 59604
406-444-5622
www.dphhs.mt.gov/

The mission of the Disability Services Division (DSD) of the Montana Department of Public Health and Human Services is to provide services that help Montanans with disabilities to live, work and fully participate in their communities.

Nebraska

2369 Nebraska Department of Health and Human Services (NHHS)
PO Box 95026
Lincoln, NE 68509-5026
402-471-3121
www.hhs.state.ne.us/

The mission of the NHHS is to help people live better lives through effective health and human services.

2370 Nebraska Health & Human Services: Medicaid and Managed Care Division
Department of Finance & Support
PO Box 95026
Lincoln, NE 68509-5026
402-471-3121
www.hhs.state.ne.us

The Finance and Support agency aligns human resources, financial resources, and information needs for the Nebraska Health and Human Services System and is the designated Title XIX (Medicaid) agency responsible for provider enrollment activities.

2371 Nebraska Health and Human Services Division: Department of Mental Health
P O Box 95026
Lincoln, NE 68509-5026
402-471-3121
www.hhs.state.ne.us

Mental health services are designed for individuals and their families who have a serious and persistent mental illness that can create lifetime disabilities, and in some cases make the individuals dangerous to themselves or others. Services are also designed for people experiencing acute, serious mental illnesses, which in some cases may cause a life threatening event such as suicide attempts. In addition, services are provided for children and to their families.

2372 Nebraska Mental Health Centers
4545 South 86th Street
Lincoln, NE 68526
402-423-6990
888-210-8064
E-mail: drness@nmhc-clinics.com
www.nmhc-clinics.com/

Dr. Matthew Nessetti, Director

We are a primary mental health care center that is truly committed to being of service to the Lincoln/Lancaster community and Greater Nebraska.

Nevada

2373 Nevada Department of Health & Human Services Health Care Financing and Policy
1100 East William Street, Suite 101
Carson City, NV 89701
775-684-3676
E-mail: techhelp@dhcfp.nv.gov
www.dhcfp.state.nv.us/

The Division of Health Care Financing and Policy works in partnership with the Centers for Medicare & Medicaid Services to assist in providing quality medical care for eligible individuals and families with low incomes and limited resources. Services are provided through a combination of traditional fee-for-service provider networks and managed care.

2374 Nevada Department of Health and Human Services
4126 Technology Way
Room 100
Carson City, NV 89706-2009
775-684-4000
E-mail: nvdhs@dhhs.nv.gov
www.www.dhhs.nv.gov

Michael J Willden, Director

The Department of Health and Human Services (DHHS) promotes the health and well-being of Nevadans through the delivery or facilitation of essential services to ensure families are strengthened, public health is protected, and individuals achieve their highest level of self-sufficiency.

2375 Nevada Division of Mental Health & Developmental Services
4126 Technology Way
2nd Floor
Carson City, NV 89706
775-684-5943
Fax: 775-684-5964
E-mail: mhdswebmaster@mhds.nv.gov
www.www.mhds.nv.gov

Harold Cook, Acting Administrator

The Nevada Division of Mental Health provides a full array of clinical services to over 24,000 consumers each year. Services include: crisis intervention, hospital care, medication clinic, outpatient counseling, residential support and other mental health services targeted to individuals with serious mental illness.

2376 Nevada Employment Training & Rehabilitation Department
500 East Third Street
Carson City, NV 89713
775-684-3849
Fax: 775-684-3850
TTY: 775-687-5353
www.nvdetr.org/

Larry Mosley, Director

The Department of Employment, Training and Rehabilitation (DETR) is comprised of four divisions with numerous bureaus programs, and services housed in offices through-out Nevada to provide citizens the state's premier source of employment, training, and rehabilitative programs.

2377 Nevada State Health Division: Bureau of Alcohol & Drug Abuse
4126 Technology Way
Carson City, NV 89706
775-684-5943
Fax: 775-684-5964
www.www.state.nv.us

Larry Mosley, Director

The mission of the Bureau of Alcohol and Drug Abuse (BADA) is to reduce the impact of substance abuse in Nevada.

2378 Northern Nevada Adult Mental Health Services
480 Galletti Way
Sparks, NV 89431-5573
775-688-2001
Fax: 775-688-2192
www.mhds.state.nv.us

The mission of Northern Nevada Adult Mental Health Services is to provide psychiatric treatment and rehabilitation services in the least restrictive setting to support personal recovery and enhance quality of life.

2379 Southern Nevada Adult Mental Health Services
6161 W Charleston Boulevard
Las Vegas, NV 89146
702-486-6000
www.mhds.state.nv.us

Larry Mosley, Director

State operated community mental health center. Provides inpatient and outpatient psychiatric services.

New Hampshire

2380 New Hampshire Department of Health & Human Services: Bureau of Community Health Services
29 Hazen Drive
Concord, NH 03301
603-271-4638
www.dhhs.state.nh.us/DHHS/BCHS/default.htm

The Bureau of Community Health Services oversees grants to community-based agencies for medical and preventive health services, sets policy, provides technical assistance and education, and carries out quality assurance activities in its programmatic areas of expertise.

2381 New Hampshire Department of Health and Human Services: Bureau of Developmental Services
105 Pleasant Street
Concord, NH 03301
603-271-5034
Fax: 603-271-5166
www.dhhs.state.nh.us/DHHS/BDS/default.htm

The NH developmental services system offers its consumers with developmental disabilities and acquired brain disorders a wide range of supports and services within their own communities. BDS is comprised of a main office in Concord and 12 designated non-profit and specialized service agencies that represent specific geographic regions of NH; the community agencies are commonly referred to as

Area Agencies. All direct services and supports to individuals and families are provided in accordance with contractual agreements between BDS and the Area Agencies.

2382 New Hampshire Department of Health and Human Services: Bureau of Behavioral Health
105 Pleasant Street
Concord, NH 03301
603-271-5000
Fax: 603-271-5058
www.dhhs.state.nh.us/DHHS/BBH/default.htm

The Bureau of Behavioral Health (BBH) seeks to promote respect, recovery, and full community inclusion for adults, including older adults, who experience a mental illness and children with an emotional disturbance. By law and rule, BBH is mandated to ensure the provision of efficient and effective services to those citizens who are most severely and persistently disabled by mental, emotional, and behavioral dysfunction. To this end, BBH has apportioned the entire state into community mental health regions. Each of the ten regions has a BBH contracted Community Mental Health Center and many regions have Peer Support Agencies.

New Jersey

2383 Juvenile Justice Commission
1001 Spruce Street
Suite 202
Trenton, NJ 08638
609-292-1400
Fax: 609-943-4611
E-mail: commission@njjjc.org
www.state.nj.us/lps/jjc/info.htm

Thomas Flanagan, Acting Executive Director

The Juvenile Justice Commission (JJC) has three primary responsibilities: the care and custody of juvenile offenders committed to the agency by the courts, the support of local efforts to plan for and provide services to at-risk and court-involved youth through County Youth Services Commissions and the state Incentive Program, and the supervision of youth on aftercare/parole.

2384 New Jersey Department of Human Services
P O Box 700
222 S Warren Street
Trenton, NJ 08625-0700
609-292-3717
www.state.nj.us/humanservices/index.shtml

Jennifer Velez, Commissioner

The New Jersey Department of Human Services (DHS) is the state's social services agency, serving more than one million of New Jersey 's most vulnerable citizens, or about one of every eight New Jersey residents. Through the work of DHS and its 13 major divisions, individuals and families in need are able to keep their lives on track, their families together, a roof over their heads, and their health protected. Human Services offers individuals and families the breathing room they need in order to find permanent solutions to otherwise daunting problems.

2385 New Jersey Division of Mental Health Services
50 East State Street
PO Box 727
Trenton, NJ 08625-0727

800-382-6717
www.state.nj.us/humanservices/dmhs

Kevin Martone, Assistant Commissioner

The Division of Mental Health Services (DMHS) serves adults with serious and persistent mental illnesses. Central to the Division's mission is the fact that these individuals are entitled to dignified and meaningful lives. With an operating budget of $588,377,000 for FY 2005 and 5,700 employees, services are available to anyone in the state who feels they need help with a mental health problem.

2386 New Jersey Division of Youth & Family Services
P O Box 717
50 East State Street, 5th Floor
Trenton, NJ 08625
609-777-2000
Fax: 609-777-2050
www.state.nj.us/humanservices/dyfs/index.html

Lisa Von Pier, Area Director

The Division of Youth and Family Services (DYFS) is New Jersey's child protection/child welfare agency within the Office of Children's Services (OCS). DYFS is responsible for investigating allegations of child abuse and neglect and if necessary arranging for the child's protection and the family's treatment. 41 local offices handle referrals and investigations statewide. The mission of the Division of Youth and Family Services is to ensure the safety, permanency, and well-being of children and to support families.

2387 New Jersey Office of Managed Care
New Jersey Department of Banking & Insurance
20 West State Street
P O Box 325
Trenton, NJ 08625
609-292-7272
800-446-7467
www.state.nj.us/dobi/managed.htm

The Office of Managed Care is responsible for: the day-to-day tasks associated with regulating HMOs; regulating certain aspects of the operations of non-HMO carriers that offer health benefits plans in New Jersey that are managed care plans; regulating the utilization management functions of non-HMO carriers that include utilization management features in the health benefits plans they offer in New Jersey; providing certification of organized delivery systems in New Jersey; and certain review functions for other managed care matters, including review of Workers' Compensation Managed Care Organization applications and renewals, and applications of organized delivery systems that seek to be licensed by the Department of Banking and Insurance.

New Mexico

2388 New Mexico Behavioral Health Collaborative
2025 S Pocheoo Street
PO Box 2348
Santa Fe, NM 87504-2348
505-827-6250
Fax: 505-827-3185
E-mail: deborah.fickling@state.nm.us
www.state.nm.us/hsd/bhdwg/

Deborah Fickling, Director

At the heart of the Collaborative's vision is the expectation that the lives of individuals with mental illness and substance use disorders ("customers") will improve, that customers and family members will have an equal voice in the decisions that affect them and their loved ones, and that those most affected by mental illness and substance abuse can recover to lead full, meaningful lives within their communities. To achieve this will require a paradigm shift not only within the service delivery culture but also within the existing customer/family member networks.

2389 New Mexico Department of Health
1190 S St. Francis Drive
Santa Fe, NM 87502
505-827-2613
Fax: 505-827-2530
www.health.state.nm.us/

The mission of the New Mexico Department of Health is to promote health and sound health policy, prevent disease and disability, improve health services systems and assure that essential public health functions and safety net services are available to New Mexicans.

2390 New Mexico Department of Human Services
PO Box 2348
Santa Fe, NM 87504
505-827-7750
Fax: 505-827-6286
E-mail: eckert@state.nm.us
www.state.nm.us/hsd/

The Department strives to provide New Mexicans access to support and services so that they may move toward self-sufficiency.

2391 New Mexico Department of Human Services: Medical Assistance Division
PO Box 2348
Santa Fe, NM 87504-2348
505-827-3100
Fax: 505-827-3185
E-mail: nmmedicaidfraud@state.nm.us
www.state.nm.us/hsd/mad/Index.html

The Medical Assistance Division (MAD) is responsible for direct administration of the New Mexico Medicaid program. Medicaid is a joint federal and state program that pays for health care to New Mexicans who are eligible for Medicaid benefits.

2392 New Mexico Health & Environment Department
1190 St. Francis Drive
Suite N4050
Santa Fe, NM 87505
800-219-6157
www.nmenv.state.nm.us/

Our mission is to provide the highest quality of life throughout the state by promoting a safe, clean and productive environment.

2393 New Mexico Kids, Parents and Families Office of Child Development: Children, Youth and Families Department
760 Motel Blvd
Suite C
Las Cruces, NM 88005

505-827-7946
Fax: 505-476-0490
E-mail: dmhaggard@cyfd.state.nm.us
www.newmexicokids.org/Family/

Dan Haggard, Director

The Children, Youth and Families Department Office of Child Development (OCD) works collaboratively with the State Department of Education, Department of Health, Department of Labor and higher education and community programs to establish a five-year plan for Early Care, Education and Family Support Professional Development. The New Mexico Professional Development Initiative supports OCD's legislative mandate to articulate and implement training and licensure requirements for individuals working in all recognized settings with children from birth to age eight.

New York

2394 New York Office of Alcohol & Substance Abuse Services
1450 Western Avenue
Albany, NY 12203-3526
518-485-1768
E-mail: communications@oasas.state.ny.us
www.oasas.state.ny.us/pio/oasas.htm

Karen M. Carpenter-Paulumbo, Commissioner

State agency responsible for funding, licensing and monitering substance abuse prevention and treatment services in New York State.

2395 New York State Department of Health Individual County Listings of Social Services Departments
Corning Tower
Empire State Plaza
Albany, NY 12237
518-447-7300
E-mail: dohweb@health.state.ny.us
www.health.state.ny.us

Provides statewide listing of departments of social services including contact information.

2396 New York State Office of Mental Health
44 Holland Avenue
Albany, NY 12229
800-597-8481
www.omh.state.ny.us/

Michael Hogan, Commissioner

Promoting the mental health of all New Yorkers with a particular focus on providing hope and recovery for adults with serious mental illness and children with serious emotional disturbances.

North Carolina

2397 North Carolina Department of Human Resources
2001 Mail Service Center
Raleigh, NC 27699-2001
919-733-2940
www.www.ncdhhs.gov/humanresources

Kathy Gruer, Director

Whether it is helping applicants find information on available jobs, providing consultation to managers and supervisors, informing current employees of benefits and services, or spearheading efforts to recruit hard-to-fill vacancies, the Division of Human Resources supports the overall mission of the Department of Health and Human Services (DHHS) to serve people.

2398 North Carolina Division of Mental Health

325 North Salisbury Street
Raleigh, NC 27601
919-733-7011
Fax: 919-508-0951
E-mail: contactdmh@ncmail.net
www.www.ncdhhs.gov/mhddsas/

Michael Moseley, Director

North Carolina will provide people with, or at risk of, mental illness, developmental disabilities and substance problems and their families the necessary prevention, intervention, treatment, services and supports they need to live successfully in communities of their choice.

2399 North Carolina Division of Social Services

325 N Salisbury Street
Albemarle Building 8th Floor
Raleigh, NC 27601
919-733-3055
Fax: 919-733-9386
E-mail: dssweb@ncmail.net
www.www.ncdhhs.gov/dss

The North Carolina Division of Social Services is dedicated to assisting and providing opportunities for individuals and families in need of basic support and services to become self sufficient and self reliant. The Division of Social Services advocates for and encourages individuals' rights to select actions appropriate to their needs.

2400 North Carolina Substance Abuse Professional Certification Board (NCSAPCB)

PO Box 10126
Raleigh, NC 27605
919-832-0975
Fax: 919-833-5743
www.ncsapcb.org

Provides guidelines for the certification of professionals in the substance abuse field of human services.

North Dakota

2401 North Dakota Department of Human Services: Medicaid Program

600 E Boulevard Avenue
Dept 325
Bismarck, ND 58505-0250
701-328-2321
Fax: 701-328-1544
E-mail: dhsmed@nd.gov
www.www.nd.gov/dhs

Pays for a wide array of medical services including mental health services for certain low-income residents of North Dakota. Anyone interested in applying for services should contact their local County Social Service Board office.

2402 North Dakota Department of Human Services: Mental Health Services Division

600 E Boulevard Avenue
Dept 325
Bismarck, ND 58505-0250

701-328-2321
Fax: 701-328-1544
E-mail: dhsmed@nd.gov
www.www.nd.gov

The Department of Human Services' Mental Health and Substance Abuse Services Division provides leadership for the planning, development, and oversight of a system of care for children, adults, and families with severe emotional disorders, mental illness, and/or substance abuse issues.

2403 North Dakota Department of Human Services Division of Mental Health and Substance Abuse Services

1237 West Divide Avenue
Suite 1C
Bismarck, ND 58501-1208
701-328-8920
800-755-2719
Fax: 701-328-8969
E-mail: dhsmhsas@nd.gov
www.www.nd.gov/dhs/services/mentalhealth

Provides leadership for the planning, development and oversight of a system of care for children, adults and families with severe emotional disorders, mental illness and/or substance abuse issues. Mental health and substance abuse services are delivered through eight Regional Human Services Centers and the North Dakota State Hospital in Jamestown.

Ohio

2404 Ohio Community Drug Board

725 East Market Street
Akron, OH 44305
330-434-4141
Fax: 330-434-7125
TDD: 330-535-4889
www.commhealthcenter.org/

The Community Health Center is committed to enhancing the quality of life by providing a diverse, holistic, patient-centered continuum of care. Our innovative and effective services include addiction treatment, behavioral and primary healthcare, wellness, prevention and housing programs that are responsive to the needs of the community. We have been serving Northeast Ohio since 1974.

2405 Ohio Department of Mental Health

30 East Broad Street
8th Floor
Columbus, OH 43215-3430
614-466-2596
877-275-6364
TTY: 614-752-9696
E-mail: uhricks@mh.state.oh.us
www.mh.state.oh.us/

Ensures high quality mental health care is available to all Ohioans, particularly individuals with severe mental illness.

Oklahoma

2406 Oklahoma Department of Human Services

PO Box 25352
2400 N Lincoln Blvd
Oklahoma City, OK 73125
405-521-3646
www.www.okdhs.org

The mission of the Oklahoma Department of Human Services is to help individuals and families in need help themselves lead safer, healthier, more independent and productive lives.

2407 Oklahoma Department of Mental Health and Substance Abuse Service (ODMHSAS)

1200 NE 13th Street
PO Box 53277
Oklahoma City, OK 73152-3277
405-522-3908
800-522-9054
Fax: 405-522-3650
TDD: 405-522-3851
www.odmhsas.org

State agency responsible for mental health, substance abuse, and domestic violence and sexual assault services.

2408 Oklahoma Healthcare Authority

4545 North Lincoln Boulevard
Suite 124
Oklahoma City, OK 73105
405-522-7300
www.ohca.state.ok.us/

Provides health and medical policy information to Medicaid consumers and providers, administers SoonerCare and other health related programs.

2409 Oklahoma Mental Health Consumer Council

3200 NW 48th
Suite 102
Oklahoma City, OK 73112
405-604-6975
888-424-1305
Fax: 405-605-8175
E-mail: consumercouncil@okmhcc.org
www.www.okmhcc.org

Consumer run statewide advocacy organization for education, empowerment, quality of life, encouragement and rights protection of persons with mental illness. Services include empowerment training, systems advocacy, peer support and jail diversion programs.

2410 Oklahoma Office of Juvenile Affairs

3812 North Santa Fe
Suite 400
Oklahoma City, OK 73118
918-530-2800
Fax: 918-530-2890
www.state.ok.us/~oja/

State agency charged with delivery of programs and services to delinquent youth. Services include delinquency prevention, diversion, counseling in both community and secure residential programs. OJA provides counseling services with counselors, social workers and psychologists, as well as contracted service providers.

Oregon

2411 Marion County Health Department

3180 Center Street NE
Suite 2100
Salem, OR 97310
503-588-5357
Fax: 503-364-6552
E-mail: health@co.marion.or.us
www.www.co.marion.or.us/

The Marion County Health Department fosters wellness, monitors health trends, and responds to community health needs.

2412 Office of Mental Health and Addiction Services Training & Resource Center

500 Summer Street Ne E86
Salem, OR 97301
503-945-5863
Fax: 503-378-8467
www.www.oregon.gov/dhs/addiction

We are a library and clearinghouse, your connection to resources for prevention and treatment of disorders related to the use of alcohol, tobacco, other drugs and problem gambling. Our goal is to provide current, accurate and timely information to professionals and the public. We also seek to promote use of research based practices and promising approaches to prevention and treatment.

2413 Oregon Commission on Children and Families

530 Center Street NE
Suite 405
Salem, OR 97301
503-373-1283
www.oregon.gov/OCCF/index.shtml

Has various support services for children and families. Includes mental counseling, education training, and community outreach programs.

2414 Oregon Department of Human Resources: Division of Health Services

800 NE Oregon Street
Portland, OR 97232
971-673-1222
Fax: 971-673-1299
TTY: 971-673-0372
www.oregon.gov/DHS/ph/about_us.shtml

Health Services administers low-income medical programs, and mental health and substance abuse services. It provides public health services such as monitoring drinking-water quality and communicable-disease outbreaks, inspecting restaurants and promoting healthy behaviors.

2415 Oregon Department of Human Services: Mental Health Services

500 Summer Street NE
Salem, OR 97301
503-945-5944
Fax: 503-378-2897
TTY: 503-945-6214
E-mail: dhs.info@state.or.us
www.oregon.gov/DHS/index.shtml

The Office of Mental Health Services oversees a continuum of services and care including crisis services, local acute care, clinic based and outpatient care, state hospital referral, supported housing and employment. Programs include Community Services; Extended Care; Quality Assurance; Medical Director; Planning and Projects Development; Mental Health Planning and Management Advisory Council; Budget, Data and Operations; Contract and Budget Coordination; and Office Operations and Support.

2416 Oregon Department of Human Services: Office of Developmental Disabilities

500 Summer Street NE
Salem, OR 97301

503-945-5944
Fax: 503-378-2897
E-mail: dhs.info@state.or.us
www.oregon.gov/DHS/index.shtml

The Office of Developmental Disability Services oversees a system of community based programs for individuals with developmental disabilities including residential care, vocational/employment assistance, family support, and crisis/diversion services. Programs include Administration, Protective Services, Contracts, Licensing and Certification, Information and Data, Training, Self-Directed Supports, Medicaid Twenty-Hour Personal Care, Employment/Alternatives to Employment, Development Team, 24-Hour Residential Facilities, Vocational Programs, Diversion/Crisis, Diagnosis and Evaluation, Medical Director, and Housing.

2417 Oregon Health Policy and Research: Policy and Analysis Unit

1225 Ferry Street Se
1st Floor
Salem, OR 97301
503-373-1824
www.oregon.gov/

Facilitates collaborative health services and research and policy analysis on issues affecting the Oregon Health Plan population and works to effectively communicate timely, quality results of health services research and analysis in the interest of informing health policy.

Pennsylvania

2418 Dauphin County Drug and Alcohol

1100 South Cameron Street
Harrisburg, PA 17104
717-635-2254
Fax: 717-635-2266

2419 Pennsylvania Bureau Drug and Alcohol Programs: Monitoring

2 Kline Plaza
Suite B
Harrisburg, PA 17104
717-783-8200
Fax: 717-787-6285
www.dsf.health.state.pa.us/health/cwp/view.asp?A=173&Q

The Bureau of Drug and Alcohol Programs was established by the Pennsylvania Drug and Alcohol Abuse Control Act and is charged with developing and implementing a comprehensive health, education, and rehabilitation program for the prevention, intervention, treatment and case management of drug and alcohol abuse and dependence. This program is implemented through grant agreements with the 49 Single County Authorities (SCAs) who, in turn, contract with private service providers. BDAP provides for central planning, management, and monitoring; the SCAs provide administrative oversight to the local contracted programs

2420 Pennsylvania Bureau of Community Program Standards: Licensure and Certification
Pennsylvania Department of Health

7th & Forster Streets
Harrisburg, PA 17120
877-724-3258
www.dsf.health.state.pa.us/health/site/default.asp

The Bureau's mission is to assure that certain healthcare providers are delivering quality services by adhering to es-

tablished minimum state and federal standards of operation. Bureau staff conduct on-site surveys to assess adherence to the standards, as well as consumer satisfaction with the services provided.

2421 Pennsylvania Bureau of Drug and Alcohol Programs: Information Bulletins

2 Kline Plaza
Suite B
Harrisburg, PA 17104
717-783-8200
Fax: 717-787-6285
www.dsf.health.state.pa.us/health/CWP/view.asp?A=173&Q

The Bureau of Drug and Alcohol Programs was established by the Pennsylvania Drug and Alcohol Abuse Control Act and is charged with developing and implementing a comprehensive health, education, and rehabilitation program for the prevention, intervention, treatment and case management of drug and alcohol abuse and dependence. This program is implemented through grant agreements with the 49 Single County Authorities (SCAs) who, in turn, contract with private service providers. BDAP provides for central planning, management, and monitoring; the SCAs provide administrative oversight to the local contracted programs

2422 Pennsylvania Department of Health: Bureau of Drug and Alcohol Programs

2 Kline Plaza
Suite B
Harrisburg, PA 17104
717-783-8200
Fax: 717-787-6285
www.dsf.health.state.pa.us/health/cwp/view.asp?A=173&Q

The Bureau of Drug and Alcohol Programs was established by the Pennsylvania Drug and Alcohol Abuse Control Act and is charged with developing and implementing a comprehensive health, education, and rehabilitation program for the prevention, intervention, treatment and case management of drug and alcohol abuse and dependence. This program is implemented through grant agreements with the 49 Single County Authorities (SCAs) who, in turn, contract with private service providers. BDAP provides for central planning, management, and monitoring; the SCAs provide administrative oversight to the local contracted programs.

2423 Pennsylvania Department of Public Welfare and Mental Health Services

PO Box 2675
Harrisburg, PA 17105
717-787-6443
www.dpw.state.pa.us/Family/MentalHealthServ/

The Department of Public Welfare is charged with numerous program areas that include all children, youth and family concerns, mental health, mental retardation, income maintenance, medical assistance and social program issues in the Commonwealth. They also license assisted living facilities and day care centers.

2424 Pennsylvania Division of Drug and Alcohol Prevention: Treatment

2 Kline Street
Suite B
Harrisburg, PA 17104
717-783-8200
Fax: 717-787-6285
www.dsf.health.state.pa.us/health/cwp/view.asp?A=173&Q

The Bureau of Drug and Alcohol Programs was established by the Pennsylvania Drug and Alcohol Abuse Control Act and is charged with developing and implementing a comprehensive health, education, and rehabilitation program for the prevention, intervention, treatment and case management of drug and alcohol abuse and dependence. This program is implemented through grant agreements with the 49 Single County Authorities (SCAs) who, in turn, contract with private service providers. BDAP provides for central planning, management, and monitoring; the SCAs provide administrative oversight to the local contracted programs.

2425 Pennsylvania Medical Assistance Programs

Health & Welfare Building
Room 515, PO Box 2675
Harrisburg, PA 17105-2675
717-787-1870
www.dpw.state.pa.us/OMAP/

Mission is to implement mandatory managed care statewide; to expand home and community based services; to improve the quality of services to consumers and providers in all our health care delivery systems; and to improve our technology infrastructure by supporting H-Net Development and re-designing MAMIS.

Rhode Island

2426 Rhode Island Department of Human Services

600 New London Avenue
Cranston, RI 02920
401-462-3019
www.dhs.state.ri.us/

Gary Alexander, Director

We are an organization of opportunity, working hand-in-hand with other resources in Rhode Island to offer a full continuum of services for families, adults, children, the elderly, those with disabilities and veterans.

2427 Rhode Island Division of Substance Abuse

14 Harrington Road
Cranston, RI 02920
401-462-2339
Fax: 401-462-6636
www.mhrh.state.ri.us/

Craig S Stenning, Executive Director

Substance Abuse Treatment and Prevention Services (SATPS) is responsible for planning, coordinating and administering a comprehensive statewide system of substance abuse, treatment and prevention activities. SATPS develops, supports and advocates for high quality, accessible, comprehensive and clinically appropriate substance abuse prevention and treatment services in order to decrease the negative effects of alcohol, tobacco and other drug use in Rhode Island, and improve the overall behavioral health of Rhode Islanders.

2428 State of Rhode Island Department of Mental Health, Retardation and Hospitals
Division of Behavioral Healthcare Services

14 Harrington Road
Cranston, RI 02920
401-462-2339
Fax: 401-462-1564
www.mhrh.state.ri.us/

Craig S Stenning, Executive Director

Our overall mission will focus on the unique needs and goals of individuals who experience a mental illness, an emotional disturbance, and/or a substance abuse or addiction problem and to prevent, whenever possible, these from ever occurring.

South Carolina

2429 LRADAC The Behavioral Health Center of the Midlands

134 North Hospital Drive
Columbia, SC 29250
800-373-0459
www.lradac.org/

Deborah Francis, President/Coo

The mission of LRADAC is to provide effective, personalized services to prevent or reduce the harm of substance use and addictions. We will provide evidence-based, best practice prevention, intervention and treatment services to the populations of Richland and Lexington Counties and others as appropriate.

2430 Mental Health Association in South Carolina

1823 Gadsden Street
Columbia, SC 29201
803-779-5363
800-375-9894
Fax: 803-779-0017
E-mail: mha@mha-sc.org

The Mental Health Association in South Carolina believes in a healthy society in which all people are accorded respect, dignity and the opportunity to achieve their full potential free from stigma and prejudice. The MHASC is dedicated to preventing mental disorders through research and achieving victory over mental illnesses through systems and individual advocacy, education and unmet service development.

2431 South Carolina Department of Alcohol and Other Drug Abuse Services

101 Executive Center Drive
Suite 215
Columbia, SC 29210
803-896-5555
Fax: 803-896-5557
E-mail: leecatoe@daodas.state.sc.us
www.daodas.state.sc.us

Lee W Catoe, Director

DAODAS is the cabinet-level department responsible for ensuring the availability of comprehensive alcohol and other drug abuse services for the citizens of South Carolina.

2432 South Carolina Department of Mental Health

2414 Bull Street
Columbia, SC 29202
803-898-8581
TTY: 864-297-5130
www.state.sc.us/dmh/

The administrative offices of the South Carolina Department of Mental Health are located in Columbia and provide support services including long-range planning, performance and clinical standards, evaluation and quality assurance, personnel management, communications, information resource management, legal counsel, financial, and procurement. In addition, the central office administers services for the hearing impaired; children, adolescents and their families; people with developmental disabilities; those needing alcohol and drug treatment; the elderly; and patients who need long-term care.

2433 South Carolina Department of Social Services

1535 Confederate Avenue Extension
P O Box 1520
Columbia, SC 29202-1520
803-898-7601
www.state.sc.us/dss/

Kathleen Hayes, State Director

The mission of the South Carolina Department of Social Services is to ensure the safety and health of children and adults who cannot protect themselves, and to assist those in need of food assistance and temporary financial assistance while transitioning into employment.

South Dakota

2434 South Dakota Department of Human Services: Division of Mental Health

E Highway 34, Hillsview Plaza
Pierre, SD 57501
605-773-5991
800-265-9684
Fax: 605-773-7076
www.state.sd.us/dhs/dmh/

Serves as the point of contact for state funded services, support and treatment for adults with severe and persistent mental illness (SPMI), and children with serious emotional disturbance (SED).

2435 South Dakota Department of Social Services Office of Medical Services

700 Governors Drive
Pierre, SD 57501
605-773-3165
Fax: 605-773-4855
E-mail: Medical@STATE.SD.US
www.state.sd.us/social/Medical/

The South Dakota Office of Medical Services covers medical care provided to low income people who meet eligibility standards either under Medicaid (Title XIX) or the Children's Health Insurance Program (CHIP). These programs are financed jointly by state and federal government and are managed by the SD Department of Social Services.

2436 South Dakota Human Services Center

3515 Broadway Avenue
PO Box 7600
Yankton, SD 57078-7600
605-668-3100
Fax: 605-668-3460
E-mail: infohsc@state.sd.us
www.www.dhs.sd.gov/hsc

Cory D. Nelson, Administrator

Provides persons who are mentally ill or chemically dependent with effective,individualized professional treatment thats enables them to achieve their highest level of personal independence in the most therapeutic environment.

Tennessee

2437 Alcohol and Drug Council of Middle Tennessee

2612 Westwood Drive
Nashville, TN 37204
615-269-0029
Fax: 615-269-0299
E-mail: mmckinney@adcmt.org
www.adcmt.org

Mary McKinney, Executive Director
Mr Boyd Smith, President

Programs of education, prevention and intervention. With a commitment to helping people find a better way.

2438 Bureau of TennCare: State of Tennessee

310 Great Circle Road
Nashville, TN 37243
800-342-3145
www.state.tn.us/tenncare/

Darin Gordon, Deputy Commissioner

On January 1, 1994, Tennessee began a new health care reform program called TennCare. This program, which required no new taxes, essentially replaced the Medicaid program in Tennessee. TennCare was designed as a managed care model. It extended coverage to uninsured and uninsurable persons who were not eligible for Medicaid.

2439 Chattanooga/Plateau Council for Alcohol and Drug Abuse

911 Pineville Road
Chattanooga, TN 37405
423-756-7644
877-282-2327
Fax: 432-756-7646
E-mail: info@cadas.org
www.cadas.org/

Welcome to CADAS, founded in 1964. The CADAS mission is to deliver the highest quality treatment, prevention, and educational services to the chemically dependent, their families, and the community at large.

2440 Memphis Alcohol and Drug Council

1430 Poplar Avenue
Memphis, TN 38104
901-274-0056

Provides referrals, alcohol and other drug prevention, intervention and treatment services. Also, regional and county school prevention coordination, and a clearinghouse for Shelby County including national data search and materials distribution.

2441 Middle Tennessee Mental Health Institute

221 Stewarts Ferry Pike
Nashville, TN 37214-3325
615-902-7400
www.state.tn.us/mental/mhs/mhs2.html

Lynn McDonald, Chief Officer

TDMHDD operates 5 Regional Mental Health Institutes (RMHIs). Lakeshore Mental Health Institute (Knoxville), Moccasin Bend Mental Health Institute (Chattanooga) and Memphis Mental Health Institute provide in-patient psychiatric services for adults; Middle Tennessee Mental Health Institute (Nashville) and Western Mental Health Institute

(Bolivar) provide in-patient psychiatric services for both adults and children/youth. Most RMHI admissions are on an emergency involuntary basis, with a variety of court-ordered inpatient evaluation and treatment services also provided. The RMHIs provide psychiatric services based upon the demonstrated and emerging best practices of each clinical discipline.

2442 Tennessee Commission on Children and Youth

710 James Robertson Parkway
9th Floor
Nashville, TN 37243-0800
615-741-2633
E-mail: linda.oneal@state.tn.us
www.state.tn.gov/tccy

Linda O'Neal, Executive Director
Pat Wade, Program Director

2443 Tennessee Department of Health

425 5th Avenue N
Cordell Hull Building, 3rd Floor
Nashville, TN 37243
651-741-3111
E-mail: TN.health@state.tn.us
www.www.health.state.tn.us

Susan Cooper, Commissioner

Provides information on a wide variety of topics including community services, health maintenance organizations, immunizations and alcohol and drug services.

2444 Tennessee Department of Health: Alcohol and Drug Abuse

425 5th Avenue N
3rd Fl
Nashville, TN 37243
615-741-1921
Fax: 615-532-2419

2445 Tennessee Department of Human Services

400 Deaderick Street
15th Floor
Nashville, TN 37243-1403
615-313-4700
Fax: 614-741-4165
E-mail: Human-Services.Webmaster@state.tn.us
www.state.tn.us/humanserv/

Gina Lodge, Commissioner

Provides information about available programs and services, such as family assistance and child support, community programs, and rehabilitation services.

2446 Tennessee Department of Mental Health and Developmental Disabilities

5th Floor Cordell Hall
425 5th Avenue North
Nashville, TN 37243
615-532-6500
E-mail: opie.tdmhdd@state.tn.us
www.state.tn.us/mental
Virginia Trotter Betts, Commissioner

Tennessee's state mental health and developmental disabilities authority. It has responsibility for system planning, setting policy and quality standards, system monitering and evaluation, disseminating public information and advocating for persons of all ages who have mental illness, serious emotional disturbance or developmental disabilities.

2447 Williamson County Council on Alcohol and Drug Prevention

1320 W Main Street
Suite 418
Franklin, TN 37064-3737
615-790-5783
Fax: 615-790-5783
E-mail: WCCADAP@USIT.NET
www.williamson-franklinchamber.com/member_detail.html

Allen Murray, Executive Director

Provides alcohol and drug treatment counseling and rehabilitation services.

Texas

2448 Austin Travis County Mental Health: Mental Retardation Center

1430 Collier Street
Austin, TX 78704
512-447-4141
E-mail: webmaster@atcmhmr.com
www.atcmhmr.com

Provides mental health, mental retardation and substance services to the Austin-Travis County community.

2449 Harris County Mental Health: Mental Retardation Authority

7011 Southwest Freeway
Houston, TX 77074
713-970-7000
www.mhmraharris.org

MHMRA of Harris County is one of the largest mental health centers in the United States, serving more than 30,000 persons in the Houston metropolitan area who suffer from mental illness and/or mental retardation. We serve the "priority population" - adults who are diagnosed with severe and persistent mental illness, children with serious

2450 Mental Health Association of Greater Dallas

624 North Good-Latimer
200
Dallas, TX 75204
214-871-2420
Fax: 214-954-0611
www.mhadallas.org

To lead, coordinate and involve the community in improving mental health by advocating for improved care and treatment of people with mental illness.

2451 Tarrant County Mental Health: Mental Retardation Services

3840 Hulen Street
North Tower
Fort Worth, TX 76107
817-569-4300
www.mhmrtc.org/

We serve the citizens in our north Texas community who face the challenges of mental illness, mental retardation, autism, addiction and early childhood developmental delays.

2452 Texas Commission on Alcohol and Drug Abuse
Texas Department of State Health Services

909 West 45th Street
Austin, TX 78758

512-206-5000
E-mail: contact@tcada.state.tx.us
www.tcada.state.tx.us/

The Department of State Health Services promotes optimal health for individuals and communities while providing effective health, mental health and substance abuse services to Texans.

2453 Texas Department of Aging and Disability Services: Mental Retardation Services
701 West 51st St.
PO Box 149030
Austin, TX 78751
512-438-3011
E-mail: mail@dads.state.tx.us
www.www.dads.state.tx.us

Adelaide Horn, Commissioner
Gordon Taylor, Cfo

State agency which works to improve the quality and efficiency of public and private services and supports for Texans with mental illnesses.

2454 Texas Department of Family and Protective Services
701 W. 51st Street
PO Box 149030
Austin, TX 78751
512-438-4800
www.dfps.state.tx.us/

Ommy Strauch, Chair

The mission of the Texas Department of Family and Protective Services (DFPS) is to protect the unprotected _ children, elderly, and people with disabilities _ from abuse, neglect, and exploitation.

2455 Texas Health & Human Services Commission
4900 N. Lamar Blvd.
Brown-Heatly Building
Austin, TX 78751-2316
512-424-6500
877-787-8999
TTY: 888-425-6889
E-mail: contact@hhsc.state.tx.us
www.hhsc.state.tx.us/

Albert Hawkins, Executive Commissioner

The Health and Human Services Commission provides leadership and direction, and fosters the spirit of innovation needed to achieve an efficient and effective health and human services system for Texans.

Utah

2456 Utah Commission on Criminal and Juvenile Justice
Utah Capitol Complex
East Office Building, Suite E330
Salt Lake City, UT 84114
801-538-1031
Fax: 801-538-1024
E-mail: mhaddon@utah.gov
www.justice.utah.gov/

Chris Mitchell, Director Research
Robert Yeates, Executive Director

The mission of the Utah Commission on Criminal and Juvenille Justice is to: establish sentencing policy for both adult and juvenile offenders; establish strategies for combatting substance abuse, illegal drug activity, and violence; promote the development of an effective and coordinated juvenile justice system; and provide services to those who have become victims of violent crime in Utah.

2457 Utah Department of Health
288 N 1460 West
Salt Lake Cty, UT 84114
801-538-6111
www.health.utah.gov/

David Sundwall, MD, Executive Director

Oversees and regulates health care services for children, seniors, the mentally ill, substance abusers, and all residents of Utah.

2458 Utah Department of Health: Health Care Financing
Box 143101
Salt Lake City, UT 84114
801-538-6406
www.health.utah.gov/medicaid

Provides information and assistance on Utah Medicaid programs including eligibility and additional contact info and links for administrators of the program.

2459 Utah Department of Human Services
120 North 200 West, Room 319
Salt Lake City, UT 84103
801-538-4001
800-662-3722
Fax: 801-538-4016
E-mail: dirdhs@utah.gov
www.dhs.utah.gov/

Lisa-Michele Church, Executive Director

Provides services for the elderly, substance abusers, people with disabilities,ed children, youthful offenders, mentally ill and others.ple with disabilities,

2460 Utah Department of Human Services: Division of Substance Abuse And Mental Health
120 N 200 W
Room 209
Salt Lake City, UT 84103
801-538-3939
Fax: 801-538-9892
E-mail: dsamhwebmaster@utah.gov
www.dsamh.utah.gov/

Dr Michael Crookston, Chair
Paula Bell, Vice Chair

The Utah State Division of Substance Abuse and Mental Health Division is the agency responsible for ensuring that substance abuse and mental health prevention and treatment services are available statewide. The Division also acts as a resource by providing general information, research, and statistics to the public regarding substances of abuse and mental health services.

2461 Utah Department of Mental Health
120 N 200 W
Room 209
Salt Lake City, UT 84103
801-538-3939
Fax: 801-538-9892
www.www.dsamh.utah.gov

Vermont

2462 State of Vermont Developmental Disabilities Services
103 South Main Street
Weeks Building
Waterbury, VT 05671-1601
802-241-2388
Fax: 802-241-1363
E-mail: AHS-dail-deptweb.master@ahs.state.vt.us
www.www.dail.vermont.gov

The State of Vermont, Department of Disabilities, Aging and Independent Living, Division of Disability and Aging Services, plans and coordinates state- and federally-funded services for people with developmental disabilities and their families within Vermont. The Division provides funding for services, systems planning, technical assistance, training, quality assurance, program monitoring and standards compliance.

2463 Vermont Department for Children and Families Economic Services Division (ESD)
103 S Main Street
Waterbury, VT 05676-1201
802-241-2880
800-287-0589
www.dsw.state.vt.us/

ESD, formerly the Department of Prevention, Assistance, Transition, and Health Access (PATH) and before that the Department of Social Welfare (DSW), administers state and federal programs such as Medicaid, Food Stamps, and Reach Up to assist eligible Vermonters in need. Our mission is to help Vermonters find a path to a better life. To this end, we take on many roles: employment coach, health insurance provider, crisis manager, career planner, champion of families, and promoter of human potential.

2464 Vermont Department of Health: Division of Mental Health Services
108 Cherry Street
Burlington, VT 05402
802-863-7200
800-464-4343
Fax: 802-865-7754
www.healthyvermonters.info/ddmhs/index.shtml

On July 1, 2004 the Department of Developmental and Mental Health Services ceased to exist as an independent department within the Agency of Human Services. Under the Agency's reorganization plan, the division of Mental Health became part of the existing Department of Health. The division of Mental Health includes adult mental health; child, adolescent, and family mental health; emergency services; and the Vermont State Hospital. The division of Developmental Services merged with the Department of Aging and Disabilities to become a new Department of Disability, Aging & Independent Living (DAIL).

Virginia

2465 Virginia Department of Medical Assistance Services
600 E Broad Street
Richmond, VA 23219
804-786-7933
TDD: 800-343-0634
E-mail: info@dmas.virginia.gov
www.www.dmas.virginia.gov

Patrick Finnerty, Director

2466 Virginia Department of Mental Health, Mental Retardation and Substance Abuse Services (DMHMRSAS)
PO Box 1797
Richmond, VA 23218-1797
804-786-3921
800-451-5544
Fax: 804-371-6638
TDD: 804-371-8977
www.dmhmrsas.virginia.gov/

DMHMRSAS provides leadership and service to improve Virginia's system of quality treatment, habilitation, and prevention services for individuals and their families whose lives are affected by mental illness, mental retardation, or substance use disorders.

2467 Virginia Department of Social Services
7 North Eight Street
Richmond, VA 23219
804-726-7000
800-552-3431
E-mail: citizen.services@dss.virginia.gov
www.dss.virginia.gov/

Promotes self-reliance, prevention, and protection by serving as a catalyst for healthy families and communities.

2468 Virginia Office of the Secretary of Health and Human Resources
Patrick Henry Building
1111 East Broad Street
Richmond, VA 23219
804-786-7765
Fax: 804-371-6984
www.hhr.virginia.gov/

The DHHR administers programs that benefit the citizens of West Virginia.

Washington

2469 Washington Department of Alcohol and Substance Abuse: Department of Social and Health Service
1115 Washington Street
Olympia, WA 98504
360-902-8400
www.www.dshs.wa.gov

The Division of Alcohol and Substance Abuse promotes strategies that support healthy lifestyles by preventing the misuse of alcohol, tobacco, and other drugs, and support recovery from the disease of chemical dependency.

2470 Washington Department of Social & Health Services
PO Box 45130
Olympia, WA 98504-5130
800-737-0617
www.www.dshs.wa.gov

The mission of DSHS is to improve the quality of life for individuals and families in need. We help people achieve safe, self-sufficient, healthy and secure lives.

2471 Washington Department of Social and Health Services: Mental Health Division
1115 Washington Street
PO Box 45320
Olympia, WA 98504-5320
800-446-0259
Fax: 360-902-0809
www.www.dshs.wa.gov/mentalhealth

The mission of the Mental Health Division is to promote recovery and safety.

West Virginia

2472 West Virginia Bureau for Behavioral Health and Health Facilities
West Virginia Department of Health and Human Resources
350 Capitol Street
Room 350
Charleston, WV 25301-3702
304-558-0627
Fax: 304-558-1008
E-mail: obhs@wvdhhr.org
www.wvdhhr.org/bhhf/

John E Bianconi, Commissioner

We ensure that positive meaningful opportunities are available for persons with mental illness, chemical dependency, developmental disabilities and those at risk. We provide support for individuals, families, and communities in assisting persons to achieve their potential and to gain greater control over the direction of their future.

2473 West Virginia Department of Health & Human Resources (DHHR)
350 Capitol Street
Room 730
Charleston, WV 25301
304-558-2974
Fax: 304-558-4194
www.wvdhhr.org/default.asp

The DHHR administers programs that benefit the citizens of West Virginia.

2474 West Virginia Department of Welfare Bureau for Children and Families
West Virginia Department of Health & Human Resources
350 Capitol Street
Room 730
Charleston, WV 25301
304-558-4069
Fax: 304-558-4623
www.wvdhhr.org/bcf/family_assistance/fs.asp

The Bureau for Children and Families provides an accessible, integrated, comprehensive quality service system for West Virginia's children, families and adults to help them achieve.

2475 West Virginia Division of Criminal Justice Services (DCJS)
1204 Kanawha Boulevard, East
Charleston, WV 25301
304-558-8814
Fax: 304-558-0391
www.wvdcjs.com/index.html

The mission of the Division of Criminal Justice Services is to assist the criminal justice and juvenile justice agencies and the local government with research and performance data, planning, funding and management of programs supported with grant funds, and to provide oversight of law enforcement training.

Wisconsin

2476 Bureau of Mental Health and Substance Abuse Services
Department of Health and Family Services
1 West Wilson Street
Room 434
Madison, WI 53707-7851
608-267-7792
Fax: 608-266-7793
E-mail: allenjb@dhfs.state.wi.us
www.www.dhfs.wisconsin.gov/MH_BCMH/

Joyce Allen, Director

The Bureau of Mental Health and Substance Abuse Services' mission is to support and improve the quality and effectiveness of mental health and substance abuse services in order to create a recovery-focused system for the people of Wisconsin.

2477 Dane County Mental Health Center
625 West Washington Avenue
Madison, WI 53703-2637
608-280-2700
Fax: 608-280-2707
E-mail: webmaster@mhcdc.org
www.mhcdc.org/

William Greer, Executive Director

The mission of the Mental Health Center of Dane County, Inc. is to provide individuals and families with high quality, community based, recovery oriented, mental health, substance abuse, and advocacy services that respect cultural differences and foster hope, strength, and self determination. We will give priority to individuals and families with high needs and low resources.

2478 Department of Health and Family Services: Southern Region
One West Wilson Street
Madison, WI 53703
608-266-1865
E-mail: webmaster@dhfs.state.wi.us
www.dhfs.state.wi.us/

The Wisconsin Department of Health and Family Services administers a wide range.

2479 University of Wisconsin Center for Health Policy and Program Evaluation
610 Walnut Street
Suite 760
Madison, WI 53726
608-263-6294
Fax: 608-262-6404
www.pophealth.wisc.edu/UWPHI/index.htm

The Institute serves as a focal point for applied public health and health policy within the University of Wisconsin-Madison School of Medicine and Public Health as well as a bridge to public health and health policy practitioners in the state. We strive to: address a broad range of real world problems of importance to government, business, providers and the public; and catalyze partnerships of inquiry between researchers and users of research and break down barriers between the academic community and public and private policy makers.

2480 Wisconsin Bureau of Health Care Financing
PO Box 7886
Madison, WI 53707-7886
800-423-1938
Fax: 800-423-1939
www.www.dhfs.wisconsin.gov/ddb

Disability decisions for Wisconsin residents are made by the Wisconsin Division of Health Care Financing, Disability Determination Bureau (DDB). Applicants who are determined to have a disability, and also meet other specific eligibility requirements, may receive monthly money payments and/or healthcare coverage for many of their medical expenses.

2481 Wisconsin Department of Health and Family Services
1 West Wilson Street
Madison, WI 53703
608-266-1865
TTY: 608-267-7371
www.www.dhfs.wisconsin.gov

The Wisconsin Department of Health and Family Services administers a wide range of services to clients in the community and at state institutions.

Wyoming

2482 Wyoming Department of Family Services
2300 Capitol Avenue
Hathaway Bldg Fl 3
Cheyenne, WY 82002-0490
307-777-7564
www.dfsweb.state.wy.us

Jacquie Bensley, Director

The mission of the Wyoming Department of Family Services is to have Families assume more responsibility for raising their own children. Communities will assume more responsibility for their own families. The Department of Family Services will facilitate both.

2483 Wyoming Department of Health: Division of Health Care Finance
401 Hathaway Bldg
Cheyenne, WY 82002
307-777-7656
866-571-0944
Fax: 307-777-7439
www.wdh.state.wy.us/main/about.html

Dr Brent Sherard, Director

The Office of Health Care Financing administers the EqualityCare (Medicaid) program, the largest of the State's public health insurance programs. The name EqualityCare reflects Wyoming's history as the Equality State as well as promoting equality of health care benefits and services for all Wyoming citizens regardless of economic status. In addition to providing Medicaid Primary Care services, the Office oversees the administration of Medicaid services provided by the following divisions within the Department: Community and Family Health, Developmental Disabilities, Mental Health, Aging, and Substance Abuse.

2484 Wyoming Mental Health Division
Wyoming State Government
6101 Yellowstone Road
Suite 20
Cheyenne, WY 82002
307-777-2432
www.www.wdh.state.wy.us

State administrative agency of the Department of Health, for mental health in Wyoming.

Professional

Accreditation & Quality Assurance

2485 American Board of Examiners in Clinical Social Work
27 Congress Street Suite 501
Shetland Park
Salem, MA 01970
978-825-9311
800-694-5285
Fax: 978-740-5395
E-mail: abe@abecsw.org
www.abecsw.org

Howard Snooks Ph.D BCD, President
Robert Booth, Executive Director
Leonard Hill MSW BCD, Vice President

Clinical Social Work certifying and standard setting organization. ABE's no cost online and CD ROM directories (both searchable/sortable) are sources used by the healthcare industry nationwide for network development and referrals. They contain verified information about the education, training, experience and practice specialties of over 11,000 Board Certified Diplomates in Clinical Social Work (BCD). Visit our website for the directory, employment resources, continuing education and other services.

2486 American Board of Examiners of Clinical Social Work Regional Offices
414 First Street E
Suite 3
Sonoma, CA 95476-2005
707-938-3233
888-279-9378
Fax: 707-938-3233
E-mail: abe@abecsw.org
www.www.abecsw.org

Howard Snooks Ph.D BCD, President
Robert Booth, Executive Director
Leonard Hill MSW BCD, Vice President

Sets national practice standards, issues an advance-practice credential, and publishes reference information about its board-certified clinicians.

2487 Brain Imaging Handbook
WW Norton & Company
500 5th Avenue
New York, NY 10110-0017
212-354-5500
800-233-4830
Fax: 212-869-0856
E-mail: npb@wwnorton.com
www.wwnorton.com/psych

The past 10 years have seen an explosion in the use of brain imaging technologies to aid treatment of medical as well as mental health conditions. MRI, CT ("CAT") scans, and PET scans are now common. This book is the first quick reference to these technologies, rich in illustrations and including discussions of which techniques are best used in particular instances of care.

2488 CARF: Commission on Accreditation of Rehabil itation Facilities
4891 E Grant Road
Tucson, AZ 85712

520-325-1044
Fax: 520-318-1129
TTY: 888-281-6531
www.carf.org

Brian J. Boom Ph.D, President/CEO
Amanda Birch, Administrator Of Operations

CARF assists organizations to improve the quality of their services, to demonstrate value, and to meet internationally recognized organizational and practice standards.

2489 Cenaps Corporation
6147 Deltona Boulevard
Spring Hill, FL 34606
352-596-8000
Fax: 352-596-8002
E-mail: info@cenaps.com
www.cenaps.com

Terence T Gorski, President
Tresa Watson, Business Manager

CENAPS is an acronym for the Center for Applied Sciences. They are a private training firm committed to providing advanced clinical skills training for the addiction and behavioral health fields.

2490 CompHealth Credentialing
PO Box 713100
Salt Lake City, UT 84171-3100
801-930-4517
800-453-3030
Fax: 801-930-4517
E-mail: info@comphealth.com
www.www.comphealth.com

Assists in analyzing the total costs involved in credentialing verifications, including some items frequently overlooked; assesses and/or develops a provider application to meet accreditation standards; can assess current credentialing files; can assist in developing policy and procedures for the verification process.

2491 Consumer Satisfaction Team
1001 Sterigere Street
Building 6
Norristown, PA 19401
610-270-3685
Fax: 610-270-9155
E-mail: watsons@cstmont
www.cstmont.com

Marge Zipin, MEd, President
Sandra F Watson, Executive Director

The central role of CST is to provide the Montgomery County Office of MH/MR/DD with information about satisfaction with the mental health services that adults are receiving and make recommendations for change.

2492 Council on Accreditation (COA) of Services for Families and Children
120 Wall Street
11th Floor
New York, NY 10005
212-797-3000
Fax: 212-797-1428
E-mail: jfulmer@coanet.org
www.coanet.org

Richard Klarberg, President/CEO
John Polsky, CFO

The Council of Accreditation of Services for Families and Children, Inc., is an independent, not-for-profit accreditor of behavioral healthcare and social service organizations in the United States and Canada. COA's mission is to promote standards, champion quality services for children, youth and families, and advocate for the value of accreditation. COA accredits programs in more than 1,000 organizations and publishes standards for the full array of community mental health services.

2493 Council on Social Work Education
1725 Duke Street
Suite 500
Alexandria, VA 22314-3457
703-683-8080
Fax: 703-683-8099
E-mail: info@cswe.org
www.cswe.org

Julia M. Watkins, PhD,, Executive Director
Nicole Demarco, Executive Assistant To Exec. Dir

A national association that preserves and enhances the quality of social work education for the purpose of promoting the goals of individual and community well being and social justice. Pursues this mission through setting and maintaining policy and program standards, accrediting bachelors and masters degree programs in social work, promoting research and faculty development, and advocating for social work education.

2494 Healtheast Behavioral Care
559 Capitol Boulevard
Saint Paul, MN 55103
651-232-3222
Fax: 651-232-6414
www.healtheast.org

Timothy H. Hanson, President/CEO
Robert D. Gill, VP Finance/CFO
Robert J. Beck, VP Medical Affairs

Assessment and referral for: Psychiatric, Inpatient, Chemical Dependancy.

2495 Joint Commission on Accreditation of Healthcare Organizations
1 Renaissance Boulevard
Oakbrook Terrace, IL 60181
630-792-5000
Fax: 630-792-5005
E-mail: customerservice@jcaho.org
www.jcaho.org

Mark Chassin, President
Mark Angood, VP/Chief Patient Safety Officer

The Joint Commission evaluates and accredits nearly 20,000 health care organizations and programs in the United States. An independent, not-for-profit organization, the Joint Commission is the nation's predominant standards-setting and accrediting body in health care. The Joint Commission has developed state-of-the-art, professionally-based standards and evaluated the compliance of health care organizations against these benchmarks.

2496 Lanstat Incorporated
270 Beckett Point Road
PO Box 1388
Port Townsend, WA 98368
360-379-8628
800-672-3166
Fax: 360-379-8949
E-mail: info@lanstat.com
www.lanstat.com

Landon Kimbrough, President
Sherry Kimbrough, VP

Provides techinical assistance in the areas of CARF accreditation, outcomes and customer satisfaction, program evaluation, policies and procedures, clinical forms and training.

2497 Med Advantage
11301 Corporate Boulevard
Suite 300
Orlando, FL 32817
407-282-5131
Fax: 407-282-9240
E-mail: info@med-advantage.com
www.med-advantage.com

Fully accredited by URAC and certified in all 11 elements by NCQA, Med Advantage is one of the oldest credentials verification organizations in the country. Over the past eight years, they have developed sophisticated computer systems and one of the largest data warehouses of medical providers in the nation, containing information on over 900,000 healthcare providers. Their system is continually updated from primary source data required to meet the standards of the URAC, NCQA and JCAHO.

2498 Mertech
PO Box 787
Norwell, MA 02061
781-659-0701
Fax: 781-659-2049
E-mail: admin-info@mertech.org
www.mertech.org

John Kopacz, Founder
Leann Johnson, Account Manager

A business development organization that specializes in helping clients capitalize on business opportunities in an efficient and effective manner to meet their goals and objectives. They have three business units: Mertech Health Care Consultants, Mertech Personal Health Improvement Program and Managed Care Information Systems.

2499 National Board for Certified Counselors
3 Terrace Way
Greensboro, NC 27403-3660
336-547-0607
Fax: 336-547-0017
E-mail: nbcc@nbcc.org
www.nbcc.org

Thomas Clawson, President/CEO
Linda Foster, Chairman Of The Board

National voluntary certification board for counselors. Certified counselors have met minimum criteria. Referral lists can be provided to consumers.

2500 National Register of Health Service Providers in Psychology
1120 G Street NW
Suite 330
Washington, DC 20005
202-783-7663
Fax: 202-347-0550
www.nationalregister.org

Morgan Sammons, President/Chair
Greg Hurley, Vice President/Vice-Chair

Nonprofit credentialing organization for psychologists; evaluates education, training, and experience of licensed psychologists. Committed to advancing psychology as a profession and improving the delivery of health services to the public.

Year Founded: 1974

2501 SAFY of America: Specialized Alternatives for Families and Youth
10100 Elida Road
Delphos, OH 45833
419-224-2279
800-532-7239
Fax: 419-224-2287
E-mail: webmaster@safy.org
www.safy.org

Druann Whitaker MS LSW LPC, CEO
John Hollenkamp, SVP Of Finance

A not-for-profit treatment foster care agency serving more than 1000 children and their families in eight states. Offers programs and services tailored to children's unique needs.

Year Founded: 1984

2502 SUPRA Management
2424 Edenborn Avenue
Suite 660
Metairie, LA 70009-6588
504-837-5557
Fax: 504-833-3466

2503 Skypek Group
2528 W Tennessee Avenue
Tampa, FL 33629-6255
813-254-3926
Fax: 813-254-3657

Computerized accreditation systems and consultation

2504 Sweetwater Health Enterprises
3939 Belt Line Road
Suite 600
Dallas, TX 75244
972-888-5638
Fax: 972-620-7351

Cherie Holmes-Henry, VP Sales/Marketing

Credentials verification organization

Associations

2505 Academy of Psychosomatic Medicine
5272 River Road
Suite 630
Bethesda, MD 20816
301-718-6520
Fax: 301-656-0989
E-mail: apm@apm.org
www.apm.org

Kristen Flemming, Academy Coordinator
Norman Wallis Ph.D, Executive Director

Represents psychiatrists dedicated to the advancement of medical science, education, and healthcare for persons with comorbid psychiatric and general medical conditions and

provides national and international leadership in the furtherance of those goals.

2506 Advanced Psychotherapy Association
319 Court House Rd
#B
Gulfport, MS 39507
228-897-7730
Fax: 228-897-2121

Karen Seymour, Contact
Philip Schaeffer, Contact

2507 Agency for Healthcare Research & Quality
540 Gaither Road
Suite 2000
Rockville, MD 20850
301-427-1364
Fax: 301-427-1875
www.ahcpr.gov

Carolyn Clancy M.D., Director

2508 Alliance for Children and Families
11700 W Lake Park Drive
Milwaukee, WI 53224-3099
414-359-1040
Fax: 414-359-1074
E-mail: pgoldberg@alliance1.org
www.www.alliance1.org

Elizabeth Carey, SVP/COO
Peter Goldberg, President/CEO
John Schmidt, CFO

National membership association representing more than three hundred forty private, nonprofit child and family-serving organizations. It's mission is to strengthen members' capacity to serve and advocate for children, families and communities.

2509 American Academy of Child & Adolescent Psychiatry
3615 Wisconsin Avenue NW
Washington, DC 20016-3007
202-966-7300
Fax: 202-966-2891
E-mail: communications@aacap.org
www.aacap.org

Robert Hendren, President
David Herzog, Secretary
William Bernet, Treasurer

Provides information on childhood psychiatric disorders.

2510 American Academy of Clinical Psychiatrists
PO Box 458
Glastonbury, CT 06033
860-635-5533
Fax: 860-613-1650
E-mail: aacp@cox.net
www.aacp.com

Carol S. North, MD, President
Charles L. Rich, MD, Vice President
Sanjay Gupta MD, Secretary/Treasurer

Practicing board-eligible or board-certified psychiatrists. Promotes the scientific practice of psychiatric medicine. Conducts educational and teaching research. Publications: Annals of Clinical Psychiatry, quarterly journal. Clinical

Psychiatry Quarterly, newsletter. Annual conference and exhibits in fall.

2511 American Academy of Medical Administrators
701 Lee Street
Suite 600
Des Plaines, IL 60016-4516
847-759-8601
Fax: 847-759-8602
E-mail: info@aameda.org
www.aameda.org

Renee S Schleicher CAE, President/CEO
Holly Estal, Director Of Education

Their mission is to advance Academy member and the field of healthcare management, and promote excellence and integrity in healthcare delivery and leadership.
Year Founded: 1957

2512 American Academy of Psychiatry and the Law (AAPL)
One Regency Drive
PO Box 30
Bloomfield, CT 06002
860-242-5450
800-331-1389
Fax: 860-286-0787
E-mail: execoff@aapl.org
www.aapl.org

Jacquelyn T Coleman, Executive Director
Jeffrey Janofsky MD, President
Kenneth Appelbaum MD, Vice President

Seeks to exchange ideas and experience in areas where psychiatry and the law overlap and develop standards of practice in the relationship of psychiatry to the law and encourage the development of training programs for psychiatrists in this area. Publications: Journal of the American Academy of Psychiatry and the Law, quarterly. Scholarly articles on forensic psychiatry. Newsletter of the American Academy of Psychiatry and Law, 3 year. Membership Directory, annual.

2513 American Academy of Psychoanalysis and Dynam ic Psychiatry
One Regency Drive
PO Box 30
Bloomfield, CT 06002
888-691-8281
Fax: 860-286-0787
E-mail: info@aapdp.org
www.aapsa.org

Jacquelyn T Coleman CAE, Executive Director
Sherry Katz-Bearnot, President
Carol Filiaci, Secretary

Founded in 1956 to provide an open forum for psychoanalysts to discuss relevant and responsible views of human behavior and to exchange ideas with colleagues and other social behavioral scientists. Aims to develop better communication among psychoanalysts and psychodynamic psychiatrists in other disiplines in science and the humanities. Meetings of the Academy provide a forum for inquiry into the phenomena of individual and interpersonal behavior. Advocates an acceptance of all relevant and responsible psychoanalytic views of human behavior, rather than adherence to one particular doctrine.

2514 American Association for Marriage and Family Therapy
112 S Alfred Street
Alexandria, VA 22314
703-838-9808
Fax: 703-838-9805
E-mail: central@aamft.org
www.aamft.org

Scott Johnson, President
Linda Schwallie, President-Elect
Douglas Sprenkle, Treasurer

The professional association for the field of marriage and family therapy. They represent the professional interests of more than 23,000 marriage and family therapists throughout the United States, Canada and abroad. They facilitate research, theory development and education. They develop standards for graduate education and training, clinical supervision, professional ethics and the clinical practice of marriage and family therapy. They host an annual national training conference each fall as well as a week-long series of continuing education institutes in the summer.

2515 American Association for Protecting Children
63 Inverness Drive E
Englewood, CO 80112
303-792-9900
Fax: 303-792-5333
www.www.americanhumane.org

Marie Belew-Wheatley, President/CEO
Bonny Reinmuth, Secretary

Leader in developing programs, policies and services to prevent the abuse and neglect of children, while strengthening families and communities and enhancing social service systems.

2516 American Association of Community Psychiatrists (AACP)
PO Box 570218
Dallas, TX 75357-0218
972-613-0985
Fax: 972-613-5532
E-mail: frda1@airmail.net
www.www.epic.pitt.edu/aacp

Wesley Sowers MD, President
Annelle Primm, Vice President
Francis Bell, Administrative Director

The mission of AACP is to inspire, empower and equip Community Psychiatrists to promote and provide quality care and to integrate practice with policies that improve the well being of individuals and communities.

2517 American Association of Chairs of Department s of Psychiatry
1594 Cumberland Street
Lebanon, PA 17042
717-270-1673
Fax: 717-270-1673
E-mail: aacdp@verizon.net
www.aacdp.org

Peter Buckley, President
Stuart Munro, Secretary/Treasurer

Represents the leaders of departments of psychiatry in all the medical schools in the United States and Canada. They are committed to promotion of excellence in psychiatric education, research and clinical care. They are also committed to advocating for health policy to create appropriate and affordable psychiatric care for all.

2518 American Association of Children's Residential Centers

11700 W Lake Park Drive
Milwaukee, WI 53224
877-332-2272
Fax: 877-362-2272
E-mail: kbehling@alliance1.org
www.aacrc-dc.org

Kari Behling, National Coordinator
Steve Elson, President

Funded by the Mental Health Community Support Program. The purpose of the association is to share information about services, providers and ways to cope with mental illnesses. Available services include referrals, professional seminars, support groups and a variety of publications.

2519 American Association of Directors of Psychiatric Residency Training

1594 Cumberland Street
Lebanon, PA 17042
717-270-1673
E-mail: aadprt@verizon.net
www.www.aadprt.org

Mark Servis, President
Lucille Meinsler, Administrative Manager

To better meet the nation's mental healthcare needs, the mission of the American Association of Directors of Psychiatric Residency Training is to promote excellence in education and training of future psychiatrists.

2520 American Association of Geriatric Psychiatry (AAGP)

7910 Woodmont Avenue
Suite 1050
Bethesda, MD 20814-3004
301-654-7850
Fax: 301-654-4137
E-mail: main@aagponline.org
www.aagpgpa.org

Christine Devries, CEO/Executive Vice President
Annie Williams, Administrative Assistant

Members are psychiatrists interested in promoting better mental health care for the elderly. Maintains placement service and speakers' bureau. Publications: AAGP Membership Directory, annual. Geriatric Psychiatry News, bimonthly newsletter. Growing Older and Wiser, covers consumer and general public information. Annual meeting and exhibits in February or March.

2521 American Association of Health Plans

601 Pennsylvania Avenue NW
South Building, Suite 500
Washington, DC 20004
202-778-3200
Fax: 202-331-7487
E-mail: ahip@ahip.org
www.aahp.org

Michael Abbott, Board Member
Richard Rivers, Board Member

The American Association of Health Plans (AAHP) is the nation's principal association of health plans, representing more than 1,000 plans that provide coverage for approximately 170 million Americans nationwide.

2522 American Association of Healthcare Consultants

5938 N Drake Avenue
Chicago, IL 60659
888-350-2242
Fax: 773-463-3552
E-mail: info@aahcmail.org
www.aahc.net

Billy Adkisson, Chairman

Serve as the preeminent credentialing, professional, and practice development organization for the healthcare consulting profession; to advance the knowledge, quality, and standards of practice for consulting to management in the healthcare industry; and to enhance the understanding and image of the healthcare consulting profession and Member Firms among its various publics.

2523 American Association of Homes and Services for the Aging

2519 Connecticut Avenue NW
Washington, DC 20008-1520
202-783-2242
Fax: 202-783-2255
E-mail: info@aahsa.org
www.aahsa.org

William Minnix, President
Katrinka Smith Sloan, COO/SVP Member Services

An association committed to advancing the vision of healthy, affordable, ethical long term care for America. The association represents 5,600 million driven, not-for-profit nursing homes, continuing care facilities and community care retirement facilities and community service organizations.

2524 American Association of Mental Health Professionals in Corrections (AAMHPC)

PO Box 160208
Sacramento, CA 95816-0208
Fax: 916-649-1080
E-mail: corrmentalhealth@aol.com

Pam Christensen, Contact

Mental health professionals working in correctional settings. Goals include improving the treatment, rehabilitation and care of the mentally ill, retarded and emotionally disturbed. Promotes research and professional education and conducts scientific meetings to advance the therapeutic community in all institutional settings including hospitals, churches, schools, industry and the family. Publications: Corrective and Social Psychiatry, quarterly. Annual conference and symposium and workshops.

2525 American Association of Pastoral Counselors

9504A Lee Highway
Fairfax, VA 22031-2303
703-385-6967
Fax: 703-352-7725
E-mail: info@aapc.org
www.aapc.org

Douglas M Ronsheim, Executive Director
Dale Kuhn, President
Joretta Marshall, Vice President

Organized in 1963 to promote and support the ministry of pastoral counseling within religious communities and the field of mental health in the United States and Canada.

2526 American Association of Pharmaceutical Scientists
2107 Wilson Boulevard
Suite 700
Arlington, VA 22201-3042
703-243-2800
Fax: 703-243-9650
www.aapspharmaceutica.com

Karen Habucky, President
John Lisack, Executive Director

The American Association of Pharmaceutical Scientists will be the premier organization of all scientists dedicated to the discovery, development and manufacture of pharmaceutical products and therapies through advances in science and technology.

2527 American Association of Retired Persons
601 E Street NW
Washington, DC 20049
202-434-2263
888-687-2277
www.aarp.org

Bill Novelli, CEO
Erik Olsen, President

AARP is a non profit membership organization of persons 50 and older dedicated to addressing their needs and interests.

2528 American Association on Mental Retardation (AAR)
AAMR
444 N Capitol Street NW
Suite 846
Washington, DC 20001-1512
800-424-3688
Fax: 202-387-2193
E-mail: dcroser@aaidd.org
www.www.aaidd.org

Doreen Croser, Executive Director
Paul Aitken, Director Finance/Administration
Bruce Appelgren, Director Of Publications

Books, pamphlets, videos of interest to those who support persons with mental and physical disabilities.

2529 American Board of Examiners in Clinical Social Work
27 Congress Street Suite 501
Shetland Park
Salem, MA 01970
978-825-9311
800-694-5285
Fax: 978-740-5395
E-mail: abe@abecsw.org
www.abecsw.org

Howard Snooks Ph.D BCD, President
Robert Booth, Executive Director
Leonard Hill MSW BCD, Vice President

Clinical social work certification and standards setting organization.

2530 American Board of Professional Psychology (ABPP)
300 Drayton Street
3rd Floor
Savannah, GA 31401
912-234-5477
800-255-7792
Fax: 912-234-5120
E-mail: office@abpp.org
www.abpp.org

Christine Maguth Nezu Ph.D, President
David Cox, Executive Officer

ABPP serves the public need by providing oversight certifying psychologists competent to deliver high quality services in various specialty areas of psychology.

2531 American Board of Psychiatry and Neurology (ABPN)
2150 E Lake Cook Road
Suite 900
Buffalo Grove, IL 60089
847-229-6500
Fax: 847-229-6600
www.abpn.com

Burton Reifler, President
Patricia Coyle, Vice President

ABPN is a nonprofit organization that promotes excellence in the practice of psychiatry and neurology through lifelong certification including compentency testing processes.

2532 American College Health Association
PO Box 28937
Baltimore, MD 21240-8937
410-859-1500
Fax: 410-859-1510
E-mail: lsacher@admin.fsu.edu
www.acha.org

Lesley Sacher, President
Doyle E Randol MS, Executive Director

Advocate and leadership organization for college and university health. Provides advocacy, education, communications, products and services as well as promotes research and culturally competent practices to enhance its members' ability to advance the health of all students and the campus community.

2533 American College of Health Care Administrators (ACHCA)
300 N Lee Street
Suite 301
Alexandria, VA 22314
703-739-7900
Fax: 703-739-7901
E-mail: mgrachek@achca.org
www.achca.org

Marianna Kern Grachek, President/CEO
Diana Buttram, COO
Anita Bell, Office Coordinator

Nonprofit membership organization which provides educational programming, certification in a variety of positions and career development. Promotes excellence in leadership among long-term health care administrators.

Year Founded: 1962

2534 American College of Healthcare Executives
One N Franklin Street
Suite 1700
Chicago, IL 60606-3529
312-424-2800
Fax: 312-424-0023
E-mail: geninfo@ache.org
www.ache.org

Alyson Pitman Giles, Chairman
David Rubenstein, Chairman-Elect

International professional society of nearly 30,000 healthcare executives. ACHE is known for its prestigious credentialing and educational programs. ACHE is also known for its journal, Journal of Healthcare Management, and magazine, Healthcare Executive, as well as groundbreaking research and career development programs. Through its efforts, ACHE works toward its goal of improving the health status of society by advancing healthcare management excellence.

2535 American College of Mental Health Administration (ACMHA)
7804 Loma del Norte Road NE
Albuquerque, NM 87109-5419
505-822-5038
E-mail: executive.director@acmha.org
www.acmha.org

Kris Ericson, Executive Director

Advancing the field of mental health and substance abuse administration and to promote the continuing education of clinical professionals in the areas of administration and policy. Publication: ACMHA Newsletter, quarterly. Annual Santa Fe Summit, conference.

Year Founded: 1979

2536 American College of Osteopathic Neurologists & Psychiatrists
28595 Orchard Lake Road
Suite 200
Farmington Hills, MI 48334
248-553-0010
Fax: 248-553-0818
E-mail: acn-aconp@msn.com
www.osteopathic.org

David Simpson, President
Sue Wesserling, Executive Director

Purpose is to promote the art and science of osteopathic medicine in the fields of neurology and psychiatry; to maintain and further elevate the highest standards of proficiency and training among osteopathic neurologists and psychiatrists; to stimulate original research and investigation in neurology and psychiatry; and to collect and disseminate the results of such work for the benefit of the members of the college, the public, the profession at large, and the ultimate benefit of all humanity.

2537 American College of Psychiatrists
122 S. Michigan Ave
Suite 1360
Chicago, IL 60603
312-662-1020
Fax: 312-662-1025
E-mail: angel@acpsych.org
www.acpsych.org

Maureen Shick, Executive Director
Angel Waszak, Administrative Assistant

Nonprofit honorary association of psychiatrists who, through excellence in their chosen fields, have been recognized for thier significant contributions to the profession. The society's goal is to promote and support the highest standards in psychiatry through education, research and clinical practice.

2538 American College of Psychoanalysts (ACPA)
PO Box 570218
Dallas, TX 75357-0218
972-613-0985
www.acopsa.org

Elise Snyder, President

Honorary, scientific and professional organization for physician psycholanalysts. Goal is to contribute to the leadership and support high standards in the practice of psychoanalysis, and understanding the relationship between mind and brain.

2539 American Counseling Association
5999 Stevenson Avenue
Alexandria, VA 22304-3302
703-823-9800
800-347-6647
Fax: 800-473-2329
TDD: 703-823-6862
E-mail: webmaster@counseling.org
www.counseling.org

Brian Canfield, President

ACA serves professional counselors in the US and abroad. Provides a variety of programs and services that support the personal, professional and program development goals of its members. ACA works to provide quality services to the variety of clients who use their services in college, community agencies, in mental health, rehabilitation and related settings. Offers a large catalog of books, manuals and programs for the professional counselor.

2540 American Counseling Association (ACA)
5999 Stevenson Avenue
Alexandria, VA 22304-3302
800-347-6647
Fax: 800-473-2829
E-mail: ryep@counseling.org
www.counseling.org

Brian Canfield, President
Richard Yep, Executive Officer

A not-for-profit, professional and educational organization that is dedicated to the growth and enhancement of the counseling profession.

Year Founded: 1952

2541 American Geriatrics Society
350 5th Avenue, Suite 801
Empire State Building
New York, NY 10118
212-308-1414
Fax: 212-832-8646
E-mail: info@americangeriatrics.org
www.americangeriatrics.org

Linda Hiddemen Barondess, Executive Vice President
Ellen Baumritter, Administrative Assistant

Nationwide, nonprofit association of geriatric health care professionals, research scientists and other concerned individuals dedicated to improving the health, independence and quality of life for all older people. Pivotal force in shaping attitudes, policies and practices regarding health care for older people.

2542 American Group Psychotherapy Association
25 E 21st Street
6th Floor
New York, NY 10010
212-477-2677
877-668-2472
Fax: 212-979-6627
E-mail: info@agpa.org
www.agpa.org

Marsha S Block CAE, CEO
Elizabeth Knight MSW CGP FAGPA, President

Interdisciplinary community that has been enhancing practice, theory and research of group therapy for over 50 years. Provides support to enhance your work as a mental health care professional, or your life as a member of a therapeutic group.

Year Founded: 1942

2543 American Health Care Association
1201 L Street NW
Washington, DC 20005
202-832-4444
Fax: 202-842-3860
www.www.ahcancal.org

Bruce Yarwood, President/CEO

Nonprofit federation of affiliated state health organizations, together representing nearly 12,000 nonprofit and for profit assisted living, nursing facility, developmentally disabled and subacute care providers that care for more than 1.5 million elderly and disabled individuals nationally. AHCA represents the long term care community at large — to government, business leaders and the general public. It also serves as a force for change within the long term care field, providing information, education, and administrative tools that enhance quality at every level.

2544 American Health Information Management Association
233 N Michigan Avenue
21st Floor
Chicago, IL 60601-5800
312-233-1100
Fax: 312-233-1090
E-mail: info@ahima.org
www.ahima.org

Becky Garris-Perry, Executive Vice President/CFO
Linda L Kloss CAE, CEO

Dynamic professional association that represents more than 46,000 specially educated health information management professionals who work throughout the healthcare industry. Health information management professionals serve the health care industry and the public by managing, analyzing and utilizing data vital for patient care and making it accessible to healthcare providers when it is needed most.

2545 American Hospital Association: Section for Psychiatric and Substance Abuse
1 N Franklin
Chicago, IL 60606-3421

312-422-3000
Fax: 312-422-4796
www.aha.org

Richard Umbdenstock, President/CEO
Stephen Ahnen, Senior Vice President

AHA represents and serves all types of hospitals, health care networks and their patients and communities. Provides education for health care leaders and is a source of information on health care issues and trends. The AHA Section for Psychiatric and Substance Abuse Services (SPSAS) provides perspective on behavioral health issues.

2546 American Managed Behavioral Healthcare Association
1101 Pennsylvania Avenue NW
6th Floor
Washington, DC 20004
202-756-7726
Fax: 202-756-7308
E-mail: info@abhw.org
www.www.abhw.org

Pamela Greenberg, President/CEO

An association of the nation's leading managed behavioral healthcare companies. Member companies are both national and regional and are collectively responsible for managing mental health and substance abuse services in the public and private sector for over 110 million individuals across the country.

2547 American Medical Association
515 N State Street
Chicago, IL 60610
312-464-5289
800-621-8335
Fax: 312-464-4184
www.ama-assn.org

Joseph Annis, Member Board Of Trustees
Peter Carmel, Member Board Of Trustees

Speaks out in issues important to patients and the nation's health. AMA policy on such issues is decided through its democratic policy making process, in the AMA House of Delegates, which meets twice a year. The House is comprised of physician delegates representing every state; nearly 100 national medical specialty societies, federal service agents, including the Surgeon General of the US; and 6 sections representing hospital and clinic staffs, resident physicians, medical students, young physicians, medical schools and international medical graduates. The AMA's envisioned future is to be a part of the professional life of every physician and an essential force for progress in improving the nation's health.

2548 American Medical Directors Association
11000 Broken Land Parkway
Suite 400
Columbia, MD 21044
410-740-9743
800-876-2632
Fax: 410-740-4572
E-mail: info@amda.com
www.amda.com

Alva Baker, President
David Brechtelsbauer, Vice President

Professional association of medical directors and physicians practicing in the long-term care continuum, dedicated to excellence in patient care by providing education, advocacy and professional development.

2549 American Medical Group Association
1422 Duke Street
Alexandria, VA 22314-3403
703-838-0033
Fax: 703-548-1890
E-mail: roconnor@amga.org
www.amga.org

Donald Fisher, President/CEO
Francis Marzoni, Secretary

Advocates for the multispecialty group practice model of health care delivery and for the patients served by medical groups, through innovation and information sharing, benchmarking and continuous striving to improve patient care.

2550 American Medical Informatics Association
4915 St. Elmo Avenue
Suite 401
Bethesda, MD 20814
301-657-1291
Fax: 301-657-1296
E-mail: mail@amia.org
www.amia.com

Sarah Ingersoll, Treasurer
Don E Detmer MD MA, President/CEO

Nonprofit membership organization of individuals, institutions and corporations dedicated to developing and using information technologies to improve health care. Our members include physicians, nurses, computer and information scientists, biomedical engineers, medical librarians, academic researchers and educators. Holds an annual syposium, 2 congresses, prints a journal and maintains a resource center.

Year Founded: 1990

2551 American Mental Health Counselors Association (AMHCA)
801 N Fairfax Street
Suite 304
Alexandria, VA 22314
703-548-6002
800-326-2642
Fax: 703-548-4775
E-mail: vmoore@amhca.org
www.amhca.org

W Mark Hamilton PhD, Executive Director
Virginia Moore, Administration

Professional counselors employed in mental health services and students. Aims to deliver quality mental health services to children, youth, adults, families and organizations and to improve the availability and quality of services through licensure and certification, training standards and consumer advocacy. Publishes an Advocate Newsletter, Journal of Mental Health Counseling, quarterly, Mental Health Brights, brochures. Annual National Conference.

2552 American Neuropsychiatric Association
700 Ackerman Road
Suite 625
Columbus, OH 43202
614-447-2077
Fax: 614-263-4366
E-mail: anpa@osu.edu
www.anpaonline.org

Fred Ovsiew MD, President
C. Edward Coffey, Treasurer

An association of professionals in neuropsychiatry and clinical neurosciences. Their mission is to promote neuroscience for the benefit of people. They work together in a collegial fashion to provide a forum for learning and provide excellent, scientific and compassionate care. They hold their annual scientific meeting in the early spring.

Year Founded: 1988

2553 American Nurses Association
8515 Georgia Avenue
Suite 400
Silver Spring, MD 20910
301-628-5000
800-274-4262
Fax: 301-628-5001
E-mail: webmaster@ana.org
www.nursingworld.org

Rebecca Patton, President

A full-service professional organization representing the nation's 2.7 million registered nurses through its 54 constituent members associations. The ANA advances the nursing profession by fostering high standards of nursing practice, promoting the economic and general welfare of nurses in the workplace, projecting a positive and realistic view of nursing, and by lobbying the Congress and regulatory agencies on health care issues affecting nurses and the public.

2554 American Pharmacists Association
1100 15th Street NW
Suite 400
Washington, DC 20005-1707
202-628-4410
Fax: 202-783-2351
E-mail: feedback@pharmacist.com
www.www.pharmacist.com

John A Gans, Executive Vice President/CEO
Winnie Landis, President

National professional society of pharmacists, formerly the American Pharmaceutical Association. Our members include practicing pharmacists, pharmaceutical students, pharmacy scientists, pharmacy technicians, and others interested in advancing the profession. Provides professional information and education for pharmacists and advocates for improved health of the American public through the provision of comprehensive pharmaceutical care.

Year Founded: 1852

2555 American Psychiatric Association (APA)
1000 Wilson Boulevard
Suite 1825
Arlington, VA 22209-3901
703-907-7300
E-mail: apa@psych.org
www.psych.org

Carol Robinowitz, President

The American Psychiatric Association is a medical specialty society comprised of over 35,000 members who work together to ensure appropriate care and effective treatment for all persons with mental disorders, including mental retardation and substance-related disorders.

2556 American Psychiatric Nurses Association
1555 Wilson Boulevard
Suite 602
Arlington, VA 22209
703-243-2443
866-243-2443
Fax: 703-243-3390
E-mail: clement.1@osu.edu
www.apna.org

Jeanne Clement, President
Dorothy Hill, Treasurer

Provides leadership to promote the psychiatric-mental health nursing profession, improve mental health care for culturally diverse individuals, families, groups and communities and shape health policy for the delivery of mental health services.

2557 American Psychiatric Publishing
1000 Wilson Boulevard
Suite 1825
Arlington, VA 22209-3901
703-907-7322
800-368-5777
Fax: 703-907-1091
E-mail: appi@psych.org
www.appi.org

Ron McMillen, Chief Executive Officer
Joan Lang, Treasurer

2558 American Psychoanalytic Association (APsaA)
309 E 49th Street
New York, NY 10017-1601
212-752-0450
Fax: 212-593-0571
E-mail: info@apsa.com
www.apsa.org

Tina Faison, Administrative Assistant
Dean Stein, Executive Director

Professional Membership Organization with approximately 3,500 members nationwide, with 43 Affiliate Societies and 29 Training Institutes. Seeks to establish and maintain standards for the training of psychoanalysts and for the practice of psychoanalysis, fosters the integration of psychoanalysis with other disciplines (psychiatry, psychology, social work), and encourages research. Publications include: Journal of the Psychoanalyst (JAPA), American Psychoanalyst, a quarterly newsletter; Ethics Case Book; and Roster. Twice a year the organization sponsors scientific meetings and exhibits.

2559 American Psychologial Association: Division of Family Psychology
750 1st Street NE
Washington, DC 20002-4242
202-336-5500
800-374-2721
E-mail: webmaster@apa.org
www.apa.org

Alan Kazdin, President

A division of the American Psychological Association. Psychologists intersted in research, teaching, evaluation, and public interest initiatives in family psychology. Seeks to promote human welfare through the development, dissemination, and application of knowledge about the dynamics, structure, and functioning of the family. Conducts research and specialized education programs.

2560 American Psychological Association
750 1st Street NE
Washington, DC 20002-4241
202-336-5500
800-374-2721
Fax: 202-336-5797
www.apa.org

Alan Kazdin, President

Scientific and professional society of psychologists. Students participate as affiliates. Works to advance psychology as a science, as a profession, and as means of promoting human welfare. Annual convention.

2561 American Psychological Association Division of Independent Practice (APADIP)
919 W Marshall Avenue
Phoenix, AZ 85013
602-246-6768
Fax: 602-246-6577
E-mail: div42apa@cox.net
www.www.division42.org

Jeannie Beeaff, Administrator
Gordon Herz, Internet Editor

Members of the American Psychological Association engaged in independent practice. Works to ensure that the needs and concerns of independent psychology practitioners are considered by the APA. Gathers and disseminates information on legislation affecting the practice of psychology, managed care, and other developments in the health care industries, office management, malpractice risk and insurance, hospital management. Offers continuing professional and educational programs. Semiannual convention, with board meeting.

2562 American Psychological Association: Applied Experimental and Engineering Psychology
750 First Street NE
Washington, DC 20002-4242
202-336-5500
www.www.apa.org/divisions/div21

James R Callan, President

A division of the American Psychological Association. Individuals whose principal fields of study, research, or work are within the area of applied experimental and engineering psychology. Promotes research on psychological factors in the design and use of environments and systems within which human beings work and live.

2563 American Psychology- Law Society (AP-LS)
AP-LS Central Office
PO Box 638
Niwot, CO 80544
303-652-9154
E-mail: div41apa@comcast.net
www.ap-ls.org

Margaret Bull Kovera, President
Brad McAuliff, Treasurer

A division of the American Psychological Association. It is an interdisciplinary organization devoted to the scholarship, practice and public service in psychology and law. Their goals include advancing the contributions of psychology to the understanding of law and legal institutions through basic and applied research; promoting the education of psychologists in matters of law and education of legal personnel in matters of psychology.

2564 American Psychosomatic Society
6728 Old McLean Village Drive
McLean, VA 22101-3906
703-556-9222
Fax: 703-556-8729
E-mail: info@psychosomatic.org
www.psychosomatic.org

William Lovallo, President
Michael Irwin, Secretary/Treasurer

A worldwide community of scholars and clinicians dedicated to the scientific understanding of the interaction of mind, brain, body and social context in promoting health and contributing to the pathogenesis, course and treatment of disease. Holds an annual meeting in a different location each year.

Year Founded: 1942

2565 American Society for Adolescent Psychiatry (ASAP)
PO Box 570218
Dallas, TX 75357-0218
972-613-0985
Fax: 972-613-5532
E-mail: info@adolpsych.org
www.adolpsych.org

Frances Bell, Executive Director
Mohan Nair, President

Psychiatrists concerned with the behavior of adolescents. Provides for the exchange of psychiatric knowledge, encourages the development of adequate standards and training facilities and stimulates research in the psychopathology and treatment of adolescents. Publications: Adolescent Psychiatry, annual journal. American Society for Adolescent Psychiatry Newsletter, quarterly. ASAP Membership Directory, biennial. Journal of Youth and Adolescence, bimonthly. Annual conference. Workshops.

Year Founded: 1967

2566 American Society for Clinical Pharmacology & Therapeutics
528 N Washington Street
Alexandria, VA 22314
703-836-6981
Fax: 703-836-5223
E-mail: info@ascpt.org
www.ascpt.org

John J Schrogie MD, President
Sharon Swan, Executive Director

Over 1,900 professionals whose primary interest is to promote and advance the science of human pharmacology and theraputics. Most of the members are physicians or other doctoral scientists. Other members are pharmacists, nurses, research coordinators, fellows in training and other professionals.

Year Founded: 1900

2567 American Society of Consultant Pharmacists
1321 Duke Street
Alexandria, VA 22314
703-739-1300
800-355-2727
Fax: 703-739-1321
E-mail: info@ascp.com
www.ascp.com

John Feather, Executive Director/CEO
Phylliss M Moret, Associate Executive Director/COO

International professional association that provides leadership, education, advocacy and resources to advance the practice of senior care pharmacy. Consultant pharmacists specializing in senior care pharmacy practice are essential participants in the health care system, ensuring that their patients medications are the most appropriate, effective, the safest possible and are used correctly. They identify, resolve and prevent medication related problems that may interfere with the goals of therapy.

2568 American Society of Group Psychotherapy & Psychodrama
301 N Harrison Street
Suite 508
Princeton, NJ 08540
609-452-1339
Fax: 732-605-7033
E-mail: asgpp@asgpp.org
www.asgpp.org

John Rasberry, President
Eduardo Garcia, Executive Director
Sue Barnum, Secretary

Fosters national and international cooperation among all concerned with the theory and practice of psychodrama, sociometry, and group psychotherapy. Promotes research and fruitful application and publication of the findings. Maintains a code of professional standards.

Year Founded: 1942

2569 American Society of Health System Pharmacists
7272 Wisconsin Avenue
Bethesda, MD 20814
301-657-3000
Fax: 301-657-1251
E-mail: Custserv@ashp.org
www.ashp.org

Henri R Manasse Jr. PhD, Executive VP/CEO
Janet Silvester, President

Thirty thousand member national professional association that represents pharmacists who practice in hospitals, health maintenance organizations, long-term care facilities, ambulatory care, home care and other components of health care systems. ASHP helps people make the best use of their medications, advances and supports the professional practice of pharmacists in hospitals and health systems and serves as their collective voice on issues related to medication use and public health.

2570 American Society of Psychoanalytic Physicians (ASPP)
13528 Wisteria Drive
Germantown, MD 20874
301-540-3197
Fax: 301-540-3511
E-mail: cfcotter@aspp.net
www.aspp.net

Christine Cotter, Executive Director

An organization of physicians established for non-profit education, scientific, and professional purposes. Its objective is to futher the study of psyhcoanalytic methods for the treatment and prevention of emotional disorders and mental illnesses. The Society provides scientific meetings to foster its aims and to share information, namely research, evaluation of treatment, dissemination of information, and to publish and recognize achievement and provide professional opportunities among its members.

Year Founded: 1985

2571 American Society of Psychopathology of Expression (ASPE)
74 Lawton Street
Brookline, MA 02446-5801
617-738-9821
Fax: 617-975-0411

Dr. Irene Jakab, President

Psychiatrists, psychologists, art therapists, sociologists, art critics, artists, social workers, linguists, educators, criminologists, writers, and historians. At least two-thirds of the members are physicians. Fosters collaboration among specialists in the United States who are interested in problems of expression and in artistic activities connected with psychiatric, sociological, and pathological research. Disseminates information about research and clinical applications in the field of psychopathology of expression. Sponsors consultations, seminars, and lectures on art therapy.

2572 American Society on Aging
833 Market Street
Suite 511
San Francisco, CA 94103
415-974-9600
800-537-9728
Fax: 415-974-0300
E-mail: info@asaging.org
www.asaging.org

Robert Stein, President/CEO
Robert Lowe, Director Of Operations

Nonprofit organization committed to enhancing the knowledge and skills of those working with older adults and their families. They produce educational programs, publications, conferences and workshops.

Year Founded: 1954

2573 Annie E Casey Foundation
701 St. Paul Street
Baltimore, MD 21202
410-547-6600
Fax: 410-547-3610
E-mail: webmail@aecf.org
www.aecf.org

Doug Nelson, President
Ralph Smith, Senior Vice President

Working to build better futures for disadvantaged children and their families in the US. The primary mission of the Foundation is to foster policies, human service reforms and community supports that more effectively meet the needs of today's vulnerable children and families.

Year Founded: 1948

2574 Association for Academic Psychiatry (AAP)
464 Commonwealth Street
#147
Belmont, MA 02478
617-393-3935
Fax: 617-393-1808
E-mail: cberney@mah.harvard.edu
www.academicpsychiatry.org

Carole Berney MA, Administrative Director
Joan Anzia, President

Focuses on education in psychiatry at every level from beginning of medical school through lifelong learning for psychiatrists and other physicians. It seeks to help psychiatrists who are interested in careers in academic psychiatry develop the skills and knowledge in teaching, research and career development that they must have to succeed. The Association provides a forum for members to exchange ideas on teaching techniques, curriculum, and other issues to work together to solve problems. It works with other professional organizations on mutual interests and objectives through committee liaison and collaborative programs.

2575 Association for Advancement of Psychoanalysis: Karen Horney Psychoanalytic Institute and Center
80 Eighth Avenue
Suite 1501
New York, NY 10011
212-741-0515
Fax: 212-366-4347
E-mail: dfmaxwell@mac.com
www.www.naap.org

Margery Quackenbush, Executive Director
Douglas Maxwell, President

Certified psychoanalysis disseminating psychoanalytic principles to the medical-psychiatric profession and the general community. Conducts scientific meetings. Maintains a consultation and referral service, placement service and speakers' bureau. Supports research programs, sponsors public educational lectures. Publications: The American Journal of Psychoanalysis, quarterly. Newsletter, semiannual. Annual Karen Horney Lecture in New York City.

2576 Association for Ambulatory Behavioral Healthcare
247 Douglas Avenue
Portsmouth, VA 23707
757-673-3741
Fax: 757-966-7734
E-mail: mickey@aabh.org
www.aabh.org

Larry Meikel, President

Powerful forum for people engaged in providing mental health services. Promoting the evolution of flexible models of responsive cost-effective ambulatory behavioral healthcare.

2577 Association for Applied Psychophysiology & Biofeedback
10200 W 44th Avenue
Suite 304
Wheat Ridge, CO 80033
303-422-8436
800-477-8892
Fax: 303-422-8894
E-mail: aapb@resourcenter.com
www.aapb.org

Alan Glaros, President
Steven Baskin, Treasurer

Their purpose is to advance the development, dissemination, and utilization of knowledge about applied psychophysiology and biofeedback to improve health and the quality of life through research, education and practice.

Year Founded: 1969

2578 Association for Behavior Analysis
1219 South Park Street
Kalamazoo, MI 49001
269-492-9310
Fax: 269-492-9316
E-mail: mail@abainternational.org
www.abainternational.org

Janet Twyman, President
Maria E Malott PhD, Executive Director

Their purpose is to develop, enhance and support the growth and vitality of behavior analysis through research, education and practice.

2579 Association for Behavioral and Cognitive Therapies
305 Seventh Avenue
16th Floor
New York, NY 10001
212-647-1890
Fax: 212-647-1865
E-mail: mebrown@abct.org
www.aabt.org

Mary Jane Eimer, Executive Director
Mary Ellen Brown, Administration/Convention

Professional, interdisciplinary organization that is concerned with the application of behavioral and cognitive sciences to understanding human behavior, developing interventions to enhance the human condition and promoting the appropriate utilization of these interventions.

2580 Association for Birth Psychology
PO Box 1398
Forestville, CA 95436
707-887-2838
Fax: 707-887-2838
E-mail: apppah@aol.com
www.birthpsychology.com

Maureen Wolfe, Executive Director
David Chamberlain, Treasurer/Website Editor

Obstetricians, pediatricians, midwives, nurses, psychotherapists, psychologists, counselors, social workers, sociologists, and others interested in birth psychology, a developing discipline concerned with the experience of birth and the correlation between the birth process and personality development. Seeks to promote communication among professionals in the field; encourage commentary, research and theory from different points of view; establish birth psychology as an autonomous science of human behavior; develop guidelines and give direction to the field. Annual conference, regional meetings, workshops.

2581 Association for Child Psychoanalysts
7820 Enchanted Hills Blvd
#A-233
Rio Rancho, NM 87144
201-825-3138
Fax: 201-825-3138
E-mail: carlaneely2@msn.com
www.childanalysis.org

Carla Elliott-Neely, President
Jim Miller, Secretary

Child psychoanalysts united to provide a forum for discussion and dissemination of information in their field. Conducts national and international scientific meetings. Publications: Abstracts, triennial. Association for Child Psychoanalysis-Newsletter, semi-annual. Membership Roster, biennial. Annual Scientific Meeting.

2582 Association for Hospital Medical Education
109 Brush Creek Road
Irwin, PA 15642
724-864-7321
866-617-4780
Fax: 724-864-6153
E-mail: info@ahme.org
www.ahme.org

Margie Kleppick, Executive Director
Charles Daschbach, President/Board Chairman

National, nonprofit professional association involved in the continuum of medical education — undergraduate, graduate, and continuing medical education. More than 600 members represent hundreds of teaching hospitals, academic medical centers and consortia nationwide. Promotes improvement in medical education to meet health care needs, serves as a forum and resource for medical education information, advocates the value of medical education in health care.

Year Founded: 1956

2583 Association for Humanistic Psychology
1516 Oak Street
#320A
Alameda, CA 94501-2947
510-769-6495
Fax: 510-769-6433
E-mail: ahpoffice@aol.com
www.ahpweb.org

Carroy Ferguson, President

Psychologists, social workers, clergy, educators, psychiatrists, and others engaged in humanistic practice. Functions as a worldwide network for the development of human sciences in ways that recognize distinctive human qualities and work toward fulfilling the innate capacities of people, both as individuals and in society. Annual midwest conference. Bimonthly magazine/newsletter.

Year Founded: 1962

2584 Association for Pre- & Perinatal Psychology and Health
PO Box 1398
Forestville, CA 95436
707-887-2838
Fax: 707-887-2838
E-mail: apppah@aol.com
www.birthpsychology.com

Maureen Wolfe, Executive Director
David Chamberlain, Treasurer/Website Editor

Forum for individuals from diverse backgrounds and disciplines interested in psychological dimensions of prenatal and perinatal experiences. Typically, this includes childbirth educators, birth assistants, doulas, midwives, obstetricians, nurses, social workers, perinatologists, pediatricians, psychologists, counselors researchers and teachers at all levels. All who share these interests are welcome to join. Quarterly journal published.

Year Founded: 1983

2585 Association for Psychoanalytic Medicine (APM)
333 Central Park West
New York, NY 10025
718-548-6088
Fax: 212-866-4817
E-mail: gsagi@mac.com
www.theapm.org

Jonah Schein, President
Edith Cooper, Secretary

A non-profit organization that is a component society of both the American Psychoanalytic Association and the International Psychoanalytic Association.

Year Founded: 1942

2586 Association for Psychological Science
1010 Vermont Avenue NW
11th Floor
Washington, DC 20005-4918
202-783-2077
Fax: 202-783-2083
E-mail: akraut@psychologicalscience.org
www.psychologicalscience.org

Alan G Kraut, Executive Director
John Cacioppo, President
Linda Bartoshuk, Secretary

Scientists and academics working for the development of the discipline of psychology and the promotion of human welfare through research and application. Educates policy makers on the role human behavior plays in societal problems. Mailing lists, on-line services, annual convention. Publishes 2 journals, a newsletter, and a book called Lessons Learned: practical advice for teaching psychology.

2587 Association for Research in Nervous and Mental Disease
1300 York Avenue, Box 171
Room F - 1231
New York, NY 10021
570-839-0296
E-mail: amgooder@ptd.net
www.arnmd.org

Dr Annlouise Goodermuth, Executive Director

Keeps practicing physicians in nuerology and psychiatry, and neuroscientists, informed about state of the art research findings of interest to these ever more related disciplines, findings that are beginning to inform the thinking and practice of neurology and psychiatry.

Year Founded: 1920

2588 Association for Women in Psychology
Florida International University
DM 212
University Park
Miami, FL 33199
305-348-2408
Fax: 305-348-3143
E-mail: awp@fiu.edu
www.awpsych.org

Suzanna Rose PhD, Director

Nonprofit scientific and educational organization committed to encouraging feminist psychological research, theory and activism. They are an organization with a history of affirming and celebrating differences, deepening challenges, and experiencing growth as feminists.

Year Founded: 1969

2589 Association for the Advancement of Psychology
PO Box 38129
Colorado Springs, CO 80937-8129
800-869-6595
Fax: 719-520-0375
E-mail: Krivard@AAPNet.org
www.AAPNet.org

Stephen M Pfeiffer PhD, Executive Officer
Karen Rivard, Administrator

Promotes the interests of all psychologists before public and governmental bodies. AAP's fundamental mission is the support of candidates for the US Congress who are sympathetic to psychology's concerns, through electioneering activities.

Year Founded: 1974

2590 Association of Black Psychologists
PO Box 55999
Washington, DC 20040-5999
202-722-0808
Fax: 202-722-5941
E-mail: abpsi_office@abpsi.org
www.abpsi.org

Dorothy Holmes, President
Pamela Hall, Secretary
Muriel Kennedy, Treasurer

Members are professional psychologists and others in associated disciplines. Aims to: enhance the psychological well-being of black people in America; define mental health in consonance with newly established psychological concepts and standards, develop policies for local, state, and national decision making that have impact on the mental health of the black community; support established black sister organizations and aid in the development of new, independent black institutions to enhance the psychological educational, cultural, and economic situation. Offers training and information on AIDS. Conducts seminars, workshops and research. Periodic conference, annual convention.

Year Founded: 1968

2591 Association of State and Provincial Psychology Boards
PO Box 241245
Montgomery, AL 36124-1245
334-832-4580
Fax: 334-269-6379
E-mail: aspbb@asppb.org
www.asppb.org

Stephen T DeMers EdD, Executive Officer
Alex Siegel, President
Martha Storie, Secretary/Treasurer

ASPPB is the association of psychology licensing boards in the United States and Canada. They create the Examination for Professional Practice in Psychology which is used in licensing boards to assess candidates for licensure and certification. They also publish training materials for training programs and for students preparing to enter the profession

Year Founded: 1961

2592 Association of University Centers on Disabilities (UACD)
1010 Wayne Avenuet
Suite 920
Silver Spring, MD 20910
301-588-8252
Fax: 301-588-2842
E-mail: aucdinfo@aucd.org
www.www.aucd.org

George Jesien, Executive Director
William Kiernan, President

A network of interdisciplinary centers advancing policy and practice for and with individuals with developmental and other disabilities, their families and communities.

2593 Association of the Advancement of Gestalt Therapy
60 Waller Avenue
White Plains, NY 10605
914-686-3477
E-mail: info@aagt.org
www.aagt.org

Peter Philippson, President
Sylvie Falschlunger, Administrative Assistant

Dynamic, inclusive, energetic nonprofit organization committed to the advancement of theory, philosophy, practice and research in Gestalt Therapy and its various applications. This includes but is not limited to personal growth, mental health, education, organization and systems development, political and social development and change, and the fine and performing arts. Their international member base includes psychiatrists, psychologists, social workers, teachers, academics, artists, writers, organizational consultants, political and social analysts, activists and students.

2594 Bazelon Center for Mental Health Law
1101 15th Street NW
Suite 1212
Washington, DC 20005
202-467-5730
Fax: 202-223-0409
E-mail: webmaster@baxelon.org
www.bazelon.org

Robert Bernstein, Executive Director
Albert Archie, Operations Manager

Provides technical support to lawyers and advocates on legal issues affecting children and adults with mental disabilities. Website has extensive legal advocacy resources and an online book store with handbooks, manuals and other publications.

2595 Behavioral Health Systems
2 Metroplex Drive
Suite 500
Birmingham, AL 35209
205-879-1150
800-245-1150
Fax: 205-879-1178
E-mail: generalwebsite@bhs-inc.com
www.bhs-inc.com

Deborah L Stephens, Founder/Chairman/CEO
Kyle Strange, Senior Vice President/COO

Provides behavioral health services to business and industry which are high quality and state of the art, cost effective and accountable, uniformly accessible over a broad geo-

graphic area and care continuum, and managed within a least restrictive treatment approach.

2596 Bonny Foundation
PO Box 39355
Baltimore, MD 21212
866-345-5465
E-mail: info@bonnyinstitute.org
www.bonnyfoundation.org

Donald Stoner, President

Nonprofit organization which provides resources and training in the therapeutic use of the arts for professional music therapists, related health professionals, and the general public. The Bonny Foundation Newsletter provides current information on applications of GIM (Guided Imagery and Music), training schedules and publications. Their GIM training program is fully accredited by the Association for Music and Imagery.

2597 CG Jung Foundation for Analytical Psychology
28 E 39th Street
New York, NY 10016-2587
212-697-6430
Fax: 212-953-3989
E-mail: info@cgjungny.org
www.cgjungny.org

Janet M Careswell, Executive Director
Maxon McDowell, President
David Rottman, Vice President

Analysts who follow the precepts of Carl G Jung, a Swiss psychologist, and any other persons interested in analytical psychology. Sponsors public lectures, films, continuing education, courses and professional seminars. Operates book service which provides publications on analytical psychology and related topics, and lectures on audio cassettes. Publishes journal, Quadrant.

Year Founded: 1962

2598 Center for Applications of Psychological Type
2815 NW 13th Street
Suite 401
Gainesville, FL 32609-2868
352-375-0160
800-777-2278
Fax: 352-378-0503
E-mail: customerservice@capt.org
www.capt.org

Nonprofit organization founded to conduct research and develop applications of the Myers-Briggs Type Indicator for the constructive use of differences. The MBTI is based on CG Jung's theory of psychological types. CAPT provides training for users of the MBTI and the Murphy-Meisgeier Type Indicator for Children, publishes and distributes books and resource materials, and maintains the Isabel Briggs Myers memorial library and the MBTI Bibliography. The MBTI is used in counseling individuals and families, to understand differences in learning styles, and for improving leadership and teamwork in organizations.

Year Founded: 1975

2599 Child Welfare League of America: Washington
2345 Crystal Drive
Suite 250
Arlington, VA 22202
703-412-2400
Fax: 703-412-2401

E-mail: wtc@cwla.org
www.cwla.org

Christine James-Brown, President/CEO

Provides two national conferences each year: Finding Better Ways and Information Technology: Tools That Work; comprehensive training programs for managers, supervisiors, foster parents, adoptive parents and direct care workers. Also provides a range of published materials and training curricula relating to all facets of child welfare service.

2600 Children's Health Council

650 Clark Way
Palo Alto, CA 94304
650-326-5530
Fax: 650-688-0206
E-mail: intake@chconline.org
www.chconline.org

Bruce Fielding, CFO Administration/Finance DIR
Bren Leisure, Secretary
Lawrence Schwab, Treasurer

Working to make a measurable difference in the lives of children who face severe or complex behavioral and developmental challenges by providing interdisciplinary educational, assessment and treatment services and professional training.

2601 Christian Association for Psychological Studies

PO Box 365
Batavia, IL 60510-0365
630-639-9478
Fax: 630-454-3799
E-mail: info@caps.net
www.caps.net

Paul Regan EdD, Executive Director

Psychologists, marriage and family therapists, social workers, educators, physicians, nurses, ministers, researchers, pastoral counselors, and rehabilitation workers and others professionally engaged in the fields of psychology, counseling, psychiatry, pastoring and related areas. Association is based upon a genuine commitment to superior clinical, pastoral and scientific enterprise in the theoretical and applied social sciences and theology, assuming persons in helping professions will be guided to professional and personal growth and a greater contribution to others in this way.

Year Founded: 1956

2602 Clinical Social Work Federation

239 N Highland Street
Arlington, VA 22201
703-522-3866
Fax: 703-522-9441
E-mail: nfscswlo@aol.com
www.cswf.org

Kevin Host, President
Sidney Grossberg, Vice President

A confederation of 31 state societies for clinical social work. The state societies are formed as voluntary associations for the purpose of promoting the highest standards of professional education and clinical practice. Each society is active with legislative advocacy and lobbying efforts for adequate and appropriate mental health services and coverage at their state and national levels of government.

2603 Commission on Accreditation of Rehabilitation Facilities

4891 E Grant Road
Tucson, AZ 85712
520-325-1044
888-281-6531
Fax: 520-318-1129
TTY: 888-281-6531
www.carf.org

Brian J Boon PhD, President/CEO
Amanda Birch, Administrator Of Operations

Promotes the quality, value and optimal outcomes through a consultative accreditation process that centers on enhancing the lives of the people served.

2604 Commonwealth Fund

One E 75th Street
New York, NY 10021
212-606-3800
Fax: 212-606-3500
E-mail: cmwf@cmwf.org
www.cmwf.org

Karen Davis, President
John Craig, COO/Executive Vice President

Private foundation that supports independent research on health and social issues and make grants to improve health care practice and policy.

2605 Community Action Partnership

1140 Connecticut Avenue
Suite 1210
Washington, DC 20036
202-265-7546
Fax: 202-265-8850
E-mail: info@communityactionpartnership.com
www.communityactionpartnership.com

Donald Mathis, President/CEO
Avril Weisman, Vice President

The national organization representing the interests of the 1,000 Community Action Agencies working to fight poverty at the local level.

Year Founded: 1971

2606 Community Anti-Drug Coalitions of America:

625 Slaters Lane
Suite 300
Alexandria, VA 22314
703-706-0560
800-542-2322
Fax: 703-706-0565
E-mail: info@cadca.org
www.cadca.org

Arthur T Dean, Chair/CEO
Addie Liles, Executive Assistant

With more than five thousand members across the country, CADCA is working to build and strengthen the capacity of community coalitions to create safe, healthy, and drug free communities. CADCA supports its members with technical assistance and training, public policy, media and marketing, conferences and special events.

2607 Corporate Counseling Associates

475 Park Avenue South
Fifth Floor
New York, NY 10016-6901

212-686-6827
800-833-8707
Fax: 212-686-6511
E-mail: info@corporatecounseling.com
www.corporatecounseling.com

Robert Levy, President
Steve Salee, SVP Consultative Services

Customized, integrated workplace solutions designed to enhance business performance by enriching employee productivity.

2608 Council of Behavioral Group Practice

1110 Mar West Street E
Tiburon, CA 94920
415-435-9821
Fax: 415-543-9821

2609 Council on Social Work Education

1725 Duke Street
Suite 500
Alexandria, VA 22314-3457
703-683-8080
Fax: 703-683-8099
E-mail: info@cswe.org
www.cswe.org

Julia M. Watkins PhD, Executive Director
Nicole Demarco, Executive Assistant To Exec. Dir

A national association that preserves and enhances the quality of social work education for the purpose of promoting the goals of individual and community well being and social justice. Pursues this mission through setting and maintaining policy and program standards, accrediting bachelors and masters degree programs in social work, promoting research and faculty development, and advocating for social work education.

Year Founded: 1952

2610 Developmental Disabilities Nurses Association

PO Box 536489
Orlando, FL 32853-6489
407-835-0642
800-888-6733
Fax: 407-426-7440
www.ddna.org

Kathy Brown, Vice President
Richanne Cunningham, Secretary

National nonprofit professional association for nurses working with individuals with developmental disabilities. Publishes a quarterly newsletter.

Year Founded: 1992

2611 Employee Assistance Professionals Association

4350 North Fairfax Drive
Suite 410
Arlington, VA 22203
703-387-1000
Fax: 703-522-4585
E-mail: ceo@eap-association.org
www.eap-association.org

John Maynard PhD, CEO
Mickey McKay, President
Jan Paul, Secretary/Treasurer

International association of approximately 5,000 members who are primarily employee assistance professionals as well as individuals in related fields such as human re-

sources, chemical dependency treatment, mental health treatment, managed behavioral health care, counseling and benefits administration. Hosts annual EAP conference.

Year Founded: 1971

2612 Employee Assistance Society of North America

2001 Jefferson Davis Highway
Suite 1004
Arlington, VA 22202-3617
703-416-0060
Fax: 703-416-0014
E-mail: easnamember@ardel.com
www.easna.org

Joseph Seoane, Director Client Relations

International group of professional leaders with competencies in such specialties as workplace and family wellness, employee benefits and organizational development. Maintains accreditation program, membership services and professional training opportunities, promotes high standards of employee assistance programs.

Year Founded: 1985

2613 Gerontoligical Society of America

1030 15th Street NW
Suite 250
Washington, DC 20005
202-842-1275
Fax: 202-842-1150
E-mail: geron@geron.org
www.geron.org

Carol Ann Schutz, Advisor
Linda Krogh Harootyan, Interim Executive Director

Nonprofit professional organization with more than 5000 members in the field of aging. GSA provides researchers, educators, practitioners and policy makers with opportunities to understand, advance, integrate and use basic and applied research on aging to improve the quality of life as one ages.

2614 Gorski-Cenaps Corporation Training & Consultation

6147 Deltona Boulevard
Spring Hill, FL 34606
352-596-8000
Fax: 352-596-8002
E-mail: info@cenaps.com
www.cenaps.com

Terence T Gorski, President
Tresa Watson, Business Manager

Cenaps provides advanced clinical skills training for the addiction behavioral health and mental health fields. Their focus is recovery and relapse prevention.

2615 Group for the Advancement of Psychiatry

PO Box 570218
Dallas, TX 75357-0218
972-613-3044
Fax: 972-613-5532
E-mail: frad1@airmail.net
www.groupadpsych.org

Frances Roton, Executive Director

An organization of nationally respected psychiatrists dedicated to shaping psychiatric thinking, public programs and clinical practice in mental health. Meets twice a year at the Renaissance Westchester Hotel in White Plains, NY.

Year Founded: 1946

2616 Health Service Providers Verified
1120 G Street NW
Suite 230
Washington, DC 20005-3801
202-783-1270
Fax: 202-783-1269

Judy Hall PhD, President

2617 Institute for the Advancement of Human Behavior (IAHB)
4370 Alpine Road
Suite 209
Portola Valley, CA 94028
650-851-8411
Fax: 650-851-0406
E-mail: staff@iahb.org
www.ibh.com

Gerry Piaget, President
Joan Piaget, Executive Director

A non-profit educational organization. They are a fully accredited sponsor of continuing education and continuing medical education for mental health, chemical dependency, and substance abuse treatment providers in the United States and Canada. Their mission is to provide high-quality clinical training to healthcare professionals as well as to companies and individuals with healthcare-related interests. They produce workshops and seminars on timely and important clinical topics conducted by scientist-practitioners who represent the state-of-the art in their chosen fields.

2618 Institute of HeartMath
14700 W Park Avenue
Boulder Creek, CA 95006
831-338-8500
Fax: 831-338-8504
E-mail: ihminquiry@heartmath.org
www.heartmath.org

Sara Paddison, President/CEO
Rollin McCarty, Executive VP/Dir. Of Research
Brian Kabaker, CFO/Dir. Sales & Marketing

Nonprofit research and education on stress, emotional physiology and heart-brain interactions. Purpose is to reduce stress, school violence, improve mental and emotional attitudes, promote harmony within facilities and communities, improve academic performance and improve workplace health and performance. Research facility provides psychometric assessments for both individual and organizational assessment as well as autonomic assessments for physiological assessment and diagnostic purposes. Education initiative currently developing curriculum for rehabilitation of incarcerated teen felons in drug and alcohol recovery program.

Year Founded: 1991

2619 Institute on Psychiatric Services: American Psychiatric Association
1000 Wilson Boulevard
Suite 1825
Arlington, VA 22209-3901
703-907-7300
E-mail: apa@psych.org
www.psych.org

Carol Robinowitz, President

Open to employees of all psychiatric and related health and educational facilities. Includes lectures by experts in the field and workshops and accredited courses on problems, programs and trends. Offers on-site Job Bank, which lists opportunities for mental health professionals. Organized scientific exhibits. Publications: Psychiatric Services, monthly journal. Annual Institute on Psychiatric Services conference and exhibits in October, Chicago, IL.

2620 Integrated Behavioral Health Consultants
7701 Park Ridge Circle
Fort Collins, CO 80528-8909
970-223-5633
Fax: 970-223-1697

Nina M Smith, President

2621 International Center for the Study of Psychiatry And Psychology (ISCPP)
1036 Park Avenue
Suite 1B
New York, NY 10028
212-861-7400
E-mail: djriccio@aol.com
www.icspp.org

Peter Breggin, Founder/Director Emeritus
Dominick Riccio PhD, Executive Director

Nonprofit research and educational network whose focus is the critical study of the mental health movement. ICSPP is completely independent and their funding consists solely of individual membership dues. Fosters prevention and treatment of mental and emotional disorders. Promotes alternatives to administering psychiatric drugs to children.

2622 International Society for Developmental Psychobiology
8181 Tezel Road
#10269
San Antonio, TX 78250
830-796-9393
866-377-4416
Fax: 830-796-9394
E-mail: isdp@isdpcentraloffice.org
www.isdp.org

Rick Richardson, Secretary
Susan Brunelli, Treasurer

Members are research scientists in the field of developmental psychobiology and biology and psychology students. Promotes research in the field of developmental psychobiology, the study of the brain and brain behavior throughout the life span and in relation to other biological proccesses. Stimulates communication and interaction among scientists in the field. Provides the editorship for the journal, Development Psychobiology. Bestows awards. Compiles statistics. Annual conference.

2623 International Society of Political Psychology
Moynihan Institute of Global Affairs
346 Eggers Hall
Syracuse University
Syracuse, NY 13244
315-443-4470
Fax: 315-443-9085
E-mail: ispp@maxwell.syr.edu
www.http://ispp.org

Bruce Dayton, Executive Director

Facilitates communication across disciplinary, geographic and political boundaries among scholars, concerned individuals in government and public posts, the communication media and elsewhere who have a scientific interest in the relationship between politics and psychological processes. ISPP seeks to advance the quality of scholarship in political psychology and to increase the usefulness of work in political psychology.

2624 International Transactional Analysis Association (ITAA)
2186 Rheem Drive #B-1
Pleasanton, CA 94588
925-600-8110
Fax: 925-600-8112
E-mail: info@itaa-net.org
www.itaa-net.org

Ken Fogleman, CFO
Lee Beer, Webmaster

A non-profit educational organization with members in over 65 countries. Its purpose is to advance the theory, methods and principles of transactional analysis.

2625 Jean Piaget Society: Society for the Study of Knowledge and Development (JPSSSKD)
Department Of Psychology
Clark University
950 Main St
Worcester, MA 01610-1477
508-793-7250
Fax: 508-793-7265
E-mail: webmaster@piaget.org
www.piaget.org

Nancy Budwig, President
Ashley Maynard, Treasurer

Scholars, teachers, and researchers interested in exploring the nature of the developmental construction of human knowledge. Purpose is to further research on knowledge and development, especially in relation to the work of Jean Piaget, a Swiss developmentalist noted for his work in child psychology, the study of human development, and the origin and growth of human knowledge. Conducts small meetings and programs.

2626 Managed Health Care Association
1299 Pennsylvania Avenue NW
Washington, DC 20004
202-218-4121
Fax: 202-478-1734

2627 Med Advantage
11301 Corporate Boulevard
Suite 300
Orlando, FL 32817-1445
407-282-5131
Fax: 407-282-9240
E-mail: info@med-advantage.com
www.med-advantage.com

Fully accredited by URAC and certified in all 11 elements by NCQA, Med Advantage is one of the oldest credentials verification organizations in the country. Over the past eight years, they have developed sophisticated computer systems and one of the largest data warehouses of medical providers in the nation, containing information on over 900,000 healthcare providers. Their system is continually updated from primary source data required to meet the standards of the URAC, NCQA and JCAHO.

2628 Medical Group Management Association
104 Inverness Terrace E
Englewood, CO 80112-5306
303-799-1111
877-275-6462
Fax: 303-643-4439
E-mail: service@mgma.com
www.mgma.com

Warren White, Secretary/Treasurer
Steve Hellebush, COO

The national membership association providing information networking and professional development for the individuals who manage and lead medical group practices.

Year Founded: 1926

2629 Mental Health Corporations of America
1876-A Eider Court
Tallahassee, FL 32308-3763
850-942-4900
Fax: 850-942-0560
E-mail: heveyd@mhca.com
www.mhca.com

Donald J Hevey, President/CEO
Tara Boyter, Director Of Communications

Membership in MHCA is by invitation only. It is the organization's intent to include in its network only the highest quality behavioral healthcare organizations in the country. Their alliance is designed to strengthen members' competitive position, enhance their leadership capabilities and facilitate their strategic networking opportunities.

2630 Mental Health Materials Center (MHMC)
PO Box 304
Bronxville, NY 10708-0304
914-337-6596
Fax: 914-779-0161

Alex Sareyan, President

Professionals of mental health and health education, seeking to stimulate the development of wider, more effective channels of communication between health educators and the public. Provides consulting services to nonprofit organizations on the implementation of their publishing operations in areas related to mental health and health. Publications: Study on Suicide Training Manual. Survival Manual for Medical Students. Books, booklets and pamphlets. Annual Meeting in New York City.

2631 National Academy of Neuropsychology (NAN)
2121 S Oneida Street
Suite 550
Denver, CO 80224-2594
303-691-3694
Fax: 303-691-5983
E-mail: office@nanonline.org
www.nanonline.org

Ruben Echemendia, President
John Meyers, Treasurer

Clinical neuropsychologists and others interested in brain-behavior relationships. Works to preserve and advance knowledge regarding the assessment and remediation of neuropsychological disorders. Promotes the development of neuropsychology as a science and profession; develops standard of practice and training guidelines for the field; fosters communication between members, represents the professional interests of members, serves as an information resource, facilitates the exchange of information among related organizations. Offers continuing education programs, conducts research.

2632 National Association For Childrens Behavioral Health

1025 Connecticut Avenue NW
Suite 1012
Washington, DC 20036-5145
202-857-9735
Fax: 202-362-5145
E-mail: cthompson@youthconnect.org
www.www.nacbh.org

Charles Thompson, President
Jim Maley, President-Elect/Vice President

To promote the availibility and delivery of appropriate and relevant services to children and adolescents with, or at risk of, serious emotional disturbances and their families. Advocate for the full array of mental health and related services necessery, the development and use of assessment and outcome tools based on functional as well as clinical indicators, and the elimination of categorial funding barriers.

2633 National Association for the Advancement of Psychoanalysis

80 Eighth Avenue
Suite 1501
New York, NY 10011-5126
212-741-0515
Fax: 212-366-4347
E-mail: dfmaxwell@mac.com
www.naap.org

Mary Quackenbush, Executive Director
Douglas Maxwell, President

Individual psychoanalysts having variety of schools of psychoanalytic thought united for the advancement of psychoanalysis as a profession. Publications: NAAP NEWS, quarterly. National Registry of Psychoanalysts, annual directory. Annual Conference.

Year Founded: 1972

2634 National Association in Women's Health Professionals

300 West Adams Street
Suite 328
Chicago, IL 60606
312-786-1468
Fax: 312-786-0376
www.nawh.org

Shirley Sachs, Executive Director

2635 National Association of Addiction Treatment Providers

313 W Liberty Street
Suite 129
Lancaster, PA 17603-2748
717-392-8480
Fax: 717-392-8481
E-mail: rhunsicker@naatp.org
www.naatp.org

Ronald J Hunsicker, President/CEO

The mission of the National Association of Addiction Treatment Providers (NAATP) is to promote, assist and enhance the delivery of ethical, effective, research-based treatment for alcoholism and other drug addictions. Provides members and the public with accurate, responsible information and other resources related to the treatment of these diseases, advocates for increased access to and availability of quality treatment for those who suffer from alcoholism and other drug addictions; works in partnership with other organizations and individuals that share NAATP's mission and goals.

Year Founded: 1978

2636 National Association of Community Health Centers

7200 Wisconsin Avenue
Suite 210
Bethesda, MD 20814
301-347-0400
Fax: 301-347-0459
www.nachc.com

Gary Wiltz, Secretary
Kauila Clark, Treasurer

A non-profit organization whose mission is to enhance and expand access to quality, community-responsive health care for America's medically underserved and uninsured. A major source for information, data, research and advocacy on key issues affecting community-based health centers and the delivery of health care. Provides education, training, technical assistance and leadership development to health center staff, boards and others to promote excellence and cost-effectiveness in health delivery practice and community board governance. Builds partnerships and linkages that stimulate public and private sector investment in the delivery of quality health care services to medically underserved communities.

2637 National Association of Nouthetic Counselors

3600 W 96th Street
Indianapolis, IN 46268-2095
317-337-9100
Fax: 317-337-9199
E-mail: info@nanc.org
www.nanc.org

Randy Patten, Executive Director
Jo Ann Pabody, Office Administrator

NANC is a fellowship of Christian counselors and laymen who have banded together to promote excellence in biblical counseling. NANC was founded in 1975 in service to Christ to address several needs in the counseling community.

Year Founded: 1975

2638 National Association of Psychiatric Health Systems

701 13th Street NW
Suite 950
Washington, DC 20005-3903
202-393-6700
Fax: 202-783-6041
E-mail: naphs@naphs.org
www.naphs.org

Jeff Borenstein, President
Debra Osteen, First Vice President

Advocates for behavioral health and represents provider systems that are committed to the delivery of responsive, accountable, and clinically effective treatment and prevention programs for children, adolescents, adults and older adults with mental and substance abuse disorders.

Year Founded: 1933

2639 National Association of School Psychologists (NASP)
4340 East West Highway
Suite 402
Bethesda, MD 20814
301-657-0270
Fax: 301-657-0275
E-mail: sgorin@naspweb.org
www.nasponline.org

Susan Gorin, Executive Director
Ted Feinberg, Assistant Executive Director

School psychologists who serve the mental health and educational needs of all children and youth. Encourages and provides opportunites for professional growth of individual members. Informs the public on the services and practice of school psychology, and advances the standards of the profession. Operates national school psychologist certification system. Sponsers children's services.

2640 National Association of Social Workers
750 First Street NE
Suite 700
Washington, DC 20002-4241
202-336-8244
800-638-8799
Fax: 202-336-8310
E-mail: membership@naswdc.org
www.socialworkers.org

Elvira Craig de Silva CSW, President
Willie Walker, Vice President

The largest membership organization of professional social workers in the world, with more than 153,000 members. NASW works to enhance the professional growth and development of its members, to create and maintain professional standards and to advance sound social policies.

2641 National Association of State Mental Health Program Directors (NASMHPD)
66 Canal Center Plaza
Suite 302
Alexandria, VA 22314
703-739-9333
Fax: 703-548-9517
E-mail: roy.praschil@nasmhpd.org
www.nasmhpd.org

Robert W Glover, Executive Director
Roy Praschil, Director Operations

State commissioners in charge of state mental disability programs for children and youth, aged, legal services, forensic services and adult services. Promotes state government agencies to deliver services to mentally disabled persons and fosters the exchange of scientific and program information in the administration of public mental health programs. Publications: Children and Youth Update, periodic. Federal Agencies, periodic newsletter. State Report, periodic newsletter.

2642 National Business Coalition Forum on Health (NBCH)
1015 18th Street NW
Suite 730
Washington, DC 20036
202-775-9300
Fax: 202-775-1569
E-mail: awebber@nbch.org
www.nbch.org

Andrew Webber, President/CEO
Maria Cornejo, Director Of Operations
Carly McKeon, Office Administrator

A national, non-profit membership organization of employer-based coalitions. Dedicated to value-based purchasing of health care services through the collective action of public and private purchasers. NCBH seeks to accelerate the nations progress towards safe, efficient, high quality health care and the improved health status of the American population.

2643 National Coalition for the Homeless
2201 P Street NW
Washington, DC 20037
202-462-4822
Fax: 202-462-4823
E-mail: info@nationalhomeless.org
www.nationalhomeless.org

A national network of people who are currenlty experiencing or have experienced homelessness, activists and advocates, community-based and faith-based service providers, and others commiited to ending homelessness.

Year Founded: 1984

2644 National Committee for Quality Assurance
1100 13th Street NW
Suite 1000
Washington, DC 20005
202-955-3500
Fax: 202-955-3599
www.ncqa.org

Margaret O'Kane, President
Greg Pawlson, Executive Vice President
Esther Emard, COO

A non-profit organization whose mission is to improve health care quality everywhere and to transform health care quality through measurement, transparency and accountability.

2645 National Council of Juvenile and Family Court Judges
PO Box 8970
Reno, NV 89507-8970
775-784-6012
Fax: 775-784-6628
E-mail: staff@ncjfcj.org
www.ncjfcj.org

Susan Carbon, President
Mary V Mentaberry, Executive Director

Their mission is to improve courts and systems practice and raise awareness of the core issues that touch the lives of many of our nation's childrens and families.

Year Founded: 1937

2646 National Council on Aging
1901 L Street NW
4th Floor
Washington, DC 20036
202-479-1200
Fax: 202-479-0735
E-mail: info@ncoa.org
www.ncoa.org

James Firman, President/CEO
Jay Greenberg, EVP For Business Development

A national network of organizations and individuals dedicated to improving the health and independence of older persons and increasing their continuing contributions to communities, society and future generations.

Year Founded: 1950

2647 National Criminal Justice Association
720 7th Street NW
Third Floor
Washington, DC 20001
202-628-8550
Fax: 202-448-1723
E-mail: info@ncja.org
www.ncja.org

David Steingraber, President
Roland Mena, Vice President

Promotes the development of justice systems in states, tribal nations, and units of local government that enhance public safety; prevent and reduce the harmful effects of criminal and delinquent behavior of victims, individuals and communities; adjudicate defendents and sanction offenders fairly and justly; and that are effective and efficient.

2648 National Eldercare Services Company
7315 Wisconsin Avenue
Suite 400 East
Bethesda, MD 20814
301-340-2851
Fax: 301-942-5832
E-mail: natleldr@bellatlantic.net
www.natl-eldercare-service.com

Rebecca Rush, Contact

An eldercare benefit management system.

2649 National Managed Health Care Congress
71 2nd Avenue
Floor 3
Waltham, MA 02451-1107
888-446-6422
Fax: 781-663-6411
www.nmhcc.com

Brings senior executives from Fortune 500 companies, hospitals, and health plans practical solutions to control costs, improve quality and increase access.

2650 National Mental Health Association
2000 N Beauregard Street
6th Floor
Alexandria, VA 22311
703-684-7722
800-969-6642
Fax: 703-684-5968
TTY: 800-433-5959
www.nmha.org

David Shern, President/CEO
Kate Gaston, VP Afiliate Services

Dedicated to improving treatments, understanding and services for adults and children with mental health needs. Working to win political support for funding for school mental health programs. Provides information about a wide range of disorders.

2651 National Nurses Association
1767 Business Center Drive
Suite 150
Reston, VA 20190
703-438-3060
877-662-6253
Fax: 703-438-3072
E-mail: info@nationalnurses.org
www.nationalnurses.org

Laurie Campbell PhD, Executive Director

Purpose is to help enhance the personal development as well as economic well being of its members. They provide services and benefits meaningful to the unique demands of the nursing professional.

Year Founded: 1984

2652 National Pharmaceutical Council
1894 Preston White Drive
Reston, VA 20191-5433
703-620-6390
Fax: 703-476-0904
E-mail: info@npcnow.com
www.npcnow.org

Karen Williams, President
Pat Adams, VP Business Operations

NPC sponsors a variety of research and education projects aimed at demonstrating that the appropriate use of pharmaceuticals improves both patient treatment outcomes and the cost effective delivery of overall health care services.

2653 National Psychological Association for Psychoanalysis (NPAP)
150 W 13th Street
New York, NY 10011-7891
212-924-7440
Fax: 212-989-7543
E-mail: info@npap.org
www.npap.org

Paul Kaiser, President
Arlyne Rochlin, Vice President

Professional society for practicing psychoanalysts. Conducts training program leading to certification in psychoanalysis. Offers information and private referral service for the public. Operates speakers' bureau. Publications: National Psychological Association for Psychoanalysis-Bulletin, biennial. National Psychological Association for Psychoanalysis-News and Reviews, semiannual. Psychoanalytic Review, bimonthly journal.

Year Founded: 1948

2654 National Register of Health Service Provider s in Psychology
1120 G Street NW
Suite 330
Washington, DC 20005

202-783-7663
Fax: 202-347-0550
www.nationalregister.org

Morgan Sammons, President/Chair
Greg Hurley, Vice President/Vice-Chair

Psychologists who are licensed or certified by a state/provincial board of examiners of psychology and who have met council criteria as health service providers in psychology.

Year Founded: 1974

2655 National Treatment Alternative for Safe Communities
1500 N Halsted
Chicago, IL 60622
312-787-0208
Fax: 312-787-9663
E-mail: information@tasc-il.org
www.tasc-il.org

Melody M Heaps, President
Peter Palanca, Vice President

TASC is a not-for-profit organization that provides behavioral health recovery management services for individuals with substance abuse and mental health disorders. They provide direct services, design model programs and build collaborative networks between public systems and community-based human service providers. TASC's purpose is to see that under-served populations gain access to the services they need for health and self-sufficiency, while also ensuring that public and private resources are used most efficiently.

2656 North American Society of Adlerian Psychology (NASAP)
NASAP
614 West Chocolate Avenue
Hershey, PA 17033
717-579-8795
Fax: 717-533-8616
E-mail: info@alfrdadler.org
www.alfredadler.org

Mel Markowski, President
Al Milliren, Vice President

NASAP is a professional organization for couselors, educators, psychologists, parent educators, business professionals, researchers and others who are interested in Adler's Individual Psychology. Membership includes journals, newsletters, conferences and training.

Year Founded: 1952

2657 Pharmaceutical Care Management Association
601 Pennsylvania Avenue NW
7th Floor
Washington, DC 20004
202-207-3610
Fax: 202-207-3623
E-mail: info@pcmanet.org
www.pcmanet.org

Mark Merritt, President/CEO
Missy Jenkins, SVP Federal Affairs

A national association representing Pharmacy Benefit Managers. They are dedicated to enhancing the proven tools and techniques that PBMs have pioneered in the marketplace and working to lower the cost of prescription drugs for more than 200 million Americans.

2658 Physicians for a National Health Program
29 E Madison
Suite 602
Chicago, IL 60602
312-782-6006
Fax: 312-782-6007
E-mail: info@pnhp.org
www.pnhp.org

Ana Malinow, President
Steffie Woolhandler, Secretary

A single issue organization advocating a universal, comprehensive Single-Payer National Health Program.

Year Founded: 1987

2659 Professional Risk Management Services
The Psychiatrists' Program
1515 Wilson Boulevard
Suite 800
Arlington, VA 22209-2402
800-245-3333
E-mail: aboutus@prms.com
www.prms.com

Martin G Tracy JD ARM, President/CEO
Joseph Detorie, Executive Vice President/CFO

Professional Risk Management Services Inc (PRMS), a managing general agent, specializes in professional liability insurance, risk management, and loss prevention services. Our goal is to protect physicians and improve patient care through the development, design, and delivery of innovative professional liability insurance programs. At PRMS, we excel at providing superior, cost effective products and services that protect and support the demands and needs of our clients, including physicians, physician groups, facilities, and organizations. A key link to the success of PRMS is our staff of dedicated legal, clinical, and insurance professionals who turn their expertise into practice.

2660 Psychiatric Society Of Informatics American Association For Technology In Psychiatry
PO Box 11
Bronx, NY 10464-0011
718-502-9469
E-mail: aatp@techpsych.org
www.www.techpsych.org

Robert Kennedy, Executive Director
Carlyle Chan, Secretary
Naakesh Dewan, President

2661 Psychohistory Forum
627 Dakota Trail
Franklin Lakes, NJ 07417
201-891-7486
E-mail: pelovitz@aol.com
www.www.cliospsyche.org

Paul H Elovitz PhD, Editor

Psychologists, psychiatrists, psychotherapists, social workers, historians, psychohistorians and others having a scholarly interest in the integration of depth psychology and history. Aids individuals in psychohistorical research. Holds lecture series. Publications: Clio's Psyche: Understanding the Why of Current Events and History, quarterly journal. Immigrant Experience: Personal Narrative and Psychological Analysis, monograph. Periodic Meeting.

2662 Psychology Society (PS)
100 Beekman Street
New York, NY 10038-1810
212-285-1872

Dr Pierre Haber, Executive Director

Professional membership is limited to psychologists who have a doctorate and are certified/licensed. Associate membership is intended for teachers and researchers as well as persons whose professional status is pending. Seeks to further the use of psychology in therapy, family and social problems, behavior modification, and treatment of drug abusers and prisoners. Encourages the use of psychology in the solution of social and political conflicts.

2663 Psychology of Religion
Doctoral Program in Clinical Psychology
750 First Street NE
Washington, DC 20002-4242
202-336-6013
Fax: 202-218-3599
E-mail: division@apa.org
www.www.apa.org/divisions/div36

Lisa Miller, President
Michael Donahue, Secretary

A division of the American Psychologial Association. Seeks to encourage and accelerate research, theory, and practice in the psychology of religion and related areas. Facilitates the dissemination of data on religious and allied issues and on the integration of these data with current psychological research, theory and practice.

2664 Psychonomic Society
1710 Fortview Road
Austin, TX 78704
512-462-2442
Fax: 512-462-1101
www.psychonomic.org

Laura Carlson, Secretary/Treasurer
Roger Mellgren, Convention Manager

Persons qualified to conduct and supervise scientific research in psychology or allied sciences; members must hold a PhD degree or its equivalent and must have published significant research other than doctoral dissertation. Promotes the communication of scientific research in psychology and allied sciences.

2665 Rapid Psychler Press
3560 Pine Grove Avenue
Suite 374
Port Huron, MI 48060
519-433-7642
888-779-2453
Fax: 888-779-2457
E-mail: rapid@psychler.com
www.psychler.com

David Robinson, Publisher

Produces books and presentation media for educating mental health professionals. Products cover a wide range of learning needs. Where possible, humor is incorporated as an educational aid to enhance learning and retention.

2666 Risk and Insurance Management Society
1065 Avenue Of The Americas
13th Floor
New York, NY 10018

212-286-9292
www.www.rims.org

Janice Ochenkowski, President/Director
Joseph Restoule, Vice President

2667 Sciacca Comprehensive Services Development
299 Riverside Drive
New York, NY 10025-5278
212-866-5935
Fax: 212-666-1942
E-mail: ksciacca@pobox.com

Kathleen Sciacca MA, Executive Director/Consultant

Provides consulting, education and training for treatment and program development for dual diagnosis of mental illness and substance disorders including severe mental illness. Materials available include manuals, videos, articles, book chapters, journals and books. Trains in Motivational Interviewing. Develops programs across the mental health and substance abuse systems.

2668 Screening for Mental Health
1 Washington Street
Suite 304
Wellesley Hills, MA 02481
781-239-0071
Fax: 781-431-7447
E-mail: smhinfo@mentalhealthscreening.org
www.mentalhealthscreening.org

Douglas G Jacobs MD, Executive Director

Nonprofit organization devoted to assisting people with undiagnosed, untreated mental illness connect with local treatment resources via national screening programs for depression, anxiety, eating disorders and alcohol problems.

2669 Sigmund Freud Archives (SFA)
23 The Hemlocks
c/o Harold P Blum, MD
Roslyn, NY 11576-1721
516-621-6850
Fax: 516-621-3014
E-mail: did2005@med.cornell.edu
www.www.library.med.cornell.edu

Harold P Blum MD, Executive Director

Psychoanalysts interested in the preservation and collection of scientific and personal writings of Sigmund Freud. Assists in research on Freud's life and work and the evolution of psychoanalytic thought. Collects and classifies all documents, papers, publications, personal correspondence and historical data written by, to, and on Freud. Transmits all materials collected to the Library of Congress. Annual meeting in New York City.

2670 Society for Pediatric Psychology (SPP)
Citadel
Department of Phychiatry
Charleston, SC 29409
843-953-5320
Fax: 843-953-6797
www.apa.org

Lori Stark, President
Christina Adams, Secretary

Dedicated to research and practice addressing the relationship between children's physical, cognitive, social, and emotional functioning and their physical well-being, including maintenance of health, promotion of positive health behaviors, and treatment of chronic and serious medical conditions. A division of the APA. Bimonthly Journal, Newletter three times a year.

2671 Society for Personality Assessment
6109H Arlington Boulevard
Falls Church, VA 22044
703-534-4772
Fax: 703-534-6905
E-mail: manager@spaonline.org
www.personality.org

Virginia Brabender, President
F. Barton Evans, Treasurer
Carol Groves Overton, Secretary

International professional trade association for psychologists, behavioral scientists, anthropologists, and psychiatrists. Promotes the study, research development and application of personality assessment.

2672 Society for Psychophysiological Research
2810 Crossroads Drive
Suite 3800
Madison, WI 53718
608-443-2472
Fax: 608-443-2474
E-mail: spr@reesgroupinc.com
www.sprweb.org

Monica Fabiani, President
Karen Quigley, Treasurer

Founded in 1960, the Society for Psychophysiological Research is an international scientific society. The purpose of the society is to foster research on the interrelationship between physiological and phychological aspects of behavior.

2673 Society for Women's Health Research
1025 Connecticut Avenue Nw
Suite 701
Washington, DC 20036
202-223-8224
Fax: 202-833-3472
E-mail: info@womenshealthresearch.org
www.womenshealthresearch.org

Phyllis Greenberger, President/CEO
Suzanne Stone, VP Finance And Administration

The nation's only not-for-profit organization whose sole mission is to improve the health of women through research. Founded in 1990, The Society advocates increased funding for research on women's health, encourages the study of sex differences that may affect the prevention, diagnosis and treatment of disease, and promotes the inclusion of women in medical research studies.

2674 Society for the Advancement of Social Psychology (SASP)
630 Convention Tower
Buffalo, NY 14202
301-405-5921
Fax: 301-314-9566
E-mail: sesp@sesp.org
www.sesp.org

Garold Stasser, Secretary
Charles Stangor, Executive Officer

Social psychologists and students in social psychology. Advances social psychology as a profession by facilitating communication among social psychologists and improving

dissemination and utilization of social psychological knowledge. Annual meeting every October.

2675 Society for the Psychological Study of Social Issues (SPSSI)
208 I Street NE
Washington, DC 20002-4340
202-675-6956
Fax: 202-675-6902
E-mail: spssi@spssi.org
www.spssi.org

Susan Dudley, Administrative Director
Anila Balkissoon, Administrative Coordinator

An international group of over 3,500 psychologists, allied scientists, students, and others who share a common interest in research on the psychological aspects of important social issues. The Society seeks to bring theory and practice into focus on human problems of the group, the community, and nations as well as the increasingly important problems that have no national boundaries.

2676 Society of Behavioral Medicine
555 East Wells Street
Suite 1100
Milwaukee, WI 53202-3823
414-918-3156
Fax: 414-276-3349
E-mail: info@sbm.org
www.sbm.org

Michael Long, Executive Director
David Wood, Associate Dir. Member Services

A non-profit organization is a scientific forum for over 3,000 behavioral and biomedical researchers and clinicians to study the interactions of behavior, physiological and biochemical states, and morbidity and mortality. SBM provides an interactive network for education and collaboration on common research, clinical and public policy concerns related to prevention, diagnosis and treatment, rehabilitation, and health promotion.

Year Founded: 1978

2677 Society of Multivariate Experimental Psychology (SMEP)
University of Virginia
102 Gilmer Hall
Department of Psychology
Charlottesville, VA 22903
804-924-0656
E-mail: shrout@psych.nyu.edu
www.smep.org

Steve West, President
Wayne Velicer, President-Elect

An organization of researchers interested in multivariate quantitative methods and their application to substantive problems in psychology. Membership is limited to 65 regular active members. SMEP oversees the publication of a research journal which publishes research articles on multivariate methodology and its use in psychological research. Annual meeting held every October.

Year Founded: 1960

2678 Society of Teachers of Family Medicine
11400 Tomahawk Creek Parkway
Suite 540
Leawood, KS 66211

913-906-6000
800-274-2237
Fax: 913-906-6096
E-mail: stmoffice@stfm.org
www.stfm.org

Stacy Brungardt, Executive Director
Angela Broderick, Deputy Executive Director

Mulitdisciplinary, medical organization that offers numerous faculty development opportunities for individuals involved in family medicine education. STFM publishes a monthly journal, hosts a web site, distributes books, coordinates CME conferences devoted to family medicine teaching and research and other activities designed to improve teaching skills of family medicine educators.

2679 Therapeutic Communities of America
1601 Connecticut Avenue NW
Suite 803
Washington, DC 20009
202-296-3503
Fax: 202-518-5475
E-mail: tca.office@verizon.net
www.therapeuticcommunitiesofamerica.org

Patrcia Beauchemin, Executive Director
Michael Harle, President
Sushma Taylor, First Vice President

National nonprofit membership association representing over 500 substance abuse treatment programs. The member agencies provide services to substance abuse clients of diverse special needs. Members provide a continuum of care including assessment, detoxification, residential care, case management, outpatient treatment, transitional housing, education, vocational and medical care.

2680 United States Psychiatric Rehabilitation Organization (USPRA)
601 Global Way
Suite 106
Linthicum, MD 21090
410-789-7054
Fax: 410-789-7675
E-mail: info@uspra.org
www.uspra.org

Marcia Granahan CAE, CEO
Dave Mank, CFO

The USPRA, formerly IAPSRS, is an organization of psychosocial rehabilitation agencies, practitioners, and interested organizations and individuals dedicated to promoting, supporting and strengthening community-oriented rehabilitation services and resources for persons with psychiatric disabilities.

2681 Wellness Councils of America
9802 Nicholas Stnue
Suite 315
Omaha, NE 68114
402-827-3590
Fax: 402-827-3594
E-mail: wellworkplace@welcoa.org
www.welcoa.org

David Hunnicutt PhD, President
Brittanie Leffelman, Director Of Operations

A national non-profit membership organization dedicated to promoting healthier life styles for all Americans, especially through health promotion initiatives at the worksite. They

publish a number of source books, a monthly newsletter, an extensive line of brochures and conducts numerous training seminars.

Year Founded: 1987

2682 WorldatWork
14040 N Northsight Boulevard
Scottsdale, AZ 85260
877-951-9191
480-951-9191
Fax: 866-816-2962
E-mail: customerrelations@worldatwork.org
www.worldatwork.org

Anne Ruddy, President
Marcia Rhodes, Media Relations

A not-for-profit professional association dedicated to knowledge leadership in compensation, benefits and total rewards. Focuses on human resources disciplines associated with attracting, retaining and motivating employees. Provides education programs, a monthly magazine, online information resources, surveys, publications, conferences, research and networking opportunities.

Year Founded: 1955

2683 Yssociation for Psychological Type
9650 Rockville Pike
Bethesda, MD 20814-3998
301-634-7450
800-847-9943
Fax: 301-634-7455
E-mail: web@aptinternational.org
www.aptinternational.org

John Lord, Executive Director
Jane Kise, President

Individuals involved in organizational development, religion, management, education and counseling, and who are interested in psychological type, the Myers-Briggs Type Indicator, and the works of Carl G Jung. Purpose is to share ideas related to the uses of MBTI and the application of personality type theory in any area; promotes research, development, and education in the field. Sponsors seminars, conferences, and training sessions on the use of psychological type.

Books

General

2684 A Family-Centered Approach to People with Mental Retardation
AAMR
444 N Capitol Street NW
Suite 846
Washington, DC 20001-1512
800-424-3688
Fax: 202-387-2193
E-mail: dcroser@aaidd.org
www.www.aaidd.org

Doren Croser, Executive Director
Paul Aitken, Director Finance/Administration
Bruce Appelgren, Director Of Publications

Outlines key principles relevant to a family-centered approach to mental retardation and identifies four components to family-centered practice. *$12.95*

53 pages ISBN 0-940898-59-4

2685 A Guide to Consent
AAMR
444 N Capitol Street NW
Suite 846
Washington, DC 20001-1512
202-387-1968
800-424-3688
Fax: 202-387-2193
E-mail: dcroser@aamr.org
www.aamr.org

Examines current consent issues and explores legal implications of self-determination topics. Focuses on critical life events for people with mental retardation and practical applications of consent law, such as adult guardianship, consent to sexual activity, program placement and home ownership, capacity for and access to legal representation, capacity and other liberty and autonomy issues. *$27.95*

125 pages ISBN 0-940898-58-6

2686 A History of Nursing in the Field of Mental Retardation
AAMR
444 N Capitol Street NW
Suite 846
Washington, DC 20001-1512
202-387-1968
800-424-3688
Fax: 202-387-2193
E-mail: dcroser@aamr.org
www.aamr.org

For nursing scholars and anyone interested in the history of the treatment of people with mental retardation. *$19.95*

205 pages ISBN 0-940898-68-3

2687 A Primer on Rational Emotive Behavior Therapy
Research Press
Dept 24 W
PO Box 9177
Champaign, IL 61826
217-352-3273
800-519-2707
Fax: 217-352-1221
E-mail: rp@researchpress.com
www.researchpress.com

Dr Windy Dryden, Author
Dennis Wiziecki, Marketing

This concise, systematic guide addresses recent developments in the theory and practice of Rational Emotive Behavior Therapy (REBT). The authors discuss rational versus irrational thinking, the ABC framework, the three basic musts that interfere wtih rational thinking and behavior, two basic biological tendencies, two fundamental human disturbances, and the theory of change in REBT. A detailed case example that includes verbatim dialogue between therapist and client illustrates the 18-step REBT treatment sequence. An appendix by Albert Ellis examines the special features of REBT. *$13.95*

114 pages ISBN 0-878224-78-5

2688 A Research Agenda for DSM-V
American Psychiatric Publishing
1000 Wilson Boulevard
Suite 1825
Arlington, VA 22209-3901

703-907-7322
800-368-5777
Fax: 703-907-1091
E-mail: appi@psych.org
www.appi.org

In the ongoing quest to improve our psychiatric diagnostic system, we are now searching for new approaches to understanding the etiological and pathophysiological mechanisms that can improve the validity of our diagnoses and the consequent power of our preventative and treatment interventions-venturing beyond the current DSM paradigm and DSM-IV framework. This volume represents a far-reaching attempt to stimulate research and discussion in the field in preparation for the start of the DSM-V process, still several years away, and to integrate information from a wide variety of sources and technologies. *$38.95*

352 pages Year Founded: 2002 ISBN 0-890422-92-3

2689 Adaptive Behavior and Its Measurement Implications for the Field of Mental Retardation
AAMR
444 N Capitol Street NW
Suite 846
Washington, DC 20001-1512
202-387-1968
800-424-3688
Fax: 202-387-2193
E-mail: dcroser@aamr.org
www.aamr.org

Integrates the concept of adaptive behavior more fully into the AAMR definition of mental retardation.

227 pages ISBN 0-940898-64-0

2690 Addressing the Specific needs of Women with Co-Occuring Disorders in the Criminal Justice System
Policy Research Associates
345 Delaware Avenue
Delmar, NY 12054
518-439-7415
800-444-7415
Fax: 518-439-7612
E-mail: gains@prainc.com
www.prainc.com

Brochure emphasizes the need for gender specific programs to meet the management needs of female offenders. For law enforcement and justice administrators.

2691 Advances in Projective Drawing Interpretation
Charles C Thomas Publisher
2600 S 1st Street
Springfield, IL 62704-4730
217-789-8980
800-258-8980
Fax: 217-789-9130
E-mail: books@ccthomas.com
www.ccthomas.com

Exceptional contributors were chosen for their pertinence, range and inventiveness. This outstanding book assembles the progress in the science and in the clinical art of projective drawings as we enter the twenty-first century. *$80.95*

476 pages Year Founded: 1997 ISBN 0-398067-43-0

2692 Advancing DSM: Dilemmas in Psychiatric Diagnosis
American Psychiatric Publishing
1000 Wilson Boulevard
Suite 1825
Arlington, VA 22209-3901
703-907-7322
800-368-5777
Fax: 703-907-1091
E-mail: appi@psych.org
www.appi.org

Presents case studies from leading clinicians and researchers that illuminate the need for a revamped system. Each chapter presents a diagnostic dilemma from clinical practice that is intriguing, controversial, unresolved and remarkable in its theoretical and scientific complexity. Chapter by chapter, Advancing DSM raises important questions about the nature of diagnosis under the current DSM system and recommends broad changes. *$41.95*
304 pages Year Founded: 2002 ISBN 0-890422-93-1

2693 Adverse Effects of Psychotropic Drugs
Gilford Press
72 Spring Street
New York, NY 10012
212-431-9800
Fax: 212-966-6708
$63.00

2694 Agility in Health Care
Jossey-Bass Publishers
350 Sansome Street
5th Floor
San Francisco, CA 94104
415-394-8677
800-956-7739
Fax: 800-605-2665
www.josseybass.com
$42.95
250 pages ISBN 0-787942-11-1

2695 American Psychiatric Glossary
American Psychiatric Publishing
1000 Wilson Boulevard
Suite 1825
Arlington, VA 22209-3901
703-907-7322
800-368-5777
Fax: 703-907-1091
E-mail: appi@psych.org
www.appi.org

Hardcover. Paperback also available. *$28.50*
224 pages Year Founded: 1994 ISBN 0-880485-26-4

2696 American Psychiatric Publishing Textbook of Clinical Psychiatry
American Psychiatric Publishing
1000 Wilson Boulevard
Suite 1825
Arlington, VA 22209-3901
703-907-7322
800-368-5777
Fax: 703-907-1091
E-mail: appi@psych.org
www.appi.org

This densely informative textbook comprises 40 scholarly, authorative chapters by an astonishing 89 experts and combines junior and senior authors alike to enhance the rich diversity and quality of clinical perspectives. *$239.00*
1776 pages Year Founded: 2002 ISBN 1-585620-32-7

2697 Americans with Disabilities Act and the Emerging Workforce
AAMR
444 N Capitol Street NW
Suite 846
Washington, DC 20001-1512
202-387-1968
800-424-3688
Fax: 202-387-2193
E-mail: dcroser@aamr.org
www.aamr.org

Presents an empirical investigation of ADA issues and their effect on the employment of people with disabilities. Filled with legal cases, court opinions, charts, and tables. *$39.95*
303 pages ISBN 0-940898-52-7

2698 Assesing Problem Behaviors
AAMR
444 N Capitol Street NW
Suite 846
Washington, DC 20001-1512
202-387-1968
800-424-3688
Fax: 202-387-2193
E-mail: dcroser@aamr.org
www.aamr.org

Shows how to conduct a functional assessment, to link assessment results to interventions, and gives an example of completed fuctional analysis. *$21.95*
44 pages ISBN 0-940898-39-X

2699 Basic Personal Counseling: Training Manual for Counslers
Charles C Thomas Publisher
2600 S 1st Street
Springfield, IL 62704-4730
217-789-8980
800-258-8980
Fax: 217-789-9130
E-mail: books@ccthomas.com
www.ccthomas.com

Contents: Becoming a Counselor; The Counseling Relationship; An Overview of Skills Training; Attending to the Client and the Use of Minimal Responses; Reflection of Feelings; Reflection of Content and Feeling; The Seeing, Hearing, and Feeling Modes; Asking Questions; Summmarizing; Exploring Options; Reframing; Confrontation; Challenging Self-Destructive Beliefs; Termination; Procedure of the Counseling Experience; The Immediacy of the Counseling Experience; The Human Personality as it Emerges in the Counseling Experience; The Angry Client; Loss and Grief Counseling; The Suicidal Client; Arrangement of the Counseling Room; Keeping Records of Counseling Sessions; Confidentiality; Supervision and Ongoing Training; and The Counselor's Own Well-Being. *$42.95*
214 pages Year Founded: 1989 ISBN 0-398055-40-8

2700 Best of AAMR: Families and Mental Retardation
AAMR
444 N Capitol Street NW
Suite 846
Washington, DC 20001-1512
202-387-1968
800-424-3688
Fax: 202-387-2193
E-mail: dcroser@aamr.org
www.aamr.org

Provides a comprehensive look at families and mental retardation in the 20th century through the eyes of some of its most respected researchers and service providers. *$59.95*

382 pages ISBN 0-940898-76-4

2701 Boundaries and Boundary Violations in Psychoanalysis
American Psychiatric Publishing
1000 Wilson Boulevard
Suite 1825
Arlington, VA 22209-3901
703-907-7322
800-368-5777
Fax: 703-907-1091
E-mail: appi@psych.org
www.appi.org

240 pages Year Founded: 2002 ISBN 1-585620-98-X

2702 Brain Calipers: Descriptive Psychopathology and the Mental Status Examination, Second Edition
Rapid Psychler Press
3560 Pine Grove Avenue
Suite 374
Port Huron, MI 48060
519-433-7642
888-779-2453
Fax: 888-779-2457
E-mail: rapid@psychler.com
www.psychler.com

David Robinson, Publisher

$34.95

ISBN 1-894328-02-7

2703 Breakthroughs in Antipsychotic Medications: A Guide for Consumers, Families, and Clinicians
WW Norton & Company
500 5th Avenue
New York, NY 10110
212-354-5500
800-233-4830
Fax: 212-869-0856
E-mail: admalmud@wwnorton.com
www.wwnorton.com/psych

Gives patients and their families needed information about the pros and cons of switching medications, possible side effects. *$ 22.95*

240 pages Year Founded: 1999 ISBN 0-393703-03-7

2704 Brief Coaching for Lasting Solutions
WW Norton & Company
500 5th Avenue
New York, NY 10110-0017
212-354-5500
800-233-4830
Fax: 212-869-0856
E-mail: npb@wwnorton.com
www.wwnorton.com/psych

Successful coaching is about finding solutions and optimizing clients' lives. Insoo Kim Berg, one of the founders of solution-focused psychotherapy, collaborates with Peter Szabo in order to show how to help clients achieve their goals by applying their therapeutic approach to coaching.

ISBN 0-393704-72-6

2705 Brief Therapy and Managed Care
Jossey-Bass Publishers
350 Sansome Street
5th Floor
San Francisco, CA 94104
415-394-8677
800-956-7739
Fax: 800-605-2665
www.josseybass.com

Provides focused, time-sensitive treatment to your patients. Pratical guidelines on psychotherapy that are conscientiously managed, appropriate, and sensitive to a client's needs. *$40.95*

443 pages ISBN 0-787900-77-X

2706 Brief Therapy with Intimidating Cases
Jossey-Bass Publishers
350 Sansome Street
5th Floor
San Francisco, CA 94104
415-394-8677
800-956-7739
Fax: 800-605-2665
www.josseybass.com

This hands-on guide shows you how to apply the proven principles of brief therapy to a range of complex psychological problems once thought to be treatable only through long-term therapy or with medication. Learn how to focus on your clients' primary complaint and understand how and in what context the undesired behavior is performed. *$34.95*

224 pages ISBN 0-787943-64-9

2707 Cambridge Handbook of Psychology, Health and Medicine
Cambridge University Press
40 W 20th Street
New York, NY 10011-4221
212-924-3900
Fax: 212-691-3239
E-mail: marketing@cup.org
www.cambridge.org

Andrew Baum, Editor

This important text collates international and interdisciplinary expertise to form a unique encyclopedic handbook to this field that will be valuable to medical practitioners as well as psychologists. *$85.00*

678 pages Year Founded: 1997 ISBN 0-521436-86-9

2708 Challenging Behavior of Persons with Mental Health Disorders and Severe Developmental Disabilities
AAMR
444 N Capitol Street NW
Suite 846
Washington, DC 20001-1512
202-387-1968
800-424-3688
Fax: 202-387-2193
E-mail: dcroser@aamr.org
www.aamr.org

Provides a valuable compendium of the current knowledge base and empirically tested treatments for individuals with severe developmental disabilities, especially when problematic patterns of behavior are evident. *$39.95*

278 pages ISBN 0-940898-66-7

2709 Changing Health Care Marketplace
Jossey-Bass Publishers
350 Sansome Street
5th Floor
San Francisco, CA 94104
415-394-8677
800-956-7739
Fax: 800-605-2665
www.josseybass.com

$35.95

366 pages ISBN 0-787902-52-7

2710 Children in Therapy: Using the Family as a Resource
WW Norton & Company
500 5th Avenue
New York, NY 10110-0017
212-354-5500
800-233-4830
Fax: 212-869-0856
E-mail: npb@wwnorton.com
www.wwnorton.com/psych

This anthology presents theoretical perspectives of five different competency-based approaches: solution-oriented brief therapy, narrative therapy, collaborative language systems therapy, internal family systems therapy, and emotionally focused family therapy.

ISBN 0-393704-85-8

2711 Clinical Dimensions of Anticipatory Mourning
Research Press
Dept 24 W
PO Box 9177
Champaign, IL 61826
217-352-3273
800-519-2707
Fax: 217-352-1221
E-mail: rp@researchpress.com
www.researchpress.com

Russell Pense, VP Marketing

Dr. Therese Rando is joined by 17 contributing authors to present the most comprehensive resource available on the perspectives, issues, interventions, and changing views associated with anticipatory mourning. *$29.95*

616 pages ISBN 0-878223-80-0

2712 Clinical Integration
Jossey-Bass Publishers
350 Sansome Street
5th Floor
San Francisco, CA 94104
415-394-8677
800-956-7739
Fax: 800-605-2665
www.josseybass.com

Learn how to create information systems that can support care coordination and management across delivery sites, develop a case management model program for multi-provider systems, and more. *$41.95*

272 pages ISBN 0-787940-39-9

2713 Cognitive Therapy in Practice
WW Norton & Company
500 5th Avenue
New York, NY 10110
212-354-5500
800-233-4830
Fax: 212-869-0856
E-mail: npd@wwnorton.com
www.wwnorton.com/psych

Basic text for graduate studies in psychotherapy, psycholgy nursing social work and counseling. *$29.00*

224 pages Year Founded: 1989 ISBN 0-393700-77-1

2714 Collaborative Therapy with Multi-Stressed Families
Guilford Publications
72 Spring Street
New York, NY 10012
212-431-9800
800-365-7006
Fax: 212-966-6708
E-mail: info@guilford.com
www.guilford.com

Written with a clear and fresh style, this is a guide to working in collaboration with clients, therapists and agencies. Experienced and beginning clinicians will appreciate a progressive approach to intricate problems. *$31.50*

358 pages Year Founded: 1999 ISBN 1-572304-90-1

2715 Communicating in Relationships: A Guide for Couples and Professionals
Research Press
Dept 24 W
PO Box 9177
Champaign, IL 61826
217-352-3273
800-519-2707
Fax: 217-352-1221
E-mail: rp@researchpress.com
www.researchpress.com

Russell Pense, VP Marketing

Addresses the behavioral, affective and cognitive aspects of communicating in relationships. The book can be used by couples as a self-help guide, by professionals as an adjunct to therapy, or as a supplementary text for related college courses. Numerous readings are interspersed with 44 exercises that provide a hands-on approach to learning. The authors outline 18 steps for developing communication skills and describe procedures for integrating the skills into relationships. *$29.95*

280 pages ISBN 0-878223-42-8

2716 Community-Based Instructional Support
AAMR
444 N Capitol Street NW
Suite 846
Washington, DC 20001-1512
202-387-1968
800-424-3688
Fax: 202-387-2193
E-mail: dcroser@aamr.org
www.aamr.org

Offers practical guidelines for applying instructional strategies for adults who are learning community-based tasks. *$12.95*

34 pages ISBN 0-940898-43-8

2717 Comprehensive Textbook of Geriatric Psychitry
WW Norton & Company
500 5th Avenue
New York, NY 10110-0017
212-354-5500
800-233-4830
Fax: 212-869-0856
E-mail: npb@wwnorton.com
www.wwnorton.com/psych

Sponsored by the American Association for Geriatric Psychiatry (AAGP), this invaluable reference covers the entire range of geriatric psychiatry, including: the ageing process; psychiatric disorders of the elderly; princpiles of diagnosis and treatment; medical-legal, ethical, and financial issues.

ISBN 0-393704-26-2

2718 Computerization of Behavioral Healthcare
Jossey-Bass Publishers
350 Sansome Street
5th Floor
San Francisco, CA 94104
415-433-1767
800-956-7739
Fax: 800-605-2665
www.josseybass.com

How computers and networked interactive information systems can help to contain costs, improve clinical outcomes, make your organizations more competitive using practical guidelines. *$27.95*

304 pages Year Founded: 1996 ISBN 0-787902-21-7

2719 Concise Guide to Marriage and Family Therapy
American Psychiatric Publishing
1000 Wilson Boulevard
Suite 1825
Arlington, VA 22209-3901
703-907-7322
800-368-5777
Fax: 703-907-1091
E-mail: appi@psych.org
www.appi.org

Developed for use in the clinical setting, presents the core knowledge in the field in a single quick-reference volume. With brief, to-the-point guidance and step-by-step protocols, it's an invaluable resource for the busy clinician. *$29.95*

240 pages Year Founded: 2002 ISBN 1-585620-77-7

2720 Concise Guide to Mood Disorders
American Psychiatric Publishing
1000 Wilson Boulevard
Suite 1825
Arlington, VA 22209-3901
703-907-7322
800-368-5777
Fax: 703-907-1091
E-mail: appi@psych.org
www.appi.org

Designed for daily use in the clinical setting, the Concise Guide to Mood Disorders is a fingertip library of the latest information, easy to understand and quick to access. This practical reference summarizes everything a clinician needs to know to diagnose and treat unipolar and bipolar mood disorders. *$29.95*

320 pages Year Founded: 2002 ISBN 1-585620-56-4

2721 Concise Guide to Psychiatry and Law for Clinicians
American Psychiatric Publishing
1000 Wilson Boulevard
Suite 1825
Arlington, VA 22209-3901
703-907-7322
800-368-5777
Fax: 703-907-1091
E-mail: appi@psych.org
www.appi.org

Katie Duffy, Marketing Assistant

Practical information for psychiatrists in understanding legal regulations, legal decisions and present managed care applications. *$29.95*

296 pages Year Founded: 1998 ISBN 0-880483-29-6

2722 Concise Guide to Psychopharmacology
American Psychiatric Publishing
1000 Wilson Boulevard
Suite 1825
Arlington, VA 22209-3901
703-907-7322
800-368-5777
Fax: 703-907-1091
E-mail: appi@psych.org
www.appi.org

Packed with practical information that is easy to access via detailed tables and charts, this pocket-sized volume (it literally fits into a lab coat or jacket pocket) is designed to be immediately useful for students, residents and clinicians working in a variety of treatment settings, such as inpatient psychiatry units, outpatient clinics, consultation-liaison services and private offices. *$29.95*

224 pages Year Founded: 2002 ISBN 1-585620-75-0

2723 Consent Handbook for Self-Advocates and Support Staff
AAMR
444 N Capitol Street NW
Suite 846
Washington, DC 20001-1512
202-387-1968
800-424-3688
Fax: 202-387-2193

E-mail: dcroser@aamr.org
www.aamr.org

Offers options for self-advocates and those for people who cannot consent on their own. *$14.95*

36 pages ISBN 0-904898-69-1

2724 Countertransference Issues in Psychiatric Treatment
American Psychiatric Publishing
1000 Wilson Boulevard
Suite 1825
Arlington, VA 22209-3901
703-907-7322
800-368-5777
Fax: 703-907-1091
E-mail: appi@psych.org
www.appi.org

Katie Duffy, Marketing Assistant

Overview of countertransference: theory and technique. *$37.50*

160 pages Year Founded: 1999 ISBN 0-880489-59-6

2725 Crisis: Prevention and Response in the Community
AAMR
444 N Capitol Street NW
Suite 846
Washington, DC 20001-1512
202-387-1968
800-424-3688
Fax: 202-387-2193
E-mail: dcroser@aamr.org
www.aamr.org

Provides a look at crisis services for people with developmental disabilities and how they impact the surrounding community. *$49.95*

240 pages ISBN 0-940898-74-8

2726 Cross-Cultural Perspectives on Quality of Life
AAMR
444 N Capitol Street NW
Suite 846
Washington, DC 20001-1512
202-387-1968
800-424-3688
Fax: 202-387-2193
E-mail: dcroser@aamr.org
www.aamr.org

Provides a ground-breaking global outlook on quality-of-life issues for people with mental retardation. *$47.95*

380 pages ISBN 0-940898-70-5

2727 Cruel Compassion: Psychiatric Control of Society's Unwanted
John Wiley & Sons
605 3rd Avenue
New York, NY 10058-0180
212-850-6000
Fax: 212-850-6008
E-mail: info@wiley.com
www.wiley.com

Demonstrates that the main problem that faces mental health policy makers today is adult dependency. A sobering look at some of our most cherished notions about our hu-

mane treatment of society's unwanted, and perhaps more importantly, about ourselves as a compassionate and democratic people. *$19.95*

264 pages Year Founded: 1994 ISBN 0-471010-12-X

2728 Culture & Psychotherapy: A Guide to Clinical Practice
American Psychiatric Publishing
1000 Wilson Boulevard
Suite 1825
Arlington, VA 22209-3901
703-907-7322
800-368-5777
Fax: 703-907-1091
E-mail: appi@psych.org
www.appi.org

Katie Duffy, Marketing Assistant

Case presentations, analysis, special issues and populations are covered. *$51.50*

320 pages Year Founded: 2001 ISBN 0-880489-55-3

2729 Cutting-Edge Medicine: What Psychiatrists Need to Know
American Psychiatric Press
1000 Wilson Boulevard
Suite 1825
Arlington, VA 22209-3901
703-907-7322
800-368-5777
Fax: 703-907-1091
E-mail: appi@psych.org
www.appi.org

Nada L Stotland, MD MPH, Editor

Offers a comprehensive overview of recent developments in cardiovascular illness, gastrointestinal disorders, transplant medicine, and premenstrual mood disorders. *$36.95*

164 pages Year Founded: 2003 ISBN 1-585620-72-6

2730 Cybermedicine
Jossey-Bass Publishers
350 Sansome Street
5th Floor
San Francisco, CA 94104
415-394-8677
800-956-7739
Fax: 800-605-2665
www.josseybass.com

A passionate plea for the use of computers for initial diagnosis and assessment, treatment decisions, and for self-care, research, prevention, and above all, patient empowerment. *$25.00*

235 pages ISBN 0-787903-43-4

2731 DRG Handbook
Dorland Healthcare Information
1500 Walnut Street
Suite 1000
Philadelphia, PA 19102
215-875-1212
800-784-2332
Fax: 215-735-3966
E-mail: info@dorlandhealth.com
www.dorlandhealth.com

Diagnosis-related groups are the building blocks of hospital reimbursement under the Medicare Prospective Payment

System. Also provides the ability to forecast and manage information at DRG-specific levels using comparison groups of like hospitals, a critical tool for both providers and payers. *$399.00*

1 per year Year Founded: 1998 ISBN 1-573721-39-5

2732 DSM: IV Diagnostic & Statistical Manual of Mental Disorders
American Psychiatric Publishing
1000 Wilson Boulevard
Suite 1825
Arlington, VA 22209-3901
703-907-7322
800-368-5777
Fax: 703-907-1091
E-mail: appi@psych.org
www.appi.com

Katie Duffy, Marketing Assistant

Focuses on clinical, research and educational findings. Practical and useful for clinicians and researchers of many orientations. Leatherbound. Hardcover and paperback also available. *$75.00*

886 pages Year Founded: 1994 ISBN 0-890420-64-5

2733 DSM: IV Personality Disorders
Rapid Psychler Press
3560 Pine Grove Avenue
Suite 374
Port Huron, MI 48060
519-433-7642
888-779-2453
Fax: 888-779-2457
E-mail: rapid@psychler.com
www.psychler.com

David Robinson, Publisher

$9.95

ISBN 1-894328-23-x

2734 Designing Positive Behavior Support Plans
AAMR
444 N Capitol Street NW
Suite 846
Washington, DC 20001-1512
202-387-1968
800-424-3688
Fax: 202-387-2193
E-mail: dcroser@aamr.org
www.aamr.org

Provides a conceptual framework for understanding, designing, and evaluating positive behavior support plans. *$21.95*

43 pages ISBN 0-940898-55-1

2735 Developing Mind: Toward a Neurobiology of Interpersonal Experience
Guilford Publications
72 Spring Street
New York, NY 10012
212-431-9800
800-365-7006
Fax: 212-966-6708
E-mail: info@guilford.com
www.guilford.com

Concise research results as to the origins of our behavior based on cognitive neuroscience.

2736 Disability at the Dawn of the 21st Century and the State of the States
AAMR
444 N Capitol Street NW
Suite 846
Washington, DC 20001-1512
202-387-1968
800-424-3688
Fax: 202-387-2193
E-mail: dcroser@aamr.org
www.aamr.org

Consumate source book on the analysis of financing services and supports for people with developmental disabilities in the United States. A detailed state-by-state analysis of public financial support for persons with MR/DD, mental illness, and physical disabilities.

512 pages ISBN 0-940898-85-3

2737 Diversity in Psychotherapy: The Politics of Race, Ethnicity, and Gender
Praeger
2727 Palisade Avenue
Suite 4H
Bronx, NY 10463-1020
718-796-0971
Fax: 718-796-0971
www.vd6@columbia.edu

Dr. Victor De La Cancela, President/CEO Salud Management

This challenging and insightful work wrestles with difficult treatment problems confronting both culturally and socially oppressed clients and psychotherapists. Case studies offer highly valuable resource material and insights into challenging perpsectives on behavioral health services. *$49.95*

224 pages Year Founded: 1993 ISBN 0-275941-80-9

2738 Doing What Comes Naturally: Dispelling Myths and Fallacies About Sexuality and People with Developmental Disabilities
High Tide Press
3650 W 183rd Street
Homewood, IL 60430
708-206-2054
888-487-7377
Fax: 708-206-2044
E-mail: managing.editor@hightidepress.com
www.hightidepress.com

Diane J Bell, Managing Editor

Uncovers misconceptions about adults whose sexual needs vary greatly, and yet are often treated as children or non-sexual people. Includes heartwarming success stories from adults Mrs. Anderson has supported, as well as suggestions for teaching and a guide to sexual incident reporting. *$19.95*

119 pages ISBN 1-892696-13-4

2739 Dynamic Psychotherapy: An Introductory Approach
American Psychiatric Publishing
1000 Wilson Boulevard
Suite 1825
Arlington, VA 22209-3901
703-907-7322
800-368-5777
Fax: 703-907-1091

E-mail: appi@psych.org
www.appi.org
Katie Duffy, Marketing Assistant
Principles and techniques. *$33.50*
229 pages Year Founded: 1990

2740 Efficacy of Special Education and Related Services
AAMR
444 N Capitol Street NW
Suite 846
Washington, DC 20001-1512
202-387-1968
800-424-3688
Fax: 202-387-2193
E-mail: dcroser@aamr.org
www.aamr.org

Provides an objective, explicit, and clear evaluation of the existing literature of special education. Also evaluates general education practices adapted and modified for special education. *$31.95*

123 pages ISBN 0-940898-51-9

2741 Electroconvulsive Therapy: A Guide
Madison Institute of Medicine
7617 Mineral Point Road
Suite 300
Madison, WI 53717-1623
608-827-2470
Fax: 608-827-2479
E-mail: mim@miminc.org
www.miminc.org

ECT is an extremely effective method of treatment for severe depression that does not respond to medication. This guidebook explains what ECT is and how it is used today to help patients overcome depression and other serious, treatment resistant psychiatric disorders. *$5.95*

19 pages

2742 Embarking on a New Century: Mental Retardation at the end of the Twentieth Century
AAMR
444 N Capitol Street NW
Suite 846
Washington, DC 20001-1512
202-387-1968
800-424-3688
Fax: 202-387-2193
E-mail: dcroser@aamr.org
www.aamr.org

This volume of 18 essays summarizes major public policy and service delivery advancements from 1975 to 2000. These changes can be summarized as a siginificant shift in many areas — from services to supports; from passive to active consumer roles; from normalization to quality. *$29.97*

265 pages

2743 Emergencies in Mental Health Practice
Guilford Publications
72 Spring Street
New York, NY 10012
212-431-9800
800-365-7006

Fax: 212-966-6708
E-mail: info@guilford.com
www.guilford.com

Focusing on acute clinical situations in which there is an imminent risk of serious harm or death to self or others, this practical resource helps clinicians evaluate and manage a wide range of mental health emergencies. The volume provides guidelines for interviewing with suicidal patients, potentially violent patients, vulnerable victims of violence, as well as patients facing life-and-death medical decisions, with careful attention to risk management and forensic issues. *$24.95*

450 pages ISBN 1-572305-51-7

2744 Essential Guide to Psychiatric Drugs
St. Martin's Press
175 5th Avenue
New York, NY 10010
212-674-5151
E-mail: webmaster@stmartins.com
www.stmartins.com

Information not found in other drug references. Lists many common drugs and not so common side effects, including drug interaction and the individual's reaction, including sexual side effects. Expert but nontechnical narrative. *$6.99*

416 pages Year Founded: 1998 ISBN 0-312954-58-1

2745 Essentials of Clinical Psychiatry: Based on the American Psychiatric Press Textbook of Psychiatry
American Psychiatric Publishing
1000 Wilson Boulevard
Suite 1825
Arlington, VA 22209-3901
703-907-7322
800-368-5777
Fax: 703-907-1091
E-mail: appi@psych.org
www.appi.org
Robert E Hales MD MBA, Editor
Stuart C Yudofsky MD, Editor

51 distinguished experts have created a compelling reference reflecting a biopsychosocial approach to patient treatment that is at once exciting and accessible. *$77.00*

1032 pages Year Founded: 1999 ISBN 0-880488-48-4

2746 Ethical Way
Jossey-Bass Publishers
350 Sansome Street
5th Floor
San Francisco, CA 94104
415-394-8677
800-956-7739
Fax: 800-605-2665
www.josseybass.com

Leads you through a maze of ethical principles and crucial issues confronting mental health professionals. *$38.95*

254 pages ISBN 0-787907-41-X

2747 Evidence-Based Mental Health Practice: A Textbook
WW Norton & Company
500 5th Avenue
New York, NY 10110-0017

212-354-5500
800-233-4830
Fax: 212-869-0856
E-mail: npb@wwnorton.com
www.wwnorton.com/psych

The specific term evidence-based medicine was introduced in 1990 to refer to a systematic approach to helping doctors to apply scientific evidence to decision-making at the point of contact with a specific consumer. As support for evidence-based medicine grows in mental health, the need to clarify its fundamental principles also increases. An essential primer for all practititioners and students who are grappling with the new age of evidence-based practice.

ISBN 0-393704-43-2

2748 Executive Guide to Case Management Strategies
Jossey-Bass Publishers
350 Sansome Street
5th Floor
San Francisco, CA 94104
415-394-8677
800-956-7739
Fax: 800-605-2665
www.josseybass.com

A guide to plan, organize, develop, improve and help case management programs reach their full potential in the clinical and financial management of care. *$58.00*

160 pages ISBN 1-556481-28-4

2749 Exemplar Employee: Rewarding & Recognizing Direct Contact Employees
High Tide Press
3650 W 183rd Street
Homewood, IL 60430
708-206-2054
888-487-7377
Fax: 708-206-2044
E-mail: managing.editor@hightidepress.com
www.hightidepress.com

Monica Regan, Managing Editor

With staff turnover as high as 90 percent in some agencies, you need to provide direct contact employees with as many incentives to excel as you can. This successful recognition program for non-management, direct contact employees is broken down and explained, with specific advice on how to implement it in your own organization from the people who developed the program. *$10.95*

48 pages ISBN 1-892696-03-7

2750 Family Approach to Psychiatric Disorders
American Psychiatric Publishing
1000 Wilson Boulevard
Suite 1825
Arlington, VA 22209-3901
703-907-7322
800-368-5777
Fax: 703-907-1091
E-mail: appi@psych.org
www.appi.org

Katie Duffy, Marketing Assistant

Examines how treatment can and should involve the family of the patient. *$67.50*

404 pages Year Founded: 1996

2751 Family Stress, Coping, and Social Support
Charles C Thomas Publisher
2600 S 1st Street
Springfield, IL 62704-4730
217-789-8980
800-258-8980
Fax: 217-789-9130
E-mail: books@ccthomas.com
www.ccthomas.com

$48.95

294 pages Year Founded: 1982 ISSN 0-398-06275-7ISBN 0-398046-92-1

2752 Family Therapy Progress Notes Planner
John Wiley & Sons
10475 Crosspoint Boulevard
Indianapolis, IN 46256
877-762-2974
Fax: 800-597-3299
E-mail: consumers@wiley.com
www.wiley.com

Extends the line into the growing field of family therapy. Included is critical information about HIPAA guidelines, which greatly impact the privacy status of patient progress notes. Helps mental health practitioners reduce the amount of time spent on paperwork by providing a full menu of pre-written progress notes that can be easily and quickly adapted to fit a particular patient need or treatment situation. *$ 49.95*

352 pages ISBN 0-471484-43-1

2753 Fifty Ways to Avoid Malpractice: A Guidebook for Mental Health Professionals
Professional Resource Press
PO Box 15560
Sarasota, FL 34277-1560
941-343-9601
800-443-3364
Fax: 941-343-9201
E-mail: orders@prpress.com
www.prpress.com

Debra Fink, Managing Editor

Offers straightforward guidance on providing legally safe and ethically appropriate services to your clients. *$18.95*

158 pages Year Founded: 1988 ISBN 0-943158-54-0

2754 First Therapy Session
Jossey-Bass Publishers
350 Sansome Street
5th Floor
San Francisco, CA 94104
415-394-8677
800-956-7739
Fax: 800-605-2665
www.josseybass.com

Presents an effective, straightforward approach for conducting first therapy sessions, showing step-by-step, how to identify client problems and help solve them within families. *$27.95*

ISBN 1-555421-94-6

2755 Five-HTP: The Natural Way to Overcome Depression, Obesity, and Insomnia
Bantam Doubleday Dell Publishing
1745 Broadway
New York, NY 10019
212-782-9000
Fax: 212-782-9700

An authorative and comprehensive guide to realizing the health benefits of 5-HTP. Explains how this natural amino acid can safely and effectively regulate low serotonin levels, which have been linked to depression, obesity, insomnia, migraines, and anxiety. 5-HTP is also a powerful antioxidant that can protect the body from free-radical damage, reducing the risk of serious illnesses such as cancer. *$11.95*

304 pages Year Founded: 1999 ISBN 0-553379-46-1

2756 Flawless Consulting
Jossey-Bass Publishers
350 Sansome Street
5th Floor
San Francisco, CA 94104
415-394-8677
800-956-7739
Fax: 800-605-2665
www.josseybass.com

This book offers advice on what to say and what to do in specific situations to see your recommendations through. *$39.95*

214 pages ISBN 0-893840-52-1

2757 Forgiveness: Theory, Research and Practice
Guilford Publications
72 Spring Street
New York, NY 10012
212-431-9800
800-365-7006
Fax: 212-966-6708
E-mail: info@guilford.com
www.guilford.com

Scholarly, up-to-date examination of forgiveness ranges many disiplines for mental health professionals. *$35.00*

334 pages Year Founded: 2000 ISBN 1-572305-10-X

2758 Foundations of Mental Health Counseling
Charles C Thomas Publisher
2600 S 1st Street
Springfield, IL 62704-4730
217-789-8980
800-258-8980
Fax: 217-789-9130
E-mail: books@ccthomas.com
www.ccthomas.com

The latest writings regarding the explosive growth of mental health counseling over the past twenty years. Leading experts discuss the past, present, and future of the field from their unique positions as practitioners, theoreticians, and educators. Major issues such as professional identity, ethics, assessment, research, and theory are joined with the contemporary problems of managed health care, insurance reimbursement, and private practice. An up-to-date resource in the field of mental health counseling. *$89.95*

446 pages Year Founded: 1996 ISBN 0-398066-69-8

2759 Fundamentals of Psychiatric Treatment Planning
American Psychiatric Publishing
1000 Wilson Boulevard
Suite 1825
Arlington, VA 22209-3901
703-907-7322
800-368-5777
Fax: 703-907-1091
E-mail: appi@psych.org
www.appi.org

Professional discussion of important basics. *$49.00*

368 pages Year Founded: 2002 ISBN 1-585620-61-0

2760 Group Involvement Training
New Harbinger Publications
5674 Shattuck Avenue
Oakland, CA 94609-1662
510-652-2002
800-748-6273
Fax: 510-652-5472
E-mail: customerservice@newharbinger.com
www.newharbinger.com

This book shows how training chronically ill mental patients in a series of structured group tasks can be used to treat the symptoms of apathy, withdrawl, poor interpersonal skills, helplessness, and the inability to structure leisure time constructively. *$24.95*

160 pages Year Founded: 1988 ISBN 0-934986-65-7

2761 Guide to Possibility Land: Fifty One Methods for Doing Brief, Respectful Therapy
WW Norton & Company
500 5th Avenue
New York, NY 10110
212-790-9456
Fax: 212-869-0856
E-mail: admalmud@wwnorton.com
www.wwnorton.com

The creator of Possibility therapy, William O'Hanlon, outlines acknowledging patient's experience and opinions about their lives while seeing that possibilites for change are explored and underlined. *$13.00*

94 pages Year Founded: 1999 ISBN 0-393702-97-9

2762 Guide to Treatments That Work
Oxford University Press/Oxford Reference
198 Madison Avenue
New York, NY 10016
212-726-6000
800-451-7556
Fax: 919-677-1303
www.oup-usa.org/orbs/

A systematic review of various treatments currently in use for virtually all of the recognized mental disorders. *$75.00*

624 pages Year Founded: 1997 ISBN 0-195102-27-4

2763 Handbook on Quality of Life for Human Service Practitioners
AAMR
444 N Capitol Street NW
Suite 846
Washington, DC 20001-1512
202-387-1968
800-424-3688

Fax: 202-387-2193
E-mail: dcroser@aamr.org
www.aamr.org

Revolutionary generic model for quality of life that integrates core domains and indicators with a cross-cultural systems prespective that can be used in all human services. *$59.95*

429 pages ISBN 0-940898-77-2

2764 Helper's Journey: Working with People Facing Grief, Loss, and Life-Threatening Illness
Research Press
Dept 24 W
PO Box 9177
Champaign, IL 61826
217-352-3273
800-519-2707
Fax: 217-352-1221
E-mail: rp@researchpress.com
www.researchpress.com

Russell Pense, VP Marketing

Written for both professional and volunteer caregivers, this unique manual provides exercises, activities and specific strategies for more successful caregiving, increased personal growth and effective stress management. The author explores the theory and practice of helping. He includes numerous case examples and verbatim disclosures of fellow caregivers that powerfully convey the joys and sorrows of the helper's journey. Cited as a "Book of the Year" by the American Journal of Nursing. *$21.95*

292 pages ISBN 0-878223-44-4

2765 High Impact Consulting
Jossey-Bass Publishers
350 Sansome Street
5th Floor
San Francisco, CA 94104
415-394-8677
800-956-7739
Fax: 800-605-2665
www.josseybass.com

Offers a new model for consulting services that shows how to produce short-term successes and use them as a springboard to larger accomplishments and, ultimately, to organization-wide continuous improvement. Also includes specific guidance to assist clients in analyzing their situation, identifying their real needs, and choosing an appropriate consultant. *$26.00*

256 pages ISBN 0-787903-41-8

2766 Home Maintenance for Residential Service Providers
High Tide Press
3650 W 183rd Street
Homewood, IL 60430
708-206-2054
888-487-7377
Fax: 708-206-2044
E-mail: managing.editor@hightidepress.com
www.hightidepress.com

Monica Regan, Managing Editor

What happens when a human service organization becomes a large, commercial landlord, not unlike a real estate firm or condominium management company? Property management for homes supporting persons with disabilities re-

quires a unique blend of human services and physical plant expertise. Provides detailed checklists for all house systems, fixtures and furnishings. Includes a discussion of maintaining an attractive residence that blends with the neighborhood. *$10.95*

42 pages ISBN 0-965374-46-7

2767 How to Partner with Managed Care
John Wiley & Sons
605 3rd Avenue
New York, NY 10058-0180
212-850-6000
Fax: 212-850-6008
E-mail: info@wiley.com
www.wiley.com

A Do It Yourself Kit for Building Working Relationships & Getting Steady Referrals.

366 pages Year Founded: 1996

2768 IEP-2005: Writing and Implementing Individualized Education Programs
Charles C Thomas Publishers
PO Box 19265
Springfield, IL 62794-9265
217-789-8980
800-258-8980
Fax: 217-789-9130
www.ccthomas.com

Purpose is to provide guidelines to develop appropriate Individualized Education Programs (IEPs) for children with disabilities based on the Individuals with Disabilities Education Act amendments of 2004 (IDEA-2004) or Pblic LAw 108-446. These guidelines are intended to result in IEPs that are streamlined, focused, and reasonably calculated to provide educational benefit. Available in paperback for $41.95. *$61.95*

302 pages Year Founded: 2006 ISBN 0-398076-24-3

2769 Improving Clinical Practice
Jossey-Bass Publishers
350 Sansome Street
5th Floor
San Francisco, CA 94104
415-394-8677
800-956-7739
Fax: 800-605-2665
www.josseybass.com

Enhance your organization's clinical decision making, and ultimately improve the quality of patient care. *$41.95*

342 pages ISBN 0-787900-93-1

2770 Improving Therapeutic Communication
Jossey-Bass Publishers
350 Sansome Street
5th Floor
San Francisco, CA 94104
415-394-8677
800-956-7739
Fax: 800-605-2665
www.josseybass.com

Improve your communication technique with this definitive guide for counselors, therapists, and caseworkers. Focuses on the four basic skills that facilitate communication in therapy: empathy, respect, authenticity, and confrontation. *$62.95*

394 pages ISBN 0-875893-08-2

2771 In Search of Solutions: A New Direction in Psychotherapy
WW Norton & Company
500 5th Avenue
New York, NY 10110-0017
212-354-5500
800-233-4830
Fax: 212-869-0856
E-mail: npb@wwnorton.com
www.wwnorton.com/psych

O'Hanlon and Weiner-Davis provide guidelines for clinicians in implementing solution-oriented language and explain how to aviod dead ends. New material bring the reader up to date on advances in this field since the book's original publication in 1989.

ISBN 0-393704-37-8

2772 Increasing Variety in Adult Life
AAMR
444 N Capitol Street NW
Suite 846
Washington, DC 20001-1512
202-387-1968
800-424-3688
Fax: 202-387-2193
E-mail: dcroser@aamr.org
www.aamr.org

Step-by-step guidelines for implementing the general-case instructional process and shows how the process can be used across a variety of activities. *$12.95*

38 pages ISBN 0-940898-43-2

2773 Independent Practice for the Mental Health Professional
Brunner/Routledge
325 Chestnut Street
Philadelphia, PA 19106
800-821-8312
Fax: 215-269-0363

Ralph H Earle PhD
Dorothy J Barnes MC

An excellent resource for beginning therapists considering private practice or for experienced therapists moving from agency or institutional settings into private practice. Offers practical, down-to-earth suggestions for practice settings, marketing and working with clients. The authors provide worksheets and examples of successful planning for the growth of a practice. *$24.95*

141 pages ISBN 0-876308-38-8

2774 Infanticide: Psychosocial and Legal Perspectives on Mothers Who Kill
American Psychiatric Publishing
1000 Wilson Boulevard
Suite 1825
Arlington, VA 22209-3901
703-907-7322
800-368-5777
Fax: 703-907-1091
E-mail: appi@psych.org
www.appi.org

Written to help remedy today's dearth of up-to-date, research-based literature, this unique volume brings together a multidisciplinary group of 17 experts who focus on the psychiatric perspective of this tragic cause of infant death. Balanced perspective on a highly emotional issue will find a wide audience among psychiatric and medical professionals, legal professionals, public health professionals and interested laypersons. *$53.50*

304 pages Year Founded: 2002 ISBN 1-585620-97-1

2775 Innovative Approaches for Difficult to Treat Populations
American Psychiatric Publishing
1000 Wilson Boulevard
Suite 1825
Arlington, VA 22209-3901
703-907-7322
800-368-5777
Fax: 703-907-1091
E-mail: appi@psych.org
www.appi.org

Katie Duffy, Marketing Assistant

Alternate methods when the usual approaches are not helpful. *$86.95*

512 pages Year Founded: 1997

2776 Insider's Guide to Mental Health Resources Online
Guilford Publications
72 Spring Street
New York, NY 10012
212-431-9800
800-365-7006
Fax: 212-966-6708
E-mail: info@guilford.com
www.guilford.com

This guide helps readers take full advantage of Internet and world-wide-web resources in psychology, psychiatric, self-help and patient education. The book explains and evaluates the full range of search tools, newsgroups, databases and describes hundreds of specific disorders, find job listings and network with other professionals, obtain needed articles and books, conduct grant searches and much more. *$ 21.95*

338 pages ISBN 1-572305-49-5

2777 Instant Psychopharmacology
WW Norton & Company
500 5th Avenue
New York, NY 10110
212-790-9456
Fax: 212-869-0856
E-mail: admalmud@wwnorton.com
www.wwnorton.com

Revision of the best selling guide to all the new medications. Straightforward book teaches non medical therapists, clients and their families how the five different classes of drugs work, advice on side effects, drug interaction warnings and much more practical information. *$18.95*

168 pages Year Founded: 2002 ISBN 0-393703-91-6

2778 Integrated Treatment of Psychiatric Disorders
American Psychiatric Publishing
1000 Wilson Boulevard
Suite 1825
Arlington, VA 22209-3901

703-907-7322
800-368-5777
Fax: 703-907-1091
E-mail: appi@psych.org
www.appi.org

Katie Duffy, Marketing Assistant

Psychodynamic therapy and medication. *$34.95*

208 pages Year Founded: 2001 ISBN 1-585620-27-0

2779 Integrating Psychotherapy and Pharmaco-therapy: Disolving the Mind-Brain Barrier
WW Norton & Company
500 5th Avenue
New York, NY 10110-0017
212-354-5500
800-233-4830
Fax: 212-869-0856
E-mail: npb@wwnorton.com
www.wwnorton.com/psych

Will help all mental health clinicians to dissolve their conceptual mind/brain barriers by recognizing the reciprocal influences of psychological and pharmacological interventions. The reader responds to thought-provoking questions and vignettes of problematic cases.

ISBN 0-393704-03-3

2780 Integrative Brief Therapy: Cognitive, Psychodynamic, Humanistic & Neurobehavioral Approaches
Impact Publishers
PO Box 6016
Atascadero, CA 93423-6016
805-466-5917
800-246-7228
Fax: 805-466-5919
E-mail: info@impactpublishers.com
www.impactpublishers.com

Thorough discussion of the factors that contribute to effectiveness in therapy carefully integrates key elements from diverse theoretical viewpoints. *$17.95*

272 pages Year Founded: 1998 ISBN 1-886230-09-9

2781 International Handbook on Mental Health Policy
Greenwood Publishing Group
88 Post Road W
PO Box 5007
Westport, CT 06880-4208
203-226-3571
Fax: 203-222-1502

Major reference book for academics and practitioners that provides a systematic survey and analysis of mental health policies in twenty representative countries. *$125.00*

512 pages Year Founded: 1993 ISBN 0-313275-67-X

2782 Interpersonal Psychotherapy
American Psychiatric Publishing
1000 Wilson Boulevard
Suite 1825
Arlington, VA 22209-3901
703-907-7322
800-368-5777
Fax: 703-907-1091
E-mail: appi@psych.org
www.appi.org

Katie Duffy, Marketing Assistant

An overview of interpersonal psychotherapy for depression, preventative treatment for depression, bulimia nervosa and HIV positive men and women. *$37.50*

156 pages Year Founded: 1998 ISBN 0-880488-36-0

2783 Introduction to Time: Limited Group Psychotherapy
American Psychiatric Publishing
1000 Wilson Boulevard
Suite 1825
Arlington, VA 22209-3901
703-907-7322
800-368-5777
Fax: 703-907-1091
E-mail: appi@psych.org
www.appi.org

Katie Duffy, Marketing Assistant

Do more with limited time and sessions. *$57.95*

317 pages Year Founded: 1997

2784 Introduction to the Technique of Psychotherapy: Practice Guidelines for Psychotherapists
Charles C Thomas Publisher
2600 S 1st Street
Springfield, IL 62704-4730
217-789-8980
800-258-8980
Fax: 217-789-9130
E-mail: books@ccthomas.com
www.ccthomas.com

A basic, simply written book, with a minimum of theory, helpful to the beginning therapist. Discuss how to conduct psychotherapy: by having a format in mind, taking a comprehensive history, and a careful, observing examination of the patient. *$34.95*

122 pages Year Founded: 1998 ISSN 0-398-06905-0ISBN 0-398069-04-2

2785 Languages of Psychoanalysis
Analytic Press
101 W Street
Hillsdale, NJ 07642-1421
201-358-9477
800-926-6579
Fax: 201-358-4700
E-mail: TAP@analyticpress.com
www.analyticpress.com

Paul E Stepansky PhD, Managing Director
John Kerr PhD, Sr Editor

A guide to understanding the full range of human discourse, especially behavioral conflicts and communicational deficits as they impinge upon the transactions of the analytic dyad. Available in hardcover. *$39.95*

224 pages Year Founded: 1996 ISBN 0-881631-86-8

2786 Leadership and Organizational Excellence
AAMR
444 N Capitol Street NW
Suite 846
Washington, DC 20001-1512
202-387-1968
800-424-3688

Fax: 202-387-2193
E-mail: dcroser@aamr.org
www.aamr.org

Examines key managerial and organizational strategies that can be used to help ensure high-quality work environments for both staff and service delivery for people with developmental disabilities. *$ 14.95*

65 pages ISBN 0-940898-78-0

2787 Life Course Perspective on Adulthood and Old Age
AAMR
444 N Capitol Street NW
Suite 846
Washington, DC 20001-1512
202-387-1968
800-424-3688
Fax: 202-387-2193
E-mail: dcroser@aamr.org
www.aamr.org

Experts in gerontology, sociology, and cognitive disability share the latest research, trends, and thoughtful insights into old age. *$19.95*

229 pages ISBN 0-940898-31-4

2788 Making Money While Making a Difference: Achieving Outcomes for People with Disabilities
High Tide Press
3650 W 183rd Street
Homewood, IL 60430
708-206-2054
888-487-7377
Fax: 708-206-2044
E-mail: managing.editor@hightidepress.com
www.hightidepress.com

Diane J Bell, Managing Editor

Unique handbook for corporations and nonprofits alike. The authors guide readers through a step-by-step process for implementing strategic alliances between nonprofit organizations and corporate partners. Learn the tenets of cause related marketing and much more. *$14.95*

231 pages ISBN 0-965374-49-1

2789 Managed Mental Health Care in the Public Sector: a Survival Manual
Brunner/Routledge
325 Chestnut Street
Philadelphia, PA 19106
800-821-8312
Fax: 215-269-0363

Manual for administrators, planners, clinicians and consumers with concepts and strategies to maneuver in public sector managed mental healthcare system. *$35.00*

410 pages Year Founded: 1996 ISBN 9-057025-37-X

2790 Managing Client Anger: What to Do When a Client is Angry with You
New Harbinger Publications
5674 Shattuck Avenue
Oakland, CA 94609-1662
510-652-2002
800-748-6273
Fax: 510-652-5472
E-mail: customerservice@newharbinger.com
www.newharbinger.com

Guide to help therapists understand their reactions and make interventions when clients express anger toward them. *$49.95*

261 pages Year Founded: 1998 ISBN 1-572241-23-3

2791 Manual of Clinical Psychopharmacology
American Psychiatric Publishing
1000 Wilson Boulevard
Suite 1825
Arlington, VA 22209-3901
703-907-7322
800-368-5777
Fax: 703-907-1091
E-mail: appi@psych.org
www.appi.org

Examines the recent changes and standard treatments in psychopharmacology. *$63.00*

736 pages Year Founded: 2002 ISBN 0-880488-65-4

2792 Mastering the Kennedy Axis V: New Psychiatric Assessment of Patient Functioning
American Psychiatric Publishing
1000 Wilson Boulevard
Suite 1825
Arlington, VA 22209-3901
703-907-7322
800-368-5777
Fax: 703-907-1091
E-mail: appi@psych.org
www.appi.org

Professional evaluation methods. *$44.00*

320 pages Year Founded: 2002 ISBN 1-585620-62-9

2793 Meditative Therapy Facilitating Inner-Directed Healing
Impact Publishers
PO Box 6016
Atascadero, CA 93423-6016
805-466-5917
800-246-7228
Fax: 805-466-5919
E-mail: info@impactpublishers.com
www.impactpublishers.com

Offers to the professional therapist a full description of the therapeutic procedures that facilitate inner-directed healing and explains the therapist's role in guiding clients' growth psychologically, physiologically and spiritually. *$27.95*

230 pages Year Founded: 1999 ISBN 1-886230-11-0

2794 Mental Disability Law: Primer, a Comprehensive Introduction
Commission on the Mentally Disabled
1800 M Street NW
Washington, DC 20036-5802
202-331-2240

An updated and expanded version of the 1984 edition provides a comprehensive overview of mental disability law. Part I of the Primer examines the scope of mental disability law, defines the key terms and offers tips on how to provide effective representation for clients. Part II reviews major federal legislative initiatives including the Americans with Disabilities Act. *$15.00*

ISBN 0-897077-98-9

2795 Mental Health Rehabilitation: Disputing Irrational Beliefs
Charles C Thomas Publisher
2600 S 1st Street
Springfield, IL 62704-4730
217-789-8980
800-258-8980
Fax: 217-789-9130
E-mail: books@ccthomas.com
www.ccthomas.com

Applicable to a wide variety of disciplines involved with therapeutic counseling of people with mental and/or physical disabilities such as rehabilitation counseling, mental health counseling, pastoral counseling, school counseling, clinical social work, clinical and counseling psychology, and behavioral science oriented medical specialities and related health and therapeutic professionals. *$36.95*

106 pages Year Founded: 1995 ISBN 0-398065-31-4

2796 Mental Health Resources Catalog
Paul H Brookes Company
PO Box 10624
Baltimore, MD 21285-0624
410-337-9580
800-638-3775
Fax: 410-337-8539
E-mail: custserv@brookespublishing.com
www.brookespublishing.com

This catalog offers practical resources for mental health professionals serving young children and their families, including school psychologists, teachers and early intervention professionals. FREE.

2 per year

2797 Mental Retardation: Definition, Classification, and Systems of Supports
AAMR
444 N Capitol Street NW
Suite 846
Washington, DC 20001-1512
202-387-1968
800-424-3688
Fax: 202-387-2193
E-mail: dcroser@aamr.org
www.aamr.org

Presents a complete system to define and diagnose mental retardation, classify and describe strengths and limitations, and plan a supports needs profile. *$79.95*

250 pages ISBN 0-940898-81-0

2798 Metaphor in Psychotherapy: Clinical Applications of Stories and Allegories
Impact Publishers
PO Box 6016
Atascadero, CA 93423-6016
805-466-5917
800-246-7228
Fax: 805-466-5919
E-mail: info@impactpublishers.com
www.impactpublishers.com

Comprehensive resource aids therapists in helping clients change distorted views of the human experience. Dozens of practical therapeutic activities involving metaphor, drama, fantasy, and meditation. *$29.95*

320 pages Year Founded: 1998 ISBN 1-886230-10-2

2799 Microcounseling
Charles C Thomas Publisher
2600 S 1st Street
Springfield, IL 62704-4730
217-789-8980
800-258-8980
Fax: 217-789-9130
E-mail: books@ccthomas.com
www.ccthomas.com

Innovations in Interviewing, Counseling, Psychotherapy, and Psychoeducation. *$91.95*

624 pages Year Founded: 1978 ISSN 0-398-06175-0ISBN 0-398037-12-4

2800 Natural Supports: A Foundation for Employment
AAMR
444 N Capitol Street NW
Suite 846
Washington, DC 20001-1512
202-387-1968
800-424-3688
Fax: 202-387-2193
E-mail: dcroser@aamr.org
www.aamr.org

Step-by-step strategy for developing a network of natural supports aimed at promoting the goals and interests of all individuals in the work setting. *$12.95*

34 pages ISBN 0-940898-65-9

2801 Negotiating Managed Care: Manual for Clinicians
American Psychiatric Publishing
1000 Wilson Boulevard
Suite 1825
Arlington, VA 22209-3901
703-907-7322
800-368-5777
Fax: 703-907-1091
E-mail: appi@psych.org
www.appi.org

Katie Duffy, Marketing Assistant

Help for professionals to successfully present a case during clinical review. *$26.95*

120 pages Year Founded: 2002 ISBN 1-585620-42-4

2802 Neurobiology of Violence
American Psychiatric Publishing
1000 Wilson Boulevard
Suite 1825
Arlington, VA 22209-3901
703-907-7322
800-368-5777
Fax: 703-907-1091
E-mail: appi@psych.org
www.appi.org

Important information on the basic science of violence, including genetics, with topics of great practical value to today's clinician, including major mental disorders and violence; alcohol and substance abuse and violence; and psychopharmacological approaches to managing violent behavior. *$69.00*

368 pages Year Founded: 2002 ISBN 1-585620-81-5

2803 Neurodevelopment & Adult Psychopathology
Cambridge University Press
40 W 20th Street
New York, NY 10011-4221
212-924-3900
Fax: 212-691-3239
E-mail: marketing@cup.org
www.cup.org

2804 Neurology for Clinical Social Work: Theory and Practice
WW Norton & Company
500 5th Avenue
New York, NY 10110-0017
212-354-5500
800-233-4830
Fax: 212-869-0856
E-mail: npb@wwnorton.com
www.wwnorton.com/psych

Social work educators Jeffrey Applegate and Janet Shapiro demystify the explosion of recent research on neurobiology and present it anew with social workers specifically in mind. Abundant case examples show clinicians how to make use of neurobiological concepts in assessment as well as in designing treatment plans and interventions. Community mental health, family service agencies, and child welfare settings are discussed.

ISBN 0-393704-20-3

2805 Neuropsychiatry and Mental Health Services
American Psychiatric Publishing
1000 Wilson Boulevard
Arlington, VA 22209-3901
703-907-7322
800-368-5777
Fax: 703-907-1091
E-mail: appi@psych.org
www.appi.org

Katie Duffy, Marketing Assistant

Cognitive therapy practices in conjunction with mental health treatment. *$79.95*

448 pages Year Founded: 1999 ISBN 0-880487-30-5

2806 Neuropsychology of Mental Disorders: Practical Guide
Charles C Thomas Publisher
2600 S 1st Street
Springfield, IL 62704-4730
217-789-8980
800-258-8980
Fax: 217-789-9130
E-mail: books@ccthomas.com
www.ccthomas.com

Discusses the advances in diverse areas such as biology, electrophysiology, genetics, neuroanatomy, pharmacology, psychology, and radiology which are increasingly important for a practical understanding of behavior and its pathology. *$70.95*

338 pages Year Founded: 1994 ISBN 0-398059-05-5

2807 New Roles for Psychiatrists in Organized Systems of Care
American Psychiatric Publishing
1000 Wilson Boulevard
Suite 1825
Arlington, VA 22209-3901
703-907-7322
800-368-5777
Fax: 703-907-1091
E-mail: appi@psych.org
www.appi.org

Katie Duffy, Marketing Assistant

Comprehensive view of opportunities, challenges and roles for psychiatrists who are working for or with new organized systems of care. Discusses the ethical dilemmas for psychiatrists in managed care settings and training and identity of the field as well as historical overviews of health care policy. *$50.00*

312 pages Year Founded: 1998 ISBN 0-880487-58-5

2808 Of One Mind: The Logic of Hypnosis, the Practice of Therapy
WW Norton & Company
500 5th Avenue
New York, NY 10110-0017
212-354-5500
800-233-4830
Fax: 212-869-0856
E-mail: admalmud@wwnorton.com
www.wwnorton.com/psych

A new approach to an old treatment, the author explains his ideas on connecting with patients in hypno and brief therapies. *$30.00*

240 pages Year Founded: 2001 ISBN 0-393703-82-7

2809 On Being a Therapist
Jossey-Bass Publishers
350 Sansome Street
5th Floor
San Francisco, CA 94104
415-394-8677
800-956-7739
Fax: 800-605-2665
www.josseybass.com

This thoroughly revised and updated edition shows you how to use the insights gained from your clients' experiences to solve your own problems, realize positive change in yourself, and become a better therapist. *$22.00*

320 pages ISBN 1-555425-55-0

2810 On the Counselor's Path: A Guide to Teaching Brief Solution Focused Therapy
New Harbinger Publications
5674 Shattuck Avenue
Oakland, CA 94609-1662
510-652-2002
800-748-6273
Fax: 510-652-5472
E-mail: customerservice@newharbinger.com
www.newharbinger.com

A teacher's guide for conducting training sessions on solution focused techniques. *$24.95*

92 pages Year Founded: 1996 ISBN 1-572240-48-2

2811 Opportunities for Daily Choice Making
AAMR
444 N Capitol Street NW
Suite 846
Washington, DC 20001-1512
202-387-1968
800-424-3688
Fax: 202-387-2193
E-mail: dcroser@aamr.org
www.aamr.org

Provides strategies for increasing choice-making opportunities for people with developmental disabilities. It describes basic principles of choice-making, shows how to teach choice-making skills to the passive learner, describes how to build in multiple choice-making opportunities within daily routines, introduces self-scheduling, and addresses common questions. *$12.95*

48 pages ISBN 0-904898-44-6

2812 Out of Darkness and Into the Light: Nebraska's Experience In Mental Retardation
AAMR
444 N Capitol Street NW
Suite 846
Washington, DC 20001-1512
202-387-1968
800-424-3688
Fax: 202-387-2193
E-mail: dcroser@aamr.org
www.aamr.org

The Nebraska model for dealing with the condition of mental retardation has been so successful that it has been emulated throughout the United States and other countries. The inspiring story of how this change occured, written by those who made it happen. It is an account of both the changing approach to those once considered less the human, and their successful movement from despondency to hope, and from patient to people. *$29.97*

267 pages

2813 Participatory Evaluation for Special Education and Rehabilitation
AAMR
444 N Capitol Street NW
Suite 846
Washington, DC 20001-1512
202-387-1968
800-424-3688
Fax: 202-387-2193
E-mail: dcroser@aamr.org
www.aamr.org

Nine-step method for identifying and weighing the importance of disparate goals and outcomes. *$31.95*

90 pages ISBN 0-940898-73-X

2814 Person-Centered Foundation for Counseling and Psychotherapy
Charles C Thomas Publisher
2600 S 1st Street
Springfield, IL 62704-4730
217-789-8980
800-258-8980
Fax: 217-789-9130
E-mail: books@ccthomas.com
www.ccthomas.com

Focusing on counseling and psychotherapy, its goals are to renew interest in the person-centered approach in the US, make a signigicant contribution to extending person-centered theory and practice, and promote fruitful dialogue and futher development of person-centered theory. Presents: the rationale for an eclectic application of person-centered counseling; the rationale and process for reflecting clients' feelings; the importance of the theory as the foundation for the counseling process; the importance of values and their influence on the counseling relationship; the modern person-centered counselor's role; and the essential characteristics of a person-centered counseling relationship.

260 pages Year Founded: 1999 ISSN 0-398-06966-2ISBN 0-398069-64-6

2815 PharmaCoKinetics and Therapeutic Moniltering of Psychiatric Drugs
Charles C Thomas Publisher
2600 S 1st Street
Springfield, IL 62704-4730
217-789-8980
800-258-8980
Fax: 217-789-9130
E-mail: books@ccthomas.com
www.ccthomas.com

$52.95

226 pages Year Founded: 1993 ISBN 0-398058-41-5

2816 Positive Bahavior Support for People with Developmental Disabilities: A Research Synthesis
AAMR
444 N Capitol Street NW
Suite 846
Washington, DC 20001-1512
202-387-1968
800-424-3688
Fax: 202-387-2193
E-mail: dcroser@aamr.org
www.aamr.org

Offers a careful analysis documenting that positive behavioral procedures can produce important change in the behavior and lives of people with disabilities. *$31.95*

108 pages ISBN 0-940898-60-8

2817 Positive Behavior Support Training Curriculum
AAMR
444 N Capitol Street NW
Suite 846
Washington, DC 20001-1512
202-387-1968
800-424-3688
Fax: 202-387-2193
E-mail: dcroser@aamr.org
www.aamr.org

Designed for training supervisors of direct support staff, as well as direct support professionals themselves in the values and practices of positive behavior support.

2818 Practical Guide to Cognitive Therapy
WW Norton & Company
500 5th Avenue
New York, NY 10110
212-790-9456
Fax: 212-869-0856

E-mail: admalmud@wwnorton.com
www.wwnorton.com

Based on highly successful workshops by the author, this book provides a framework to apply cognitive therapy model to office practices. *$22.95*

200 pages Year Founded: 1991 ISBN 0-393701-05-0

2819 Practical Psychiatric Practice Forms and Protocols for Clinical Use
American Psychological Publishing
1400 K Street NW
Washington, DC 20005
202-682-6262
800-368-5777
Fax: 202-789-2648
E-mail: appi@psych.org
www.appi.org

Katie Duffy, Marketing Assistant

Designed to aid psychiatrists in organizing their work. Provides rating scales, model letters, medication tracking forms, clinical pathology requests and sample invoices. Handouts on disorders and medication are provided for patients and their families. Spiralbound. *$47.50*

312 pages Year Founded: 1998 ISBN 0-880489-43-X

2820 Practice Guidelines for Extended Psychiatric Residential Care: From Chaos to Collaboration
Charles C Thomas Publisher
2600 S 1st Street
Springfield, IL 62704-4730
217-789-8980
800-258-8980
Fax: 217-789-9130
E-mail: books@ccthomas.com
www.ccthomas.com

Patrick W Corrigan, Author/Editor
Stanley McCracken, Author/Editor
Joseph Mehr, Author/Editor

Presents a set of practice guidelines that represent state-of-the-art treatments for consumers of extended residential care. Written for line-level staff charged with the day-to-day services: psychiatrists, psychologists, social workers, activity therapists, nurses, and psychiatric technicians who work closely with consumers in residential programs and program administrators who have immediate responsibility for supervising treatment teams. *$47.95*

176 pages Year Founded: 1995 ISSN 0-398-06536-5 ISBN 0-398065-35-7

2821 Primer of Brief Psychotherapy
WW Norton & Company
500 5th Avenue
New York, NY 10110
212-790-9456
Fax: 212-869-0856
E-mail: admalmud@wwnorton.com
www.wwnorton.com

Positive guide to brief therapy is a task oriented aid with emphasis on the first session and details of procedures afterward. *$ 19.55*

160 pages Year Founded: 1995 ISBN 0-393701-89-1

2822 Primer of Supportive Psychotherapy
Analytic Press
101 W Street
Hillsdale, NJ 07642-1421
201-358-9477
800-926-6579
Fax: 201-358-4700
E-mail: TAP@analyticpress.com
www.analyticpress.com

Paul E Stepansky PhD, Managing Director
John Kerr PhD, Sr Editor

Focuses on the rationale for and techniques of supportive psychotherapy as a form of dyadic intervention distinct from expressive psychotherapies. The realities, ironies, conundrums and opporturities of the therapeutic encounter are vividly portrayed in scores of illustrative dialogues drawn from actual treatments. Among the topics covered are how to provide reassurance in the realistic way, how to handle requests for advice, the role of praise and reinforcement, the appropriate use of reframing techniques and of modeling, negotiating patients' concerns about medication and other collateral forms of treatment. *$45.00*

296 pages Year Founded: 1997 ISBN 0-881632-74-0

2823 Psychiatric Disorders In Current Medical Diagnosis and Treatment
Stamford: Appleton & Lange
www.stamford.com

Stuart J Eisendrath, Author
Stepehn J McPhee, Editor
Year Founded: 1997

2824 Psychiatry in the New Millennium
American Psychiatric Publishing
1000 Wilson Boulevard
Suite 1825

703-907-7322
800-368-5777
Fax: 703-907-1091
E-mail: appi@psych.org
www.appi.org

Katie Duffy, Marketing Assistant

Keeping the standards and utilizing advances in diagnosis and treatment. *$66.50*

352 pages Year Founded: 1999 ISBN 0-880489-38-3

2825 Psychoanalysis, Behavior Therapy & the Relational World
American Psychological Association
750 1st St NE
Washington, DC 20002-4241
202-336-5647
Fax: 202-216-7610
www.apa.org

Carolyn Valliere, Marketing Specialist

2826 Psychoanalytic Therapy as Health Care Effectiveness and Economics in the 21st Century
Analytic Press
101 W Street
Hillsdale, NJ 07642-1421
201-358-9477
800-926-6579

Fax: 201-358-4700
E-mail: TAP@analyticpress.com
www.analyticpress.com

Paul E Stepansky PhD, Managing Director
John Kerr PhD, Sr Editor

Drawing on a wide range of clinical and empirical evidence, authors argue that contemporary psychoanalytic approaches are applicable to seriously distressed persons in a variety of treatment contexts. Failure to include such long term therapies within health care delivery systems, they conclude, will deprive many patients of help they need, and help from which they can benefit in enduring ways that far transcend the limited treatment goals of managed care. Available in hardcover. *$ 49.95*

312 pages Year Founded: 1999 ISBN 0-881632-02-3

2827 Psychological Aspects of Women's Health Care
American Psychiatric Press
1000 Wilson Boulevard
Suite 1825
Arlington, VA 22209-3901
703-907-7322
800-368-5777
Fax: 703-907-1091
E-mail: appi@psych.org
www.appi.org

Nada L Stotland, MD MPH, Editor
Donna E Stewart, MD FRCPC, Editor

The Interface Between Psychiatry and Obstetrics and Gynecology, Second Edition. Discussion from major leaders in the specialties of psychiatry and obstetrics/gynecology covering every major area of contemporary concern. Issues in pregnancy, gynecology, and general issues such as reproductive choices, breast disorders, violence, lesbian health care, and the male perspective are included. *$77.00*

672 pages Year Founded: 2001 ISBN 0-880488-31-X

2828 Psychologists' Desk Reference
Oxford University Press/Oxford Reference Book Society
198 Madison Avenue
New York, NY 10016
212-726-6000
800-451-7556
Fax: 919-677-1303
www.oup-usa.org/orbs/

For the practicing psychologist; easily accessible, current information on almost any topic by some of the leading thinkers and innovators in the field. *$65.00*

672 pages Year Founded: 1998 ISBN 0-195111-86-9

2829 Psychoneuroendocrinology: The Scientific Basis of Clinical Practice
American Psychiatric Publishing
1000 Wilson Boulevard
Suite 1825
Arlington, VA 22209-3901
703-907-7322
800-368-5777
Fax: 703-907-1091
E-mail: appi@psych.org
www.appi.org

Applications of scientific research.

752 pages Year Founded: 2003 ISBN 0-880488-57-3

2830 Psychopharmacology Desktop Reference
Manisses Communications Group
208 Governor Street
Providence, RI 02906
401-831-6020
800-333-7771
Fax: 401-861-6370
E-mail: manissescs@manisses.com
www.manisses.com

Karienne Stovell, Editor

Covers medications for all types of mental disorders. Provides detailed information on all the latest drugs as well as colored photographs of the different kinds of drugs. Helps you spot side effects and avoid drug interactions. Includes revealing case studies and outcomes data. *$159.00*

ISBN 1-864937-69-1

2831 Psychopharmacology Update
Manisses Communications Group
208 Governor Street
Providence, RI 02906
401-831-6020
800-333-7771
Fax: 401-861-6370
E-mail: manissescs@manisses.com
www.manisses.com

Karienne Stovell, Editor

Offers psychopharmacology advice for general practitioners and nonprescribing professionals in the mental health field. Covers child psychopharmacology and street drugs. Contains case reports. Recurring features include news of research and book reviews. *$147.00*

12 per year ISSN 1068-5308

2832 Psychosocial Aspects of Disability
Charles C Thomas Publishers
PO Box 19265
Springfield, IL 62794-9265
217-789-8980
800-258-8980
Fax: 217-789-9130
www.ccthomas.com

This expanded and updated new edition continues the theme of the first and second editions of emphasizing that attitudinal barriers create environmental barriers for persons with disabilities. The new edition is improved as a primary introductory text or a supplemental text for student helping professionals with the addition of chapters on employment, understanding ethnic groups, concepts, theories, therapies, and issues for the twenty-first century. Available in paperback for $55.95. *$75.95*

424 pages Year Founded: 2004 ISBN 0-398074-86-0

2833 Psychotherapist's Duty to Warn or Protect
Charles C Thomas Publisher
2600 S 1st Street
Springfield, IL 62704-4730
217-789-8980
800-258-8980
Fax: 217-789-9130
E-mail: books@ccthomas.com
www.ccthomas.com

Alan R Felthous, Author

$47.95

194 pages Year Founded: 1989 ISBN 0-398055-46-7

**2834 Psychotherapist's Guide to Cost Containment:
How to Survive and Thrive in an Age of
Managed Care**
Sage Publications
2455 Teller Road
Thousand Oaks, CA 91320
805-499-9774
800-818-7243
Fax: 800-583-2665
E-mail: info@sagepub.com
www.sagepub.com

$23.50

Year Founded: 1998 ISBN 0-803973-81-0

2835 Psychotherapy Indications and Outcomes
American Psychiatric Publishing
1000 Wilson Boulevard
Suite 1825
Arlington, VA 22209-3901
703-907-7322
800-368-5777
Fax: 703-907-1091
E-mail: appi@psych.org
www.appi.org

Katie Duffy, Marketing Assistant

Clinical approaches to different symptoms. *$66.50*

416 pages Year Founded: 1999 ISBN 0-880487-61-5

2836 Psychotropic Drug Information Handbook
Lexi-Comp
1100 Terex Road
Hudson, OH 44236-3771
330-650-6506
800-837-5394
Fax: 330-656-4307
www.lexi.com

Concise handbook, designed to fit into your lab coat, is a
current and portable psychotropic drug reference with 150
drugs and 35 herbal monographs. Perfect companion to
Drug Information Handbook for Psychiatry. *$38.75*

1 per year ISBN 1-591951-15-1

2837 Psychotropic Drugs: Fast Facts
WW Norton & Company
500 5th Avenue
New York, NY 10110-0017
212-354-5500
800-233-4830
Fax: 212-869-0856
E-mail: npb@wwnorton.com
www.wwnorton.com/psych

Now in its third edition, Psychotropic Drugs: Fast Facts
continues to present valuable information in a clear and accessible format. The book organizaes and presents data clinicians need to choose the right treatment for common
psychiatric problems and to anticipate and deal with problems that arise in treatment.

ISBN 0-393703-01-0

2838 Quality of Life: Volume II
AAMR
444 N Capitol Street NW
Suite 846
Washington, DC 20001-1512
202-387-1968
800-424-3688
Fax: 202-387-2193
E-mail: dcroser@aamr.org
www.aamr.org

Focuses on how the concepts and research on quality of life
can be applied to people with mental retardation. *$19.95*

267 pages ISBN 0-940898-41-1

2839 Questions of Competence
Cambridge University Press
40 W 20th Street
New York, NY 10011-4221
212-924-3900
Fax: 212-691-3239
E-mail: marketing@cup.org
www.cup.org

**2840 Reaching Out in Family Therapy: Home Based,
School, and Community Interventions**
Guilford Publications
72 Spring Street
New York, NY 10012
212-431-9800
800-365-7006
Fax: 212-966-6708
E-mail: info@guilford.com
www.guilford.com

Practical framework for clinicians using multisystems intervention. *$27.00*

244 pages Year Founded: 2000 ISBN 1-572305-19-3

**2841 Recognition and Treatment of Psychiatric
Disorders: Psychopharmacology Handbook for
Primary Care**
American Psychiatric Publishing
1000 Wilson Boulevard
Suite 1825
Arlington, VA 22209-3901
703-907-7322
800-368-5777
Fax: 703-907-1091
E-mail: appi@psych.org
www.appi.org

Provides the primary care physician with practical and
timely strategies for screening and treating patients who
have psychiatric disorders. Includes an overview of the epidemiology, pathophysiology, presentation, diagnostic criteria and screening tests for common psychiatric disorders
including anxiety, mood, substance abuse, somatization and
eating disorders, as well as insomnia, dementia and schizophrenia. *$35.00*

324 pages

2842 Recognition of Early Psychosis
Cambridge University Press
40 W 20th Street
New York, NY 10011-4221
212-924-3900
Fax: 212-691-3239

E-mail: marketing@cup.org
www.cup.org

2843 Review of Psychiatry
American Psychiatric Publishing
1000 Wilson Boulevard
Suite 1825
Arlington, VA 22209-3901
703-907-7322
800-368-5777
Fax: 703-907-1091
E-mail: appi@psych.org
www.appi.org

Katie Duffy, Marketing Assistant

Cognitive therapy, repressed memories and obsessive-compulsive disorder across the life cycle. *$59.95*

928 pages Year Founded: 1997 ISBN 0-880484-43-8

2844 Sandplay Therapy: Step By Step Manual for Physchotherapists of Diverse Orientations
WW Norton & Company
500 5th Avenue
New York, NY 10110
212-790-9456
Fax: 212-869-0856
E-mail: admalmud@wwnorton.com
www.wwnorton.com

Change often occurs on a non-verbal level. This book is for psychotherapists with alternative methods. *$35.00*

256 pages Year Founded: 2000 ISSN 70319-3

2845 Selecting Effective Treatments: a Comprehensive, Systematic, Guide for Treating Mental Disorders
Jossey-Bass Publishers
350 Sansome Street
5th Floor
San Francisco, CA 94104
800-956-7739
Fax: 800-605-2665
www.josseybass.com

$39.95

416 pages Year Founded: 1998 ISBN 0-787943-07-X

2846 Social Work Dictionary
National Association of Social Workers
750 1st Street NE
Suite 700
Washington, DC 20002-4241
202-408-8600
800-638-8799
Fax: 202-336-8312
E-mail: press@naswdc.org
www.naswpress.org

Paula Delo, Executive Editor, NASW Press

More than 8,000 terms are defined in this essential tool for understanding the language of social work and related disciplines. The resulting reference is a must for every human services professional. *$34.95*

620 pages Year Founded: 1999 ISBN 0-871012-98-7

2847 Strategic Marketing: How to Achieve Independence and Prosperity in Your Mental Health Practice
Professional Resource Press
PO Box 15560
Sarasota, FL 34277-1560
941-343-9601
800-443-3364
Fax: 941-343-9201
E-mail: orders@prpress.com
www.prpress.com

Debra Fink, Managing Editor

Presents ways to reshape your practice to capitalize on new opportunities for success in today's healthcare marketplace. *$21.95*

152 pages Year Founded: 1997 ISBN 1-568870-31-0

2848 Supports Intensity Scale
AAMR
444 N Capitol Street NW
Suite 846
Washington, DC 20001-1512
202-387-1968
800-424-3688
Fax: 202-387-2193
E-mail: dcroser@aamr.org
www.aamr.org

Designed to help you plan meaningful supports for adults with mental retardation. Consists of a comprehensive scoring system that measures the needs of persons with mental retardation in 57 key life activities based on 7 areas of competence. *$125.00*

128 pages

2849 Surviving & Prospering in the Managed Mental Health Care Marketplace
Professional Resource Press
PO Box 15560
Sarasota, FL 34277-1560
941-343-9601
800-443-3364
Fax: 941-343-9201
E-mail: orders@prpress.com
www.prpress.com

Debra Fink, Managing Editor

Includes examples of different managed care models, extensive references, and checklists. Offers examples of the typical steps in providing outpatient treatment in a managed care milieu, and other extremely useful resources. *$14.95*

106 pages Year Founded: 1994 ISBN 1-568870-04-3

2850 Suzie Brown Intervention Maze
High Tide Press
3650 W 183rd Street
Homewood, IL 60430
708-206-2054
888-487-7377
Fax: 708-206-2044
E-mail: managing.editor@hightidepress.com
www.hightidepress.com

Diane J Bell, Managing Editor

Suzie Brown, age 25, has severe developmental disabilities. She lives in a staffed house for six adults, where you work as a team. She has major communication difficulties, is prone to self-injurous behavior, and no longer responds to all the usual calming methods. What can you do? This workbook offers a practical blueprint for group decision making. Each option page presents a new scenario and ideas for moving forward. Decision logs keep track of decisions as they are made. The binder format allows for easy photocopying. *$69.99*

ISBN 1-892696-09-6

2851 Teaching Buddy Skills to Preschoolers
AAMR
444 N Capitol Street NW
Suite 846
Washington, DC 20001-1512
202-387-1968
800-424-3688
Fax: 202-387-2193
E-mail: dcroser@aamr.org
www.aamr.org

Shows how the rewards of social interactions must outweigh the costs to encouraging friendships between pre-schoolers with and without disabilities. *$12.95*

40 pages ISBN 0-940898-45-4

2852 Teaching Goal Setting and Decision-Making to Students with Developmental Disabilities
AAMR
444 N Capitol Street NW
Suite 846
Washington, DC 20001-1512
202-387-1968
800-424-3688
Fax: 202-387-2193
E-mail: dcroser@aamr.org
www.aamr.org

Link four basic steps of goal setting and decision making to twelve instructional principles that engage students in activities. *$12.95*

34 pages ISBN 0-940898-97-7

2853 Teaching Practical Communication Skills
AAMR
444 N Capitol Street NW
Suite 846
Washington, DC 20001-1512
202-387-1968
800-424-3688
Fax: 202-387-2193
E-mail: dcroser@aamr.org
www.aamr.org

Discusses strategies for teaching students to request their preferences, protest non-preferred activities, and clarify misunderstandings. *$12.95*

30 pages ISBN 0-940898-42-X

2854 Teaching Problem Solving to Students with Mental Retardation
AAMR
444 N Capitol Street NW
Suite 846
Washington, DC 20001-1512
202-387-1968
800-424-3688
Fax: 202-387-2193

E-mail: dcroser@aamr.org
www.aamr.org

Gives clear teaching strategies for social problem-solving, including role-playing, modeling, and training sequences. *$12.95*

30 pages ISBN 0-940898-62-4

2855 Teaching Self-Management to Elementary Students with Developmental Disabilities
AAMR
444 N Capitol Street NW
Suite 846
Washington, DC 20001-1512
202-387-1968
800-424-3688
Fax: 202-387-2193
E-mail: dcroser@aamr.org
www.aamr.org

This book will help you design and implement self-management systems for elementary students with disabilities including self-monitoring and self-evaluation. *$12.95*

51 pages ISBN 0-940898-48-9

2856 Teaching Students with Severe Disabilities in Inclusive Settings
AAMR
444 N Capitol Street NW
Suite 846
Washington, DC 20001-1512
202-387-1968
800-424-3688
Fax: 202-387-2193
E-mail: dcroser@aamr.org
www.aamr.org

Presents student-specific strategies for teaching students with severe disabilities in inclusive settings. Strategies include how to write IEPs in inclusive settings; effective scheduling; planning for adaptations of objectives; materials, responses, and settings; and anticipating the need for support. *$12.95*

50 pages ISBN 0-940898-49-7

2857 Textbook of Family and Couples Therapy: Clinical Applications
American Psychiatric Publishing
1000 Wilson Boulevard
Suite 1825
Arlington, VA 22209-3901
703-907-7322
800-368-5777
Fax: 703-907-1091
E-mail: appi@psych.org
www.appi.org

Blending theoretical training and up-to-date clinical strategies. It's a must for clinicians who are currently treating couples and families, a major resource for training future clinicians in these highly effective therapeutic techniques. *$63.00*

448 pages Year Founded: 2002 ISBN 0-880485-18-3

2858 The Special Education Consultant Teacher
Charles C Thomas Publishers
PO Box 19265
Springfield, IL 62794-9265

217-789-8980
800-258-8980
Fax: 217-789-9130
www.ccthomas.com

This book is intended for special education teachers and other professionals providing special education services with information, guidelines and suggestions relating to the role and responsibilities of the special education consultant teacher. Available in paperback for $ 45.95. *$67.95*

330 pages Year Founded: 2004 ISBN 0-398075-10-7

2859 Theory and Technique of Family Therapy
Charles C Thomas Publisher
2600 S 1st Street
Springfield, IL 62704-4730
217-789-8980
800-258-8980
Fax: 217-789-9130
E-mail: books@ccthomas.com
www.ccthomas.com

Charles P Barnard, Author
Ramon Garrido Corrales, Author

Contents: The Family as an Interactional System; The Family as an Intergenerational System; A Model for the Therapeutic Relationship in Family Theory, The Therapeutic Process and Related Concerns; Therapeutic Intervention Techniques and Adjuncts; Marital Group and Multiple Family Therapy; Counseling at Two Critical Stages of Family Development, Formation and Termination of Marriage. Useful information for students and practitioners of family therapy, social workers, the clergy, psychiatrists, psychologists, counselors, and related professionals. *$55.95*

352 pages Year Founded: 1981 ISBN 0-398038-59-7

2860 Thesaurus of Psychological Index Terms
American Psychological Association Database Department/PsycINFO
750 1st Street NE
Washington, DC 20002-4241
202-336-5650
800-374-2722
Fax: 202-336-5633
TDD: 202-336-6123
E-mail: psycinfo@apa.org
www.apa.org/psycinfo

Reference to the PsycINFO database vocabulary of over 5,400 descriptors. Provides standardized working to represent each concept for complete, efficient and precise retrieval of psychological information and is updated regularly. 9th edition published 2001. *$60.00*

379 pages ISBN 1-557987-75-0

2861 Three Spheres: Psychiatric Interviewing Primer
Rapid Psychler Press
3560 Pine Grove Avenue
Suite 374
Port Huron, MI 48060
519-433-7642
888-779-2453
Fax: 888-779-2457
E-mail: rapid@psychler.com
www.psychler.com

David Robinson, Publisher

$16.95

ISBN 0-968032-49-4

2862 Through the Patient's Eyes
Jossey-Bass Publishers
350 Sansome Street
5th Floor
San Francisco, CA 94104
415-394-8677
800-956-7739
Fax: 800-605-2665
www.josseybass.com

Jennifer Daley, Editor
Thomas Delbanco, Editor

Learn how providers can improve their ability to meet patient's needs and enhance the quality of care by bringing the patient's perspective to the design and delivery of health services. *$36.95*

347 pages ISBN 7-555425-44-5

2863 Tools of the Trade: A Therapist's Guide to Art Therapy Assessments
Charles C Thomas Publishers
PO Box 19265
Springfield, IL 62794-9265
217-789-8980
800-258-8980
Fax: 217-789-9130
www.ccthomas.com

Provides critical reviews of art therapy tests along with some new reviews of assessments and updated research in the field. Comprehensive in the approach to consider reliability and validity evidence provided by test authors. Available in paperback for $35.95. *$53.95*

256 pages Year Founded: 2004 ISBN 0-398075-21-2

2864 Total Quality Management in Mental Health and Mental Retardation
AAMR
444 N Capitol Street NW
Suite 846
Washington, DC 20001-1512
202-387-1968
800-424-3688
Fax: 202-387-2193
E-mail: dcroser@aamr.org
www.aamr.org

Describes how this leadership philosophy helps an organization identify and achive quality outcomes for all its customers. *$14.95*

64 pages ISBN 0-940898-67-5

2865 Training Families to do a Successful Intervention: A Professional's Guide
Hazelden
15251 Pleasant Valley Road
PO Box 176
Center City, MN 55012-0176
651-213-2121
800-328-9000
Fax: 651-213-4590
E-mail: customersupport@hazelden.org
www.hazelden.org

Helps professionals explain basic intervention concepts and give clients step-by-step instructions. *$15.95*

152 pages ISBN 1-562461-16-8

2866 Transition Matters-From School to Independence
Resources for Children with Special Needs
116 E 16th Street
5th Floor
New York, NY 10003
212-677-4650
Fax: 212-254-4070
E-mail: info@resourcesnyc.org
www.resourcesnyc.org

This new guide and directory to the transition from school to adult life for youth with disabilities takes you through the systems involved and covers rights, entitlements, options, and programs. More than 1000 organization descriptions cover college, specialized education, job training, supported work, indpendent living and much more. In collaboration with New York Lawyers for the Public Interest. *$35.00*

ISBN 0-967836-56-5

2867 Treating Complex Cases: Cognitive Behavioral Therapy Approach
John Wiley & Sons
605 3rd Avenue
New York, NY 10058-0180
212-850-6000
Fax: 212-850-6008
E-mail: info@wiley.com
www.wiley.com

Amy Bazarnik, Conventions Coordinator

2868 Treatment of Complicated Mourning
Research Press
Dept 24 W
PO Box 9177
Champaign, IL 61826
217-352-3273
800-519-2707
Fax: 217-352-1221
E-mail: rp@researchpress.com
www.researchpress.com

Russell Pense, VP Marketing

This is the first book to focus specifically on complicated mourning, often referred to as pathological, unresolved or abnormal grief. It provides caregivers with practical therapeutic strategies and specific interventions that are necessary when traditional grief counseling is unsufficient. The author provides critically important information on the prediction, identification, assessment, classification and treatment of complicated mourning. *$39.95*

768 pages ISBN 0-878223-29-0

2869 Treatments of Psychiatric Disorders
American Psychiatric Publishing
1000 Wilson Boulevard
Suite 1825
Arlington, VA 22209-3901
703-907-7322
800-368-5777
Fax: 703-907-1091
E-mail: appi@psych.org
www.appi.org

Katie Duffy, Marketing Assistant

Examines customary approaches to the major psychiatric disorders. Diagnostic, etiologic and therapeutic issues are clearly addressed by experts on each topic. *$307.00*

2800 pages Year Founded: 1995 ISBN 0-880487-00-3

2870 Using Computers In Educational and Psychological Research
Charles C Thomas Publishers
PO Box 19265
Springfield, IL 62794-9265
217-789-8980
800-258-8980
Fax: 217-789-9130
www.ccthomas.com

This book has been designed to assist researchers in the social sciences and education fields who are interested in learning how information technologies can help them successfully navigate the research process. Most researchers are familiar with the use of programs like SPSS to analyze data, but many are not aware of other ways informaiton technologies can support the research process. This book is available in paperback for $44.95. *$69.95*

274 pages Year Founded: 2006 ISBN 0-398076-16-2

2871 Values Clarification for Counselors
Charles C Thomas Publisher
2600 S 1st Street
Springfield, IL 62704-4730
217-789-8980
800-258-8980
Fax: 217-789-9130
E-mail: books@ccthomas.com
www.ccthomas.com

Gordon M Hart, Author

How Counselors, Social Workers, Psychologists, and Other Human Service Workers Can Use Available Techniques. *$24.95*

104 pages Year Founded: 1978 ISBN 0-398038-47-3

2872 What Psychotherapists Should Know About Disability
Guilford Publications
72 Spring Street
New York, NY 10012
212-431-9800
800-365-7006
Fax: 212-966-6708
E-mail: info@guilford.com
www.guilford.com

Available in alternate formats for people with disabilities, this guide confronts biases and relates the human dimesions of disability. Stereotypes and discomfort can get in the way of even a well intentioned therapist, this helps achieve a clearer professional relationship with clients of special need. *$35.00*

368 pages Year Founded: 1999 ISBN 1-572302-27-5

2873 Where to Start and What to Ask: An Assessmen t Handbook
WW Norton & Company
500 5th Avenue
New York, NY 10110-0017
212-354-5500
800-233-4830
Fax: 212-869-0856
E-mail: npb@wwnorton.com
www.wwnorton.com/psych

As a life raft for beginners and their supervisors, provides all the necessary tools for garnering information from clients. Offers a framework for thinking about that information and formulating a thorough assessment, helps neophytes organize their approach to the initial phase of treatment.

ISBN 0-393701-52-2

2874 Where to Start and What to Ask: Assessment Handbook
WW Norton & Company
500 5th Avenue
New York, NY 10110
212-790-9456
Fax: 212-869-0856
E-mail: admalmud@wwnorton.com
www.wwnorton.com

Framework for gathering information from the client and using that information to formulate an accurate assessment. *$15.95*

Year Founded: 1993 ISSN 70152-2

2875 Women's Mental Health Services: Public Health Perspecitive
Sage Publications
2455 Teller Road
Thousand Oaks, CA 91320
805-499-9774
800-818-7243
Fax: 800-583-2665
E-mail: info@sagepub.com
www.sagepub.com

Paperback, hardcover also available. *$29.95*

Year Founded: 1998 ISBN 0-761905-09-X

2876 Workbook: Mental Retardation
AAMR
444 N Capitol Street NW
Suite 846
Washington, DC 20001-1512
202-387-1968
800-424-3688
Fax: 202-387-2193
E-mail: dcroser@aamr.org
www.aamr.org

Presents key components from a practical point of view. *$29.95*

64 pages ISBN 0-940898-82-9

2877 Working with the Core Relationship Problem in Psychotherapy
Jossey-Bass Publishers
350 Sansome Street
5th Floor
San Francisco, CA 94104
415-394-8677
800-956-7739
Fax: 800-605-2665
www.josseybass.com

Learn to reveal, understand, and use the core relationship problem, which is formed from earliest childhood and creates an image of the self in relation to others so it can aid in understanding the underlying conflict that repeatedly plays out in a client's behavior. *$39.95*

256 pages ISBN 0-787943-01-0

2878 Writing Behavioral Contracts: A Case Simulation Practice Manual
Research Press
Dept 24 W
PO Box 9177
Champaign, IL 61826
217-352-3273
800-519-2707
Fax: 217-352-1221
E-mail: rp@researchpress.com
www.researchpress.com

Dr William J DeRiski, Author
Dennis Wiziecki, Marketing

The most difficult aspect of using contingency contracting is designing a contract acceptable to and appropriate for all involved parties. This unusually versatile book improves contract-writing skills through practice with typical cases. Valuable for social workers, mental health professionals and educators. *$11.95*

94 pages ISBN 0-878221-23-9

2879 Writing Psychological Reports: A Guide for Clinicians
Professional Resource Press
PO Box 15560
Sarasota, FL 34277-1560
941-343-9601
800-443-3364
Fax: 941-343-9201
E-mail: orders@prpress.com
www.prpress.com

Debra Fink, Managing Editor

Presents widely accepted structured format for writing psychological reports. Numerous useful suggestions for experienced clinicians, and qualifies as essential reading for all clinical psychology students. *$21.95*

158 pages Year Founded: 2002 ISBN 1-568870-76-0

Adjustment Disorders

2880 Ambiguous Loss: Learning to Live with Unresolved Grief
Harvard University Press
79 Garden Street
Cambridge, MA 02138
800-405-1619
Fax: 800-406-9145
E-mail: CONTACT_HUP@harvard.edu
www.hup.harvard.edu

$22.00

192 pages Year Founded: 1999 ISBN 0-674017-38-2

2881 Attachment and Interaction
Jessica Kingsley
47 Runway Drive
Suite G
Levittown, PA 19057-4738
215-269-0400
Fax: 215-269-0363
www.taylorandfrancis.com

Available in paperback. *$29.95*

238 pages Year Founded: 1998 ISBN 1-853025-86-0

2882 Body Image: Understanding Body Dissatisfaction in Men, Women and Children
Routledge
2727 Palisade Avenue
Suite 4H
Bronx, NY 10463-1020
718-796-0971
Fax: 718-796-0971
www.vdg@columbia.edu
$75.00

208 pages Year Founded: 1998 ISBN 0-415147-84-0

Alcohol/Substance Abuse & Dependence

2883 Addiction Treatment Homework Planner
John Wiley & Sons
10475 Crosspoint Boulevard
Indianapolis, IN 46256
877-762-2974
Fax: 800-597-3299
E-mail: consumers@wiley.com
www.wiley.com

Helps clients suffering from chemical and nonchemical addictions develop the skills they need to work through problems. *$ 49.95*

370 pages ISBN 0-471274-59-3

2884 Addiction Treatment Planner
John Wiley & Sons
10475 Crosspoint Boulevard
Indianapolis, IN 46256
877-762-2974
Fax: 800-597-3299
E-mail: consumers@wiley.com
www.wiley.com

Provides all the elements necessary to quickly and easily develop formal treatment plans that satisfy the demands of HMOs, managed care companies, third-party payers, and state and federal review agencies. *$49.95*

384 pages ISBN 0-471418-14-5

2885 Addictive Behaviors Across the Life Span
Sage Publications
2455 Teller Road
Thousand Oaks, CA 91320
805-499-9774
800-818-7243
Fax: 800-583-2665
E-mail: info@sagepub.com
www.sagepub.com

Leading scholars, researchers and clinicians in the field of addictive behavior provide and examination of drug dependency from a life span perspective in this authoritative volume. Four general topic areas include: etiology; early intervention; integrated treatment; and policy issues across the life span. Other topics include biopsychosocial perspectives on the intergenerational transmission of alcoholism to children and reducing the risks of addictive behaviors. *$59.95*

358 pages Year Founded: 1993 ISBN 0-803950-78-0

2886 Addictive Thinking: Understanding Self-Deception
Health Communications
292 Fernwood Avenue
Edison, NJ 08837
732-346-0027
Fax: 732-346-0442
www.hcomm.com

Exposes the irrational and contradictory patterns of addictive thinking, and shows how to overcome them and barriers they create; low self-esteem and relapse.

140 pages ISBN 1-568381-38-7

2887 Adolescents, Alcohol and Drugs: A Practical Guide for Those Who Work With Young People
Charles C Thomas Publisher
2600 S 1st Street
Springfield, IL 62704-4730
217-789-8980
800-258-8980
Fax: 217-789-9130
E-mail: books@ccthomas.com
www.ccthomas.com
$41.95

210 pages Year Founded: 1988 ISBN 0-398053-93-6

2888 Adolescents, Alcohol and Substance Abuse: Reaching Teens through Brief Interventions
Guilford Press
72 Spring Street
New York, NY 10012
212-431-9800
800-365-7006
Fax: 212-966-6708
E-mail: info@guilford.com
www.guilford.com

Reviews a range of empirically supported approaches to dealing with the growing problems of substance use and abuse among young people. While admission to specialized treatment programs is relatively rare in today's health care climate, there are many opportunities for brief interventions. Brief interventions also allow the clinician to work with the teen on his or her home turf, emphasize autonomy and personal responsibility, and can be used across the full range of teens who are engaging in health risk-behavior.

350 pages ISBN 1-572306-58-0

2889 American Psychiatric Press Textbook of Substance Abuse Treatment
American Psychiatric Publishing
1000 Wilson Boulevard
Suite 1825
Arlington, VA 22209-3901
703-907-7322
800-368-5777
Fax: 703-907-1091
E-mail: appi@psych.org
www.appi.org

Katie Duffy, Marketing Assistant

Comprehensive view of basic science and psychology underlying addiction and coverage of all treatment modalities. New topics include the neurobiology of alcoholism, stimulants, marijuana, opiates and hallucinogens, club drugs, and addiction in women. *$95.00*

608 pages Year Founded: 1999 ISBN 0-880488-20-4

2890 An Elephant in the Living Room: Leader's Guide for Helping Children of Alcoholics
Hazelden
15251 Pleasant Valley Road
PO Box 176
Center City, MN 55012-0176
651-213-2121
800-328-9000
Fax: 651-213-4590
www.hazelden.org

Marion H Typpo PhD, Co-Author
Jill M Hastings PhD, Co-Author

Practical guidance for education and health professionals who help young people cope with a family member's chemical dependency. *$9.95*

129 pages ISBN 1-568380-34-8

2891 Assessing Substance Abusers with the Million Clinical Multiaxial Inventory
Charles C Thomas Publishers
PO Box 19265
Springfield, IL 62794-9265
217-789-8980
800-258-8980
Fax: 217-789-9130
www.ccthomas.com

The construct validity of a psychological test is assessed by a multitrai-multimethod nomothetic matrix, which means that the psychometric properties of an assessment instrument are studied with a variety of populations and in a variety of settings and weighed against a variety of other measures that purportedly assess the same construct. This concept implies that a test might have strong validity with some populations and weak validity with others, and this is the central theme of this book. Also, the book comes in paperback for only $26.95. *$ 46.95*

164 pages Year Founded: 2005 ISBN 0-398075-91-3

2892 Before It's Too Late: Working with Substance Abuse in the Family
WW Norton & Company
500 5th Avenue
New York, NY 10110
212-790-9456
Fax: 212-869-0856
E-mail: admalmud@wwnorton.com
www.wwnorton.com

Sometimes, the problem a patient or the family of the patient's root cause to the problem they seek help for, is actually substance abuse. How to present the problem, and step-by-step models for working with families dealing with substance abuse are examined. *$ 23.95*

224 pages Year Founded: 1989 ISBN 0-393700-68-2

2893 Behind Bars: Substance Abuse and America's Prison Population
Center on Addiction at Columbia University
633 3rd Avenue
19th Floor
New York, NY 10017-6706
212-841-5200
Fax: 212-956-8020
www.casacolumbia.org

Steven Belenko

Results of a three year study of American prisons and the reason drugs are responible for the booming prison population and escalating costs. *$25.00*

Year Founded: 1998

2894 Blaming the Brain: The Truth About Drugs and Mental Health
Free Press
866 3rd Avenue
New York, NY 10022-6221
212-832-2101
800-323-7445
Fax: 800-943-9831
www.simonsays.com

Exposes weaknesses inherent in the scientific arguments supporting the theory that biochemical imbalances are the main cause of mental illness. It discusses how the accidental discovery of mood-altering drugs stimulated an interest in psychopharmacology. *$25.00*

320 pages Year Founded: 1998 ISBN 0-684849-64-X

2895 Building Bridges: States Respond to Substance Abuse and Welfare Reform
Center on Addiction at Columbia University
633 3rd Avenue
19th Floor
New York, NY 10017-6706
212-841-5200
Fax: 212-956-8020
www.casacolumbia.org

Prepared in partnership with the American Public Human Services Association, this two year study among the front line workers in the nation's welfare offices, job training programs and substance abuse agencies reveals what they find works and does not work in helping clients. *$15.00*

Year Founded: 1999

2896 CASAWORKS for Families: Promising Approach to Welfare Reform and Substance-Abusing Women
Center on Addiction at Columbia University
633 3rd Avenue
19th Floor
New York, NY 10017-6706
212-841-5200
Fax: 212-956-8020
www.casacolumbia.org

Designed for TANF recipients, this promising approach to welfare reform is used in 11 cities and nine states. *$5.00*

2897 Clinician's Guide to the Personality Profiles of Alcohol and Drug Abusers: Typological Descriptions Using the MMPI
Charles C Thomas Publisher
2600 S 1st Street
Springfield, IL 62704-4730
217-789-8980
800-258-8980
Fax: 217-789-9130
E-mail: books@ccthomas.com
www.ccthomas.com

Donald J Tosi, Author
Dennis M Eshbaugh, Author
Michael A Murphy, Author

$39.95

156 pages Year Founded: 1993 ISSN 0-399-06463-6ISBN 0-398058-85-7

2898 Critical Incidents: Ethical Issues in Substance Abuse Prevention and Treatment
Hazelden
15251 Pleasant Valley Road
PO Box 176
Center City, MN 55012-0176
651-213-2121
800-328-9000
Fax: 651-213-4590
www.hazelden.com

Two hundred critical situations for health care professionals to sharpen their decision-making skills about everyday ethical dilemmas that arise in their field. *$17.95*

276 pages ISBN 0-938475-03-7

2899 Dangerous Liaisons: Substance Abuse and Sex
Center on Addiction at Columbia University
633 3rd Avenue
19th Floor
New York, NY 10017-6706
212-841-5200
Fax: 212-956-8020
www.casacolumbia.org

An intensive report on the dangerous and sometimes life-threatening connection between alcohol, drug abuse and sexual activity. Parents, guidance professionals and others will find this useful. *$22.00*

170 pages Year Founded: 1999

2900 Determinants of Substance Abuse: Biological, Psychological, and Environmental Factors
Kluwer Academic/Plenum Publishers
233 Spring Street
New York, NY 10013
212-620-8000
Fax: 212-463-0742
www.kluweronline.com

Hardcover. *$90.00*

454 pages Year Founded: 1985 ISBN 0-306418-73-8

2901 Drug Information for Teens: Health Tips about the Physical and Mental Effects of Substance Abuse
Omnigraphics
615 Giswold
Detroit, MI 48226
313-961-1340
Fax: 313-961-1383
E-mail: info@omnigraphics.com
www.omnigraphics.com

Provides students with facts about drug use, abuse, and addiction. It describes the physical and mental effects of alcohol, tobacco, marijuana, ecstasy, inhalants and many other drugs and chemicals that are often abused. It includes information about the process that leads from casual use to addiction and offers suggestions for resisting peer pressure and helping friends stay drug free.

452 pages ISBN 0-780804-44-9

2902 Empowering Adolesent Girls
WW Norton & Company
500 5th Avenue
New York, NY 10110
212-790-9456
Fax: 212-869-0856
E-mail: admalmud@wwnorton.com
www.wwnorton.com

Strategies and activities for professionals who work with adolesent girls (teachers, counselors, therapists) to offer support and encouagement through the Go Girls program. *$32.00*

256 pages Year Founded: 2001 ISSN 70347-9

2903 Ethics for Addiction Professionals
Hazelden
15251 Pleasant Valley Road
PO Box 176
Center City, MN 55012-0176
651-213-2121
800-328-9000
Fax: 651-213-4590
www.hazelden.org

The first on ethics written by and for addiction professionals that addresses complex issues such as patient confidentiality versus mandatory reporting, clinician relapse, personal and social relationships with clients and other important related issues. *$14.95*

60 pages ISBN 0-894864-54-8

2904 Hispanic Substance Abuse
Charles C Thomas Publisher
2600 S 1st Street
Springfield, IL 62704-4730
217-789-8980
800-258-8980
Fax: 217-789-9130
E-mail: books@ccthomas.com
www.ccthomas.com

Addresses the concerns of students and professionals who work with Hispanics. Brings together current research on this problem by well-known experts in the fields of alcohol and drug abuse. Useful for scholars and researchers, practitioners in the human services, and the general public. There is shown the extent of substance abuse problems in Hispanic communities, the differences between the Hispanic subgroups and the casual factors that are involved. There are detailed strategies for prevention and the necessary approaches to treatment. *$57.95*

258 pages Year Founded: 1993 ISSN 0-398-06274-9ISBN 0-398058-49-0

2905 Jail Detainees with Co-Occurring Mental Health and Substance Use Disorders
Policy Research Associates
345 Delaware Avenue
Delmar, NY 12054
518-439-7415
800-444-7415
Fax: 518-439-7612
E-mail: gains@prainc.com
www.prainc.com

Brief report that discusses the issue of keeping federal benefits for jail detainees.

2906 Love First: A New Approach to Intervention for Alcoholism and Drug Addiction
Hazelden
15245 Pleasant Valley Road
PO Box 11-CO 3
Center City, MN 55012-0011
651-213-4000
800-257-7810
Fax: 651-213-4411
www.hazelden.org

A straightforward, simple and practical resource written specifically for families seeking to help a loved one struggling with substance addiction.

280 pages ISBN 1-568385-21-8

2907 Malignant Neglect: Substance Abuse and America's Schools
Center on Addiction at Columbia University
633 3rd Avenue
19th Floor
New York, NY 10017-6706
212-841-5200
Fax: 212-956-8020
www.casacolumbia.org

Six years of exhaustive research of focus groups, schools, parents and professionals. Findings of the costs of drug abuse in dollars, student behavior, truancy and more.
$22.00

117 pages Year Founded: 2001

2908 Missed Opportunity: National Survey of Primary Care Physicians and Patients on Substance Abuse
Center on Addiction at Columbia University
633 3rd Avenue
19th Floor
New York, NY 10017-6706
212-841-5200
Fax: 212-956-8020
www.casacolumbia.org

Findings and recomendations based on a CASA report that revealed 94% of primary care physicians fail to diagnose symptoms of alcohol abuse in adult patients, and 41% of pediatricians missed a diagnosis of drug abuse when presented with a classic description of a teenage patient with these symptoms. The report also sheds light on the fact that many physicians feel unprepared to diagnose substance abuse and have little confidence in the effectiveness of treatments available. *$22.00*

Year Founded: 2000

2909 Narrative Means to Sober Ends: Treating Addiction and Its Aftermath
Guilford Publications
72 Spring Street
New York, NY 10012
212-431-9800
800-365-7006
Fax: 212-966-6708
E-mail: info@guilford.com
www.guilford.com

This eloquently written volume illuminates the devastating power of addiction and describes an array of innovative approaches to facilitating clients' recovery. Demonstrated are creative ways to help clients explore their relationship to drugs and alcohol, take the first steps toward sobriety and develop meaningful ways of living without addiction.
$37.95

386 pages ISBN 1-572305-66-5

2910 No Place to Hide: Substance Abuse in Mid-Size Cities and Rural America
Center on Addiction at Columbia University
633 3rd Avenue
19th Floor
New York, NY 10017-6706
212-841-5200
Fax: 212-956-8020
www.casacolumbia.org

Surprisingly to some, young people in smaller cities and rural areas are more likely to use many forms of illegal substances. Tobacco use is also higher away from the major cities. The findings on other statistics of drugs and rural adolescent and teenager use are included. *$10.00*

Year Founded: 2000

2911 No Safe Haven: Children of Substance-Abusing Parents
Center on Addiction at Columbia University
633 3rd Avenue
19th Floor
New York, NY 10017-6706
212-841-5200
Fax: 212-956-8020
www.casacolumbia.org

Jeanne Reid, Author
Peggy Macchetto, Author
Susan Foster, Author

Comprehensive report with shattering facts and figures reveals the impact of substance abuse on parenting skills and child neglect. The number of children affected by their parent's substance abuse driven behavior has more than doubled in the last ten years, greater than the rise in children's overall population. This report calls for a reworking of the child welfare system, and provides guidelines to when the child should be permanently remove from the home.
$22.00

Year Founded: 1999

2912 Non Medical Marijuana: Rite of Passage or Russian Roulette?
Center on Addiction at Columbia University
633 3rd Avenue
19th Floor
New York, NY 10017-6706
212-841-5200
Fax: 212-956-8020
www.casacolumbia.org

The most recent numbers available find that more teens from 19 years old and younger enter treatment for marijuana abuse than for any other drug, including alcohol. Many teens also have a problem with secondary drugs. This report released by CASA at Columbia University, concludes that non medical marijuana is indeed a dangerous substance. *$20.00*

Year Founded: 1999

2913 Perfect Daughters
Health Communications
292 Fernwood Avenue
Edison, NJ 08837
732-346-0027
Fax: 732-346-0442
www.hcomm.com

Identifies what differentiates the adult daughters of alcoholics from other women. Adult daughters of alcoholics operate from a base of harsh and limiting views of themselves and the world. Having learned that they must function perfectly in order to avoid unpleasant situations, these women often assume responsibility for the failures of others. They are drawn to chemically dependent men and are more likely to become addicted themselves. This book collects the thoughts, feelings and experience of twelve hundred perfect daughters, offering readers an opportunity to explore their own life's dynamics and thereby heal and grow.

350 pages ISBN 1-558749-52-7

2914 Principles of Addiction Medicine
American Society of Addiction Medicine
4601 N Park Avenue
Suite 101, Upper Arcade
Chevy Chase, MD 20815
301-987-9278
800-844-8948
E-mail: email@asam.com
www.asam.org

James F Callahan DPA, Executive VP/CEO

Textbook on the basic and clinical science of prevention and treatment of alcohol, nicotine, and other drug dependencies and addictions. *$155.00*

1338 pages ISBN 1-880425-04-0

2915 Proven Youth Development Model that Prevents Substance Abuse and Builds Communities
Center on Addiction at Columbia University
633 3rd Avenue
19th Floor
New York, NY 10017-6706
212-841-5200
Fax: 212-956-8020
www.casacolumbia.org

How-to manual developed with nine years of research. The program is a collaboration of local school, law enforcement, social service and health teams to help high risk youth between the ages of 8 - 13 years old and their families prevent substance abuse and violent behavior. Used in 23 urban and rural communities in 11 states and the District of Columbia. *$50.00*

79 pages Year Founded: 2001

2916 Psychological Theories of Drinking and Alcoholism
Guilford Publications
72 Spring Street
New York, NY 10012
212-431-9800
800-365-7006
Fax: 212-966-6708
E-mail: info@guilford.com
www.guilford.com

Multidisciplinary approach discusses biological, pharmacological and social factors that influence drinking and alcoholism. Contributors review established and emerging approaches that guide research into the psychological processes influencing drinking and alcoholism. *$47.95*

460 pages Year Founded: 1999 ISBN 1-572304-10-3

2917 Relapse Prevention Maintenance: Strategies in the Treatment of Addictive Behaviors
Guilford Publications
72 Spring Street
New York, NY 10012
212-431-9800
800-365-7006
Fax: 212-966-6708
E-mail: info@guilford.com
www.guilford.com

Research on relapse prevention to problem drinking, smoking, substance abuse, eating disorders and compulsive gambling. Analyzes factors that may lead to relapse and offers practical techniques for maintaining treatment gains. *$55.00*

558 pages Year Founded: 1985 ISBN 0-898620-09-0

2918 Relapse Prevention Maintenance: Strategies in the Treatment of Addictive Behaviors
Guilford Publications
72 Spring Street
New York, NY 10012
212-431-9800
800-365-7006
Fax: 212-966-6708
E-mail: info@guilford.com
www.guilford.com

Research on relapse prevention to problem drinking, smoking, substance abuse, eating disorders and compulsive gambling. Analyzes factors that may lead to relapse and offers practical techniques for maintaining treatment gains. *$55.00*

558 pages Year Founded: 1985 ISBN 0-898620-09-0

2919 So Help Me God: Substance Abuse, Religion and Spirituality
Center on Addiction at Columbia University
633 3rd Avenue
19th Floor
New York, NY 10017-6706
212-841-5200
Fax: 212-956-8020
www.casacolumbia.org

Results of a 2 year study, finding that spirituality has enormous power to potentially lower the risks of substance abuse. When this is combined with professional treatment, an individual's religion helps greatly with recovery. *$10.00*

Year Founded: 2001

2920 Solutions Step by Step: Substance Abuse Treatment Manual
WW Norton & Company
500 5th Avenue
New York, NY 10110
212-790-9456
Fax: 212-869-0856
E-mail: admalmud@wwnorton.com
www.wwnorton.com

Quick tips, questions and examples focusing on successes that can be experienced helping substance abusers help themselves. *$ 25.00*

192 pages Year Founded: 1997 ISSN 70251-0

2921 Substance Abuse and Learning Disabilities: Peas in a Pod or Apples and Oranges?
Center on Addiction at Columbia University
633 3rd Avenue
19th Floor
New York, NY 10017-6706
212-841-5200
Fax: 212-956-8020
www.casacolumbia.org

Report originating from a conference in 1999 sponsored by CASA, the relationship between learning disabilities that are not addressed, and possible substance abuse by these same children is examined. Attention Deficit/Hyperactivity Disorder and Conduct Disorder and the link to substance abuse is also considered. *$10.00*

00 pages

2922 Substance Abuse: A Comprehensive Textbook
Lippincott Williams & Wilkins
PO Box 1600
Hagerstown, MD 21741-1600
301-714-2300
800-638-3030
Fax: 301-824-7390
www.lww.com

$162.00

956 pages Year Founded: 1997 ISBN 0-683181-79-3

2923 Teens and Alcohol: Gallup Youth Survey Major Issues and Trends
Mason Crest Publishers
370 Reed Road
Suite 302
Broomall, PA 19008
866-627-2665
Fax: 610-543-3878
E-mail: gbrffr@masoncrest.com
www.masoncrest.com

Eighty-seven percent of high school seniors have tried alcohol and, according to a Gallup Youth Survey, 27 percent of teenagers say it is very easy for them to get alcoholic beverages. Alcohol is a contributor to the three leading causes of death for teens and young adults: automobile crashes, homicide and suicides.

112 pages ISBN 1-590847-23-7

2924 Therapeutic Communities for Addictions: Reading in Theory, Research, and Practice
Charles C Thomas Publisher
2600 S 1st Street
Springfield, IL 62704-4730
217-789-8980
800-258-8980
Fax: 217-789-9130
E-mail: books@ccthomas.com
www.ccthomas.com

George De Leon, Author
James T Ziegenfuss Jr, Author

Contents: The Therapeutic Community (TC) for Substance Abuse; Democratic TCs or Programmatic TCs or Both?;

Motivational Aspects of Heroin Addicts in TCs; A Sociological View of the TC; Psychodynamics of TCs for Treatment of Heroin Addicts; Britain and the Psychoanalytic Tradition in TCs; TC Research; Outcomes of Drug Abuse Treatment; 12-Year Follow-up Outcomes, College Training in a TC; Client Evaluations of TCs and Retention; Side Bets and Secondary Adjustments; Measuring Program Implementation; The TC Looking Ahead; TCs within Prisons; Uses and Abuses of Power and Authority. *$51.95*

282 pages Year Founded: 1986 ISBN 0-398052-06-9

2925 Treating Substance Abuse: Part 1
American Counseling Association
5999 Stevenson Avenue
Alexandria, VA 22304-3300
800-422-2648
Fax: 703-823-0252
TDD: 703-823-6862
E-mail: webmaster@counseling.org
www.counseling.org

The first of a two-volume set presents up-to-date findings on the treatment of alcoholism and addiction to cocaine, caffeine, hallucinogens, and marijuana. Techniques and case examples are offered from a variety of approaches, including motivational enhancement therapy, marriage and family therapy as well as cognitive-behavioral. *$26.95*

280 pages ISBN 1-886330-48-4

2926 Treating Substance Abuse: Part 2
American Counseling Association
5999 Stevenson Avenue
Alexandria, VA 22304-3300
800-422-2648
Fax: 703-823-0252
E-mail: webmaster@counseling.org
www.counseling.org

For treating select populations of substance-abusing clients, including those with disabilities, psychiatric disorders, schizophrenia and major depression. Also serves adolescents, older adults, pregnant women and clients whose addictions affect their ability to function in the workplace. *$29.95*

311 pages ISBN 1-886330-49-2

2927 Treating the Alcoholic: Developmental Model of Recovery
John Wiley & Sons
605 3rd Avenue
New York, NY 10058-0180
212-850-6000
Fax: 212-850-6008
E-mail: info@wiley.com
www.wiley.com

376 pages Year Founded: 1985

2928 Under the Rug: Substance Abuse and the Mature Woman
Center on Addiction at Columbia University
633 3rd Avenue
19th Floor
New York, NY 10017-6706
212-841-5200
Fax: 212-956-8020
www.casacolumbia.org

Discusses the fact that millions of mature women are robbed of a healthy and longer lifespan due to a substance abuse problem that they discreetly hide. Their reluctance to get help costs them and the health systems billions. *$25.00*

Year Founded: 1998

2929 Understanding Psychiatric Medications in the Treatment of Chemical Dependency and Dual Diagnoses
Charles C Thomas Publisher
2600 S 1st Street
Springfield, IL 62704-4730
217-789-8980
800-258-8980
Fax: 217-789-9130
E-mail: books@ccthomas.com
www.ccthomas.com

Designed to address coexisting chemical dependency and psychiatric disorder (dual diagnoses) and specifically to focus on the appropriate role of psychotropic medications in the treatment of dual diagnonsis patients. The text presents a comprehensive overview of psychiatric medication treatment for dual diagnoses that speaks to a broad professional audience while being sensitive to the values and beliefs of the chemical dependents. *$39.95*

134 pages Year Founded: 1995 ISSN 0-398-05964-0ISBN 0-398059-63-2

2930 Your Drug May Be Your Problem: How and Why to Stop Taking Pyschiatric Medications
Perseus Books Group
550 Central Avenue
Boulder, CO 80301
800-386-5656
Fax: 720-406-7336
E-mail: westview.orders@perseusbooks.com
www.perseusbooksgroup.com

In a very short time, a doctor may prescribe a drug which an individual may take for months, years, even the rest of their lives. This book provides up-to-date, descriptions of the pros and cons of taking psychiatric medication, dangers involved, and explains a safe method of withdrawl if needed. *$17.00*

288 pages Year Founded: 2000 ISBN 0-738203-48-3

Anxiety Disorders

2931 Anxiety Disorders: A Scientific Approach for Selecting the Most Effective Treatment
Professional Resource Press
PO Box 15560
Sarasota, FL 34277-1560
941-343-9601
800-443-3364
Fax: 941-343-9201
E-mail: orders@prpress.com
www.prpress.com

Debra Fink, Managing Editor

Presents descriptive and empirical information on the differential diagnosis of DSM-IV and DSM-III-R categories of anxiety disorders. Explicit decision rules are provided for developing treatment plans based on both scientific research and clinical judgement. *$14.95*

114 pages Year Founded: 1994 ISBN 1-568870-00-0

2932 Applied Relaxation Training in the Treatment of PTSD and Other Anxiety Disorders
New Harbinger Publications
5674 Shattuck Avenue
Oakland, CA 94609-1662
510-652-2002
800-748-6273
Fax: 510-652-5472
E-mail: customerservice@newharbinger.com
www.newharbinger.com

Comes with a one hundred five minute video tape and a 52 page paperback manual. *$100.00*

Year Founded: 1998 ISBN 1-889287-08-3

2933 Assimilation, Rational Thinking, and Suppression in the Treatment of PTSD and Other Anxiety Disorders
New Harbinger Publications
5674 Shattuck Avenue
Oakland, CA 94609-1662
510-652-2002
800-748-6273
Fax: 510-652-5472
E-mail: customerservice@newharbinger.com
www.newharbinger.com

Comes with two videotapes and a ninety four page paperback manual. *$150.00*

Year Founded: 1998 ISBN 1-889287-06-7

2934 Client's Manual for the Cognitive Behavioral Treatment of Anxiety Disorders
New Harbinger Publications
5674 Shattuck Avenue
Oakland, CA 94609-1662
510-652-2002
800-748-6273
Fax: 510-652-5472
E-mail: customerservice@newharbinger.com
www.newharbinger.com

$10.00

106 pages Year Founded: 1994 ISBN 1-889287-99-7

2935 Cognitive Therapy
American Psychiatric Publishing
1000 Wilson Boulevard
Suite 1825
Arlington, VA 22209-3901
703-907-7322
800-368-5777
Fax: 703-907-1091
E-mail: appi@psych.org
www.appi.org

Katie Duffy, Marketing Assistant

Cognitive therapy for anxiety, substance abuse, personality, eating and mental disorders. *$37.50*

176 pages Year Founded: 1997 ISBN 0-880484-45-4

2936 Gender Differences in Mood and Anxiety Disorders: From Bench to Bedside
American Psychiatric Publishing
1000 Wilson Boulevard
Suite 1825
Arlington, VA 22209-3901

703-907-7322
800-368-5777
Fax: 703-907-1091
E-mail: appi@psych.org
www.appi.org

Katie Duffy, Marketing Assistant

Gender differences in neuroimaging. Discusses women, stress and depression, sex differences in hypothalamic-pituitary-adrenal axis regulation, modulation of anxiety by reproductive hormones. Questions if hormone replacement and oral contraceptive therapy induce or treat mood symptoms. *$37.50*

224 pages Year Founded: 1999 ISBN 0-880489-58-8

2937 Generalized Anxiety Disorder: Diagnosis, Treatment and Its Relationship to Other Anxiety Disorders
American Psychiatric Publishing
1000 Wilson Boulevard
Suite 1825
Arlington, VA 22209-3901
703-907-7322
800-368-5777
Fax: 703-907-1091
E-mail: appi@psych.org
www.appi.org

Katie Duffy, Marketing Assistant

Historical introduction, diagnosis, classification and differential diagnosis. Relationship with depression, panic and OCD. Treatments. *$74.95*

96 pages Year Founded: 1998 ISBN 1-853176-59-1

2938 Integrative Treatment of Anxiety Disorders
American Psychiatric Publishing
1000 Wilson Boulevard
Suite 1825
Arlington, VA 22209-3901
703-907-7322
800-368-5777
Fax: 703-907-1091
E-mail: appi@psych.org
www.appi.org

Katie Duffy, Marketing Assistant

Up-to-date look at combined pharmacotherapy and cognitive behavioral therapy in the treatment of anxiety disorders. *$41.50*

320 pages Year Founded: 1995 ISBN 0-880487-15-1

2939 Long-Term Treatments of Anxiety Disorders
American Psychiatric Publishing
1000 Wilson Boulevard
Suite 1825
Arlington, VA 22209-3901
703-907-7322
800-368-5777
Fax: 703-907-1091
E-mail: appi@psych.org
www.appi.org

Katie Duffy, Marketing Assistant

Treatment of anxiety disorders encapsulating important advances made over the past two decades. *$56.00*

464 pages Year Founded: 1996 ISBN 0-880486-56-2

2940 Overcoming Agoraphobia and Panic Disorder
New Harbinger Publications
5674 Shattuck Avenue
Oakland, CA 94609-1662
510-652-2002
800-748-6273
Fax: 510-652-5472
E-mail: customerservice@newharbinger.com
www.newharbinger.com

A twelve to sixteen session treatment. *$11.95*

88 pages Year Founded: 1998 ISBN 1-572241-46-2

2941 Panic Disorder: Clinical Diagnosis, Management and Mechanisms
American Psychiatric Publishing
1000 Wilson Boulevard
Suite 1825
Arlington, VA 22209-3901
703-907-7322
800-368-5777
Fax: 703-907-1091
E-mail: appi@psych.org
www.appi.org

Katie Duffy, Marketing Assistant

Novel and important new discoveries for biological research together with up to date information for the diagnosis and treatment for the practicing clinician. *$75.00*

264 pages Year Founded: 1998 ISBN 1-853175-18-8

2942 Panic Disorder: Theory, Research and Therapy
John Wiley & Sons
605 3rd Avenue
New York, NY 10058-0180
212-850-6000
Fax: 212-850-6008
E-mail: info@wiley.com
www.wiley.com

364 pages Year Founded: 1989

2943 Phobias: Handbook of Theory, Reseach and Treatment
John Wiley & Sons
605 3rd Avenue
New York, NY 10058-0180
212-850-6000
Fax: 212-850-6008
E-mail: info@wiley.com
www.wiley.com

Provides an up-to-date summary of current knowledge of phobias. Psychological treatments available for specific phobias have been refined considerably in recent years. This extensive handbook acknowledges these treatments and includes the description and nature of prevalent phobias, details of symptoms, prevalence rates, individual case histories, and a brief review of of our knowledge of the etiology of phobias.

470 pages Year Founded: 1995

2944 Practice Guideline for the Treatment of Patients with Panic Disorder
American Psychiatric Publishing
1000 Wilson Boulevard
Suite 1825
Arlington, VA 22209-3901

703-907-7322
800-368-5777
Fax: 703-907-1091
E-mail: appi@psych.org
www.appi.org
Katie Duffy, Marketing Assistant

Summarizes data, evaluation of the patient for coexisting mental disorders and issues specific to the treatment of panic disorders in children and adolescents. *$22.50*

160 pages Year Founded: 1998 ISBN 0-890423-11-3

2945 Shy Children, Phobic Adults: Nature and Treatment of Social Phobia
American Psychiatric Publishing
1000 Wilson Boulevard
Suite 1825
Arlington, VA 22209-3901
703-907-7322
800-368-5777
Fax: 703-907-1091
E-mail: appi@psych.org
www.appi.org
Katie Duffy, Marketing Assistant

Describes the similiarities and differences in the syndrome across all ages. Draws from the clinical, social and developmental literatures, as well as from extensive clinical experience. Illustrates the impact of developmental stage on phenomenology, diagnoses and assessment and treatment of social phobia. *$39.95*

321 pages Year Founded: 1998 ISBN 1-557984-61-1

2946 Social Phobia: Clinical and Research Perspectives
American Psychiatric Publishing
1000 Wilson Boulevard
Suite 1825
Arlington, VA 22209-3901
703-907-7322
800-368-5777
Fax: 703-907-1091
E-mail: appi@psych.org
www.appi.org
Katie Duffy, Marketing Assistant

Comprehensive and practice guide for mental health professionals who encounter individuals with social phobia. *$48.00*

384 pages Year Founded: 1995 ISBN 0-880486-53-8

2947 Treating Anxiety Disorders
Jossey-Bass Publishers
350 Sansome Street
5th Floor
San Francisco, CA 94104
415-394-8677
800-956-7739
Fax: 800-605-2665
www.josseybass.com
$30.95

288 pages ISBN 0-787903-16-7

2948 Treating Anxiety Disorders with a Cognitive
New Harbinger Publications
5674 Shattuck Avenue
Oakland, CA 94609-1662

510-652-2002
800-748-6273
Fax: 510-652-5472
E-mail: customerservice@newharbinger.com
www.newharbinger.com

Behavioral Exposure Based Approach and the Eye Movement Technique comes with a fifty eight minute videotape and a fifty one page paperback manual. *$100.00*

Year Founded: 1998 ISBN 1-889287-02-4

2949 Treating Panic Disorder and Agoraphobia: A Step by Step Clinical Guide
New Harbinger Publications
5674 Shattuck Avenue
Oakland, CA 94609-1662
510-652-2002
800-748-6273
Fax: 510-652-5472
E-mail: customerservice@newharbinger.com
www.newharbinger.com

Treatment program covering breath control training, changing automatic thoughts and underlying beliefs. *$49.95*

296 pages Year Founded: 1997 ISBN 1-572240-84-9

Asperger's Syndrome

2950 Asperger Syndrome Diagnostic Scale (ASDS)
Pro-Ed
8700 Shoal Creek Boulevard
Austin, TX 78757-6897
800-897-3202
Fax: 800-397-7633
E-mail: feedback@proedinc.com
www.proedinc.com
Brenda Myles
Stacey Bock
Richard Simpson

The ASDS is a quick, easy-to-use rating scale that helps determine whether a child has Asperger Syndrome. Anyone who knows the child or youth well can complete the scale. Parents, teachers, siblings, paraeducators, speech-language pathologists, psychologists, psyciatrists and other professionals can answer the 50 yes/no items in 10 to 15 minutes. *$100.00*

2951 Children and Youth with Asperger Syndrome
Program Development Associates
PO Box 2038
Syracuse, NY 13220-2038
315-452-0643
Fax: 315-452-0710
E-mail: info@disabilitytraining.com
www.disabilitytraining.com

Classroom teachers now get special information to accommodate students with Asperger Syndrome, who display symptoms similar to, but milder than, autism. Strategies include research-based instructional, behavioral and environmental modifications. *$35.95*

200 pages

ADHD

2952 ADHD in Adolesents: Diagnosis and Treatment
Guilford Publications
72 Spring Street
New York, NY 10012
212-431-9800
800-365-7006
Fax: 212-966-6708
E-mail: info@guilford.com
www.guilford.com

Practical reference with a down to earth approach to diagnosing and treatment of ADHD in adolesents. A structured intervention program with guidelines to using educational, psycholgical and medical components to help patients.

461 pages   Year Founded: 1999 ISBN 1-572305-45-2

2953 ADHD in Adulthood: Guide to Current Theory, Diagnosis and Treatment
Johns Hopkins University Press
2715 North Charles Street
Baltimore, MD 21218-4363
410-516-6900
800-537-5487
Fax: 410-516-6968
www.press.jhu.edu

Discusses how ADHD manifests itself in adult life and answers popular questions posed by physicians and by adults with ADHD. Provides health professionals with a practical approach for treatment and diagnosis in adult ADHD patients. *$49.95*

392 pages   Year Founded: 1999 ISBN 0-801861-41-1

2954 All About ADHD: Complete Practical Guide for Classroom Teachers
ADD WareHouse
300 NW 70th Avenue
Suite 102
Plantation, FL 33317
954-792-8100
800-233-9273
Fax: 954-792-8545
E-mail: sales@addwarehouse.com
www.addwarehouse.com

Brings together both the art and science of effective teaching for students with ADHD using the Parallel Teaching Model as the base for blending behavior management and teaching, particularly in regular classroom settings.

2955 Attention Deficit Disorder ADHD and ADD Syndromes
Pro-Ed Publications
8700 Shoal Creek Boulevard
Austin, TX 78757-6816
512-451-3246
800-897-3202
Fax: 800-397-7633
E-mail: info@proedinc.com
www.proedinc.com

This book enters its third edition with even more complete explanations of how ADHD and ADD interfere with: class-room learning, behavior at home, job performance, and social skills development. *$ 19.00*

216 pages   Year Founded: 1998 ISBN 0-890797-42-0

2956 Attention Deficit Disorder and Learning Disabilities: Realities, Myths and Controversial Treatments
ADD WareHouse
300 NW 70th Avenue
Suite 102
Plantation, FL 33317
954-792-8100
800-233-9273
Fax: 954-792-8545
E-mail: sales@addwarehouse.com
www.addwarehouse.com

Designed to help parents and professionals recognize symptoms of learning disabilities and attentional disorders. Covers in detail conventional treatments that have been scientifically validated plus more controversial methods of treatment such as orthomolecular therapies, amino acid supplementation, dietary interventions, EEG biofeedback, cognitive therapy and visual training. *$13.00*

240 pages

2957 Attention Deficit/Hyperactivity Disorder
American Psychiatric Publishing
1000 Wilson Boulevard
Suite 1825
Arlington, VA 22209-3901
703-907-7322
800-368-5777
Fax: 703-907-1091
E-mail: appi@psych.org
www.appi.org

Clinical Guide to Diagnosis and Treatment for Health and Mental Health Professionals making the proper diagnosis, and treatment strategies. *$29.95*

298 pages   Year Founded: 1999 ISBN 0-880489-40-5

2958 Attention-Deficit Hyperactivity Disorder: A Handbook for Diagnosis and Treatment
Guilford Publications
72 Spring Street
New York, NY 10012
212-431-9800
800-365-7006
Fax: 212-966-6708
E-mail: info@guilford.com
www.guilford.com

This second edition incorporates the latest finding on the nature, diagnosis, assessment and treatment of ADHD. Includes select chapters by seasoned colleagues covering their respective areas of expertise and providing clear guidelines for practice in clinical, school and community settings. *$56.95*

602 pages   Year Founded: 1998 ISBN 1-572302-75-5

2959 Attention-Deficit/Hyperactivity Disorder in the Classroom
Pro-Ed Publications
8700 Shoal Creek Boulevard
Austin, TX 78757-6816
512-451-3246
800-897-3202

Fax: 800-397-7633
E-mail: info@proedinc.com
www.proedinc.com

Provides educators with a complete guide on how to deal effectively with students with attention deficits in their classroom. Emphasizes practical applications for teachers to use that will facilitate the success of students, both academically and socially, in a school setting. *$29.00*

291 pages Year Founded: 1998 ISBN 0-890796-65-3

2960 Family Therapy for ADHD: Treating Children, Adolesents and Adults
Guilford Publications
72 Spring Street
New York, NY 10012
212-431-9800
800-365-7006
Fax: 212-966-6708
E-mail: info@guilford.com
www.guilford.com

ADHD affects the entire family. This book helps the clinician evaluate its impact on marital dynamics, parent/sibling/child relationships and the complex treatment of ADHD in a larger context. Includes session by session plans and clinical material. *$32.95*

270 pages Year Founded: 1999 ISBN 1-572304-38-3

2961 How to Operate an ADHD Clinic or Subspecialty Practice
ADD WareHouse
300 NW 70th Avenue
Suite 102
Plantation, FL 33317
954-792-8100
800-233-9273
Fax: 954-792-8545
E-mail: sales@addwarehouse.com
www.addwarehouse.com

This book goes beyond academic discussions of ADHD and gets down to how to establish and manage an ADHD practice. In addition to practice guidelines and suggestions, this guide presents a compendium of clinic forms and letters, interview formats, sample reports, tricks of the trade and resource listings, all of which will help you develop or refine your clinic/counseling operation. *$65.00*

325 pages

2962 Medications for Attention Disorders and Related Medical Problems: A Comprehensive Handbook
ADD WareHouse
300 NW 70th Avenue
Suite 102
Plantation, FL 33317
954-792-8100
800-233-9273
Fax: 954-792-8545
E-mail: sales@addwarehouse.com
www.addwarehouse.com

ADHD and ADD are medical conditions and often medical intervention is regarded by most experts as an essential component of the multimodal program for the treatment of these disorders. This text presents a comprehensive look at medications and their use in attention disorders. *$37.00*

420 pages

2963 Parenting a Child With Attention Deficit/Hyperactivity Disorder
Pro-Ed Publications
8700 Shoal Creek Boulevard
Austin, TX 78757-6816
512-451-3246
800-897-3202
Fax: 800-397-7633
E-mail: info@proedinc.com
www.proedinc.com

Offers proven parenting approaches for helping children between the ages of 5-11 years improve their behavior. *$29.00*

150 pages Year Founded: 1999 ISBN 0-890797-91-9

2964 Pretenders: Gifted People Who Have Difficulty Learning
High Tide Press
3650 W 183rd Street
Homewood, IL 60430
708-206-2054
888-487-7377
Fax: 708-206-2044
E-mail: managing.editor@hightidepress.com
www.hightidepress.com

Monica Regan, Managing Editor

Profiles of 8 adults with dyslexia and/or ADD with whom the author has worked. Informative, fascinating, at times heartbreaking, but ultimately inspiring. *$24.50*

177 pages ISBN 1-892696-06-1

Autistic Disorder

2965 Asperger Syndrome: a Practical Guide for Teachers
ADD WareHouse
300 NW 70th Avenue
Suite 102
Plantation, FL 33317
954-792-8100
800-233-9273
Fax: 954-792-8545
E-mail: sales@addwarehouse.com
www.addwarehouse.com

A clear and concise guide to effective classroom practice for teachers and support assistants working with children with Asperger Syndrome in school. The authors explain characteristics of children with Asperger Syndrome, discuss methods of assessment and offer practical strategies for effective classroom interventions. *$24.95*

90 pages

Cognitive Disorders

2966 Geriatric Mental Health Care: A Treatment Guide for Health Professionals
Guilford Publications
72 Spring Street
New York, NY 10012
212-431-9800
800-365-7006
Fax: 212-966-6708
E-mail: info@guilford.com
www.guilford.com

Designed for mental health practitioners and primary care providers without advanced training in geriatric psychiatry. Covers depression, anxiety, the dementias, psychosis, mania, sleep disturbances, personality and pain disorders, adapting principles, sexuality, elder issues, alcohol and substance abuse, suicide risk, consultation, legal and ethic issues, exercise and much more. *$39.00*

347 pages ISBN 1-572305-92-4

2967 Guidelines for the Treatment of Patients with Alzheimer's Disease and Other Dementias of Late Life
American Psychiatric Publishing
1000 Wilson Boulevard
Suite 1825
Arlington, VA 22209-3901
703-907-7322
800-368-5777
Fax: 703-907-1091
E-mail: appi@psych.org
www.appi.org

Katie Duffy, Marketing Assistant

Diagnosis and treatment strategies. *$22.50*

40 pages Year Founded: 1995 ISBN 0-890423-04-0

2968 Loss of Self: Family Resource for the Care of Alzheimer's Disease and Related Disorders
WW Norton & Company
500 5th Avenue
New York, NY 10110
212-790-9456
Fax: 212-869-0856
E-mail: admalmud@wwnorton.com
www.wwnorton.com

How to help a relative and also meet a family's own needs during the long and tragic period of care involved with Alzheimer's Disease. Challenges are more than medical and can be emotional, involve family conflict, sexuality, abuse, and eventually, dealing with death. As well as the emotional challenges, the latest treatments, drugs and diagnosis information, plus causes and preventative measures are included. *$27.95*

432 pages Year Founded: 2001 ISBN 0-393050-16-5

2969 Neurobiology of Primary Dementia
American Psychiatric Publishing
1000 Wilson Boulevard
Suite 1825
Arlington, VA 22209-3901
703-907-7322
800-368-5777
Fax: 703-907-1091
E-mail: appi@psych.org
www.appi.org

Katie Duffy, Marketing Assistant

Study of aging and Alzheimer's. Contains investigations of the basic neurobiologic aspects of the etiology of dementia, clear discussions of the diagnostic process with regard to imaging and other laboratory tests, psychopharmacologic treatment and genetic counseling. *$61.50*

440 pages Year Founded: 1998 ISBN 0-880489-15-4

2970 Strange Behavior Tales of Evolutionary Neurolgy
WW Norton & Company
500 5th Avenue
New York, NY 10110-0017
212-354-5500
800-233-4830
Fax: 212-869-0856
E-mail: webmaster@wwnorton.com
www.wwnorton.com

Both educational and entertaining, the author presents an array of people with unusual problems who have one thing in common, brain disorder. Carefully constructed, this book outlines the functioning of the brain and evolution of language skills. *$13.95*

256 pages Year Founded: 2001 ISBN 0-393321-84-3

2971 The New Handbook of Cognitive Therapy Techniques
WW Norton & Company
500 5th Avenue
New York, NY 10110-0017
212-354-5500
800-233-4830
Fax: 212-869-0856
E-mail: npb@wwnorton.com
www.wwnorton.com/psych

Describes, explains, and demonstrates over a hundred cognitive therapy techniques, offering for each the theorretical basis, a thumbnail description of the method, case examples, and resources for further information.
ISBN 0-393703-13-4

Conduct Disorder

2972 Behavioral Risk Management
Jossey-Bass Publishers
350 Sansome Street
5th Floor
San Francisco, CA 94104
415-394-8677
800-956-7739
Fax: 800-605-2665
www.josseybass.com

Learn to identify potential mental health and behavioral problems on the job and apply effective intervention strategies for behavioral risk. *$41.95*

432 pages ISBN 0-787902-20-9

2973 Beyond Behavior Modification: Cognitive-Behavioral Approach to Behavior Management in the School
Pro-Ed Publications
8700 Shoal Creek Boulevard
Austin, TX 78757-6816
512-451-3246
800-897-3202
Fax: 800-397-7633
E-mail: info@proedinc.com
www.proedinc.com

Focuses on traditional behavior modification, and presents a social learning theory approach. *$39.00*

643 pages Year Founded: 1995 ISBN 0-890796-63-7

2974 Effective Discipline
Pro-Ed Publications
8700 Shoal Creek Boulevard
Austin, TX 78757-6816
512-451-3246
800-897-3202
Fax: 800-397-7633
E-mail: info@proedinc.com
www.proedinc.com

Designed to provide principals, counselors, teachers, and college students preparing to become educators with information about research-based techniques that reduce or eliminate school behavior problems. Provides the knowledge to prevent discipline problems, identify specific behaviors that disrupt the environment, match interventions with behavioral infractions, implement a variety of intervention tactics, and evaluate the effectiveness of the intervention program. *$28.00*

220 pages Year Founded: 1993 ISBN 0-890795-79-7

2975 Helping Parents, Youth, and Teachers
Understand Medications for Behavioral and
Emotional Problems
American Psychiatric Press
1000 Wilson Boulevard
Suite 1825
Arlington, VA 22209-3901
703-907-7322
800-368-5777
Fax: 703-907-1091
E-mail: appi@psych.org
www.appi.org

Katie Duffy, Marketing Assistant

Valuable resource for anyone involved in evaluating psychiatric disturbances in children and adolescents. Provides a compilation of information sheets to help promote the dialogue between the patient's family, caregivers and the treating physician. *$39.95*

196 pages Year Founded: 1999 ISBN 0-880487-94-1

2976 Inclusion Strategies for Students with Learning
and Behavior Problems
Pro-Ed Publications
8700 Shoal Creek Boulevard
Austin, TX 78757-6816
512-451-3246
800-897-3202
Fax: 800-397-7633
E-mail: info@proedinc.com
www.proedinc.com

Provides the components necessary to implement successful inclusion by presenting the experience of those directly impacted by inclusion: an individual with a disability; parents of a student with a disbility; teachers who implement inclusion; and researchers of best practices. Integrates theory and practice in an easy, how-to manner. *$36.00*

416 pages Year Founded: 1997 ISBN 0-890796-98-X

2977 Outrageous Behavior Mood: Handbook of
Strategic Interventions for Managing
Impossible Students
Pro-Ed Publications
8700 Shoal Creek Boulevard
Austin, TX 78757-6816

512-451-3246
800-897-3202
Fax: 800-397-7633
E-mail: info@proedinc.com
www.proedinc.com

This handbook is for educators who have had success in managing difficult students. Introduces such methods as planned confusion, disruptive word pictures, unconscious suggestion, double-bind predictions, off the wall interpretations, and even some straight faced paradoxical assignments. *$26.00*

154 pages Year Founded: 1999 ISBN 0-890798-17-6

Depression

2978 A Woman Doctor's Guide to Depression
Hyperion
www.hyperionbooks.com

Includes information on what depression feels like and how it affects daily life, women's unique risks of developing depression throughout the life cycle from puberty to menopause and current treatment strategies and their risks and benefits, preventive measures and warning signs. *$9.95*

176 pages Year Founded: 1997 ISBN 0-786881-46-1

2979 Active Treatment of Depression
WW Norton & Company
500 5th Avenue
New York, NY 10110
212-790-9456
Fax: 212-869-0856
E-mail: admalmud@wwnorton.com
www.wwnorton.com

A candid discussion on depression and effective, hopeful therapy strategies. *$35.00*

272 pages Year Founded: 2001 ISSN 70322-3

2980 Antidepressant Fact Book: What Your Doctor
Won't Tell You About Prozac, Zoloft, Paxil,
Celexa and Luvox
Perseus Books Group
550 Central Avenue
Boulder, CO 80301
800-386-5656
Fax: 720-406-7336
E-mail: westview.orders@perseusbooks.com
www.perseusbooksgroup.com

What antidepressants will and won't treat, documented side and withdrawl effects, plus what parents need to know about teenagers and antidepressants. The author has been a medical expert in many court cases invloving the use and misuse of psychoactive drugs. *$13.00*

240 pages Year Founded: 2001 ISBN 0-738204-51-X

2981 Antipsychotic Medications: A Guide
Madison Institute of Medicine
7617 Mineral Point Road
Suite 300
Madison, WI 53717-1623
608-827-2470
Fax: 608-827-2479
E-mail: mim@miminc.org
www.miminc.org

A number of medications are available today to treat schizophrenia and other illnesses that may lead to psychotic behaviors. This concise guide covers antipsychotic medications available today and provides information about correct dosing and possible side effects. *$5.95*

39 pages

2982 Brief Therapy for Adolescent Depression
Professional Resource Press
PO Box 15560
Sarasota, FL 34277-1560
941-343-9601
800-443-3364
Fax: 941-343-9201
E-mail: orders@prpress.com
www.prpress.com

Debra Fink, Managing Editor

Useful book for practicing clinicians and advanced students interested in building new skills for working with depressed young people. Written from the perspective that adaptations of cognitive therapy are necessary when working with adolescents both because of the difference in thinking (relative verses absolute) between adults and adolescents, and because adolescents are deeply embedded in their families of origin and effective treatment rarely can be conducted without intervening with the family. Includes detailed clinical vignettes to illustrate key principles and techniques of this treatment model. *$13.95*

112 pages Year Founded: 1997 ISBN 1-568870-28-0

2983 Cognitive Therapy of Depression
Guilford Publications
72 Spring Street
New York, NY 10012
212-431-9800
800-365-7006
Fax: 212-966-6708
E-mail: info@guilford.com
www.guilford.com

Shows how psychotherapists can effectively treat depressive disorders. Case examples illustrate a wide range of strategies and techniques. Chapter topics include the role of emotions in cognitive therapy, application of behavioral techniques and cognitive therapy and antidepressant medications. Hardcover. Paperback also available. *$ 46.95*

425 pages Year Founded: 1979 ISBN 0-898620-00-7

2984 Concise Guide to Women's Mental Health
American Psychiatric Publishing
1000 Wilson Boulevard
Suite 1825
Arlington, VA 22209-3901
703-907-7322
800-368-5777
Fax: 703-907-1091
E-mail: appi@psych.org
www.appi.org

Katie Duffy, Marketing Assistant

Examines the biological, psychological, and sociocultural factors that influence a woman's mental health and often contribute to psychiatric disorders. Supplies clinicians with important information on gender related differences on differential diagnosis, case formulation and treatment planning. Topics include premenstrual dysphoric disorder, hormonal contraception and effects on mood, psychiatric disorders in pregnancy, postpartum psychiatric disorders and perimenopause and menopause. *$21.95*

187 pages Year Founded: 1997 ISBN 0-880483-43-1

2985 Depression & Antidepressants
Madison Institute of Medicine
7617 Mineral Point Road
Suite 300
Madison, WI 53717-1623
608-827-2470
Fax: 608-827-2479
E-mail: mim@miminc.org
www.miminc.org

A concise, up-to-date guide to the wide range of medications available today for the treatment of depression. *$5.95*

48 pages ISBN 1-890802-19-0

2986 Depression in Context: Strategies for Guided Action
WW Norton & Company
500 5th Avenue
New York, NY 10110
212-790-9456
Fax: 212-869-0856
E-mail: admalmud@wwnorton.com
www.wwnorton.com

Description of Behavioral Activation, a new treatment for Depression. *$32.00*

224 pages Year Founded: 2001 ISSN 70350-9

2987 Evaluation and Treatment of Postpartum Emotional Disorders
Professional Resource Press
PO Box 15560
Sarasota, FL 34277-1560
941-343-9601
800-443-3364
Fax: 941-343-9201
E-mail: orders@prpress.com
www.prpress.com

Debra Fink, Managing Editor

Teaches how to recognize and treat postpartum emotional disorders. Procedures for clinical assessment, psychotherapeutic interventions, and medical - psychiatric treatments are described. *$ 13.95*

110 pages Year Founded: 1997 ISBN 1-568870-24-8

2988 Handbook of Depression
Guilford Publications
72 Spring Street
New York, NY 10012
212-431-9800
800-365-7006
Fax: 212-966-6708
E-mail: info@guilford.com
www.guilford.com

Brings together well-known authorities who address the need for a comprehensive review of the most current information available on depression. Surveys current theories and treatment models, covering both what the MD and non-MD needs to know. *$65.00*

628 pages Year Founded: 1995 ISBN 0-898628-41-5

2989 Interpersonal Psychotherapy
American Psychiatric Publishing
1000 Wilson Boulevard
Suite 1825
Arlington, VA 22209-3901
703-907-7322
800-368-5777
Fax: 703-907-1091
E-mail: appi@psych.org
www.appi.org

Katie Duffy, Marketing Assistant

An overview of interpersonal psychotherapy for depression, preventative treatment for depression, bulimia nervosa and HIV positive men and women. *$26.00*

156 pages Year Founded: 1998 ISBN 0-880488-36-0

2990 Postpartum Mood Disorders
American Psychiatric Publishing
1000 Wilson Boulevard
Suite 1825
Arlington, VA 22209-3901
703-907-7322
800-368-5777
Fax: 703-907-1091
E-mail: appi@psych.org
www.appi.org

Katie Duffy, Marketing Assistant

$38.50

280 pages Year Founded: 1999 ISBN 0-880489-29-4

2991 Premenstrual Dysphoric Disorder: A Guide
Madison Institute of Medicine
7617 Mineral Point Road
Suite 300
Madison, WI 53717-1623
608-827-2470
Fax: 608-827-2479
E-mail: mim@miminc.org
www.miminc.org

This new 41 page booklet explains what Premenstrual Dysphoric Disorder (PMDD) is, how it is diagnosed, how it differs from PMS, and how it is treated. Anyone seeking information about PMDD and its treatments will find this concise guide of great benefit in their search for accurate, up-to-date information. *$5.95*

41 pages

2992 Scientific Foundations of Cognitive Theory and Therapy of Depression
John Wiley & Sons
605 3rd Avenue
New York, NY 10058-0180
212-850-6000
Fax: 212-850-6008
E-mail: info@wiley.com
www.wiley.com

A synthesis of decades of research and practice, this semminal book presents and critically evaluates this scientific and emprical status of co author Aaron Beck's revised cognitive theory and therapy of depression. The authors explore the evolution of cognitive theory and therapy of depression and discuss the future directions for the treatment of depression.

400 pages Year Founded: 1999

2993 Symptoms of Depression
John Wiley & Sons
605 3rd Avenue
New York, NY 10058-0180
212-850-6000
Fax: 212-850-6008
E-mail: info@wiley.com
www.wiley.com

336 pages Year Founded: 1993

2994 Treating Depressed Children: A Therapeutic Manual of Proven Cognitive Behavioral Techniques
New Harbinger Publications
5674 Shattuck Avenue
Oakland, CA 94609-1662
510-652-2002
800-748-6273
Fax: 510-652-5472
E-mail: customerservice@newharbinger.com
www.newharbinger.com

A full twelve session treatment program incorporates cartoons and role playing games to help children recognize emotions, change negative thoughts, gain confidence and learn crucial interpersonal skills. *$49.95*

160 pages Year Founded: 1996 ISBN 1-572240-61-X

2995 Treating Depression
Jossey-Bass Publishers
350 Sansome Street
5th Floor
San Francisco, CA 94104
415-394-8677
800-956-7739
Fax: 800-605-2665
www.josseybass.com

$27.95

244 pages ISBN 0-787915-85-8

2996 Treatment of Recurrent Depression
American Psychiatric Publishing
1000 Wilson Boulevard
Suite 1825
Arlington, VA 22209-3901
703-907-7322
800-368-5777
Fax: 703-907-1091
E-mail: appi@psych.org
www.appi.org

Katie Duffy, Marketing Assistant

Five topics covered are, Lifetime Impact of Gender on Recurrent Major Depressive Disorder in Women, Treatment Stategies, Prevention of Recurrences in Bipolar Patients, Potential Applications and Updated Recommendations. *$29.95*

208 pages Year Founded: 2001 ISBN 1-585620-25-4

Dissociative Disorders

2997 Dissociative Identity Disorder: Diagnosis, Clinical Features, and Treatment of Multiple Personality
John Wiley & Sons
605 3rd Avenue
New York, NY 10058-0180

212-850-6000
Fax: 212-850-6008
E-mail: info@wiley.com
www.wiley.com

Comprehensive and interesting, this account of the history of MPD dispells many myths and presents new insight into the treatment of MPD. Perfect for sexual abuse clinics, child abuse agencies, correctional facilities and clinicians of all fields. *$64.50*

Year Founded: 1996 ISBN 0-471132-65-9

2998 Handbook of Dissociation: Theoretical, Empirical, and Clinical Perspectives
Kluwer Academic/Plenum Publishers
233 Spring Street
New York, NY 10013
212-620-8000
Fax: 212-463-0742
www.kluweronline.com

Covers both current and emerging theories, research and treatment of dissociative phenomena. Discusses historic, epidemiologic, phenomenologic, etiologic, normative and cross-cultural dimensions of dissociation, providing an empirical foundation for the last chapters. Eight case studies apply dissociation theory and research to specific treatment modalities. *$132.00*

615 pages Year Founded: 1996 ISBN 0-306451-50-6

Eating Disorders

2999 Biting The Hand That Starves You: Inspiring Resistance to Anorexia/Bulimia
WW Norton & Company
500 5th Avenue
New York, NY 10110-0017
212-354-5500
800-233-4830
Fax: 212-869-0856
E-mail: npb@wwnorton.com
www.wwnorton.com/psych

Details a unique way of thinking and speaking about anorexia/bulimia (a/b), by having conversations with insiders in which the problem is viewed as an external influence rather than a part of the person. Coercion is sidestepped in favor of practices that are collaborative, accountable, and spirit-nurturing.

ISBN 0-393703-37-1

3000 Drug Therpay and Eating Disorders
Mason Crest Publishers
370 Reed Road
Suite 302
Broomall, PA 19008
610-543-6200
866-627-2665
Fax: 610-543-3878
E-mail: dtaylor@masoncrest.com
www.masoncrest.com

Provides a clear, concise account of the history, symptoms, and current treatment of anorexia nervosa and bulimia nervosa. It is estimated the eating disorders affect five million Americans each year, and many more millions among other nations.

ISBN 1-590845-65-X

3001 Handbook of Treatment for Eating Disorders
Guilford Publications
72 Spring Street
New York, NY 10012
212-431-9800
800-365-7006
Fax: 212-966-6708
E-mail: info@guilford.com
www.guilford.com

Includes coverage of binge eating and examines pharmacological as well as therapeutic approaches to eating disorders. Presents cognitive behavioral, psychoeducational, interpersonal, family, feminist, group and psychodynamic approaches, as well as the basics of pharmacological management. Features strategies for handling sexual abuse, substance abuse, concurrent medical conditions, personality disorder, prepubertal eating disorders and patients who refuse therapy. *$56.95*

540 pages Year Founded: 1997 ISBN 1-572301-86-4

3002 Interpersonal Psychotherapy
American Psychiatric Publishing
1000 Wilson Boulevard
Suite 1825
Arlington, VA 22209-3901
703-907-7322
800-368-5777
Fax: 703-907-1091
E-mail: appi@psych.org
www.appi.org

Katie Duffy, Marketing Assistant

An overview of interpersonal psychotherapy for depression, preventative treatment for depression, bulimia nervosa and HIV positive men and women. *$26.00*

156 pages Year Founded: 1998 ISBN 0-880488-36-0

3003 Sexual Abuse and Eating Disorders
200 E Joppa Road
Suite 207
Baltimore, MD 21286
410-825-8888
888-825-8249
Fax: 410-337-0747
E-mail: sidran@sidran.org
www.sidran.org

This is the first book to explore the complex relationship between sexual abuse and eating disorders. Sexual abuse is both an extreme boundary violation and a disruption of attachment and bonding; victims of such abuse are likely to exhibit symptoms of self injury, including eating disorders. This volume is a discussion of the many ways that sexual abuse and eating disorders are related, also has accounts by a survivor of both. Investigates the prevalence of sexual abuse among individuals with eating disorders. Also examines how a history of sexual violence can serve as a predictor of subsequent problems with food. Looks at related social factors, reviews trauma based theories, more controversial territory and discusses delayed memory versus false memory. *$34.95*

228 pages

Factitious Disorder

3004 Munchausen Syndrome by Proxy: Issues in Diagnosis and Treatment
Lexington Books
4501 Forbes Boulevard
Suite 200
Lanham, MD 20706
301-459-3365
www.lexingtonbooks.com

AV Levin, Editor
MS Sheridan, Editor

Reference/Resource material for professionals.

Year Founded: 1995

3005 Munchausen by Proxy Syndrome: Misunderstood Child Abuse
Sage Publications
2455 Teller Road
Thousand Oaks, CA 91320
800-818-7243
www.sagepub.com

Teresa F Parnell
Deborah O Day

Professional reference/resource book

Year Founded: 1998

3006 Munchausen by Proxy: Identification, Intervention, and Case Management
Haworth Press
10 Alice Street
Binghamton, NY 13904
800-429-6784
Fax: 800-895-0582
E-mail: getinfo@haworthpress.com
www.haworthpress.com

Louisa J Lasher, Author
Mary S Sheridan, Author

A step-by-step guide to help identify and manage cases of this unique form of child maltreatment. *$59.95*

384 pages Year Founded: 2004 ISBN 0-789012-17-0

Gender Identification Disorder

3007 Gender Loving Care
WW Norton & Company
500 5th Avenue
New York, NY 10110
212-790-9456
Fax: 212-869-0856
E-mail: admalmud@wwnorton.com
www.wwnorton.com

Understanding and treating gender identity disorder, especially transexuals, who may feel stuck in the wrong-sexed body. *$ 25.00*

196 pages Year Founded: 1999 ISBN 0-393703-40-5

3008 Homosexuality and American Psychiatry: The Politics of Diagnosis
Princeton University Press
Princeton University
Princeton, NJ 08544
800-777-4726
Fax: 800-999-1958
www.pup.princeton.edu
$18.00

249 pages Year Founded: 1987 ISBN 0-691028-37-0

3009 Identity Without Selfhood
Cambridge University Press
40 W 20th Street
New York, NY 10011-4221
212-924-3900
Fax: 212-691-3239
E-mail: marketing@cup.org
www.cup.org

Mariam Fraser

Situated at the crossroads of feminism, queer theory and poststructuralist debates around identity, this is a book that shows how key Western concepts such as individuality constrain attempts to deconstruct the self and prevent bisexuality being understood as an identity. *$64.95*

226 pages Year Founded: 1999

3010 Principles and Practice of Sex Therapy
Guilford Publications
72 Spring Street
New York, NY 10012
212-431-9800
800-365-7006
Fax: 212-966-6708
E-mail: info@guilford.com
www.guilford.com

Many new developments in theory, diagnosis and treatment of sexual disorders have occured in the past decade. The authors set clear guidlines for assessment and treatment with fresh clinical material. A text for professionals and students in a wide range of mental health fields; sexual disorders, male and female, paraphilias, gender identity disorders, vasoactive drugs and more are covered. *$50.00*

518 pages Year Founded: 2000 ISBN 1-572305-74-6

3011 Psychoanalytic Therapy & the Gay Man
Analytic Press
101 W Street
Hillsdale, NJ 07642-1421
201-358-9477
800-926-6579
Fax: 201-358-4700
E-mail: TAP@analyticpress.com
www.analyticpress.com

Paul E Stepansky PhD, Managing Director
John Kerr PhD, Sr Editor

Explores of the subjectivities of gay men in psychoanalytic psychotherapy. It is a vitally human testament to the richly varied inner experiences of gay men. Offers that sexual identity, which encompass a spectrum of possibilities for any gay man, must be addressed in an atmosphere of honest encounter that allows not only for exploration of conflict and dissasociation but also for restitutive conformation of the patient's right to be himself. Available in hardcover. *$55.00*

384 pages Year Founded: 1998 ISBN 0-881632-08-2

3012 Transvestites and Transsexuals: Toward a Theory of Cross-Gender Behavior
Kluwer Academic/Plenum Publishers
233 Spring Street
New York, NY 10013

212-620-8000
Fax: 212-463-0742
www.kluweronline.com

This book proposes a theory of transvestism and transexualism presented with a large amount of important raw data collected from interviews with one hundred ten transvestites and thirty five of their wives. *$54.00*

266 pages Year Founded: 1988 ISBN 0-306428-78-4

Impulse Control Disorders

3013 Abusive Personality: Violence and Control in Intimate Relationships
Guilford Publications
72 Spring Street
New York, NY 10012
212-431-9800
800-365-7006
Fax: 212-966-6708
E-mail: info@guilford.com
www.guilford.com

A study of domestic violence, especially male perpetrators. *$26.95*

214 pages Year Founded: 1998 ISBN 1-572303-70-0

3014 Coping With Self-Mutilation: a Helping Book for Teens Who Hurt Themselves
Rosen Publishing Group
29 E 21st Street
New York, NY 10010-6209
800-237-9932
Fax: 888-436-4643
E-mail: info@rosenpub.com
www.rosenpublishing.com

Examines the reasons for this phenomenon, and ways one might seek help. *$17.95*

Year Founded: 1999 ISBN 0-823925-59-5

3015 Dealing with Anger Problems: Rational-Emotive Therapeutic Interventions
Professional Resource Press
PO Box 15560
Sarasota, FL 34277-1560
941-343-9601
800-443-3364
Fax: 941-343-9201
E-mail: orders@prpress.com
www.prpress.com

Debra Fink, Managing Editor

Demonstrates ways to apply rational-emotive therapy techniques to help your clients control their anger. Offers step-by-step anger control treatment program that includes a variety of cognitive, emotive, and behavioral homework assignments, and procedures for modifying behaviors and facilitating change. *$11.95*

68 pages Year Founded: 1990 ISBN 0-943158-59-1

3016 Domestic Violence 2000: Integrated Skills Program for Men
WW Norton & Company
500 5th Avenue
New York, NY 10110
212-790-9456
Fax: 212-869-0856

E-mail: admalmud@wwnorton.com
www.wwnorton.com

Various theories are examined to deal with this difficult social problem. For group classes. *$23.20*

224 pages Year Founded: 1999 ISSN 70314-2

3017 Sex Murder and Sex Aggression: Phenomenology Psychopathology, Psychodynamics and Prognosis
Charles C Thomas Publisher
2600 S 1st Street
Springfield, IL 62704-4730
217-789-8980
800-258-8980
Fax: 217-789-9130
E-mail: books@ccthomas.com
www.ccthomas.com

By Eugene Revitch, Robert Wood Johnson School of Medicine, Piscataway, New Jersey, and Louis B Schlesinger, New Jersey Medical School, Newark. With a foreword by Robert R Hazelwood. Contents: The Place of Gynocide and Sexual Aggression in the Classification of Crime; Catathymic Gynocide; Compulsive Gynocide; Psychodynamics, Psychopathology and Differential Diagnosis; Prognostic Considerations. *$43.95*

152 pages Year Founded: 1989 ISSN 0-398-06346-XISBN 0-398055-56-4

3018 Teaching Behavioral Self Control to Students
Pro-Ed Publications
8700 Shoal Creek Boulevard
Austin, TX 78757-6816
512-451-3246
800-897-3202
Fax: 800-397-7633
E-mail: info@proedinc.com
www.proedinc.com

Demonstrates how teachers, counselors and parents can help children of all ages and ability levels to modify their own behavior. Clear step-by-step methods describe how common childhood problems can be solved by helping children become more responsible and independent. *$ 21.00*

122 pages Year Founded: 1995 ISBN 0-890796-17-3

Obsessive Compulsive Disorder

3019 Current Treatments of Obsessive-Compulsive Disorder
American Psychiatric Publishing
1000 Wilson Boulevard
Suite 1825
Arlington, VA 22209-3901
703-907-7322
800-368-5777
Fax: 703-907-1091
E-mail: appi@psych.org
www.appi.org

Helps clinicians better match treatment approaches with each patients unique needs.

Year Founded: 01 ISBN 0-880487-79-8

3020 Motivational Interviewing: Prepare People to Change Addictive Behavior
Hazelden
15251 Pleasant Valley Road
PO Box 176
Center City, MN 55012-0176
651-213-2121
800-328-9000
Fax: 651-213-4590
www.hazelden.org

William K Miller, Co-Author
Stephen Rollnick, Co-Author

A key resource for clinical psychologists, social workers and chemical dependency counselors for mastering interviewing skills and working with resistant clients. *$21.95*

348 pages ISBN 0-898624-69-X

3021 Obsessive-Compulsive Disorder: Contemporary Issues in Treatment
Lawrence Erlbaum Associates
10 Industrial Avenue
Mahwah, NJ 07430-2262
201-825-3200
800-926-6577
Fax: 201-236-0072
E-mail: orders@erlbaum.com
www.erlbaum.com

Hardcover.

Year Founded: 00 ISBN 0-805828-37-0

3022 Obsessive-Compulsive and Related Disorders in Adults: a Comprehensive Clinical Guide
Cambridge University Press
40 W 20th Street
New York, NY 10011-4221
212-924-3900
Fax: 212-691-3239
E-mail: marketing@cup.org
www.cup.org

The author challenges the current implicit models used in alcohol problem prevention and demonstrates an ecological perspective of the community as a complex adaptive systems composed of interacting subsystems. This volume represents a new and sensible approach to the prevention of alcohol dependence and alcohol-related problems. *$65.00*

380 pages Year Founded: 1999 ISBN 0-521559-75-8

3023 Overcoming Obsessive-Compulsive Disorder
New Harbinger Publications
5674 Shattuck Avenue
Oakland, CA 94609-1662
510-652-2002
800-748-6273
Fax: 510-652-5472
E-mail: customerservice@newharbinger.com
www.newharbinger.com

A fourteen session treatment. *$11.95*

72 pages Year Founded: 1998 ISBN 1-572241-29-2

3024 Treatment of Obsessive Compulsive Disorder
Guilford Publications
72 Spring Street
New York, NY 10012
212-431-9800
800-365-7006

Fax: 212-966-6708
E-mail: info@guilford.com
www.guilford.com

Provides everything the mental health professional needs for working with clients who suffer from obsessions and compulsions. Supplies background by describing in detail up-to-date clinically relevant information and a step-by-step guide for conducting behavioral treatment. *$39.95*

224 pages Year Founded: 1993 ISBN 0-898621-84-4

Personality Disorders

3025 Bad Boys, Bad Men: Confronting Antisocial Personality Disorder
Oxford University Press
198 Madison Avenue
New York, NY 10016
212-726-6000
800-451-7556
Fax: 919-677-1303
www.oup-usa.org

This book examines the mental condition characterized by a serial pattern of bad behavior. Draws on case studies, scientific data, and current events. *$25.00*

256 pages Year Founded: 1999 ISBN 0-195121-13-9

3026 Biological Basis of Personality
Charles C Thomas Publisher
2600 S 1st Street
Springfield, IL 62704-4730
217-789-8980
800-258-8980
Fax: 217-789-9130
E-mail: books@ccthomas.com
www.ccthomas.com

H J Eysenck, Author

$70.95

420 pages Year Founded: 1977 ISBN 0-398005-38-9

3027 Biology of Personality Disorders
American Psychiatric Publishing
1000 Wilson Boulevard
Suite 1825
Arlington, VA 22209-3901
703-907-7322
800-368-5777
Fax: 703-907-1091
E-mail: appi@psych.org
www.appi.org

Katie Duffy, Marketing Assistant

Content topics include neurotransmitter function in personality disorders, new biological researcher strategies for personality disorders, the genetics psychobiology of the seven - factor model of personality disorders, and significance of biological research for a biopsychosocial model of personality disorders. *$25.00*

166 pages Year Founded: 1998 ISBN 0-880488-35-2

3028 Borderline Personality Disorder: A Therapist Guide to Taking Control
WW Norton & Company
500 5th Avenue
New York, NY 10110

212-354-5500
800-233-4830
Fax: 212-869-0856
E-mail: npb@wwnorton.com
www.wwnorton.com/psych

From identification to relapse prevention, this guide helps therapists manage a patient's treatment for the rather complex problem of Borderline Personality Disorder, an often difficult and sometimes life threatening condition. *$27.50*

224 pages Year Founded: 2002 ISBN 0-393703-52-5

3029 Borderline Personality Disorder: Tailoring the Psychotherapy to the Patient
American Psychiatric Publishing
1000 Wilson Boulevard
Suite 1825
Arlington, VA 22209-3901
703-907-7322
800-368-5777
Fax: 703-907-1091
E-mail: appi@psych.org
www.appi.org

Katie Duffy, Marketing Assistant

$34.00

256 pages Year Founded: 1996 ISBN 0-880486-89-9

3030 Cognitive Therapy for Personality Disorders: a Schema-Focused Approach
Professional Resource Press
PO Box 15560
Sarasota, FL 34277-1560
941-343-9601
800-443-3364
Fax: 941-343-9201
E-mail: orders@prpress.com
www.prpress.com

Debra Fink, Managing Editor

A guide to treating the most difficult cases in your practice: personality disorders and other chronic, self - defeating problems. Contains rationale, theory, practical applications, and active cognitive behavioral techniques. *$13.95*

96 pages Year Founded: 1999 ISBN 1-568870-47-7

3031 Cognitive Therapy of Personality Disorders
Guilford Publications
72 Spring Street
New York, NY 10012
212-431-9800
800-365-7006
Fax: 212-966-6708
E-mail: info@guilford.com
www.guilford.com

Focuses on the use of cognitive therapy to treat people with personality disorders who do not usually engage in therapy. Emanates the research and practical experience of Beck and his associates and is the first to focus specifically on this diverse and clinically demanding population. Case vignettes are used throughout. *$43.00*

396 pages Year Founded: 1990 ISBN 0-989624-34-7

3032 Dealing With the Problem of Low Self-Esteem: Common Characteristics and Treatment
Charles C Thomas Publisher
2600 S 1st Street
Springfield, IL 62704-4730
217-789-8980
800-258-8980
Fax: 217-789-9130
E-mail: books@ccthomas.com
www.ccthomas.com

Robert P Rugel, Author

Considers the practice of psychotherapy from the self-esteem perspective. Describes the common characteristics of low self-esteem that are manifested in clients with diverse problems; focuses on the functions the therapist performs in addressing these characteristics. The third is to consider the modalities of treatment through which the therapist delivers these therapeutic functions. *$ 48.95*

228 pages Year Founded: 1995 ISSN 0-398-05951-9ISBN 0-398059-36-5

3033 Disorders of Personality: DSM-IV and Beyond
John Wiley & Sons
605 3rd Avenue
New York, NY 10058-0180
212-850-6000
Fax: 212-850-6008
E-mail: info@wiley.com
www.wiley.com

Clarifies the distinctions between the vast array of personality disorders and helps clinicians make accurate diagnoses; thoroughly updated to incorporate the recent change in the DSM - IV. Guides the clinicians throught the intricate maze of personality disorders, with special attention on changes in their conceptualization over the last decade. *$85.00*

Year Founded: 1995 ISBN 0-471011-86-X

3034 Group Exercises for Enhancing Social Skills & Self-Esteem
Professional Resource Press
PO Box 15560
Sarasota, FL 34277-1560
941-343-9601
800-443-3364
Fax: 941-343-9201
E-mail: orders@prpress.com
www.prpress.com

Debra Fink, Managing Editor

Includes exercises for enhancing self-esteem utilizing proven social, emotional, and cognitive skill-building techniques. These exercises are useful in therapeutic, psychoeducational, and recreational settings. *$24.95*

150 pages Year Founded: 1996 ISBN 1-568870-20-5

3035 Personality Characteristics of the Personality Disordered
John Wiley & Sons
605 3rd Avenue
New York, NY 10058-0180
212-850-6000
Fax: 212-850-6008
E-mail: info@wiley.com
www.wiley.com

340 pages Year Founded: 1995

3036 Personality Disorders and Culture: Clinical and Conceptual Interactions
John Wiley & Sons
605 3rd Avenue
New York, NY 10058-0180
212-850-6000
Fax: 212-850-6008
E-mail: info@wiley.com
www.wiley.com

Discusses two of the most timely and complex areas in mental health, personality disorders and the impact of cultural variables. Treading on the timeless nature - nurture debate, it suggests that social variables have a dramatic impact on the definition, development, and manifestation of personality disorders.

310 pages Year Founded: 1998

3037 Personality and Stress: Individual Differences in the Stress Process
John Wiley & Sons
605 3rd Avenue
New York, NY 10058-0180
212-850-6000
Fax: 212-850-6008
E-mail: info@wiley.com
www.wiley.com

302 pages Year Founded: 1991

3038 Psychotherapy for Borderline Personality
John Wiley & Sons
605 3rd Avenue
New York, NY 10058-0180
212-850-6000
Fax: 212-850-6008
E-mail: info@wiley.com
www.wiley.com

Based on the work of a research team, this manual offers techniques and strategies for treating patients with Borderline Personality Disorder using Transference Focused Psychology. Provides therapists with an overall strategy for treating BPD patients and helpful tactics for working with individual patients on a session by session basis.

400 pages Year Founded: 1999

3039 Role of Sexual Abuse in the Etiology of Borderline Personality Disorder
200 E Joppa Road
Suite 207
Baltimore, MD 21286
410-825-8888
888-825-8249
Fax: 410-337-0747
E-mail: sidran@sidran.org
www.sidran.org

Presenting the latest generation of research findings about the impact of traumatic abuse on the development of BPD. This book focuses on the theoretical basis of BPD, including topics such as childhood factors associated with the development, the relationship of child sexual abuse to dissociation and self mutilation, severity of childhood abuse, borderline symptoms and family environment. Twenty six contributors cover every aspect of BPD as it relates to childhood sexual abuse. *$42.00*

248 pages

3040 Shorter Term Treatments for Borderline Personality Disorders
New Harbinger Publications
5674 Shattuck Avenue
Oakland, CA 94609-1662
510-652-2002
800-748-6273
Fax: 510-652-5472
E-mail: customerservice@newharbinger.com
www.newharbinger.com

This guide offers approaches designed to help clients stabilize emotions, decrease vulnerability and work toward a more adaptive day to day functioning. *$49.95*

184 pages Year Founded: 1997 ISBN 1-572240-92-X

3041 Treating Difficult Personality Disorders
Jossey-Bass Publishers
350 Sansome Street
5th Floor
San Francisco, CA 94104
415-394-8677
800-956-7739
Fax: 800-605-2665
www.josseybass.com

In this essential resource, experts in the field provide the most current information for the successful assessment and clinical treatment of this challenging client population. This book presents flexible treatment options for clients suffering from borderline, narcissistic, and antisocial personality disorders. *$28.95*

288 pages ISBN 0-787903-15-9

Post Traumatic Stress Disorder

3042 Body Remembers: Psychophysiology of Trauma and Trauma Treatment
WW Norton & Company
500 5th Avenue
New York, NY 10110
212-790-9456
Fax: 212-869-0856
E-mail: admalmud@wwnorton.com
www.wwnorton.com

Unites traditional verbal therapy and body oriented therapies for Post Traumatic Stress Disorder patients, as memories sometimes present in a physical disorder. *$30.00*

224 pages Year Founded: 2000 ISSN 70327-4

3043 Brief Therapy for Post Traumatic Stress Disorder
John Wiley & Sons
605 3rd Avenue
New York, NY 10058-0180
212-850-6000
Fax: 212-850-6008
E-mail: info@wiley.com
www.wiley.com

Discusses a new and exciting treatment technique that has proven to be more effective than the widely used direct theraputic exposure technique. Fills the growing need for a step by step practical treatment manual for PTSD using Traumatic Incident Reduction. It is an ideal companion to training workshops.

192 pages Year Founded: 1998

3044 Cognitive Processing Therapy for Rape Victims
Sage Publications
2455 Teller Road
Thousand Oaks, CA 91320
805-499-9774
800-818-7243
Fax: 800-583-2665
E-mail: info@sagepub.com
www.sagepub.com

Information regarding the assessment and treatment of rape victims. Discusses disorders that result from rape and add to a victim's suffering such as post traumatic stress, depression, poor self-esteem, interpersonal difficulties and sexual dysfunction. *$46.00*

192 pages Year Founded: 1993 ISBN 0-803949-01-4

3045 Concise Guide to Brief Dynamic Psychotherapy
American Psychiatric Publishing
1000 Wilson Boulevard
Suite 1825
Arlington, VA 22209-3901
703-907-7322
800-368-5777
Fax: 703-907-1091
E-mail: appi@psych.org
www.appi.org

Katie Duffy, Marketing Assistant

Seven brief psychodynamic therapy models including supportive, time - limited, interpersonal, time - limited dynamic, short term dynamic for post traumatic stress disorder and brief dynamic for substance abuse. *$21.00*

224 pages Year Founded: 1997 ISBN 0-880483-46-6

3046 Does Stress Damage the Brain? Understanding Trauma-Related Disorders from a Mind-Body Perspective
WW Norton & Company
500 5th Avenue
New York, NY 10110-0017
212-354-5500
800-233-4830
Fax: 212-869-0856
E-mail: npb@wwnorton.com
www.wwnorton.com/psych

Shows that extreme stress may result in lasting damage to the brain, especially a part of the brain involved in memory. This new neurobiological understanding of the relation between cognitive problems and trauma has many important implications for both self-understanding of trauma survivors and for the treatment of the effects of trauma.

ISBN 0-393704-74-2

3047 Effective Treatments for PTSD: Practice Guidelines from the International Society for Traumatic Stress Studies
Guilford Publications
72 Spring Street
New York, NY 10012
212-431-9800
800-365-7006
Fax: 212-966-6708
E-mail: info@guilford.com
www.guilford.com

Developed under the auspices of the PTSD Treatment Guidelines Task Force of the International Society for Trau-

matic Stress Studies, this comprehensive volume brings together leading authorities on psychological trauma to offer best practice guidelines for the treatment of PTSD. Approaches covered include acute interventions, cognitive-behavior therapy, pharmacotherapy, EMDR, group therapy, psychodynamic therapy, impatient treatment, psychosocial rehabilitation, hypnosis, creative therapies, marital and family treatment. *$42.00*

388 pages ISBN 1-572305-84-3

3048 Even from a Broken Web: Brief, Respectful Solution Oriented Therapy for Sexual Abuse and Trauma
WW Norton & Company
500 5th Avenue
New York, NY 10110
212-354-5500
800-233-4830
Fax: 212-869-0856
E-mail: npb@wwnorton.com
www.wwnorton.com/psych

Recent years have shown more people than ever coming to therapy with the after affects of sexual abuse. The authors provide therapists solution oriented treatment that considers a person's inner healing abilities. This method is less traumatic and disruptive to the patient's life than traditional therapies. *$16.95*

208 pages Year Founded: 2002 ISBN 0-393703-94-0

3049 Eye Movement Desensitization and Reprocessing: Basic Principles, Protocols, and Procedures
Guilford Publications
72 Spring Street
New York, NY 10012
212-431-9800
800-365-7006
Fax: 212-966-6708
E-mail: info@guilford.com
www.guilford.com

Reviews research and development, discusses theoretical constructs and possible underlying mechanisms, and presents protocols and procedures for treatment of adults and children with a range of presenting complaints. Material is applicable for victims of sexual abuse, crime, combat and phobias. *$45.00*

398 pages Year Founded: 1995 ISBN 0-898629-60-8

3050 Group Treatments for Post-Traumatic Stress Disorder
Brunner/Routledge
325 Chestnut Street
Philadelphia, PA 19106
800-821-8312
Fax: 215-269-0363
www.brunner-routledge.com

Contains contributions from renowned PTSD experts who provide group treatment to trauma survivors. It reviews the state-of-the-art applications of group therapy for such survivors of trauma as rape victims, combat veterans, adult survivors of childhood abuse, motor vehicle accident survivors, survivors of disaster, homicide witnesses and disaster relief workers. *$34.95*

216 pages ISBN 0-876309-83-X

3051 Life After Trauma: Workbook for Healing
Guilford Publications
72 Spring Street
New York, NY 10012
212-431-9800
800-365-7006
Fax: 212-966-6708
E-mail: info@guilford.com
www.guilford.com

Useful exercises for clinicians and trauma survivors, very empowering. *$17.95*

352 pages Year Founded: 1999 ISBN 1-572302-39-9

3052 Memory, Trauma and the Law
WW Norton & Company
500 5th Avenue
New York, NY 10110
212-790-9456
Fax: 212-869-0856
E-mail: admalmud@wwnorton.com
www.wwnorton.com

Professionals need to be informed of memory in the legal context to avoid malpractice liability suits. Recovered memory research, trauma treatment and the controversy of false memory in some cases are covered. *$100.00*

960 pages Year Founded: 1998 ISSN 70254-5

3053 Overcoming Post-Traumatic Stress Disorder
New Harbinger Publications
5674 Shattuck Avenue
Oakland, CA 94609-1662
510-652-2002
800-748-6273
Fax: 510-652-5472
E-mail: customerservice@newharbinger.com
www.newharbinger.com

An eleven to twenty four session treatment. *$11.95*

95 pages Year Founded: 1998 ISBN 1-572241-47-0

3054 PTSD in Children and Adolesents
American Psychiatric Publishing
1000 Wilson Boulevard
Suite 1825
Arlington, VA 22209-3901
703-907-7322
800-368-5777
Fax: 703-907-1091
E-mail: appi@psych.org
www.appi.org

Katie Duffy, Marketing Manager

Mental health and other professionals who work with Post Traumatic Stress Disorder and the young people who suffer from it will find discussions of evaluation, biological treatment strategies, the need for an integrated approach to juvenile offenders who suffer from PTSD and more. *$29.95*

208 pages Year Founded: 2001

3055 Perturbing the Organism: The Biology of Stressful Experience
University of Chicago Press
5801 S Ellis
Chicago, IL 60637
773-702-7700
Fax: 773-702-9756

E-mail: marketing@press.uchicago.edu
www.press.uchicago.edu

Critical analysis of the entire range of research and theory on stress in animals and humans, from the earliest studies in the 30's to present day. Includes empirical and conceptual advances of recent years, but also supplies a new working definition of stressful experience. Hardcover. *$40.50*

358 pages Year Founded: 1992 ISBN 0-226890-41-4

3056 Post Traumatic Stress Disorder
New Harbinger Publications
5674 Shattuck Avenue
Oakland, CA 94609-1662
510-652-2002
800-748-6273
Fax: 510-652-5472
E-mail: customerservice@newharbinger.com
www.newharbinger.com

Includes techniques for managing flashbacks, anxiety attacks, nightmares, insomnia, and dissociation; working through layers of pain; and handling survivor guilt, secondary wounding, low self esteem, victim thinking, anger, and depression. *$49.95*

384 pages Year Founded: 1994 ISBN 1-879237-68-7

3057 Post Traumatic Stress Disorder: Complete Treatment Guide
200 E Joppa Road
Suite 207
Baltimore, MD 21286
410-825-8888
888-825-8249
Fax: 410-337-0747
E-mail: sidran@sidran.org
www.sidran.org

For clinicians who want to work more effectively with trauma survivors, this textbook provides a step by step description of PTSD treatment strategies. Includes chapters on definitions, diagnostic criteria and the biochemistry of PTSD. Reflects a generalized 'ideal' structure of the healing process. Includes cognitive and behavioral techniques for managing flashbacks, anxiety attacks, sleep disturbances and dissociation; a comprehensive program for working through deeper layers of pain; plus PTSD related problems such as survivor guilt, secondary wounding, low self esteem, victim thinking, anger and depression. Presents trauma issues clearly for both general audiences and trauma professionals. *$49.95*

345 pages

3058 Posttraumatic Stress Disorders in Children and Adolescents Handbook
WW Norton & Company
500 5th Avenue
New York, NY 10110-0017
212-354-5500
800-233-4830
Fax: 212-869-0856
E-mail: npb@wwnorton.com
www.wwnorton.com/psych

The 15 chapters gathered here address different aspects of childhood and adolescent trauma-some consider a distinct therapeutic situation (abuse and neglect), others pertain to standard clinical procedure (assessment), and still others focus on complex research issues (neurobiology and genetics of PSTD).

ISBN 0-393704-12-2

3059 Rebuilding Shattered Lives: Responsible Treatment of Complex Post-Traumatic and Dissociative Disorders
John Wiley & Sons
605 3rd Avenue
New York, NY 10058-0180
212-850-6000
Fax: 212-850-6008
E-mail: info@wiley.com
www.wiley.com

The most up-to-date, integrative and emperically sound account of trauma theory and practice availible. Based on more than a decade of clinical research and treatment experience at the Harvard Medical School, this comprehensive and nontechnical text offers a stage oriented approach to understanding and treating complex and difficult traumatized patients, integrating modern trauma theory with traditional theraputic interventions. *$47.50*

256 pages Year Founded: 1998 ISBN 0-471247-32-4

3060 Remembering Trauma: Psychotherapist's Guide to Memory & Illusion
John Wiley & Sons
605 3rd Avenue
New York, NY 10058-0180
212-850-6000
Fax: 212-850-6008
E-mail: info@wiley.com
www.wiley.com

Amy Abzarnik, Conventions Coordinator

3061 Standing in the Spaces: Essays on Clinical Process, Trauma, and Dissociation
Analytic Press
101 W Street
Hillsdale, NJ 07642-1421
201-358-9477
800-926-6579
Fax: 201-358-4700
E-mail: TAP@analyticpress.com
www.analyticpress.com

Paul E Stepansky PhD, Managing Director
John Kerr PhD, Sr Editor

Bromberg's essays are delightfully unpredictable, as they strive to keep the reader continually abreast of how words can and cannot capture the subtle shifts in relatedness that characterize the clinical process. Radiating clinical wisdom infused with compassion and wit, Standing in the Spaces, is a classic destined to be read and reread by anlysts and therapists for decades to come. *$55.00*

376 pages Year Founded: 1998 ISBN 0-881632-46-5

3062 The Body Remembers Casebook: Unifying Methods and Models in the Treatment of Trauma and PTSD
WW Norton & Company
500 5th Avenue
New York, NY 10110-0017
212-354-5500
800-233-4830
Fax: 212-869-0856
E-mail: npb@wwnorton.com
www.wwnorton.com/psych

Emphasizes the importance of tailoring every trauma therapy to the particular needs of each individual client. Each varied and complex case is approached with a combination of methods ranging from traditional psychodynamic approaches and applications of attachment theory to innovative trauma methods including EMDR and Levine's SIBAM model.

ISBN 0-393704-00-9

3063 The Body Remembers: The Psychphysiology of Trauma and Trauma Treatment
WW Norton & Company
500 5th Avenue
New York, NY 10110-0017
212-354-5500
800-233-4830
Fax: 212-869-0856
E-mail: npb@wwnorton.com
www.wwnorton.com/psych

There is tremendous value in understanding the psychophysiology of trauma and knowing what to do about its manifestations. This book illuminates psychophysiology, casting light on the impact of trauma on the body and the phenomenon of somatic memory. Presents principles and non-touch techniques for giving the body its due.

ISBN 0-393703-27-4

3064 The Pathology of Man: A Study of Human Evil
Charles C Thomas Publishers
PO Box 19265
Springfield, IL 62794-9265
217-789-8980
800-258-8980
Fax: 217-789-9130
www.ccthomas.com

Deals with a topic that is both timely and of enduring importance. Expected to be a unique and important contribution that responds to the concerns of students and professionals in a wide range of diciplines. A comprehensive and solid study of the multi-casual nature of phonomenon that, until now, has been treated almost exclusively in terms of religion, myth, symbolism, moral philosophy, and ethics. Available in paperback for $53.95. *$73.95*

376 pages Year Founded: 2005 ISBN 0-398075-57-3

3065 The Trauma Spectrum: Hidden Wounds and Human Resiliency
WW Norton & Company
500 5th Avenue
New York, NY 10110-0017
212-354-5500
800-233-4830
Fax: 212-869-0856
E-mail: npb@wwnorton.com
www.wwnorton.com/psych

Scaer, a neurologist with over 30 years experience working with car accident victims, extends the conceptual and practical horizons of trauma treatment, redefining trauma as a continuum of variably negative life events occuring over a lifespan-including "little traumas" such as car accidents, risky medical interventions, childhood abuse and neglect, and social discrimination and poverty-that shape every aspect of our existence.

ISBN 0-393704-66-1

3066 Transforming Trauma: EMDR
WW Norton & Company
500 5th Avenue
New York, NY 10110
212-790-9456
Fax: 212-869-0856
E-mail: admalmud@wwnorton.com
www.wwnorton.com

Has helped thousands of people dealing with abuse histories or recent traumatic events. The author has a unique perspective, as she is both a client of EMDR and a therapist. *$14.95*

288 pages Year Founded: 1996 ISSN 31757-9

3067 Trauma Response
WW Norton & Company
500 5th Avenue
New York, NY 10110
212-790-9456
Fax: 212-869-0856
E-mail: admalmud@wwnorton.com
www.wwnorton.com

Different causes of psychological trauma and modes of recovery. *$22.36*

240 pages Year Founded: 1993

3068 Traumatic Events & Mental Health
Cambridge University Press
40 W 20th Street
New York, NY 10011-4221
212-924-3900
Fax: 212-691-3239
E-mail: marketing@cup.org
www.cup.org

Psychosomatic Disorders

3069 Anatomy of a Psychiatric Illness: Healing the Mind and the Brain
American Psychiatric Publishing
1000 Wilson Boulevard
Suite 1825
Arlington, VA 22209-3901
703-907-7322
800-368-5777
Fax: 703-907-1091
E-mail: appi@psych.org
www.appi.org

Katie Duffy, Marketing Assistant

  $22.95

232 pages Year Founded: 1993

3070 Concise Guide to Neuropsychiatry and Behavioral Neurology
American Psychiatric Publishing
1000 Wilson Boulevard
Suite 1825
Arlington, VA 22209-3901
703-907-7322
800-368-5777
Fax: 703-907-1091
E-mail: appi@psych.org
www.appi.org

Katie Duffy, Marketing Assistant

Provides brief synopsis of the major neuropsychiatric and neurobehavioral syndromes, discusses their clinical assessment, and provides guidelines for management. *$21.00*

368 pages Year Founded: 1995 ISBN 0-880483-43-1

3071 Concise Guide to Psychodynamic Psychotherapy: Principles and Techniques in the Era of Managed Care
American Psychiatric Publishing
1000 Wilson Boulevard
Suite 1825
Arlington, VA 22209-3901
703-907-7322
800-368-5777
Fax: 703-907-1091
E-mail: appi@psych.org
www.appi.org

Katie Duffy, Marketing Assistant

Thoroughly updated coverage of all the major principles and important issues in psychodynamic psychotherapy and issues not commonly addressed in the standard training curriculum, including the office setting, suicidal and dangerous patients, and what to do when the therapist makes an error. *$21.00*

272 pages Year Founded: 1998 ISBN 0-880483-47-4

3072 Functional Somatic Syndromes
Cambridge University Press
40 W 20th Street
New York, NY 10011-4221
212-924-3900
Fax: 212-691-3239
E-mail: marketing@cup.org
www.cup.org

3073 Manual of Panic: Focused Psychodynamic Psychotherapy
American Psychiatric Publishing
1000 Wilson Boulevard
Suite 1825
Arlington, VA 22209-3901
703-907-7322
800-368-5777
Fax: 703-907-1091
E-mail: appi@psych.org
www.appi.org

Katie Duffy, Marketing Assistant

A psychodynamic formulation applicable to many or most patients with Axis 1 panic disorders. *$28.00*

112 pages Year Founded: 1997 ISBN 0-880488-71-9

3074 Overcoming Specific Phobia
New Harbinger Publications
5674 Shattuck Avenue
Oakland, CA 94609-1662
510-652-2002
800-748-6273
Fax: 510-652-5472
E-mail: customerservice@newharbinger.com
www.newharbinger.com
  $9.95

72 pages Year Founded: 1998 ISBN 1-572241-15-2

3075 Somatization, Physical Symptoms and Psychological Illness
American Psychiatric Publishing
1000 Wilson Boulevard
Suite 1825
Arlington, VA 22209-3901
703-907-7322
800-368-5777
Fax: 703-907-1091
E-mail: appi@psych.org
www.appi.org

Katie Duffy, Marketing Assistant

$99.95

351 pages Year Founded: 1990 ISBN 0-632028-39-4

3076 Somatoform Dissociation: Phenomena, Measurem ent, and Theoretical Issues
WW Norton & Company
500 5th Avenue
New York, NY 10110-0017
212-354-5500
800-233-4830
Fax: 212-869-0856
E-mail: npb@wwnorton.com
www.wwnorton.com/psych

In this first North Americacn edition of his work, Nijenhuis expands upon his theory of somatoform dissociation by providing two new chapters-one on dissociation and the re-call of sexual abuse and a second on the phycometric characteristics of the Traumatic Experiences Checklist (TEC).

ISBN 0-393704-60-2

3077 Somatoform and Factitious Disorders
American Psychiatric Publishing
1000 Wilson Boulevard
Suite 1825
Arlington, VA 22209-3901
703-907-7322
800-368-5777
Fax: 703-907-1091
E-mail: appi@psych.org
www.appi.org

Katie Duffy, Marketing Assistant

Consise yet thorough, this book covers Factitious disorders, Somatization disorder, Conversion disorder, Hypochondriasis and Body dysmorphic disorder. Explores the latest on these conditions and emphasises the need for further research to improve patient treament and understanding. $29.95

208 pages Year Founded: 2001 ISBN 1-585620-29-7

Schizophrenia

3078 Behavioral High-Risk Paradigm in Psychopathology
Springer-Verlag New York
175 5th Avenue
New York, NY 10010-2485
212-460-1500
800-777-4643
Fax: 212-533-3503
E-mail: custserv@springer-ny.com
www.springer-ny.com

Examines both traditional clinical research on psychopathology and psychophysiological research on psychopathology, with an emphasis on risk for schizophrenia and for mood disorders. Complementing treatments of risk for psychopathology in other sources which emphasize either genetic factors or large-scale psychosocial factors, chapters focus on research in specific areas of each disorder. Hardcover. *$98.00*

304 pages Year Founded: 1995 ISBN 0-387945-04-0

3079 Cognitive Therapy for Delusions, Voices, and Paranoia
John Wiley & Sons
605 3rd Avenue
New York, NY 10058-0180
212-850-6000
Fax: 212-850-6008
E-mail: info@wiley.com
www.wiley.com

A cognitive view of delusions and voices. The practice of therapy and the problem of engagement.

230 pages Year Founded: 1995

3080 Delusional Beliefs
John Wiley & Sons
605 3rd Avenue
New York, NY 10058-0180
212-850-6000
Fax: 212-850-6008
E-mail: info@wiley.com
www.wiley.com

Unique collection of ideas and empirical data provided by leading experts in a variety of disciplines. Each offers perspectives on questions such as: What criteria should be used to identify, describe and classify delusions? How can delusional individuals be identified? What distinguishes delusions from normal beliefs? *$95.00*

352 pages Year Founded: 1988 ISBN 0-471836-35-4

3081 Families Coping with Schizophrenia: Practitioner's Guide to Family Groups
John Wiley & Sons
605 3rd Avenue
New York, NY 10058-0180
212-850-6000
Fax: 212-850-6008
E-mail: info@wiley.com
www.wiley.com

294 pages Year Founded: 1995

3082 Practice Guideline for the Treatment of Patients with Schizophrenia
American Psychiatric Publishing
1000 Wilson Boulevard
Suite 1825
Arlington, VA 22209-3901
703-907-7322
800-368-5777
Fax: 703-907-1091
E-mail: appi@psych.org
www.appi.org

Katie Duffy, Marketing Assistant

$22.00

146 pages Year Founded: 1997

3083 Schizophrenia Revealed: From Nuerons to Social Interactions
WW Norton & Company
500 5th Avenue
New York, NY 10110
212-354-5500
800-233-4830
Fax: 212-869-0856
E-mail: admalmud@wwnorton.com
www.wwnorton.com/psych

Helps explain some of the former mysteries of Schizophrenia that are now possible to study through advances in neuroscience. *$ 10.80*

Year Founded: 1979 ISBN 0-398704-48-1

Sexual Disorders

3084 Assessing Sex Offenders: Problems and Pitfalls
Charles C Thomas Publishers
PO Box 19265
Springfield, IL 62794-9265
217-789-8980
800-258-8980
Fax: 217-789-9130
www.ccthomas.com

This book reviews the scientific evidence relevant to assessing the recidivism risk of sex offenders. Too often, the issues detailed in these chapters have been overlooked and/or misinterpreted. As a result, the likelihood of psychologists misusing and abusing scientific data when assessing sex offenders whould not be underestimated. The text identifies numerous instances of such misuse and abuse. Paperback is available for $41.95. *$61.95*

266 pages Year Founded: 2004 ISBN 0-398075-02-6

3085 Erectile Dysfunction: Integrating Couple Therapy, Sex Therapy and Medical Treatment
WW Norton & Company
500 5th Avenue
New York, NY 10110
212-790-9456
Fax: 212-869-0856
E-mail: admalmud@wwnorton.com
www.wwnorton.com

Helpful to marriage and couple therapists, very up to date and encompassing, with simple and professional writing. *$30.00*

208 pages Year Founded: 2000 ISSN 70330-4

3086 Hypoactive Sexual Desire: Integrating Sex and Couple Therapy
WW Norton & Company
500 5th Avenue
New York, NY 10110
212-790-9456
Fax: 212-869-0856
E-mail: admalmud@wwnorton.com
www.wwnorton.com

Discussion of treating the couple, not the individual with lack of desire, the authors include distinguishing between organic and psychogenic problems plus how to combine relational and sex therapy. Although lack of desire is one of the most common problems couples face, it is one of the most challenging to treat. *$30.00*

288 pages Year Founded: 2002 ISSN 70344-4

Suicide

3087 Assessment and Prediction of Suicide
Guilford Publications
72 Spring Street
New York, NY 10012
212-431-9800
800-365-7006
Fax: 212-966-6708
E-mail: info@guilford.com
www.guilford.com

Comprehensive reference volume that includes contributions from top suicide experts of the current knowledge in the field of suicide. Covers concepts and theories, methods and quantification, in-depth case histories, specific single predictors applied to the case histories and comorbidity. *$90.00*

697 pages Year Founded: 1992 ISBN 0-898627-91-5

3088 Comprehensive Textbook of Suicidology
Guilford Publications
72 Spring Street
New York, NY 10012
212-431-9800
800-365-7006
Fax: 212-966-6708
E-mail: info@guilford.com
www.guilford.com

This volume presents an authoritative overview of current scientific knowledge about suicide and suicide prevention. Multidisciplinary and comprehesive in scope, the book provides a solid foundation in theory, research and clinical applications. Topics covered include the classification and prevalence of suicidal behaviors, psychiatric and medical factors, ethical and legal issues in intervention as well as the social, cultural and gender context of suicide. *$70.00*

650 pages ISBN 1-572305-41-X

3089 Practical Art of Suicide Assessment: A Guide for Mental Health Professionals and Substance Abuse Counselors
John Wiley & Sons
10475 Crosspoint Boulevard
Indianapolis, IN 46256
877-862-2974
800-597-3299
Fax: 800-597-3299
E-mail: consumers@wiley.com
www.wiley.com

Covers the critical elements of suicide assessment, from risk factor analysis to evaluating clients with borderline personality disorders or psychotic process.

316 pages ISBN 0-471237-61-2

3090 Suicide From a Psychological Prespective
Charles C Thomas Publisher
2600 S 1st Street
Springfield, IL 62704-4730
217-789-8980
800-258-8980
Fax: 217-789-9130
E-mail: books@ccthomas.com
www.ccthomas.com
$39.95

142 pages Year Founded: 1988 ISBN 0-398057-09-5

3091 Teens and Suicide
Mason Crest Publishers
370 Reed Road
Suite 302
Broomall, PA 19008
866-627-2665
Fax: 610-543-3878
www.masoncrest.com

Suicide is the third-leading cause of death among adolescents in the United States; in a recent study by The Gallup Organization, 47 percent of teenagers between the ages of 13 and 17 said they know someone who has tried to take their own lives. This volume examines the cause of teen-age suicide and explores such issues as teens and guns as well as suicide rates among minorities.

3092 Treatment of Suicidal Patients in Managed Care
American Psychiatric Publishing
1000 Wilson Boulevard
Suite 1825
Arlington, VA 22209-3901
703-907-7322
800-368-5777
Fax: 703-907-1091
E-mail: appi@psych.org
www.appi.org

Katie Duffy, Marketing Assistant

Suicide is an all too common cause of death and preventable, but the managed care concerns of cost control with rapid diagnosis and treatment of depression puts the clinician in a dilemma. This book guides the professional with advice on knowing who to contact, and getting more of what is needed from the patient's managed care provider. *$39.00*

240 pages Year Founded: 2001 ISBN 0-880488-28-x

Pediatric & Adolescent Issues

3093 Adolescents in Psychiatric Hospitals: A Psychodynamic Approach to Evaluation and Treatment
Charles C Thomas Publisher
2600 S 1st Street
Springfield, IL 62704-4730
217-789-8980
800-258-8980
Fax: 217-789-9130
E-mail: books@ccthomas.com
www.ccthomas.com

A short history of adolescent inpatient psychiatry and its clinical methods, and a month-long, running account of the morning meetings of a typical inpatient ward. For trainees in child and adolescent psychiatry, nurses, social workers, administrators, and psychologists working in the field of adolescent inpatient psychiatry. *$32.95*

208 pages Year Founded: 1998 ISBN 0-398068-60-7

3094 Adolesent in Family Therapy: Breaking the Cycle of Conflict and Control
Guilford Publications
72 Spring Street
New York, NY 10012
212-431-9800
800-365-7006
Fax: 212-966-6708

E-mail: info@guilford.com
www.guilford.com

Family relationships that are troubled can be catalysts for change. A guide to treating a wide range of parent/adolesent problems with straightforward advice. *$19.95*

336 pages Year Founded: 1998 ISBN 1-572305-88-6

3095 At-Risk Youth in Crises
Pro-Ed Publications
8700 Shoal Creek Boulevard
Austin, TX 78757-6816
512-451-3246
800-897-3202
Fax: 800-397-7633
E-mail: info@proedinc.com
www.proedinc.com

This edition has updated material in the chapters covering divorce, loss, abuse, severe depression and suicide. *$31.00*

268 pages Year Founded: 1994 ISBN 0-890795-74-6

3096 Attachment, Trauma and Healing: Understanding and Treating Attachment Disorder in Children and Families
200 E Joppa Road
Suite 207
Baltimore, MD 21286
410-825-8888
888-825-8249
Fax: 410-337-0747
E-mail: sidran@sidran.org
www.sidran.org

An in depth look at the causes of attachment disorder, explains the normal development of attachment, examines the research in this area and present treatment plans. Numerous appendices include a sample intake packet, two brief day in the life accounts of children with attachment disorder, assessment guides, treatment plans and references. *$34.95*

313 pages

3097 Basic Child Psychiatry
American Psychiatric Publishing
1000 Wilson Boulevard
Suite 1825
Arlington, VA 22209-3901
703-907-7322
800-368-5777
Fax: 703-907-1091
E-mail: appi@psych.org
www.appi.org

Katie Duffy, Marketing Assistant

$46.95

416 pages Year Founded: 1995 ISBN 0-632037-72-5

3098 Behavior Modification for Exceptional Children and Youth
Pro-Ed Publications
8700 Shoal Creek Boulevard
Austin, TX 78757-6816
512-451-3246
800-897-3202
Fax: 800-397-7633
E-mail: info@proedinc.com
www.proedinc.com

An authoritative textbook for courses in behavior modification. Serves as a practical, comprehensive reference work for clinicians working with people with disabilities and behavior problems. *$37.00*

296 pages Year Founded: 1993 ISBN 1-563720-42-6

3099 Behavior Rating Profile
Pro-Ed Publications
8700 Shoal Creek Boulevard
Austin, TX 78757-6816
512-451-3246
800-897-3202
Fax: 800-397-7633
E-mail: info@proedinc.com
www.proedinc.com

Provides different evaluations of a student's behavior at home, at school, and in interpersonal relationships from the varied perpsectives of parents, teachers, peers, and the target students themselves. Identifies students whose behavior is perceived to be deviant, the settings in which behavior problems are prominent, and the persons whose perceptions of student's behavior are different from those of other respondents. *$194.00*

Year Founded: 1990

3100 Behavioral Approach to Assessment of Youth with Emotional/Behavioral Disorders
Pro-Ed Publications
8700 Shoal Creek Boulevard
Austin, TX 78757-6816
512-451-3246
800-897-3202
Fax: 800-397-7633
E-mail: info@proedinc.com
www.proedinc.com

This new book addresses one of the most challenging aspects of special education: evaluating students referred for suspected emotional/behavioral disorders. Geared to the practical needs and concerns of school-based practitioners, including special education teachers, school psychologists and social workers. *$44.00*

729 pages Year Founded: 1996 ISBN 0-890796-25-4

3101 Behavioral Approaches: Problem Child
Cambridge University Press
40 W 20th Street
New York, NY 10011-4221
212-924-3900
Fax: 212-691-3239
E-mail: marketing@cup.org
www.cup.org

3102 Candor, Connection and Enterprise in Adolesent Therapy
WW Norton & Company
500 5th Avenue
New York, NY 10110
212-790-9456
Fax: 212-869-0856
E-mail: admalmud@wwnorton.com
www.wwnorton.com

Suggestions and troubleshooting for therapists dealing with uncooperative adolesent patients. Avoiding the appearence of trying too hard, dialogues that seem to go nowhere, and gaining the faith of a child who may not appreciate efforts on their behalf. *$35.00*

208 pages Year Founded: 2001 ISSN 70356-8

3103 Child Friendly Therapy: Biophysical Innovations for Children and Families
WW Norton & Company
500 5th Avenue
New York, NY 10110
212-790-9456
Fax: 212-869-0856
E-mail: admalmud@wwnorton.com
www.wwnorton.com

Family centered treatment for children. Suggestions and case studies, therapy room set up and session structure, multi sensory skill building leading to a fresh understanding of often misunderstood children. Family members can be incorporated to work as a team to help with therapy. *$32.00*

256 pages Year Founded: 2002 ISSN 70355-X

3104 Child Psychiatry
American Psychiatric Publishing
1000 Wilson Boulevard
Suite 1825
Arlington, VA 22209-3901
703-907-7322
800-368-5777
Fax: 703-907-1091
E-mail: appi@psych.org
www.appi.org

Katie Duffy, Marketing Assistant

Provides the essential facts and concepts for everyone involved in child psychiatry, the book includes 200 questions and answers for trainees approaching professional examinations. *$46.95*

336 pages Year Founded: 1987 ISBN 0-632038-85-3

3105 Child Psychopharmacology
American Psychiatric Publishing
1000 Wilson Boulevard
Suite 1825
Arlington, VA 22209-3901
703-907-7322
800-368-5777
Fax: 703-907-1091
E-mail: appi@psych.org
www.appi.org

Katie Duffy, Marketing Assistant

Includes: Tic disorders and obsessive-compulsive disorder; Attention-deficit/hyperactivity disorder; Children and adolescents with psychotic disorders; Affective disorders in children and adolescents; Anxiety disorders; Eating disorders. *$26.00*

200 pages ISBN 0-880488-33-6

3106 Child and Adolescent Mental Health Consultation in Hospitals, Schools and Courts
American Psychiatric Publishing
1000 Wilson Boulevard
Suite 1825
Arlington, VA 22209-3901
703-907-7322
800-368-5777
Fax: 703-907-1091
E-mail: appi@psych.org
www.appi.org

Katie Duffy, Marketing Assistant

Leading experts present a practical guide for mental health professionals. *$38.50*

316 pages Year Founded: 1993 ISBN 0-880484-18-7

3107 Child and Adolescent Psychiatry: Modern Approaches
American Psychiatric Publishing
1000 Wilson Boulevard
Suite 1825
Arlington, VA 22209-3901
703-907-7322
800-368-5777
Fax: 703-907-1091
E-mail: appi@psych.org
www.appi.org

Katie Duffy, Marketing Assistant
ISBN 0-632028-21-1

3108 Child-Centered Counseling and Psychotherapy
Charles C Thomas Publisher
2600 S 1st Street
Springfield, IL 62704-4730
217-789-8980
800-258-8980
Fax: 217-789-9130
E-mail: books@ccthomas.com
www.ccthomas.com

Topics include an introduction to child-centered counseling, counseling as a three-phase process, applying the reflective process, phase three alternatives, counseling through play, consultation, and professional issues. It represents the status of child-centered counseling which also indentifies ideas which can influence its future. *$62.95*

262 pages Year Founded: 1995 ISSN 0-398-06522-5ISBN 0-398065-21-7

3109 Childhood Behavior Disorders: Applied Research and Educational Practice
Pro-Ed Publications
8700 Shoal Creek Boulevard
Austin, TX 78757-6816
512-451-3246
800-897-3202
Fax: 800-397-7633
E-mail: info@proedinc.com
www.proedinc.com

Provides the balance of theory, research and practical relevance needed by students in graduate and undergraduate introductory courses, as well as practicing teachers and other professionals. *$ 39.00*

550 pages Year Founded: 1998 ISBN 0-890797-19-6

3110 Childhood Disorders
Brunner/Routledge
325 Chestnut Street
Philadelphia, PA 19106
800-821-8312
Fax: 215-269-0363
www.brunner-routledge.com

Provides an up-to-date summary of the current information about the psychological disorders of childhood as well as their causes, nature and course. Together with discussion and evaluation of the major models that guide psychological thinking about the disorders. Gives detailed consider-

ation of the criteria used to make the diagnoses, a presentation of the latest research findings on the nature of the disorder and an overview of the methods used and evaluations conducted for the treatment of the disorders. *$26.95*

240 pages ISBN 0-863776-09-4

3111 Childs Work/Childs Play
135 Dupont Street
PO Box 760
Plainview, NY 11803-0760
800-962-1141
Fax: 800-262-1886
E-mail: info@childswork.com
www.childswork.com

Catalog of books, games, toys and workbooks relating to child development issues such as recognizing emotions, handling uncertainty, bullies, ADD, shyness, conflicts and other things that children may need some help navigating.

3112 Clinical & Forensic Interviewing of Children & Families
Jerome M Sattler
PO Box 3557
La Mesa, CA 91944-3557
619-460-3667
Fax: 619-460-2489
www.sattlerpublisher.com

3113 Clinical Application of Projective Drawings
Charles C Thomas Publisher
2600 S 1st Street
Springfield, IL 62704-4730
217-789-8980
800-258-8980
Fax: 217-789-9130
E-mail: books@ccthomas.com
www.ccthomas.com

On its way to becoming the classic in the field of projective drawings, this book provides a grounding in fundamentals and goes on to consider differential diagnosis, appraisal of psychological resources as treatment potentials and projective drawing usage in therapy. *$65.95*

688 pages Year Founded: 1980 ISBN 0-398007-68-3

3114 Clinical Child Documentation Sourcebook
John Wiley & Sons
605 3rd Avenue
New York, NY 10058-0180
212-850-6000
Fax: 212-850-6008
E-mail: info@wiley.com
www.wiley.com

This easy to use resource offers child psychologists and therapists a full array of forms, inventories, checklists, client handouts, and clinical records essential to a successful practice in either and organizational or clinical setting. *$49.95*

256 pages Year Founded: 1999 ISBN 0-471291-11-0

3115 Cognitive Behavior Therapy Child
Cambridge University Press
40 W 20th Street
New York, NY 10011-4221
212-924-3900
Fax: 212-691-3239

3116 Concise Guide to Child and Adolescent Psychiatry
American Psychiatric Publishing
1000 Wilson Boulevard
Suite 1825
Arlington, VA 22209-3901
703-907-7322
800-368-5777
Fax: 703-907-1091
E-mail: appi@psych.org
www.appi.org

Katie Duffy, Marketing Assistant

Topics include evaluation and treatment planning, axis I disorders usually first diagnosed in infancy, childhood or adolescence, attention deficit and disruptive behavior disorders, developmental disorders, special clinical circumstances, psychopharmacology, and psychosocial treatments. *$21.95*

400 pages Year Founded: 1998 ISBN 0-880489-05-7

3117 Counseling Children with Special Needs
American Psychiatric Publishing
1000 Wilson Boulevard
Suite 1825
Arlington, VA 22209-3901
703-907-7322
800-368-5777
Fax: 703-907-1091
E-mail: appi@psych.org
www.appi.org

Katie Duffy, Marketing Assistant
$29.95

224 pages Year Founded: 1997 ISBN 0-632041-51-

3118 Creative Therapy with Children and Adolescents
Impact Publishers
PO Box 6016
Atascadero, CA 93423-6016
805-466-5917
800-246-7228
Fax: 805-466-5919
E-mail: info@impactpublishers.com
www.impactpublishers.com

Encourages creativity in therapy, assists therapists in talking with children to facilitate change. From simple ideas to fresh innovations, the activities are to be used as tools to supplement a variety of therapeutic approaches, and can be tailored to each child's needs. *$21.95*

192 pages Year Founded: 1999 ISBN 1-886230-19-6

3119 Defiant Teens
Guilford Publications
72 Spring Street
New York, NY 10012
212-431-9800
800-365-7006
Fax: 212-966-6708
E-mail: info@guilford.com
www.guilford.com

Guidelines for best practices in working with families and their teenaged children.

250 pages Year Founded: 1999 ISBN 1-572304-40-5

3120 Developmental Therapy/Developmental Teaching
Pro-Ed Publications
8700 Shoal Creek Boulevard
Austin, TX 78757-6816
512-451-3246
800-897-3202
Fax: 800-397-7633
E-mail: info@proedinc.com
www.proedinc.com

Constance Quirk, Editor

Provides extensive applications for teachers, counselors, parents and other adults concerned about the behavior and emotional stability of children and teens. The focus is on helping children and youth to cope effectively with the stresses of comtemporary life, with an emphasis on the positive effects adults can have on students when they adjust strategies to the social emotional needs of children. *$41.00*

398 pages Year Founded: 1996 ISBN 0-890796-64-5

3121 Enhancing Social Competence in Young Students
Pro-Ed Publications
8700 Shoal Creek Boulevard
Austin, TX 78757-6816
512-451-3246
800-897-3202
Fax: 800-397-7633
E-mail: info@proedinc.com
www.proedinc.com

Addresses conceptual and practical issues of providing social competence-enhancing interventions for young students in schools, based on research findings. Summarizes recent advances in social skills programming for at-risk students and prevention interventions for all students. Discussions of developmental issues of childhood maladjustment, intervention strategies, implementation issues and assessment/evaluation issues are provided. *$28.00*

281 pages Year Founded: 1995 ISBN 0-890796-20-3

3122 Group Therapy With Children and Adolescents
American Psychiatric Publishing
1000 Wilson Boulevard
Suite 1825
Arlington, VA 22209-3901
703-907-7322
800-368-5777
Fax: 703-907-1091
E-mail: appi@psych.org
www.appi.org

Explores a major treatment modality often used with adult populations and rarely considered for child and adolescent treatments. With contributions from international experts, this book looks at the effectiveness of treatment and cost of group therapy as it applies to this particular age group. *$52.00*

400 pages ISBN 0-880484-06-3

3123 Handbook of Child Behavior in Therapy and in the Psychiatric Setting
John Wiley & Sons
605 3rd Avenue
New York, NY 10058-0180

212-850-6000
Fax: 212-850-6008
E-mail: info@wiley.com
www.wiley.com
512 pages Year Founded: 1994

3124 Handbook of Infant Mental Health
Guilford Publications
72 Spring Street
New York, NY 10012
212-431-9800
800-365-7006
Fax: 212-966-6708
E-mail: info@guilford.com
www.guilford.com

Included are chapters on neurobiology, diagnostic issues, parental mental health issues and family dynamics. *$60.00*

588 pages Year Founded: 2000 ISBN 1-572305-15-0

3125 Handbook of Parent Training: Parents as Co-Therapists for Children's Behavior Problems
John Wiley & Sons
605 3rd Avenue
New York, NY 10058-0180
212-850-6000
Fax: 212-850-6008
E-mail: info@wiley.com
www.wiley.com

This completely revised handbook shows professionals who work with troubled children how to teach parents to become co-therapists. It presents various techniques and behavior modification skills that will help parents to better relate, communicate, and respond to their child. Updates are provided on such problems as noncompliance, ADHD, and conduct disorder, and a new section on special needs parents which includes adolescent mothers, aggressive parents, substance abusing parents, and more.

594 pages Year Founded: 1994

3126 Handbook of Psychiatric Practice in the Juvenile Court
American Psychiatric Press
1000 Wilson Boulevard
Suite 1825
Arlington, VA 22209-3901
703-907-7322
800-368-5777
Fax: 703-907-1091
E-mail: appi@psych.org
www.appi.org

Katie Duffy, Marketing Assistant

Examines the role that psychiatrists and other mental health professionals are asked to play when children, adolescents, and their families end up in court. *$12.95*

198 pages ISBN 0-890422-33-8

3127 Helping Parents, Youth, and Teachers Understand Medications for Behavioral and Emotional Problems
American Psychiatric Publishing
1000 Wilson Boulevard
Suite 1825
Arlington, VA 22209-3901

703-907-7322
800-368-5777
Fax: 703-907-1091
E-mail: appi@psych.org
www.appi.org

Katie Duffy, Marketing Assistant

Valuable resource for anyone involved in evaluating psychiatric disturbances in children and adolescents. Provides a compilation of information sheets to help promote the dialogue between the patient's family, caregivers, and the treating physician. *$39.95*

196 pages Year Founded: 1999 ISBN 0-880487-94-1

3128 How to Teach Social Skills
Pro-Ed Publications
8700 Shoal Creek Boulevard
Austin, TX 78757-6816
512-451-3246
800-897-3202
Fax: 800-397-7633
E-mail: info@proedinc.com
www.proedinc.com

$8.00

ISBN 0-890797-61-7

3129 In the Long Run... Longitudinal Studies of Psychopathology in Children
American Psychiatric Publishing
1000 Wilson Boulevard
Suite 1825
Arlington, VA 22209-3901
703-907-7322
800-368-5777
Fax: 703-907-1091
E-mail: appi@psych.org
www.appi.org

$29.95

224 pages Year Founded: 1999 ISBN 0-873182-11-1

3130 Infants, Toddlers and Families: Framework for Support and Intervention
Guilford Publications
72 Spring Street
Department 4E
New York, NY 10012-9902
Fax: 212-966-6708
E-mail: exam@guilford.com
www.guilford.com

Examines the complex development in a child's first 3 years of life. Instead of preaching or judging, this book acknowledges the challenges facing all families, especially vulnerable ones, and offers straightforward advice. *$28.95*

204 pages Year Founded: 1999 ISBN 1-572304-87-1

3131 Interventions for Students with Emotional Disorders
Pro-Ed Publications
8700 Shoal Creek Boulevard
Austin, TX 78757-6816
512-451-3246
800-897-3202
Fax: 800-397-7633
E-mail: info@proedinc.com
www.proedinc.com

This graduate textbook for special education students advocates an eclectic approach toward teaching children with social adjustment problems. Provides how-to information for implementing various techniques to successfully enhance positive sociobehavioral development in children with emotional disorders. *$36.00*

212 pages Year Founded: 1991 ISBN 0-890792-96-8

3132 Interviewing Children and Adolesents: Skills and Strategies for Effective DSM-IV Diagnosis
Guilford Publications
72 Spring Street
New York, NY 10012
212-431-9800
800-365-7006
Fax: 212-966-6708
E-mail: info@guilford.com
www.guilford.com

Guide to developmentally appropriate interviewing. *$45.00*

482 pages Year Founded: 99 ISBN 1-572305-01-0

3133 Interviewing the Sexually Abused Child
American Psychiatric Publishing
1000 Wilson Boulevard
Suite 1825
Arlington, VA 22209-3901
703-907-7322
800-368-5777
Fax: 703-907-1091
E-mail: appi@psych.org
www.appi.org

Katie Duffy, Marketing Assistant

A guide for mental health professionals who need to know if a child has been sexually abused. Presents guidelines on the structure of the interview and covers the use of free play, toys, and play materials by focusing on the investigate interview of the suspected victim. *$15.00*

80 pages Year Founded: 1993 ISBN 0-880486-12-0

3134 Learning Disorders and Disorders of the Self in Children and Adolesents
WW Norton & Company
500 5th Avenue
New York, NY 10110
212-790-9456
Fax: 212-869-0856
E-mail: admalmud@wwnorton.com
www.wwnorton.com

Clinicians who work with learning disabled children need to understand the complex, integrated framework of learning and self image problems. Specific problems and treatments are discussed. *$32.00*

332 pages Year Founded: 2001 ISSN 70377-0

3135 Living on the Razor's Edge: Solution-Oriented Brief Family Therapy with Self-Harming Adolesents
WW Norton & Company
500 5th Avenue
New York, NY 10110
212-790-9456
Fax: 212-869-0856
E-mail: admalmud@wwnorton.com
www.wwnorton.com

Research supported stategies and a therapy model for self harming adolescents and their families to devlop a closer and more meaningful relationships. *$25.60*

320 pages Year Founded: 2002 ISSN 70335-5

3136 Making the Grade: Guide to School Drug Prevention Programs
Drug Strategies
1616 P Street NW
Washington, DC 20036
202-289-9070
Fax: 202-414-6199
E-mail: dspoilcy@aol.com
www.drugstrategies.org

Updated and expanded from the 1996 original, this guide to drug prevention programs in America helps parents and educators make informed decisions with often limited budgets. *$14.95*

3137 Manual of Clinical Child and Adolescent Psychiatry
American Psychiatric Publishing
1000 Wilson Boulevard
Suite 1825
Arlington, VA 22209-3901
703-907-7322
800-368-5777
Fax: 703-907-1091
E-mail: appi@psych.org
www.appi.org

Katie Duffy, Marketing Assistant

Addresses current issues such as cost containment, insurance complications, and legal and ethical issues, as well as neuropsychology, alcohol, and substance abuse, and mental retardation and genetics. *$42.50*

528 pages ISBN 0-880485-28-0

3138 Mental Affections Childhood
Cambridge University Press
40 W 20th Street
New York, NY 10011-4221
212-924-3900
Fax: 212-691-3239
E-mail: marketing@cup.org
www.cup.org

$30.00

185 pages Year Founded: 1991

3139 Myth of Maturity: What Teenagers Need from Parents to Become Adults
WW Norton & Company
500 5th Avenue
New York, NY 10110
212-790-9456
Fax: 212-869-0856
E-mail: admalmud@wwnorton.com
www.wwnorton.com

Debunking outdated and misguided ideas about maturity, the author discusses the amount of support teens need from their parents, what is too much for independence, or not enough. *$24.95*

256 pages Year Founded: 2001 ISBN 0-393049-42-6

3140 Narrative Therapies with Children and Adolescents
Guilford Publications
72 Spring Street
New York, NY 10012
212-431-9800
800-365-7006
Fax: 212-966-6708
E-mail: info@guilford.com
www.guilford.com

Many renowned, creative contributors collaborate to bring this professional resource to the shelf. Transcripts of case examples, using many different methods and mediums are shown to engage children of different perspectives and ages. This book can serve as a text for child/adolesent psychotherapy, or is a useful guide for mental health professionals. *$39.95*

469 pages Year Founded: 1997 ISBN 1-572302-53-4

3141 National Survey of American Attitudes on Substance Abuse VI: Teens
Center on Addiction at Columbia University
633 3rd Avenue
19th Floor
New York, NY 10017-6706
212-841-5200
Fax: 212-956-8020
www.casacolumbia.org

Results of the sixth annual CASA National Survey of teens 12 - 17 years old reveals that parents that are more involved with their children's activities and have house rules and expectations can greatly influence teen behavior choices. Other statistics about availability of illegal substances and who may use them. *$22.00*

3142 No-Talk Therapy for Children and Adolescents
WW Norton & Company
500 5th Avenue
New York, NY 10110
212-790-9456
Fax: 212-869-0856
E-mail: admalmud@wwnorton.com
www.wwnorton.com

Creative approach to treatment of young people who cannot respond to conversation based therapy. Seemingly sullen patients can be helped to find a voice of their own. *$.27*

288 pages Year Founded: 1999 ISSN 70286-3

3143 Ordinary Families, Special Children: Systems Approach to Childhood Disability
Guilford Publications
72 Spring Street
New York, NY 10012
212-431-9800
800-365-7006
Fax: 212-966-6708
E-mail: info@guilford.com
www.guilford.com

Families, including siblings and grandparents are impacted by the special needs of a child's disability. The authors explore personal accounts that shape a family's response to childhood disability and how they come to adapt these unique needs to a satisfactory lifestyle. Available in hardcover and paperback. *$35.00*

324 pages Year Founded: 1999 ISBN 1-572301-55-4

3144 Outcomes for Children and Youth with Emotional and Behavioral Disorders and their Families
Pro-Ed Publications
8700 Shoal Creek Boulevard
Austin, TX 78757-6816
512-451-3246
800-897-3202
Fax: 800-397-7633
E-mail: info@proedinc.com
www.proedinc.com

This new book addresses one of the most challenging aspects of serving children and youth with emotional and behavioral disorders-evaluating the outcomes of the services you've provided. Also includes information on such topics as: child and family outcomes, system level anaylsis, case study analysis, cost analysis, cultural diversity, managed care, and consumer satisfaction. *$44.00*

730 pages Year Founded: 1998 ISBN 0-890797-50-1

3145 Pediatric Psychopharmacology: Fast Facts
WW Norton & Company
500 5th Avenue
New York, NY 10110-0017
212-354-5500
800-233-4830
Fax: 212-869-0856
E-mail: npb@wwnorton.com
www.wwnorton.com/psych

This new title in the Fast Facts series, full of up-to-date and authoritative infomration, is a critical resource for all health care professionals, including psychiatrists, prescribing psychologists, psychotherapists, pediatricians, family practice physicians, pediatric neurologists, nurse practitioners, and allied mental health professionals. Clear explanations of clinical directions for the prescriber and nonprescriber alike.

ISBN 0-393704-61-0

3146 Play Therapy with Children in Crisis: Individual, Group and Family Treatment
Guilford Publications
72 Spring Street
New York, NY 10012
212-431-9800
800-365-7006
Fax: 212-966-6708
E-mail: info@guilford.com
www.guilford.com

$45.00

506 pages Year Founded: 1999 ISBN 1-572304-85-5

3147 Power and Compassion: Working with Difficult Adolescents and Abused Parents
Guilford Publications
72 Spring Street
New York, NY 10012
212-431-9800
800-365-7006
Fax: 212-966-6708
E-mail: info@guilford.com
www.guilford.com

Useful as a supplemental text, or for mental health professionals dealing with aggressive teenagers and their parents.

Pragmatic guide to help demoralized parents be more understanding, but more decisive. *$16.95*

196 pages Year Founded: 1999 ISBN 1-572304-70-7

3148 Practical Charts for Managing Behavior
Pro-Ed Publications
8700 Shoal Creek Boulevard
Austin, TX 78757-6816
512-451-3246
800-897-3202
Fax: 800-397-7633
E-mail: info@proedinc.com
www.proedinc.com

$29.00

160 pages Year Founded: 1998 ISBN 0-890797-36-6

3149 Psychological Examination of the Child
John Wiley & Sons
605 3rd Avenue
New York, NY 10058-0180
212-850-6000
Fax: 212-850-6008
E-mail: info@wiley.com
www.wiley.com

279 pages Year Founded: 1991

3150 Psychotherapies with Children and Adolescents
American Psychiatric Publishing
1000 Wilson Boulevard
Suite 1825
Arlington, VA 22209-3901
703-907-7322
800-368-5777
Fax: 703-907-1091
E-mail: appi@psych.org
www.appi.org

Katie Duffy, Marketing Assistant

Illustrated with case histories and demonstrates how psychoanalytic techniques can be modified to meet the therapeutic needs of children and adolescents in specific clinical situations. *$47.50*

346 pages ISBN 0-880484-06-3

3151 Safe Schools/Safe Students: Guide to Violence Prevention Stategies
Drug Strategies
1616 P Street NW
Washington, DC 20036
202-289-9070
Fax: 202-414-6199
E-mail: dspoilcy@aol.com
www.drugstrategies.org

Practical assistance in rating over 84 violence prevention programs for classroom use, helps examine school policies and possible changes for student protection. *$14.95*

3152 Severe Stress and Mental Disturbance in Children
American Psychiatric Publishing
1000 Wilson Boulevard
Suite 1825
Arlington, VA 22209-3901
703-907-7322
800-368-5777
Fax: 703-907-1091

E-mail: appi@psych.org
www.appi.org

Katie Duffy, Marketing Assistant

Uniquely blends current research and clinical data on the effects of severe stress on children. Each chapter is written by international experts in their field. *$69.95*

708 pages ISBN 0-880486-57-0

3153 Structured Adolescent Pscyhotherapy Groups
Professional Resource Press
PO Box 15560
Sarasota, FL 34277-1560
941-343-9601
800-443-3364
Fax: 941-343-9201
E-mail: orders@prpress.com
www.prpress.com

Debra Fink, Managing Editor

Provides specific techniques for use in the beginning, middle, and end phase of time-limited structured psychotherapy groups. Offers concrete suggestions for working with hard to reach and difficult adolescents, providing feedback to parents, and dealing with administrative, legal, and ethical issues. Examples of pre/post evaluation forms, therapy contracts, evaluation feedback letters, parent response forms, therapist rating scales, co-therapist rating forms, problem identification forms, supervision and session records, client and patient handouts, and specific group exercises. Solidly anchored to research on the curative factors in group therapy, this book includes empirical data, references, theoretical formulations and examples of group sessions. *$19.95*

164 pages Year Founded: 1994 ISBN 0-943158-74-5

3154 Textbook of Child and Adolescent Psychiatry
American Psychiatric Publishing
1000 Wilson Boulevard
Suite 1825
Arlington, VA 22209-3901
703-907-7322
800-368-5777
Fax: 703-907-1091
E-mail: appi@psych.org
www.appi.org

Katie Duffy, Marketing Assistant

Includes chapter on changes in DSM-IV classification and discusses the latest research and treatment advances in the areas of epidemiology, fenetics, developmental neurobiology, and combined treatments. A special section covers essential issues such as HIV and AIDS, gender identity disorders, physical and sexual abuse, and substance abuse, for the child and adolescent psychiatrist. *$140.00*

960 pages ISBN 1-882103-03-3

3155 Textbook of Pediatric Neuropsychiatry
American Psychiatric Publishing
1000 Wilson Boulevard
Suite 1825
Arlington, VA 22209-3901
703-907-7322
800-368-5777
Fax: 703-907-1091
E-mail: appi@psych.org
www.appi.org

Katie Duffy, Marketing Assistant

Comprehensive textbook on pediatric medicine. *$175.00*
1632 pages Year Founded: 1998 ISBN 0-880487-66-6

3156 Through the Eyes of a Child
WW Norton & Company
500 5th Avenue
New York, NY 10110
212-354-5500
800-233-4830
Fax: 212-869-0856
E-mail: npb@wwnorton.com
www.wwnorton.com/psych

Comprehensive and helpful, this book helps therapists work with children and parents in the application of EMDR with children. *$ 37.00*

288 pages Year Founded: 1999 ISSN 70287-1ISBN 0-393702-87-1

3157 Treating Depressed Children: A Therapeutic Manual of Proven Cognitive Behavior Techniques
New Harbinger Publications
5674 Shattuck Avenue
Oakland, CA 94609-1662
510-652-2002
800-748-6273
Fax: 510-652-5472
E-mail: customerservice@newharbinger.com
www.newharbinger.com

Program incorporating cartoons and role playing games to help children recognize emotions, change negative thoughts, gain confidence, and learn interpersonal skills. *$49.94*

160 pages Year Founded: 1996 ISBN 1-572240-61-

3158 Treating the Aftermath of Sexual Abuse: a Handbook for Working with Children in Care
Child Welfare League of America
440 First Street NW
Third Floor
Washington, DC 20001-2085
202-638-2952
Fax: 202-638-4004
www.cwla.org

A handbook for working with children in care who have been sexually abused. The authors review the impact of sexual abuse on a child's physical and emotional development and describe the effect of abuse on basic life experiences. Paperback. *$18.95*

176 pages Year Founded: 1998 ISBN 0-878686-93-2

3159 Treating the Tough Adolesent: Family Based Step by Step Guide
Guilford Publications
72 Spring Street
New York, NY 10012
212-431-9800
800-365-7006
Fax: 212-966-6708
E-mail: info@guilford.com
www.guilford.com

Model for effective family therapy, with reproducible handouts. *$35.00*

320 pages Year Founded: 1998 ISBN 1-572304-22-7

3160 Troubled Teens: Multidimensional Family Therapy
WW Norton & Company
500 5th Avenue
New York, NY 10110
212-790-9456
Fax: 212-869-0856
E-mail: admalmud@wwnorton.com
www.wwnorton.com

Based on 17 years of research, this treatment manual is for therapists who work with youth referred for substance abuse and behavior counseling. Treatment involves drug counseling, family and individual sessions and interventions. People or systems of influence outside the family are also considered. *$35.00*

320 pages Year Founded: 2002 ISBN 0-393703-40-1

3161 Understanding and Teaching Emotionally Disturbed Children and Adolescents
Pro-Ed Publications
8700 Shoal Creek Boulevard
Austin, TX 78757-6816
512-451-3246
800-897-3202
Fax: 800-397-7633
E-mail: info@proedinc.com
www.proedinc.com

Shows how diverse theoretical perspectives translate into practice by exploring forms of therapy and types of interventions currently employed with children and adolescents. *$41.00*

620 pages Year Founded: 1993 ISBN 0-890795-75-4

3162 Ups & Downs: How to Beat the Blues and Teen Depression
Price Stern Sloan Publishing
www.penguingroup.com

Andy Cooke, Illustrator

This book discusses how to recognize depression in teens and what to do about it. Informal, yet informative, using quotes and case studies representing typical young people who are dealing with mood swings, eating disorders and problems at school or at home. The book also demystifies therapy and advises readers on how to seek help, particularly if they, or their friends, have suicidal thoughts. Reading level ages nine to twelve. *$4.99*

90 pages Year Founded: 1999 ISBN 0-843174-50-1

3163 Working with Self-Harming Adolescents: A Collaborative, Strengths-Based Therapy Approach
WW Norton & Company
500 5th Avenue
New York, NY 10110-0017
212-354-5500
800-233-4830
Fax: 212-869-0856
E-mail: npb@wwnorton.com
www.wwnorton.com/psych

A unique approach to this illness combines flexability, compassion, and candor. His integration of the family in these treatments demonstrates the complex interplay between self-harming teens and their parents, peers, communities, and culture. Originally published in hardcover as Living on the Razor's Edge.

ISBN 0-393704-99-8

3164 Youth Violence: Prevention, Intervention, and Social Policy
American Psychiatric Publishing
1000 Wilson Boulevard
Suite 1825
Arlington, VA 22209-3901
703-907-7322
800-368-5777
Fax: 703-907-1091
E-mail: appi@psych.org
www.appi.org

Katie Duffy, Marketing Assistant

Based on more than a decade of clinical research and treatment experience, this comprehensive and non-technical book offers a stage-oriented approach to understanding and treating complex and difficult traumatized patients, integrating modern trauma theory with traditional therapeutic interventions. *$48.50*

336 pages Year Founded: 1998 ISBN 0-880488-09-3

Conferences & Meetings

3165 AAMA Annual Conference
American Academy of Medical Administrators
701 Lee Street
Suite 600
Des Plaines, IL 60016-4516
847-759-8601
Fax: 847-759-8602
E-mail: info@aameda.org
www.aameda.org

Renee S Schleicher, President/CEO
Merle Hedland, Meeting Planner

Learn the newest trends in healthcare administration; focus on your area of specialty or broaden your knowledge; become energized with new information and contacts in your field; and return to your organization ready to implement new ideas anad face new challenges.

3166 AMA's Annual Medical Communications Conferen ce
American Medical Association
515 N State Street
Chicago, IL 60610-4325
800-621-8335
www.ama-assn.org

Ronald M Davis, President

Provides hands-on communications training and hear from top-level medical communicators, government leaders and national journalists

3167 American Academy of Child and Adolescent Psychiatry (AACAP): Annual Meeting
3615 Wisconsin Avenue NW
Washington, DC 20016-3007
202-966-7300
Fax: 202-966-2891
E-mail: communications@aacap.org
www.aacap.org

Robert Hendren, President
David Herzog, Secretary
William Bernet, Treasurer

Professional society of physicians who have completed an additional five years of stimulate and advance medical contributions to the knowledge and treatment of psychiatric illnesses of children and adolescents. Annual meeting.

3168 American Academy of Addiction Psychiatry: Annual Meeting
7301 Mission Road
Suite 252
Prairie Village, KS 66208-3075
913-262-6161
Fax: 913-262-4311
E-mail: info@aaap.org
www.aaap.org

Michael H Hendel MD, President

3169 American Academy of Psychiatry & Law Annual Conference
American Academy of Psychiatry & Law
1 Regency Drive
PO Box 30
Bloomfield, CT 06002
860-242-5450
800-331-1389
Fax: 860-286-0787
E-mail: execoff@aapl.org
www.aapl.org

Jacquelyn T. Coleman, Executive Director
Jeffrey Janofsky MD, President
Kenneth Appelbaum MD, Vice President

3170 American Academy of Psychoanalysis Preliminary Meeting
American Academy of Psychoanalysis and Dynamic Psychiatry
One Regency Drive
PO Box 30
Bloomfield, CT 06002
888-691-8281
Fax: 860-286-0787
E-mail: info@aapdp.org
www.aapsa.org

Jacquelyn T Coleman CAE, Executive Director
Sherry Katz-Bearnot, President
Carol Filiaci, Secretary

Annual meeting, Toronto, Canada.

3171 American Association of Children's Residential Center Annual Conference
American Association of Children's Residential Centers
11700 W Lake Park Drive
Milwaukee, WI 53224
877-332-2272
Fax: 877-362-2272
E-mail: kbehling@alliance1.org
www.aacrc-dc.org

Kari Behling, National Coordinator
Steve Elson, President

Funded by the Mental Health Community Support Program. The purpose of the association is to share information about services, providers and ways to cope with mental illnesses. Available services include referrals, professional seminars, support groups and a variety of publications.

3172 American Association of Geriatric Psychiatry Annual Meetings
7910 Woodmont Avenue
Suite 1050
Bethesda, MD 20814-3004
301-654-7850
Fax: 301-654-4137
E-mail: main@aagponline.org
www.aagpgpa.org

Christine Devries, CEO/Executive Vice President
Annie Williams, Administrative Assistant

Annual Meeting: March, Puerto Rico

3173 American Association of Health Care Consultants Annual Fall Conference
American Association of Health Care Consultants
5938 Drake Avenue
Chicago, IL 60659
888-350-2242
Fax: 773-463-3552
E-mail: info@aahcmail.org
www.aahc.net

Billy Adkisson, Chairman

Association hosts an Annual Fall Conference: October.

3174 American Association of Homes & Services for the Aging Annual Convention
American Association of Homes & Services for the Aging
2519 Connecticute Avenue NW
Washington, DC 20008-1520
202-783-2242
Fax: 202-783-2255
E-mail: info@aahsa.org
www.aahsa.org

William Minnix, President
Katrinka Smith Sloan, COO/SVP Member Services

3175 American Association on Intellectual and Dev elopmental Disabilities Annual Meeting
444 N Capitol Street NW
Suite 846
Washington, DC 20001-1512
202-387-1968
800-424-3688
Fax: 202-387-2193
E-mail: maria@aaidd.org
www.aaidd.org

Doreen M Croser, Executive Director
Maria A Alfaro, Meeting Planner/We Manager

Provides the opportunity of networking with old friends and colleagues, and is a wonderful opportunity to welcome students and new disability professionals to our Association.
$445.00

3176 American Board of Disability Analysts Annual Conference
Park Plaza Medical Building
345 24th Avenue North
Nashville, TN 37203
E-mail: americanbd@aol.com
www.americandisability.org

3177 American College of Health Care Administrators: ACHCA Annual Meeting
300 N Lee Street
Suite 301
Alexandria, VA 22314
703-739-7900
Fax: 703-739-7901
E-mail: mgrachek@achca.org
www.achca.org

Marianna Kern Grachek, President/CEO
Diana Buttram, COO
Anita Bell, Office Coordinator

Professional society for nearly 6,300 administrators in long-term care, assisted living and subacute care. Their mission is to be the premier organization serving as a catalyst to empower administrators who will define professionalism throughout the continuum of care.

3178 American College of Healthcare Executives Educational Events
American College of Healthcare Executives
One N Franklin Street
Suite 1700
Chicago, IL 60606-3529
312-424-2800
Fax: 312-424-0023
E-mail: geninco@ache.org
www.ache.org

Alyson Pitman Giles, Chairman
David Rubenstein, Chairman-Elect

3179 American College of Psychiatrists Annual Meeting
122 S. Michigan Ave
Suite 1360
Chicago, IL 60603
312-662-1020
Fax: 312-662-1025
E-mail: angel@acpsych.org
www.acpsych.org

Maureen Shick, Executive Director
Angel Waszak, Administrative Assistant

Nonprofit honorary association of psychiatrists who, through excellence in their chosen fields, have been recognized for their significant contributions to the profession. The society's goal is to promote and support the highest standards in psychiatry through education, research and clinical practice. Annual Meeting in February.

3180 American Group Psychotherapy Association Annual Conference
American Group Psychotherapy Association
25 E 21st Street
6th Floor
New York, NY 10010
212-477-2677
877-668-2472
Fax: 212-979-6627
E-mail: info@agpa.org
www.agpa.org

Marsha S Block, CEO
Elizabeth Knight, President

Educational conference with a changing annual focus. February.

Year Founded: 1942

3181 American Health Care Association Annual Convention
1201 L Street NW
Washington, DC 20005
202-842-4444
Fax: 202-842-3860
www.www.ahcancal.org

Bruce Yarwood, President/CEO

Exhibits and educational workshops from the nonprofit federation of affiliated state health organizations, together representing nearly 12,000 nonprofit and for profit assisted living, nursing facility, developmentally disabled and sub-acute care providers that care for more than 1.5 million elderly and disabled individuals nationally. AHCA represents the long term care community at large — to government, business leaders and the general public. It also serves as a force for change within the long term care field, providing information, education, and administrative tools that enhance quality at every level.

3182 American Health Information Management Association Annual Exhibition and Conference
233 N Michigan Avenue
21st Floor
Chicago, IL 60601-5800
312-233-1100
Fax: 312-233-1090
E-mail: info@ahima.org
www.ahima.org

Linda Kloss, CEO
Becky Garris-Perry, Executive Vice President/CFO

Exhibits, business and educational conferences of the dynamic professional association that represents more than 46,000 specially educated health information management professionals who work throughout the healthcare industry. Health information management professionals serve the health care industry and the public by manageing, analyzing and utilizing data vital for patient care and making it accessible to healthcare providers when it is needed most.

3183 American Society for Adolescent Psychiatry: Annual Meeting
PO Box 570218
Dallas, TX 75357-0218
972-613-0985
Fax: 972-613-5532
E-mail: info@adolpsych.org
www.adolpsych.org

Mohan Nair, President
Frances Bell, Executive Director

Feature presentations by prominent members of the professional community, exhibits, workshops, receptions, award ceremony and installation of officers. Annual meeting held in March.

3184 Annual Early Childhood Conference: Effective Relationship-Based Practices in Promoting Positive Child Outcomes
Lincoln Center Campus
Lowenstein Bldg (12th Fl-Pres'l Loun)
113 West 60th Street
New York, NY 10023-7414
www.losninisservices.com/training/fordham_2006/index.h

Annual conference brings together experts on best practices in relationship-based approaches in working with young children and families with special needs, especially those with pervasive developmental disorders and autistic disorder.

3185 Annual Meeting & Medical-Scientific Conference
American Society of Addiction Medicine
4601 N Park Avenue
Upper Arcade #101
Chevy Chase, MD 20815
301-656-3920
Fax: 301-656-3815
E-mail: email@asam.org
www.asam.org

Michael Miller, President
Eileen McGrath, Executive Vice President

Goal is to present the most up-to-date information in the addictions field. to attain this goal, program sessions will focus on the latest developments in research and treatment issues and will tanslate them into clinically useful knowledge. Through a mix of symposia, courses, workshops, didactic lectures, and paper and poster presentations based on submitted abstracts, participants will have an opportunity to interact with experts in their field.

3186 Annual Santa Fe Psychiatric Symposium
Psychiatry Department
University of Arizona
Campbell Ave, PO Box 245002
Tucson, AZ 85724-5002
520-626-6254
Fax: 520-626-2004
www.psychiatry.arizona.edu

Designed to meet the educational needs of physicians (psychiatrists, family practitioners, general practitioners), psychologists, nurse practitioners, physician assistants, nurses and other health care professionals. Each half-day will provide practical and clinically relevant information for day-to-day problems. Morning lectures will be followed by panel discussions.

3187 Annual Summit on International Managed Care Trends
Academy for International Health Studies
273 Hebron Avenue
Glastonbury, CT 06033
860-430-1388
Fax: 860-430-1420
www.aihs.com

Bruce A Pollack, President

Global healthcare meeting; 500 people, 47 nations attended previous summits.

3188 Association for Ambulatory Behavioral Healthcare: Training Conference
247 Douglas Avenue
Portsmouth, VA 23707
703-673-3741
Fax: 757-966-7734
E-mail: mickey@aabh.org
www.aabh.org

Larry Meikel MBA, President

Powerful forum for people engaged in providing mental health services. Promoting the evolution of flexible models of responsive cost-effective ambulatory behavioral healthcare.

3189 Association of Black Psychologists Annual Convention

PO Box 55999
Washington, DC 20040-5999
202-722-0808
Fax: 202-722-5941
E-mail: abpsi_office@abpsi.org
www.abpsi.org

Dorothy Holmes, President
Pamela Hall, Secretary
Muriel Kennedy, Treasurer

Feature presentations, exhibits and workshops held over a four day period focusing on the unique concerns of Black professionals.

3190 Georgia Psychological Society First Annual Conference
GPS Proposals

1500 North Patterson Street
Department of Psychology, VSU
Valdosta, GA 31698-0100
E-mail: blbrowne@valdosta.edu or crtalor@valdosta.edu
www.georgiapsychologicalsociety.org

Proposals for symposia, papers, posters and workshops on topics in all areas of psychology are invited. Proposals should not exceed 500 words, and each proposal must include a summary that is no longer than 50 words.

3191 Institute for Advancement of Human Behavior

4370 Alpine Road
Suite 209
Portola Valley, CA 94028-7927
650-851-8411
800-258-8411
Fax: 650-851-0406
E-mail: staff@iahb.org
www.ibh.com

Gerry Piaget, President
Joan Piaget, Executive Director

Host 10-15 meetings a year. Representing the cutting edge in professional education.

3192 NADD Annual Conference & Exhibit Show
National Association for the Dually Diagnosed

132 Fair Street
Kingston, NY 12401
845-331-4336
800-331-5362
Fax: 845-331-4569
E-mail: info@thenadd.org
www.thenadd.org

Robert J Fletcher, Founder/CEO

3193 NAMI National Convention
National Alliance on Mental Illness

2107 Wilson Boulevard
Suite 300
Arlington, VA 22201-3042
703-524-7600
800-950-6264
Fax: 703-524-9094
TDD: 703-516-7227

E-mail: info@nami.org
www.nami.org

Michael J Fitzpatrick, Executive Director

Join the thousands who will gather to explore strategy and tactics to improve the lives of people who live with mental illnesses.

3194 National Multicultural Conference and Summit

Brakins Consulting & Psychological Svs
13805 60th Avenue North
Phymouth, MN 55446
www.multiculturalsummit.com

The mission is to convene students, practitioners, and scholars in psychology and related fields to inform and inspire multicultural research and practice.

3195 Traumatic Incident Reduction Workshop
E-Productivity-Services.Net

Division of 21st Century Enterprises
13 NW Barry Rd PMB 214
Kansas City, MO 64155-2728
816-468-4945
Fax: 816-468-6656
E-mail: nld@espn.net
www.espn.net

Nancy L Day, Certifien Trauma Specialist

Defines the Conditioned Response Phenomena, establishes a safe environment, analyzes and applies the Unblocking technique to resolve issues relating to emotionally charged persons, places, things and situations, and analyzes and applies Traumatic Incident Reduction (TIR) to resolve known and unknown past traumatic experiences and the unwanted feelings, emotions, sensations, attitutdes and pain associated with them.

3196 YAI/National Institute for People with Disabilities

460 W 34th Street
New York, NY 10001-2382
212-273-6100
www.yai.org

Joel M Levy, CEO
Philip H Levy, President/COO

Consulting Services

3197 American Society of Addiction Medicine

4601 N Park Avenue
Upper Arcade #101
Chevy Chase, MD 20815
301-656-3920
Fax: 301-656-3815
E-mail: email@asam.org
www.asam.org

Michael Miller, President
Eileen McGrath, Executive Vice President

Increase access to and improve the quality of addictions treatment. Educate physicians, medical and osteopathic, and the public.

3198 Info Management Associates

1595 Lincoln Highway
Edison, NJ 08817
732-572-2253
800-572-2256

Fax: 732-572-3039
E-mail: info@imasys.com
www.imasys.com

Gail Willis, IMA Service
Art Erickson, IMA Helpdesk

Custom software applications for a variety of industries, with a special focus on systems and services for human services organizations.

3199 MHM Services

1593 Spring Hill Road
Suite 610
Vienna, VA 22182
703-749-4600
800-416-3649
Fax: 703-749-4604
www.mhm-services.com

Michael Pinkert, Founder/Chairman/CEO
Steve Wheeler, President/COO

National specialist in providing on-site mental health services to correctional systems, including state and local prison, jails and juvenile detention centers. Also is a leader in the management of behavioral health programs in the community

3200 Mental Health Consultants

1878 Sugar Bottom Road
Furlong, PA 18925-1525
215-345-6838
Fax: 215-345-8488
www.mhconsultants.com

Edward Haaz, President

Workplace behavioral specialty network in southeastern Pennsylvania and New Jersey. 850+ licensed professionals/trainers, 45 inpatient and alternative care facilities under contract. Provides Employee Assistance Services on a case rate or capitated basis. In addition, MHC offers the following workplace services: employee education workshops/seminars, executive coaching, team building, communication enhancement, trauma intervention, critical incident stress debriefing, workplace behavioral assessments, risk management assessments.

3201 River Valley Behavioral Health

1100 Walnut Street
Owensboro, KY 42302
270-689-6500
800-737-0696
E-mail: info@rvbh.com
www.www.rvbh.com

Professional management company for behavioral health and mental retardation/developmental disability service providers; offering training, evaluation, substance abuse, supported employment, community support, case management, professional placement, and organizational management. Training topics include consumer advocacy, juvenile justice, elder abuse, and estate planning for people with disabilities.

Periodicals & Pamphlets

3202 AACAP News
AACAP
3615 Wisconsin Avenue NW
Washington, DC 20016-3007

202-966-7300
Fax: 202-966-2891
E-mail: communications@aacap.org
www.aacap.org

Robert Hendren, President
David Herzog, Secretary
William Bernet, Treasurer

The American Academy of Child and Adolescent Psychiatry, (AACAP) publishes a newsletter which focuses events within the Academy, child and adolescent psychiatrists, and AACAP members.

36-64 pages 6 per year

3203 AAMI Newsletter
Arizona Alliance for the Mentally Ill (NAMI Arizona)
2210 N 7th Street
Phoenix, AZ 85006
602-244-8166
800-626-5022
Fax: 602-244-9264
E-mail: namiaz@namiaz.org
www.namiaz.org

Diane McVicker, President
Cheryl Weiner, Educutive Director

Provides support, education, research, and advocacy for individuals and families affected by mental illness. Reports on legislative updates, conventions, psychiatry/psychological practices, and activities of the alliance. Newsletter with membership. *$10.00*

8 pages 4 per year

3204 AAPL Newsletter
American Academy of Psychiatry and the Law
One Regency Drive
PO Box 30
Bloomfield, CT 06002-0030
860-242-5450
800-331-1389
Fax: 860-286-0787
E-mail: execoff@aapl.org
www.aapl.org

Jacquelyn T. Coleman, Executive Director
Jeffrey Janofsky MD, President
Kenneth Appelbaum MD, Vice President

Newsletter that discusses psychiatry as it relates to the law. Recurring features include recent legal cases, legislative updates, letters to the editor, notices of publications available, news of educational opportunities, job listings, a calendar of events, and editorial columns. *$25.00*

20 pages 3 per year

3205 AJMR-American Journal on Mental Retardation
AAMR
444 N Capitol Street NW
Suite 846
Washington, DC 20001-1512
202-387-1968
800-424-3688
Fax: 202-387-2193
E-mail: dcroser@aamr.org
www.aamr.org

Provides updates on the latest program advances, current research, and information on products and services in the developmental disabilities field. *$10.50*

24 per year ISSN 0047-6765

3206 APA Monitor
American Psychological Association
750 1st Street NE
Washington, DC 20002-4242
202-336-5500
800-374-2721
Fax: 202-336-6103
E-mail: letters.monitor@apa.org
www.apa.org/monitor

Magazine of the American Psychological Association.

12 per year ISSN 1529-4978

3207 ARC News
Association for Retarded Citizens-Pennsylvania
1617 Bald Eagle Avenue
S Williamsport, PA 17702-7034
570-326-6997

Publicizes work of the Association, which is committed to securing for all people with mental retardation the opportunity to choose and realize their goals; promotes reducing the incidence and limiting the consequence of mental retardation through education, research, advocacy, and the support of family, friends, and the community; provides leadership in the field and strives for development of necessary human and financial resources to succeed.

4 pages 12 per year

3208 ASAP Newsletter
American Society for Adolescent Psychiatry
PO Box 570218
Dallas, TX 75357-0218
972-613-0985
Fax: 972-613-5532
E-mail: info@adolpsych.org
www.adolpsych.org

Mohan Nair, President
Frances Bell, Executive Director

Contains articles about adolescent psychiatry and society news. Recurring features include news of research, a calendar of events, and book reviews. *$10.00*

16-20 pages 4 per year

3209 Advocate: Autism Society of America
Autism Society of America
7910 Woodmont Avenue
Suite 300
Bethesda, MD 20814-3067
301-657-0881
800-328-8476
Fax: 301-657-0869
www.autism-society.org

Reports news and information of national significance for individuals, families, and professionals dealing with autism. Recurring features include personal features and profiles, research summaries, government updates, book reviews, statistics, news of research, and a calendar of events.

32-36 pages 6 per year ISSN 0047-9101

3210 Alcohol & Drug Abuse Weekly
John Wiley & Sons
111 River Street
Hoboken, NJ 07030-5774
201-748-6000
Fax: 201-748-6088
www.wiley.com

48-issue subsrciption offers significant news and analysis of federal and state policy developments. A resource for directors of addiction treatment centers, managed care executives, federal and state policy makers and healthcare consultants. Topics include the latest findings in treatment and prevention; funding and survival issues for providers; the impact of state and federal policy on treatment and prevention; working under managed care; and co-occurring disorders.

8 pages 48 per year Year Founded: 1992 ISSN 1042-1394

3211 American Association of Community Psychiatrists (AACP)
PO Box 570218
Dallas, TX 75357-0218
972-613-0985
Fax: 972-613-5532
E-mail: frda1@airmail.net
www.www.wpic.pitt.edu/aacp

Wesley Sowers MD, President
Annelle Primm, Vice President
Francis Bell, Administrative Director

Psychiatrists and psychiatry residents practicing in community mental health centers or similar programs that provide care to the mentally ill regardless of their ability to pay. Addresses issues faced by psychiatrists who practice within CMHCs. Publications: AACP Membership Directory, annual. Community Psychiatrist, quarterly newsletter. Annual meeting, in conjunction with American Psychiatric Association in May. Annual meeting, in conjunction with Institute on Hospital and Community in fall.

4 per year

3212 American Institute for Preventive Medicine
American Institute for Preventive Medicine Press
30445 Northwestern Highway
Suite 350
Farmington Hills, MI 48334-3107
248-539-1800
800-345-2476
Fax: 248-539-1808
E-mail: aipm@healthy.net
www.healthylife.com

Don R Powell, President
Sue Jackson, VP

AIPM is an internationally renowned developer and provider of wellness programs and publications that address both mental and physical health issues. It works with over 11,500 corporations, hospitals, MCOs, universities, and goverment agencies to reduce health care costs, lower absenteeism, and improve productivity. The Institute has a number of publications that address mental health issues, including stress management, depression, self - esteem, and EAP issues.

Year Founded: 1999

3213 Association for Child Psychoanalysis Newsletter
Association for Child Psychoanalysis
320 Glendale Drive
Chapel Hill, NC 27514-5914
919-967-5819
Fax: 919-929-0988
E-mail: brinich@unc.edu

Paul Brinich, Editor

Discusses child analysis methods, child psycholanalysis training, and the treatment and education of children throughout the world. Recurring features include news of members and the Association and announcements of research training programs, meetings, lectures, and committees concerned with child psychoanalysis.

24-36 pages 2 per year ISSN 1077-0305

3214 Behavioral Health Industry News
Open Minds
163 York Street
Gettysburg, PA 17325-1933
717-334-1329
877-350-6463
Fax: 717-334-0538
E-mail: openminds@openminds.com
www.openminds.com

Provides information on marketing, financial, and legal trends in the delivery of mental health and chemical dependency benefits and services. Recurring features include interviews, news of research, a calendar of events, job listings, book reviews, notices of publications available, and industry statistics. *$185.00*

12 pages 12 per year ISSN 1043-3880

3215 Behavioral Health Management
PO Box 20179
Cleveland, OH 44120
216-391-9100
Fax: 216-391-9200
www.behavioral.net

Richard Peck, Editorial Director
Douglas J Edwards, Managing Editor

Informs decision makers in managed behavioral healthcare organizations, provider groups, and treatment centers of the ever-changing demands of their field. The magazine publishes analyses, editorials, and organizations case studies to give readers the information they need for best practices in a challenging marketplace.

3216 Brown University: Child & Adolescent Psychopharmacology Update
John Wiley & Sons
111 River Street
Hoboken, NJ 07030-5744
201-748-6000
Fax: 201-748-6088
E-mail: jbsubs@wiley.com
www.www.wiley.com

Monthly newsletter that gives information on children and adolescent's unique psychotropic medication needs. Delivers updates on new drugs, their uses, typical doses, side effects and interactions, examines generic vs. name brand drugs, reports on new research and new indications for existing medications. Each issue also includes case studies, references for future reading, industry news notes, abstracts

of current research and a patient psychotropic medication handout. *$190.00*

12 per year ISSN 1527-8395

3217 Brown University: Digest of Addiction Theory and Application (DATA)
John Wiley & Sons
111 River Street
Hoboken, NJ 07030-5774
201-748-6000
Fax: 201-748-6088
E-mail: jbsubs@wiley.com
www.www.wiley.com

Monthly synopsis of critical research developments in the treatment and prevention of alcoholism and drug abuse, including dozens of research abstracts chosen from over 75 medical journals. *$129.00*

8 pages 12 per year ISSN 1040-6328

3218 Brown University: Geriatric Psychopharmacology Update
John Wiley & Sons
111 River Street
Hoboken, NJ 07030-5774
201-748-6000
Fax: 201-748-6088
E-mail: jbsubs@wiley.com
www.www.wiley.com

This monthly report is an easy way to keep up to date on the newest breakthroughs in geriatric medicine that have an impact on psychiatric practice. *$190.00*

12 per year ISSN 1529-2584

3219 Brown University: Psychopharmacology Update
John Wiley & Sons
111 River Street
Hoboken, NJ 07030-5774
201-748-6000
Fax: 201-748-6088
www.www.wiley.com

Each issue examines the pros and cons of specific drugs, drug-drug interactions, side effects, street drugs, warning signs, case reports and more. *$199.00*

12 per year ISSN 1608-5308

3220 Bulletin of Menninger Clinic
Guilford Publications
72 Spring Street
New York, NY 10012
785-380-5000
800-288-3950
Fax: 785-273-8625
www.menninger.edu

W Walter Meninger, Editor

Valuable, practical information for clinicans. Recent topical issues have focused on rekindling the psychodynamic vision, treatment of different clinical populations with panic disorder, and treatment of complicated personality disorders in an era of managed care. All in an integrated, psychodynamic approach. *$75.00*

ISSN 0025-9284

3221 Bulletin of Psychological Type
Association for Psychological Type
9650 Rockville Pike
Bethesda, MD 20814-3998
301-634-7450
800-847-9943
Fax: 301-634-7455
E-mail: web@aptinternational.org
www.aptinternational.org

John Lord, Executive Director
Jane Kise, President

Provides information on regional, national, and international events to keep professionals up-to-date in the study and application of psychological type theory and the Myers-Briggs Type Indicator. Contains announcements of training workshops; international, national, and regional conferences; and awards, along with articles on issues directly related to type theory.

3222 Capitation Report
National Health Information
PO Box 15429
Atlanta, GA 30333-0429
404-607-9500
800-597-6300
Fax: 404-607-0095
www.nhionline.net

NHI publishes specialized, targeted information for health care executives on a variety of topics from capitation to disease management.

3223 Child and Adolescent Psychiatry
American Academy of Child and Adolescent Psychiatry
3615 Wisconsin Avenue NW
Washington, DC 20016-3007
202-966-7300
Fax: 202-966-2891
E-mail: communications@aacap.org
www.aacap.org

Robert Hendren, President
David Herzog, Secretary
William Bernet, Treasurer

Journal focusing on today's psychiatric research and treatment of the child and adolescent. *$175.00*

12 per year   ISSN 0890-8567

3224 Chronicle
Association for the Help of Retarded Children (AHRC)
200 Park Avenue South
New York, NY 10003-1503
212-780-2500
Fax: 212-777-5893
E-mail: ahrcnyc@ahrcnyc.org
www.ahrcnyc.org

Covers developmental disabilities, includes legislation and entitlements updates, field news, accessing information and services, advocacy issues, and current research. Recurring features include interviews, news of research, a calendar of events, reports of meetings, book reviews, and notices of publications available.

16-28 pages   4 per year

3225 Clinical Psychiatry News
International Medical News Group
12230 Wilkins Avenue
Rockville, MD 20852-1834
301-816-8700
877-524-9335
Fax: 301-816-8712
E-mail: cpsnews@elsevier.com
www.imng.com

A leading independent newspaper for the Psychiatrist.

3226 Clinical Psychiatry Quarterly
AACP
PO Box 458
Glastonbury, CT 06033
860-633-5045
Fax: 860-633-6023
E-mail: info@aacp.com
www.aacp.com

Informs members of of news and events. Recurring features include letters to the editor, news of research, a calendar of events, reports of meetings, and book reviews.

4 per year

3227 Couples Therapy in Managed Care
Haworth Press
10 Alice Street
Binghamton, NY 13904-1580
607-722-5857
800-429-6784
Fax: 607-722-1424
E-mail: getinfo@haworthpressinc.com
www.haworthpress.com

Provides social workers, psychologists and counselors with an overview of the negative effects of the managed care industry on the quality of marital health care.

ISBN 7-890078-86-6

3228 Development & Psychopathology
Cambridge University Press
40 W 20th Street
New York, NY 10011-4221
212-924-3900
Fax: 212-691-3239
E-mail: marketing@cup.org
www.cup.org

This multidisciplinary journal is devoted to the publication of original, empirical, theoretical and review papers which address the interrelationship of normal and pathological development in adults and children. It is intended to serve and intergrate the emerging field of developmental psychopathology which strives to understand patterns of adaptation and maladaptation throughout the lifespan. This journal is of vital interest to psychologists, psychiatrists, social scientists, neuroscientists, pediatricians and researchers. *$66.00*

4 per year   ISSN 0954-5794

3229 Developmental Brain Research
Customer Support Department
PO Box 945
New York, NY 10159-0945
212-633-3730
888-437-4636
Fax: 212-633-3680
www.elsevier.com

ISSN 0165-3806

3230 Disability Funding Week
CD Publications
8204 Fenton Street
Silver Spring, MD 20910-4509
301-588-6380
800-666-6380
Fax: 301-588-6385
E-mail: cdpubs@clark.net
www.cdpublications.com

Wayne Welch, Editor

Up to date news for mental health professionals. *$ 259.00*

14-18 pages 24 per year Year Founded: 1992 ISSN 1069-1359

3231 EAPA Exchange
Employee Assistance Professionals Association
2101 Wilson Boulevard
Arlington, VA 22201-3062
703-522-6272
Fax: 703-522-4585

3232 ETR Associates
Health Education, Research, Training Curriculum
4 Carbonero Way
Scotts Valley, CA 95066
831-438-4060
800-321-4407
Fax: 831-438-4284
www.etr.org

John Henry Ledwith, National Sales Director

Publishes a complete line of innovative materials covering the full spectrum of health education topics, including maternal/child health, HIV/STD prevention, risk and injury prevention, self esteem, fitness and nutrition, college health, and wellness education, engaging in both extensive training and research endeavors and a comprehensive K-12 health curriculum.

3233 Employee Benefits Journal
International Foundation of Employee Benefit Plans
PO Box 69
Brookfield, WI 53008-0069
414-786-6700
Fax: 414-786-8670
E-mail: marybr@ifebp.org
www.ifebp.org

Contains articles on all aspects of employee benefits and related topics. *$70.00*

32-48 pages 4 per year ISSN 0361-4050

3234 Exceptional Parent
PO Box 5446
Pittsfield, MA 01203-5446
201-634-6550
800-372-7368
Fax: 740-389-6845
www.eparent.com

Magazine for parents and professionals involved in the care and development of children and young adults with special needs, including physical disabilities, developmental disabilities, mental retardation, autism, epilepsy, learning dis-

abilities, hearing/vision impairments, emotional problems, and chronic illnesses. *$36.00*

12 per year

3235 Focal Point: Research, Policy and Practice in Children's Mental Health
Regional Research Institue-Portland State University
PO Box 751
Portland, OR 97207-0751
503-725-4040
800-628-1696
Fax: 503-725-4180
E-mail: rtcpubs@pdx.edu
www.rtc.pdx.edu

Janet Walker, Editor

Features information on research, interventions, organizations, strategies, and conferences to aid families that have children with emotional, mental, and/or behavioral disorders.

24 pages

3236 Forty Two Lives in Treatment: a Study of Psychoanalysis and Psychotherapy
Guilford Publications
72 Spring Street
New York, NY 10012
212-431-9800
800-365-7006
Fax: 212-966-6708
E-mail: info@guilford.com
www.guilford.com

Comprehensive results of the study of 42 patients undergoing psychoanalysis and analytic psychotherapy. *$79.95*

784 pages Year Founded: 1986 ISBN 0-898623-25-1

3237 From the Couch
Behavioral Health Record Section-AMRA
919 N Michigan Avenue
Suite 1400
Chicago, IL 60611-1692
312-787-2672
Fax: 312-787-5926

From the couch, the newsletter for the Behavioral Health Record section of the American Medical Record Association, covers aspects of the medical records industry that pertain to mental health records.

4 per year

3238 Frontiers of Health Services Management
American College of Healthcare Executives
1 N Franklin Street
Chicago, IL 60606-3529
312-424-2800
Fax: 312-424-0023
E-mail: hap1@ache.org
www.ache.org

Audrey Kaufman, Assistant Director
Janet Davis, Acquisitions Editor

Enhanced by special access to today's healthcare leaders. Frontiers provides you with the cutting edge insight you want. Each quarterly issue engages you in a vigorous debate on a hot healthcare topic. One stimulating article leads the debate, followed by commentaries and perspectives from recognized experts. Unique combination of opinion, practice and research stimulate you to develop new management strategies. *$70.00*

4 per year   ISSN 0748-8157

3239   General Hospital Psychiatry: Psychiatry, Medicine and Primary Care
Elsevier Science
725 Concord Avenue
Suite 4200
Cambridge, MA
617-661-3544
Fax: 617-661-4800
E-mail: don_lipsitt@hms.harvard.edu
www.elsevier.com

Journal that explores the linkages and interfaces between psychiatry, medicine and primary care. As a peer-reviewed journal, it provides a forum for communication among professionals with clinical, academic and research interests in psychiatry's essential function in the mainstream of medicine. *$195.00*

84 pages 6 per year   ISSN 01638343

3240   Geriatrics
Advanstar Communications
7500 Old Oak Boulevard
Cleveland, OH 44130-3343
440-243-8100
Fax: 440-891-2733
E-mail: arossetti@advanstar.com
www.geri.com

David Briemer, Sales Manager
Rich Ehrlich, Associate Publisher

Peer-reviewed clinical journal for primary care physicians who care for patients age 50 and older.

100 pages 12 per year

3241   Group Practice Journal
Amerian Medical Group Association
1422 Duke Street
Alexandria, VA 22314-3403
703-838-0033
Fax: 703-548-1890
E-mail: roconnor@amga.org
www.amga.org

Francis Marzoni, Secretary
Donald Fisher, President/CEO

Penned by healthcare professionals, articles in the Group Practice Journal give a view from the trenches of modern medicine on a wide variety of topics, including innovative disease management and clinical best practices. Readers look to the publication to learn strategies and solutions from peers in the profession, healthcare thought leaders, and industry experts.

10 per year

3242   Harvard Mental Health Letter
Harvard Health Publications
10 Shattuck Street
Suite 612
Boston, MA 02115-6011
617-432-1485
Fax: 617-432-1506
E-mail: mental_health@hms.harvard.edu
www.health.harvard.edu

Delivers information on current thinking and debate on mental health issues that concern professionals and layment a like. In the ever-changing and complex field of mental health care, the newsletter has become a trusted source for psychiatrists, psychologists, social workers and therapists of all kinds. *$59.00*

8 pages 12 per year Year Founded: 1983 ISSN 08843783

3243   Harvard Review of Psychiatry
Taylor and Francis
01650 Toebben Drive
Independence, KY 41051
800-634-7064
Fax: 800-248-4724

An authoritative source for scholarly reviews and perspectives on important topics in psychiatry. Founded by the Harvard Medical School's Department of Psychiatry, the Harvard Review of Psychiatry features review papares that summarize and synthesize the key literature in a scholarly and clinically relevant manner. *$185.00*

6 per year

3244   Health & Social Work
National Association of Social Workers
750 1st Street NE
Suite 700
Washington, DC 20002-4241
202-336-8236
Fax: 202-336-8312
www.naswdc.org

Articles cover research, policy, specialized servies, quality assurance, inservice training and other topics that affect the delivery of health care services. *$125.00*

3245   Health Data Management
Faulkner & Gray
11 Penn Plaza
New York, NY 10001-2006
212-967-7000
Fax: 212-239-4993

3246   Health Grants & Contracts Weekly
Capitol Publications
1101 K Street
Suite 444
Alexandria, VA 22314
703-583-4100
Fax: 703-739-6517

Provides information on health-related project opportunities in research, training and service

3247   IABMCP Newsletter
IABMCP
3208 N Academy Boulevard, Suite 160
Colorado Springs, CO 80917
719-597-5959
Fax: 719-597-0166
E-mail: iabmcp@att.net

The International Academy of Behavioral Medicine, Counseling, and Psychotherapy, (IABMCP) publishes research articles in the field of behavioral medicine, 'the systematic application of various principles of behavioral science to health care problems.' Contains news of the Academy and its members. Recurring features include book reviews, letters to the editor, and a calendar of events. *$60.00*

4-8 pages 4 per year

3248 Insider
Alliance for Children and Families
1701 K Street NW
Suite 200
Washington, DC 20006-1523
202-223-3447
Fax: 202-331-7476
E-mail: policy@alliance1.org
www.alliance1.org

Carmen Delgado Votaw, Sr VP
Peter Goldberg, President/CEO
Thomas Harney, VP Membership

Alliance for Children and Families' tool for providing
members with accurate and up-to-date information on current legislation, issues the Alliance is advocating on Capitol
Hill, summaries of how proposed bills will affect member
organizations and the people they serve, and suggestions for
local advocacy efforts.

3249 International Drug Therapy Newsletter
Lippincott Williams & Wilkins
351 W Camden Street
Baltimore, MD 21201-7912
410-528-8517
800-882-0483
Fax: 410-528-4312
E-mail: korourke@lww.com
www.lww.com

Newsletter that focuses on psychotropic drugs, discussing
individual drugs, their effectiveness, and history. Examines
illnesses and the drugs used to treat them, studies done on
various drugs, their chemical make-up, and new developments and changes in drugs. *$149.00*

8 pages ISSN 0020-6571

3250 International Journal of
Neuropsychopharmacology
Cambridge University Press
40 W 20th Street
New York, NY 10011-4221
212-924-3900
Fax: 212-691-3239
E-mail: marketing@cup.org
www.cup.org

3251 International Journal of Aging and Human
Developments
Baywood Publishing Company
26 Austin Avenue
Box 337
Amityville, NY 11701
631-691-1270
800-638-7819
Fax: 631-691-1770
E-mail: baywood@baywood.com
www.baywood.com

$218.00

8 per year Year Founded: 1973 ISSN 0091-4150

3252 International Journal of Health Services
Baywood Publishing Company
26 Austin Avenue
Box 337
Amityville, NY 11701
631-691-1270
800-638-7819

Fax: 631-691-1770
E-mail: baywood@baywood.com
www.baywood.com

$160.00

4 per year Year Founded: 1970

3253 International Journal of Psychiatry in Medicine
Baywood Publishing Company
26 Austin Avenue
Box 337
Amityville, NY 11701
631-691-1270
800-638-7819
Fax: 631-691-1770
E-mail: baywood@baywood.com
www.baywood.com

$160.00

4 per year Year Founded: 1970 ISSN 0091274

3254 Journal of AHIMA
American Health Information Management
Association
233 N Michigan Avenue
21st Floor
Chicago, IL 60601-5800
312-233-1100
Fax: 312-233-1090
E-mail: info@ahima.org
www.ahima.org

Linda Kloss, CEO
Becky Garris-Perry, Executive Vice President/CFO

Monthly magazine with articles, news and event
annoucements from the nonprofit federation of affiliated
state health organizations, together representing nearly
12,000 nonprofit and for profit assisted living, nursing facility, developmentally disabled and subacute care providers that care for more than 1.5 million elderly and disabled
individuals nationally.

3255 Journal of American Health Information
Management Association
American Health Information Management
Association
233 N Michigan Avenue
21st Floor
Chicago, IL 60601-5800
312-233-1100
Fax: 312-233-1090
E-mail: info@ahima.org
www.ahima.org

Linda Kloss, CEO
Becky Garris-Perry, Executive Vice President/CFO

3256 Journal of American Medical Information
Association
Hanley & Befus
210 S 13th Street
Philadelphia, PA 19107-5467
215-546-4656

3257 Journal of Drug Education
Baywood Publishing Company
26 Austin Avenue
Box 337
Amityville, NY 11701

631-691-1270
800-638-7819
Fax: 631-691-1770
E-mail: info@baywood.com
www.baywood.com

$160.00

4 per year Year Founded: 1970

3258 Journal of Education Psychology
American Psychological Association
750 1st Street NE
Washington, DC 20002-4241
202-336-5510
800-374-2721
Fax: 202-336-5502
TDD: 202-336-6123
TTY: 202-336-6123
E-mail: order@apa.org
www.apa.org/books

Carole Beal, Associate Editor

$102.00

4 per year ISSN 0022-0663

3259 Journal of Emotional and Behavioral Disorders
Pro-Ed Publications
8700 Shoal Creek Boulevard
Austin, TX 78757-6816
512-451-3246
800-897-3202
Fax: 800-397-7633
E-mail: info@proedinc.com
www.proedinc.com

Lisa Tippett, Managing Production Editor

An international, multidisciplinary journal featuring articles on research, practice and theory related to individuals with emotional and behavioral disorders and to the professionals who serve them. Presents topics of interest to individuals representing a wide range of disciplines including corrections, psychiatry, mental health, counseling, rehabilitation, education, and psychology. *$39.00*

64 pages 4 per year ISSN 1063-4266

3260 Journal of Intellectual & Development Disability
Taylor & Francis Publishing
875 Massachusetts Avenue
Suite 81
Cambridge, MA 02139-3067
215-625-8900
Fax: 215-269-0363
www.taylorandfrancis.com

3261 Journal of Neuropsychiatry and Clinical Neurosciences
American Neuropsychiatric Association
700 Ackerman Road
Suite 625
Columbus, OH 43202
614-447-2077
Fax: 614-263-4366
E-mail: anpa@osu.edu
www.www.anpaonline.org

Fred Ovsiew MD, President
C. Edward Coffey, Treasurer

Official publication of the organization and a benefit of membership. Our mission is to apply neuroscience for the benefit of people. Three core values have been identified for the association: advancing knowledge of brain-behavior relationships, providing a forum for learning, and promoting excellent, scientific and compassionate health care.

3262 Journal of Positive Behavior Interventions
Pro-Ed Publications
8700 Shoal Creek Boulevard
Austin, TX 78757-6816
512-451-3246
800-897-3202
Fax: 800-397-7633
E-mail: info@proedinc.com
www.proedinc.com

Lisa Tippett, Managing Production Editor

Deals with principles of positive behavioral support in school, home, and community settings for people with challenges in behavioral adaptation. *$39.00*

64 pages 4 per year ISSN 1098-3007

3263 Journal of Practical Psychiatry
Williams & Wilkins
351 W Camden Street
Baltimore, MD 21201-7912
410-528-4000
Fax: 410-528-4312

3264 Journal of the American Medical Informatics Association
American Medical Informatics Association
4915 St. Elmo Avenue
Suite 401
Bethesda, MD 20814-6052
301-657-1291
Fax: 301-657-1296
E-mail: mail@amia.org
www.amia.org

Don Detmer, President/CEO
Sarah Ingersoll, Treasurer

JAMIA is a bi-monthly journal that presents peer-reviewed articles on the spectrum of health care informatics in research, teaching, and application. *$212.00*

3265 Journal of the American Psychiatric Nurses Association
Sage Publishing
2455 Teller Road
Thoasand Oaks, CA 91320
805-499-9774
800-818-7243
Fax: 805-499-0871
E-mail: journals@sagepub.com
www.sagepub.com

Karen Frachau Stein PhD, Editor

Official Journal of the American Psychiatric Nurses Association *$128.00*

ISSN 1078-3903

3266 Journal of the American Psychoanalytic Association
Analytic Press
101 W Street
Hillsdale, NJ 07642-1421

201-358-9477
800-926-6579
Fax: 201-358-4700
E-mail: TAP@analyticpress.com
www.analyticpress.com

Paul E Stepansky PhD, Managing Director
John Kerr PhD, Sr Editor

JAPA is one of the preeminent psychoanalytic journals. Recognized for the quality of its clinical and theoretical contributions, JAPA is now a major publication source for scientists and humanists whose work elaborates, applies, critiques or impinges on psychoanalysis. Topics include child psychoanalysis and the effectiveness of the intensive treatment of children, boundary violations, problems of memory and false memory syndrome, the concept of working through, the scientific status of psychoanalysis and the relevance or irrevance of infant observation for adult analysis. *$115.00*

300 pages 4 per year Year Founded: 1952 ISSN 0003-0651

3267 Journal of the International Neuropsychological Society
Cambridge University Press
40 W 20th Street
New York, NY 10011-4221
212-924-3900
Fax: 212-691-3239
E-mail: marketing@cup.org
www.cup.org

3268 Key
National Mental Health Consumers Self-Help
1211 Chestnut Street
Lobby 100
Philadelphia, PA 19107-4114
215-751-1810
800-553-4539
Fax: 215-636-6310
TTY: 215-751-9655
E-mail: info@mhselfhelp.org
www.mhselfhelp.org

Violet Phillips, Editor

Provides information for consumers of mental health services/psychiatric survivors on mental health issues, including advocacy and alternative mental health services. *$15.00*

12 pages 4 per year

3269 Managed Care Strategies
Managed Care Strategies & Psychotherapy Finances
13901 US Highway 1
Suite 5
Juno Beach, FL 33408-1612
561-624-1155
Fax: 561-624-6006

3270 Mayo Clinic Health Letter
Mayo Clinic
200 1st Street SW
Rochester, MN 55905-0002
507-284-2511
Fax: 507-266-0230
E-mail: healthletter@mayo.edu
www.mayoclinic.com

Helping our subscribers achieve healthier lives by providing useful, easy to understand health information that is timely and of broad interest.

ISSN 0741-6245

3271 Medical Psychotherapist
Americal Board of Medical Psychotherapists & Psychodiagnosticians
345 24th Avenue N
Suite 201
Nashville, TN 32703-1520
615-327-2984
Fax: 615-327-9235

Official newsletter of the American Board of Medical Psychotherapists and Psychodiagnosticians.

3272 Medications
National Institute of Mental Health
6001 Executive Boulevard
Room 8184
Bethesda, MD 20892-9663
866-615-6464
Fax: 301-443-4279
TTY: 301-443-8431
E-mail: nimhinfo@nih.gov
www.nimh.nih.gov

This booklet is designed to help mental health patients and their families understand how and why medications can be used as part of the treatment of mental health problems.

36 pages

3273 Mental & Physical Disability Law Reporter
American Bar Association
740 15th Street NW
9th Floor
Washington, DC 20005-1022
202-662-1570
Fax: 202-662-1032
TTY: 202-662-1012
E-mail: CMPDL@abanet.org
www.abanet.org/disability

Amy Allbright, Managing Editor
Renee Dexter, Production/Marketing Manager

Contains bylined articles and summaries of federal and state court opinions and legislative developments addressing persons with mental and physical disabilities.

6 per year Year Founded: 1976 ISSN 0883-7902

3274 Mental Health Aspects of Developmental Disabilities
Psych-Media
PO Box 57
Bear Creek, NC 27207-0057
336-581-3700
Fax: 336-581-3766
E-mail: mhdd@amji.net
www.mhaspectsofdd.com

Margaret Zwilling, Managing Editor
Linda Vollmoeller, Assistant Managing Editor

A practical clinical reference for the hands on clinician. This is a peer-reviewed journal covering the diagnosis, treatment and rehabilitation needs of persons with developmental disabilities. *$ 58.00*

40 pages 4 per year ISSN 1057-3291

3275 Mental Health Law Reporter
Business Publishers
8737 Colesville Road
Suite 1100
Silver Spring, MD 20910-3956
301-587-6300
800-274-6737
Fax: 301-587-1081
E-mail: jbond@bpinews.com
www.bpinews.com

Nancy Biglin, Director Marketing

Summary of court cases pertaining to mental health professionals. *$273.00*

12 per year   ISSN 0741-5141

3276 Mental Health Report
Business Publishers
8737 Colesville Road
Suite 1100
Silver Spring, MD 20910-3928
301-587-6300
800-274-6737
Fax: 301-587-4530
E-mail: jbond@bpinews.com
www.bpinews.com

Nancy Biglin, Director Marketing

Independent, inside Washington coverage of mental health administration, legislation and regulation, state policy plus research and trends. *$396.00*

26 per year   ISSN 0191-6750

3277 Mental Health Views
CD Publications
8204 Fenton Street
Silver Spring, MD 20910-4509
301-588-6380
Fax: 301-588-6385

3278 Mental Health Weekly
Manisses Communications Group
PO Box 9758
Providence, RI 02940-9758
401-831-6020
800-333-7771
Fax: 401-861-6370
E-mail: manissescs@manisses.com
www.manisses.com

William Kanapaux, Managing Editor

Economic and policy issues for mental health professionals. *$499.00*

48 per year   ISSN 10581103

3279 Mental Retardation
AAMR
444 N Capitol Street NW
Suite 846
Washington, DC 20001-1512
202-387-1968
800-424-3688
Fax: 202-387-2193
E-mail: dcroser@aamr.org
www.aamr.org

Newsletter that provides information on the latest program advances, current research, and information on products and services in the developmental disabilities field. Free with membership.

24 per year   ISSN 0895-8033

3280 Mentally Disabled and the Law
William S Hein & Company
1285 Main Street
Buffalo, NY 14209-1911
716-882-2600
800-828-7571
Fax: 716-883-8100

Offers information on treatment rights, the provider-patient relationship, and the rights of mentally disabled persons in the community. *$80.00*

3281 NAMI Advocate
National Alliance for the Mentally Ill
200 N Glebe Road
Suite 1015
Arlington, VA 22203-3728
703-524-7600
800-950-6264
Fax: 703-524-9094
TDD: 703-516-7227
E-mail: frieda@nami.org
www.nami.org

Newsletter that provides information on latest research, treatment, and medications for brain disorders. Reviews status major policy and legislation at federal, state, and local levels. Recurring features include interviews, news of research, news of educational opportunities, book reviews, politics, legal issues, and columns titled President's Column, Ask the Doctor, and News You Can Use. Included as NAMI membership benefit.

24-28 pages   24 per year

3282 NAMI Beginnings
National Alliance on Mental Illness
2107 Wilson Boulevard
Suite 300
Arlington, VA 22201-3042
703-524-7600
800-950-6264
Fax: 703-524-9094
TDD: 703-516-7227
E-mail: david@nami.org
www.nami.org

David Todd, Director of Publications

A publication dedicated to the Young Minds of America from the Child and Adolescent Action Center, a free newsletter about children and adolescents living with mental illnesses.

4 per year

3283 NASW News
National Association of Social Works
750 1st Street NE
Suite 700
Washington, DC 20002-4241
202-336-8236
Fax: 202-336-8312

3284 News & Notes
AAMR
444 N Capitol Street NW
Suite 846
Washington, DC 20001-1512
202-387-1968
800-424-3688
Fax: 202-387-2193
E-mail: dcroser@aamr.org
www.aamr.org

Doreen Croser, Executive Director

Covers legislative, program, and research developments of
interest to the field, as well as international news, Association activities, job ads and other classifieds and upcoming
events.

3285 Newsletter of the American Psychoanalytic
Association
Analytic Press
101 W Street
Hillsdale, NJ 07642-1421
201-358-9477
800-926-6579
Fax: 201-358-4700
E-mail: TAP@analyticpress.com
www.analyticpress.com

Paul E Stepansky PhD, Managing Director
John Kerr PhD, Sr Editor

A scholarly and clinical resource for all analytic practitioners and students of the field. Articles and essays focused
on contemporary social, political and cultural forces as they
relate to the practice of psychoanalysis, regular interviews
with leading proponents of analysis, essays and reminis-
cences that chart the evolution of anlaysis in America. The
newsletter publishes articles that are rarely if ever found in
the journal literature. Sample copies available. *$29.50*

4 per year

3286 North American Society of Adlerian Psychology
Newsletter
NASAP
614 W Chocolate Avenue
Hershey, PA 17033
717-579-8795
Fax: 717-533-8616
E-mail: nasap@msn.com
www.alfredadler.org

Becky LaFountain, Administrator

Relates news and events of the North American Society of
Alderian Psychology and regional news of affiliated associations. Recurring features include lists of courses and workshops offered by affiliated associations, reviews of new
publications in the field, professional employment opportunities, a calendar of events, and a column titled President's
Message. *$20.00*

8 pages   24 per year   ISSN 0889-9428

3287 ORTHO Update
American Orthopsychiatric Association
2001 Beauregard Street
12th Floor
Alexandria, VA 22311
703-797-2584
Fax: 703-684-5968

E-mail: amerortho@aol.com
www.amerortho.org

Intended for members of the Association, who are concerned with the early signs of mental and behavioral disorder and preventive psychiatry. Provides news notes and
feature articles on the trends, issues and events that concern
mental health, as well as Association news.

6-16 pages   3 per year

3288 Open Minds
Behavioral Health Industry News
10 York Street
Suite 200
Gettysburg, PA 17325-2301
717-334-1329
Fax: 717-334-0538
E-mail: openminds@openminds.com
www.openminds.com

Provides information on marketing, financial, and legal
trends in the delivery of mental health and chemical dependency benefits and services. Recurring features include
interviews, news of research, a calendar of events, job listings, book reviews, notices of publications available, and
industry statistics. *$185.00*

12 pages   12 per year   ISSN 1043-3880

3289 Professional Counselor
3201 SW 15th Street
Deerfield Beach, FL 33442
954-360-0909
800-851-9100
Fax: 954-360-0034
www.professionalcounselor.com

The number one publication serving the addictions and
mental health fields.

3290 Provider Magazine
American Health Care Association
1201 L Street NW
Washington, DC 20005
202-842-4444
Fax: 202-842-3860
www.www.ahcancal.org

Bruce Yarwood, President/CEO

Of interest to the professionals who work for the nearly
12,000 nonprofit and for profit assisted living, nursing facility, developmentally disabled and subacute care providers that care for more than 1.5 million elderly and disabled
individuals nationally. Provides information, education, and
administrative tools that enhance quality at every level.

3291 PsycINFO News
American Psychological Association Database
Department/PsycINFO
750 1st Street NE
Washington, DC 20002-4241
202-336-5650
800-374-2722
Fax: 202-336-5633
TDD: 202-336-6123
TTY: 202-336-6123
E-mail: psycinfo@apa.org
www.apa.org/psycinfo

Free newsletter that keeps you up to date on enhancements
to PsycINFO products.

4 per year

3292 PsycSCAN Series
PsycINFO/American Psychological Association
750 1st Street NE
Washington, DC 20002-4242
202-336-5650
800-374-2722
Fax: 202-336-5633
TDD: 202-336-6123
E-mail: psycinfo@apa.org
www.apa.org/psycinfo

Quarterly current awareness print publications in the fields of clinical, developmental, and applied psychology, as well as learning disorders/mental retardation and behavior analysis and therapy. Contains relevant citations and abstracts from the PsycINFO database. PyscScan: Psychopharmacology is an electronic only publication.

4 per year

3293 Psych Discourse
Association of Black Psychologists
PO Box 55999
Washington, DC 20040-5999
202-722-0808
Fax: 202-722-5941
E-mail: admin@abpsi.org
www.abpsi.org

Halford Fairchild, Editor

Publishes news of the Association. Recurring features include editorials, news of research, letters to the editor, a calendar of events, and columns titled Social Actions, Chapter News, Publications, and Members in the News. *$110.00*

32-64 pages 12 per year Year Founded: 1969 ISSN 1091-4781

3294 Psychiatric News
American Psychiatric Publishing
1000 Wilson Boulevard
Suite 1825
Arlington, VA 22209-3901
703-907-7322
800-368-5777
Fax: 703-907-1091
E-mail: appi@psych.org
www.appi.org

Katie Duffy, Marketing Assistant

Psychiatric News is the official newspaper for the American Psychiatric Association. It is published twice a month and mailed to all APA members as a member benefit as well as to about 2,000 subscribers.

3295 Psychiatric Rehabilitation Journal
International Association of Psychosocialogy
10025 Gover
Columbia, MD 21044
410-730-5965

3296 Psychiatric Times
Continuing Medical Education
2801 McGaw Avenue
Irvine, CA 92614-5835
949-250-1008
800-993-2632
Fax: 949-250-0445

E-mail: pt@mhsource.com
www.psychiatrictimes.com

John Schwartz MD, Editor-in-Chief

Allows you to earn CME credit every month with a clinical article, as well as keeping you up to date on the current news in the field. *$54.95*

12 per year

3297 Psychiatry Drug Alerts
MJ Powers & Company
65 Madison Avenue
Ssite 220
Morristown, NJ 07960-7307
973-898-1200
800-875-0058
Fax: 973-898-1201
E-mail: psych@alertpubs.com
www.alertpubs.com

Jenny Marie DeJesus, Circulation Manager

Discusses drugs used in the psychiatric field, including side effects and risks. *$63.00*

8 pages 12 per year ISSN 0894-4873

3298 Psychiatry Research
Customer Support Department
PO Box 945
New York, NY 10159-0945
212-633-3730
888-437-4636
Fax: 212-633-3680
www.elsevier.nl/locate/psychres
ISSN 0165-1781

3299 Psychohistory News
International Psychohistorical Assocation (IPA)
34 Plaza Street E
Suite 1109
Brooklyn, NY 11238-5061
718-638-1414

Includes news of Association events, conference announcements, events in the psychohistorical field, and interviews and reviews. *$15.00*

8-10 pages 4 per year

3300 Psychological Abstracts
PsycINFO/American Psychological Association
750 1st Street NE
Washington, DC 20002-4242
202-336-5650
800-374-2722
Fax: 202-336-5633
TDD: 202-336-6123
E-mail: psycinfo@apa.org
www.apa.org/psycinfo

Print index containing citations and abstracts for journal articles, books, and book chapters in psychology and related disciplines. Annual indexes.

12 per year

3301 Psychological Assessment Resources
PO Box 998
Odessa, FL 33556-0998
813-968-3003
Fax: 813-968-2598

3302 Psychological Science Agenda
Science Directorate-American Psychological Association
750 1st Street NE
Washington, DC 20002-4241
202-336-6000
800-374-2721
Fax: 202-336-5953
E-mail: science@apa.org
www.apa.org/science/psa/psacover.html

This newsletter disseminates information on scientific psychology, including news on activities of the Association and congressional and federal advocacy efforts of the Directorate. Recurring features include reports of meetings, news of research, notices of publications available, interviews, and the columns titled Science Directorate News, On Behalf of Science, Science Briefs, Announcements, and Funding Opportunities.

16-20 pages   6 per year   ISSN 1040-404X

3303 Psychology Teacher Network Education Directorate
750 1st Street NE
Washington, DC 20002-4241
202-336-6021
Fax: 202-336-5962
E-mail: jrg.apa@email.apa.org

Provides descriptions of experiments and demonstrations aimed at introducing topics as a basis for classroom lectures or discussion. Recurring features include news and announcements of courses, workshops, funding sources, and meetings; reviews of teaching aids; and reports of innovative programs or curricula occurring in schools, interviews and brief reports from prominent psychologists. *$15.00*

16 pages   5 per year

3304 Psychophysiology
Cambridge University Press
40 W 20th Street
New York, NY 10011-4221
212-924-3900
Fax: 212-691-3239
E-mail: marketing@cup.org
www.cup.org

3305 Psychosomatic Medicine
American Psychosomatic Society
6728 Old McLean Village Drive
McLean, VA 22101-3906
703-556-9222
Fax: 703-556-8729
E-mail: info@psychosomatic.org
www.psychosomatic.org

Michael Irwin, Secretary/Treasurer
William Lovallo, President

News and event annoucements, examines the scientific understanding of the interrelationships among biological, psychological, social and behavioral factors in human health and disease, and the integration of the fields of science that separately examine each.

3306 Psychotherapy Bulletin
American Psychological Association
750 First Street NE
Washington, DC 20002-4242

202-336-5500
800-374-2721
Fax: 202-336-5708
www.apa.org

Recurring features include letters to the editor, news of research, reports of meetings, news of educational opportunities, committee reports, legislative issues, and columns titled Washington Scene, Finance, Marketing, Professional Liability, Medical Psychology Update, and Substance Abuse. *$8.00*

50 pages   4 per year

3307 Psychotherapy Finances
Managed Care Strategies & Psychotherapy Finances
13901 US Highway 1
Suite 58979
Juno Beach, FL 33408-1612
561-624-1155
800-869-8450
Fax: 561-624-6006

3308 Research and Training for Children's Mental Health-Update
University of South Florida
13301 Bruce B Downs Boulevard
Florida Mental Health Institute
Tampa, FL 33612-3807
813-974-4661
Fax: 813-974-6257
www.rtckids.fmhi.usf.edu

Services and research on children with emotional disorders.

2 per year

3309 Smooth Sailing
Depression and Related Affective Disorders Association
600 N Wolfe Street
John Hopkins Hospital Meyer 3-181
Baltimore, MD 21287-7381
Fax: 410-614-3241
www.med.jhu.edu/drada/

Outreach to students and parents through schools.

4 per year

3310 Social Work
National Association of Social Works
750 1st Street NE
Suite 700
Washington, DC 20002-4241
202-336-8236
Fax: 202-336-8312

3311 Social Work Abstracts
National Association of Social Works
750 1st Street NE
Suite 700
Washington, DC 20002-4241
202-336-8236
Fax: 202-336-8312

3312 Social Work Research
National Association of Social Works
750 1st Street NE
Suite 700
Washington, DC 20002-4241

202-336-8236
Fax: 202-336-8312

3313 Social Work in Education
National Association of Social Works
750 1st Street NE
Suite 700
Washington, DC 20002-4241
202-336-8236
Fax: 202-336-8312

3314 Society for Adolescent Psychiatry Newsletter
PO Box 570218
Dallas, TX 75357-0218
972-613-0985
Fax: 972-613-5532
E-mail: info@adolpsych.org
www.adolpsych.org

Frances Bell, Executive Director
Mohan Nair, President

Puts psychiatrists in touch with an informed cross-section of the profession from all over North America. Dedicated to education development and advocacy of adolescents and the adolescent psychiatric field.

3315 World Federation for Mental Health Newsletter
World Federation for Mental Health
PO Box 16810
Alexandria, VA 22302-0810
703-838-7525
Fax: 703-519-7648
E-mail: info@wfmh.com
www.wfmh.com

Gwen Dixon, Office Administrator

World-wide mental health reports. Education and advocacy on mental health issues. Working to protect the human rights of those defined as mentally ill.

8 pages 1 per year Year Founded: 1984

Testing & Evaluation

3316 Assessment and Treatment of Anxiety Disorders in Persons with Mental Retardation
NADD
132 Fair Street
Kingston, NY 12401
845-331-4336
800-331-5362
Fax: 845-331-4569
E-mail: info@thenadd.org
www.www.thenadd.org

Robert Fletcher, CEO

Anxiety disorders as a group are the commonest mental health disorders seen in the general population, as they probably also are in people with developmental disorders. This upgraded version of a book first published in 1996 describes issues of diagnosis and treatment of various anxiety disorders, and includes modalities for staff training in those conditions. *$19.95*

ISBN 1-572560-01-0

3317 Assessment of Neuropsychiatry and Mental Health Services
American Psychiatric Publishing
1000 Wilson Boulevard
Suite 1825
Arlington, VA 22209-3901
703-907-7322
800-368-5777
Fax: 703-907-1091
E-mail: appi@psych.org
www.www.appi.org

Robert Pursell, Marketing

Examines the importance of an integrated approach to neuropsychiatric conditions and looks at ways to overcome the difficulties in assessing medical disorders in psychiatric populations. Addresses neuropsychiatric disorders and their costs and implications on policy. *$94.00*

448 pages Year Founded: 1999 ISBN 0-880487-30-5

3318 Attention-Deficit/Hyperactivity Disorder Test: a Method for Identifying Individuals with ADHD
Pro-Ed Publications
8700 Shoal Creek Boulevard
Austin, TX 78757-6897
512-451-3246
800-897-3202
Fax: 800-397-7633
E-mail: info@proedinc.com
www.proedinc.com

An effective instrument for identifying and evaluating attention - deficit disorders in persons ages three to twenty-three. Designed for use in schools and clinics, the test is easily completed by teachers, parents and others who are knowledgeable about the referred individual. *$110.00*

Year Founded: 1995

3319 Behavioral and Emotional Rating Scale
Pro-Ed Publications
8700 Shoal Creek Boulevard
Austin, TX 78757-6897
512-451-3246
800-897-3202
Fax: 800-397-7633
E-mail: info@proedinc.com
www.proedinc.com

Helps to measure the personal strengths of children ages five through eighteen. Contains 52 items that measure five aspects of a child's strength: interpersonal strength, involvement with family, intrapersonal strength, school functioning, and affective strength. Provides overall strength score and five subtest scores. Identifies individual behavioral and emotional strengths of children, the areas in which individual strengths need to be developed, and the goals for individual treatment plans. *$165.00*

Year Founded: 1998

3320 CPP Incorporated
1055 Joaquin Rd
2nd Floor
Mountain View, CA 94043
650-969-8901
800-624-1765
Fax: 650-969-8608
E-mail: custserv@cpp.com
www.cpp.com

3321 Childhood History Form for Attention Disorders
ADD WareHouse
300 NW 70th Avenue
Suite 102
Plantation, FL 33317
954-792-8100
800-233-9273
Fax: 954-792-8545
E-mail: websales@addwarehouse.com
www.addwarehouse.com

This form is completed by parents prior to a history taking session. It is designed to be used in conjunction with standardized assessment questionaires utilized in the evaluation of attention disorders. 25 per package. *$45.00*

10 pages

3322 Children's Depression Inventory
ADD WareHouse
300 NW 70th Avenue
Suite 102
Plantation, FL 33317
954-792-8100
800-233-9273
Fax: 954-792-8545
E-mail: websales@addwarehouse.com
www.addwarehouse.com

A self-report, symptom-oriented scale which requires at least a first grade reading level and was designed for school-aged children and adolescents. The CDI has 27 items, each of which consists of three choices. Quickscore form scoring make the inventories easy and economical to administer. The profile contains the following five factors plus a total score normed according to age and sex: negative mood, interpersonal problems, ineffectiveness, anhedonia and negative self-esteem. Contains ten items and provides a general indication of depressive symptoms. *$148.00*

3323 Clinical Evaluations of School Aged Children
Professional Resource Press
PO Box 15560
Sarasota, FL 34277-1560
800-443-3364
Fax: 941-343-9201
www.prpress.com

This book delineates the specific symptoms and behaviors associated with each DSM - IV diagnostic syndrome and provides an exceptionally well designed system for communicating diagnostic findings with great clarity when working with parents and professionals from different disciplines. *$34.95*

376 pages Year Founded: 1998 ISBN 1-568870-27-2

3324 Clinical Interview of the Adolescent: From Assessment and Formulation to Treatment Planning
Charles C Thomas Publisher
2600 S 1st Street
Springfield, IL 62704
217-789-8980
800-258-8980
E-mail: books@ccthomas.com
www.ccthomas.com

Thomas Fagan, Author

This book addresses the process of interviewing troubled and psychologically disturbed adolescents who are seen in hospital settings, schools, courts, clinics, and residential facilities. Interviews with adolescents, younger children or adults should follow a logical, sequential and integrated procedure, accomplishing diagnostic closure and the development of a treatment formulation. The nine chapters cover the theoretical and developmental concerns of adolescence; the initial referral; meeting with parents; the therapist; getting acquainted; getting to the heart of the matter; making order out of disorder; the reasons and rationale for the behavior problems. *$59.95*

234 pages Year Founded: 1997 ISBN 0-398067-79-1

3325 Concise Guide to Assessment and Management of Violent Patients
American Psychiatric Publishing
1000 Wilson Boulevard
Suite 1825
Arlington, VA 22209-3901
703-907-7322
800-368-5777
Fax: 703-907-1091
E-mail: appi@psych.org
www.appi.org

Kenneth Tardiff MD MPH

Written by an expert on violence, this edition provides current information on psychopharmacology, safety of clinicians and how to deal with threats of violence to the clinician. *$32.95*

180 pages Year Founded: 1996 ISBN 0-880483-44-X

3326 Conducting Insanity Evaluations
Guilford Publications
72 Spring Street
New York, NY 10012
800-365-7006
Fax: 212-966-6708
E-mail: info@guilford.com
www.guilford.com

Robert Matloff, President

Great resource for both psychologists and lawyers. Covers legal standards and their applications to clinical work. Mental health professionals who evaluate defendants or consult to courts on criminal matters will find this a useful resource. *$50.00*

342 pages Year Founded: 2000 ISBN 1-572305-21-5

3327 Conners' Rating Scales
Pro-Ed Publications
8700 Shoal Creek Boulevard
Austin, TX 78757-6897
512-451-3246
800-897-3202
Fax: 800-397-7633
E-mail: info@proedinc.com
www.proedinc.com

Conner's Rating Scales are a result of 30 years of research on childhood and adolescent psychopathology and problem behavior. This revision adds a number of enhancements to a set of measures that has long been the standard instruments for the measurement of attention-deficit/hyperactivity disorder in children and adolescents. *$153.00*

Year Founded: 1997

3328 Depression and Anxiety in Youth Scale
Pro-Ed Publications
8700 Shoal Creek Boulevard
Austin, TX 78757-6897
512-451-3246
800-897-3202
Fax: 800-397-7633
E-mail: info@proedinc.com
www.proedinc.com

A unique battery of three norm-referenced scales useful in identifying major depressive disorder and overanxious disorders in children and adolescents. *$150.00*

Year Founded: 1994

3329 Diagnosis and Treatment of Multiple Personality Disorder
Guilford Publications
72 Spring Street
New York, NY 10012
800-365-7006
Fax: 212-966-6708
E-mail: info@guilford.com
www.guilford.com

Robert Matloff, President

Comprehensive and integrated approach to a complex psychotherapeutic process. From first interview to crisis management to final post-integrative treatment each step is systematically reviewed, with detailed instructions on specific diagnostic and therapeutic techniques and examples of clinical applications. Specially geared to the needs of therapists, novice or expert alike, struggling with their first MPD case. *$48.00*

351 pages Year Founded: 1989 ISBN 0-898621-77-1

3330 Diagnosis and Treatment of Sociopaths and Clients with Sociopathic Traits
New Harbinger Publications
5674 Shattuck Avenue
Oakland, CA 94609
800-748-6273
Fax: 510-652-5472
E-mail: customerservice@newharbinger.com
www.newharbinger.com

Debra Benueniste, Author

This text presents a full course of treatment, with special attention to safety issues and other concerns for different client populations in a range of treatment settings. *$49.95*

208 pages Year Founded: 1996 ISBN 1-572240-47-4

3331 Diagnostic Interview Schedule for Children: CDISC
Columbia DISC Development Group
Columbia University
1051 Riverside Drive, Unit 78
New York, NY 10032
212-543-5298
Fax: 212-543-1000
E-mail: jjwebsite@childpsycho.columbia.edu

David Shaffer MD, Executive Director

Automated diagnostic interview assessing 34 common child and adolescent mental health disorders, using DSM-IV criteria. A valuable aid to research, as well as clinical and school assessments.

3332 Draw a Person: Screening Procedure for Emotional Disturbance
Pro-Ed Publications
8700 Shoal Creek Boulevard
Austin, TX 78757-6897
512-451-3246
800-897-3202
Fax: 800-397-7633
E-mail: info@proedinc.com
www.proedinc.com

Helps identify children and adolescents ages six through seventeen who have emotional problems and require further evaluation. *$140.00*

Year Founded: 1991

3333 Functional Assessment and Intervention: Guide to Understanding Problem Behavior
High Tide Press
3650 W 183rd Street
Homewood, IL 60430
708-206-2054
800-469-9461
www.hightidepress.com

These experienced practitioners in behavior analyses provide a hands-on, practical approach to recognizing, analyzing, understanding and modifying problem behaviors. Learn the fundamentals of functional assessment and behavior management. *$12.95*

62 pages ISBN 1-892696-31-2

3334 Handbook of Psychological Assessment
John Wiley & Sons
605 3rd Avenue
4th Floor
New York, NY 10158
800-225-5945
E-mail: info@wiley.com
www.wiley.com

Gary Groth-Marnat, Author

Classic, revised and new psychological tests are all considered for validity and overall reliability in the light of current clinical thought and scientific development. The new edition has expanded coverage of neuropsychological assessment and reports on assessment and treatment planning in the age of managed care. *$95.00*

862 pages Year Founded: 1997 ISBN 0-471419-79-6

3335 Harvard Medical School Guide to Suicide Assessment and Intervention
Jossey-Bass Publishers
989 Market Street
San Francisco, CA 94103
415-433-1740
Fax: 415-433-0499
www.www.wiley.com

The definitive guide for helping mental health professionals determine the risk for suicide and appropriate treatment strategies for suicidal or at-risk patients. *$85.00*

736 pages ISBN 0-787943-03-7

3336 Health Watch
28 Maple Avenue
Medford, MA 02155
800-643-2757
www.healthwatch.cc

On site performer of preventative health screening services and disease risk management programming. Specializing in point of care testing, we perform fast and accurate health screening tests and services to assist in indentifying participant's risk for developing future disease.

Year Founded: 1987

3337 Scale for Assessing Emotional Disturbance
Pro-Ed Publications
8700 Shoal Creek Boulevard
Austin, TX 78757-6897
512-451-3246
800-897-3202
Fax: 800-397-7633
E-mail: info@proedinc.com
www.proedinc.com

Helps you identify children and adolescents who qualify for the federal special education category Emotional Disturbance. *$100.00*

Year Founded: 1998

3338 Screening for Brain Dysfunction in Psychiatric Patients
Charles C Thomas Publisher
2600 S 1st Street
Springfield, IL 62704
217-789-8980
800-258-8980
E-mail: books@ccthomas.com
www.ccthomas.com

This book presents how medical diseases can be misdiagnosed as psychiatric disorders and how clinicians without extensive training in the neurosciences can do a competent job of screening psychiatric clients for possible brain disorders. The research cited in this book, dating back to the 1890's, establishes beyond a doubt that such misdiagnoses are more common than most clinicians would guess. This book focuses on one type of medical condition that is likely to be misdiagnosed: brain injuries and illnesses. *$36.95*

148 pages Year Founded: 1998 ISBN 0-398069-21-2

3339 Sexual Dysfunction: Guide for Assessment and Treatment
Guilford Publications
72 Spring Street
New York, NY 10012
800-365-7006
Fax: 212-966-6708
E-mail: info@guilford.com
www.guilford.com

Designed as a succinct guide to contemporary sex therapy, this book provides an empirically based overview of the most common sexual dysfunctions and a step-by-step manual for their assessment and treatment. Provides a biopsychosocial model of sexual function and dysfunction and describes the authors' general approach to management of sexual difficulties. *$25.00*

212 pages Year Founded: 1991 ISBN 0-898622-07-7

3340 Social-Emotional Dimension Scale
Pro-Ed Publications
8700 Shoal Creek Boulevard
Austin, TX 78757-6897

512-451-3246
800-897-3202
Fax: 800-397-7633
E-mail: info@proedinc.com
www.proedinc.com

A rating scale for teachers, counselors, and psychologists to screen age 5 1/2 through 18 1/2 who are at risk for conduct disorders, behavior problems, or emotional disturbance. It assesses physical/fear reaction, depressive reaction, avoidance of peer interaction, avoidance of teacher interaction, aggressive interaction, and inappropriate behaviors. *$149.00*

Year Founded: 1986

3341 Test Collection at ETS
Educational Testing Service
Brigham Library
Rosedale Road
Princeton, NJ 08541
609-921-9000
Fax: 609-734-5410
www.www.ets.org

Linda Savadge, Professional Associate/Intermed.

Provides 1,200 plus tests available in microfiche or downloadable for reaserch.

Training & Recruitment

3342 Ackerman Institute for the Family
149 E 78th Street
New York, NY 10075
212-879-4900
Fax: 212-744-0206
E-mail: ackerman@ackerman.org
www.ackerman.org

Marcia Steinberg CSW, Director Training

A not-for-profit agency devoted to the treatment and study of families and to the training of family therapists. One of the first training institutions in the United States committed to promoting family functioning and family mental health, Acker is dedicated to helping all families at all stages of family life.

3343 Active Intervention
735 Whitney Avenue
Gretna, LA 70056
504-367-5766

3344 Alfred Adler Institute (AAI)
594 Broadway
Suite 1213
New York, NY 10012
212-254-1048
Fax: 212-254-8271
E-mail: director@alfredadler-ny.org
www.alfredadler-ny.org

Offers training in psychotherapy and analysis to psychiatrists, psychologists, social workers, teachers, clergymen and other related professional persons. Conducts three-year program to provide an understanding of the dynamics of personality and interpersonal relationships and to teach therapeutic methods and techniques. Presents the theory of Individual Psychology as formulated by Alfred Adler. Publications: Journal of Individual Psychology, quarterly. Annual meeting. Semi-annual seminar.

3345 Alliance Behavioral Care: University of Cincinnati Psychiatric Services
222 Piedmont Avenue
Suite 8800
Cincinnati, OH 45219-4218
513-475-8622
800-926-8862
www.alliance-behavioral.com

A regional managed behavioral healthcare organization committed to continuously improving the resources and programs that serve their members and providers. Their goal is to provide resources that improve the well-being of those they serve and to integrate the behavioral healthcare within the overall healthcare systems.

3346 Alton Ochsner Medical Foundation, Psychiatry Residency
1514 Jefferson Highway
New Orleans, LA 70121
504-842-3260
Fax: 504-842-3193
E-mail: gme@ochsner.org
www.www.ochsner.org

Michael Finan, Program Director

3347 American Academy of Child and Adolescent Psychiatry
3615 Wisconsin Avenue NW
Washington, DC 20016-3007
202-966-7300
Fax: 202-966-2891
E-mail: communications@aacap.org
www.aacap.org

Robert Hendren, President
David Herzog, Secretary
William Bernet, Treasurer

Training programs in child and adolescent psychiatry.

3348 American College of Healthcare Executives
One N Franklin Street
Suite 1700
Chicago, IL 60606-3529
312-424-2800
Fax: 312-424-0023
E-mail: geninfo@ache.org
www.ache.org

Alyson Pitman Giles, Chairman
David Rubenstein, Chairman-Elect

International professional society of nearly 30,000 healthcare executives. ACHE is known for its prestigious credentialing and educational programs. ACHE is also known for its journal, Journal of Healthcare Management, and magazine, Healthcare Executive, as well as groundbreaking research and career development programs. Through its efforts, ACHE works toward its goal of improving the health status of society by advancing healthcare management excellence.

3349 American College of Women's Health Physicians
1100 E Woodfield Road
Suite 520
Schaumburg, IL 60173
847-517-7402
Fax: 847-517-7229
E-mail: info@acwhp.org
www.acwhp.org

The mission of ACWHP is to advance women-centered healthcare.

3350 Andrus Children's Center
Julia Dyckman Andrus Memorial
1156 N Broadway
Yonkers, NY 10701
914-965-3700
Fax: 914-965-3883
www.andruschildren.org

Nancy Woodruff Ment, President/CEO

Vision is to "give opportunity to youth." A private, non-profit community agency that provides assessment, treatment, education and preventive services for children and their families in residential, day and other restorative programs. Mission is to serve families, without regard to background or financial status, who have or are at risk for developing behavioral health problems. A highly qualified and caring staff uses established techniques and innovative programs to accomplish these purposes.

3351 Asian Pacific Development Center for Human Development
1825 York Street
Denver, CO 80206
303-393-0304
www.apdc.org

A community-based non-profit organization that serves the needs of a growing population of Asian American and Pacific Islander residents throughout Colorado. APDC operates a licensed Community Mental Health Clinic and a multicultural Interpreters Bank.

Year Founded: 1980

3352 Behavioral Healthcare Center
464 Commonwealth Street
#147
Belmont, MA 02478
617-393-3935
Fax: 617-393-1808
E-mail: cberney@mah.harvard.edu
www.www.academicpsychiatry.org

Carole Berney, Administrative Director
Joan Anzia, President

A behavorial health facility providing consultation in psychiatry, psychopharmacology and psychotherapy to primary care physicians and their patients.

3353 Behavioral Medicine and Biofeedback Consultants
150 SW 12th Avenue
Suite 330
Pompano Beach, FL 33069
954-783-5100
Fax: 954-783-5176
E-mail: behmed@aol.com
www.www.behavioralmedicine.com

3354 Brandeis University/Heller School
415 South Street
Waltham, MA 02454-9110

781-736-2000
www.brandeis.edu

3355 Breining Institute College for the Advanced Study of Addictive Disorders
8894 Greenback Lane
Orangevale, CA 95662-4019
916-987-0662
Fax: 916-907-9384
E-mail: college@breining.edu
www.breining.edu

Kathy Breining, Dean of Students

The mission of Breining Institute faculty and staff is to ensure a consistent standard of higher education, training, testing and certification of professionals working in the field of addictions.

Year Founded: 1986

3356 Brown Schools Behavioral Health System
PO Box 150459
Austin, TX 78715
800-848-9090

3357 California Institute of Behavioral Sciences
701 Welch Road
Suite 203
Palo Alto, CA 94304
650-325-1501

Sanjay Jasuja MD, Medical Director

Provides the following services for children, adolescents, adults and families on national and international level: Objective testing and comprehensive treatment for ADHD/ADD, depression, manic depressive disorder or Bipolar disorder, anxiety disorders, including obsessive compulsive disorder, panic attacks, phobias, post-traumatic stress disorder, Tourette's syndrome, stuttering, psychopharmacology, stress and anger control, violence and workplace issues, learning and behavior problems, and parenting support groups.

3358 Cambridge Hospital: Department of Psychiatry
1493 Cambridge Street
Cambridge, MA 02139
617-665-1000

3359 Center for Health Policy Studies
10440 Little Patuxent Parkway
10th Floor
Columbia, MD 21044
410-715-9400

3360 Children and Adolescents with Emotional and Behavioral Disorders
Virginia Commonwealth University, Medical College
PO Box 980489
Richmond, VA 23298-0489
804-828-4393

Cynthia R Eillis MD, Program Chair

3361 College of Health and Human Services: SE Missouri State
901 S National Ave
Springfield, MO 65897
417-836-4176
www.www.missouristate.edu

3362 College of Southern Idaho
315 Falls Avenue
PO Box 1238
Twin Falls, ID 83303
208-732-6221
800-680-0274
Fax: 208-736-4705
E-mail: info@csi.edu
www.csi.edu

Jerry Beck, President
Jerry Gee, Executive VP/CAO

Addiction Studies

3363 Colonial Services Board
1657 Merrimac Trail
Williamsburg, VA 23185
757-220-3200
www.www.colonialcsb.org

MR and substance abuse

3364 Columbia Counseling Center
900 St. Andrews Road
Columbia, SC 29210
803-731-4708
www.www.columbiacouncelingcenter.com

3365 Copper Hills Youth Center
5899 Rivendell Drive
West Jordan, UT 84088
801-561-3377
800-776-7116
Fax: 801-569-3274
www.www.copperhillsyouthcenter.com

3366 Corphealth
1300 Summit Avenue
6th Floor
Fort Worth, TX 76102-4414
817-332-2519
800-240-8388
Fax: 817-335-9100
E-mail: businessdevelopment@corphealth.com
www.corphealth.com

Patrick D Gotchen II, President/CEO
Brae Jacobson, COO
Michael Baker, CFO

Privately owned and managed behavioral health care company which serves its customers by facilitating the resolution of behavioral health problems in a manner which balances the needs of purchasers, patients and providers. Provides services that bring added value to insurers and health plans while delivering quality care for their members and customers.

3367 Counseling Services
18 W Colony Plaza
Suite 250
Durham, NC 27705-5582
919-493-2674
Fax: 919-493-1923

3368 Daniel Memorial Institute
3725 Belfort Road
Jacksonville, FL 32216-5899
904-296-1055
Fax: 904-296-1953

3369 Daniel and Yeager Healthcare Staffing Solutions
6767 Old Madison Pike
Suite 690
Huntsville, AL 35806
800-955-1919
Fax: 256-551-1075
www.dystaffing.com

Setting the standard for excellence in health care staffing.

3370 Department of Psychiatry: Dartmouth University
Dartmouth Medical School
Lebanon, NH 03756
603-650-5834
Fax: 603-650-5842

3371 Distance Learning Network
111 Boal Ave
Boalsburg, PA 16827
814-466-7808

Eric Porterfield, Director

Broadcast and multimedia company dedicated solely to meeting the medical education and communications needs of physicians through the use of both traditional and innovative media formats. More than 150,000 physicians, nurses and pharmacists turn to DLN each year for their medical education.

Year Founded: 1996

3372 Downstate Mental Hygiene Association
370 Lenox Road
Brooklyn, NY 11226-2206
718-287-4806

3373 East Carolina University Department of Psychiatric Medicine
600 Moye Boulevard
Room 4E-98
Greenville, NC 27834
252-744-3772
Fax: 252-744-3815

3374 Eastern County Mental Health Center
100 West Laurel
Sheridan County Courthouse
Plentywood, MT 59254
406-765-2550
Fax: 406-228-4553

Mental health and chemical dependency help for over 17 counties in Montana.

3375 Emory University School of Medicine, Psychology and Behavior
1440 Clifton Road NE
Atlanta, GA 30322
404-727-5640
Fax: 404-727-0473

3376 Emory University: Psychological Center
532 Kilgo Circle
Atlanta, GA 30322
404-727-7438
Fax: 404-727-0372
E-mail: psych@emory.edu
www.psychology.emory.edu

Nonprofit community clinic providing low cost counseling and psychological testing services for children and adults.

3377 Fletcher Allen Health Care
111 Colchester Avenue
Burlington, VT 05401
802-847-0000
www.fahc.org

Fletcher Allen Health Care is both a community hospital and, in partnership with the University of Vermont, the state's academic health center. Their mission is to improve the health of the people in the communities they serve by integrating patient care, education and research in a caring environment.

3378 Genesis Learning Center (Devereux)
430 Allied Drive
Nashville, TN 37211
615-832-4222

3379 George Washington University
2121 1 Street
Washington, DC 20052
202-994-1000
www.www.gwu.edu

3380 Harper House: Change Alternative Living
2940 E Eight Mile Road
Detroit, MI 48234
313-891-4976

3381 Haymarket Center, Professional Development
932 W Washington
Chicago, IL 60607
312-226-7984
Fax: 312-226-8048
E-mail: info@hcenter.org
www.www.hcenter.org

Raymond Soucek, President
Donald Musil, Executive Vp

Drug and alcohol treatment programs.

3382 Heartshare Human Services
12 Metro Tech Center
29th Floor
Brooklyn, NY 11201
718-422-4200
E-mail: info@heartshare.org
www.www.heartshare.org

Ralph A. Subbiondo, Chairman
William R. Guarinello, President/ Ceo
Mia Higgins, Executive Vp
Lynette Fernandez, Assistant Comptroller

A nonprofit human services agency dedicated to improving the lives of people in need of special services and support.

3383 Hillcrest Utica Psychiatric Services
1120 S Utica Street
South Physician Bldg Suite 1000
Tulsa, OK 74120
918-579-2912
www.www.hillcrest.com

3384 Institute for Behavioral Healthcare
4370 Alpine Road
Suite 209
Portola Valley, CA 94028
650-851-8411
800-258-8411
Fax: 650-851-0406
E-mail: staff@iahb.org
www.iahb.org

Gerry Piaget, President
Joan Piaget, Executive Director

Non-profit educational organization that is a fully accredited sponsor of continuing education and continuing medical education for mental health, chemical dependency, and substance abuse treatment providers in the United States and Canada. Mission is to provide high-quality training to healthcare professionals as well as to companies and individuals with healthcare-related interests.

3385 Jacobs Institute of Women's Health
2021 K Street
Nw Suite 800
Washington, DC 20006
202-530-2376
Fax: 202-296-0025
E-mail: whieditor@gwu.edu
www.www.jiwh.org

Richard Mauery, Managing Staff Director

Working to improve health care for women through research, dialogue and information dissemination. Mission is to identify and study women's health care issues involving the interaction of medical and social systems; facilitate informed dialogue and foster awareness among consumers and providers alike; and promote problem resolution, interdisciplinary coordination and information dissemination at the regional, national and international levels.

3386 Jefferson Drug/Alcohol
833 Chestnut East
Suite 210
Philadelphia, PA 19107
215-955-6912
www.www.jeffersonhospital.org/psychiatry

Michael Vergare MD, Chair Dpt Psychiatry/Human Bhvr

Provides clinical and consultation services to Thomas Jefferson University Hospital and its medical community. In addition, its staff focuses special attention on the consultation and treatment of the most common psychiatric problems of anxiety, depression, insomnia, substance abuse, eating disorders and sleep disorders.

3387 John A Burns School of Medicine Department of Psychiatry
1356 Lusitana Street
Floor 4
Honolulu, HI 96813
808-586-2900
Fax: 808-586-2940
www.www.jabsom.hawaii.edu

Naleen Andrade, Chair

Medical School Programs and Residency Programs, general, geriatric, addictive and, child and adolescent.

3388 Langley Porter Psych Institute at UCSF Parnassus Campus
401 Parnassus Avenue
San Francisco, CA 94143
415-476-7500
Fax: 415-476-7320

3389 Laurelwood Hospital and Counseling Centers
35900 Euclid Avenue
Willoughby, OH 44094
440-953-3000
800-438-4673
www.laurelwoodhospital.net

Full-service behavioral healthcare system-(comprehensive outpatient and inpatient services).

3390 Life Science Associates
1 Fenimore Road
Bayport, NY 11705-2115
631-472-2111
Fax: 631-472-8146
E-mail: lifesciassoc@pipeline.com
www.lifesciassoc.home.pipeline.com

Publishes over fifty computer programs for individuals impaired by head trauma and stroke. Also produces EDS, a software/hardware system for assessing driving.

3391 Locumtenens.com
3650 Mansell Road
Suite 310
Alpharetta, GA 30022
800-930-0748
www.locumtenens.com

Richard M Jackson, CEO
David Roush, President/COO
Harrison L Rogers Jr, MD, Medical Director

Specializing in temporary and permanant placement of psychiatrists. Physicians tell us where and when they want to work and locumtenens.com will find a jop that fits those needs.

3392 MCG Telemedicine Center
1120 15th Street
Augusta, GA 30912
706-721-0211
E-mail: decisionsupport@mcg.edu
www.www.mcg.edu

Daniel W. Rahn, President

Involved in the delivery of mental health services via telemedicine. In addition, the Telemedicine Center maintains the Georgia Mental Health Network website, a comprehensive listing of mental health resources in the State.

3393 MCW Department of Psychiatry and Behavioral Medicine
8701 Watertown Plank Road
Milwaukee, WI 53226
414-456-8296
Fax: 414-456-6506
E-mail: webmaster@mcw.edu
www.www.mcw.edu

3394 Management Recruiters of Washington, DC
12520 Prosperity Drive
Suite 320
Silver Spring, MD 20904

301-625-5100
Fax: 301-625-3001
E-mail: info@mr-twg.com
www.www.mr-twg.com

Frank Black Jr., Partner,President
John Marty, Managing Director

3395 Marsh Foundation

1229 Lincoln Highway
PO Box 150
Van Wert, OH 45891
419-238-1695
Fax: 419-238-1747
E-mail: marshfound@embarqmail.com
www.marshfoundation.org

Jeff Grothouse, Executive Secretary/Treasurer
Terry Geiger, Coordinator

Nonprofit center serving children and families with special emphasis in juvenile sex offender population. Services include individual therapy, group therapy, case management and diagnostic assessment.

3396 Masters of Behavioral Healthcare Management
California School of Professional Psychology

Los Angeles Campus
1000 South Fremont Avenue, Unit 5
Alhambra, CA 91803
626-284-2777
866-825-5426
TDD: 800-585-5087
www.alliant.edu

Geoffrey Cox PhD, President

Offers industry-specific training to mid-management and supervisory personnel employed in behavioral healthcare organizations.

3397 Medical College of Georgia

1120 15th Street
Augusta, GA 30912
706-721-0211
www.www.mcg.edu

Daniel W Rahn, President

The mission of the Medical College of Georgia is to improve health and resuce the burden of illness in society by discovering, disseminating, and applying knowledge of human health and disease.

3398 Medical College of Ohio, Psychiatry

3000 Arlington Avenue
Toledo, OH 43614
419-383-4117
Fax: 419-383-6140

Mission is to improve the human condition through the creation, dissemination and application of knowledge using wisdom and compassion as our guides.

3399 Medical College of Pennsylvania

3300 Henry Avenue
Philadelphia, PA 19129
215-842-6000

A tertiary care educational facility that reaches out to a regional referral base for select specialty services while continuing to offer primary and secondary service to the residents of its immediate community.

3400 Medical College of Virginia

Division of Substance Abuse Medic
PO Box 980109
Richmond, VA 23298-0109
804-828-3584

3401 Medical College of Wisconsin

8701 Watertown Plank Road
Milwaukee, WI 53226
414-456-8296
Fax: 414-456-6633
www.www.mcw.edu

3402 Medical Doctor Associates

145 Technology Parkway NW
Norcross, GA 30092
770-246-9191
800-780-3500
Fax: 770-246-0882
www.mdainc.com

Ken Shumard, Founder
Mike Pretiger, Cfo

Committed to providing the most complete staffing services available to the healthcare industry. The family of services offered by Medical Doctor Associates includes Locum Tenens, Contract, and Permanent Placement staffing for physicians, allied health and rehabilitation staffing, and credentials verification and licensing services.

3403 Medical University of South Carolina Institute of Psychiatry, Psychiatry Access Center

171 Ashley Avenue
Charleston, SC 29425
843-792-2300
www.www.musc.edu

3404 Meharry Medical College

1005-David B Todd Boulevard
Nashville, TN 37208
615-327-6000

3405 Menninger Division of Continuing Education
Menninger Clinic Department of Research

2801 Gessner Drive
Houston, TX 77080
713-275-5000
800-351-9058
Fax: 713-275-5107
www.menninger.edu

Ian Aitken, President/CEO
Lynn Bodenhamer, Executive Assistant

The international psychiatric center of excellence, restoring hope to each person through innovative programs in treatment, research and education.

3406 NEOUCOM-Northeastern Ohio Universities College of Medicine

4209 State Route 44
PO Box 95
Rootstown, OH 44272
800-686-2511
www.neoucom.edu

Mission is to graduate qualified physicians who are passionate about serving their communities. All of our graduates, regardless of specialty, have a solid background in community and public health. NEOUCOM strives to improve the quality of health care throughout northeast Ohio by instilling in each graduate the desire to serve the public and the highest ideals of the medical profession.

3407 Nathan S Kline Institute for Psychiatric Research
140 Old Orangeburg Road
Orangeburg, NY 10962
845-398-5500
Fax: 845-398-5510
E-mail: webmaster@nki.rfmh.org
www.rfmh.org/nki

Research programs in Alzheimers disease, analytical psychopharmacology, basic and clinical neuroimaging, cellular and molecular neurobiology, clinical trial data management, co-occuring disorders and many other mental health studies.

3408 National Association of Alcholism and Drug Abuse Counselors
901 N Washington Street
Suite 600
Alexandria, VA 22314-1535
703-741-7686
800-548-0497
E-mail: ncac@naadac.org
www.naadac.org

NAADAC is the only professional membership organization that serves counselors who specialize in addiction treatment. With 14,000 members and 47 state affiliates representing more than 80,000 addiction counselors, it is the nation's largest network of alcoholism and drug abuse treatment professionals. Among the organization's national certifacation programs are the National Certified Addiction Counselor and the Masters Addiction Counselor designations.

3409 National Association of School Psychologists
4340 E West Highway
Suite 402
Bethesda, MD 20814
301-657-0270
866-331-6277
Fax: 301-657-0275
www.nasponline.org

3410 New York University Behavioral Health Programs
530 1st Avenue
Suite 7D
New York, NY 10016
212-263-7419
Fax: 212-263-7460
www.med.nyu.edu/nyubhp

David Ginsburg MD, Director

Outpatient psychiatry group for Tisch Hospital at NYU Medical Center. Our multidisciplinary team of licensed psychiatrists and social workers offers you the most up-to-date and scientifically validated treatments.

3411 Nickerson Center
7025 N Lombard Street
Portland, OR 97203
503-289-9071

3412 Northwestern University Medical School Feinberg School of Medicine
710 North Lakeshore Drive
Chicago, IL 60611
312-908-8262
Fax: 312-908-5070
E-mail: clinpsych@northwestern.edu
www.clinpsych.northwestern.edu

Mark A Reinecke PhD, Chief Division Psychology

The Mental Health Services and Policy Program is a multidisciplinary research/educational program on the development and implementation of outcomes management technology.

3413 Ochester Psychological Service
1924 Copper Oaks Circle
Blue Springs, MO 64015
816-224-6500

Jeffery L Miller PhD, Psychologist/Owner

Offers a full range of outpatient mental health services including individuals, couples and family therapy. Offers psychological testing and evaluation. Adults, adolescents and children served.

3414 Onslow County Behavioral Health
165 Center Street
Jacksonville, NC 28546
910-219-8000
www.www.ocbhs.org

3415 PRIMA A D D Corp.
13140 Coit RoadRoad
Suite 500
Dallas, TX 75240
972-386-8599

Prima ADD Corp specializes in the diagnosis and treatment of Attention-Deficit/Hyperactivity Disorder (ADHD). We treat children and adults. Services include: psychological assessment (including intellectual, achievement and pesonality testing), counseling, coaching and consultation. We also carry books and CD's concerning ADHD.

3416 Parent Child Center
2001 W Blue Heron Blvd
W Palm Beach, FL 33407
561-841-3500
Fax: 561-844-3577
E-mail: information@parent-childcenter.org
www.www.parent-childcenter.org

3417 Penelope Price
Cindy Hide
4281 MacDuff Plaza
Dublin, OH 43016
614-793-0165
www.penelope.com

3418 Penn State Hershey Medical Center
500 University Drive
Hershey, PA 17033
717-531-8080
www.www.hmc.psu.edu

3419 Pepperdine University, Graduate School of Education and Psychology
6100 Center Drive
Los Angeles, CA 90045
310-568-5600
800-347-4849
www.www.gsep.pepperdine.edu

Andrew Benton, President

Offers graduate degree programs designed to prepare psychologists, marriage and family therapists, and mental health practitioners. Many programs accommodate a full-time work schedule with evening and weekend classes available in a trimester schedule. The average class size is 15. There are five educational centers in southern California and three community counseling clinics available to the surrounding community.

3420 Pittsburgh Health Research Institute
600 Forbes Avenue
Pittsburgh, PA 15282-0001

3421 Postgraduate Center for Mental Health
138 E 26th Street
5th Floor
New York, NY 10010-1843
212-576-4168
E-mail: crichards@pgcmh.org
www.www.pgcmh.org

Information on mental health.

3422 Pressley Ridge Schools
530 Marshall Avenue
Pittsburgh, PA 15214
412-321-6995
Fax: 412-321-5313
www.pressleyridge.org

B Scott Finnell PhD, President/CEO
Scott Erickson, Executive VP/CfO

Provides an array of social services, special education programs, and mental health services for troubled children and their families in Delaware, Maryland, Ohio, Pennsylvania, Virginia, Washngton, DC and West Virginia as well as worldwide.

3423 Professional Horizons, Mental Health Service
PO Box 20078
Fountain Hills, AZ 85269
602-246-3311
Fax: 602-482-0156

3424 Psych-Med Association, St. Francis Medical
2616 Wilmington Road
New Castle, PA 16105
724-652-2323

3425 PsychTemps
2404 Auburn Avenue
Cincinnati, OH 45219
513-651-9500
888-651-8367
Fax: 513-651-9558
E-mail: info@psychtemps.com
www.psychtemps.com

Holly D Dorna MA LPCC, President/CEO

Specialized recruiting and staffing company that fills temporary, permanent, and temp-to-hire job placement for the behavioral healthcare field.

3426 Psychiatric Associates
2216 W Alto Road
Kokomo, IN 46902
765-453-9338

3427 Psychological Associates-Texas
10609 Grant Road
Houston, TX 77070
281-469-6395

3428 Psychological Center
135 Oakland Street
Pasadena, CA 91101
626-584-5500

3429 Psychological Diagnostic Services
10850 E Traverse Highway
Suite 2204
Traverse City, MI 49684-1363
616-947-6634
Fax: 616-947-3340

3430 Psychology Department
Bowling Green University
Bowling Green, OH 43403
419-372-2835
Fax: 419-372-6013

3431 QuadraMed Corporation
12110 Sunset Hills Road
Reston, VA 20190
703-709-2300
800-393-0278
Fax: 703-709-2490
E-mail: boardofdirectors@quadramed.com
www.quadramed.com

3432 Regional Research Institute for Human Services of Portland University
1600 Sw 4th Ave
Suite 900
Portland, OR 97201
503-725-4040
Fax: 503-725-4180
www.rri.pdx.edu

3433 Research Center for Children's Mental Health, Department of Children and Family
University of South Florida
13301 Bruce B Downs Boulevard
Tampa, FL 33612
813-974-4640
Fax: 813-974-7743
www.www.cfs.fmhi.usf.edu

The center conducts research, synthesized and shared existingknowledge, provided training and consultation, and served as a resource for other researchers, policy makers, administrators in the public system, and organizations representing parents, consumers, advocates, professional societies and practitioners.

3434 River City Mental Health Clinic
2265 Como Avenue
Suite 201
Saint Paul, MN 55108
651-646-8985
Fax: 651-646-3959
www.www.rivercityclinic.com

Psychotherapy and assessment for all ages.

3435 Riveredge Hospital
8311 W Roosevelt
Forest Park, IL 60130
708-771-7000
Fax: 708-209-2280
www.psysolutions.com

Mark R Russell, Chairman/CEO

Striving to foster an environment that demonstrates compassion and caring with timely and effective communication through comprehensive behavioral health care services of clinical excellence.

3436 Riverside Center
PO Box 2259
671 Sw Main
Winston, OR 97496
541-679-6129
www.www.riversidecenter.org

3437 Rockland Children's Psychiatric Center
599 Convent Road
Orangeburg, NY 10962
845-680-4000
Fax: 845-680-8905
E-mail: rocklandcpc@omh.state.ny.us
www.omh.state.ny.us/omhweb/facilities/rcpc/facility.ht

RCPC is a JCAHO accredited children's psychiatric center. We provide inpatient care to youngsters 10 - 18 years of age from the lower Hudson Valley. An array of local, school-based outpatient services are available in each of the seven counties in the area.

3438 Rosemont Center
2440 Dawnlight Avenue
Columbus, OH 43211
614-471-2626
800-753-0424
Fax: 614-478-3234
www.rosemont.org

Robert Marx, Ceo
Kate Tesoriero, Director Of Development

Provides for the physical, emotional, mental and spiritual well being of our community's most troubled young people and their families. the caring people of rosemont offer a more comprehensive program to address a wider range of cases and ages than other central Ohio mental health providers.

3439 SAFY of America
10100 Elida Road
Delphos, OH 45833
419-224-2279
800-532-7239
Fax: 419-224-2287
E-mail: webmaster@safy.org
www.safy.org

Druann Whitaker MS LSW LPC, CEO
John Hollenkamp, SVP of Finance

3440 Schneider Institute for Health Policy
The Heller School for Social Policy & Management
Brandeis University
415 South Street, Mailstop 035
Waltham, MA 02454-9110
781-736-3900
Fax: 781-736-3905
E-mail: colnon@brandeis.edu
www.sihp.brandeis.edu

Stanley S Wallack, Executive Director

Committed to developing an objective, university-based entity capable of providing research assistance to the Federal government on the major problems it faced in financing and delivering care to the elderly, disabled and poor. Our role has always been to solve complex health care problems, and to link research studies to policy change.

3441 School of Nursing, UCLA
PO Box 951702
Los Angeles, CA 90095-1702
310-825-7181
Fax: 310-267-0330
E-mail: sonsaff@sonnet.ucla.edu
www.nursing.ucla.edu

Rene Dennis, Director Development

3442 Southern Illinois University School of Medicine:
Department of Psychiatry
PO Box 19621
Springfield, IL 62794
217-545-2155
www.siumed.edu

3443 Southern Illinois University School of Medicine
SIU School of Medicine
PO Box 19621
Springfield, IL 62794
217-545-8000
www.www.siumed.edu

Stephen M Soltys MD, Pfr/Chair Dpt. of Psychiatry
Philip Pan MD, Division Chief

Provides high quality clinical treatment,outstanding teaching and solid efforts in research and community service.

3444 St. Francis Medical Center
400 45th Street
Pittsburgh, PA 15201
412-622-4343

3445 St. Joseph Behavioral Medicine Network
861 Corporate Drive
Suite 103
Lexington, KY 40503
859-224-2022

3446 St. Louis Behavioral Medicine Institute
1129 Macklind Avenue
Saint Louis, MO 63110
314-534-0200
877-245-2688
www.slbmi.com

Offers exceptional quality, result-focused treatment. Have remained true to our commitment of providing excellence in clinical care and customer service. We offer comprehensive treatment plans to meet the individual needs of children, adolescents, adults, older adults, and their families suffering from emotional and behavioral problems.

3447 Stonington Institute
75 Swantown Hill Road
N Stonington, CT 06359
860-535-1010
800-832-1022
E-mail: andrea.keeney@uhsinc.com
www.stoningtoninstitute.com

Andrea Keeney, Director Admissions

3448 Success Day Training Program
Skills Unlimited
2060-3 Ocean Ave
Ronkonkoma, NY 11779
631-580-5319
Fax: 631-580-5394
E-mail: success@skillsunlimited.org
www.www.skillsunlimited.org

SUCCESS is a socialization, recreation and prevocational day program for persons with chronic mental illness. Transportation is provided for attendees from Islip, Babylon, and Brookhaven townships. There is no cost to consumers. An evening and weekend program is also available to Islip residents.

3449 Topeka Institute for Psychoanalysis
PO Box 829
Topeka, KS 66601
800-288-3950

A training facility for health care professionals, the Topeka Institute for Psychoanalysis has the tripartite mission of promoting research to expand the knowledge base in its field of expertise; providing didactic education and clinical supervision to trainees; and caring for patients in need of its services through a low-fee clinic.

3450 Training Behavioral Healthcare Professionals: Higher Learning in an Era of Managed Care
Wiley Europe and Jossey-Bass Publications
1110 Mar Street
Suite E
Tiburon, CA 94920
415-435-9821
Fax: 415-435-9092
www.wileyeurope.com

Identifies best practices and a model curriculum for training the next generation of behavioral healthcare providers. *$ 32.95*

208 pages Year Founded: 1997 ISBN 0-787907-95-2

3451 Training Behavioral Healthcare Professionals
Jossey-Bass Publishers
350 Sansome Street
5th Floor
San Francisco, CA 94104
800-956-7739

Provides text on strategies for training mental health professionals in the skills necessary for providing services in a framework of limited resources. *$46.00*

180 pages Year Founded: 1997 ISBN 0-787907-95-2

3452 UCLA Neuropsychiatric Institute and Hospital
700 Westwood Plaza
Los Angeles, CA 90024
310-825-0511
www.npi.ucla.edu/institute.html

Multidisciplinary institute of human neurosciences, and is unifying focus of scholarly activity at UCLA in this area. Scientific advances recent decades have shown the value in approaches that cut across traditional academic departments, and which emphasize interdisciplinary collaborations.

3453 UCSF-Department of Psychiatry, Cultural Competence
1001 Potrero Avenue
San Francisco, CA 94110-3518
415-206-8984

3454 USC Psychiatry and Psychology Associates
1640 Marengo Street
Suite 510
Los Angeles, CA 90033

3455 USC School of Medicine
Health Sciences Campuses
Name/Department USC
Los Angeles, CA 90089
323-442-1100
www.usc.edu/schools/medicine/

3456 Ulster County Mental Health Department
239 Golden Hill Lane
Kingston, NY 12401
845-340-4000
www.co.ulster.ny.us/mentalhealth

Marshall Beckman MPA, Director

Responsible for planning, funding and monitoring of community mental health, mental retardation/developmental disability and alcohol and substance abuse services in Ulster County.

3457 Union County Psychiatric Clinic
117 Roosevelt Avenue
Plainfield, NJ 07060
908-412-9792

3458 University Behavioral Healthcare
671 Hoes Lane
Piscataway, NJ 08855
800-969-5300
www.www.ubhc.umdnj.edu

3459 University of California at Davis Psychiatry and Behavioral Sciences Department
2315 Stockton Boulevard
Sacramento, CA 95817
916-734-2011
www.ucdmc.ucdavis.edu/psychiatry

Offers opportunities for students and faculty for clinical and research applications in all aspects of psychiatry and behavioral sciences.

3460 University of Cincinnati College of Medical Department of Psychiatry
231 Albert Sabin Way
Medical Sciences Building/Ml 0559
Cincinnati, OH 45267
513-558-4274
Fax: 513-558-0187
www.psychiatry.uc.edu
Caleb Adler, Contact

Researches eating disorders, bipolar disorder, and chemical dependency.

3461 University of Colorado Health Sciences Center
4200 E 9th Avenue
Box A-080
Denver, CO 80262
303-315-8832
877-472-2586
Fax: 303-315-7729
E-mail: alumni@uchsc.edu
www.www.uchsc.edu

3462 University of Connecticut Health Center
263 Farmington Avenue
Farmington, CT 06030
860-679-2000
TDD: 860-679-2242
www.www.uchc.edu

3463 University of Iowa Hospital
200 Hawkins Drive
Iowa City, IA 52242
319-356-6161
800-777-8442
TDD: 319-356-4999
E-mail: uihc-webcomments@uiowa.edu
www.uihealthcare.com

3464 University of Kansas Medical Center
3901 Rainbow Boulevard
Kansas City, KS 66160
913-588-5000
TDD: 913-588-7963
www.kumc.edu

Barbara Atkinson, Executive Vice Chancellor

An integral and unique component of the University of Kansas and the Kansas Board of Regents system, is composed of the School of Medicine, the School of Nursing, the School of Allied Health, the University of Kansas Hospital, and a Graduate School. KU Medical Center is a complex institution whose basic functions include research, education, patient care, and community service involving multiple constituencies at state and national levels.

3465 University of Kansas School of Medicine
1010 N. Kansas
Wichita, KS 67214
316-293-2635
E-mail: kusmw@kumc.edu
www.wichita.kumc.edu

3466 University of Louisville School of Medicine
Abell Administration Center
323 E. Chestnut Street
Louisville, KY 40292

502-852-1499
E-mail: meddean@louisville.edu
www.louisville.edu/medschool

Mission is to be a vital component in the University of Louisville's quest to become a premier, nationally recognized metropolitan research university, to excel in the education of physicians and scientists for careers in teching, research, patient care and community service, and to bring the fundamental discoveries of our basic and clinical scientists to the bedside.

3467 University of Maryland Medical Systems
701 W Pratt Street
Suite 388
Baltimore, MD 21201
410-328-6600
www.www.umm.edu

3468 University of Maryland School of Medicine
655 West Baltimore Street
Baltimore, MD 21201-1559
410-706-7410
Fax: 410-706-0235
www.medschool.umaryland.edu

E Albert Reece, Dean/Vp Medical Affairs

Dedicated to providing excellence in biomedical education, basic and clinical research, quality patient care and service to improve the health of the citizens of Maryland and beyond.

3469 University of Massachusetts Medical Center
55 Lake Avenue N
Worcester, MA 01655
508-856-8989
www.umassmed.edu

Mission is to serve the people of the commonwealth through national distinction in health sciences, education, research, public service and clinical care.

3470 University of Miami - Department of Psychology
PO Bo 248185
Coral Gables, FL 33124-0751
305-284-2814
Fax: 305-284-3402
E-mail: webmaster@psy.miami.edu
www.psy.miami.edu

A facility that publishes approximately 100 journal articles, chapters, and books, and make numerous convention presentations, invited addresses, and colliquia.

3471 University of Michigan
400 E Eisenhower Parkway
Ann Arbor, MI 48108
734-764-1817
E-mail: info@umich.edu
www.umich.edu

3472 University of Minnesota Fairview Health Systems
2450 Riverside Ave
Minneapolis, MN 55454
612-273-3000
TTY: 612-672-7300
www.www.university.fairview.org

Mission is to improve the health of the communities we serve. We commit our skills and resources to the benefit of the whole person by providing the finest in healthcare, while addressing the physical, emotional and spiritual needs of individuals and their families. Pledge to support the research and education efforts of our partner, the University of Minnesota, and its tradition of excellence.

3473 University of Minnesota, Family Social Science
290 McNeal Hall
1985 Buford Avenue
Saint Paul, MN 55108
612-625-1900
Fax: 612-625-4227
E-mail: fsosinfo@umn.edu
www.www.fsos.cehd.umn.edu

Mission is to enhance the well-being of diverse families in a changing world through teaching, research, and outreach.

3474 University of New Mexico, School of Medicine Health Sciences Center
Ofc of the Executive VP for Health Svs
MSC09 5300 1 University Of New Mexico
Albuquerque, NM 87131-5001
505-272-5849
Fax: 505-272-3601
www.hsc.unm.edu

Paul B Roth MD, Exec VP, Dean School of Medicine

Established in 1994, the University of New Mexico Health Sciences Center is the largest academic health complex in the state. Located on the University of New Mexico campus in Albuquerque, New Mexico, the HSC combines its four mission area-education, research, patient care and partnership-the provide New Mexicans with the highest level of health care.

3475 University of North Carolina School of Socia l Work
Behavioral Healthcare Resource Institute
301 Pittsboro Street
Cb # 3550
Chapel Hill, NC 27599
919-843-3018
E-mail: bhrinstitute@listserv.unc.edu
www.behavioralhealthcareinstitute.org

3476 University of North Carolina, School of Medicine
4030 Bondurant Hall
Cb# 7000
Chaple Hill, NC 27599
919-962-8331
E-mail: admissions@med.unc.edu
www.med.unc.edu

Mission is to improve the health of North carolinians and others whom we serve. We will accomplish this by achieving excellence and providing leadership in the interrelated areas of patient care, education, and research.

3477 University of Pennsylvania Health System
399 S 34th Street
Suite 2002 Penn Tower
Philadelphia, PA 19104
215-662-2560
Fax: 215-349-8312
www.uphs.upenn.edu

3478 University of Pennsylvania, Department of Psychiatry
PENN Behavioral Health
1019 Blockley Hall
423 Guardian Drive
Philadelphia, PA 19104-6021
215-662-2560
Fax: 215-573-6410
E-mail: vdongen@mail.med.upenn.edu
www.www.uphs.upenn.edu

3479 University of Tennessee Medical Group: Department of Medicine and Psychiatry
135 N Pauline Street
Memphis, TN 38105
901-448-4572
Fax: 901-448-1684
E-mail: jgreen41@utmem.edu
www.www.utmem.edu/psych

James A. Greene, Professor/Interim Chair

3480 University of Texas Medical Branch Managed Care
301 University Boulevard
Galveston, TX 77555
409-772-1506
800-228-1841
Fax: 409-772-6216
E-mail: public.affairs@utmb.edu
www.www.utmb.edu

3481 University of Texas, Southwestern Medical Center
5323 Harry Hines Boulevard
Dallas, TX 75390
214-648-3111
Fax: 214-648-8955
www.utsouthwestern.edu

3482 University of Texas-Houston Health Science Center
7000 Fannin
Suite 1200
Houston, TX 77030
713-500-4472
Fax: 713-500-3026
www.uth.tmc.edu

A comprehensive health sciences health science university composed of six schools, an institute of molecular medicine and a psychiatric center. UTHSC-H's mission is to treat, cure and prevent disease now and in the future of educating health science professionals; discovering and translating advances in socials and biomedical sciences; and modeling the best practices in clincal care.

3483 University of Utah Neuropsychiatric
501 Chipeta Way
Salt Lake City, UT 84108
801-583-2500
E-mail: sarah.latta@hsc.utah.edu
www.uuhsc.utah.edu/uni

Sarah Latta, Contact

Located in the University's Research Park, is a full service 90-bed psychiatric hospital providing mental health and substance abuse treatment. Services include inpatient, day treatment, intensive outpatient, and ooutpatient services for children, adolescents and adults. Confidential assessments, referrals, and intervention education are available.

3484 Wake Forest University
1834 Wake Forest Road
Winston Salem, NC 27106
336-758-5255

3485 Wayne University-University of Psychiatric Center-Jefferson: Outpatient Mental Health for Children, Adolescents and Adults
2751 E Jefferson Avenue
Suite 436 Upc Jefferson
Detroit, MI 48207
313-577-3031
E-mail: rmarcian@med.wayne.edu
www.www.brain.wayne.edu/rocco/rocco.htm

Rocco Marciano, Director Of Clinical Programs

The University Psychiatric Centers' Early Childhood Intervention (ECI) provides services to preschool children with emotional and behavioral problems and their families. The program works to increase parental understanding of the child's developmental and emotional issues. this is achieved through education, support, and the observation of child management techniques. The program places a strong emphasis on family involvement and preventing more serious difficulties later in the child's life.

3486 West Jefferson Medical Center
1101 Medical Center Boulevard
Marrero, LA 70072
504-347-5511
www.wjmc.org

Nancy Casssagne, Interim Ceo

Not-for-profit community hospital on the West Bank of Jefferson Parish. Continues to strengthen its community base while maintaining its mission and values. Dedicated to considerate and respectful quality healthcare, the institution welcomes patient, family, and visitor feedback regarding programs, services, and community needs.

3487 Western Psychiatric Institute and Clinic
3811 Ohara Street
Pittsburgh, PA 15213
412-624-2100
877-624-4100
www.www.upmc.com

A national leader in the diagnosis, management, and treatment of mental health and addictive disorders. Providing the most comprehensive range of behavioral health services available today, but also shaping tomorrow's behavioral health care through clinical innovation, research, and education.

3488 Wordsworth
3905 Ford Road
Philadelphia, PA 19131
215-643-5400
E-mail: info@wordsworth.org
www.wordsworth.org

Madeleine Kessler, Community Relations

The mission of Wordsworth, a not-for-profit institution, is to provide quality education, treatment and care to children and families with special needs.

Year Founded: 1952

3489 Yale University School of Medicine: Child Study Center
230 S Frontage Road
New Haven, CT 06520
203-785-2513
www.info.med.yale.edu/chldstdy

Fred Volkmar, Director

Provides a comprehensive range of in-depth diagnostic and treatment services for children with psychiatric and developmental disorders. These services include specialized developmental evaluations for children ages zero-four, and psychological and psychiatric evaluations for children 5-18. Individualized treatment plans following evaluation make use for a range of theraputic interventions, including psychotherapy, group therapy, family therapy, psycho-pharmacological treatment, parent counseling, consultation and service planning. Immediate access for children needing to be seen within 24 hours and walk-in service is also available.

Video & Audio

3490 Asperger's Diagnostic Assessment with Dr. Tony Attwood
Program Development Associates PO Box 2038
Syracuse, NY 13220-2038
315-452-0643
Fax: 315-452-0710
E-mail: info@disabilitytraining.com
www.disabilitytraining.com

New from acclaimed autism expert Dr. Tony Attwood, this 4-hour DVD set with program guide offers diagnostic characteristics of Asperger's Syndrome in children and adults, patient interviews and impacts on girls. An essential guide for Child Psychologists, Special Ed teachers and Parents. *$129.95*

3491 Cognitive Behavioral Assessment
New Harbinger Publications
5674 Shattuck Avenue
Oakland, CA 94609-1662
510-652-2002
800-748-6273
Fax: 510-652-5472
E-mail: customerservice@newharbinger.com
www.newharbinger.com

A videotape that guides three clients through PAC (Problem, Antecedents, Consequences) method of cognitive behavioral assessment. *$49.95*

ISBN 1-572243-15-5

3492 Couples and Infertility - Moving Beyond Loss
Guilford Publications
72 Spring Street
New York, NY 10012
212-431-9800
800-365-7006
Fax: 212-966-6708
E-mail: info@guilford.com
www.guilford.com

A VHS video explores the biological and resulting psychological and social issues of infertility. *$95.00*

Year Founded: 1995 ISBN 1-572302-86-0

3493 Educating Clients about the Cognitive Model
New Harbinger Publications
5674 Shattuck Avenue
Oakland, CA 94609-1662
510-652-2002
800-748-6273
Fax: 510-652-5472
E-mail: customerservice@newharbinger.com
www.newharbinger.com

Videotape that helps three clients understand their symptoms as they work toward developing a working contract to begin cognitive restructing. *$49.95*

ISBN 1-572243-19-8

3494 Gender Differences in Depression: Marital Therapy Approach
Guilford Publications
72 Spring Street
New York, NY 10012
212-431-9800
800-365-7006
Fax: 212-966-6708
E-mail: info@guilford.com
www.guilford.com

Male-female treatment team is shown working with a markedly depressed couple to improve communication and sense of well being in their marriage. *$85.50*

Year Founded: 1996 ISBN 1-572302-87-9

3495 Group Work for Eating Disorders and Food Issues
American Counseling Association
5999 Stevenson Avenue
Alexandria, VA 22304-3300
800-422-2648
Fax: 703-823-0252
www.counseling.org

A plan for working with high school and college age females who are at risk for eating disorders. This video provides a method for identifying at-risk clients, a session-by-session desciption of the group, exercises and information on additional resources. *$89.95*

Year Founded: 1995 ISSN 79801

3496 Help This Kid's Driving Me Crazy - the Young Child with Attention Deficit Disorder
Pro-Ed Publications
8700 Shoal Creek Boulevard
Austin, TX 78757-6816
512-451-3246
800-897-3202
Fax: 800-397-7633
E-mail: info@proedinc.com
www.proedinc.com

This videotape provides information about the behavior and special needs of young children with ADD and offers suggestions on fostering appropriate behaviors. *$89.00*

3497 I Love You Like Crazy: Being a Parent with Mental Illness
Mental Illness Education Project
PO Box 470813
Brookline Village, MA 02247-0244
617-562-1111
800-343-5540

Fax: 617-779-0061
E-mail: miep@tiac.net
www.miepvideos.org

Christine Ledoux, Executive Director

In this videotape, eight mothers and fathers who have mental illness discuss the challenges they face as parents. Most of these parents have faced enormous obstacles from homelessness, addictions, legal difficulties and hospitalizations, yet have maintained a positive and loving relationship with their children. The tape introduces issues of work, fear, stigma, relationships with children and the rest of the family, with professionals, and with the community at large. Discounted price for families/consumers. *$79.95*

Year Founded: 1999

3498 Inner Health Incorporated
Christopher Alsten, PhD
1260 Lincoln Avenue
San Diego, CA 92103-2322
619-299-7273
800-283-4679
Fax: 619-291-7753
E-mail: sleepenhancement@aol.com

Provides a series of prerecorded therapeutic audio programs for anxiety, insomnia and chemical dependency, both for adults and children. Developed over a 15 year period by a practicing psychiatrist and recording engineer they employ state-of-the-art 3-D sound technologies and the latest relaxation and psychological techniques (but no stimulants). Clients include: US Air Force, US Navy, National Institute of Health, National Institute of Aging and various psychiatric and chemical dependency facilities and companies with shiftworkers.

3499 Know Your Rights: Mental Health Private Practice & the Law
American Counseling Association
5999 Stevenson Avenue
Alexandria, VA 22304-3300
800-347-6647
Fax: 703-823-0252
E-mail: webmaster@counseling.org
www.counseling.org

Whether you are in private practice or are thinking about opening your own practice, this forum lead by national experts, offers answers to important questions and provides invaluable information for every practitioner. Helps to orientate practitioners on the legally permissible boundaries, legal liabilities that are seldom known and how to respond in the face of legal action. *$145.00*

ISSN 79062

3500 Life Is Hard: Audio Guide to Healing Emotional Pain
Impact Publishers
PO Box 6016
Atascadero, CA 93423-6016
805-466-5917
800-246-7228
Fax: 805-466-5919
E-mail: info@impactpublishers.com
www.impactpublishers.com

In a very warm and highly personal style, psychologist Preston offers listeners powerful advice — realistic, practical, effective, on dealing with the emotional pain life often inflicts upon us. *$11.95*

Year Founded: 1996 ISBN 0-915166-99-2

3501 Life Passage in the Face of Death, Volume I: A Brief Psychotherapy
American Psychiatric Publishing
1000 Wilson Boulevard
Suite 1825
Arlington, VA 22209-3901
703-907-7322
800-368-5777
Fax: 703-907-1091
E-mail: appi@psych.org
www.appi.org

A senior psychoanalyst demonstrates the extraordinary impact of a very brief dynamic psychotherapy on a patient in a time of crisis — the terminal illness and death of a spouse. We not only meet the patient and observe the therapy, but our understanding is guided by the therapist's ongoing explanation of the process. He vividly illustrates concepts such as transference, clarification, interpretation, insight, denial, isolation and above all the relevance of understanding the past for changing the present. This unique opportunity to see a psychotherapy as it is conducted will be of immense value for all mental health clinicians and trainees.

3502 Life Passage in the Face of Death, Volume II : Psychological Engagement of the Physically Ill Patient
American Psychiatric Publishing
1000 Wilson Boulevard
Suite 1825
Arlington, VA 22209-3901
703-907-7322
800-368-5777
Fax: 703-907-1091
E-mail: appi@psych.org
www.appi.org

Ongoing explanation of therapy from a recognized expert. Valuable to clinicians and students alike.

3503 Medical Aspects of Chemical Dependency The Neurobiology of Addiction
Hazelden
15251 Pleasant Valley Road
PO Box 176
Center City, MN 55012-0176
651-213-2121
800-328-9000
Fax: 651-213-4590
www.hazelden.org

This interactive curriculum helps professionals educate clients in treatment and other settings about medical effects of chemical use and abuse. The program includes a video that explains body and brain changes that can occur when using alcohol or other drugs, a workbook that helps clients apply the information from the video to their own situations, a handbook that provides in-depth information on addiction, brain chemistry and the physiological effects of chemical dependency and a pamphlet that answers critical questions clients have about the medical effects of chemical dependency. Total price of $244.70, available to purchase separately. Program value packages available for $395.00, with 25 workbooks, two handbooks, two video and 25 pamphlets. *$225.00*

Year Founded: 2003 ISBN 1-568389-87-6

3504 Mental Illness Education Project
PO Box 470813
Brookline Village, MA 02447-0813
617-562-1111
800-343-5540
Fax: 617-779-0061
E-mail: info@miepvideos.org
www.miepvideos.org

Christine Ledoux, Executive Director

Engaged in the production of video-based educational and support materials for the following specific populations: people with psychiatric disabilities; families, mental health professionals, special audiences, and the general public. The Project's videos are designed to be used in hospital, clinical and educational settings, and at home by individuals and families.

3505 Personality and Stress Center for Applications of Psychological Type
2815 NW 13th Street
Suite 401
Gainesville, FL 32609-2868
352-375-0160
800-777-2278
Fax: 352-378-0503
E-mail: customerservice@capt.org
www.catp.org

Alecia Perkins, Director Customer Service

Humorous and energetic presentation of the use of type and rational-emotive therapy concepts in stress management. The authors share years of experience using this model in a hospital setting. Useful to the counselor, educator, or anyone working with stress management. *$11.00*

audio pages Year Founded: 1989

3506 Physicians Living with Depression
American Psychiatric Publishing
1000 Wilson Boulevard
Suite 1825
Arlington, VA 22209-3901
703-907-7322
800-368-5777
Fax: 703-907-1091
E-mail: appi@psych.org
www.appi.org

Michael F Myers MD, Producer
Katie Duffy, Marketing Assistant

Designed to help doctors see the signs of depression in their fellow physicians and to alert psychiatrists to the severity of the illness in their physician patients, the tape contains two fifteen-minute interviews, one with an emergency physician and one with a pediatrician. *$25.00*

ISBN 0-890422-78-8

3507 Rational Emotive Therapy
Research Press
Dept 26 W
PO Box 9177
Champaign, IL 61826
217-352-3273
800-519-2707
Fax: 217-352-1221

E-mail: rp@researchpress.com
www.researchpress.com
Dennis Wiziecki, Marketing
Dr Albert Ellis, Author

This video illustrates the basic concepts of Rational Emotive Therapy (RET). It includes demonstrations of RET procedures, informative discussions and unstaged counseling sessions. Viewers will see Albert Ellis and his colleagues help clients overcome such problems as guilt, social anxiety, and jealousy. Also, Dr. Ellis shares his perspectives on the evolution of RET. *$195.00*

3508 Solutions Step by Step - Substance Abuse Treatment Videotape
WW Norton & Company
500 5th Avenue
New York, NY 10110
212-790-9456
Fax: 212-869-0856
E-mail: admalmud@wwnorton.com
www.wwnorton.com

Quick tips, questions and examples focusing on successes that can be experienced helping substance abusers help themselves. *$ 100.00*

Year Founded: 1997 ISSN 70260-X

3509 Testing Automatic Thoughts with Thought Records
New Harbinger Publications
5674 Shattuck Avenue
Oakland, CA 94609-1662
510-652-2002
800-748-6273
Fax: 510-652-5472
E-mail: customerservice@newharbinger.com
www.newharbinger.com

Videotape that helps a client explore the hot thoughts that contribute to depression. *$49.95*

ISBN 1-572243-17-1

Web Sites

3510 www.aacap.org
American Academy of Child and Adolescent Psychiatry

Represents over 6,000 child and adolescent psychiatrists, brochures availible online which provide concise and up-to-date material on issues ranging from children who suffer from depression and teen suicide to stepfamily problems and child sexual abuse.

3511 www.aan.com
American Academy of Neurology

Provides information for both professionals and the public on neurology subjects, covering Alzheimer's and Parkinson's diseases to stroke and migraine, includes comprehensive fact sheets.

3512 www.aapb.org
Association for Applied Psychophysiology and Biofeedback

Represents clinicians interested in psychopsysiology or biofeedback, offers links to their mission statement, membership information, research, FAQ about biofeedback, conference listings, and links.

3513 www.abecsw.org
American Board of Examiners in Clinical Social Work
Fax: 978-740-5395

Information about the American Board of Examiners, credentialing, and ethics.

3514 www.about.com
About.Com

Network of comprehensive Web sites for over 600 mental health topics.

3515 www.abpsi.org
American Association of Black Psychologists

Includes information about the Association's history and objectives, contact and member information, upcoming events, and publications of interest.

3516 www.ama-assn.org
American Medical Association

Offers a wide range of medical information and links, full-text abstracts of each journal's current and past articles.

3517 www.americasdoctor.com
AmericasDoctor.com

Center researching for new medicine.

3518 www.apa.org
American Psychological Association

Information about journals, press releases, professional and consumer information related to the psychological profession; resources include ethical principles and guidelines, science advocacy, awards and funding programs, testing and assessment information, other on-line and real world resources.

3519 www.apna.org
American Psychiatric Nurses Association

Includes membership information, contact information, organizational information, announcements and related links.

3520 www.appi.org
American Psychiatric Publishing Inc

Informational site about mental disorders, 'Lets Talk Facts' brochure series.

3521 www.apsa.org
American Psychoanalytic Asssociation

Includes searchable bibliographic database containing books, reviews and articles of a psychoanalytical orientation, links and member information.

3522 www.assc.caltech.edu
Association for the Scientific Study of Consciousness

Electronic journal dedicated to interdisciplinary exploration on the nature of consciousness and its relationship to the brain, congitive science, philosophy, psychology, physics, neuroscience, and artificial intelligence.

3523 www.blarg.net/~charlatn/voices
Compilation of Writings by People Suffering from Depression

3524 www.bpso.org
BPSO-Bipolar Significant Others

3525 www.bpso.org/nomania.htm
How to Avoid a Manic Episode

3526 www.cape.org
Cape Cod Institute

Offers symposia every summer for keeping mental health professionals up-to-date on the latest developments in psychology, treatment, psychiatry, and mental health, outlines available workshops, links and other relevant information.

3527 www.chadd.org
CHADD

Peg Nichols, Director Communications

National non-profit organization representing children and adults with attention deficit/hyperactivity disorder (AD/HD).

3528 www.cnn.com/Health
CNN Health Section

Updated with health and mental health-related stories three to four times weekly.

3529 www.compuserve.com
IQuest/Knowledge Index

On-line research and database information provider.

3530 www.counseling.com
American Counseling Association

Hosts information about the American Counseling Association, membership, legislative and news updates, a conference and workshop calendar, and links to related resources and publications.

3531 www.counselingforloss.com
Counseling for Loss and Life Changes

Look under articles for reprints of writings and links.

3532 www.cyberpsych.org
CyberPsych

Hosts the American Psychoanalyists Foundation, American Association of Suicideology, Society for the Exploration of Psychotherapy Intergration, and Anxiety Disorders Association of America. Also subcategories of the anxiety disorders, as well as general information, including panic disorder, phobias, obsessive compulsive disorder (OCD), social phobia, generalized anxiety disorder, post traumatic stress disorder, and phobias of childhood. Book reviews and links to web pages sharing the topics.

3533 www.factsforhealth.org
Madison Institute of Medicine

Resource to help identify, understand and treat a number of medical conditions, including social anxiety disorder and posttraumatic stress disorder.

3534 www.geocities.com
Have a Heart's Depression Home

Several fine essays and seven triggers for suicide.

3535 www.geocities.com/enchantedforest/1068
Bipolar Kids Homepage

Set of links.

3536 www.goaskalice.columbia.edu
GoAskAlice/Healthwise Columbia University

Oriented toward students, information on sexuality, sexual health, general health, alcohol and other drugs, fitness and nutrition, emotional wellbeing and relationships.

3537 www.grieftalk.com/help1.html
Grief Journey

Short readings for clients.

3538 www.habitsmart.com/cogtitle.html
Cognitive Therapy Pages

Offers accessible explanations.

3539 www.healthgate.com/
HealthGate

On-line reference and database information service, $.75/record.

3540 www.healthtouch.com
Healthtouch Online

Healthtouch Online is a resource that brings together valuable information from trusted health organizations.

3541 www.healthy.net
HealthWorld Online

Consumer-oriented articles on a wide range of health and mental health topics, including: Welcome Center, QuickN'Dex, Site Search, Free Medline, Health Conditions, Alternative Medicine, Referral Network, Health Columns, Global Calendar, Discussion, Cybrarian, Professional Center, Free Newsletter, Opportunities, Healthy Travel, Homepage, Library, University, Marketplace, Health Clinic, Wellness Center, Fitness Center, News Room, Association Network, Public Health, Self Care Central, and Nutrition Center.

3542 www.helix.com
Helix MEDLINE: GlaxoSmithKline

Helix is an Education, Learning and Information exchange. Developed especially for healthcare practitioners by GlaxoSmithKline, HELIX is a premire source of on-line education and professional resources on a range of therapeutic and practice-management issues.

3543 www.human-nature.com/odmh
On-line Dictonary of Mental Health

Global information resource and research tool. It is compiled by Internet mental health resource users for Internet mental health resource users, and covers all the disciplines contributing to our understanding of mental health.

3544 www.infotrieve.com
Infotrieve Medline Services Provider

Infotrieve is a library services company offering full-service document delivery, databases on the web and a variety of tools to simplify the process of identifying, retrieving and paying for published literature.

3545 www.intelihealth.com
InteliHealth

3546 www.krinfo.com
DataStar/Dialog

Information provider: reference and databases.

3547 www.lollie.com/blue/suicide.html
Comprehensive Approach to Suicide Prevention

Readings for anyone contemplating suicide.

3548 www.mayohealth.org/mayo
Mayo Clinic Health Oasis Library

Healthcare library and resources.

3549 www.med.jhu.edu/drada/creativity.html
Creativity and Depression and Manic-Depression

3550 www.med.nyu.edu/Psych/index.html
NYU Department of Psychiatry

General mental health information, screening tests, reference desk, continuing educations in psychiatry program, interactive testing in psychiatry, augmentation of antidepressants, NYU Psychoanalytic Institute, Psychology Internship Program, Internet Mental Health Resources links.

3551 www.medinfosource.com
CME, Medical Information Source

Medical information and education, fully accredited for all medical specialties.

3552 www.medscape.com
Medscape

Oriented toward physicians and medical topics, but also carries information relevant to the field of psychology and mental health.

3553 www.medweb.emory.edu/MedWeb/
MedWeb Emory University Health Sciences Center Library

Hundreds of links for mental health, psychology, and pscyhiatry. Recognized nationally for clinical, educational and research programs, and its hospitals and professional schools are ranked among the top in the nation. Webpage includes General Information Links, Emory Healthcare, Schools and Research Centers, Libraries and Research Tools, Health Sciences Communications Office, Employment Opportunities, Frequently Requested Contact Information, and much more.

3554 www.members.aol.com/dswgriff
Now Is Not Forever: A Survival Guide

Print out a no-suicide contract, do problem solving, and other exercises.

3555 www.mentalhealth.com/book
Schizophrenia: A Handbook for Families

Mostly unique information.

3556 www.mentalhealth.com/p20-grp.html
Manic-Depressive Illness

Click on Bipolar and then arrow down to Booklets.

3557 www.mentalhealth.com/story
How to Help a Person with Depression

Valuable family education.

3558 www.metanoia.org/suicide/
If You Are Thinking about Suicide...Read This First

Excellent suggestions, information and links for the suicidal.

3559 www.mhsource.com
CME Mental Health InfoSource

Mental health information and education, fully accredited for all medical specialties.

3560 www.mhsource.com/
CME Psychiatric Time

Select articles published online from the Psychiatric Times, topics relevant to all mental health professionals.

3561 www.mindfreedom.org
Support Coalition Human Rights & Psychiatry Home Page

Support Coalition is an independent alliance of several dozen grassroots groups in the USA, Canada, Europe, New Zealand; has used protests, publications, letter-writing, e-mail, workshops, Dendron News, the arts and performances. Led by psychiatric survivors, and open to the public, membership is open to anyone who supports its mission and goals.

3562 www.mirror-mirror.org/eatdis.htm
Mirror, Mirror

Relapse prevention for eating disorders.

3563 www.moodswing.org/bdfaq.html
Bipolar Disorder Frequently Asked Questions

Excellent for those newly diagnosed.

3564 www.naphs.org
National Association of Psychiatric Health Systems

The NAPHS advocates for behavioral health and represents provider systems that are committed to the delivery of responsive, accountable and clinically effective prevention, treatment and care for children, adolescents and adults with mental and substance use disorders.

3565 www.naswdc.org/
National Associaton of Social Workers

Central resource for clinical social workers, includes information about the federation, a conference and workshop calender, information on how to subscribe to social worker mailing lists, legislative and news updates, links to state agencies and social work societies, and publications.

3566 www.ndmda.org/justmood.htm
Just a Mood...or Something Else

A brochure for teens.

3567 www.nimh.nih.gov
National Institute of Mental Health (NIMH)

The mission of NIMH is to diminish the burden of mental illness through research of the biological, behavioral, clinical, epidemiological, economic, and social science aspects of mental illnesses.

3568 www.nmha.org
National Mental Health Association

Dedicated to promoting mental health, preventing mental disorders and achieving victory over mental illness through advocacy, education, research and service. NMHA's collaboration with the National GAINS Center for People with Co-Occuring Disorders in the Justice System has produced the Justice for Juveniles Initiative. This program battles to reform the juvenile justice system so that the inmates mental needs are addressed. Envisions a just, humane and healthy society in which all people are accorded respect, dignity and the opportunity to achieve their full potential free from stigma and prejudice.

3569 www.oclc.org
EPIC

On-line reference and database information provider, $40/hour (plus connection fees) and $.75/record.

3570 www.oznet.ksu.edu/library/famlf2/
Family Life Library

3571 www.pace-custody.org
Professional Academy of Custody Evaluators

Nonprofit corporation and membership organization to acknowledge and strengthen the professionally prepared comprehensive custody evaluation; psychologicals legal knowledge base, assessment procedures, courtroom testimony, provides continuing education courses, conferences, conventions and seminars.

3572 www.paperchase.com
PaperChase

Searches may be conducted through a browsable list of topics, search engine recognizes queries made in natural language.

3573 www.parenthoodweb.com
Blended Families

Resolving conflicts.

3574 www.planetpsych.com
Planetpsych.com

Learn about disorders, their treatments and other topics in psychology. Articles are listed under the related topic areas. Ask a therapist a question for free, or view the directory of professionals in your area. If you are a therapist sign up for the directory. Current features, self-help, interactive, and newsletter archives.

3575 www.positive-way.com/step.htm
Stepfamily Information

Introduction and tips for stepfathers, stepmothers and re-married parents.

3576 www.psych.org
American Psychiatric Association

A medical specialty society recognized world-wide. Its 40,500 US and international physicians specializing in the diagnosis and treatment of mental and emotional illness and substance use disorders.

3577 www.psychcentral.com
Psych Central

Personalized one-stop index for psychology, support, and mental health issues, resources, and people on the Internet.

3578 www.psychcrawler.com
American Psychological Association

Indexing the web for the links in psychology.

3579 www.psychology.com/therapy.htm
Therapist Directory

Therapists listed geographically plus answers to frequently asked questions.

3580 www.psycom.net/depression.central.html
Dr. Ivan's Depression Central

Medication-oriented site.

3581 www.recovery-inc.com
Recovery

Describes the organizations approach.

3582 www.reutershealth.com
Reuters Health

Relevant and useful clinical information on mental disorders, news briefs updated daily.

3583 www.save.org
SA/VE - Suicide Awareness/Voices of Education

3584 www.schizophrenia.com
Schizophrenia.com

Offers basic and in-depth information, discussion and chat.

3585 www.schizophrenia.com/ami
Alliance for the Mentally Ill

Information on mental disorders, reducing the stigmatization of them in our society today, and how you can be more active in your local community. Includes articles, press information, media kits, mental disorder diagnostic and treatment information, coping issues, advocacy guides and announcements.

3586 www.schizophrenia.com/newsletter
Schizophrenia.com

Comprehensive psychoeducational site on schizophrenia.

3587 www.shpm.com
Self-Help and Psychology Magazine

General psychology and self-help magazine online, offers informative articles on general well being and psychology topics. Features Author of the Month, Breaking News Stories of the Month, Most Popular Pages, What's Hot, Departments, and Soundoff (articles and opinion page). This online compendium of hundreds of readers and professionals.

3588 www.shpm.com/articles/depress
Placebo Effect Accounts for Fifty Percent of
Improvement

3589 www.siop.org
Society for Industrial and Organizational
Psychology

Home to the Industrial-Organizational Pyschologist newsletter, links and resources, member information, contact information for doctoral and master's level program in I/O
psychology, and announcements of various events and conferences.

3590 www.stepfamily.org/tensteps.htm
Ten Steps for Steps

Guidelines for stepfamilies.

3591 www.stepfamilyinfo.org/sitemap.htm
Stepfamily in Formation

3592 www.usatoday.com
USA Today

'Mental Health' category includes news and in-depth reports.

3593 www.webmd.com
WebMD

3594 www.wingofmadness.com
Wing of Madness: A Depression Guide

Accurate information, advice, support, and personal experiences.

Workbooks & Manuals

3595 Activities for Adolescents in Therapy
Charles C Thomas Publisher
2600 S 1st Street
Springfield, IL 62704-4730
217-789-8980
800-258-8980
Fax: 217-789-9130
E-mail: books@ccthomas.com
www.ccthomas.com

In this practical resource manual, professionals will find
more than 100 therapeutic group activities for use in counseling troubled adolescents. This new edition provides spe-
cifics on establishing an effective group program while, at
the same time, outlining therapeutic activities that can be
used in each phase of a therapy group. Step-by-step instructions have been provided for setting up, planning and facilitating adolescent groups with social and emotional
problems. The interventions provided have been designed
specifically for initial, middle and termination phases of
group. $39.95 *$46.95*

264 pages Year Founded: 1998 ISBN 0-398068-07-0

3596 Activities for Children in Therapy: Guide for
Planning and Facilitating Therapy with
Troubled Children
Charles C Thomas Publisher
2600 S 1st Street
Springfield, IL 62704-4730
217-789-8980
800-258-8980

Fax: 217-789-9130
E-mail: books@ccthomas.com
www.ccthomas.com

Provides the mental health professional with a wide variety
of age-appropriate activities which are simultaneously fun
and therapeutic for the five-to-twelve-year-old troubled
child. Activities have been designed as enjoyable games in
the context of therapy. Provides a comprehensive listing of
books with other therapeutic intervention ideas,
bibliotherapy materials, assessment scales for evaluating
youngsters, and a sample child assessment for individual
therapy. For professionals who provide counseling to children, such as social workers, psychologists, guidance counselors, speech/language pathologists, and art therapists.
$52.95

302 pages Year Founded: 1999 ISBN 0-398069-71-9

3597 Chemical Dependency Treatment Planning
Handbook
Charles C Thomas Publisher
2600 S 1st Street
Springfield, IL 62704-4730
217-789-8980
800-258-8980
Fax: 217-789-9130
E-mail: books@ccthomas.com
www.ccthomas.com

Provides the entry-level clinician with a broad data base of
treatment planning illustrations from which unpretentious
treatment plans for the chemically dependent client can be
generated. They are simple, largely measurable, and purposefully with language that is cognizant of comprehen-
sion and learning needs of clients. It will be of interest to
drug and alcohol counselors. *$29.95*

174 pages Year Founded: 1997 ISBN 0-398067-76-7

3598 Clinical Manual of Supportive Psychotherapy
American Psychiatric Publishing
1000 Wilson Boulevard
Suite 1825
Arlington, VA 22209-3901
703-907-7322
800-368-5777
Fax: 703-907-1091
E-mail: appi@psych.org
www.appi.org

Katie Duffy, Marketing Assistant

New approaches and ideas for your practice. *$64.00*

362 pages Year Founded: 1993

3599 Comprehensive Directory: Programs and
Services for Children with Disabilities and
Their Families
Resources for Children with Special Needs
116 E 16th Street
Fifth Floor
New York, NY 10003
212-677-4550
Fax: 212-254-4070
E-mail: info@resourcesnyc.org
www.resourcesnyc.org

This directory includes up-to-date information about agencies, schools, after-school social, recreational and cultural
programs, camps and summer programs, family support
and respite services, plus legal, advocacy, medical, evalua-

tion, diagnostic, therapeutic services- and much more. This directory lists services taught cover your child's needs at every age, from early intervention through vocational and job-training programs. Everything you need to know to provide support and assistance to children. *$55.00*

ISBN 0-967836-51-4

3600 Concise Guide to Laboratory and Diagnostic Testing in Psychiatry
American Psychiatric Publishing
1000 Wilson Boulevard
Suite 1825
Arlington, VA 22209-3901
703-907-7322
800-368-5777
Fax: 703-907-1091
E-mail: appi@psych.org
www.appi.org

Katie Duffy, Marketing Assistant

Basic strategies for applying laboratory testing and evaluation. *$19.50*

176 pages Year Founded: 1989 ISBN 0-880483-33-4

3601 Creating and Implementing Your Strategic Plan: Workbook for Public and Nonprofit Organizations
Jossey-Bass Publishers
1110 Mar Street
Suite E
Tiburon, CA 94920
415-435-9821
Fax: 415-435-9092
www.josseybass.com

Step-by-step workbook to conducting strategic planning in public and nonprofit organizations. *$30.00*

192 pages Year Founded: 2004 ISBN 0-787967-54-8

3602 Handbook for the Study of Mental Health
Cambridge University Press
40 W 20th Street
New York, NY 10011-4221
212-924-3900
Fax: 212-691-3239
E-mail: marketing@cup.org
www.cup.org

Offers the first comprehensive presentation of the sociology of mental health illness, including original, contemporary contributions by experts in the relevant aspects of the field. Divided into three sections, the chapters cover the general perspectives in the field, the social determinants of mental health and current policy areas affecting mental health services. Designed for classroom use in sociology, social work, human relations, human services and psychology. With its useful definitions, overview of the historical, social and institutional frameworks for understanding mental health and illness, and nontechnical style, the text is suitable for advanced undergraduate or lower level graduate students. *$90.00*

694 pages Year Founded: 1999 ISBN 0-521561-33-7

3603 Handbook of Clinical Psychopharmacology for Therapists
New Harbinger Publications
5674 Shattuck Avenue
Oakland, CA 94609-1662

510-652-2002
800-748-6273
Fax: 510-652-5472
E-mail: customerservice@newharbinger.com
www.newharbinger.com

This newly revised classic includes updates on new medications, and expanded quick reference section, and new material on bipolar illness, the treatment of psychosis, and the effect of severe trauma. *$55.95*

264 pages Year Founded: 2005 ISBN 1-572240-94-6

3604 Handbook of Constructive Therapies
Jossey-Bass Publishers
350 Sansome Street
5th Floor
San Francisco, CA 94104
415-394-8677
800-956-7739
Fax: 800-605-2665
www.josseybass.com

Learn techniques that focus on the strengths and resources of your clients and look to where they want to go rather than where they have been. *$64.00*

500 pages Year Founded: 1998 ISBN 0-787940-44-5

3605 Handbook of Counseling Psychology
John Wiley & Sons
605 3rd Avenue
New York, NY 10058-0180
212-850-6000
Fax: 212-850-6008
E-mail: info@wiley.com
www.wiley.com

Provides a cross-disciplinary survey of the entire field and offers analysis of important areas of counseling psychology activity. the book elaborates on future directions for research, highlighting suggestions that may advance knowledge and stimulate further inquiry. Specific advice is presented from the literature in counseling psychology and related disciplines to help improve one's counseling practice. *$ 120.00*

880 pages Year Founded: 2000 ISBN 0-471254-58-4

3606 Handbook of Managed Behavioral Healthcare
Jossey-Bass Publishers
350 Sansome Street
5th Floor
San Francisco, CA 94104
415-394-8677
800-956-7739
Fax: 800-605-2665
www.josseybass.com

A comprehensive curriculum to understanding managed care. *$43.00*

240 pages Year Founded: 1998 ISBN 0-787941-53-0

3607 Handbook of Medical Psychiatry
Mosby
11830 Westline Industrial Drive
Saint Louis, MO 63146
314-872-8370
800-325-4177
Fax: 314-432-1380

This large-format handbook covers almost every psychiatric, neurologic and general medical condition capable of causing disturbances in thought, feeling, or behavior and includes almost every psychopharmacologic agent available in America today. *$61.95*

544 pages Year Founded: 1996 ISBN 0-323029-11-6

3608 Handbook of Mental Retardation and Development
Cambridge University Press
40 W 20th Street
New York, NY 10011-4221
212-924-3900
Fax: 212-691-3239
E-mail: marketing@cup.org
www.cup.org

This book reviews theoretical and empirical work in the developmental approach to mental retardation. Armed with methods derived from the study of typically developing children, developmentalists have recently learned about the mentally retarded child's own development in a variety of areas. These now encompass many aspects of cognition, language, social and adaptive functioning, as well as of maladaptive behavior and psychopathology. In addition to a focus on individuals with mental retardation themselves, other ecological factors have influenced developmental approaches to mental retardation. Comprised of twenty seven chapters on various aspects of development, this handbook provides a comprehensive guide to understanding mental retardation. *$80.00*

764 pages Year Founded: 1998

3609 Handbook of Psychiatric Education and Faculty Development
American Psychiatric Publishing
1000 Wilson Boulevard
Suite 1825
Arlington, VA 22209-3901
703-907-7322
800-368-5777
Fax: 703-907-1091
E-mail: appi@psych.org
www.appi.org

Katie Duffy, Marketing Assistant

Putting education to work in the real world. *$68.50*

496 pages Year Founded: 1999 ISBN 0-880487-80-1

3610 Handbook of Psychiatric Practice in the Juvenile Court
American Psychiatric Publishing
1000 Wilson Boulevard
Suite 1825
Arlington, VA 22209-3901
703-907-7322
800-368-5777
Fax: 703-907-1091
E-mail: appi@psych.org
www.appi.org

Katie Duffy, Marketing Assistant

How your practice can work with the court system, so your patients can get the help they need. *$27.95*

198 pages Year Founded: 1992 ISBN 0-890422-33-8

3611 Living Skills Recovery Workbook
Elsevier Science
11830 Westline Industrial Drive
St. Louis, MO 63146

314-453-7010
800-545-2522
Fax: 314-453-7095
E-mail: orders@bhusa.com or custserv@bhusa.com
www.bh.com

Katie Hennessy, Medical Promotions Coordinator

Provides clinicians with the tools necessary to help patients with dual diagnoses acquire basic living skills. Focusing on stress management, time management, activities of daily living, and social skills training, each living skill is taught in relation to how it aids in recovery and relapse prevention for each patient's individual lifestyle and pattern of addiction.

224 pages ISBN 0-750671-18-1

3612 On the Client's Path: A Manual for the Practice of Brief Solution - Focused Therapy
New Harbinger Publications
5674 Shattuck Avenue
Oakland, CA 94609-1662
510-652-2002
800-748-6273
Fax: 510-652-5472
E-mail: customerservice@newharbinger.com
www.newharbinger.com

Provides everything you need to master the solution - focused model. *$49.95*

157 pages Year Founded: 1995 ISBN 1-572240-21-0

3613 Relaxation & Stress Reduction Workbook
New Harbinger Publications
5674 Shattuck Avenue
Oakland, CA 94609-1662
510-652-2002
800-748-6273
Fax: 510-652-5472
E-mail: customerservice@newharbinger.com
www.newharbinger.com

Matthew McKay, Editor

Details effective stress reduction methods such as breathing exercises, meditation, visualization, and time management. Widely reccomended by therapists, nurses, and physicians throughout the US, this fourth edition has been substantially revised and updated to reflect current research. Line drawings and charts. *$19.95*

276 pages Year Founded: 2005 ISBN 1-879237-82-2

3614 Skills Training Manual for Treating Borderline Personality Disorder, Companion Workbook
Guilford Publications
72 Spring Street
New York, NY 10012
212-431-9800
800-365-7006
Fax: 212-966-6708
E-mail: info@guilford.com
www.guilford.com

A vital component in Dr. Linehan's comprehensive treatment program, this step-by-step manual details precisely how to implement the skills training procedures and includes practical pointers on when to use the other treatment strategies described. It includes useful, clear-cut handouts that may be readily photocopied. *$27.95*

180 pages Year Founded: 1993 ISBN 0-898620-34-1

3615 Step Workbook for Adolescent Chemical Dependency Recovery
American Psychiatric Publishing
1000 Wilson Boulevard
Suite 1825
Arlington, VA 22209-3901
703-907-7322
800-368-5777
Fax: 703-907-1091
E-mail: appi@psych.org
www.appi.org

Katie Duffy, Marketing Assistant

Strategies for younger patients in your practice. *$ 62.00*

72 pages Year Founded: 1990 ISBN 0-882103-00-9

3616 Stress Management Training: Group Leader's Guide
Professional Resource Press
PO Box 15560
Sarasota, FL 34277-1560
941-343-9601
800-443-3364
Fax: 941-343-9201
E-mail: orders@prpress.com
www.prpress.com

This practical guide will help you define the concept of stress for group members and teach them various intervention techniques ranging from relaxation training to communication skills. Includes specific exercises, visual aids, stress response index, stress analysis form and surveys for evaluating program effectiveness. *$13.95*

96 pages Year Founded: 1990 ISBN 0-943158-33-8

3617 Stress Owner's Manual: Meaning, Balance and Health in Your Life
Impact Publishers
PO Box 6016
Atascadero, CA 93423-6016
805-466-5917
800-246-7228
Fax: 805-466-5919
E-mail: info@impactpublishers.com
www.impactpublishers.com

Offers specific solutions: maps, checklists and rating scales to help you assess your life; dozens of stress buffer activities to help you deal with stress on the spot; life-changing strategies to prepare you for a lifetime of effective stress management. *$15.95*

224 pages Year Founded: 2003 ISBN 1-886230-54-4

3618 Therapist's Workbook
Jossey-Bass Publishers
350 Sansome Street
5th Floor
San Francisco, CA 94104
415-394-8677
800-956-7739
Fax: 800-605-2665
www.josseybass.com

This workbook nourishes and challenges counselors, guiding them on a journey of self-reflection and renewal. *$35.00*

192 pages Year Founded: 1999 ISBN 0-787945-23-4

3619 Treating Alcohol Dependence: a Coping Skills Training Guide
Guilford Publications
72 Spring Street
New York, NY 10012
212-431-9800
800-365-7006
Fax: 212-966-6708
E-mail: info@guilford.com
www.guilford.com

Treatment program based on a cognitive-social learning theory of alcohol abuse. Presents a straight-forward treatment strategy that copes with how to stop drinking and provides the training skills to make it possible. *$21.95*

240 pages Year Founded: 1989 ISBN 0-898622-15-8

3620 Uniquity
PO Box 10
Galt, CA 95632-0010
209-745-2111
800-521-7771
Fax: 209-745-4430
E-mail: uniquity@uniquitypsych.com
www.uniquitypsych.com

Reuven E Epstein, Owner

Mail order and internet supplier of mental health materials, anger tools, play therapy, foster care, adoption, attachment, group therapy, child abuse and more.

Directories & Databases

3621 AAHP/Dorland Directory of Health Plans
Dorland Healthcare Information
1500 Walnut Street
Suite 1000
Philadelphia, PA 19102
215-875-1212
800-784-2332
Fax: 215-735-3966
E-mail: info@dorlandhealth.com
www.dorlandhealth.com

Paperback, published yearly. *$215.00*

3622 American Academy of Child and Adolescent Psychiatry - Membership Directory
3615 Wisconsin Avenue NW
Washington, DC 20016-3007
202-966-7300
800-333-7636
Fax: 202-966-2891
E-mail: communications@aacap.org
www.aacap.org

Robert Hendren, President
David Herzog, Secretary
William Bernet, Treasurer

$30.00

179 pages 2 per year

3623 American Academy of Psychoanalysis and Dynam ic Psychiatry
American Academy of Psychoanalysis and Dynamic Psychiatry
One Regency Drive
PO Box 30
Bloomfield, CT 06002

888-691-8281
Fax: 860-286-0787
E-mail: info@aapdp.org
www.aapsa.org

Jacquelyn T Coleman CAE, Executive Director
Sherry Katz-Bearnot, President
Carol Filiaci, Secretary

The journal of the American Academy of Psychoanalysis and Dynamic Psychiatry. Publishes articles by members and other authors who have a significant contribution to make to the community of scholars or practitioners interested in a psychodynamic understanding of human behavior. *$50.00*

70 pages

3624 American Network of Community Options and Resources-Directory of Members
ANCOR
1101 King Street
Suite 380
Alexandria, VA 22314
703-535-7850
Fax: 703-535-7860
E-mail: ancor@ancor.org
www.ancor.org

Covers 650 agencies serving people with mental retardation and other developmental disabilities. *$25.00*

179 pages 1 per year

3625 American Psychiatric Association-Membership Directory
Harris Publishing
2500 Westchester Avenue
Suite 400
Purchase, NY 10577
800-326-6600
Fax: 914-641-3501
www.bcharrispub.com

$59.95

816 pages

3626 American Psychoanalytic Association - Roster
American Psychological Association
750 1st Street NE
Washington, DC 20002-4241
202-336-5500
800-374-2721
Fax: 202-336-5568
E-mail: webmaster@apa.org
www.apa.org

$40.00

194 pages

3627 American Society of Psychoanalytic Physicians: Membership Directory
13528 Wisteria Drive
Germantown, MD 20874
301-540-3197
Fax: 301-540-3511
E-mail: cfcotter@aspp.net
www.aspp.net

Christine Cotter, Executive Director

Directory of member psychoanalysts and psychoanalytically oriented phychiatrists and physicians and others interested in the field.

15 pages 1 per year

3628 Association for Advancement of Behavior Therapy: Membership Directory
305 Seventh Avenue
16th Floor
New York, NY 10001-6008
212-647-1890
Fax: 212-647-1890
E-mail: mebrown@aabt.org
www.aabt.org

Mary Jane Eimer, Executive Director
Mary Ellen Brown, Administration/Convention
Rosemary Park, Membership Services

Covers over 4,500 psychologists, psychiatrists, social workers and other interested in behavior therapy. *$50.00*

240 pages 2 per year

3629 At Health Incorporated
1370 116th Avenue NE, Suite 206
Eastview Professional Building
Bellevue, WA 98004-3825
425-451-4399
888-284-3258
Fax: 425-451-7399
E-mail: support@athealth.com
www.athealth.com

John E Cebhart III, CEO
John L Miller MD, CMIO

Mental health information, directory of mental health practitioners and treatment facilities, and online continuing education for mental health professionals and other healthcare providers.

3630 Behavioral Measurement Database Services
PO Box 110287
Pittsburgh, PA 15232-0787
412-687-6850
Fax: 412-687-5213
E-mail: bmds@aol.com

Service health and psychosocial instruments, a database of over 75,000 records on measurement instruments enriching the health and psychosocial sciences. Records include questionnaires, interview schedules, vignettes/scenarios, coding schemes, and other scales, checklists, indexes, and tests in medicine, nursing, public health, psychology, social work, sociology, and communicaiton. Also provides copies of selected instruments cited in the HAPI database through its instrument delivery service. Contact Ovid Technologies 1-800-950-2035

3631 CARF Directory of Organizations with Accredited Programs
Rehabilitation Accreditation Commission
4891 E Grant Road
Tucson, AZ 85712
520-325-1044
Fax: 520-318-1129
TTY: 888-281-6531
www.carf.org

Brian J. Boom, President/CEO
Amanda Birch, Administrator Of Operations

Covers about three thousand organizations in seven thousand locations offering more than eighteen hundred medical rehabilitation, behavioral health, and employment and community support services that have been accredited by CARF. *$100.00*

200 pages 1 per year Year Founded: 1999

3632 Case Management Resource Guide
Dorland Healthcare Information
1500 Walnut Street
Suite 1000
Philadelphia, PA 19102
215-875-1212
800-784-2332
Fax: 215-735-3966
E-mail: info@dorlandhealth.com
www.dorlandhealth.com

Extensive directory of healthcare services used by case managers, discharge planners, managed care contracting staff, sales and marketing professionsal, search firms and information and referral agencies. $175 for four-volume set or $49 for each regional edition.

1 per year

3633 Case Management Resource Guide (Health Care)
Dorland Healthcare Information
1500 Walnut Street
Suite 1000
Philadelphia, PA 19102
215-875-1212
800-784-2332
Fax: 215-735-3966
E-mail: info@dorlandhealth.com
www.dorlandhealth.com

In four volumes, over 110,000 health care facilities and support services are listed, including homecare, rehabilitation, psychiatric and addiction treatment programs, hospices, adult day care and burn and cancer centers.

5,200 pages 1 per year ISBN 1-880874-84-9

3634 Case Manager Database
Dorland Healthcare Information
1500 Walnut Street
Suite 1000
Philadelphia, PA 19102
215-875-1212
800-784-2332
Fax: 215-735-3966
E-mail: info@dorlandhealth.com
www.dorlandhealth.com

Largest database of information on case managers in US, especially of case managers who work for health plans and health insurers. Covers over 15,000 case managers and includes detailed data such as work setting and clinical specialty, which can be used to carefully target marketing communications. $2500 for full database, other prices available.

3635 Community Mental Health Directory
Department of Community Health
320 S Walnut
Suite 6
Lansing, MI 48913-0001
517-373-3740
Fax: 517-335-3090
www.mdch.state.mi.us

Covers about 51 public community mental health services and programs in Michigan.

20 pages 2 per year

3636 Complete Directory for People with Disabilities
Grey House Publishing
185 Millerton Road
PO Box 860
Millerton, NY 12546
518-789-8700
800-562-2139
Fax: 518-789-0545
E-mail: books@greyhouse.com
www.www.greyhouse.com

Leslie Mackenzie, Publisher
Laura Mars-Proietti, Editor

This one-stop annual resource provides immediate access to the latest products and services available for people with disabilities, such as Periodicals & Books, Assistive Devices, Employment & Education Programs, Camps and Travel Groups. *$165.00*

1200 pages ISBN 1-592370-07-1

3637 Complete Learning Disabilities Directory
Grey House Publishing
185 Millerton Road
PO Box 860
Millerton, NY 12546
518-789-8700
800-562-2139
Fax: 518-789-0545
E-mail: books@greyhouse.com
www.www.greyhouse.com

Leslie Mackenzie, Publisher
Laura Mars-Proietti, Editor

This annual resource includes information about Associations & Organizations, Schools, Colleges & Testing Materials, Government Agencies, Legal Resources and much more. *$195.00*

745 pages ISBN 1-930956-79-7

3638 Complete Mental Health Directory
Grey House Publishing
185 Millerton Road
PO Box 860
Millerton, NY 12546
518-789-8700
800-562-2139
Fax: 518-789-0545
E-mail: books@greyhouse.com
www.www.greyhouse.com

Leslie Mackenzie, Publisher
Laura Mars-Proietti, Editor

This bi-annual directory offers understandable descriptions of 25 Mental Health Disorders as well as detailed information on Associations, Media, Support Groups and Mental Health Facilities. *$165.00*

800 pages ISBN 1-592370-46-2

3639 **DSM-IV Psychotic Disorders: New Diagnostic Issue**
American Psychiatric Publishing
1000 Wilson Boulevard
Suite 1825
Arlington, VA 22209-3901
703-907-7322
800-368-5777
Fax: 703-907-1091
E-mail: appi@psych.org
www.appi.org

Nancy Andreasen, Moderator
Katie Duffy, Marketing Assistant

Updates on clinical findings. *$39.95*
Year Founded: 1995

3640 **Detwiler's Directory of Health and Medical Resources**
Dorland Healthcare Information
1500 Walnut Street
Suite 1000
Philadelphia, PA 19102
215-875-1212
800-784-2332
Fax: 215-735-3966
E-mail: info@dorlandhealth.com
www.dorlandhealth.com

An invaluable guide to healthcare information sources. This directory lists information on over 2,000 sources of information on the medical and healthcare industry. *$195.00*
1 per year Year Founded: 1999 ISBN 1-880874-57-1

3641 **Directory for People with Chronic Illness**
Grey House Publishing
185 Millerton Road
Millerton, NY 12546
518-789-8700
800-562-2139
Fax: 518-789-0545
E-mail: books@greyhouse.com
www.www.greyhouse.com

Leslie MacKenzie, Publisher
Laura Mars-Proietti, Editor

This bi-annual resource provides a comprehensive overview of the support services and information resources available for people diagnosed with a chronic illness. Includes 12,000 entries. *$165.00*
1200 pages ISBN 1-592370-81-0

3642 **Directory of Developmental Disabilities Services**
Nebraska Health and Human Services System
PO Box 94728
Department of Services
Lincoln, NE 68509-4728
402-471-2851
800-833-7352
Fax: 402-479-5094

Covers agencies and organizations that provide developmental disability services and programs in Nebraska.
28 pages

3643 **Directory of Health Care Professionals**
Dorland Healthcare Information
1500 Walnut Street
Suite 1000
Philadelphia, PA 19102
215-875-1212
800-784-2332
Fax: 215-735-3966
E-mail: info@dorlandhealth.com
www.dorlandhealth.com

Helps you easily locate the key personnel and facilities you want by hospital name, system head-quarters, or job title. Valuable for locating industry professionals, recruiting, networking, and prospecting for industry business. *$299.00*
1 per year Year Founded: 1998 ISBN 1-573721-40-9

3644 **Directory of Hospital Personnel**
Grey House Publishing
185 Millerton Road
PO Box 860
Millerton, NY 12546
518-789-8700
800-562-2139
Fax: 518-789-0545
E-mail: books@greyhouse.com
www.greyhouse.com

Leslie MacKenzie, Publisher
Laura Mars-Proietti, Editor

Best annual resource for researching or marketing a product or service to the hospital industry. Includes 6,000 hospitals and over 80,000 key contacts. *$275.00*
2400 pages ISBN 1-592370-26-8

3645 **Directory of Physician Groups & Networks**
Dorland Healthcare Information
1500 Walnut Street
Suite 1000
Philadelphia, PA 19102
215-875-1212
800-784-2332
Fax: 215-735-3966
E-mail: info@dorlandhealth.com
www.dorlandhealth.com

This directory offers the most comprehensive and current data on these fast-changing organizations. Includes valuable lists and rankings such as the top 200 group practices, plus, five industry experts provide exclusive reviews of current dynamics and trends in the physician marketplace. *$349.00*

3646 **Directory of Physician Groups and Networks**
Dorland Healthcare Information
1500 Walnut Street
Suite 1000
Philadelphia, PA 19102
215-875-1212
800-784-2332
Fax: 215-735-3966
E-mail: info@dorlandhealth.com
www.dorlandhealth.com

Reference tool with over 4,000 entries covering IPAs, PHOs, large medical group practices with 20 or more physicians, MSOs and PPMCs. Paperback, published yearly. *$345.00*
Year Founded: 1998 ISBN 1-880874-50-4

3647 Dorland's Medical Directory
Dorland Healthcare Information
1500 Walnut Street
Suite 1000
Philadelphia, PA 19102
215-875-1212
800-784-2332
Fax: 215-735-3966
E-mail: info@dorlandhealth.com
www.dorlandhealth.com

Contains expanded coverage of healthcare facilities with profiles of 616 group practices, 661 hospitals and 750 rehabilitation, subacute, hospice and long term care facilities. *$699.00*

1 per year ISBN 1-880874-82-2

3648 Drug Information Handbook for Psychiatry
Lexi-Comp
1100 Terex Road
Hudson, OH 44236-3771
330-650-6506
800-837-5394
Fax: 330-656-4307
www.lexi.com

Katie Seabeck, Marketing

Written specifically for mental health professionals. Addresses the fact that mental health patients may be taking additional medication for the treatment of another medical condition in combination with their psychtropic agents. With that in mind, this book contains information on all drugs, not just the psychotropic agents. Specific fields of information contained within the drug monograph include Effects on Mental Status and Effects on Psychiatric Treatment. *$38.75*

1 per year ISBN 1-591951-14-3

3649 HMO & PPO Database & Directory
Dorland Healthcare Information
1500 Walnut Street
Suite 1000
Philadelphia, PA 19102
215-875-1212
800-784-2332
Fax: 215-735-3966
E-mail: info@dorlandhealth.com
www.dorlandhealth.com

Delivers comprehensive and current information on senior-level individuals at virtually all US HMOs and PPOs at an affordable price. *$400.00*

3650 HMO/PPO Directory
Grey House Publishing
185 Millerton Road
PO Box 860
Millerton, NY 12546
518-789-8700
800-562-2139
Fax: 518-789-0545
E-mail: books@greyhouse.com
www.greyhouse.com

Leslie MacKenzie, Publisher
Laura Mars-Proetti, Editor

This annual resource provides detailed information about health maintenance organizations and preferred provider organizations nationwide. *$275.00*

500 pages ISBN 1-592370-22-5

3651 Innovations in Clinical Practice: Source Book - Volumes 4-20
Professional Resource Press
PO Box 15560
Sarasota, FL 34277-1560
941-343-9601
800-443-3364
Fax: 941-343-9201
E-mail: orders@prpress.com
www.prpress.com

Debra Fink, Managing Editor

Provides a comprehensive source of practical information and applied techniques that can be put to immediate use in your practice. *$64.95*

524 pages Year Founded: 1999

3652 Medi-Pages On-Line Directory
Medi-Pages
719 Main Street
Niagara Falls, NY 14301-1703
716-284-4277
800-554-6661
Fax: 716-284-4401
E-mail: marilyn@medipages.com
www.medipages.com

Marilyn Gould, Executive Assistant

On-line service covers more than 1.5 million listings of hospitals, nursing homes, clinics, home healthcare providers, HMOs, PPOs, CPOs, health associations, professional associations, federal government agencies, international health organizations, medical libraries, hospital management companies, case managers, HFCA offices, AT&T numbers as well as an online medical product locater.

3653 Medical & Healthcare Marketplace Guide Directory
Dorland Healthcare Information
1500 Walnut Street
Suite 1000
Philadelphia, PA 19102
215-875-1212
800-784-2332
Fax: 215-735-3966
E-mail: info@dorlandhealth.com
www.dorlandhealth.com

Contains valuable data on pharmaceutical, medical advice, and clinical and non-clinical healthcare service companies worldwide. *$499.00*

3654 Mental Health Directory
Office of Consumer, Family & Public Information
5600 Fishers Lane, Room 15-99
Center For Mental Health Services
Rockville, MD 20857-0002
301-443-2792
Fax: 301-443-5163

Covers hospitals, treatment centers, outpatient clinics, day/night facilities, residential treatment centers for emotionally disturbed children, residential supportive programs such as halfway houses, and mental health centers offering mental health assistance. *$23.00*

468 pages

3655 **National Association of Psychiatric Health Systems: Membership Directory**
325 Seventh Street NW
Suite 625
Washington, DC 20004-2802
202-393-6700
Fax: 202-783-6041
E-mail: naphs@naphs.org
www.naphs.org

Mark Covall, Executive Director
Carole Szpak, Director Communications

Contact information of professional groups working to co-ordinate a full spectrum of treatment services, including in-patient, residential, partial hospitalization and outpatient programs as well as prevention and management services. *$32.10*

48 pages 1 per year Year Founded: 1933

3656 **National Directory of Medical Psychotherapists and Psychodiagnosticians**
345 24th Avenue N
Park Plaza Medical Building Suite 201
Nashville, TN 37203-1595
615-327-2984
Fax: 615-327-9235
E-mail: americanbd@aol.com

Includes the following: Disability Analysis in Practice: Fundamental Framework for an Interdisciplinary Science, and The Disability Handbook: Tools for Independent Practice. *$45.00*

240 pages 1 per year

3657 **National Register of Health Service Providers in Psychology**
1120 G Street NW
Suite 330
Washington, DC 20005
202-783-7663
Fax: 202-347-0550
www.nationalregister.org

Morgan Sammons, President/Chair
Greg Hurley, Vice President/Vice-Chair

Psychologists who are licensed or certified by a state/pro-vincial board of examiners of psychology and who have met council criteria as health service providers in psychol-ogy.

Year Founded: 1974

3658 **National Registry of Psychoanalysts**
National Association for the Advancement of Psychoanalysis
80 8th Avenue
Suite 1501
New York, NY 10011-5126
212-741-0515
Fax: 212-366-4347
E-mail: dfmaxwell@mac.com
www.naap.org

Mary Quackenburh, Executive Director
Douglas Maxwell, President

NAAP provides information to the public on psychoanaly-sis. Publishes quarterly NAAP News, annual Registry of Psychoanalysts. *$ 15.00*

175 pages

3659 **Patient Guide to Mental Health Issues: Desk Chart**
Lexi-Comp
1100 Terex Road
Hudson, OH 44236-3771
330-650-6506
800-837-5394
Fax: 330-656-4307
www.lexi.com

Katie Seabeck, Marketing

Designed specifically for healthcare professionals dealing with mental health patients. Combines eight of our popular Patient Chart titles into one, convienient desktop presenta-tion. This will assist in explaining the most common mental health issue to your patients on a level that they will under-stand. *$38.75*

1 per year ISBN 1-591950-54-6

3660 **PsycINFO Database**
PsycINFO, American Psychological Association
750 1st Street NE
Washington, DC 20002-4242
202-336-5650
800-374-2722
Fax: 202-336-5633
TDD: 202-336-6123
E-mail: psycinfo@apa.org
www.apa.org/psychinfo

PsycINFO is a database that contains citations and summa-ries of journal articles, book chapters, books, dissertations and technical reports in the field of psychology and the psy-chological aspects of related disciplines, such as medicine, psychiatry, nursing, sociology, education, pharmacology, physiology, linguistics, anthropology, business and law. Journal coverage, spanning 1887 to present, includes inter-national material from 1,800 periodicals written in over 30 languages. Current chapter and book coverage includes worldwide English language material published from 1987 to present. Over 75,000 references are added annually through weekly updates.

52 per year

3661 **Rating Scales in Mental Health**
Lexi-Comp
1100 Terex Road
Hudson, OH 44236-3771
330-650-6506
800-837-5394
Fax: 330-656-4307
www.lexi.com

Ideal for clinicians as well as administrators, this title pro-vides an overview of over 100 recommended rating scales for mental health assessment. This book is also a great tool to assist mental healthcare professionals determine the ap-propriate psychiatric rating scale when assessing their cli-ents. *$38.75*

1 per year ISBN 1-591950-52-X

3662 **Roster: Centers for the Developmentally Disabled**
Nebraska Health and Human Services
301 Centennial Mall S
Lincoln, NE 68509-5007
402-471-4363
Fax: 402-471-0555

TDD: 070-119-99
www.2.hhs.state.ne.us/

Joann Erickson RN, Program Manager

Covers approximately 160 licensed facilities in Nebraska
for the developmentally disabled.

40 pages 1 per year

3663 Roster: Health Clinics
Nebraska Health and Human Services
301 Centennial Mall S
Lincoln, NE 68509
402-471-4363
Fax: 402-471-0555
www.2.hhs.state.ne.us/

Joann Erickson RN, Section Administrator

Covers approximately 90 licensed health clinic facilities in
Nebraska.

11 pages 1 per year

3664 Roster: Substance Abuse Treatment Centers
Nebraska Health and Human Services
301 Centennial Mall S
Lincoln, NE 68509-5007
402-471-4363
Fax: 402-471-0555
www.2.hhs.state.ne.us/

Joann Erickson RN, Program Manager

Covers approximately 56 licensed substance abuse treatment centers in Nebraska.

12 pages 1 per year

Publishers

Books

3665 Active Parenting Publishers

1955 Vaughn Road NW
Suite 108
Kennesaw, GA 30144-7808
770-429-0565
800-825-0060
Fax: 770-429-0334
E-mail: cservice@activeparenting.com
www.activeparenting.com

Delivers quality education programs for parents, children and teachers to schools, hospitals, social service organizations, churches and corporate market. Innovator in the educational market.

3666 American Psychiatric Publishing (APPI)

1000 Wilson Boulevard
Suite 1825
Arlington, VA 22209
703-907-7322
800-368-5777
Fax: 703-907-1091
E-mail: appi@psych.org
www.appi.org

Ron McMillen, CEO
Joan Lang, Treasurer

Publisher of books, journals, and multi-media on psychiatry, mental healths and behavioral science. Offers authoratative, up-to-date and affordable information geared toward psychiatrists, other mental health professionals, psychiatric residents, medical students and the general public.

3667 Analytic Press

10 Industrial Avenue
Mahwah, NJ 07430
201-258-2200
Fax: 201-760-3735
www.analyticpress.com

Publishes works of substance and originality that constitute genuine contributions to their respective disciplines and professions.

3668 Baker and Taylor

2550 West Tyvola Road
Suite 300
Charlotte, NC 28217
704-998-3100
800-775-1800
www.btol.com

Richard Willis, Chairman/President/CEO
Robert Agres, Executive VP/CFO

Provides quality information and entertainment services. Worldwide distributor of books, videos, music and games in all disciplines.

3669 Brookes Publishing

PO Box 10624
Baltimore, MD 21285-0624
410-337-9580
800-638-3775
Fax: 410-337-8539

E-mail: custserv@brookespublishing.com
www.brookespublishing.com

Paul H Brookes, President
Melissa A Behm, Vice President

Publishes highly respected resources in early childhood, early interventions, inclusive and special education, developmental disabilities, learning disabilities, communication and language, behavior, and mental health

3670 Brookline Books/Lumen Editions

34 University Road
Brookline, MA 02445
617-734-6772
Fax: 617-734-3952
www.brooklinebooks.com

Publishes books on learning disabilities, study skills, self-advocacy for the disabled, early childhood intervention, and more, in readable language that reaches beyond the academic community.

3671 Brunner-Routledge Mental Health

270 Madison Avenue
New York, NY 10016
800-634-7064
www.routledgementalhealth.com

The Routledge imprint publishes books and journals on clinical psychology, psychiatry, psychoanalysis, analytical psychology, psychotherapy, counseling, mental health and other professional subjects.

3672 Bull Publishing Company
Bull Publishing Company

PO Box 1377
Boulder, CO 80306
800-676-2855
Fax: 303-545-6354
E-mail: jim.bullpubco@comcast.net
www.bullpub.com

Jim Bull, Publisher

Publisher of books focused on addressing the growing need for sound health information and good advice.

3673 Cambridge University Press

40 West 20th Street
New York, NY 10011-4221
212-924-3900
Fax: 212-691-3239
www.cambridge.org/americas

Printing and publishing house that is an integral part of the University and has similar charitable objectives in advancing knowledge, education, learning and research.

3674 Charles C Thomas Publishers

2600 South First Street
PO Box 19265
Springfield, IL 62704-9265
217-789-8980
800-258-8980
Fax: 217-789-9130
E-mail: books@ccthomas.com
www.ccthomas.com

Producing a strong list of specialty titles and textbooks in the biomedical sciences. Also very active in producing books for the behavioral sciences, education and special education, speech language and hearing, as well as rehabilitation and long-term care. One of the largest producers of books in all areas of criminal justice and law enforcement.

3675 Crossroad Publishing
481 Eighth Avenue
Suite 1550
New York, NY 10001
212-868-1801
Fax: 212-868-2171
E-mail: ask@crossroadspublishing.com
www.cpcbooks.com

Publishes words of thoughtfulness and hope. A leading independent publishing house.

3676 EBSCO Publishing
10 Estes Street
Ipswich, MA 01938
978-356-6500
800-653-2726
Fax: 978-356-6565
www.epnet.com

Robert Preston, Medical Inside Sales Manager
Daniel Boutchie, Inside Sales Representative
Jeffery Greaves, Inside Sales Representative

EBSCO Publishing offers electronic access to a variety of health data: full text databases containing aggregate journals, access to publishers' electronic journals, and the citational databases produced by the American Psychiatric Association to name just a few. Offers a free, nonobligation, on-line trial.

3677 Family Experiences Productions
PO Box 5879
Austin, TX 78763
512-494-0338
Fax: 512-494-0340
E-mail: info@fepi.com
www.fepi.com

R Geyer, Executive Producer

Consumers Health videos; available individually, or in large volume (private branded) for health providers to give to patients, professionals, staff. Postpartum Emotions, Parenting Preschoolers, Facing Death (5-tape series) and teen grief English and Spanish.

ISSN 1-930772-00-9

3678 Fanlight Productions
4196 Washington Street
Boston, MA 02131
617-469-4999
800-937-4113
Fax: 617-469-3379
E-mail: info@fanlight.com
www.fanlight.com

Distributor of innovative film and video works on the social issues of our time, with a special focus on healthcare, mental health, profesional ethics, aging and gerontology, disabilites, the workplace, and gender and family issues.

3679 Franklin Electronic Publishers
Frankling Electronic Publishers
1 Franklin Plaza
Burlington, NJ 08016
609-239-4333
800-266-5626

Fax: 609-387-1787
www.franklin.com

Publishes materials for healthcare.

3680 Free Spirit Publishing
217 Fifth Avenue North
Suite 200
Minneapolis, MN 55401-1299
612-338-2068
866-703-7322
Fax: 612-337-5050
www.freespirit.com

Publisher of learning tools that support young people's social and emotional health. Known for unique understanding of what young adults want and need to know to navigate life successfully.

3681 Greenwood Publishing Group
88 Post Road West
Westport, CT 06881
203-226-3571
E-mail: webmaster@greenwood.com
www.greenwood.com

Publisher of reference titles, academic and general interest books, texts, books for librarians and other profesionals, and electronic resources.

3682 Guilford Publications
72 Spring Street
New York, NY 10012
212-431-9800
800-365-7006
Fax: 212-966-6708
E-mail: info@guilford.com
www.guilford.com

Seymour Weingarten, Editor-In-Chief

Publisher of books, periodicals, software and audiovisual programs in mental health, education, and the social sciences.

Year Founded: 1973

3683 Gurze Books
PO Box 2238
Carisbad, CA 92015
760-434-7533
800-756-7533
Fax: 760-434-5476
E-mail: mylo@gurze.net
www.gurze.com

Publishing company that specializes in resources and education on eating disorders. Offers high quality materials on understanding and overcoming eating disorders of all kinds.

3684 Harper Collins Publishers
10 East 53rd Street
New York, NY 10022
212-207-7000
www.harpercollins.com

A subsidiary of News Corporation, Harper Collins produces literary and commercial fiction, business books, children's books, cookbooks, mystery, romance, reference, religious, healthcare and spiritual books.

3685 Harvard University Press
79 Garden Street
Cambridge, MA 02138

401-531-2800
800-405-1619
Fax: 800-531-2800
E-mail: contact_hup@harvard.edu
www.hup.harvard.edu

Publishes material on varied topics including healthcare.

3686 Haworth Press
10 Alice Street
Binghamton, NY 13904
607-722-5857
800-429-6784
Fax: 800-895-0582
E-mail: getinfo@haworthpress.com
www.haworthpress.com

Publishers of library science, social work and human services, gerontology and aging, marketing, gay/lesbian/bisexual studies, and additional subject fields.

3687 Hazelden
CO3 PO Box 11
Center City, MN 55012-0011
651-213-4200
800-257-7810
Fax: 651-213-4590
E-mail: info@hazelden.org
www.hazelden.org

A nonprofit organization that helps people transform their lives by providing the highest quality treatment and continuing care services, education, research, and publishing products available today.

3688 Health Communications
3201 sW 15th Street
Deerfield Beach, FL 33442
954-360-0909
800-441-5569
Fax: 954-360-0034
www.hci-online.com

Original publisher of informational pamphlets for the recovery community; publishes inspiration, soul/spirituality, relationships, recovery/healing, women's issues and self-help material.

3689 High Tide Press
3650 W 183rd Street
Homewood, IL 60430
708-206-2054
800-469-9461
Fax: 708-206-2044
www.hightidepress.com

Art Dykstra, Executive Director
Steve Baker, Director

Provides high quality books, training materials and seminars to people working in the field of human services. Seek to provide the best resources in developmental, mental and learning disabilities, as well as psychology, leadership and management.

3690 Hogrefe & Huber Publishers
218 Main Street
Suite 485
Kirkland, WA 98033
866-823-4726
Fax: 617-354-6875

E-mail: info@hhpub.com
www.hhpub.com

Publisher of journals and books of all different variety titles including healthcare.

3691 Hope Press
800-321-4039
Fax: 626-358-3520
E-mail: dcomings@mail.earthlink.net
www.hopepress.com

Specializes in the publication of books on Tourette Syndrome, Attention Deficit Hyperactivity Disorder (ADHD, ADD), Conduct Disorder, Oppositional Defiant Disorder and other psychological, psychiatric and behavioral problems.

3692 Hyperion Books
77 West 66th Street
11th Floor
New York, NY 10023
Fax: 212-456-1980
www.hyperionbooks.com

Publishes general-interest fiction and nonfiction books for adults including healthcare titles. Includes the Miramax, ESPN Books, ABC Daytime Press, Hyperion East and Hyperion Audiobooks.

3693 Impact Publishers
PO Box 6016
Atascadero, CA 93423-6016
E-mail: info@impactpublishers.com
www.impactpublishers.com

Produces a select list of psychology and self improvement books and audio-tapes for adults, children, families, organizations, and communities. Written by highly respected psychologists and other human service professionals.

3694 Jason Aronson Publishers
4501 Forbes Blvd
Suite 200
Lanham, MD 20706
301-459-3366
800-462-6420
Fax: 301-429-5748
www.aronson.com

Publisher of highly regarded books in psychotherapy. Dedicated to publishing professional, scholarly works by respected and gifted authors.

3695 Jerome M Sattler Publisher
PO Box 3557
La Mesa, CA 91944-3557
619-460-3667
Fax: 619-460-2489
E-mail: sattlerpublisher@sbcglobal.net
www.sattlerpublisher.com

Publishes books that represent the cutting edge of clinical assessment of children and families. Designed for students in training as well as for practitioners ans clinicians.

3696 Jessica Kingsley Publishers
116 Pentonville Road
London
N1 9JB,
E-mail: post@jkp.com
www.jkp.com

Wholly independent company, committed to publishing books for professional and general readers in a range of subjects including the autism spectrum, social work, and the arts therapies. Recent titles include mental health, counseling, palliative care, and practical theology.

3697 John Wiley & Sons
111 River Street
Hoboken, NJ 07030-5774
201-748-6000
Fax: 201-748-6088
E-mail: custserv@wiley.com
www.wiley.com

A global publisher of print and electronic products, specializing in scientific, technical, and medical books and journals professional and consumer books and subscription services; also textbooks and other educational materials for undergraduate and graduate students as well as lifelong learners.

3698 Johns Hopkins University Press
2715 North Charles Street
Baltimore, MD 21218
410-516-6900
E-mail: webmaster@jhupress.jhu.edu
www.press.jhu.edu/index.html

Publishes 58 scholarly periodicals and more than 200 new books each year. A leading online provider of scholarly journals, bringing more than 250 periodicals to the desktops of 9 million students, scholars, and others worldwide.

3699 Jossey-Bass
111 River Street
Hoboken, NJ 07030-5774
201-748-6000
Fax: 201-748-6088
E-mail: custserv@wiley.com
www.wiley.com

Jossey-Bass publishes books, periodicals, and other media to inform and inspire those interested in developing themselves, their organizations and their communities. The publications feature the work of some of the world's best-known authors in leadership, business, education, religion and spirituality, parenting, nonprofit, public health and health administration, conflict resolution and relationships.

3700 Lawrence Erlbaum Associates
10 Industrial Avenue
Mahwah, NJ 07430-2262
201-258-2200
800-926-6579
Fax: 201-236-0072
www.erlbaum.com

An international academic publisher and distributor of a full range of books, journals, and software, as well as electronic media. Dedicated to providing quality scholarship and knowledge that will contribute to each representative field, including healthcare, and offer promising new direction for teachers, researchers, and practitioners.

3701 Lexington Books
4501 Forbes Blvd
Suite 200
Lanham, MD 20706
301-459-3366
800-462-6420

Fax: 301-429-5748
www.lexingtonbooks.com

John Sisk, Publisher

Publisher of specialized new work by established and emerging scholars, including material for the healthcare community.

3702 Lippincott Williams & Wilkins
530 Walnut Street
Philadelphia, PA 19106-3621
215-521-8300
Fax: 215-521-8902
www.lww.com

Publishes specialized publications and software for physicians, nurses, students and specialized clinicians. Products include drug guides, medical journals, nursing journals, medical textbooks and medical pda software.

3703 Love Publishing
9101 East Kenyon Avenue
Suite 2200
Denver, CO 80237
303-221-7333
Fax: 303-221-7444
E-mail: lpc@lovepublishing.com
www.lovepublishing.com

Publishes books that offer therapy options to children of all ages, adults, and adolescents.

3704 Mason Crest Publishers
370 Reed Road
Suite 302
Broomall, PA 19008
866-627-2665
Fax: 610-543-3878
www.masoncrest.com

Publishes core-related materials for grades K-12. Current catalog includes many titles for health care and mental health curriculums.

3705 Nelson Thornes
Delta Place
27 Berth Road
Cheltenham Glos GL53 7TH, UK
124-226-7100
www.nelsonthornes.com

Leading educational publisher of books, CD-Rom and electronic teaching and learning resources, formed through the merger of two UK publishing businesses — Thomas Nelson and Stanley Thornes.

3706 New Harbinger Publications
5674 Shattuck Avenue
Oakland, CA 94609
800-748-6273
Fax: 510-652-5472
www.newharbinger.com

Matt McKay, Co-Founder
Patrick Fanning, Co-Founder

Publisher of self-help books that teach the reader skills they could use to significantly improve the quality of their lives.

Year Founded: 1973

3707 New World Library
14 Pamaron Way
Nopvato, CA 94949
415-884-2100
800-972-6657
Fax: 415-884-2199
www.newworldlibrary.com

Publishes books and audios that inspire and challenge us to improve the quality of our lives and our world.

3708 New York University Press
838 Broadway
3rd Floor
New York, NY 10003-4812
212-998-2575
800-996-6987
Fax: 212-995-3833
E-mail: information@nyupress.org
www.nyupress.nyu.edu

Steve Maikowski, Director
Eric Zinner, Editor-In-Chief

Publishes approximately 100 new books each year, and enjoys a backlist of over 1500 titles that includes health care and academic materials.

3709 Omnigraphics
615 Griswold
PO Box 624
Detroit, MI 48226
800-234-1340
Fax: 800-875-1340
E-mail: info@omnigraphics.com
www.omnigraphics.com

Fred Ruffner, Co-Founder
Peter Ruffner, Co-Founder

Quality reference resources for libraries and schools.
Year Founded: 1985

3710 Oxford University Press
2001 Evans Road
Cary, NC 27513
919-677-0977
800-445-9714
Fax: 919-677-1303
E-mail: custserv.us@oup.com
www.oup.com

Publishes works that further Oxford University's objective of excellence in research, scholarship, and education, including titles in the health care and mental health field.

3711 Penguin Group
345 Hudson Street
New York, NY 10014
212-741-0100
Fax: 212-463-9814
www.us.penguingroup.com

Publishes under a wide range of prominent imprints and trademarks, among them Berkeley Books, Dutton, Grosset & Dunlap, New American Library, Penguin, Philomel, G.P. Putnam's Sons, Riverhead Books, Viking and Frederick Warne. Includes a variety of titles in health care and mental health subjects.

3712 Perseus Books Group
1094 Flex Drive
Jackson, TN 38301

800-371-1669
Fax: 800-453-2884
E-mail: perseus.orders@perseusbooks.com
www.perseusbooksgroup.com

Titles include science, public issues, military history, modern maternity, health care and mental health.

3713 Princeton University Press
41 William Street
Princeton, NJ 08540-5237
609-258-4900
Fax: 609-258-6305
www.pup.princeton.edu

Independent publisher with close connection to Princeton Unviersity. Fundamental mission is to disseminate through books, journals, and electronic media, with both academia and society at large on a variety of social issues, including health care and mental health.

3714 Pro-Ed Publications
8700 Shoal Creek Blvd
Austin, TX 78757-6897
800-897-3202
Fax: 800-397-7633
E-mail: feedback@proedinc.com
www.proedinc.com

Leading publisher of nationally standardized tests, resource and reference texts, curricular and therapy materials, and professional journals covering: speech, language and hearing; psychology and counseling; special education including developmental disabilities, rehabilitation, and gifted education; early childhood intervention; and occupational and physical therapy.

3715 Professional Resource Press
Professional Resource Press
PO Box 15560
Sarasota, FL 34277-1560
941-343-9601
800-443-3364
Fax: 941-343-9201
E-mail: orders@prpress.com
www.prpress.com

Debra Fink, Managing Editor

Publisher of books, continuing education programs and other applied resources for mental health professionals, including psychologists, psychiatrists, clinical social workers, counselors, OTs, and recreational therapists.

3716 Rapid Psychler Press
3560 Pine Grove Avenue
Suite 374
Port Huron, MI 48060
888-779-2453
Fax: 888-779-2457
E-mail: rapid@psychler.com
www.psychler.com

Produces textbooks and presentation graphics for use in mental health education (mainly psychiatry). Products are thoroughly researched and clinically oriented. Designed by students, instructors and clinicians.

3717 Research Press Publishers
Department 26W
PO Box 9177
Champaign, IL 61826

217-352-3273
800-519-2707
Fax: 217-352-1221
E-mail: rp@researchpress.com
www.researchpress.com

Publishes books and videos in school counseling, special education, psychology, counseling and therapy, parenting, death and dying, and developmental disabilities.

3718 Riverside Publishing

425 Spring Lake Drive
Itasca, IL 60143-2079
630-467-7000
800-323-9540
Fax: 630-467-7192
www.riverpub.com

Dedicated to providing society with the finest professional testing products and services available. Division of Houghton Mifflin Company.

3719 Sage Publications

2455 Teller Road
Thousand Oaks, CA 91320
800-818-7243
E-mail: info@sagepub.com
www.sagepub.com

An independent international publisher of journals, books, and electronic media, known for commitment to quality and innovation in scholarly, educational and professional markets.

3720 Sidran Institute

200 East Joppa Road
Suite 207
Towson, MD 21286
410-825-8888
Fax: 410-337-0747
E-mail: sidran@sidran.org
www.sidran.org

Leader in traumatic stress education and advocacy. Devoted to helping people who have experienced traumatic life events by publishing books and educational materials on traumatic stress and dissociative conditions.

3721 Simon & Schuster

100 Front Street
Riverside, NJ 08075
Fax: 800-943-9831
www.simonsays.com

Jack Romanos, President/CEO

Leader in the field of general interest publishing, providing consumers worldwide with a diverse range of quality books and multimedia products across a wide variety of genres and formats, including health care and mental health.

3722 Springer Science and Business Media

233 Spring Street
New York, NY 10013
212-460-1500
Fax: 212-460-1575
E-mail: service-ny@springer.com
www.springer-ny.com

Derek Haank, CEO
Martin Mos, COO

Develops, manages and disseminates knowledge through books, journals and the internet in a variety of subjects, including health care and mental health.

3723 St. Martin's Press

175 Sth Avenue
New York, NY 10010
212-677-7456
Fax: 212-674-6132
www.stmartins.com

Publishes 700 titles a year, including those titles in a variety of health care and mental health subjects.

3724 Taylor & Francis Group

325 Chestnut Street
Suite 800
Philadelphia, PA 19106
800-354-1420
Fax: 215-625-8914
E-mail: beverley.acreman@tandf.co.uk
www.taylorandfrancis.com

Publishes more than 1000 journals and 1800 new books each year with a books backlist in excess of 20,000 specialty titles. Providers of quality information and knowledge that enable our customers to perform their jobs efficiently, continue their education, and help contribute to the advancement of their chosen markets.

3725 Therapeutic Resources

PO Box 16814
Cleveland, OH 44116
888-331-7114
Fax: 440-331-7118
E-mail: contact@therapeuticresources.com
www.therapeuticresources.com

Publishers of a variety of titles including ADD/ADHD, Alzheimer/Dimentia, Anger Management, Autism/PDD, Bereavement/Adjustment Disorders, Substance Abuse and more.

3726 Time Warner Bookmark

1271 Avenue of the Americas
New York, NY 10020
800-759-0190
Fax: 800-331-1664

Formerly known as Time Warner Trade Publishing, consists of Warner Books and its various imprints: the Mysterious Press, Warner Vision, Warner Business Books, Aspect, Warner Faith, and Little, Brown and Company. Includes a variety of titles in health care and mental health.

3727 Underwood Books

PO Box 1919
Nevada City, CA 95959
800-788-3123
E-mail: contact@underwoodbooks.com
www.underwoodbooks.com

A publisher specializing in fantasy art, science fiction, and self-help/health related titles.

3728 University of California Press

2120 Berkeley Way
Berkeley, CA 94704-1012
510-642-4247
Fax: 510-643-7127

E-mail: askucp@ucpress.edu
www.ucpress.edu

Distinguished university press that enriches lives around
the world by advancing scholarships in the humanities, social sciences, and natural sciences.

3729 University of Chicago Press

1427 East 60th Street
Chicago, IL 60637
773-702-7700
Fax: 773-702-9756
E-mail: marketing@press.uchicago.edu
www.press.uchicago.edu

Holds an obligation to disseminate scholarship of the highest standard and to publish serious works that promote education, foster public understanding, and enrich cultural life.

3730 University of Minnesota Press

111 Third Avenue South
Suite 290
Minneapolis, MN 55401
612-627-1970
Fax: 612-627-1980
E-mail: ump@umn.edu
www.upress.umn.edu

Publisher of groundbreaking work in social and cultural
thought, critical theory, race and ethnic studies, urbanism,
feminist criticism, and media studies.

3731 WW Norton

500 Fifth Avenue
New York, NY 10110
212-354-5500
Fax: 212-869-0856
www.wwnorton.com

Publishing house owned by its employees, and publishes
books in fiction, nonfiction, poetry, college, cookbooks, art,
and professional subjects, including health care and mental
health.

3732 Woodbine House

6510 Bells Mill Road
Bethesda, MD 20817
301-897-3570
800-843-7323
www.woodbinehouse.com

Publishes special needs books for parents, children, teachers and professionals.

Facilities

3733 Ancora Psychiatric Hospital
202 Spring Garden Road
Ancora, NJ 08037-9699
609-561-1700
Fax: 609-561-2509
E-mail: donna.ingram@dhs.state.nj.us
www.state.nj.us/humanservices/pfnurses/ancora.htm

Donna Ingram, Contact

Provides quality comprehensive psychiatric, medical and
rehabilitative services that encourage maximun patient independence and movement towards community reintegration with an enviroment that is safe and caring.

3734 Brainerd Regional Human Services Center
1777 Highway 18 E
Brainerd, MN 56401-7389
218-828-2201

Harcey G Cakdwell, Contact

Alabama

3735 Bryce Hospital
200 University Boulevard
Tuscaloosa, AL 35401-1294
205-759-0750
Fax: 205-759-0845

David L Bennett, Director

3736 Greil Memorial Psychiatric Hospital
2140 Upper Wetumpka Road
Montgomery, AL 36107-1398
334-262-0363

Susan P Chambers MPA, Contact

Greil Hospitalis a 50-bed acute care psychiatric hospital located in Montgomery, the capital city. Fully accredited by
the Joint Commission on Accreditation of Healthcare Organizations and certified by Medicare, Greil services as a regional facility for 11 counties in central Alabama. The
hospital's facilities are among the newest and most recently
renovated in the Alabama Mental Health system.

**3737 Mary Starke Harper Geriatric Psychiatry
Center**
201 University Boulevard
Tuscaloosa, AL 35402
205-759-0900
Fax: 205-759-0931

Beverly White, Contact

3738 North Alabama Regional Hospital
Highway 31 S
Decatur, AL 35609
256-560-2200

Kay V Greenwood, Contact

3739 Searcy Hospital
Coy Smith Highway
PO Box 1001
Mount Vernon, AL 35660
251-662-6700

John T Bartlett, Contact

3740 Taylor Hardin Secure Medical Facility
1301 Jack Warner Parkway NE
Tuscaloosa, AL 35405-1098
205-556-7060

James F Reddoch Jr, JD, Facility Director

Alaska

3741 Alaska Psychiatric Institute
2800 Providence Drive
Anchorage, AK 99508-4677
907-269-7100
Fax: 907-269-7251
www.hss.state.al.us/dbh/API/default.htm

Ron Adler, Director/CEO
R Duane Hopson MD, Medical Director

In partnership with individuals, their families and the community, natural network and providers, API's Alaska Recovery Center provides therapeutic services which assist
individuals to achieve a personal level of satisfaction and
success in their recovery.

Arizona

3742 Arizona State Hospital
2500 East Van Buren
Phoenix, AZ 85008-6079
602-244-1331
Fax: 602-220-6292
www.azdhs.gov/azsh/

John C Cooper, CEO

The mission of the Arizona State Hospital is to restore and
enhance the mental health of persons requiring psychiatric
services in a safe and therapeutic environment

3743 Southwest Behavorial Health Services
3450 North 3rd Street
Phoenix, AZ 85012
602-265-8338
E-mail: ifno@sbhservices.org
www.sbhservices.org

Inspire people to feel better and reach their potential.

Arkansas

3744 Arkansas State Hospital
4313 West Markham Street
Little Rock, AR 72205-4096
501-686-9000
Fax: 501-686-9182
www.arkansas.gov/dhhs/dmhs/ar_state_hospital.htm

Charles Smith, Administrator
Albert Kittrell, MD, Medical Director

The Arkansas State Hospital is a psychiatric inpatient
treatment facility for those with mental or emotional disorders which includes 90 beds for acute psychiatric admission; a 60-bed forensic treatment services program which
offers assistance to circuit courts throughout the state; a
16-bed adolescent treatment program for youth 13-18; and
a program for juvenile sex offenders.

3745 Center for Outcomes Research and Effectiveness
4301 W Markham Street
Little Rock, AR 72204-1773
501-660-7550
Fax: 501-660-7543
E-mail: kramerteresal@uams.edu
www.uams.edu

I Dodd Wilson MD

California

3746 ANKA Behavioral Health
1875 Willow Pass Road
Suite 300
Concord, CA 94520
925-825-4700
Fax: 925-825-2610
www.ankabhs.org

Michael Jacquemet-Barrington, President/CEO
Chris Withrow, Deputy CEO/Exec VP
Maryann Silva, Corporate Compliance Officer

Offers comprehensive services and programs designed to promote a client's overall wellness and to attain an enhanced quality of life.

3747 Atascadero State Hospital
10333 El Camino Real
Atascadero, CA 93422
805-468-2000
Fax: 805-468-6011
www.dmh.ca.gov

Jon Demorales, Executive Director

The staff members of Atascadero State Hospital (ASH) proudly serve the people of the State of California by providing protection for the community, expert evaluations for the courts, and state-of-the-science psychiatric recovery services for individuals referred to us from across the state.

3748 Augustus F Hawkins Community Mental Health Center
Los Angeles County Department of Mental Health
1720 E 120th Street
Los Angeles, CA 90059-3097
310-668-4186

James C Allen, Deputy Director

Provides community and client crisis intervention, case management, community promotion and outpatient services. Clinical facilities for professional field training.

3749 Campobello Chemical Dependency Treatment Services
3250 Guerneville Road
Santa Rosa, CA 95404
707-579-4066
800-806-1833
www.campobello.org

William Twitchell, Owner/CEO
Kathy Leigh Willis, Executive Director

Innovative chemical dependency treatment center with the belief in the 12 step self-help programs of Alcoholics Anonymous, Narcotics Anonymous and Al-Anon for friends and family.

3750 Changing Echoes
7632 Pool Station Road
Angels Camp, CA 95222
800-633-7066
www.changingechoes.com

Established as a social model chemical dependency facility with the intent to render high-quality treatment for affordable prices to men and women who suffer from the disease of addiction.

Year Founded: 1989

3751 Combined Addicts and Professionals Services CAPS/Residential Unit
398 South 12th Street
San Jose, CA 95112
408-294-5425
www.capsrecovery.net

Timmie Kase, Information Services

Providing individualized substance abuse treatment and recovery services. Provides a continuum of care to help clients' transition from one level of intensity to another.

3752 Comeback Treatment Centers
803 South Gilbert Street
Anaheim, CA 92804
714-628-9307
Fax: 714-628-0311
E-mail: director@comebacktreatment.com
www.comebacktreatment.com

Bart Allen, Executive Director

Provides a family atmosphere, intimate and caring. Provides social integration, and all aspects of home life to provides the best support.

3753 Department of Mental Health Vacaville Psychiatric Program
PO Box 2297
Vacaville, CA 95696
707-449-6597
Fax: 707-453-7047
www.dmh.ca.gov/services_and_programs/State_Hospitals

Victor Brewer, Executive Director

The mission of Vacaville Psychiatric Program is to provide quality mental health evaluation and treatment to inmate-patients. This is accomplished in a safe and therapeutic environment, and as part of a continuum of care.

3754 Exodus Recovery Center
3828 Delmas Terrace
Tower 6
Culver City, CA 90231
310-836-7000
800-829-3923
E-mail: lezlie@exodusrecovery.com
www.exodusrecovery.com

David Murphy, Founder

Mission is that we believe that chemically dependent men and women can achieve freedom from the bondage of drugs and alcohol. Teaching patients and their families that the devastation of addiction can be overcome. Produce personal action plans that can produce a lifetime of recovery.

3755 Family Service Agency
123 W Gutierrez Street
Santa Barbara, CA 93101-3424

805-965-1001
Fax: 805-965-2178
E-mail: hr@fsacares.org
www.fsacares.org

William EG Batty III, Executive Director
Jeff Hurley, Program Director

A non-profit human service agency whose programs help people help themselves. FSA services prevent family breakdown, intervene effectively where problems are known to exist and help individuals and families build on existing strengt

3756 Filipino American Service Group
135 N Park View Street
Los Angeles, CA 90026-5215
213-487-9804
Fax: 213-487-9806
E-mail: fasgi@fasgi.org
www.fasgi.org

Susan E Dilkes, Executive Director
Bernie Targa, Program Director
Bryan Jones, Case Manager

FASGI's chartered mission is to empower the underserved through culturally- and linguistically-competent care, advocacy, social services, education, social action and research.

Year Founded: 1981

3757 Fremont Hospital
Psychiatric Solutions
39001 Sundale Drive
Fremont, CA 94538
510-796-1100
www.fremonthospital.com

Joey A Jacobs, President/CEO/Chairman

A private, modern 96-bed behavioral healthcare facility that provides services to adolescents (ages 12-17) and adults.

3758 Life Steps Pasos de Vida
1431 Pomeroy Road
Arroyo Grande, CA 93420
805-481-2505
800-530-5433
www.lifestepsfoundation.org

Virginia Franco, Founder/CEO
Allen C Haile, President

Develops innovative programs that target underserved populations. Goal is to help participants develop healthy lifestyles free of alcohol and drugs.

3759 Lincoln Child Center
4368 Lincoln Avenue
Oakland, CA 94602
510-531-3111
Fax: 510-530-8083
E-mail: info@lincolncc.org
www.lincolncc.org

Christine Stoner-Mertz, President/CEO
Toni Taylor, Chief Program Officer

Enables vulnerable and emotionally troubled children and their families to lead independent and fulfilling live

3760 Merit Behavioral Care of California
California Department of Managed Health Care
300 Continental Blvd.
Suite 240
El Segundo, CA 92045
310-726-7090
800-424-1565
Fax: 650-742-0988
E-mail: FAVivaldo@magellanhealth.com
www.dmhc.ca.gov/mcp/details.asp?id=137

Lucinda Ehnes, Director
G Lewis Chartrand Jr, Chief Deputy Director

The people of the Department of Managed Health Care work toward an affordable, accountable and robust managed care delivery system that promotes healthier Californians. Through leadership and partnership, the Department shares responsibility with everyone in managed care to ensure aggressive prevention and high quality health care, as well as cost-effective regulatory oversight.

3761 Metropolitan State Hospital
11401 Bloomfield Avenue
Norwalk, CA 90650
562-863-7011
Fax: 562-929-3131
TDD: 562-863-1743

Sharon Smith Nevins, Executive Director

3762 Mills-Peninsula Hospital: Behavioral Health
1783 El Camino Real
Burlingame, CA 94010-3205
650-696-5909
www.mills-peninsula.org/behavioralhealth

Community hospital mental health and chemical dependency care. Our team is uniquely qualified to evaluate, diagnose and treat a wide range of behavioral conditions.

3763 Napa State Hospital
California Department of Mental Health
2100 Napa-Vallejo Highway
Napa, CA 94558-6293
707-253-5000
Fax: 707-253-5379
TDD: 707-253-5768
E-mail: nshcontact@dmhnsh.state.ca.us
www.dmh.ca.gov/Statehospitals/Napa/default.asp

Ed Foulk Ed.D., Executive Director

Napa State Hospital assists each individual in achieving his/her highest potential for independence and quality of life, leading to recovery and integrating safely and successfully into society.

3764 New Life Recovery Centers
782 Park Avenue
Suite 1
San Jose, CA 95126
408-297-1182
866-894-6572
Fax: 408-297-7450
www.newliferecoverycenters.com

Kevin Richardson, Founder
Gary Ruble, Founder

Strives to provide our clients with the very best services available. We value our employees as our greatest asset, while collectively and continuously working to adopt and implement the latest and most effective medical, clinical, and social model treatment modalities.

3765 Northridge Hospital Medical Center
18300 Roscoe Boulevard
Northridge, CA 91325-4167
818-885-8500
www.northridgehospital.org/

Tracey Veal, VP

Northridge Hospital Medical Center offers a comprehensive Behavioral Health program for both adults and adolescents.

3766 Orange County Mental Health
822 Town & Country Road
Orange, CA 92868-4712
714-547-7559
Fax: 717-543-4431
E-mail: info@mhaoc.org
www.mhaoc.org

The Mental Health Association of Orange County is a non-profit organization dedicated to improving the quality of life of Orange County residents impacted by mental illness through direct service, advocacy, education and information dissemination.

3767 PacifiCare Behavioral Health PO Box 31053 Laguna Hills, CA 92654-1053
800-999-9585
www.pbhi.com

Richard J Kelliher PsyD, Clinical Director

Provides behavioral health services to children, adolescents, adults, and seniors.

3768 Patton State Hospital
California Department of Mental Health
3102 E Highland Avenue
Patton, CA 92369
909-425-7000
TDD: 909-862-5730
www.dmh.ca.gov/Statehospitals/Patton/default.asp

Octavio C Luna, Executive Director

Patton State Hospital's mission is to empower forensic and civilly committed individuals to recover from mental illness utilizing Recovery principles and evidenced based practices within a safe, structured, and secure environment.

3769 Phoenix Programs Inc
1401 West 4th Street
Antioch, CA 94509
925-778-3750
www.phoenixprograms.org

Michael Jacquemet-Barrington, President/CEO
Chris Withrow, Executive VP/DCEO

Offers an array of services and programs designed to promote overall wellness while making it possible for all to obtain a higher quality of life.

3770 Presbyterian Intercommunity Hospital Mental Health Center
12401 Washington Boulevard
Whittier, CA 90602-1099
562-698-0811
www.whittierpres.com

Offers an inpatient program for those with a variety of mental disorders.

3771 South Coast Medical Center
31872 S Coast Highway
Laguna Beach, CA 92651
949-499-1311
E-mail: info@southcoastmedcenter.com
www.southcoastmedcenter.com

3772 Twin Town Treatment Centers
4388 E Katella Avenue
Los Alamitos, CA 90720
562-594-8844
Fax: 562-493-1280
www.twintowntreatmentcenters.com

Robert Tyler, Program Administrator

Mission is to introduce new solutions for people who find that chemically induced coping no longer works.

3773 Walden House Transitional Treatment Center
520 Townsend Street
San Francisco, CA 94103
415-554-1100
TDD: 415-431-1067
www.waldenhouse.org

Rod Libbey, CEO
Vitka Eisen, COO

A national leader in developing strategies to help addicts recover and maintain their lives.

Colorado

3774 Centennial Mental Health Center
211 W Main Street
Sterling, CO 80751-3142
970-522-4549
Fax: 970-522-9544
E-mail: webmaster@centennialmhc.org
www.centennialmhc.org

John Klein, Executive Director

A non-profit organization dedicated to providing the highest quality comprehensive mental health services to the rural communities of northeastern Colorado.

3775 Colorado Mental Health Institute at Fort Logan
3520 West Oxford Avenue
Denver, CO 80236
303-866-7066
Fax: 303-866-7088
www.cdhs.state.co.us/cmhifl

Keith LaGrenade MD, Hospital Director

The mission of the Colorado Mental Health Institute at Fort Logan is to provide the highest quality mental health services to persons of all ages with complex, serious and persistent mental illness within the resources available.

3776 Colorado Mental Health Institute at Pueblo
1600 West 24th Street
Pueblo, CO 81003
719-546-4000
Fax: 719-546-4484
www.cdhs.state.co.us/cmhip

John DeQuardo MD, Superintendent

Provides quality mental health services focused on sustaining hope and promoting recovery.

3777 Emily Griffith Center
PO Box 95
Larkspur, CO 80118
303-681-2400
Fax: 303-681-2401
www.www.emilygriffith.com

Howard Shiffman, CEO
Beth Miller, Deputy Director/COO
John Smrcka, Program Director

Provides troubled children the environment and opportunities to become healthy, participating and productive members of society.

Connecticut

3778 Cedarcrest Hospital
525 Russell Road
Newington, CT 06111-1595
860-666-4613
Fax: 860-666-7642
E-mail: thomas.kirk@po.state.ct.us
www.dmhas.state.ct.us/aboutdmhas.htm

Susan Graham, CEO
Richard Stillson Ph.D, Director of Psychology
Thomas A Kirk Jr, Commissioner

The mission of Cedarcrest Hospital is to improve the quality of life of the people of Connecticut by providing an integrated network of comprehensive, effective and efficient mental health and addiction services that foster self-sufficiency, dignity and respect.

3779 Connecticut Valley Hospital General Psychiatric Division
PO Box 351
Middletown, CT 06457-7023
860-262-5529

Thomas A Kirk, Commissioner
Pat Rehem, Deputy Commissioner
Garrell S Mullaney, CEO

The mission of Connecticut Valley Hospital is to improve the quality of life of the people of Connecticut by providing an integrated network of comprehensive, effective and efficient mental health services that foster self-sufficiency, dignity and respect.

3780 Daytop Residential Services Division
425 Grant Street
Bridgeport, CT 06610
203-337-9943
Fax: 203-337-9986
www.aptfoundation.org/daytop.htm

Nancy Moak, Intake Services

Long-term substance abuse treatment facility based on the Therapeutic Community model. Combines current research and treatment methods with traditional therapeutic community concepts.

3781 Greater Bridgeport Community Mental Health Center
1635 Central Avenue
PO Box 5117
Bridgeport, CT 06610-2700
203-551-7400
Fax: 203-551-7446

James M LeHene MPH, Contact

3782 High Watch Farm
62 Carter Road
Kent, CT 06757
860-927-3772
Fax: 860-927-1840
E-mail: admissions@highwatchfarm.com
www.highwatchfarm.com

Janina J Kean, President/CEO

A spiritually nurturing environment dedicated to providing treatment to alcohol and substance dependent individuals based on the 12-step principles of Alcoholics Anonymous.

3783 Jewish Family Service
733 Summer Street
Suite 602
Stamford, CT 06901
203-921-4161
Fax: 203-921-4169
www.ctjfs.org

Matt Greenberg, Executive Director
Isrella Knopf, LMSW, Director Senior Services
Eve Moskowitz LCSW, Clinical Services Director

Offers a wide range of innovative programs designed to address contemporary problems and issues through counseling and therapy, crisis intervention, Jewish Family Life Education, Depression, Aging and senior mental health, Obsessions and compulsions.

Year Founded: 1978

3784 Klingberg Family Centers
370 Linwood Street
New Britain, CT 06052-1998
860-224-9113
Fax: 860-832-8221
E-mail: markj@klingberg.org
www.klingberg.org

Mark H Johnson, VP

To uphold, preserve and restore families in a therapeutic environment, valuing the absolute worth of every child, while adhering to the highest ethical principles in accordance with our Judaeo-Christian heritage.

3785 McCall Foundation
58 High Street
PO Box 806
Torrington, CT 06790
860-496-2107
E-mail: mccallfoundation@snet.net
www.northwestunitedway.org/mccall.htm

Provides outpatient, partial hospital, intensive outpatient, residential, parenting and prevention programs for substance abusers and/or their family members; and helps to reduce area substance abuse in the local community. Funding is provided by the United Way.

3786 Mountainside Treatment Center
PO Box 717
Canaan, CT 06018
860-824-1397
800-762-5433
Fax: 860-824-5691
E-mail: admissions@mountainside.org
www.mountainside.org

Program is based on strategies and principles that promote healing and enhance the quality of life. Through the utilization of Motivational Interviewing, Directional Therapy, Gender-Specific Groups, the 12-Step Principles and Adventure Based Initiatives, individuals qwill encounter, confront and experience the challenges of recovery.

3787 Silver Hill Hospital

208 Valley Road
New Canaan, CT 06840
203-966-3561
800-899-4455
Fax: 203-801-2395
E-mail: info@silverhillhospital.org
www.silverhillhospital.org

Sigurd H Ackerman, President/Medical Director
Elizabeth Moore, Chief Operating Officer

A nationally recognized, independent, not-for-profit psychiatric hospital that is focused exclusively on providing patients the best possible treatment of psychiatric illnesses and substance use disorders, in the best possible environment.

Year Founded: 1931

Delaware

3788 Delaware State Hospital

1901 N Dupont Highway
New Castle, DE 19720
302-577-4000

Jiro Shimono, Contact

District of Columbia

3789 St. Elizabeth's Hospital

2700 Martin Luther King Jr Avenue SE
Washington, DC 20032-2698
202-645-5489
Fax: 202-645-5697

Dr Patrick J Canavan Psy.D., Contact

Florida

3790 Archways-A Bridge To A Brighter Future

919 NE 13th Street
Fort Lauderdale, FL 33304
954-763-2030
Fax: 954-763-9847
E-mail: intake@archways.org
www.archways.org

A not-for-profit, privately-governed organization whose mission is to provide quality comprehensive behavioral health care to individuals and families who are in need of improving their quality of life.

3791 Fairwinds Treatment Center

1569 South Fort Harrison
Clearwater, FL 33765
727-449-0300
800-226-0300
E-mail: fairwinds@fairwindstreatment.com
www.fairwindstreatment.com

M.K. El-Yousef, Medical Director
Thomas H Lewis, Clinical Director

As a dually licensed psychiatric and substance abuse center, reaches far beyond standard treatment to offer medical services for substance abuse, eating disorders, and emotional/mental health issues.

3792 First Step of Sarasota

1726 18th Street
Sarasota, FL 34234
941-366-5333
800-266-6866
www.fsos.org

David Beesley, President/CEO
Brenda Asher, CFO

Provides high quality, affordable substance abuse treatment and recovery programs on Florida's Gulf Coast. Offers a variety of programs including a medical detox, residential and outpatient services for adolescents, adults and families.

3793 Florida State Hospital

100 N Main Street
Chattahoochee, FL 32324
850-663-7536

Robert B Williams, Contact

3794 G Pierce Wood Memorial Hospital

5847 SE Highway 31
Arcadia, FL 33821-9627
863-494-3323

Myers R Kurtz, Contact

3795 Gateway Community Services

555 Stockton Street
Jacksonville, FL 32204
904-387-4661
www.gatewaycommunity.com

Gary Powers, CEO
Laura Dale, CFO
Randy Jennings, Sr VP Operations

Provides a full continuum of care that delivers effective treatment and rehabilitation services to individuals suffering from alcoholism, substance abuse and related mental health problems.

3796 Genesis House Recovery Residence

4865 40th Way South
Lake Worth, FL 33461
561-439-4070
800-737-0933
E-mail: genesishouse@yahoo.com
www.genesishouse.net

James Dodge, Program Director
Kathryn Shafer, Clinical Director

Works closely with both local and out of state courts. Provides the suffering person with a safe, secure, professional environment to glean the care, answers and support they so desperately need in their lives.

3797 Manatee Glens

391 6th Avenue W
Bradenton, FL 34205
941-741-3111
Fax: 941-741-3112
www.manateeglens.com

Mary Ruiz, CEO/President
Deborah Kostroun, COO
John Denaro, CFO
Dr Jose Zaglul, CMO

Helps families in crisis with mental health and addictions services and supports the community through prevention and recovery.

3798 Manatee Palms Youth Services
4480 51st Street W
Bradenton, FL 34210-2855
941-792-2222
Fax: 941-795-4359
www.psysolutions.com/facilities/manatee

Rose Cota, Admissions Director
Timothy Macsuga, Business Development Director

Committed to providing the highest quality comprehensive mental health care and education services for at-risk children, adolescents, families and our community.

3799 New Horizons of the Treasure Coast
4500 W Midway Road
Ft Pierce, FL 34981
772-468-5600
www.nhtcinc.org

John Romano, President/CEO
Dr Charles Buscema, Medical Director

To improve the quality of life in the community through the provision of accessible, person-centered behavioral health resources.

3800 North Florida Evaluation and Treatment Center
1200 NE 55th Boulevard
Gainesville, FL 32641-2759
352-375-8484
Fax: 352-955-2094
www.dcf.state.fl.us/institutions/nfetc/welcome.shtml

William S Baker, Administrator

Dedicated to serving you while fulfilling our responsibilities for safety, security and a positive, caring environment.

3801 North Star Centre
9033 Glades Road
Boca Raton, FL 33434
561-361-0500
E-mail: info@northstar-centre.com
www.northstar-centre.com

Ira Kaufman, Executive Director
Randi Katz, Administrative Assistant

A uniquely comprehensive facility dedicated to restoring your sense of emotional and physical well being.

3802 Northeast Florida State Hospital
7487 South State Road 121
MacClenny, FL 32063
904-259-6211
Fax: 904-259-7101
www.dcf.state.fl.us/institutions/nefsh

Steve Kennedy, Administrator

To provide comprehensive mental health treatment services to ensure a timely transition to the community.

3803 Renaissance Manor
1401 16th Street
Sarasota, FL 34236-2519
941-365-8645

Heather Eller, Administrator

Community based assisted living facility with a limited mental health license, specializes in serving adults with neuro-biological disorders and mood disorders along with other special mental health needs. Our not-for-profit organization is a program designed to encourage positive mental health while meeting the various interest of our residents.

3804 Seminole Community Mental Health Center
237 Fernwood Blvd
Fern Park, FL 32730
407-831-2411
Fax: 407-831-0195
E-mail: scmhc@scmhc.com
www.scmhc.com

A private, nonprofit organization whose goal is to provide comprehensive, biopsychosocial rehabilitation programming in the areas of mental health and substance abuse.

3805 South Florida Evaluation and Treatment Center
2200 NW 7th Avenue
Miami, FL 33127-2491
305-637-2500

Cheryl Brantley, Contact

3806 South Florida State Hospital
800 East Cypress Drive
Pembroke Pines, FL 33025
954-392-3000
www.sfsh.org/

Jorge A Diminicis, President

As one of the nation's first new comprehensive public mental health facilities in many years, the South Florida State Hospital campus was specifically designed to support the role recovery process. The distinctly non-institutional atmosphere not only improves the mental healthcare experience for persons served and their families, it also plays an integral role in their treatment and recovery.

3807 Starting Place
2057 Coolidge Street
Hollywood, FL 33020
954-925-2225
Fax: 954-921-1845
www.startingplace.org

Sheldon Shaffer, CEO

Licensed agency that provides therapeutic, prevention and intervention services as well as rehabilitative and educational counseling to all person affected by substance abuse and mental illness so that they may lead productive drug-free lives.

3808 Suncoast Residential Training Center/Developmental Services Program
Goodwill Industries-Suncoast
10596 Gandy Boulevard
St. Petersburg, FL 33733
727-523-1512
Fax: 727-563-9300
E-mail: gw.marketing@goodwill-suncoast.com
www.goodwill-suncoast.org

R Lee Waits, President/CEO
Deborah A Passerini, VP Operations

A large group home which serves individuals diagnosed as mentally retarded with a secondary diagnosed of psychiatric difficulties as evidenced by problem behavior. Providing residential, behavioral and instructional support and services that will promote the development of adaptive, socially appropriate behavior, each individual is assessed to determine, socialization, basic academics and recreation. The primary intervention strategy is applied behavior analysis. Professional consultants are utilized to address the medical, dental, psychiatric and pharmacological needs of ech individual. One of the most popular features is the active community integration component of SRTC. Program customers attend an average of 15 monthly outings to various community events.

3809 The Transition House

1224 12 Street
St Cloud, FL 34769
407-891-1551
E-mail: counselor@thetransitionhouse.org
www.thetransitionhouse.org

The adress above is the men's house. The address for the women's house is: 505 N Clyde Street Kissimmee, FL 34741. All other information is the same. Mission is to provide a milieu of comprehensive educational, health, prevention and human services to Central Florida's most disenfranchised populations.

3810 Turning Point of Tampa

6227 Sheldon Road
Tampa, FL 33615
813-882-3003
800-397-3006
Fax: 813-885-6974
www.tpoftampa.com

Darren Rothschild, Medical Director
Robin Piper, Clinical Director/CEO
Michelle Ratcliff, Owner

Provides high-quality, 12 step based addiction treatment programs specifically designed to be cost effective; to continually monitor and evaluate industry research and our own outcome data in an effort to develop our own programming.

3811 University Pavilion Psychiatric Services

7425 N University Drive
Tamarac, FL 33321-2901
954-722-9933
www.uhmchealth.com

Offers psychiatric services on an inpatient and outpatient basis for all individuals.

3812 Willough Healthcare System

9001 Tamiami Trail East
Naples, FL 34113
239-775-4500
800-722-0100
E-mail: info@thewilloughatnaples.com
www.thewilloughatnaples.com/

James O'Shea, Administrator

Specializes in the treatment of eating disorders and chemical dependency.

Georgia

3813 Candler General Hospital: Rehabilitation Unit

5353 Reynolds Street
Savannah, GA 31405-6013
912-819-6000
www.www.sjchs.org

Paul P Hinchey, President/CEO

Our vision is to set the standards of excellence in the delivery of health care throughout the regions we serve. Candler Hospital is an affiliate of St. Joseph's/Candler, the largest health care system in Southeast Georgia and the only faith based health system in Savannah. Candler Hospital is the second oldest continuously operating hospitals in the United States and the oldest hospital in Georgia.

3814 Central State Hospital

620 Broad Street
Milledgeville, GA 31062
478-445-4128
Fax: 478-445-6034
E-mail: info@centralstatehospital.org
www.centralstatehospital.org

Marvin Bailey, Chief Executive Officer
Scott Van Sant, Chief Medical Officer
Lee Ann Molini, Director of Nursing

Central State Hospital (CSH) is Georgia's largest facility for persons with mental illness and developmental disabilities. The scope of our services is extensive and includes: short-stay acute treatment for consumers with mental illness; residential units and habilitation programs for individuals with developmental disabilities; recovery programs for consumers requiring longer stays; and specialized skilled and ICF nursing centers. Some of our programs serve primarily our central Georgia region while other programs serve many counties throughout the state.

3815 Georgia Regional Hospital at Atlanta

3073 Panthersville Road
Decatur, GA 30034-3838
404-243-2110
Fax: 404-212-4628
E-mail: grha@dhr.state.ga.us
www.atlantareg.dhr.state.ga.us/

Ronald C Hogan, Chief Executive Officer
Gwen Skinner, Director

Located on 174 Acres in DeKalb County, Georgia Regional Hospital/Atlanta operates 366 licensed, accredited inpatient beds in five major program areas: Adult Mental Health, Adolescent Mental Health, Child Mental Health, Forensic Services, and Developmental Disabilities. In addition, GRH/Atlanta also offers inpatient and outpatient Dental Services and an Outpatient Forensic Evaluation Program for juveniles and adults. Finally, GRH/Atlanta operates the Fulton County Collaborative Crisis Service System which provides mobile crisis and residential services to adults experiencing mental health problems in Fulton County.

3816 Georgia Regional Hospital at Augusta

3405 Old Savannah Road
Augusta, GA 30906-3897
706-792-7019
Fax: 706-792-7041

Ben Waker EdD, Contact

3817 Georgia Regional Hospital at Savannah

1915 Eisenhower Drive
PO Box 13607
Savannah, GA 31416-0607
912-356-2045

Douglas Osborne, Contact

3818 Northwest Georgia Regional Hospital
1305 Redmond Circle
Rome, GA 30165
706-295-6246
www.nwgrh.dhr.state.ga.us

Thomas Muller, Clinical Director
Karl H Schwarzkopf, Administrator

3819 Southwestern State Hospital
400 Pinetree Boulevard
Thomasville, GA 31799-6859
912-227-3032
Fax: 912-227-2883

David Sofferin, Contact

3820 West Central Georgia Regional Hospital
PO Box 12435
Columbus, GA 31917-2432
706-568-5204
E-mail: wcgrh@dhr.state.ga.us
www.wcgrh.org

Mission is to treat customers with respect and dignity while providing comprehensive, person-centered behavioral healthcare.

Hawaii

3821 Hawaii State Hospital
45-710 Keaahala Road
Kaneohe, HI 96744-3597
808-247-2191

Marvin O Saint Clair, Contact

Idaho

3822 Children of Hope Family Hospital
PO Box 2353
Boise, ID 83701
208-658-8013
E-mail: drharper@afo.net
www.chfhosp.dmi.net

Rev Anthony R Harper PhD, Founder

3823 State Hospital North
300 Hospital Drive
Orofino, ID 83544-9034
208-476-4511
Fax: 208-476-7898

Debra Manfull, Contact

3824 State Hospital South
700 E Alice Street
PO Box 400
Blackfoot, ID 83221-0400
208-785-8401
Fax: 208-785-8448

Raymond Laible, Contact

Illinois

3825 Advocate Ravenswood Hospital Medical Center
2025 Windsor Avenue
Oakbrook, IL 60523
603-572-9393
Fax: 630-990-4752
www.advocatehealth.com

Provides a comprehensive array of services for inpatient (Adult, Adolescent, Substance Abuse), Partial Hospital, Intensive Outpatient, Psychological Rehabilitation, Emergency-Crisis, Assertive Community Outreach, Case Management, Program for Deaf and Hard of Hearing at multiple sites on the Northside of Chicago.

3826 Alexian Brothers Bonaventure House
825 W Wellington Avenue
Chicago, IL 60657
773-327-9921
E-mail: info@abam.org
www.bonaventurehouse.org

Merrill Kenna, CEO
Marty Hansen, Director Programs/Services

Offers adult men and women with HIV/AIDS-who are homeless or at-risk for homelessness- a chance to rebuild and reclaim their lives. Bonaventure House has a wide array of on-site supportive services-case management, occupational therapy, recovery, and spiritual care-most residents are able to return to independent life in the community within a 24-month period.

3827 Alton Mental Health Center
4500 College Avenue
Alton, IL 62002-5099
618-474-3209
Fax: 618-474-4800

Thomas H Johnson, Contact

3828 Andrew McFarland Mental Health Center
901 Southwind Road
Springfield, IL 62703-5195
217-786-6994

G. Scott Viniard, Hospital Administrator

3829 Chester Mental Health Center
Chester Road
Chester, IL 62233-0031
618-826-4571

Stephen Hardy PhD, Contact

3830 Choate Mental Health and Development Center
1000 N Main Street
Anna, IL 62906-1699
618-833-5161

Tom Richards, Contact

3831 Cornell Interventions Lifeworks
1611 Jefferson Street
Joliet, IL 60435
815-730-7521
Fax: 815-730-7524
www.cornellcompanies.com

James E Hyman, Chairman/President/CEO

Provides outpatient addiction counseling, education and life skills services to adolescents and adults.

3832 Delta Center
1400 Commercial Avenue
Cairo, IL 62914
618-734-2665
Fax: 618-734-1999
TTY: 618-734-1350
E-mail: delta1@midwest.net
www.deltacenter.org

A non-profit mental health center, substance abuse counseling facility, and also provides various community services to Alexander and Pulaski County, Illinois

3833 Elgin Mental Health Center
750 S State Street
Elgin, IL 60123-7692
847-742-1040

Nancy Staples, Contact

3834 FHN Family Counseling Center
421 W Exchange Street
Freeport, IL 61032-4866
815-599-7300

3835 Franklin-Williamson Human Services
1307 W Main Street
Marion, IL 62959
618-997-5336
www.fwhs.org

A place where people with mental, emotional, behavioral, family, developmental or substance abuse problems can get help. Our programs help people learn to prevent problems, acquire new skills, develop abilities and adjust to community life.

3836 H Douglas Singer Mental Health Center
4402 N Main Street
Rockford, IL 61103-1278
815-987-7096

Angelo Campagna, Contact

3837 Habilitative Systems
415 S Kilpatrick Avenue
Chicago, IL 60644-4923
773-261-2252
Fax: 773-854-8300
TDD: 773-854-8364
E-mail: hsi@habilitative.org
www.habilitative.org

Donald J Dew, President/CEO
Joyce Wade, VP Finance
Karen Barbee-Dixon, EdD, COO

To provide integrated human services to children, adults, families, and persons with disabling conditions that help them to achieve their highest level of self-sufficiency

Year Founded: 1978

3838 Harriet Tubman Women and Children Treatment Facility Residential Program
11352 South State Street
Chicago, IL 60628
773-785-4955

Primary focus is the mix of mental health and substance abuse services. Providing residential long-term treatment which is longer than 30 days.

3839 John J Madden Mental Health Center
1200 S 1st Avenue
Hines, IL 60141
708-338-7202

Patricia Madden, Contact

3840 John R Day and Associates
3716 W Brighton Avenue
Peoria, IL 61615-2938
309-692-7755
Fax: 306-692-7755

3841 Keys To Recovery
100 North River Road
Des Plaines, IL 60016
847-298-9355
www.keystorecovery.org

Philip Kolski, Director
Debra Ayanian, Nurse Manager

A leading Alcoholism and Drug Treatment Center in the Midwest, providing innovative and effective Alcoholism and Drug Treatment.

3842 Lifelink Bensenville
331 S York Road
Suite 206
Bensenville, IL 60106-2600
630-766-5800
Fax: 630-521-8856

Rev Carl Zimmerman, President/CEO
Michael Oliver, VP

Health and human organization providing quality programs and services to people of all generations, cultures, religions, genders, and socio-economic status.

Year Founded: 1895

3843 MacNeal Hospital
3231 South Euclid Avenue
Berwyn, IL 60402
708-783-3094
888-622-6325
TTY: 708-783-3058
E-mail: inf@macnealfp.com
www.macnealfp.com/hospital.htm

Donna Lawlor MD, Program Director
Davis Yang, Center Director
John Gong, Clinical Faculty
Edward C Foley MD, Director Of Research

The MacNeal Family Practice Residency Program was one of the first family practice programs in the country and the first in Illinois. We have continue a progressive tradition in all aspects of our curriculum. Our program is at the forefront of contemporary family medicine offering diverse academic and clinical opportunites and building on the innovative ideas of our residents.

3844 McHenry County Mental Health Board
620 Dakota Street
Crystal Lake, IL 60012
815-455-2828
Fax: 815-455-2925
www.mc708.org

Sandy Lewis, Executive Director
Robert Lesser, Deputy Director

To provide leadership and ensure the prevention and treatment of mental illness, developmental disabilities and chemical abuse by coordinating, developing, and contracting for quality services for all citizens of McHenry County, Illinois

3845 Metro Child and Adolescent Network
Chicago Read MHC Annex
4200 North Oak Park Avenue
Chicago, IL 60634-1457
773-794-4010

James Brunner MD, Hospital Administrator
Randy Thompson, Medical Director
Thomas Simpatico MD, Facility Director

An important psychiatric hospital which is part of the Department of Human Services of the State of Illinois. Provides comprehensive psychiatric inpatient services for adults in cooperation with a broad spectrum of community mental health service providers.

3846 Pfeiffer Treatment Center and Health Research Institute
4575 Weaver Parkway
Warrenville, IL 60555-4039
630-505-0300
866-504-6076
Fax: 630-836-0667
E-mail: info@hriptc.org
www.hriptc.org

Scott Filer, MPH, Executive Director
Allen Lewis MD, Medical Director
William Walsh, PhD, Research/Found Dir/Co-Founder

A not-for-profit, outpatient medical facility for children, teens and adults seeking a biochemical assessment and treatment for their symptons caused by a biochemical imbalance, or to support health and promote wellness. PTC physician precribes individualized program of vitamins, minerals, and amino acids to address the patient's unique biochemical needs. Common conditions: anxiety, ADHA, autism spectrum disorder, post traumatic stress syndrome, depression, bipolar disorder, schozophrenia and Alzheimer's disease.

3847 Salem Children's Home
15161 N 400 E Road
Flanagan, IL 61740
815-796-4561
Fax: 815-796-4565
E-mail: info@salemranch.com
www.salemhome.com

Salem Children's Home is a Christian organization which provides a variety of individualized services of superior quality to meet the spiritual, social, educational, emotional and psyical needs of boys and their families. We gladly accept the responsibility to provide this care in a personal, nurtuing manner to reconcile familes, develop positive self-images and build healthy relationships among those we serve.

3848 Sonia Shankman Orthogenic School
1365 E 60th Street
Chicago, IL 60637-2890
773-834-2728
Fax: 773-702-1304
www.orthogenicschool.uchicago.edu

Henry J Roth PhD, Executive Director

A coeducational residential treatment program for children and adolescents in need of support for emotional issues which cause the student to act in disruptive ways and experience unfulfilling social and educational experiences

3849 Stepping Stones Recovery Center
1621 Theodore Street
Joliet, IL 60435
815-744-4555
E-mail: info@steppingstonestreatment.com
www.steppingstonestreatment.com

Dedicated to providing effective treatment for persons suffering from the illness of addiction to alcohol and/or other drugs, even if these persons are unable to pay for the cost of such services.

3850 Tinley Park Mental Health Center
7400 W 183rd Street
Tinely Park, IL 60477-3695
708-614-4000

Janice Thomas, Contact

3851 Transitions Mental Health Rehabilitation
805 19th Street
PO Box 4238
Rock Island, IL 61204-4238
309-793-4993
Fax: 309-793-9053
E-mail: transitions@revealed.net
www.transrehab.org

Transitions is dedicated to promoting, enhancing, and improving the health, recovery, and well-being of individuals, families, and the community impacted by mental health issues.

3852 Way Back Inn-Grateful House
1915 W Roosevelt Road
Braodview, IL 60155
708-344-3301
E-mail: frankl@waybackinn.org
www.waybackinn.org

Frank Lieggi, Executive Director
Anita Pindiur, Clinical Director

Provides a high level clinical treatment program specializing in addressing the needs of men and women suffering from both chemical dependence (Alcohol and Drugs) and also Gambling Dependence.

3853 Wells Center
1300 Lincoln Avenue
Jacksonville, IL 62650
217-243-1871
TDD: 217-243-0470
E-mail: bcarter@wellscenter.org
www.wellscenter.org

B Carter, Information Services

Mission has been to improve the health and welfare of individuals and families affected by the ause of alcohol and other substances and by mental health issues. Dedicates its efforts to providing levels of care and support services in settings approval to the individual needs of the patient.

3854 White Oaks Companies of Illinois
130 Richard Pryor Place
Peoria, IL 61605
309-671-8960
800-475-0257
E-mail: whiteoaks@fayettecompanies.org
www.whiteoaks.com

Non profit agency offering comprehensive, state-of-the-art chemical dependency services, individually designed for each client.

Indiana

3855 Community Hospital Anderson
1515 N Madison Avenue
Anderson, IN 46011
765-298-4242
Fax: 765-298-5848
www.communityanderson.com

William C VanNess II MD, President and CEO

The mission of Community Hospital is to serve the medical, health and human service needs to the people in Anderson-Madison County and contiguous counties with compassion dignity, repect and excellence. Service, although focused on injury, illness and disease will also embrace prevention, education and alternative systems of health care delivery.

3856 Crossroad: Fort Wayne's Children's Home
2525 Lake Avenue
Fort Wayne, IN 46805-5457
260-484-4153
800-976-2306
Fax: 260-484-2337
www.crossroad-fwch.org

Randy Rider, President/CEO
Mick Thiel, Chief Program Officer
A Wayne Burton, CFO

A not-for-profit treatment center for emotionally troubled youth.

3857 Hamilton Center
620 Eighth Avenue
Terre Haute, IN 47804
812-231-8323
www.hamiltoncenter.org

David Fee, President
Richard Pittelkow, Vice President
Cary Sparks, Treasurer
Virginia Gilman, Secretary

Provides the full continuum of psychological health and addiction services to children, adolescents, adults and families.

3858 Indiana Family Support Network, MHA Indiana
55 Monument Circle
Suite 455
Indianapolis, IN 46204-2918
317-638-3501
800-555-6424
Fax: 317-638-3401
E-mail: mha@mentalhealthassociation.com
www.nmha.org

Elizabeth Jewell

The National Mental Association is dedicated to promoting mental health, preventing mental disorders and achieving victory over mental illnesses through advocacy, education, research and service.

3859 Parkview Hospital Rehabilitation Center
2200 Randilla Drive
Ft. Wayne, IN 46805
260-373-6450
888-480-5151
Fax: 260-373-4548
E-mail: paulette.fisher@parkview.com
www.parkview.com

Paulette Fisher RN, CRRN, Admissions Specialist

31 bed inpatient rehabilitation unit serving a wide variety of diagnoses. CARF accredited for both comprehensive and B1 programs. Outpatient services are offered at several sites throughout the community.

3860 Richmond State Hospital
498 NW 18th Street
Richmond, IN 47374
765-966-0511
www.richmondstatehospital.org

Jeff Butler, Superintendent

A public behavioral health facility operated by the State of Indiana that provides psychiatric and chemical dependency treatment to citizens on a state wide basis.

3861 Universal Behavioral Service
820 Fort Wayne Avenue
Indianapolis, IN 46204-1309
317-684-0442
Fax: 317-684-0679

Iowa

3862 Cherokee Mental Health Institute
1251 W Cedar Loop
Cherokee, IA 51012-1599
712-225-1698

Tom Deiker PhD, Contact

3863 Clarinda Mental Health Treatment Complex
1800 N 16th Street
PO Box 338
Clarinda, IA 51632-1165
712-542-2161

Mark Lund, Contact

3864 Four Seasons Counseling Clinic
2015 West Bay Drive
Muscatine, IA 52761-4003
563-263-3869
Fax: 563-263-3869

3865 Independence Mental Health Institute
2277 Iowa Avenue
Independence, IA 50644
319-334-2583

Bhasker Dave MD, Contact

3866 Mount Pleasant Mental Health Institute
1200 E Washington Street
Mount Pleasant, IA 52641-1898
319-385-7231
Fax: 319-385-8465

John Mathes, Contact

Kansas

3867 Larned State Hospital
Route 3
Box 89
Larned, KS 67550-9365
316-285-2131
Fax: 316-285-4357
www.srskansas.org/LSH/default.html

Mark Schutter, Superintendent

3868 Osawatomie State Hospital
PO Box 500
Osawatomie, KS 66064-0500
913-755-7000
Fax: 913-755-2637

Gregory Valentine, Superintendent

JCAHO accredited state psychiatric hospital.

3869 Prairie View
1901 E First Street
Newton, KS 67114
316-284-6400
800-362-0180
www.www.pvi.org

Jessie Kaye, CEO

A behavioral and mental health facility which consists of the main campus in Newton that consists of outpatient services, a 38-bed inpatient hospital and various other divisions of our organization. Also maintain outpatient offices in Hutchinson, KS; Marion, KS; McPherson, KS; along with two outpatient offices in Wichita, KS.

Year Founded: 1954

3870 Rainbow Mental Health Facility
2205 W 36th Avenue
Kansas City, KS 66103-2198
913-785-5800
www.kumc.edu/rainbow

Roz Underdahl, Contact

3871 Via Christi Research
1100 N St. Francis Street
Suite 300
Wichita, KS 67214-2878
316-291-4774
800-362-0070
Fax: 316-291-7975

Laurie Labarca, Interim President/CEO
Joe Carrithers, PhD, Research Operations Director

Provide people with mental health conditions such as depression, suicidal thoughts, schizophrenia or dementia have a unique set of needs. They receive highly skilled, compassionate treatment.

Kentucky

3872 ARH Psychiatric Center
102 Medical Center Drive
Hazard, KY 41701-9429
606-439-1331
Fax: 606-439-6701

Wendy Morris, Contact

3873 Central State Hospital
10510 LaGrange Road
Louisville, KY 40223-1228
502-253-7000

Paula Tamee-Cook, Contact

3874 Cumberland River Regional Board
PO Box 568
Corbin, KY 40702-0568
606-528-7010
www.cumberlandriver.com/crccc.html

For children with emotional, behavioral and/or mental challenges.

3875 Eastern State Hospital
627 W Fourth Street
Lexington, KY 40508-1294
859-246-7000
E-mail: mjdaniluk@bluegrass.org
www.www.bluegrass.org

Mike Daniluk, Hospital Director

3876 Kentucky Correctional Psychiatric Center
1612 Dawkins Road
PO Box 67
La Grange, KY 40031-0067
502-222-7161
Fax: 502-222-7798

Gregory Taylor, Contact

3877 Our Lady of Bellefonte Hospital
St. Christopher Drive
Ashland, KY 41101
606-833-2273
www.olbh.com

3878 Western State Hospital
2400 Russeville Road
PO Box 2200
Hopkinsville, KY 42240-3017
270-889-6025
Fax: 502-886-4487

Steven Wiggins, Contact

Louisiana

3879 Central Louisiana State Hospital
242 West Shamrock Avenue
PO Box 5031
Pineville, LA 71361-5031
318-484-6200
Fax: 318-484-6501
E-mail: clshmail@dhh.state.la.us
www.dhh.state.la.us

Thomas L Davis, Facility Director

The free-standing inpatient facility of Area C - Mental Health Services. The mission of Area C is to provide a comprehensive, integrated continuum of care (system of services) for adults with serious mental illness and children/youth with serious emotional/behavioral disturbance in need, in accordance with state and national accrediting organizations' standards for service access, quality, outcome, and cost.

3880 East Division Greenwell Springs Campus
PO Box 549
Greenwell Springs, LA 70739
225-261-2730
Fax: 225-261-9080

Mark Anders, Contact

3881 Eastern Louisiana Mental Health System
PO Box 498
Jackson, LA 70748
225-634-0100
Fax: 225-634-5827

Mark Anders, Contact

3882 Forensic Division
PO Box 888
Jackson, LA 70748
225-634-0100
Fax: 225-634-5827

Mark Anders, Contact

3883 Medical Center of LA: Mental Health Services
1532 Tulane Avenue
New Orleans, LA 70140
504-568-2869

William Malone, Contact

3884 New Orleans Adolescent Hospital
210 State Street
New Orleans, LA 70118
504-897-3400
Fax: 504-896-4959
www.dhh.louisiana.gov

Provides a fully integrated hospital and community based continuum of mental health services for children and adolescents, with serious emotional and behavioral problems, residing in Louisiana.

3885 River Oaks Hospital
1525 River Oaks Road W
New Orleans, LA 70123
504-734-1740
800-366-1740
Fax: 504-733-7020
E-mail: kim.epperson@uhsinc.com
www.riveroakshospital.com

A private psychiatric facility for adults, adolescents and children.

3886 Southeast Louisiana Hospital
23515 Highway 190
PO Box 3850
Mandeville, LA 70470-3850
985-626-6300
Fax: 985-626-6658
www.dhh.louisiana.gov

Patricia Gonzalez, Facility Director

Maine

3887 Dorthea Dix Psychiatric Center
656 State Street
PO Box 926
Bangor, ME 04402-0920

207-941-4000
E-mail: larry.larson@maine.gov
www.maine.gov/dhhs/ddpc/home.html

N Lawrence Ventura, Contact

DDPC is a 100 bed psychiatric hospital serving two-thirds of the State's geographic area that provides services for people with severe mental illness.

3888 Good Will-Hinckley Homes for Boys and Girls
PO Box 159
Hinckley, ME 04944
207-238-4000
Fax: 207-453-2515
E-mail: info@gwh.org
www.gwh.org

John Willey, Secretary
David Kimball, Chairman

Provides a home for the reception and support of needy boys and girls who are in needs maintaining and operates a school for them; attends to the physical, industrial, moral and spiritual development of those who shall be placed in its care.

3889 Riverview Psychiatric Center
250 Arsenal Street
11 SHS
Augusta, ME 04333-0011
207-624-4600
Fax: 207-287-6123
www.maine.gov/dhhs/riverview/index.shtml

David Proffitt, Superintendent

Acute care psychiatric hospital owned and operated by the state of Maine.

3890 Spring Harbor Hospital
123 Andover Road
Westbrook, ME 04092
207-761-2200
888-524-0080
www.springharbor.org

Dennis King, CEO
Rick Hamley, COO
Girard Robinson, Chief Medical Officer

Southern Maine's premier provider of inpatient services for individuals who experience acute mental illness or dual disorders issues.

Maryland

3891 Clifton T Perkins Hospital Center
8450 Dorsey Run Road
PO Box 1000
Jessup, MD 20794-9414
410-724-3002
Fax: 410-724-3002
www.dhmh.state.md.us/perkins/

Sheilah Davenport, JD,MS,RN, CEO

3892 Crownsville Hospital Center
1520 Crownsville Road
Crownsville, MD 21032
410-729-6000
800-937-0938
Fax: 410-729-6800
TDD: 410-987-0416

Ron Hendler, Contact

3893 Eastern Shore Hospital Center
5262 Woods Road
Cambridge, MD 21613-0800
410-221-2300
Fax: 410-221-2534

Mary K Noren, Contact

3894 John L. Gildner Regional Institute for Children and Adolescents
15000 Broschart Road
Rockville, MD 20850-3392
301-251-6800
Fax: 301-309-9004
www.dhmh.state.md.us/jlgrica/

Thomas E. Pukalski, CEO
Claudette Bernstein, Medical Director
Debra K. VanHorn, Director of Comm. Res. & Dev.

John L. Gildner Regional Institute for Children and Adolescents (JLG-RICA) is a community-based, public residential, clinical, and educational facility serving children and adolescents with severe emotional disabilities. The program is designed to provide residential and day treatment for students in grades 5-12. JLG-RICA's goal is to successfully return its students to an appropriate family, community, and academic or vocational setting that will lead to happy and successful lives.

3895 Kennedy Krieger Institute
707 North Broadway
Baltimore, MD 21205
443-923-9200
E-mail: info@kennedykrieger.org
www.kennedykrieger.org

Gary W Goldstein MD, President

Dedicated to improving the lives of children and adolescents with pediatric developmental disabilities through patient care, special education, research, and professional training.

3896 Laurel Regional Hospital
7300 Van Dusen Road
Laurel, MD 20707-9266
301-725-4300
Fax: 410-792-2270
www.www.laurelregionalhospital.org

Douglas Shepherd, President

Laurel Regional Hospital is a full-service community hospital serving northern Prince George's County and Montgomery, Howard, and Anne Arundel Counties with 146 beds and 670 employees.

3897 RICA: Baltimore
605 S Chapel Gate Lane
Baltimore, MD 21229-3999
410-368-7800
877-203-5179
E-mail: pmakris@dhmh.state.md.us

Penny Makris, Contact

3898 RICA: Southern Maryland
9400 Surratts Road
Cheltenham, MD 20623-1324

301-372-1840
Fax: 301-372-1906
www.pgcps.org/~rica/

Mary Sheperd, Contact

3899 Sheppard Pratt at Ellicott City
4100 College Avenue
PO Box 0836
Ellicott City, MD 21043-5506
410-465-3322
800-883-3322
Fax: 410-465-1988
www.taylorhealth.com

To provide personal, high quality mental health services for your family, by our family of health care professionals.

3900 Spring Grove Hospital Center
Wade Avenue
Catonsville, MD 21228
410-402-6000
Fax: 410-402-7094

David Helsel MD, Contact

3901 Springfield Hospital Center
6655 Sykesville Road
Sykesville, MD 21784
410-970-7000
800-333-7564
E-mail: shc_admin@dhmh.state.md.us
www.dhmh.state.md.us/springfield

Paula Langmead, CEO
Janice Bowen, COO
Jonathan Book, Clinical Director

A regional psychiatric hospital operated by the State of Maryland, Department of Health and Mental Hygiene, Mental Hygiene Administration.

3902 Thomas B Finan Center
10102 Country Club Road
PO Box 1722
Cumberland, MD 21502-8339
301-777-2240
Fax: 301-777-2364

Judy Hott, Contact

3903 Upper Shore Community Mental Health Center
Scheeler Road #330
PO Box 229
Chestertown, MD 21620-0229
410-778-6800
888-784-0137
Fax: 410-778-1648
E-mail: lloughry@dhmh.state.md.us
www.www.dhmh.state.md.us

Lori A Loughry, Contact

3904 Walter P Carter Center
630 W Fayette Street
Baltimore, MD 21201-1585
410-209-6201
www.dhmh.state.md.us/carter

Archie Wallace, Contact

Massachusetts

3905 Arbour-Fuller Hospital
200 May Street
S Attleboro, MA 02703-5515
508-761-8500
800-828-3934
TTY: 800-974-6006
E-mail: arbourhealth@mindspring.com
www.arbourhealth.com

Gary Gilberti, CEO
Frank Kahr MD, Medical Director
Judith Merel, Director Marketing

Psychiatric hospital providing services to adults, adolesents and adults with developmental disabilities.

3906 Baldpate Hospital
83 Baldpate Road
Georgetown, MA 01833
978-352-2131
www.baldpate.com

3907 Berkshire Center
18 Park Street
Lee, MA 01238
413-243-2576
www.www.berkshirecenter.org

Michael McManmon, Executive Director

3908 Choate Health Management
23 Warren Avenue
Woburn, MA 01801-4979
781-933-6700
Fax: 781-469-5013

3909 Concord Family and Adolescent Services
A Division of Justice Resource Institute, Inc
380 Massachusetts Avenue
Acton, MA 01720
978-263-3006
Fax: 978-263-3088
www.jri.org

Gregory Canfield, Executive Director

Provides professional residential schools, group home, residence for homeless teens, alternative, therapeutic high school, education and parenting programs for children, adults and families throughouth Massachusetts.

3910 First Connections and Healthy Families
A Division of Justice Resource Institute, Inc
111 Old Road to NAC
Concord, MA 01742
978-287-0221
www.jri.org

Ellen Weistein, Director

First Conneections provides resources, education and support to families with children birth through age three. First Connections is dedicated to providing quality, comprehensive parenting support services to a diverse communities seeking resources to compliment and enrich their parenting experience.

3911 Grip Project
A Division of Justice Resource Institute, Inc
174 Central Square
Suite 433
Lowell, MA 01850

978-458-3622
www.jri.org

Rachel McNamara, Program Director

A by teens, for teens young people's program with residential services as a foundation. Grip serves young people, ages 16-20, who are homeless or aging out of foster-care/group homes and are committed to being independent. There is a separate residence for young women and men, both located in Lowell, MA.

3912 Littleton Group Home
A Division of Justice Resource Institute, Inc
22 King Street
Littleton, MA 01460
978-952-6809
www.jri.org

Donna Grisi, Program Director

Prepares young men, ages 13-18 for independent living by helping them to live respectful, dignified and increasingly responsible lives. The young men participate in after school activities and have daily access to the community.

3913 Meadowridge Pelham Academy
A Division of Justice Resource Institute, Inc
13 Pelham Road
Lexington, MA 02421
781-274-6800
www.jri.org

Andre Solomita, Program Director

A residential treatment program that focuses on the special challenges of adolescent girls with emotional and behavioral difficulties.The students, between the ages of 12-22, have typically experienced trauma and poor functioning in their personal, educational and/or family life.

3914 Meadowridge Walden Street School
A Division of Justice Resource Institute, Inc
148 Walden Street
Concord, MA 01742
978-369-7611
www.jri.org

Kari Beserra, Program Director

A residential school program that focuses on the challenges and special needs of adolescent females age 12-22 whom are coping with educational, emotional and behavioral difficulties.

3915 New England Home for Little Wanderers
271 Huntington Avenue
Boston, MA 02115
617-267-3700
888-466-3321
Fax: 617-267-8142
www.thehome.org

Joan Wallace-Benjamin, President/CEO
Susan P Curnan, VP Opeations/Outcomes
Kenneth E Hamberg, Executive VP/CFO

To ensure the healthy, emotional, mental and social development of children at risk, their families and communities.

3916 Sleep Disorders Unit of Beth Israel Hospital
330 Brookline Avenue
Boston, MA 02215

617-667-7000
Fax: 617-667-1134
www.bidmc.harvard.edu/home.asp
Jean K Matheson MD, Contact

Provides testing and treatment for those with sleep disorders and offers educational workshops, plus support for their families.

3917 Taunton State Hospital
PO Box 4007
Taunton, MA 02780-0997
508-977-3000

Katherine Chmiel, Contact

3918 Victor School
A Division of Justice Resource Institute, Inc
380 Massachusetts
Acton, MA 01720
978-266-1991
www.jri.org

Wendy Rosenblum, Program Director

A private, co-ed, therapeutic day school for students in grades 8-12 with a school philosophy that children learn when they can. Provides innovative and specialized educational and emotional support and treatment.

3919 Westboro State Hospital
Lyman Street
PO Box 288
Westboro, MA 01581-0288
508-616-2100
Fax: 508-616-2875

Joel Skolnick, COO

Michigan

3920 Caro Center
2000 Chambers Road
Caro, MI 48723-9296
989-673-3191

Rose Laskowski, Hospital Director

3921 E Lansing Center for Family
425 W Grand River Avenue
E Lansing, MI 48823-4201
517-332-8900

Provides mental health treatment.

3922 Hawthorn Center
18471 Haggerty Road
Northville, MI 48167
248-349-3000
Fax: 248-349-9552
www.michigan.gov/mdch

Dr Shobhana Joshi, Director

To provide high quality inpatient mental health services to emotionally disturbed children and adolescents.

3923 Kalamazoo Psychiatric Hospital
1312 Oakland Drive
PO Box A
Kalamazoo, MI 49008
269-337-3000

James J Coleman EdD, Contact

3924 Mount Pleasant Center
1400 W Pickard
Mount Pleasant, MI 48858
989-773-7921

George Garland, Contact

3925 Northpointe Behavioral Healthcare Systems
715 Pyle Drive
Kingsford, MI 49802-4456
906-774-0522
Fax: 906-774-1570
E-mail: info@nbhs.org
www.nbhs.org

Northpointe strives to improve the well being of individuals and families through the delivery of excellent person-centered mental health services.

3926 Samaritan Counseling Center
29887 W Eleventh Mile Road
Farmington Hills, MI 48336-1309
248-474-4701
E-mail: info@samaritancounselingmichigan.com
www.samaritancounselingmichigan.com

Dr. Wesley L Brun, Executive Director

Provides professional therapeutic counseling and educational services to all God's people seeking wholeness through emotional and spiritual growth.

3927 Walter P Ruther Psychiatric Hospital
30901 Palmer Road
Westland, MI 48186-5389
734-722-4500

Norma Joses MD, Contact

3928 Westlund Child Guidance Clinic
3253 Congress Avenue
Saginaw, MI 48602-3199
989-793-4790

Provides mental health services.

Minnesota

3929 Fergus Falls Regional Treatment Center
1400 N Union Avenue
Fergus Falls, MN 56537-1200
218-739-7200

Michael Ackley, Contact

3930 Metro Regional Treatment Center: Anoka
3300 4th Avenue N
Anoka, MN 55303-1119
763-576-5500
Fax: 763-712-4013

Judith Krohn, Contact

3931 St. Peter Regional Treatment Center
100 Freeman Drive
Saint Peter, MN 56082-1599
507-931-7100
TDD: 507-931-7825

Larry Te Brake, Forensic Site Director
Jim Behrends, Regional Administrator

3932 Willmar Regional Treatment Center
1550 Highway 71 NE
Willmar, MN 56201
320-231-5100

Sandra J Butturff, Site Director

Mississippi

3933 East Mississippi State Hospital
PO Box 4128, W Station
Meridian, MS 39304
601-482-6186
Fax: 601-483-5543
www.emsh.state.ms.us

Charles Carlisle, Director

To provide a continuum of behavioral health and long term care services for adults and adolescents in a caring, compassionate environment in which ethical principles guide decision making and resources are used responsibly and creatively.

3934 Mississippi State Hospital
PO Box 157-A
Whitfield, MS 39193
601-351-8018
E-mail: info@msh.state.ms.us
www.msh.state.ms.us

Facilitates improvement in the quality of life for Mississippians who are in need of psychiatric, chemical dependency or nursing home suvices by rehabilitating to the least restrictive environment utilizing a reange of psychiatric and medical services that reflect the accepted standard of care and are in compliance with statutory and regulatory guidlelines.

3935 North Mississippi State Hospital
1937 Briar Ridge Road
Tupelo, MS 38804
662-690-4200
Fax: 662-690-4261

Paul A Callens PhD, Contact

3936 South Mississippi State Hospital
823 Highway 589
Purvis, MS 39475
601-351-0100
www.smsh.state.ms.us

Wynona Winfield, Director

Provides the highest quality acute psychiatric care for adults who live in southern Mississippi

Missouri

3937 Edgewood Children's Center
330 N Gore Avenue
Saint Louis, MO 63119-1699
314-968-2060
Fax: 314-968-8308
E-mail: info@eccstl.org
www.eccstl.org

Wayne Crull, President/CEO
Latriece N Kimbrough, CFO

Provides compassionate care and treatmetn to restore children and strengthen families through intensive therapy, special education, case management and support services.

3938 Hyland Behavioral Health System
10020 Kennerly Road
Sappington, MO 63128-2106
314-525-7200
800-525-2032

Adult and pediatric psychiatric inpatient/partial services located at St. Anthony's Medical Center.

3939 Northwest Missouri Psychiatric Rehabilitation Center
3505 Frederick Avenue
Saint Joseph, MO 64506-2914
816-387-2300

Mary Attebury, COO

Inpatient care for long-term psychiatric/adult.

3940 Southeast Missouri Mental Health Center
1010 W Columbia Street
Farmington, MO 63640
573-218-6792
E-mail: cynthia.forsyth@dmh.mo.gov
www.dmh.missouri.gov/southeast

Melissa Ring, COO

People shall receive services focusing on strenghts and promoting opportunities beyond the limitations of mental illness.

3941 Western Missouri Mental Health Center
1000 E 24th Street
Kansas City, MO 64108
816-512-7000
www.dmh.missouri.gov/wmmhc

Offers services in alcoholism, drug, family, group and individual counseling, crisis intervention, group psychiatric therapy, and suicide prevention as well as hospital inpatient care, mental health aftercare and psychiatric care.

Nebraska

3942 Norfolk Regional Center
1700 N Victory Road
PO Box 1209
Norfolk, NE 68702-1209
402-370-3400
Fax: 402-370-3194

William Gibson, CEO
TyLynne Bauer, Facility Operating Officer

A progressive 120-bed state psychiatric hospital providing specialized psychiatric care to adults.

Nevada

3943 Behavioral Health Options: Sierra Health Services
2724 N Tenaya Way
Las Vegas, NV 89128
877-393-6094
www.sierrahealth.com

Anthony M Marlon, Chairman/CEO

to manage behavioral health services in the private and public sectors on a national basis, creating value for our customers, including brokers, employers, members, providers and shareholders

3944 Northern Nevada Adult Mental Health Services
480 Galletti Way
Sparks, NV 89431-5574
775-688-2001
Fax: 775-688-2052

David Rosin MD, Contact

3945 Southern Nevada Adult Mental Health Services
6161 W Charleston Boulevard
Las Vegas, NV 89146
702-486-6000
Fax: 702-486-6248

Jim Northrop PhD, Contact

New Hampshire

3946 Hampstead Hospital
218 E Road
Hamptead, NH 03841
603-229-5311
Fax: 603-329-4746
www.hampsteadhospital.com

Provides a full range of psychiatric and chemical dependency services for children, adolescents, adults and the elderly.

3947 New Hampshire State Hospital
36 Clinton Street
Concord, NH 03301-2359
603-271-5200
Fax: 603-271-5395

a state operated, publicly funded hospital providing a range of specialized psychiatric services. NHH advocates for and provides services that support an individual's recovery.

New Jersey

3948 Ann Klein Forensic Center
Stuyvesant Avenue
PO Box 7717
W Trenton, NJ 08628
609-633-0900
Fax: 609-633-0971
E-mail: mhs.affc-infoline@dhs.state.nj.us
www.state.nj.us/humanservices/pfnurse/ak-forensic.htm

A 200-bed psychiatric hospital serving a unique population that requires a secured environment. The facility provides care and treatment to individuals suffering from mental illness who are also within the legal system.

3949 Arthur Brisbane Child Treatment Center
Route 524
Farmingdale, NJ 07727
732-938-7803
Fax: 732-938-3102
E-mail: judy.gnad@dhs.state.nj.us
www.stae.nj.us/humanservices/pfnurses/brisbane.htm

Judy Gnad, Contact

A state-run facility for the treatment of youth between the ages of eleven and seventeen who require post acute psychiatric care.

3950 Greystone Park Psychiatric Hospital Greystone Park, NJ 07950
973-292-4096
Fax: 973-993-8782

E-mail: william.lanni@dhs.state.nj.us
www.state.nj.us/humanservices/pfnurses/greystone.htm

William Lanni, Contact

A 550 bed psychiattric hospital.

3951 Jersey City Medical Center Behavioral Health Center
50 Baldwin Avenue
Jersey City, NJ 07304
201-915-2000

3952 Senator Garrett Hagedorn Psychiatric Hospital
200 Sanitarium Road
Glen Gardner, NJ 08826-3291
908-537-3169
Fax: 908-537-3121
E-mail: jdecker@state.nj.us
www.state.nj.us/humanservices/pfnurse/hagedorn.htm

A 288 bed psychiatric hospital that provides quality interdisciplinary psychiatric services that maximize potential and community reintegration within a safe and caring environment.

New Mexico

3953 Life Transition Therapy
110 Delgado Street
Santa Fe, NM 87501
505-982-4183
800-547-2574
Fax: 505-982-9219
E-mail: info@lifetransition.com
www.lifetransition.com

Sabina Schultze, Therapist
Ralph Steele, Founder

To eliminate the fear, ignorance and conditioning that fuel racism and social injustice within the individual as well as in relationships, families, communities, and the world at large.

3954 New Mexico State Hospital
3695 Hot Springs Boulevard
Las Vegas, NM 87701-9575
505-454-2100
Fax: 505-454-2346

Felix Alderete, Contact

3955 Northern New Mexico Rehabilitation Center Las Vegas Medical Center
PO Box 1388
Las Vegas, NM 87701-1388
505-454-5100

Felix Alderete, Contact

3956 Sequoyah Adolescent Treatment Center
3405 W Pan American Freeway NE
Albuquerque, NM 87107
505-222-0355
www.health.state.nm.us/satc/SATCWeb.html

A 36 bed residential treatment center whose purpose is to provide care, treatment, and reintegration into society for adolescents who are violent or who have a history of violence and have a mental disorder and who are amenable to treatment.

New York

3957 Arms Acres
75 Seminary Hill Road
Carmel, NY 10512
845-225-3400
888-227-4641
Fax: 845-704-6182
www.armsacres.com

Patrice Wallace-Moore, CEO
Sultan Niazi, CFO
Michele Saari, Health Information Management

A private health care system providing high quality, cost-effective care to those suffering from alcoholism and chemical dependency and to the many whose lives are affected by the diseases of addiction.

3958 Berkshire Farm Center and Services for Youth
13640 State Route 22
Canaan, NY 12029-3504
518-781-4567
Fax: 518-781-4577
E-mail: info@berkshirefarm.org
www.berkshirefarm.org

Harith R Flagg, CEO

Mission is to strengthen children and their families so they can lives safely, independently and productively within their home communities.

3959 Bronx Children's Psychiatric Center
1000 Waters Place
Bronx, NY 10461-2799
718-239-3600
Fax: 718-826-4858
E-mail: bronxchildrens@omh.state.ny.us
www.omh.state.ny.us/omhweb/facilities/bcpc/facility.ht

3960 Bronx Psychiatric Center
1500 Waters Place
Bronx, NY 10461-2796
718-862-3300
Fax: 718-826-4858
E-mail: bronxpc@omh.state.ny.us
www.omh.state.ny.us/omhweb/facilities/brpc/facility.ht

A 360 bed facility that has three impatient services and a comprehensive outpatient program.

3961 Brooklyn Children's Center
1819 Bergen Street
Brooklyn, NY 11233-4513
718-221-4500
Fax: 718-221-4581
E-mail: bcc@omh.state.ny.us
www.omh.state.ny.us/omhweb/facilities/bkpc/facility.ht

Provides high quality comprehensive individualized mental health treatment services to serious emotionally disturbed children and adolescents in Brooklyn, and to continuously strive to improve the quality of those services.

3962 BryLin Hospitals
1263 Delaware Avenue
Buffalo, NY 14209
716-886-8200
800-727-9546
Fax: 716-889-1986

E-mail: info@brylin.com
www.brylin.com

Provides inpatient psychiatric services for children, adolescents, adults and geriatric patients. Outpatient services are offered to persons experiencing substance abuse problems.

3963 Buffalo Psychiatric Center
400 Forest Avenue
Buffalo, NY 14213
716-885-2261
Fax: 716-885-0937
E-mail: bufflopc@omh.state.ny.us
www.omh.state.ny.us/omhweb/facilities/bupc/facility.ht

Provides psychiatric quality inpatient, outpatient, residential, vocational, and wellness services to adults with serious mental illnesses

3964 Cabrini Medical Center
227 East 19th Street
New York, NY 10003
212-995-6000
E-mail: info@cabrininy.org
www.cabrininy.org

Voluntary hospital, sponsored by the Missionary Sisters of the Sacred Heart of Jesus that seeks to promote the teachings of the Gospel and of its foundress, St. Frances Xavier Cabrini.

3965 Capital District Psychiatric Center
75 New Scotland Avenue
Albany, NY 12208-3474
518-447-9611
Fax: 518-434-0041
www.omh.state.ny.us/omhweb/facilities/cdpc/facility.ht

Provides inpatient psychiatric treatment and rehabilitation to patients who have been diagnosed with serious and persistenet mental illnesses and for whom brief or short-term treatment in a community hospital mental health unit has been unable to provide sympton stability.

3966 Central New York Psychiatric Center
PO Box 300
Marcy, NY 13404-0300
315-765-3600
Fax: 315-765-3629
E-mail: cnypc@omh.state.ny.us
www.omh.state.ny.us/omhweb/facilities/cnpc/facility.ht

A comprehensive mental health service delivery system providing a full range of care and treatment to persons incarcerated in the New York State and county correctional system.

3967 Cornerstone of Rhinebeck
500 Milan Hollow Road
Rhinebeck, NY 12572
845-266-3481
800-266-4410
Fax: 245-266-8335
E-mail: admin@cornerstoneny.com
www.cornerstoneny.com

Provides inpatient chemical dependency treatment and offers a comprehensive range of inpatient and outpatient treatment services for alcohol and substance abuse.

3968 Creedmoor Psychiatric Center
79-25 Winchester Boulevard
Queens Village, NY 11427
718-264-4000
Fax: 718-264-3627
E-mail: crpc_info@omh.state.ny.us
www.omh.state.ny.us/omhweb/facilities/crpc/facility.ht

Kathleen Iverson, Executive Director

Provides a continuum of inpatient, outpatient and related psychiatric services with inpatient hospitalization at the main campus and five outpatient sites in the boroughs of Queens.

3969 Elmira Psychiatric Center
100 Washington Street
Elmira, NY 14901-2898
607-737-4711
Fax: 607-737-0158
E-mail: elmirapc@omh.state.ny.us
www.omh.state.ny.us/omhweb/facilities/elpc/facility.ht

Provides a wide array of comprehensive psychiatric services.

3970 Freedom Ranch
PO Box 24
Lakemont, NY 14857
607-243-8126
800-842-8679
E-mail: 14jd@freedomvillageusa.com
www.freedomvillageusa.com

Dr Fletcher Brothers, Founder

An extension of Freedom Village, Freedom Ranch offers a residential program for men 21 and older with substance abuse and emotional problems. Freedom Ranch is a faith-based program seeking to help men become productive members of society.

3971 Freedom Village USA
PO Box 24
Lakemont, NY 14857
607-243-8126
800-842-8679
E-mail: 14jd@freedomvillageusa.com
www.freedomvillageusa.com

Dr Fletcher Brothers, Founder

A not-for-profit residential campus for troubled teens. Offers a faith-based approach to teenagers in crisis or at risk. Students are required to make a voluntary one-year commitment to the program. Freedom Village has an 80% success rate with troubled teenagers.

3972 Gift of Life Home
PO Box 24
Lakemont, NY 14857
607-243-8126
800-842-8679
E-mail: 14jd@freedomvillageusa.com
www.freedomvillageusa.com

Dr Fletcher Brothers, Founder

An affiliate program of Freedom Village, USA, a residential program for troubled teenagers, the Gift of Life Home offers pregnant girls a safe haven, a place of refuge, where they can come and have their baby while transforming their life as well. Freedom Village is a faith-based alternative to other residential placements.

3973 Graham-Windham Services for Children and Families: Manhattan Mental Health Center
151 W 136th Street
Lenox & 7th Avenue
New York, NY
212-368-4100
E-mail: info@graham-windham.org

Offers mental health services to children from birth through 18 years and their families: individual, family and group therapy, psychiatric evaluation and medication management, psychological assessment. Family support services program offering advocacy, support and referrals to families with seriously emotionally disturbed children.

3974 Greater Binghamton Health Center
425 Robinson Street
Binghamton, NY 13904-1755
607-724-1391
Fax: 607-773-4387
E-mail: binghamton@omh.state.ny.us
www.omh.state.ny.us/omhweb/facilities/bipc/facility.ht

Provides comprehensive outpatient and inpatient services for adults and children who are seriously mentally ill.

3975 Hope House
517 Western Avenue
Albany, NY 12203
518-482-4673
Fax: 518-482-0873
E-mail: information@hopehouseinc.org
www.hopehouseinc.org

Don Smith, Executive Director
Mathhew Kawola, Dir Human Resources/Quality Ass.

Started helping the community in need of education, intervention and treatment for the persons affected by substance abuse.

3976 Hudson River Psychiatric Center
10 Ross Circle
Poughkeepsie, NY 12601-1078
845-452-8000
Fax: 845-452-8040
www.omh.state.ny.us/omhweb/facilities/hrpc/facility.ht

Serves the seriously and persistently mentally ill through inpatient care for 150 patients, including psychotherapy, psychoeducation groups, medication and a range of rehabilitation activities.

3977 Hutchings Psychiatric Center
620 Madison Street
Syracuse, NY 13210-2319
315-426-3600
Fax: 315-426-3603
www.omh.state.ny.us/omhweb/facilities/hupc/facility.ht

A comprehensive, community-based mental health facility providing an integrated network of inpatient and outpatient services for children and adults residing in the Central New York Region.

3978 Kingsboro Psychiatric Center
681 Clarkson Avenue
Brooklyn, NY 11203-2199
718-221-7700
Fax: 718-221-7206
E-mail: kingsboro@omh.state.ny.us
www.omh.state.ny.us/omhweb/facilities/kbpc/facility.ht

Provides competent compassionate psychiatric care to people with serious mental illness with a purpose of reintegrating them to the community.

3979 Kirby Forensic Psychiatric Center
600 E 125th Street
New York, NY 10035
646-672-5800
Fax: 646-672-6893
E-mail: kirbypc@omh.state.ny.us
www.ohm.state.ny.us/omhweb/facilities/krpc/facility.ht

A maximum security hospital of the New York State Office of Mental Health that provides secure treatment and evaluation for the forensic patients and courts of New York City and Long Island.

3980 Liberty Resources
1065 James Street
Suite 200
Syracuse, NY 13203
315-425-1004
E-mail: info@liberty-resource.org
www.liberty-resource.org

Carl Coyle, CEO
Michael Sayles, President

Provides residential and non-residential services to individuals and families, our present array of services include Mental Health; Mental Retardation and Developmental Disabilities; services for individuals living with HIV/AIDS, families and youth involved in the child welfare system, domestic violence services; services to persons in recovery; and diversified case management services.

3981 Manhattan Psychiatric Center
600 E 125th Street
New York, NY 10035-6098
646-672-6767
Fax: 646-672-6446
E-mail: mpcinfo@omh.state.ny.us
www.omh.state.ny.us/omhweb/facilities/mapc/facility.ht

Offers inpatient and outpatient treatment for adults with mental illness.

3982 Mid-Hudson Forensic Psychiatric Center
Box 158, Route 17-M
New Hampton, NY 10958
845-374-3171
Fax: 845-374-3961
E-mail: midhudsonfpc@omh.state.ny.us
www.omh.state.ny.us/omhweb/facilities/mhpc/facility.ht

A secure adult psychiatric center that provides a comprehensive program of evaluation, treatment, and rehabilitation for patients admitted by court order.

3983 Middletown Psychiatric Center
122 Dorothea Dix Drive
Middletown, NY 10940-6198
845-342-5511
Fax: 845-342-4975
E-mail: midokmw@lmh.state.ny.us
www.omh.state.ny.us/omhweb/facilities/mipc/facility.ht

Offers contemporary treatment for adults with complex mental illnesses.

3984 Mohawk Valley Psychiatric Center
1400 Noyes at York
Utica, NY 13502-3802
315-738-3800
Fax: 315-738-4414
E-mail: mvpc@omh.state.ny.us
www.omh.state.ny.us/omhweb/facilities/mvpc/facility.ht

Provides quality, individualized psychiatric treatment and rehabilitation services that promote recovery.

3985 Nathan S Kline Institute
140 Old Orangeburg Road
Orangeburg, NY 10962
845-398-5500
Fax: 845-398-5510
E-mail: webmaster@nki.rfmh.org
www.rfmh.org/nki

Harold S Koplewicz MD, Director
Jerome Levine MD, Deputy Director

As one of our nation's premier centers of excellence in mental health research, a broad range of studies are conducted at NKI, including basic, clinical, and services research. All of our work is intended to improve care for people suffering from these complex, psychobiologically-based, severely disabling mental disorders.

3986 New York Psychiatric Institute
1051 Riverside Drive
New York, NY 10032
212-543-5000
www.nyspi.org

Jeffrey Lieberman, Chairman

3987 Odyssey House
95 Pine Street
New York, NY 10005
212-361-1600
Fax: 212-361-1666
E-mail: info@odysseyhouseinc.org
www.odysseyhouseinc.org

Peter Provet, President

Develops innovative treatment models to ensure that our systems take into account current research, utilizing what works most effectively to help these individuals overcome their difficulties and build a stable, producitve, drug-free life.

3988 Pahl Transitional Apartments
559-565 Sixth Avenue
Troy, NY 12182
518-237-9891
Fax: 518-237-9409
E-mail: michael_kennedy@pahlinc.org
www.pahlinc.org

Michael Kennedy, Clinical Director

A 9-12 month residential, chemical dependency treatment facility for males ages 16-25. The goal for the residents is to learn the skills necessary for long-term recovery and independent living.

3989 Phoenix House
164 West 74th Street
New York, NY 10023
212-595-5810
www.phoenixhouseusa.org

Mitchell S Rosenthal, President

Reclaims disordered lives, encourages individual responsibility, positive behavior, and personal growth, also strengthens families and communities, and safeguards public health. Also, promotes a drug-free society through prevention, treatment, education and training, research, and advocacy.

3990 Pilgrim Psychiatric Center
998 Crooked Hill Road
West Brentwood, NY 11717-1087
631-761-3500
Fax: 631-761-2600
E-mail: pilgriminfo@omh.state.ny.us
www.omh.state.ny.us/omhweb/facilities/pgpc/facility.ht

Provides excellent, integrated care in evaluation, treatment, crisis intervention, rehabilitation, support, and self help/empowerment service to individuals with serious psychiatric illness.

3991 Queens Children's Psychiatric Center
74-03 Commonwealth Boulevard
Bellerose, NY 11426
718-264-4500
Fax: 718-740-0968
E-mail: queenscpc@omh.state.ny.us
www.omh.state.ny.us/omhweb/facilities/qcpc/facility.ht

Serves seriously emotionally disturbed children and adolescents from the ages of 5 through 18 in a range of programs including Inpatient hospitalization, outpatient clinic treatment, intensive case management, homemaker services and community education and consultation services.

3992 Rochester Psychiatric Center
1111 Elmwood Avenue
Rochester, NY 14620-3972
585-241-1200
Fax: 585-241-1424
TTY: 585-241-1982
E-mail: rochesterpc@omh.state.ny.us
www.omh.state.ny.us/omhweb/facilities/ropc/facility.ht

Provides quality comprehensive treatment and rehabilitation services to people with psychiatric disabilities working toward recovery.

3993 Rockland Children's Psychiatric Center
599 Convent Road
Orangeburg, NY 10962-1199
845-680-4000
800-597-8481
Fax: 845-680-8905
E-mail: rocklandcpc@omh.state.ny.us
www.omh.state.ny.us/omhweb/facilities/rcpc/facility.ht

A psychiatric hospital exclusively for children and adolescents

3994 Rockland Psychiatric Center
140 Old Orangeburg Road
Orangeburg, NY 10962
845-359-1000
Fax: 845-359-3143
E-mail: rocklandpc@omh.state.ny.us
www.omh.state.ny.us/omhweb/facilities/rppc/facility.ht

Provides treatment, rehabilitation, and support to adults 18 and older with severe and complex mental illness.

3995 Sagamore Children's Psychiatric Center
197 Half Hollow Road
Dix Hills, NY 11746
631-370-1700
Fax: 631-370-1714
E-mail: scisdcc@omh.state.ny.us
www.omh.state.ny.us/omhweb/facilities/scpc/facility.ht

Programs for youngsters and their families include inpatient hospitalization, day hospitalization, day treatment, outpatient clinic treatment, mobile mental health team crisis services, information and referral, and community consultation and training.

3996 Samaritan Village
138-02 Queens Blvd
Briarwood, NY 11435
718-206-2000
800-532-4357
Fax: 718-657-6982
www.samaritanvillage.org

Mission is to eliminate the devastating impact of substance abuse on individuals, families and communities by helping addicted men and women take responsibility for their own recovery.

3997 South Beach Psychiatric Center
777 Seaview Avenue
Staten Island, NY 10305-3499
718-667-2300
Fax: 718-667-2344
E-mail: sbcsmss@omh.state.ny.us
www.omh.state.ny.us/omhweb/facilities/sbpc/facility.ht

Provides intermediate level inpatient services to persons living in western Brooklyn, southern Staten Island, and Manhattan south of 42nd street.

3998 St. Lawrence Psychiatric Center
1 Chimney Point Drive
Ogdensburg, NY 13669
315-541-2001
Fax: 315-541-2013
E-mail: slpcinfo@omh.state.ny.us
www.omh.state.ny.us/omhweb/facilities/slpc/facility.ht

3999 Veritas Villa
5 Ridgeview Road
Kerhonkson, NY 12446
845-626-3555
Fax: 845-626-3840
E-mail: info@veritasvilla.com
www.veritasvilla.com

Jim Cusack, Founder

Inpatient rehabilitation and wellness center

4000 Western New York Children's Psychiatric Center
1010 E & W Road
W Seneca, NY 14224
716-677-7000
Fax: 716-675-6455
E-mail: westernnewyorkcpc@omh.state.ny.us
www.omh.state.ny.us/omhweb/facilities/wcpc/facility.ht

Jed Cohen, Contact

Provides high quality, comprehensive behavioral health care services to seriously emotionally disturbed children and adolescents, and to partner with their families throughout the continuum of care.

North Carolina

4001 Broughton Hospital
1000 S Sterling Street
Morganton, NC 28655
828-433-2111
E-mail: BH.Information@NCMail.net
www.broughtonhospital.org

Dr Art Robarge, Interim Hospital Director/CEO

4002 Central Regional Hospital
1003 12th Street
Butner, NC 27509-1626
919-575-7100
www.dhhs.state.nc.us/mhddsas/centralhospital/index.htm

Formed by the merger of Dorothea Dix Hospital and John Umstead Hospital. Services include adult psychiatric services, clinical research services, child and adolescent services, medical services, and geropsychiatric services.

4003 Cherry Hospital
201 Stevens Mill Road
Goldsboro, NC 27530-1057
919-731-3204
www.cherryhospital.org

Jerry Edwards, Contact

4004 Dorthea Dix Hospital
820 S Boylan Avenue
Raleigh, NC 27603-2176
919-733-5540
Fax: 919-715-0707
www.dhhs.state.nc.us/mhddsas/DIX/

Mike Pedneau, Contact

North Dakota

4005 North Dakota State Hospital
2605 Circle Drive
Jamestown, ND 58401-6905
701-253-3650
Fax: 701-253-3999
TTY: 701-253-3880
www.nd.gov/humanservices/locations/statehospital

Alex Schweitzer EdD, Contact

Ohio

4006 Appalachian Behavioral Healthcare System
Athens Campus
100 Hospital Drive
Athens, OH 45701-2301
740-594-5000
800-372-8862

Don W Mobley, CEO
Mark McGee MD, CCO
Kelly Douglas-Markins, Hospital Manager

40 Bed inpatient psychiatric facility.

4007 Central Behavioral Healthcare
5965 Renaissance Place
Toledo, OH 43623

419-882-5678
www.centralbehavioralhealthcare.com

Kerry C Buhk PhD, Clinical Psychologist

Provides patients with a broad range of high-quality behavioral healthcare in a professional and personal matter.

4008 Clermont Counseling Center
4 Cecelia Drive
Amelia, OH 45102
513-947-7025
800-732-9805
Fax: 513-947-7055
TTY: 513-947-0333

Patricia Burke, Executive Director

Provides comprehensive mental health services to adults and families who are confronted with emotional difficulties, family and relationship problems or abuse and mental illness.

Year Founded: 1973

4009 Hannah Neil Center for Children
301 Obetz Road
Columbus, OH 43207-4092
614-491-5784
E-mail: suzan@worldofchildren.org

Randy Copas, Director

The Hannah Neil Center for Children serves children who suffer from severe behavioral and emotional difficulties.

4010 Heartland Behavioral Healthcare
3000 Erie Street S
Massillon, OH 44648-0540
330-833-3135
Fax: 330-833-6564

G Eric Carpenter, MPA, CEO

4011 Medina CFIT
Heartland Behavioral Healthcare
3076-A Remsen Road
Medina, OH 44256
330-722-0750
Fax: 330-723-0068

Charles Johnston, Contact

4012 Millcreek Children's Services
6600 Paddock Road
PO Box 16006
Cincinnati, OH 45237-3983
513-948-3983

Peter Steele, Contact

4013 Northcoast Behavioral Healthcare System
Cleveland Campus
1708 Southpoint Drive
Cleveland, OH 44109-1999
216-787-0500

George P Gintoli, Contact

4014 Northcoast Behavioral Healthcare System
Northfield Campus
PO Box 305
Northfield, OH 44067-0305
330-467-7131
Fax: 330-467-2420

George P Gintoli, Contact

4015 Northwest Psychiatric Hospital
930 S Detroit Avenue
Toledo, OH 43614-2701
419-381-1881

Terrance Smith, Contact

4016 Sagamore Children's Services: Woodside CSN
Woodside CSN
419 Main Avenue SW
Warren, OH 44481
330-742-2593

Charles Johnston, Contact

4017 Twin Valley Behavioral Healthcare
Dayton Campus, 2611 Wayne Avenue
Dayton, OH 45420-1800
937-258-0440
Fax: 937-258-6218
TDD: 937-258-6257

Robert Short, CEO

State operated BHD serving severley mentally ill adults in partnership with the community.

4018 Twin Valley Psychiatric System
Columbus Campus, 2200 W Broad Street
Columbus, OH 43223-1295
614-752-0333

James Ignelzi, Chief Executive Officer

Oklahoma

4019 Griffin Memorial Hospital
900 E Main Street
PO Box 151
Norman, OK 73070-0151
405-321-4880
Fax: 405-522-8320

Don Bowen, Contact

4020 Northwest Center for Behavioral Health
1222 10th Street
Woodward, OK 73801
580-571-3233
Fax: 580-256-8609
www.odmhsas.org

Trudy Hoffman, Contact

Comprehensive regional behavioral health center.

4021 Oklahoma Forensic Center
PO Box 69
Vinita, OK 74301-0069
918-256-7841
Fax: 918-256-4491

William Burkett, Contact

4022 Oklahoma Youth Center
320 12th Avenue
PO Box 1008
Norman, OK 73071-1008
405-364-9004
Fax: 405-573-3804

Paul Bouffard, Contact

4023 Willow Crest Hospital
130 A Street Southwest
Miami, OK 74354
918-542-1836
www.willowcresthospital.com

Oregon

4024 Blue Mountain Recovery Center
2600 Westgate
Pendleton, OR 97801
541-276-0810
Fax: 541-278-2209

Kerry Kelly, Contact

4025 Oregon State Hospital: Portland
1121 NE 2nd Avenue
Portland, OR 97232
503-731-8620
www.oregon.gov/dhs/mentalhealth/osh/main.shtml

Maynard Hammer, Interim Superintendent

4026 Oregon State Hospital: Salem
2600 Center Street NE
Salem, OR 97301
503-945-2800
www.oregon.gov/dhs/mentalhealth/osh/main.shtml

Maynard Hammer, Interim Superintendent

4027 St. Mary's Home for Boys
16535 SW Tualatin Valley Highway
Beaverton, OR 97006-5199
503-649-5651
E-mail: reception@stmaryshomeforboys.org
www.stmaryshomeforboys.org

Founded in 1889 as an orphanage for abandoned and way-ward children, today St. Mary's is a private, non-profit organization that offers comprehensive residential, day treatment and mental health services to at-risk boys between the ages of 10 and 17 who are emotionally disturbed and/or disruptive behavior disordered.

Pennsylvania

4028 Allentown State Hospital
1600 Hanover Avenue
Allentown, PA 18103-2498
610-740-3400

Gregory Smith, Contact

4029 Center For Prevention and Rehabilitation
26 Conneaut Lake Road
Greenville, PA 16125-2167
724-588-3001

4030 Clarks Summit State Hospital
1451 Hillside Drive
Clarks Summit, PA 18411-9505
570-587-7250

Thomas P Comerford Jr, Contact

4031 Craig Academy
751 N Negley Avenue
Pittsburg, PA 15206

412-361-2801
Fax: 412-536-5675
www.craigacademy.org

Operates a psychiatric partial day program and private elementary, middle, and high school programs.

4032 MHNet
1060 First Avenue
Suite 201
King of Prussia, PA 19406
888-638-7491
E-mail: edwynl@integra-ease.com
www.integra-ease.com

Wesley J Brockhoeft, PhD, President/CEO
Peter Harris, MD, Corporate Medical Director
Robert Wilson, CFO
Richard T Wright, SVP Business Development

MHNet is an outgrowth of the Center for Individual and Family Counseling, a multi-disciplinary outpatient treatment clinic with a full spectrum behavioral health organization with national service delivery capability.

Year Founded: 1981

4033 Mayview State Hospital
1601 Mayview Road
Bridgeville, PA 15017-1599
412-257-6200

Shirley Dumpman MPH, Contact

4034 Montgomery County Project SHARE
538 Dekalb Street
Norristown, PA 19401
610-272-7997
800-688-4226
E-mail: mcps@mhasp.org
www.mhasp.org

Victor Witherspoon, Director

Serving people with mental health disabilities in Montgomery County.

Year Founded: 1988

4035 National Mental Health Self-Help Clearinghouse
1211 Chestnut Street
Suite 1207
Philadephia, PA 19017
215-751-1810
800-553-4539
Fax: 215-636-6312
www.mhselfhelp.org

Joseph Rogers, Executive Director

A national consumer technical assistance center, has played a major role in the development of the mental health consumer movement.

Year Founded: 1986

4036 Norristown State Hospital
1001 Sterigere Street
Norristown, PA 19401-5399
610-313-1000
Fax: 610-313-1013

Gerald P Kent, CEO

4037 Renfrew Center Foundation
475 Spring Lane
Philadelphia, PA 19128
877-367-3383
Fax: 215-482-2695
E-mail: foundation@renfrew.org
www.renfrew.org

Susan Ice MD, VP/Medical Director

A tax-exempt, nonprofit organization advancing the education, prevention, research, and treatment of eating disorders.

4038 State Correctional Institution at Waymart Forensic Treatment Center
PO Box 256
Waymart, PA 18472-0256
570-488-5811
Fax: 570-488-2558

Stephen A Zoburt PhD, Contact

4039 Torrance State Hospital
PO Box 111
Torrance, PA 15779-0111
724-459-4511

Richard Stillwagon, Contact

4040 Warren State Hospital
33 Main Drive
N Warren, PA 16365-5099
814-723-5500
Fax: 814-726-4119

Carmen Ferranto, Contact

4041 Wernersville State Hospital
PO Box 300
Wernersville, PA 19565-0300
610-678-3411
Fax: 610-670-4101

Kenneth Ehrhart, Contact

Rhode Island

4042 Butler Hospital
345 Blackstone Boulevard
Providence, RI 02906
401-455-6200
E-mail: info@butler.org
www.butler.org

John J Hynes, President/CEO

Rhode Island's only private, nonprofit psychiatric and substance abuse hospital for adults, adolescents, children and seniors.

4043 Gateway Healthcare
249 Roosevelt Avenue
Suite 205
Pawtucket, RI 02860
401-724-8400
Fax: 401-724-8488
E-mail: developmentoffice@gatewayhealth.org
www.gatewayhealth.org

Richard Leclerc, Presiden
Scott W DiChristofero, VP Finance
Stephen Chabot MD, Medical Director

To promote resiliency and to assist people in their recovery from mental health, substance abuse, and behavioral and emotional disorder

4044 Groden Center

86 Mount Hope Avenue
Providence, RI 02906
401-274-6310
Fax: 401-421-3280
E-mail: grodencenter@grodencenter.org
www.grodencenter.org

Peggy Stocker, Admissions Coordinator

Groden Center has been providing day and residential treatment and educational services to children and youth who have developmental and behavioral difficulties and their families. By providing a broad range of individualized services in the most normal and least restrictive settings possible, children and youth learn skills that will help them engage in typical experiences and interact more successfully with others. Education and treatment take place in Groden Center classrooms, in the student's homes, and in the community with every effort made to maintain typical family and peer relationships. Call or visit our web site for more information about the Center and the publications and materials we have available.

Year Founded: 1976

South Carolina

4045 CM Tucker Jr Nursing Care Center

2200 Harden Street
Columbia, SC 29203
803-737-5300
www.state.sc.us/dmh/cmtucker_dowdy

Laura W Hughes, RN, BSN, MPH, Director

Provides excellence in resident care in an environment of concern and compassion that is respectful to others, adaptive to change and accountable for outcome.

4046 Earle E Morris Jr Alcohol & Drug Treatment Center

610 Faison Drive
Columbia, SC 29203
803-935-7100
www.state.sc.us/dmh/morris_village

Provides effective treatment of chemical dependence through comprehensive evaluation, safe detoxification, and state-of-the-art treatment servies.

4047 G Werber Bryan Psychiatric Hospital

220 Faison Drive
Columbia, SC 29203
803-935-7140
Fax: 803-935-7110
www.state.sc.us/dmh/bryan

A 277 bed short term intensive care facility that serves adult and geriatric patients ages 16 years and older. Provides therapeutic services in a warm and nurturing environment for individuals in crisis.

4048 James F Byrnes Medical Center

2100 Bull Street
Box 119
Columbia, SC 29202-0119
803-254-9325
Fax: 803-734-0779

Jaime E Condom MD, Contact

4049 Patrick B Harris Psychiatric Hospital

130 Highway 252
PO Box 2907
Anderson, SC 29622-2907
864-231-2600
Fax: 864-225-3297
www.patrickbharrispsychiatrichospital.com

John Fletcher, CEO

Provides intensive, short-term, psychiatric diagnostic and treatment services on a 24 hour, emergency voluntary and involuntary basis.

4050 South Carolina State Hospital

2100 Bull Street
Columbia, SC 29202
803-898-2038

Jaime E Condon MD, Contact

Psychiatric hospital

4051 William S Hall Psychiatric Institute

1800 Colonial Drive
PO Box 202
Columbia, SC 29292-0202
803-898-1693

Dalmer Sercy, Contact

South Dakota

4052 South Dakota Human Services Center

3515 Broadway Avenue
PO Box 7600
Yankton, SD 57078-7600
605-668-3100
Fax: 605-668-3460
www.dhs.sd.gov/hsc

Cory Nelson, Administrator

Tennessee

4053 Cherokee Health Systems

2018 Weestern Avenue
Koxville, TN 37921
865-544-0406
Fax: 865-934-6780
www.cherokeehealth.com

Dr Dennis Freeman, CEO

Uses an integrated model to provide behavioral health and primary care services in a community-based setting.

Year Founded: 1960

4054 Lakeshore Mental Health Institute

5908 Lyons View Drive
Knoxville, TN 37919-7598
865-584-1561

Lee Thomas, Chief Officer

4055 Memphis Mental Health Institute

951 Court Avenue
Memphis, TN 38103
901-577-1800

Dr Jeanne West-Freeman, Interim Chief Officer

4056 Middle Tennessee Mental Health Institute
221 Stewarts Ferry Pike
Nashville, TN 37214-3325
615-902-7400

Lynn McDonald, Chief Officer

4057 Moccasin Bend Mental Health Institute
Moccasin Bend Road
Chattanooga, TN 37405
423-265-2271

William Ventress, Chief Officer

4058 Three Springs LEAPS
Three Springs
PO Box 297
Centerville, TN 37033
931-729-5040
Fax: 931-729-9525

Robert Moore, Director Admissions
Susan Hardy, Program Administrator
Glenn Drew, Program Director

The 90-day outdoor therapeutic program near Centerville, Tennessee is accredited by JCAHO. Boys ages 13-17 just beginning to have difficulty with behavioral issues, substance abuse, and school difficulties will be considered for admission. The program offers intensive adventure based bimonthly trips such as canoeing, hiking, and mountain biking. Family therapy modules are offered to family members. Specialty groups for such issues as grief or substance abuse are offered. The boys attend the private SACS accredited school on campus. Price: $180 per diem; $16,200 for 90 days. Work with some third-party payors.

4059 Western Mental Health Institute
Highway 64 W
Bolivar, TN 38074
731-228-2000

Roger Pursley, Chief Officer

4060 Woodridge Hospital
403 State of Franklin Road
Johnson City, TN 37604
423-928-7111
800-346-8899
www.msha.com/Facility.cfm?id=479

Dr. Donald W Larkin, Administrator
Kim Cudebec, Clinical Director

Texas

4061 Austin State Hospital
4110 Guadalupe Street
Austin, TX 78751
512-452-0381
Fax: 512-419-2163
www.dshs.state.tx.us/mhhospitals/AustinSH/default.shtm

Carl Schock, Superintendent

Provides adult psychiatric services, specialty adult services and child and adolescent psychiatric services.

4062 Big Spring State Hospital
1901 N Highway 87
Big Spring, TX 79721
432-267-8213
Fax: 432-268-7263

E-mail: edward.moughon@dshs.state.tx.us
www.dshs.state.tx.us/mhhospital/bigspringssh/default

Edward Moughon, Superintendent

A 195-bed psychiatric hospital that provides hospitalization for people 18 years of age and older with psychiatric illnesses in a 57-county area in West Texas and the Texas Panhandle.

4063 Choices Adolescent Treatment Center
4521 Karnack Hwy
Marshall, TX 75670
903-938-4455
800-638-0880
E-mail: choices@sydcom.net
www.choicestreatment.com

Choices residential treatment program focuses on adolescents which abuse substances and addresses related psychiatric disorders.

4064 Dallas Metrocare Services
1380 Riverbend Drive
Dallas, TX 75247
214-743-1200
Fax: 214-630-3642
www.dallasmetrocare.com

James G Baker, CEO

Serves the neighbors with developmental or mental health challenges by helping them find lives that are meaningful and satisfying

4065 El Paso Psychiatric Center
4615 Alameda Avenue
El Paso, TX 79905
915-532-2202
Fax: 915-534-5587
E-mail: zulema.carrillo@dshs.state.tx.us
www.dshs.state.tx.us/mhhospitals/elpasopc/default.shtm

Zulema C Carrillo, CEO

A 74-bed psychiatric hospital that provides hospitalization to the citizens of far West Texas.

4066 Green Oaks Behavioral Healthcare Service
7808 Clodus Fields Drive
Dallas, TX 75251
972-991-9504
Fax: 972-789-1865
www.greenoakspsych.com

Committed to developing and emulating the latest, most effective clinical practices always, and, in all things, to promote dignity, holding compassion and respect for patients and their families as the absolute standard.

4067 Homeward Bound
233 West 10th Street
Dallas, TX 75208
214-941-3500
E-mail: ddenton@homewardboundinc.org
www.homewardboundinc.org

Douglas Denton, Executive Director

Offers chemical dependence treatment for the indigent population anad those referred by the criminal justice system, local hospitals and private practitioners.

4068 Jewish Family and Children's Services
12500 NW Military Highway
Suite 250
San Antonio, TX 78231-1871
210-302-6920

Jennifer Rosenblatt, President
Frank J Villani, Executive Director
LaDina Epstein, Associate Director

To strengthen community values, promote human dignity and enhance self-sufficiency of individuals and families through social, psychological, health educaitonal and financial support programs.

Year Founded: 1974

4069 Kerrville State Hospital
721 Thompson Drive
Kerrville, TX 78028-5154
830-896-2211
Fax: 830-792-4926
www.dshs.state.tx/us/mhhospitals/kerrvillesh/default.s

Stephen Anfinson, Superintendent

provides care for persons with major mental illnesses who need the safety, structure, and resources of an in-patient setting

4070 La Hacienda Treatment Center Hunt, TX 78024
800-749-6160
E-mail: info@lahacienda.com
www.lahacienda.com

Provides treatment for alcoholism and other chemical dependencies

4071 Laurel Ridge Treatment Center
17720 Corporate Woods Drive
San Antonio, TX 78259
210-491-9400
Fax: 210-491-3550
www.psysolutions.com

A psychiatric hospital offering a comprehensive continuum of behavioral healthcare services including acute programs for children, adolescents and adults and residential treatment for children and adolescents.

4072 Macon W Freeman Center
1401 Columbus Avenue
Waco, TX 76703
254-753-8251
Fax: 254-753-5881
E-mail: dworley@thefreemancenter.org
www.thefreemancenter.org

Tim Martindale, Medical Director
Gerald Elliot, Program Manager

Provides a chemical free environment in which professional guidance and peer support allow each client to work toward achievement of individualized treatment goals.

4073 New Horizons Ranch and Center
PO Box 549
Goldthwaite, TX 76844
915-938-5518
www.newhorizonsinc.com

To provide an environment where children, families and staff are able to heal and grow through caring relationships and unconditional love and acceptance.

4074 North Texas State Hospital: Vernon Campus
4730 College Drive
Vernon, TX 76385
940-552-9901
Fax: 940-553-2500
E-mail: jamese.smith@dshs.state.tx.us
www.dshs.state.tx.us/mhhospitals/default.shtm

James E Smith, Superintendent

4075 North Texas State Hospital: Wichita Falls Campus
6515 Lake Road
Wichita Falls, TX 76307-0300
940-692-1220
Fax: 940-689-5538
E-mail: jamese.smith@dshs.state.tx.us
www.dshs.state.tx.usmhhospitals/northtexassh/default

James E Smith, Superintendent

4076 Rio Grande State Center
1401 South Rangerville
Harlingen, TX 78551-2668
956-364-8000
Fax: 956-364-8497
www.dshs.state.tx.us/mhhospitals/riograndesc/default

Sonia Hernandez-Keeble, Superintendent

The only public provider south of San Antonio, Texas that offers healthcare, inpatient mental health services and long term mental retardation services.

4077 Rusk State Hospital
805 North Dickinson Drive
Rusk, TX 75785
903-683-3421
Fax: 903-683-7101
E-mail: ted.debbs@dshs.state.tx.us
www.dshs.state.tx.us/mhhospitals/rusksh/default.shtm

Ted Debbs, Superintendent

An inpatient hospital providing psychiatric treatment and care for citizens primarily from the East Texas region.

4078 San Antonio State Hospital
6711 South New Braunfels
Suite 100
San Antonio, TX 78223-3006
210-532-8811
Fax: 210-531-7876
E-mail: robert.arizpe@dshs.state.tx.us
www.dshs.state.tx.us/mhhospitals/sanantoniosh/default

Robert Arizpe, Superintendent

Provides intensive inpatient diagnostic, treatment, rehabilitative, and referral servious for seriously mentally ill persons from South Texas regardless of their financial status.

4079 Shades of Hope Treatment Center
PO Box 639
Buffalo Gap, TX 79508
800-588-4673
www.shadesofhope.com

Tennie McCarty, Founder/CEO

A residential and outpatient all-addictions treatment center specializing in the intensive treatment of eating disorders.

4080 Starlite Recovery Center
230 Mesa Verde Drive East
PO Box 317
Center Point, TX 78010
866-220-1626
Fax: 830-634-2532
E-mail: info@starliterecovery.com
www.starliterecovery.com

Kirk Kureska, Executive Director

Provides the highest quality of care in a cost-effective manner, insuring that our valued clients receive treatment that will allow them to return to a productive way of life.

4081 Terrell State Hospital
1200 East Brin
Terrell, TX 75160
972-524-6452
Fax: 972-551-8053
www.dshs.state.tx.us/mhhospitals/terrellsh/default.sht

A 316 bed, Joint Commission accredited and Medicare certified, psychiatric inpatient hospital, that is responsible for providing services for individuals with mental illnesses residing within a 19 county, 12,052 square mile service region, with a population of over 3 million.

4082 University of Texas Harris County Psychiatri c Center
2800 S MacGregor Way
Houston, TX 77021
713-741-5000
Fax: 713-741-5939
www.http://hcpc.uth.tmc.edu

Robert Guynn MD, Executive Director

Delivers a comprehensive program of psychiatric services to children, adolescents and adults suffering from mental illness.

4083 Waco Center for Youth
3501 N 19th Street
Waco, TX 76708
254-756-2171
Fax: 254-745-5398
E-mail: eddie.greenfield@dshs.state.tx.us
www.dshs.state.tx.us/mhhospitals/wacocenterforyouth/

Eddie Greenfield, Director

A psychiatric residential treatment facility that serves teen-agers, ages 13 through 17, with emotional difficulties and/or behavioral problems.

Utah

4084 Utah State Hospital
1300 E Center Street
Provo, UT 84606-3554
801-344-4400
Fax: 801-344-5398
E-mail: jgierisch@utah.gov
www.ush.utah.gov

provides excellent care in a safe and respectful environment to promote hope and quality of life for individuals with mental illness

Vermont

4085 Brattleboro Retreat
Anna Marsh Lane
PO Box 803
Brattleboro, VT 05301
802-257-7785
Fax: 802-258-3791
www.bratretreat.org

Robert E Simpson Jr, President/CEO

A not-for-profit health services organization which, above all else, is committed to assisting individuals to improve their health and functioning.

4086 Spring Lake Ranch
1169 Spring Lake Road
Cuttingville, VT 05738
802-492-3322
Fax: 802-492-3331
E-mail: springlakeranch@mindspring.com
www.springlakeranch.org

Offers an alternative therapeutic treatment program for adults with mental illness and/or substance abuse. Our work program and community life help residents grow and recover in the beautiful Green Mountains of Vermont. Our goal is to help people move from hospitalization or period of crisis to an independent life.

Year Founded: 1932

4087 Vermont State Hospital
103 South Main Street
Waterbury, VT 05671-2501
802-241-1000
www.state.vt.us/dmh

Bertold Francke MD, Contact

Virginia

4088 Catawba Hospital
5525 Catawba Hospital Drive
Catawba, VA 24070-2115
540-375-4201
800-451-5544
www.catawba.dmhmrsas.virginia.gov

Jack L Wood, Director

To support the continuous process of recovery by providing quality psychiatric services to those individuals entrusted to our care

4089 Central State Hospital
26317 West Washington Street
PO Box 4030
Petersburg, VA 23803
804-524-7000
www.csh.dmhmrsas.virginia.gov/default.htm

to provide state of the art mental health care and treatment to forensic and civilly committed patients in need of a structured, secure environment. The major components of the hospital's mission include Evaluation, Treatment, Protection, and Disposition

4090 Commonwealth Center for Children and Adolesc ents
PO Box 4000
Staunton, VA 24402-4000
540-332-2100
Fax: 540-332-2201

William J Tuell, Contact

4091 Dominion Hospital
2960 Sleepy Hollow Road
Falls Church, VA 22044
703-536-2000
Fax: 703-533-9650
www.dominionhospital.com

Offers individuals and families hope and help. Treats children, adolescents and adults who suffer from debilitating disorders such as anxiety, panic, depression, delusions, eating disorders, schizophrenia, school refusal, and self-injurious behavior.

4092 Eastern State Hospital
4601 Ironbound Road
Williamsburg, VA 23188-2652
757-253-5241
Fax: 757-253-5065

John M Favret, Contact

4093 Hiram W Davis Medical Center
PO Box 4030
Petersburg, VA 23803-0030
804-524-7344

David A Rosenquist, Contact

4094 Northern Virginia Mental Health Institute
3302 Gallows Road
Falls Church, VA 22042
703-207-7100
Fax: 703-207-7160
www.nvmhi.dmhmrsas.virginia.gov

Lynn DeLacy, Facility Director

Actively promoting recovery of individuals with serious mental illness through the use of safe, efficient, and effective treatment

4095 Piedmont Geriatric Hospital
5001 East Patrick Henry Highway
PO Box 427
Burkeville, VA 23922-0427
434-767-4401
Fax: 434-767-4500
E-mail: steve.herrick@pgh.dmhmrsas.virginia.gov
www.pgh.dmhmrsas.virginia.gov

Stephen Herrick, Director

A 135-bed psychiatric hospital that provides recovery based MH services to enable the elderly to thrive in the community.

4096 Southern Virginia Mental Health Institute
382 Taylor Drive
Danville, VA 24541
434-799-6220
Fax: 434-773-4274
E-mail: naomi.gibson@svmhi.dmhmrsas.virginia.gov
www.svmhi.dmhmrsas.virginia.gov

To be an inpatient mental health service provider within our Regional Service Area that responds to the patient's and area needs.

4097 Southwestern Virginia Mental Health Institute
340 Bagley Circle
Marion, VA 24354-3390

276-783-1200
www.swvmhi.dmhmrsas.virginia.gov/default.htm

4098 Western State Hospital
1301 Richmond Avenue
Staunton, VA 24401
540-332-8000
Fax: 540-332-8144
www.wsh.dmhmrsas.virginia.gov

Jack Barber, Hospital

Western State Hospital is a state psychiatric hospital which is licensed and operated by the Virginia Department of Mental Health, Mental Retardation, and Substance Abuse Services. Provides safe and effective individualized treatment in a recovery focused environment.

Washington

4099 Child Study & Treatment Center
8805 Steilacoom Boulevard SW
Lakewood, WA 98498-4771
253-756-2504
800-283-8639
Fax: 253-756-3911
www.dshs.wa.gov/mentalhealth/cstc.shtml

Kristin Steinmetz, Quality Improvement Director

Treats children from age 5 to 17 who can not be served in less restrictive setting within the community.

4100 Eastern State Hospital
Maple Street
PO Box 800
Medical Lake, WA 99022-0800
509-299-3121
Fax: 509-299-7015
E-mail: eshinfo@dshs.wa.gov
www.dshs.wa.gov/mentalhealth/esh.shtml

Shirley Maike, Information Coordinator

Eastern State Hospital is a key partner in assisting adults with psychiatric illness in their recovery through expert inpatient treatment whenever needs exceed community resources.

4101 Ryther Child Center
2400 NE 95th Street
Seattle, WA 98115-2426
206-525-5050
Fax: 206-525-9795
TDD: 800-883-6388
www.ryther.org

Lee Grogg, Executive Director/CEO

Offers and develops safe places and opportunities for children, youth and families to heal and grow so that they can reach their highest potential.

4102 Western State Hospital
9601 Steilacoom Boulevard SW
Tacoma, WA 98498-7213
253-582-8900
Fax: 253-756-2879
www.dshs.wa.gov/mentalhealth/wsh.shtmk

Kris Flowers, Public Information Officer

West Virginia

4103 Highland Hospital
300 56th Street SE
Charleston, WV 25304
304-926-1600
800-250-3806
www.highlandhosp.com

Our mission is to identify and respond to mental health needs, and promote physical, social emotional and intellectual well-being.

4104 Mildred Mitchell-Bateman Hospital
1530 Norway Avenue
PO Box 448
Huntington, WV 25705-1358
304-525-7801
800-644-9318
www.wvs.state.wv.us/newhh

Mary Beth Carlisle, CEO

Provides inpatient psychiatric treatment for the adult citizens of southern West Virginia.

4105 Weirton Medical Center
601 Colliers Way
Weirton, WV 26062
304-797-6000
www.weirtonmedical.com

Weirton Medical Center is a 238 bed, non-profit, acute-care, general community hospital located in the city of Weirton in Brooke County, West Virginia. Weirton Medical Center offers health care services to the residents of West Virginia, Ohio and Pennsylvania.

4106 William R Sharpe, Jr Hospital
936 Sharpe Hospital Road
Weston, WV 26452-8550
304-269-1210
Fax: 304-269-6235

Kevin P Stalnaker, CEO

Wisconsin

4107 Bellin Psychiatric Center
301 E St. Joseph Street
PO Box 23725
Green Bay, WI 54301-2241
920-433-3630
E-mail: Isroet@bellin.org
www.bellin.org/psych

4108 Mendota Mental Health Institute
301 Troy Drive
Madison, WI 53704
608-301-1000
Fax: 608-301-1358
www.dhfs.wisconsin.gov/mh_mendota

A psychiatric hospital operated by the Wisconsin Department of Health and Family Services, Division of Disability and Elder Services, specializes in serving patients with complex psychiatric conditions, often combined with certain problem behaviors.

4109 Wheaton Franciscan Healthcare: Elmbrook Memo rial
19333 W North Avenue
Brookfield, WI 53045-4198

262-785-2000
Fax: 262-785-2485
www.mywheaton.org

4110 Winnebago Mental Health Institute
1300 South Drive
PO Box 9
Winnebago, WI 54985-0009
920-235-4910
Fax: 920-237-2043
TDD: 888-241-9438
www.dhfs.wisconsin.gov/mh_winnebago

Winnebago Mental Health Institute (WMHI) serves as a specialized component in a community-based mental health delivery system.

Wyoming

4111 Wyoming State Hospital
831 Highway 150 South
Evanston, WY 82930-5341
307-789-3464
www.health.wyo.gov/statehospital/index.html

Pablo Hernandez MD, Administrator

A center for treatment, rehabilitation and recovery.

Clinical Management

Management Companies

4112 ABE American Board of Examiners in Clinical Social Work
27 Congress Street Suite 501
Shetland Park
Salem, MA 01970
978-825-9311
800-694-5285
Fax: 978-740-5395
E-mail: abe@abecsw.org
www.abecsw.org

Howard Snooks Ph.D BCD, President
Robert Booth, Executive Director
Leonard Hill MSW BCD, Vice President

The American Board of Examiners in Clinical Social Work (ABE) sets national practice standards, issues an advanced-practice credential, and publishes reference information about its board-certified clinicians

4113 ACORN Behavioral Care Management Corporation
134 N Narberth Avenue
Narberth, PA 19072-2299
610-664-8350
800-223-7050

4114 APOGEE
489 Devon Park Drive
Suite 301
Wayne, PA 19087
610-337-3200
877-337-3200
Fax: 610-337-2337
E-mail: info@apogeeinsgroup.com
www.apogeeinsgroup.com

Debbie Ballard, Agency Administrator
Chris Hoxie, Account Executive

4115 Academy of Managed Care Providers
1945 Palo Verde Avenue
Suite 202
Long Beach, CA 90815-3445
562-682-3559
800-297-2627
Fax: 562-799-3355
E-mail: membership@academymcp.org
www.academymcp.org

Dr. John Russell, President
William Adams, Advisory Board Member

National organization of clinicans and MCO professionals. Provides many services to members including continuing education, diplomate certification, notification of panel openings and practice opportunities, newsletter, group health insurance and many other benefits.

4116 Access Behavioral Care
117 S 17th Street
Suite 900
Philadelphia, PA 19103-5009
215-567-3638
Fax: 215-567-5572

4117 Action Healthcare Management
6245 N. 24th Parkway
Suite 112
Phoenix, AZ 85016
602-265-0681
800-433-6915
Fax: 602-265-0202
E-mail: jeanr@actionhealthcare.com
www.actionhealthcare.com

Action Healthcare Management has been an independent healthcare management company offering a full range of services that can be tailored to meet your organization's needs-from pre-certification and utilization review, management of high risk pregnancy and workers' compensation cases, to cases involving serious illness, catastrophic injury and cases requiring transplants. AHM works within your budget to assure provision of quality, affordable healthcare, negotiation of provider agreements and cost containment in the structuring of quality utilization management plans. In today's complicated healthcare system, Action Healthcare Management is a partner to both your organization and your insured. We're by your side, every step of the way.

4118 Adanta Group-Behavioral Health Services
259 Parkers Mill Road
Somerset, KY 42501
606-678-2768
Fax: 606-678-5296
E-mail: klworley@adanta.org
www.adanta.org

Cathy Epperson, CEO

Adanta is composed of three major divisions which include Human Development Services, Clinical Services and the Regional Prevention Center. While each division is responsible for providing separate and distinct services, each relies on the expertise and resources available within the overall corporation. The three major divisions are made up of many smaller specialized areas, each of which include many professionals, staff and support personnel who take great pride in the quality of their work. Their professional skills, combined with time, energy and caring, have yielded and continue to yield positive results and many success stories across the region.

4119 Adult Learning Systems
1954 S Industrial Highway
Suite A
Ann Arbor, MI 48104
734-668-7447
Fax: 734-668-2772

Sherri Turner, Contact

4120 Aetna-US HealthCare
151 Farmington Avenue
Hartford, CT 06156
860-273-0123
800-323-9930
www.aetna.com

Ronald Williams, Chairman/CEO

4121 Aldrich and Cox
3075 Southwestern Boulevard
Suite 202
Orchard Park, NY 14127
716-675-6300
Fax: 716-675-2098

E-mail: cox@aldrichandcox.com
www.aldrichandcox.com

Charles Cox, President
Herbert Cox, Chairman
James Hood Jr, Exec. VP/ Secretary

Aldrich and Cox provides independent, fee-based Risk Management, Insurance and Employee Benefit Consulting services to a wide range of clientele.

4122 Alliance Behavioral Care

222 Piedmont Avenue
Suite 8800
Cincinnati, OH 45219-4218
513-475-8622
800-926-8862
E-mail: allen.daniels@uc.edu
www.alliance-behavioral.com

Allen Daniels, CEO

Alliance Behavioral Care is a regional managed behavioral healthcare organization located in Cincinnati, Ohio. They are committed to continuously improving the resources and programs that serve their members and providers. Their goal is to provide resources that improve the well-being of those they serve and to integrate the behavioral healthcare within the overall healthcare systems.

4123 Alliance For Community Care

2001 The Alameda
San Jose, CA 95126
408-261-7777
Fax: 408-248-6520

4124 Allina Hospitals & Clinics Behavioral Health Services

2925 Chicago Avenue
Minneapolis, MN 55407
612-262-5000
800-877-7878
www.allina.com

Richard Pettingill, President/CEO
Michael McAnder, CFO

Provides clinically and geographically integrated care delivery. Innovative programs and services across comprehensive continuum of care. Practicing guideline development, outcomes data and quality managment programs to enhance care delivery.

4125 AmeriChoice

8045 Leesburg Pike, Ste.650
Wanamaker Building
Vienna, VA 22182
703-506-3555
Fax: 212-898-7967
E-mail: webmaster@americhoice.com
www.americhoice.com

4126 American Managed Behavioral Healthcare Association

1101 Pennsylvania Avenue NW
6th Floor
Washington, DC 20004
202-756-7726
Fax: 202-756-7308
E-mail: info@abhw.org
www.abhw.org

Pamela Greenberg, President/CEO

A non-profit trade association representing the nation's leading managed behavioral healthcare organizations. These organizations collectively manage mental health and substance abuse services for its over 100 million individuals.

Year Founded: 1994

4127 Analysis Group Economics

1 Brattle Square
Suite 5
Cambridge, MA 02138-3723
617-349-2100
Fax: 617-864-3742

Provides economic and financial consulting to law firms, corporations and government agencies. Specializing in antitrust, intellectual property, health care, energy, telecommunications and security analysis.

4128 Aon Consulting Group

200 East Randolph Street
Chicago, IL 60601
312-381-1000
www.aon.com

Gregory Case, President/CEO

Aon Corporation is a leading provider of risk management services, insurance and reinsurance brokerage, human capital and management consulting, and specialty insurance underwriting.

4129 Arizona Center For Mental Health PHD

5070 N 40th Street
Suite 200
Phoenix, AZ 85018
602-954-6700

4130 Arthur S Shorr and Associates

4710 Deseret Drive
Woodland Hills, CA 91364-3720
818-225-7055
800-530-5728
Fax: 818-225-7059
E-mail: arthur@arthurshorr.com
www.arthurshorr.com

Arthur Shorr, President
Nancy Daniels, Senior Consultant-Principal

Consultants to Health Care Providers

4131 Associated Counseling Services

8 Roberta Drive
Dartmouth, MA 02748
508-992-9376

Douglas Riley, Contact

4132 Barbanell Associates

3629 Sacramento Street
San Francisco, CA 94118
415-929-1155

4133 Barry Associates

6807 Knotty Pine Drive
Chapel Hill, NC 27517
919-490-8474
Fax: 765-381-1100
E-mail: info@barryonline.com
www.barry-online.com

John S Barry MSW MBA, President

Provides technical assistance services to behavioral health and social service organizations in the areas of performance measurement, survey research, program evaluation, compensation system design and other selected human resource management areas.

4134 Behavioral Health Care
6801 S Yosemite Street #201
Centennial, CO 80112-1411
303-889-4805
Fax: 303-889-4808
E-mail: bhi@bhicares.org
www.bhicares.org

Julie Holtz, Chief Executive Officer
Joe Pastor M.D., Medical Director

BHI is committed to excellence in mental health service delivery. They strive to promote recovery by focusing on the unique needs, strengths and hopes of consumers and families.

4135 Behavioral Health Care Consultants
12 Windham Lane
Beverly, MA 01915
978-921-5968
Fax: 978-921-5968
E-mail: mkatzenstein@bhcconsult.com
www.bhcconsult.com

Michael L Katzenstein CHC CHE, President

4136 Behavioral Health Management Group
1025 Main Street
Suite 708
Wheeling, WV 26003
304-232-7232
Fax: 304-232-7245
E-mail: user655349@aol.com

Carol Jarrett, Practice Manager

They offer a wide range of services for men, women, adolescents, and children. The professional staff specializes in mental and emotional disorders, marital and family counseling, group therapy, vocational counseling, alcohol and substance abuse, academic adjustment counseling, psychological testing, biofeedback, and hypnotherapy.

4137 Behavioral Health Partners
2200 Century Parkway NE
Suite 675
Atlanta, GA 30345
404-315-9325
Fax: 404-315-0786

Management consultants to integrated delivery systems, professional practices and public mental health agencies as well as the developers of Connex-a behavioral health software package enabling health care systems, MCOs and EAPs to manage financial, clinical and contract information. Specialize in tailoring partnerships with health care organizations that positively impact the delivery of behavioral health services in their communities.

4138 Behavioral Health Services
2925 Chicago Avenue
Minneapolis, MN 55407
612-262-5000
www.allina.com

Richard Pettingill, President/CEO
Mary Foarde, General Counsel/Corp Secretary

Provides clinically and geographically integrated delivery system, innovative programs and services across comprehensive continuum of care, practice guidelines development, outcomes data and quality management programs to enhance care delivery systems.

4139 Behavioral Health Systems
2 Metroplex Drive
Suite 500
Birmingham, AL 35209
205-879-1150
800-245-1150
Fax: 205-879-1178
E-mail: generalwebsite@bhs-inc.com
www.bhs-inc.com

Deborah L Stephens, Founder/Chairman/CEO
Kyle Strange, Senior Vice President/COO

Provides managed psychiatric and substance abuse and drug testing services to more than 20,000 employees nationally through a network of 7,600 providers.

4140 Berkowitz Chassion and Sklar
9911 W Pico Blvd
Suite 685W
Los Angeles, CA 90035
310-659-3823

Elaine D Chaisson, Contact

4141 Broward County Healthcare Management
4175 Davie Road
Second Floor
Davie, FL 33314
954-327-8750
Fax: 954-327-8773
www.broward.org/healthcare/hmi00100.htm

4142 Brown Consulting
121 N Erie Street
Toledo, OH 43604
419-241-8547
800-495-6786
Fax: 419-241-8689
E-mail: info@danbrownconsulting.com
www.danbrownconsulting.com

Daniel Brown, President/CEO
David Galbraith, CFO

Provides a full range of consulting services to behavioral healthcare providers. Has relationships with national, regional and state behavioral healthcare organizations.

Year Founded: 1987

4143 CAFCA
1120 Lincoln Street
Suite 701
Denver, CO 80203
720-570-8402
Fax: 720-570-8408
E-mail: info@cafca.net
www.cafca.net

Skip Barber, Executive Director
Arnie Goldstein, President
Jerry Yager, Vice President

The services provided by member agencies include: adoption, alcohol and drug treatment, day treatment, education, family support and preservation, foster care, group homes, independent living, kinship care, mental health treatment and counseling, pregnancy counseling, residential care at all levels, services for homeless and runaway youth, services for sexually reactive youth, sexual abuse services and transitional living.

4144 CBCA
10900 Hampshire Avenue S
Bloomington, MN 55438-2306
952-829-3500
800-824-3882
Fax: 952-946-7694
E-mail: info@cbca.com
www.cbca.com

Kenneth Di Bella, CEO

Provides total health plan management including 24 hours a day, seven days a week patient access and demand management, care management, behavioral health care management, disease management and disability workers' compensation management, all supported by QualityFIRST clinical decision guidelines. These services are electronically integrated with HRM's national provider networks and electronic claims management. HRM's clients include HMOs, hospital systems, insurance and self-insured plans, workers' compensation and disability plans and Medicare/Medicaid plans throughout the US, Canada and New Zealand.

4145 CBI Group
310 Busse Highway
#369
Park Ridge, IL 60068
847-292-6676
Fax: 847-823-0740
E-mail: jlemmer@cbipartners.com
www.cbipartners.com

4146 CIGNA Behavioral Care
11095 Viking Drive
Suite 350
Eden Prairie, MN 55344
800-334-8925
www.apps.cignabehavioral.com/home.html

Keith Dixon, President/CEO

Provides behavioral care benefit management, EAPs, and work/life programs to consumers through health plans offered by large U.S. employers, national and regional HMOs, Taft-Hartley trusts and disability insurers.

Year Founded: 1974

4147 CIGNA Corporation
1 Liberty Place
Philadelphia, PA 19192
215-761-8362
Fax: 215-761-5602
www.cigna.com

Provides group accident, life, and disability insurance, as well as behavioral health, vision and dental coverage.

4148 Calland and Company
2296 Henderson Mill Road
Suite 222
Atlanta, GA 30345
770-270-9100
Fax: 770-270-9300
E-mail: bob@callandcompany.com
www.callandcompany.com

Bob Calland, President
Beth Farrens, VP Of Recruiting

Concentrates in the areas of innovative and diverse healthcare businesses, including multi-site providers, managed care information technology, alternate delivery, employee benefits, contract management services, internet(content, B2B and B2C), occupational health, specialty care, rehabilitation, practice management, and other uniquely defined professional service businesses.

4149 Cameron and Associates
6100 Lake Forrest Drive
Suite 550
Atlanta, GA 30328
404-843-3399
800-334-6014
Fax: 404-843-3572
www.caiquality.com

William Cameron, Founder

Assists troubled employees and their dependents in resolving personal problems in order to provide their employer a level of acceptable job performance and efficiency, and to provide a safe working environment for all employees.

4150 Carewise
1501 4th Avenue
Suite 700
Seattle, WA 98101
206-749-1100
800-755-2136
Fax: 206-749-1125
www.www.shps.com

Rishabh Mehrotra, President/CEO
John McCarty, Executive Vice President/CFO

4151 Casey Family Services
127 Church Street
New Haven, CT 06510
203-401-6900
Fax: 203-401-6901
E-mail: info@caseyfamilyservices.org
www.caseyfamilyservices.org

Raymond L Torres, Executive Director
Michael Brennan, Co-Chairman
Year Founded: 1976

4152 Center for Health Policy Studies
40 Beaver Street
Albany, NY 12207-1511
518-426-4315
Fax: 518-426-4316

Jack Knowlton, Executive Vice President

4153 Center for the Advancement of Health
2000 Florida Avenue NW
Suite 210
Washington, DC 20009-1231
202-387-2829
Fax: 202-387-2857
E-mail: cfah@cfah.org
www.cfah.org

Maulik Joshi, Treasurer
Jessie Gruman, President

4154 Centers for Mental Healthcare Research
5800 W 10th Street
Suite 605
Little Rock, AR 72204-1773
501-660-7559
Fax: 501-660-7542
E-mail: kramerteresal@uams.edu
www.uams.edu

4155 Century Financial Services
185 NW Spanish River Boulevard
Boca Raton, FL 33431-4227
407-362-0111

4156 Children's Home of the Wyoming Conference, Quality Improvement
1182 Chenango Street
Binghamton, NY 13901
607-772-6904
800-772-6904
E-mail: info@chowc.org
www.www.chowc.org

Robert Houser, President/CEO
Patricia Giglio, CFO/Chief Admin. Officer

Child care agency referred to various departments of social services, court systems, school systems for children who are at risk, have trouble in the home, or have been abused or abandoned.

4157 ChoiceCare
655 Eden Park Drive, Suite 400
Grand Baldwin Building
Cincinnati, OH 45202-6000
513-241-1400
800-543-7158
Fax: 513-684-7461
www.choicecare.com

4158 College Health IPA
7711 Center Avenue
Suite 300
Huntington Beach, CA 92647-3067
562-467-5555
800-779-3825
Fax: 562-402-2666
E-mail: info@chipa.com
www.chipa.com

Randy Davis, President/CEO
Kevin Gardiner, VP Of Financial Operations

Culturally sensitive mental health referral service.

4159 College of Dupage
425 Fawell Boulevard
Glen Ellyn, IL 60137
630-942-2800
Fax: 630-790-2686
www.www.cod.edu

4160 College of Southern Idaho
315 Falls Avenue
PO Box 1238
Twin Falls, ID 83303
208-733-9554
800-680-0274
Fax: 208-736-4743
E-mail: info@csi.edu
www.csi.edu

Jerry Beck, President
Jerry Gee, Executive VP/CAO

4161 Columbia Hospital M/H Services
2201 45th Street
W Palm Beach, FL 33407
561-842-6141
Fax: 561-844-8955
www.columbiahospital.com

Valerie Jackson, CEO
Oon Soo Ung, CFO
Brenda Logan, CNO

250-bed acute-care facility with dedicated psychiatry, emergency psychiatry, geriatric psychiatry, inpatient and outpatient psychiatry, and partial day psychiatry units and programs.

4162 ComPsych
455 N City Front Plaza Drive
NBC Tower
Chicago, IL 60611-5532
312-595-4000
800-755-3050
Fax: 312-595-4029
E-mail: mpaskell@compsych.com
www.compsych.com

Richard Chaifetz, Chairman/CEO

Worlwide leader in guidance resources, including employee assistance programs, managed behavioral health, work-life, legal, financial, and personal convenience services. ComPsych provides services worldwide covering millions of individuals. Clients range from Fortune 100 to smaller public and private concerns, government entities, health plans and Taft-Hartley groups. Guidance Resources transforms traditionally separate services into a seamless integration of information, resources and creative solutions that address personal life challenges and improve workplace productivity and performance.

4163 Comprehensive Care Corporation
3405 W. Martin Luther King Jr. Blvd
Suite 101
Tampa, FL 33607
813-288-4808
Fax: 813-288-4844
E-mail: info@comprehensivecare.com
www.comprehensivecare.com

John Hill, President/CEO
Robert Landis, Chairman/CFO/Treasurer

Offers a flexible system of services to provide comprehensive, compassionate and cost-effective mental health and substance abuse services to managed care organizations both public and private. CompCare is committed to providing state-of-the-art comprehensive care management services for all levels and phases of behavioral health care.

4164 Comprehensive Center For Pain Management
7053 W Central Avenue
Toledo, OH 43617
419-843-1370
877-446-6724
Fax: 419-843-1362
E-mail: ccpminfo@cc4pm.com
www.www.cc4pm.com

4165 Contact Behavioral Health Services
4645 E Cotton Center Blvd
Building 1
Phoenix, AZ 85040-8884
602-657-1464
Fax: 602-689-0193
www.contactbhs.com

Jay Roundy, CEO
James Johnson, COO

Contact offers a comprehensive employee assistance program (EAP) with enhanced worklife options, a managed behavioral health care program, and an interested EAP and managed care program.

4166 Corphealth
1300 Summit Avenue
6th Floor
Fort Worth, TX 76102-4414
817-332-2519
800-240-8388
Fax: 817-335-9100
E-mail: businessdevelopment@corphealth.com
www.corphealth.com

Patrick Gotcher II, President/CEO
Brae Jacobson, COO
Michael Baker, CFO

4167 Corporate Health Systems
15153 Technology Drive
Suite B
Eden Prairie, MN 55344
952-939-0911
Fax: 952-939-0990
www.corpsyhealthsys.com

Benefits consulting firm to partner with clients to find the most flexible and comprehensive benefits packages for their investments.

4168 Counseling Associates
109 High Street
Salisbury, MD 21801
410-546-1692
888-546-1692
Fax: 410-548-9056
E-mail: tim@catherapy.com
www.catherapy.com

Anne Bass, Executive Director

Provides therapeutic counseling to help individuals lead productive and fulfilled lives.

4169 Covenant Home Healthcare
3615 19th Street
Lubbock, TX 79410
806-725-1011
www.covenanthealth.org/Services/homehealth.htm

Melinda Clark, CEO

Provides quality home care to patients when hospitalization may be unneccessary, or when the length of stay may be shorter than expected.

4170 Coventry Health Care of Iowa
211 Lake Drive
Newark, DE 19702
515-225-1234
800-752-7242
Fax: 302-283-6788
www.chciowa.com

4171 Creative Health Concepts
305 Madison Avenue
Suite 2022
New York, NY 10165
212-697-7207
Fax: 212-697-3509
E-mail: info@creativegroupny.com
www.www.creativegroupny.com

Ira Gottlieb, President/CEO
Harry Blair, Vice Chairman

4172 Cypruss Communications
430 Myrtle Ave
Suite A
Fort Lee, NJ 07024
201-735-7730
800-750-5231
E-mail: peterm@cypruss.com
www.cypruss.com

Peter Miller, VP/CFO

4173 DD Fischer Consulting
8105 White Oak Road
Quincy, IL 62305
217-656-3000

4174 DML Training and Consulting
4228 Boxelder Place
Davis, CA 95618
530-753-4300
Fax: 530-753-7500
E-mail: info@dmlmd.com
www.dmlmd.com

David Mee-Lee, Founder

4175 Deloitte and Touche LLP Management Consulting
1700 Market Street
Philadelphia, PA 19103-3984
215-246-2300
Fax: 215-569-2441
www.deloitte.com

Barry Salzberg, CEO
Sharon Allen, Chairman Of The Board

4176 DeltaMetrics
600 Public Ledger Building
150 S Independence Mall West
Philadelphia, PA 19106-3475
215-399-0988
800-238-2433
Fax: 215-399-0989
www.deltametrics.com

Jack Durell, President/CEO
John Cacciola, Senior Vice President

National research, evaluation, and consulting organization dedicated to the improvement of substance abuse and other behavioral health care treatment.

4177 Diversified Group Administrators
6345 Flank Drive
PO Box 6250
Harrisburg, PA 17112

717-652-8040
800-877-6490
Fax: 717-652-8328
E-mail: jhoellman@dgatpa.com
www.dgatpa.com

James Hoellman, Contact

4178 Dorenfest Group
455 N Cityfront Plaza Drive
NBC Tower Suite 2725
Chicago, IL 60610-5555
312-464-3000
Fax: 312-467-0541
E-mail: info@dorenfest.com
www.dorenfest.com

Sheldon Dorenfest, CEO

4179 Dougherty Management Associates Health Strategies
9 Meriam Street
Suite 4
Lexington, MA 02420-5312
781-863-8003
800-817-7802
Fax: 781-863-1519
E-mail: mail@dmahealth.com
www.dmahealth.com

Richard H Dougherty, President

Providing the public and private sectors with superior management consulting services to improve healthcare delivery systems and manage complex organizational change.

4180 Dupage County Health Department
111 North County Farm Road
Wheaton, IL 60187
630-682-7400
TDD: 630-932-1447
www.www.dupagehealth.org

Maureen McHugh, Executive Director

4181 Echo Management Group
15 Washington Street
PO Box 2150
Conway, NH 03818
603-447-8600
800-635-8209
Fax: 603-447-8680
E-mail: info@echoman.com
www.echoman.com

John Raden, CEO

Provides financial, clinical, and administrative software applications for behavioral health and social service agencies; comprehensive, fully-intergrated Human Service Information System is a powerful management tool that enables agencies to successfully operate their organizations within the stringent guidelines of managed care mandates. Provides implementation planning, training, support and systems consulting services.

4182 Elon Homes for Children
1717 Sharon Road West
Charlotte, NC 28210
704-369-2500
Fax: 404-688-2960
E-mail: info@elonhomes.org
www.elonhomes.org

Frederick Grosse, President/CEO

4183 Employee Assistance Professionals
1234 Summer Street
Stamford, CT 06905-5510
203-977-2446

4184 Employee Benefit Specialists
9351 Grant Street
Suite 300
Denver, CO 80229
303-280-1215
Fax: 303-280-1821
E-mail: cfankhouser@clickebs.com
www.clickebs.com

Alan Curtis, Chairman/CEO
Curtis Fankhouser, President

4185 Employee Network
1040 Vestal Parkway E
Vestal, NY 13850
607-754-1048
800-364-4748
Fax: 607-754-1629
www.eniweb.com

Gene Raymondi, Founder/CEO

4186 Entropy Limited
345 South Great Road
Lincoln, MA 01773
781-259-8901
Fax: 781-259-1255
E-mail: clientservices@entropylimited.com
www.entropylimited.com

Uses pattern recognition, statistics, and computer simulation to track past behavior, see current behavior and predict future behavior. Used by insuranch companies and the healthcare industry.

4187 Essi Systems
70 Otis Street
San Francisco, CA 94103
415-252-8224
800-252-3774
Fax: 415-252-5732
E-mail: essi@essisystems.com
www.essisystems.com

Esther Orioli, CEO
Karen Trocki, Research Director

4188 Ethos Consulting
3219 E Camelback Road
Suite 515
Phoenix, AZ 85018
480-296-3801
Fax: 480-664-7270
E-mail: conrad@ethosconsulting.com
www.ethosconsulting.com

Conrad Prusak, President
Julie Prusak, CEO

4189 Evaluation Center at HSRI
2336 Massachusetts Avenue
Cambridge, MA 02140
617-876-0426
Fax: 617-492-7401

E-mail: sjohniken@hsri.org
www.hsri.org
Sebrina Johniken, Office Manager

4190 FCS
1711 Ashley Circle
Suite 6
Bowling Green, KY 42104-5801
502-782-9152
800-783-9152
Fax: 270-782-1055
E-mail: admin@fcspsy.com
www.fcspsy.com

Bob Toth, President
Brian Browning, VP Of Client Services

4191 FPM Behavioral Health: Corporate Marketing
1276 Minnesota Avenue
Winter Park, FL 32789-4833
407-647-1781

4192 Family Managed Care
5745 Essen Lane
Suite 100
Baton Rouge, LA 70810
225-215-2100
E-mail: webmaster@calaishealth.com
www.calaishealth.com

Leslie Yander, Director Human Resources
Tuan Nguyen, Information Services

Provider of managed behavioral healthcare and employee assistance programs.

4193 Findley, Davies and Company
300 Madison Avenue
Suite 1000
Toledo, OH 43604-1596
419-255-1360
Fax: 419-259-5685
www.findleydavies.com

Marc E Stockwell, Market Leader

4194 First Consulting Group
111 W Ocean Boulevard
4th Floor
Long Beach, CA 90802-4632
562-624-5200
800-345-0957
Fax: 562-432-5774
www.fcg.com

Larry Ferguson, CEO
Thomas Watford, COO/CFO

4195 First Corp-Health Consulting
38 W Fulton Street
Suite 300
Grand Rapids, MI 49503-2644
616-676-3258
Fax: 616-676-0846
www.corphealth.com

Patrick Gotcher, President and CEO
Brae Jacobson, Chief Operating Officer
Year Founded: 1989

4196 Fowler Healthcare Affiliates
2000 Riveredge Parkway
Suite 920
Atlanta, GA 30328
770-261-6363
800-784-9829
Fax: 770-261-6361
www.fowler-consulting.com

Frances Fowler, President

Developed innovative solutions for managing cost of high cost patients.

4197 Freedom To Fly
27871 Medical Center Road
Ste. 285
Mission Viejo, CA 92691
949-364-1833

4198 Full Circle Programs
70 Skyview Terrace
San Rafael, CA 94903
415-499-3320
Fax: 415-499-1542
E-mail: dmeshel@fc-fi.org
www.fullcircleprograms.org

David Meshel, Contact

Activley disseminates knowledge through training and technical assistace, advocating for policies that support best practices, services and outcome for children and families.

Year Founded: 1971

4199 GMR Group
755 Business Center Drive
Suite 250
Horsham, PA 19044
215-653-7401
Fax: 215-653-7982
E-mail: webmaster@gmrgroup.com
www.gmrgroup.com

Baron Ginnetti, President/CEO
Thomas Bishop, Vice President/COO

Provides strategic and tactical solutions to the marketing and sales challenges their clients face in the managed healthcare environment.

4200 Garner Consulting
630 North Rosemead Blvd
Suite 300
Pasadena, CA 91107
626-351-2300
Fax: 626-371-0447
E-mail: info@garnerconsulting.com
www.garnerconsulting.com

John Garner, CEO
Gerti Reagan Garner, President

Provides innovative consultation, which produces immediate, bottom line results and long term value.

4201 Gaynor and Associates
111 Whitney Avenue
New Haven, CT 06510
203-865-0865
Fax: 203-865-0093

Mark Gaynor LCSW, Principle

Clinical social work provider, EAP services, and clinical practice.

4202 Geauga Board of Mental Health, Alcohol and Drug Addiction Services
13244 Ravenna Road
Chardon, OH 44024-9012
440-285-2282
Fax: 440-285-9617
E-mail: info@geauga.org
www.geauga.org

James Adams, Executive Director/CEO

4203 Glazer Medical Solutions
PO Box 121
Beach Plum Lane
Menemsha, MA 02552
508-645-9635
Fax: 308-645-3212
E-mail: glazermedicalsol@aol.com
www.glazmedsol.com

William Glazer, President/Founder

4204 HCA Healthcare
1 Park Plaza
Nashville, TN 37203
615-344-9551
www.www.hcahealthcare.com

Richard Bracken, President/CEO

4205 HPN Worldwide
119 W Vallette Street
Elmhurst, IL 60126
630-941-9030
Fax: 630-941-9064
E-mail: info@hpn.com
www.hpn.com

Bob Gorsky, Founder/President

Year Founded: 1983

4206 HSP Verified
1120 G Street NW
Suite 330
Washington, DC 20005-3801
202-783-1270
Fax: 202-783-1269

Judy Hall, President

Offers comprehensive, innovative credential verification services designed to help you find that precious time. It relieves health care providers and management of tedious administrative activities-leaving time and resources to focus on quality health care. Provides valuable information and cultivates alliances between cutting edge health care organizations/plans and qualified health care providers.

4207 Hays Group
1133 20th Street NW
Suite 450
Washington, DC 20036
202-263-4000
Fax: 202-263-4001
E-mail: info@hayscompanies.com
www.haysgroup.com

4208 Health Alliance Plan
2850 W Grand Boulevard
Detroit, MI 48202
313-872-8100
800-422-4641
TDD: 313-664-8000
www.hap.org

Francine Parker, President and CEO
Ronald Berry, Senior Vice President/CFO

4209 Health Capital Consultants
9666 Olive Boulevard
Suite 375
Saint Louis, MO 63132-3025
314-994-7641
800-394-8258
Fax: 314-991-3435
E-mail: solutions@healthcapital.com
www.healthcapital.com

Robert Cimasi, President

4210 Health Decisions
409 Plymouth Road
Suite 220
Plymouth, MI 48170
734-451-2230
Fax: 734-451-2835
www.healthdecisions.com

Si Nahra, Founder/President

4211 Health Management Associates
5811 Pelican Bay Boulevard
Suite 500
Naples, FL 34108-2710
239-598-3131
www.hma-corp.com

Burke Whitman, President/CEO
Robert Farnham, Senior Vice President/CFO

4212 Health Systems Research
1200 18th Street NW
Suite 700
Washington, DC 20036
202-828-5100
Fax: 202-728-9469
www.hsrnet.com

Lincoln Smith, President/CEO
Mark Kielb, Senior Vice President/CFO

4213 HealthPartners
2701 University Avenue SE
Minneapolis, MN 55414-3233
612-627-3500
Fax: 612-627-3535
TTY: 612-627-3584
www.healthpartners.com

Mary Brainerd, President/CEO

4214 Healthcare America
1201 Claridge Road
Glenside, PA 19038-7537
610-940-1658

4215 Healthcare Value Management Group
3200 Highland Avenue
Downers Grove, IL 60515

630-737-7900
www.www.firsthealth.com

Ronald Blaine Faulkner, COO

Consulting practice providing information technology, operations and provider contracting consultitative services.

4216 Healthcare in Partnership
3230 73rd Avenue SE
Mercer Island, WA 98040-3415
206-232-6300
Fax: 206-236-8110
E-mail: mhrnllc@comcast.net

Lawrence Jacobson, Member At Large

Health care consulting including managed care contract negotiation, IPA development, provider support. Specializes in behavioral health.

4217 Healthwise
2601 N Bogus Basin Road
Boise, ID 83702
541-389-2711
800-706-9646
Fax: 541-388-3832
www.healthwise.org

Donald Kemper, Chairman/CEO
Jim Giuffre, President/COO

4218 Healthy Companies
2101 Wilson Boulevard
Suite 1002
Arlington, VA 22201
703-351-9901
www.healthycompanies.com

James Owen Mathews, President
Eric Sass, COO
Robert Rosen, Chairman/CEO

4219 HeartMath
14700 W Park Avenue
Boulder Creek, CA 95006-9318
831-338-8500
Fax: 831-338-8504
E-mail: ihminquiry@heartmath.org
www.heartmath.com

HeartMath's Freze-Framer Interactive Learning System is an innovative approach to stress relief based on learning to change the heart rhythm pattern and create physiological coherence in the body. The Freeze-Framer has been widely used with clients to help them develop internal awareness, self-recognition and emotional management skills. Clients can learn to prevent stress by becoming aware of when the stress response starts and stopping it in the moment and taking a more active role in preventing stress, managing the emotions associated with stress, creating better health and improving performance.

4220 Helms & Company
1 Pillsbury Street
Suite 200
Concord, NH 03301
603-225-6633
Fax: 603-225-4739
E-mail: info@helmsco.com
www.www.helmsco.com

Michael Degnan, CEO

They are a New Hampshire based behavioral health management company offering managed behavioral healthcare services, community service programs, and employee assistance programs for health care insurers, members, employers and their employees.

4221 Horizon Behavioral Services
2941 South Lake Vista Drive
Lewisville, TX 75067
800-931-4646
Fax: 972-420-8252
www.horizoncare.net

Robert A Lefton, President

Provider of national managed care, utilization management and employee assistance programs. Horizon will work in collaboration with HMOs, insurance companies, employers and hospitals to develop seamless, cost-effective managed care services including practitioner panel formation, information system development, utilization management services, EAPs, outcomes measurement systems and sales and marketing functions.

4222 Horizon Management Services
PO Box 1623
Ventura, CA 93002-1623
805-644-1560
Fax: 805-644-0484

Neal Andrews, President

Consultants, business planning, corporate strategies, marketing and public relations.

4223 Horizon Mental Health Management
2941 South Lake Vista Drive
Lewisville, TX 75067
800-931-4646
Fax: 972-420-8252
E-mail: cindy.novak@horizonhealth.com
www.horizonhealthcorp.com

Cindy Novak, Contact

Inpatient, outpatient, partial hospitalization and home health psychiatric programs.

4224 Human Affairs International
10150 Centennial Parkway
Sandy, UT 84070
801-256-7000
Fax: 801-256-7669

4225 Human Behavior Associates
1350 Hayes Street
Suite B-100
Benicia, CA 94510
707-747-0117
800-937-7770
Fax: 707-747-6646
E-mail: jameswallace@callhba.com
www.callhba.com

James B Wallace, President
Yolanda Calderon, Operations Manager

National provider of employee assistance programs, managed behavioral healthcare services, critical incident debriefing services, conflict mediation and organizational consultation. Maintains a network of 6500 licensed mental health care providers and 650 hospitals, treatment centers.

4226 Human Services Research Institute
2336 Massachusetts Avenue
Cambridge, MA 02140
617-876-0426
Fax: 617-492-7401
E-mail: sjohniken@hsri.org
www.hsri.org

Sebrina Johniken, Office Manager

4227 Hyde Park Associates
1515 E 52nd Place
3rd Floor
Chicago, IL 60615
773-493-8212
Fax: 773-955-2166

Robert Ramierez, Contact

4228 IHC Behavioral Health Network
36 S State Street
Floor 22
Salt Lake City, UT 84111
801-442-2000
Fax: 801-442-3821
E-mail: contactus@intermountainmail.org
www.intermountainhealthcare.org

Kem Gardner, Chairman
Kent Murdock, Vice Chairman

4229 Insurance Management Institute
6 Stafford Court
Mount Holly, NJ 08060-3281
609-267-8998
Fax: 609-267-2472
E-mail: TIMInstitute@aol.com
www.timinstitute.com

Michael C Hill, Management Consultant/Author

4230 Interface EAP
10370 Richmond Avenue
Suite 1100
Houston, TX 77042
713-781-3364
Fax: 713-784-0425
E-mail: info@ieap.com
www.ieap.com

Fred Newman, CEO
Tina Pace, CFO

4231 Interim Physicians
1040 Crown Pointe Pkwy
Ste. 120
Atlanta, GA 30338
800-226-6347
Fax: 800-353-5714
E-mail: info@interimphysicians.com
www.interimphysicians.com

Jane Hinton, Vice President Of Operations
Michael Slupecki, CFO/Treasurer

4232 Interlink Health Services
4660 Belknap Court
Suite 209
Hillsboro, OR 97124
503-640-2000
800-599-9119
Fax: 503-640-2028

E-mail: administration@interlinkhealth.com
www.interlinkhealth.com

Sherrie Simmons, Director Of Operations
Scott Ray, SVP/General Counsel

4233 JM Oher and Associates
10 Tanglewild Plaza
Suite 100
Chappaqua, NY 10514
914-238-0607
Fax: 914-238-3161

Jim Oher, Founder

4234 JS Medical Group
Two Penn Center Plaza
Suite 200
Philadelphia, PA 19102-1706
215-854-6446
Fax: 215-893-8909
E-mail: information@jsmg.com
www.jsmg.com/main

4235 Jeri Davis Marketing Consultants
PO Box 770534
Memphis, TN 38177
901-763-0696
E-mail: inquiries@jeridavisinternational.com
www.jeridavisinternational.com

Jeri Davis, Founder/President

4236 John Maynard and Associates
258 Spruce Street
Suite 1000
Boulder, CO 80302
303-444-6300
E-mail: ceo@eap-association.org

4237 Johnson, Bassin and Shaw
8630 Fenton Street
12th Floor
Silver Spring, MD 20910-3803
301-495-1080
Fax: 301-587-4352
E-mail: info@jbsinternational.com
www.jbs.biz

Jerri Shaw, President
Gail Bassin, Chair Of The Board/Treasurer

4238 Juniper Healthcare Containment Systems
20283 State Road
Suite 400
Boca Raton, FL 33498
516-829-4670
Fax: 516-829-4691
www.www.junipergroup.com

4239 KAI Associates
6001 Montrose Road
Suite 920
Rockville, MD 20852-4801
301-770-2730
Fax: 301-770-4183
E-mail: kai@kai-research.com
www.kai-research.com

Selma Kunitz, President
Rene Kozloff, Executive Vice President

4240 Kushner and Company
1050 17th Street NW
Suite 810
Washington, DC 20036
202-887-0958
E-mail: info@kushnerco.com
www.kushnerco.com

Gary Kushner, President

4241 Lake Mental Health Consultants
54 Hospital Drive
Osage Beach, MO 65065
573-348-8000
www.www.lakeregional.com

Michael Henze, CEO
Vicki Franklin, SVP Of Operations/COO

4242 Legacy Consulting Insurance Services
811 W. Fremont Street
Suite B
Stockton, CA 95203
209-546-0402
Fax: 209-546-0824
E-mail: charless@legacyconsult.com
www.legacyconsult.com

Charlynn Harless, President/CEO

4243 Lewin Group
3130 Fairview Park Drive
Suite 800
Falls Church, VA 22042
703-269-5500
Fax: 703-269-5501
E-mail: lisa.chimento@lewin.com
www.lewin.com

Lisa Chimento, Executive Vice President

4244 Lifelink Corporation
331 S York Road
Suite 206
Bensenville, IL 60106-2600
630-766-3570
www.lifelink.org

Timothy Rhodes, President/CEO

Provides therapy services in Spanish for children, families and couples. Offers substance abuse treatment and educational groups for men who batter in English and Spanish. Provides comprehensive services to Latina victims of domestic violence and their children in Spanish.

4245 Lifespan Care Management Agency
600 Frederick Street
Santa Cruz, CA 95062
831-469-4900
Fax: 831-469-4950
E-mail: info@lifespancare.com
www.lifespancare.com

Becky Peters, CEO
Pamela Goodman, President

Comprehensive care management for adults who need care.

4246 MCF Consulting
25 Bragg Drive
Lake Meade, PA 17316
717-259-6631
Fax: 717-259-6537
E-mail: mcfconsulting@pa.aldelphia.net

Mark C Fox, President

MCF Consulting has demonstrated accomplishments in: developing managed care and management service organization (MSO) capabilities; managed Medicaid strategic planning efforts; Information System analysis and design contracts; product development projects; pricing and product positioning; business plan and marketing plan development; proposal development; organizational change; and creating joint ventures and partnerships. Clients have included managed care firms, provider groups, hospital systems, state and county governments and diverse contract agencies.

4247 MCG Telemedicine Center
1120 15th Street
EA - 100
Augusta, GA 30912
706-721-6616
Fax: 706-721-7270
E-mail: ekhasanshina@mail.mcg.edu
www.mcg.edu/telehealth

Max Stachura, Director
Brenda Starnes, Center Manager

Involved with the delivery of mental health services via telemedicine. In addition, the Telemedicine Center maintains the Georgia Mental Health Network website, a comprehensive listing of mental health resources in the State.

4248 MCW Department of Psychiatry and Behavioral Medicine
8701 Watertown Plank
Milwaukee, WI 53226
414-456-8990
Fax: 414-456-6299
E-mail: aodya@mcw.edu
www.www.mcw.edu

Laura Roberts, Chair

4249 MMHR
2550 University Avenue W
Suite 4358
Saint Paul, MN 55114-1096
651-647-1900
Fax: 651-647-1861
E-mail: tquesnell@hmr.net
www.mentalhealthinc.com

Tim Quesnell, Administrator

4250 MSI International
245 Peachtree Center Avenue
Suite 2500
Atlanta, GA 30303
404-659-5050
800-511-0383
Fax: 404-659-7139
E-mail: wayne-whatley@msi-intl.com
www.msi-intl.com

Eric Lindberg, President/CEO
Mike Didomenico, Vice President

4251 Magellan Health Service
6950 Columbia Gateway Drive
Columbia, MD 21046-3308

410-964-3222
800-458-2740
Fax: 410-953-1251
www.magellanhealth.com

Rene Lerer, President/CEO
Mark Demilio, CFO

Provides members with high quality, clinically appropriate, affordable health care which is tailored to each individual's needs.

4252 Magellan Public Solutions
222 Berkeley Street
Suite 1350
Boston, MA 02116-3733
617-661-2851
800-947-0071
Fax: 617-790-4848

4253 Managed Care Concepts
PO Box 812032
Boca Raton, FL 33481-2032
561-750-2240
800-899-3926
Fax: 561-750-4621
E-mail: info@theemployeeassistanceprogram.com
www.theemployeeassistanceprogram.com

Beth Harrell, Corporate Contacts Director
Ginger Minnelonica, Administrative Assistant

Provides comprehensive EAP services to large and small companies in the United States and parts of Canada. Also provides child/elder care referrals, drug free workplace program services, consultation and training services.

4254 Managed Care Consultants
11461 N 109 Way
Scottsdale, AZ 85259-3029
480-391-2992

4255 Managed Health Network
503 Canal Boulevard
Port Richmond, CA 94804
415-491-7200
800-327-2133
TDD: 800-735-2929
E-mail: mhnfeedback@mhn.com
www.mhn.com

Steven Sell, President/CEO
Juanell Hefner, COO

Provides high-quality, cost-effective behavioral health care services to the public sector.

4256 Managed Healthcare Consultants
1907 London Lane
Wilmington, NC 28405
910-256-6196

Daniel Patterson, Contact

4257 Managed Networks of America
905 E Horseshoe Court
Virginia Beach, VA 23451
757-425-2173
E-mail: mnamerica@aol.com
www.mnamerica.com

Management services that include strategic and business plan development, new corporate formations and contractual affiliations, product and infrastructure development, implementation, and management. Organizes cost effective provider networks which include a full continuum of care and services while supplying the necessary clinical, administrative, and financial systems to enable effective management of populations across varied geographic areas.

4258 Maniaci Insurance Services
500 Silver Spur Road
Suite 121
Palos Verdes, CA 90275
310-541-4824
866-541-4824
Fax: 310-377-2016
E-mail: mail@maniaciinsurance.com
www.maniaciinsurance.com

Eric Maniaci, Vice President
Dan Maniaci, President
Kristy Maniaci, Director Of Operations

4259 Marin Institute
24 Belvedere Street
San Rafael, CA 94901
415-456-5692
Fax: 415-456-0491
E-mail: info@marininstitute.org
www.marininstitute.org

Annan Paterson, President
Julio Rodriguez, Vice President
Larry Meredith, Treasurer

4260 Mayes Group
PO Box 399
Saint Peters, PA 19470
610-469-6900
Fax: 610-469-6088

Abby Mayes, President/Founder

Retained executive search firm that specializes exclusively in managed care/behavioral healthcare since 1982. Offices in Pennsylvania and Florida.

Year Founded: 1982

4261 McGladery and Pullen CPAs
3600 American Blvd W.
Third Floor
Bloomington, MN 55431-4502
888-214-1416
www.mcgladrey.com

4262 McGraw Hill Healthcare Management
1221 Avenue of the Americas
New York, NY 10020-1095
212-512-2000
E-mail: customer.service@mcgraw-hill.com
www.www.mcgraw-hill.com

Harold McGraw III, Chairman/President/CEO
Robert Bahash, Executive Vice President/CFO

4263 McKesson HBO and Company
5995 Windwrad Parkway
Alphretta, GA 30005
404-338-6000
www.http://www.mckesson.com

John Hammergren, Chairman/CEO

4264 Mellon HR Solutions
2100 N Central Road
Fort Lee, NJ 07024-7558
201-592-1300
www.drs.dreyfus.com

4265 Menninger Care Systems
4006 Belt Line Road
Suite 205
Addison, TX 75001
800-866-7242
Fax: 972-931-1938
E-mail: servicenow@mhnet.com
www.www.mhneteap.com

Wesley Brockhoeft, President/CEO
Robert Wilson, CFO

4266 Mental Health Network
Stonebridge Plaza I
9606 N MoPac Expressway, Suite 600
Austin, TX 78759
512-347-7900
Fax: 512-347-1810
www.www.mhnet.com

Wesley Brockhoeft, President/CEO
Robert Wilson, CFO

Health care management and solutions company providing employee assistance programs (EAP), work life programs, managed behavioral health care and consulting services.

4267 Mercer Consulting
200 Clarendon Street
Boston, MA 02116
617-450-6000
Fax: 617-450-6010
www.www.mercer.com

M. Michele Burns, Chairman/CEO
Tom Elliott, Chief Operating Officer

4268 Meridian Resource Corporation
1401 Enclave Parkway
Suite 300
Houston, TX 77077
281-597-7000
Fax: 281-597-8880
www.tmrc.com

Dale Breaux, Vice President Of Operations
Lloyd Delano, SVP/Chief Accounting Officer
Michael Mayell, President/COO

4269 Mesa Mental Health
PO Box 90607
Albuquerque, NM 87199-0607
505-816-6791
800-333-8829
Fax: 505-816-6702
E-mail: chr@mesamentalhealth.com
www.mesamentalhealth.com

4270 Mihalik Group
1300 W Belmont
Suite 500
Chicago, IL 60657
773-929-4276
Fax: 773-929-4466
E-mail: zorinag@themihalikgroup.com
www.themihalikgroup.com

Zorina Granjean, Contact

4271 Milliman, Inc
1099 18th Street
Suite 3100
Denver, CO 80202-1931
303-299-9400
Fax: 303-299-9018
www.milliman.com

Pat Grannan, President/CEO

Assist plans and payors in measuring and analyzing their healthcare costs arising from behavioral health conditions, identifying specific value opportunities, and designing innovative ways to obtain increased quality and value from behavioral health care delivery.

4272 Murphy-Harpst-Vashti
740 Fletcher Street
Cedartown, GA 30125-3249
770-748-1500
Fax: 770-749-1094
E-mail: contact@murphyharpst.org
www.murphyharpst.org

Joanne Simmons, President/CEO
Emily Saltino, VP Of Development

4273 NASW JobLink
750 First Street NE
Suite 700
Washington, DC 20002-4241
202-408-8600
E-mail: membership@naswdc.org
www.naswdc.org/joblinks/default.asp

Elvira Craig De Silva, President
Willie Walker, Vice President

4274 National Empowerment Center
599 Canal Street
Lawrence, MA 01840
978-685-1494
800-769-3728
Fax: 978-681-6426
E-mail: info4@power2u.org
www.power2u.org

Dan Fisher, Executive Director

Consumer/survivor/ex-patient run organization that carries a message of recovery, empowerment, hope and healing to people who have been diagnosed with mental illness.

4275 Network Behavioral Health
275 North Street
Harrison, NY 10528-1524
914-967-6500
888-224-2273
Fax: 914-925-5175

4276 New Day
49 Music Square W
Suite 502
Nashville, TN 37203
615-321-5577
Fax: 615-321-5566
E-mail: info@seniorhealthinc.com
www.www.seniorhealthinc.com

William Kaupas, VP Of Business Development
Kerri Kelley Frye, Vice President/CFO

quality, low cost standards in diagnosing and treating psychiatric conditions.

4277 New England Psych Group
10 Langley Road
Suite 305
Newton Center, MA 02459
617-527-4055
Fax: 617-527-2571

4278 Newbride Consultation
280 Madison Avenue
Suite 1004
New York, NY 10016
516-665-7889
E-mail: info@couplesandfamilies.com
www.www.couplesandfamilies.com

Cari Sans, Founder And Director

4279 Northpointe Behavioral Healthcare Systems
715 Pyle Drive
Kingsford, MI 49802-4456
906-774-9522
Fax: 906-774-1570
E-mail: info@nbhs.org
www.nbhs.org

Karen Raether, Chairperson
Anastasia Babladelis, Secretary

Michigan Community Mental Health agency serving Dickinson, Menominee and Iron counties. Provides a full spectrum of managed behavioral healthcare services to the chronically mentally ill and developmentally disabled. A corporate services division provides employee assistance programs both in Michigan and outside the state.

4280 Oklahoma Mental Health Consumer Council
3200 NW 48th Street
Suite 102
Oklahoma City, OK 73112
405-604-6975
888-424-1305
Fax: 405-605-8175
E-mail: consumercouncil@okmhcc.org
www.www.okmhcc.org

Larry Kelley, President
Jerry Risenhoover, Vice President

4281 One Hundred Top Series
Dorland Healthcare Information
1500 Walnut Street
Suite 1000
Philadelphia, PA 19102
215-875-1212
800-784-2332
Fax: 215-735-3966
E-mail: info@dorlandhealth.com
www.dorlandhealth.com

A leader in health and managed care business information.
$495.00

Year Founded: 1999

4282 Optimum Care Corporation
30011 Ivy Glenn Drive
Suite 219
Laguna Niguel, CA 92677

949-495-1100
Fax: 949-495-4316
www.optimumcare.com

Edward Johnson, Chairman/CEO

4283 Options Health Care
240 Corporate Boulevard
Norfolk, VA 23502-4948
757-459-5100
Fax: 757-892-5729
www.optionshealthcare.com

Barbara Hill, Chief Executive Officer
Michele Alfano, Chief Operating Officer

Specializes in creating innovative services for a full range of at-risk and administrative services only benefits, including behavioral health programs, customized provider and facility networks, utilization and case management, EAPs and youth services.

4284 PMHCC
123 S Broad Street
23rd Floor
Philadelphia, PA 19109
215-546-0300
Fax: 215-790-4975
E-mail: PMHCCExecOffice@pmhcc.org
www.pmhcc.org

Donald Brown, President
Jay Centifanti, Treasurer

4285 PRO Behavioral Health
7600 E Eastman Avenue
Ste. 500
Denver, CO 80231
303-695-8007
888-687-6755
Fax: 303-695-0100
E-mail: webmaster@probh.com
www.probh.com

Martin Dubin, Senior Vice President
Theodore Wirecki, Chair

A managed behavioral health care company dedicated to containing psychiatric and substance abuse costs while providing high-quality health care. Owned and operated by mental health care professionals, PRO has exclusive, multi-year contracts with HMOs and insurers on both coasts and in the Rocky Mountain region.

4286 PSC
1147 Starmount Court
Suite B
Bel Air, MD 21015-5650
410-569-6106
Fax: 410-569-6364

4287 PSIMED Corporation
725 Town & Country
Suite 200
Orange, CA 92868
714-689-1544
E-mail: response@arbormed.com
www.psimed-ambs.com

Suzanne Beals, Contact

4288 Paris International Corporation
185 Great Neck Rd
Ste. 305
Great Neck, NY 11021-3326
516-487-2630
Fax: 516-466-6255
E-mail: info@parisintl.com
www.www.parisintl.com

4289 Pearson
5601 Green Valley Drive
Bloomington, MN 55437
952-681-3000
800-627-7271
Fax: 800-632-9011
E-mail: pearsonassessments@pearson.com
www.www.pearsonassessments.com

pearson is a publisher of assessment tools and instructional materials in the special needs behavior management, speech, language, and mental health markets. Among their numerous products are the MMPI-2, million inventories, BASC-2, BASC monitor for ADHD, vineland adaptive behavior scales(vineland II) and the Peabody picture vocabulary test (PPVT-4).

4290 Persoma Management
2540 Monroeville Blvd
Monroeville, PA 15146
412-823-5155
Fax: 412-823-8262
www.persoma.com

Lynn Baughman, Staff Member
Richard Heil Jr., Staff Member

4291 Perspectives
20 N Clark Street
Suite 2650
Chicago, IL 60602
800-456-6327
800-866-7556
Fax: 312-558-1570
E-mail: info@perspectivesltd.com
www.www.perspectivesltd.com

Bernie Dyme, President

4292 Philadelphia Health Management
260 S Broad Street
18th Floor
Philadelphia, PA 19102-5085
215-985-2500
Fax: 215-985-2550
E-mail: info@phmc.org
www.phmc.org

Richard Cohen, President/CEO
John Loeb, Senior Vice President

4293 Pinal Gila Behavioral Health Association
2066 W Apache Trail
Suite 116
Apache Junction, AZ 85220-3733
480-982-1317
800-982-1317
Fax: 480-982-7320
E-mail: info@pgbha.org
www.pgbha.org

Sandie Smith, President
Bryan Chambers, Vice President

4294 Porter Novelli
75 Varick Street
6th Floor
New York, NY 10013
212-601-8000
Fax: 212-601-8101
E-mail: chris.lynch@porternovelli.com
www.porternovelli.com

Chris Lynch, Director Business Development
Gloria Ketenbaum, VP Of Marketing/Public Relations

4295 Posen Consulting Group
5328 Fairway Ct
W Bloomfield, MI 48323
248-661-0663
Fax: 248-661-6279

4296 Practice Management Resource Group
4100 Redwood Road #283
Oakland, CA 94619-2363
708-623-8200
Fax: 708-507-2932
E-mail: info@medicalpmrg.com
www.medicalpmrg.com

Ron Rosenberg, President/Founder

4297 Pragmatix
5650 Greenwood Plaza Boulevard
Suite 250A
Greenwood Village, CO 80111-2309
303-779-0812
Fax: 303-779-1335

4298 Preferred Mental Health Management
401 E. Douglas
Suite 300
Wichita, KS 67202
800-264-7496
E-mail: info@pmhm.com
www.pmhm.com

Les Ruthven, President/CEO

Offers managed care services and EAP services.

4299 Prime Care Consultants
297 Knollwood Road
White Plains, NY 10607
914-686-6891
800-933-8629
Fax: 914-682-7518
www.thevirtualbriefcase.com

4300 ProAmerica Managed Care
PO Box 202008
Arlington, TX 76006-8008
817-436-5172
800-523-3669
Fax: 817-436-5391
www.proamerica.com

Nancy Connaway, Chief Executive Officer
Ken Weithers, Chief Financial Officer
Kelly Robinson, Chief Information Officer

4301 ProMetrics CAREeval
480 American Avenue
King of Prussia, PA 19406
610-265-6344
Fax: 610-265-8377
E-mail: admin@prometrics.com
www.prometrics.com

Marc Duey, President

A joint venture formed by Father Flanagan's Home (Boys Town), Susquehanna Pathfinders and ProMetrics Consulting. These organizations combine years of experience as service providers and technical resource developers. Provides innovative ways to collect, store and analyze service outcome data to improve the effectiveness of your services.

4302 ProMetrics Consulting & Susquehanna PathFinders
480 American Avenue
King of Prussia, PA 19406-1405
610-265-6344
Fax: 610-265-8377
E-mail: admin@prometrics.com
www.prometrics.com

Marc Duey, President

4303 Process Strategies Institute
1418 D MacCorkle Ave SW
Charleston, WV 25303
304-348-1288
www.www.highlandhospital.net

Dave McWatters, Chief Executive Officer

4304 Professional Risk Management Services
1515 Wilson Boulevard
Suite 800
Arlington, VA 22209-2402
800-245-3333
E-mail: tracy@prms.com
www.prms.com

Martin Tracy, President/CEO
Joseph Detorie, Executive Vice President/CFO

4305 Professional Services Consultants
1147 Starmount Court
Suite B
Bel Air, MD 21015-5650
410-569-6106
Fax: 410-569-6364
E-mail: psc@netgsi.com
www.netgsi.com/~psc.

Professional Services Consultants (PSC), a unique nationally-recognized management consulting company, assists behavioral health care programs with policies, procedures, accreditation, licensure, reimbursement, documentation, infection control, credentialing, performance improvement, legal, risk management and employment issues. The PSC Healthcare Consultant is a subscription newsletter bringing you the latest on accreditation, licensure and management issues affecting health care. PSC's benchmarking system (NBN) provides an easy, low-cost approach to state-of-the-art outcome measurement. Call for more information. *$ 99.00*

4306 Providence Behavioral Health Connections
10300 SW Eastridge Street
Portland, OR 97225-5004

503-216-4984

4307 Psy Care
4550 Kearny Villa Road
Suite 116
San Diego, CA 92123
858-279-1223
www.www.psycare.org

James Adams, Board Certified Psychiatrist
Lauren Beauchamp, Psychologist

4308 PsycHealth
922 Davis Street
Evanston, IL 60201
847-864-4961
800-753-5456
Fax: 847-864-9930
E-mail: administration@psychealthltd.com
www.www.psychealthltd.com

Madeleine Gomez, President

Specialists providing mental health services, managed care and referrals.

4309 Psychiatric Associates
PO Box 6504
Kokomo, IN 46904
765-453-9338
Fax: 765-455-2710

Alok Sarda M.D., Contact

4310 Psycho Medical Chirologists
11612 Lockwood Drive
Suite 103
Silver Spring, MD 20904-2314
301-681-6614

Robert F Spiegel, Director

4311 Public Consulting Group
148 State Street
10th Floor
Boston, MA 02109
617-426-2026
800-210-6113
Fax: 617-426-4632
www.pcgus.com

William Mosakowski, President/CEO

4312 Pyrce Healthcare Group
7325 Greenfield Street
River Forest, IL 60305
708-383-7700
Fax: 708-383-7746
E-mail: phg-inc@ix.netcom.com
www.home.netcom.com

Janice M Pyrce, President/Founder

A national consulting firm, founded in 1990, with a focus on behavioral health. The firm specializes in strategic planning, market research, integrated delivery systems, business development, retreat facilitation and management/organizational development. PHG offers significant depth of resources, with direct involvement of experienced senior staff. Clients include hospitals, healthcare systems, academic medical centers, human service agencies, physician/allied practices, professional/trade associations and investor groups. The firm has over 200 organizations with locations in over 40 states.

4313 QualChoice Health Plan
6000 Parkland Boulevard
Cleveland, OH 44124-6119
440-460-0668
800-358-7311
Fax: 261-460-4006
E-mail: behavioral@qualchoice.com
www.qualchoice.com

4314 Quinco Behavioral Health Systems
720 N Marr Road
Columbus, IN 47201
812-379-2341
800-266-2341
Fax: 812-376-4875
E-mail: quincobhs@quincoinc.com
www.quincobhs.org

Robert S Dyer, CEO

Nonprofit mental health care provider serving south central Indiana. 24 hour crisis line and full continuum of mental health services.

4315 REC Management
1640 Powers Ferry Road SE
Suite 350
Marietta, GA 30067-5491
770-955-7715
Fax: 770-956-9325

4316 Salud Management Associates
2727 Palisade Avenue
Suite 4H
Riverdale, NY 10463-1020
718-796-0971
800-765-1209
Fax: 718-796-0971
www.vd6@columbia.edu

Dr. Victor De La Cancela, President/CEO

Clinical Psychology and Community Health Services. Bilingual Spanish-English culturally competent providers, trainers and organizational consultants.

4317 Sandra Fields-Neal and Associates
535 S Burdick Street
Suite 165
Kalamazoo, MI 49007-5261
269-381-5213

Sandra Fields-Neal, President/CEO

4318 Sarmul Consultants
1 Strawberry Hill Court
Stamford, CT 06902-2548
203-327-1596
Fax: 203-325-1639

4319 Schafer Consulting
602 Hemlock Road
Coraopolis, PA 15108
724-695-0652
E-mail: ask@schaferconsulting.com
www.www.schaferconsulting.com

Steve Schafer, President

4320 Scheur and Associates
1 Gateway Center
Suite 810
Newton, MA 02458
617-969-7500
Fax: 617-969-7508
E-mail: webmaster@scheur.com
www.scheur.com

Barry Scheur, President

4321 Sciacca Comprehensive Service Development for MIDAA
299 Riverside Drive
New York, NY 10025-5278
212-866-5935
Fax: 212-666-1942
E-mail: ksciacca@pobox.com

Kathleen Sciacca MA, Executive Director/Consultant

Provides consulting, education, and training for treatment and program development for dual diagnosis of mental illness and substance disorders including severe mental illness. Materials available include manuals, videos, articles, book chapters, journals, and books. Trains in Motivational Interviewing.

4322 Seelig and Company: Child Welfare and Behavioral Healthcare
140 E 45th Street
19th Floor
New York, NY 10017
212-655-3500
Fax: 212-655-3535
www.seelig.com

4323 Sheppard Pratt Health Plan
6501 N Charles Street
Baltimore, MD 21285
410-938-3000
Fax: 410-938-4099
E-mail: info@sheppardpratt.org
www.sheppardpratt.org

Steven Sharfstein, President/CEO
Diana Ramsay, Executive Vice President/COO

4324 Shueman and Associates
PO Box 90024
Pasadena, CA 91109-5024
626-585-8248

4325 Skypek Group
2528 W Tennessee Avenue
Tampa, FL 33629-6255
813-254-3926
Fax: 813-254-3926

4326 Specialized Alternatives for Families & Youth of America (SAFY)
10100 Elida Road
Delphos, OH 45833
419-224-2279
800-532-7239
Fax: 419-224-2287
E-mail: webmaster@safy.org
www.safy.org

Druann Whitaker MS LSW LPC, CEO
John Hollenkamp, SVP Of Finance

Not-for-profit managerial service organization providing a full continuum of quality care to families and youth across the nation.

4327 Specialized Therapy Associates
83 Summit Avenue
Hackensack, NJ 07601
201-488-6678
Fax: 201-488-6224
E-mail: stadocs@hotmail.com
www.www.specializedtherapy.com

Vanessa Gourdine, Director
Linda Mack, Assistant Director

4328 St. Anthony Behavioral Medicine Center, Behavioral Medicine
1000 N Lee Avenue
Oklahoma City, OK 73102
405-272-7000
800-227-6964
Fax: 405-272-6208
E-mail: st_anthony@ssmhc.com
www.www.saintsok.com

4329 Suburban Research Associates
107 Chesley Drive
Unit 4
Media, PA 19063
610-891-7200
E-mail: mmcnichol@suburbanresearch.com
www.suburbanresearch.com

Shivkumar Hatti, CEO

4330 Sue Krause and Associates
15 Jutland Road
Binghamton, NY 13903
607-771-8009

Sue Krause, Contact

4331 Supportive Systems
25 Beachway Drive
Suite C
Indianapolis, IN 46224
317-788-4111
800-660-6645
E-mail: staff@supportivesystems.com
www.supportivesystems.com

Pamela Ruster ACSW LCSW, President/CEO

4332 TASC
1500 N Halsted Street
Chicago, IL 60622
312-787-0208
Fax: 312-787-9663
E-mail: information@tasc-il.org
www.www.tasc.org

Melody Heaps, President
Pamela Rodriguez, Executive Vice President
Roy Fesmire, Vice President/CFO

4333 The Kennion Group Inc
1200 Corporate Drive
Suite G-50
Birmingham, AL 35242
205-972-0110
800-645-8058

Fax: 205-969-1199
www.www.kennion.com

W. Hal Shepherd, President/CEO

4334 Towers Perrin Integrated Heatlh Systems Consulting
335 Madison Avenue
New York, NY 10017-4605
212-309-3400
www.towersperrin.com

Mark Mactas, Chairman/CEO
Maureen Breakiron-Evans, CFO

Managed behavorial health care consultants specializing in strategy and operations, clinical effectiveness, actuarial and reimbursement and human resources for both the provider and the payer sides.

4335 United Behavioral Health
425 Market Street
27th Floor
San Francisco, CA 94105
800-888-2998
www.www.unitedbehavioralhealth.com

Gregory Bayer, CEO
Rhonda Robinson-Beale, Chief Medical Officer

4336 University of North Carolina School of Social Work, Behavioral Healthcare
Tate-Turner-Kuralt Building
325 Pittsboro Street Cb#3550
Chapel Hill, NC 27599-3550
919-962-1225
Fax: 919-962-0890
E-mail: ssw@unc.edu
www.http://ssw.unc.edu

4337 Value Health
525 Knotter Dr
Cheshire, CT 06410
203-272-3856

4338 ValueOptions
240 Corporate Blvd
Norfolk, VA 23502
757-459-5100
www.valueoptions.com

Barbara Hill, CEO
Michele Alfano, COO

Designs and operates innovative administrative and full-risk services for a wide range of behavioral health and chemical dependency programs, Medicaid, child welfare and other human services, and Employee Assistance Programs. Develops collaborative relationships with government agencies, community providers, consumer groups, health plans, insurers, and others to foster a deeper understanding of the needs of the various populations they serve. Develops child welfare programs based upon the principles of managed care.

4339 ValueOptions Jacksonville Service Center
10199 Southside Blvd
Building 100 Suite 300
Jacksonville, FL 32256
800-700-8646
www.valueoptions.com

Barbara Hill, Chief Executive Officer
E. Paul Dunn Jr., Chief Financial Officer
Michele D Alfano, Chief Operating Officer

4340 Vanderveer Group
520 Virginia Drive
Fort Washington, PA 19034-2795
215-283-5373
Fax: 215-646-5547

4341 Vasquez Management Consultants
100 S Greenleaf Avenue
Gurnee, IL 60031-3378
847-249-1900
800-367-7378
Fax: 847-249-2772
www.vmceap.com

4342 Vedder Price
222 N LaSalle Street
Chicago, IL 60601
312-609-7500
Fax: 312-609-5005
E-mail: kwendrickx@vedderprice.com
www.vedderprice.com

Kristie Wendrickx-Powell, Business Development Manager
Richard Thomas, Director Of Finance

4343 VeriCare
47415 Viewridge Avenue
Suite 230
San Diego, CA 92123
858-454-3610
800-257-8715
Fax: 800-819-1655
E-mail: contactus@vericare.com
www.www.vericare.com

David Flaugh, President/CEO
Thomas Cooper, Chairman Of The Board

4344 VeriTrak
179 Niblick Road
Suite 149
Paso Robles, CA 93446-4845
800-370-2440
E-mail: support@veritrak.com
www.veritrak.com

4345 Verispan
114 Melrich Road
Suite A
Cranbury, NJ 08512
609-235-3300
Fax: 609-235-3400
www.kwsp.com

Wayne Yetter, CEO
Peter Bird, Senior Vice President

4346 Virginia Beach Community Service Board
Pembroke 6
Suite 208
Virginia Beach, VA 23462
757-437-5770
Fax: 804-490-5736

4347 Watson Wyatt Worldwide
15303 Ventura Boulevard
Suite 700
Sherman Oaks, CA 91403-3197
818-906-2631
Fax: 808-906-2097

4348 Webman Associates
4 Brattle Street
Cambridge, MA 02138
617-864-6769

4349 WellPoint Behavioral Health
9655 Graniteridge Drive
Sixth Floor
San Diego, CA 92123
800-728-9498
www.wellpointbehavioral.com

Laurie Wright, VP EAP/Employer Based Products

4350 William M Mercer
133 Peachtree Street NE
3700 Georgia Pacific Center
Atlanta, GA 30305
404-521-2200
Fax: 404-523-1458

Michael Brase, MD, Medical Director

4351 Working Press
Pensions, Benefits & Compensators Employer
1223 Wilshire Boulevard
Suite 933
Santa Monica, CA 90405-3538
310-314-8600

Software Companies

4352 ACC
12500 San Pedro
Suite 460
San Antonio, TX 78216-2867
210-545-1010
800-880-4222
E-mail: acc@foxmed.com
www.foxmed.com

Greg Schipper, President Clinics/Grp Practices

ACC markets practice management software, FOXMed Pro and MedPro for Windows, through a network of independent dealers. These systems fully automate billing and claims for small to medium sized practices.

4353 ACS Healthcare Solutions
5225 Auto Club Drive
Dearborn, MI 48126
248-386-8300
Fax: 248-386-8301
www.www.superiorconsultants.com

We focus on the unique needs of your healthcare business through out diversified service offerings.

4354 AHMAC
140 Allens Creek Road
Rochester, NY 14618
800-638-0890
E-mail: sales@ahmac.com
www.www.hewitsoftware.com

CareManager is a microcomputer based system targeted at small to medium sized HMOs, PPOs and PHOs as well as vertical markets such as Medicaid and managed mental health. Easily customized to meet the needs and requirements of the client.

4355 AIMS
485 Underhill Boulevard
Syosset, NY 11791
516-496-7700
Fax: 516-496-7069

Ann Elbirt, Marketing Administration Mgr

Provider of systems for payers and providers. AIMS client centered, integrated care systems respond to payer cost containment strategies. The system features clinical integrity, outcome-oriented service plans with integrated notes and documentation.

4356 AMCO Computers
750 W Golden Grove Way
Covina, CA 91722-3255
626-859-6292

Medical consultants, business computing consulting, computer software.

4357 ASP Software
1031 E Duane Avenue
Suite M
Sunnyvale, CA 94086-2625
408-733-7831
800-822-7832
Fax: 408-738-0617

MEDx was designed with the belief that your practice management system should be easy to use.

4358 Accreditation Services
PO Box 73270
Metairie, LA 70033-3270
504-469-4285
Fax: 504-467-7688
E-mail: sales@mail.accreditationservices.com
www.accreditationservices.com

Glen E Philmon, Sr, Chairman

Multiple software programs dedicated to the support of health care industry's needs for training, continuing education, work order processing and inventory control and the various demands placed upon the system by regulatory boards. Services are completely confidential and available for almost every department of the hospital, nursing home, ICF/MR facilities and many others. Each software program can be customized to be site-specific.

4359 Accumedic Computer Systems
11 Grace Avenue
Suite 401
Great Neck, NY 11021
516-466-6800
800-765-9300
Fax: 516-466-6880
www.accumedic.com

Medical practice management software and healthcare information systems (HCIS) solutions.

4360 Adam Software
1600 RiverEdge Parkway
Suite 100
Atlanta, GA 30328
770-980-0888
www.www.adam.com

Provides products to connect consumers and their families to trustworthy and relevant health information.

4361 Advanced Data Systems
700 Mount Hope Avenue
Suite 101
Bangor, ME 04401
207-947-4494
800-779-4494
Fax: 207-947-0650
E-mail: info@adspro.com
www.adspro.com

Advanced Data Systems (ADS) is a New England-based software developer and reseller of accounting information systems with over 23 years of experience. We specialize in developing, implementing and supporting administrative software. As a complement to our software we also provide technical services. Advanced Data Systems is your "total accounting solution".

4362 Agilent Technologies
5301 Stevens Creek Blvd
Santa Clara, CA 95051
650-752-5000
408-345-8886
Fax: 408-345-8474
www.agilent.com/healthcare

Clinical measurement and diagnostic solutions for healthcare organizations.

4363 American Medical Software
PO Box 236
Edwardsville, IL 62025-0236
618-692-1300
800-423-8836
Fax: 618-692-1809
E-mail: sales@americanmedical.com
www.americanmedical.com

Practice management software for billing, electronic claims, appointments and electronic medical records.

4364 American Psychiatric Press Reference Library CD-ROM
American Psychiatric Publishing
1000 Wilson Boulevard
Suite 1825
Arlington, VA 22209-3901
703-907-7322
800-368-5777
Fax: 703-907-1091
E-mail: appi@psych.org
www.appi.org

$395.00

Year Founded: 1998

4365 Anasazi Software
9831 S 51st Street
Suite C117
Phoenix, AZ 85044

800-651-4411
E-mail: sales@anasazisoftware.com
www.anasazisoftware.com

Developed by and for behavioral healthcare and social service professionals, helps you provide the best care possible to your clients.

4366 Andrew and Associates

PO Box 9226
Winter Haven, FL 33883-9226
813-299-4767

William F Andrew, PE, President

IT consulting and clinical IS for computer based patient records.

4367 Aries Systems Corporation

200 Sutton Street
N Andover, MA 01845
978-975-7570
Fax: 978-975-3811
E-mail: kfinder@kfinder.com
www.kfinder.com

Lyndon Holmes, President

Provides technical innovations that empower all of the participants in the knowledge retrieval chain: publishers, database developers, librarians.

4368 Ascent

Ruby Creek Road
PO Box 230
Naples, ID 83847
208-267-3626
800-974-1999
Fax: 208-267-2295
E-mail: claudia.peterson@uhsinc.com

4369 Askesis Development Group

One Chatham Center
112 Washington Place Ste 300
Pittsburgh, PA 15219
412-803-2400
Fax: 412-803-2099
E-mail: info@askesis.com
www.askesis.com

Askesis Development Group's PsychConsult is a complete informatics solution for behavioral health organizations: inpatient or outpatient behavioral health facilities, managed care organizations, and provider networks. PsychConsult is Windows NT based, and Y2K compliant. ADG development is guided by the PsychConsult Consortium, a collaborative effort of leading institutions in behavioral health.

4370 Assist Technologies

2501 N Hayden Road
Suite 104
Scottsdale, AZ 85257
480-874-9400
Fax: 480-874-9414
E-mail: info@assistek.com
www.assistek.com

The Touch Outcomes Collector system greatly increase the quality of questionnaire data collected in clinical trials, which results in more usable data to support FDA claims.

4371 Austin Travis County Mental Health Mental Retardation Center

1430 Collier Street
Austin, TX 78704
512-447-4141
www.atcmhmr.com

Provides mental health, mental retardation and substance services to the Austin-Travis County community.

4372 Aware Resources

PO Box 247
Munroe Falls, OH 44262
330-475-0060
800-254-1532
Fax: 330-475-0066
E-mail: info@awareresources.com
www.awareresources.com

Susan Searl, RN, President

Provides behavior management consultation, staff training and client counseling.

4373 BOSS Inc

2639 N Downer Avenue
Suite 9
Milwaukee, WI 53211
800-964-4789
E-mail: bmiller@healthcareboss.com
www.healthcareboss.com

Bob Miller, President

Practice management software that is easy to use and is in more than 29,000 practices nationally. Outcome management software products for social workers and hospitals. *$1499.00*

Year Founded: 1986

4374 Beaver Creek Software

525 SW 6th Street
Corvallis, OR 97333-4323
541-752-5039
800-895-3344
Fax: 541-752-5221
E-mail: sales@beaverlog.com
www.beaverlog.com

"The THERAPIST" practice management and billing software for Windows operating systems comes in Pro and EZ versions. The EZ version is powerful yet simple to use and is tailored to needs of smaller offices. The Pro version is designed to handle the complex needs of busy practices. Use Pro to create HIPAA compliant electronic insurance claims. Both versions let you have an unlimited number of providers at no additional cost. *$249.00*

Year Founded: 1989

4375 Behavioral Health Advisor
McKesson Clinical Reference Systems

335 Interlocken Parkway
Broomfield, CO 80021
800-782-1334
www.www.mckesson.com

The Behavioral Health Advisor software program provides consumer health information for more than 600 topics covering pediatric and adult mental illness, disorders and behavioral problems. Includes behavioral health topics from the American Academy of Child and Adolescent Psychiatry. Many Spanish translations available. *$4.75*

Year Founded: 1998

4376 Behaviordata
20833 Stevens Creek Boulevard
Suite 100
Cupertino, CA 95014
408-342-0600
800-627-2673
Fax: 408-342-0617
www.www.behaviordat.com

Diana Sullivan Everstine, Contact
Dr David Nichols, Contact

4377 Bellefaire Jewish Children's Bureau
22001 Fairmount Boulevard
Shaker Heights, OH 44118
216-932-2800
www.bellefairejcb.org

Adam G Jacobs PhD, Executive Vp
Larry Pollock, President

A nonprofit mental health agency committed to serving the needs of children, youth and their families through an array of child welfare and behavioral health services. Provides its services without regard to race, religion, sex or national origin.

4378 BetaData Systems
3137 E Greenlee Road
Tucson, AZ 85716
520-917-1028
Fax: 520-733-5659
E-mail: sales@betadata.net
www.www.betadata.net

Providing computer software, hardware, consulting, service, and support to the industry.

Year Founded: 1978

4379 Body Logic
PO Box 162101
Austin, TX 78716-2101
512-327-0050
Fax: 512-307-6770

designs and consults information technology solutions for clinical delivery.

4380 Bull HN Information Systems
296 Concord Road
Billerica, MA 01821
978-294-6000
Fax: 978-294-7999
www.www.bull.us/usa.html

Provides solutions and services to key markets, including the public sector, finance, manufacturing, and telecommunications.

4381 Business Objects
3030 Orchard Parkway
San Jose, CA 95134
408-953-6000
800-527-0580
Fax: 408-953-6001
www.businessobjects.com

Our software helps organizations gain better insight into their business, improving decision making and enterprise performance.

Year Founded: 1990

4382 CASCAP
678 Massachusetts Avenue
Floor 10
Cambridge, MA 02139
617-492-5559
Fax: 617-492-6928
TTY: 617-234-2992
E-mail: info@cascap.org
www.cascap.org

Michael Haran, CEO

Committed to improving the quality of life for members of the community who may be disadvantaged by poverty, disability, or age. Our purpose is to help thos we serve achieve optimal levels of personal autonomy and community integration.

Year Founded: 1973

4383 CLARC Services
3500 Tamiami Trail
Port Charlotte, FL 33952
800-246-5488
E-mail: dclaise@clarc.com
www.www.clarc.com

Dave Claise, Sales Manager

Computer consultancy which provides software, software training and support, custom programming, modifications to packaged products and education. We help your business with hardware and software installation and setup as well as data migration, integration and data conversion. Creators of Mental Health Organizational System Interface (MHOSI).

Year Founded: 1989

4384 CSI Software
3333 Richmond
2nd Floor
Houston, TX 77098
713-942-7779
800-247-3431
Fax: 713-942-7731
E-mail: sales@csisoftwareusa.com
www.csisoftwareusa.com

CSI Software designs software for the membership industry utilizing the most sophisticated software technologies, coupled with unsurpassed and experience and support.

4385 Cardiff Software: Vista
3220 Executive Ridge
Vista, CA 92081
760-936-4500
Fax: 760-936-4800
E-mail: info@verity.com
www.cardiff.com

Provider of adaptive business process management (BPM) and content capture solutions. Cardiff enables organizations to capture data from electronic and paper sources and adapt to existing processes by managing structured, exception and people driven actions.

4386 Center for Clinical Computing
350 Longwood Avenue
Boston, MA 02115-5726
617-732-5925

4387 Center for Health Policy Studies
10400 Little Patuxent Parkway
Suite 10
Columbia, MD 21044
410-715-9400
www.heritage.org

Robert E Moffit, PhD, Director

Provides thorough analyses and develops major policy prescriptions to address matters of affordability, insurance, and quality of care.

4388 Ceridian Corporation
3311 E Old Shackopee Road
Minneapolis, MN 55425
612-853-8100
www.www.ceridian.com

A computer services and manufacturing company.

Year Founded: 1957

4389 Chartman Software
PO Box 551
Santa Barbara, CA 93102
805-563-5363

A complete electronic patient chart management solution.

4390 Cincom Systems
55 Merchant Street
Cincinnati, OH 45246
513-612-2769
800-224-6266
E-mail: info@cincom.com
www.cincom.com

Cincom provides software and service solutions that help our clients create, manage and grow relationships with their customers through adaptive e-business information systems.

4391 Client Management Information System
WilData Systems Group
255 Bradenton Avenue
Dublin, OH 43017
614-734-4719
800-860-4222
Fax: 614-734-1063
E-mail: cmis@wildatainc.com
www.wildatainc.com

Complete software package designed as a total solution for the information and reporting requirements of behavioral health care centers, drug and alcohol abuse centers, human service organizations and family service agencies. CMIS is easy to use with graphical user input screens allowing point and click capabilities under Microsoft Windows.

4392 CliniSphere version 2.0
Facts and Comparisons
77 Westport Plaza
Suite 450
Saint Louis, MO 63146
314-216-2100
800-223-0554
www.www.factsandcomparisons.com

Access to all information in a clinical drug reference library, by drug, disease, side-effects; thousands of drugs (prescription, OTC, investigational) all included; contains information from Drug Facts and Comparisons, most defin-

itive and comprehensive source for comparative drug information.

4393 Clinical Nutrition Center
7555 E Hampden Avenue
Suite 301
Denver, CO 80231
303-750-9454
Fax: 303-750-1996
www.www.clinicalnutritioncenter.com

James Berry, MD, Founder/Practice Consultant

Our programs are based on the latest development in the field of nutrition, weight loss and weight control, behavior modification.

4394 Compu-Care Management and Systems
3737 Executive Center Drive
Austin, TX 78731
512-219-8025

Application service provider for the behavioral health industry dedicated to helping providers meet their goals for efficiency and productivity.

4395 CompuLab Healthcare Systems Corporation
PO Box 11739
Fort Lauderdale, FL 33339
800-266-7852
E-mail: webmaster@compulab.com
www.compulab.com

For the development of innovative computer technology and data processing systems in a variety of industries.

4396 Computer Transition Services
3223 S Loop
Suite 556
Lubbock, TX 79423
806-793-8961
Fax: 806-793-8968
www.ctsinet.com

Improve the life and business success of clients by providing integrated solutions and professional services to meet their technological and organizational needs.

4397 Control-0-Fax Corporation
3070 W Airline Highway
Waterloo, IA 50704-0778
800-553-0070
800-344-7777
E-mail: info@controlofax.com
www.controlfax.com

Our product offering includes printed forms, clinical records, color-coded filing, chart management and four-color promotional printing. Additional services include file conversion, print and mail services and a complete array of EDI applications.

4398 CoolTalk
Netscape Communicatons
PO Box 7050
Mountain View, CA 94039-7050
650-254-1900
800-784-3348
Fax: 650-528-4124
www.netscape.com

Jim Barksdale, President/CEO

Intergrated telephone application, allows connected users to draw or sketch ideas cooperatively onto the same area on each person's computer screen.

4399 Cornucopia Software
PO Box 6111
Albany, CA 94706
510-528-7000
E-mail: supportstaff@practicemagic.com
www.practicemagic.com

Providers of Practice MAGIC, the billing and practice management software that counts for your psychotherapy practice.

4400 Creative Computer Applications
26115 Mureau Road
Suite A
Calabasas, CA 91302-3128
818-880-6700
800-437-9000
Fax: 818-880-4398
www.ccainc.com

Bruce M Miller, Chairman
Steven M Besbeck, President/CEO
William Blair, VP Sales
Douglas A Collie, Imaging Product Manager

Develop, assemble, market, install and service computer based clinical information systems and products which automate the acquisition and management of clinical data for the healthcare industry.

4401 Creative Socio-Medics Corporation
3500 Sunrise Highway
Suite D122
Great River, NY 11751
631-968-2000
Fax: 631-968-2123

Creative has pioneered delivery of information systems to the health and human services industry.

4402 DB Consultants
198 Tabor Road
PO Box 580
Ottsville, PA 18942
610-847-5065
Fax: 610-847-2298
E-mail: sales@dbconsultants.com
www.dbconsultants.com

AS/PC includes electronic claims submission. Healtcare professionals rely on AS/PC every day to help them provide quality care.

4403 DST Output
2600 Sw Blvd
Kansas City, MO 64108
816-221-1234
800-441-7587
E-mail: sales_marketing@dstoutput.com
www.www.dstoutput.com

Steve Towle, President/CEO
Frank Delfer, CTO
Jim Reinert, EVP Business Development

Providing a customer communications solution offering myriad benefits to healthcare payor organizations, including the ability to manage both inbound and outbound communications; ensure document control and content compliance;

integrate data from portal entry; distribute data, information, and material to the right place and audience with integrity.

4404 DataMark
2305 Presidents Drive
Salt Lake City, UT 84120
801-886-2002
800-279-9335
Fax: 801-886-0102
E-mail: info@datamark.com
www.www.datamark.com

Dedicated to providing innovative solutions that work to ease administrative burdens through automation, improved data capture, reduced duplication of effort and improved reporting capabilities: Custom Software Development, Data Analysis, Data Capture, Reporting, Statistic Anslysis.

4405 DeltaMetrics
600 Public Ledger Building
150 South Independence Mall West
Philadelphia, PA 19106-3475
215-399-0988
Fax: 215-399-0989
www.deltametrics.com

Jack Durell, MD, President/CEO

DeltaMetrics is now assisting treatment agencies to design and implement programs of Continuous Quality Improvement (CQI) within their systems of care.

4406 Distance Learning Network
111 Boal Ave
Boalsburg, PA 16827
814-466-7808

Eric Porterfield, Director

Broadcast and multimedia company dedicated solely to meeting the medical education and communications needs of physicians through the use of both traditional and innovative media formats. More than 150,000 physicians, nurses and pharmacists turn to DLN each year for their medical education.

Year Founded: 1996

4407 Docu Trac
20140 Scholar Drive
Suite 218
Hagerstown, MD 21742
301-766-4130
800-850-8510
Fax: 301-766-4097
E-mail: sales@quicdoc.com
www.quicdoc.com

Offering Quic Doc clinical documentation software, a comprehensive software system designed specifically for behavioral healthcare providers.

Year Founded: 1993

4408 DocuMed
3518 West Liberty Road
Ann Arbor, MI 48103
800-321-5595
E-mail: info@documed.com
www.documed.com

DocuMed 2002 is a comprehensive system for automated documentation of physician/patient encounters in ambulatory settings for solo practitioners or multiple physician groups.

4409 E Services Group
7340 Executive Way
Suite M
Frederick, MD 21704
301-698-1900
Fax: 301-698-1909
E-mail: sales@esrv.com
www.www.esrv.com

Our primary focus is on finding that perfect marriage of savvy business logic and technologies so that our healthcare IT applications solve the real world business problems of our clients.

4410 EAP Technology Systems
PO Box 1650
Yreka, CA 96097
800-755-6965
E-mail: information@eaptechnology.com
www.www.eaptechnology.com

Provider of technologies that automate work flow and enhance the business value of Employee Assistance Programs.

4411 Echo Group
519 17th Street
Suite 400
Oakland, CA 94612-1532
603-447-8600
800-635-8209
Fax: 603-447-8680
E-mail: info@echoman.com
www.echoman.com

Kenneth Fu, President

Echo Group has been helping behavioral healthcare organizations to succeed in their missions of healing.

4412 Eclipsys Corporation
1750 Clint Moore Road
Boca Raton, FL 33487
561-322-4321
www.www.eclipsys.com

R Andrew Eckert, President/CEO

Eclipsys empowers healthcare organizations to improve patient safety, financial strength, operational efficiency and customer satisfaction through innovative information software and service solutions.

Year Founded: 1995

4413 Electronic Healthcare Systems
Ehs One Metroplex Drive
Suite 500
Birmingham, AL 35209
205-871-1031
888-879-7302
Fax: 205-871-1185
E-mail: marketing@ehsmed.com
www.ehsmed.com

EHS develops and markets system solutions to a select group of physicians who are leading the way to clinical excellence and practice efficiency trhough automation.

Year Founded: 1995

4414 Emedeon Practice Services
2202 N West Shore Boulevard
Suite 300
Tampa, FL 33607-5749
877-932-6301
E-mail: lynne.durham@sage.com
www.www.sagehealth.com

Lynne Durham, Contact

Provides comprehensive systems that include all aspects of billing, scheduling, electronic data interchange(EDI), electronic health records(EHR), and enterprise data management with advanced reporting solutions.

4415 Entre Technology Services
2727 Central Ave
Billings, MT 59102
406-256-5700
Fax: 406-256-0201
www.www.entremt.com

Mike Keene, Contact

Computer Networking.

4416 Experior Corporation
5710 Coventry Lane
Fort Wayne, IN 46804
260-432-2020
800-595-2020
Fax: 260-432-4753
E-mail: sales@experior.com
www.www.experior.com

Experior provides Innovative Information systems to practice management and ASC marketplace. Out products, SurgeOn and EMS provide scheduling, case costing and billing.

4417 Facts Services
1575 San Ignacio Avenue
Suite 406
Coral Gables, FL 33146
305-284-7400
Fax: 305-661-6710
E-mail: sales@factsservices.com
www.factsservices.com

Provides fully automated and integrated software and hardware solutions for employee benefit administration, specializing in claims and encounter processing, risk management and managed care systems.

4418 Family Services of Delaware County
600 N Olive Street
Media, PA 19063
610-566-7540
Fax: 610-566-7677
www.www.fcsdc.org

Tracy Segal, Director Development

The Where to Turn Database is the most comprehensive listing of Non-Profit Human Service programs in the Delaware County area, the Young Resources Database is a condensed version of the above.

4419 First Data Bank
1111 Bayhill Drive
San Bruno, CA 94066
650-588-5454
800-633-3453

Fax: 650-588-4003
www.www.firstdatabank.com

James L Wilson, EVP

Provides thousands of drug knowledge base implementations ranging from pharmacy dispensing and claims processing to emerging applications including computerized physician order entry (CPOE), electronic health records (EHR), e-Prescribing and electronic medication administration records (EMAR).

4420 Gelbart and Associates

423 S Pacific Coast Highway
Suite 102
Redondo Beach, CA 90277
310-792-1823
Fax: 310-540-8904
www.gelbartandassociates.com

Robert Cutrow, Contact

Comprehensive Psychological and Psychiatric services for individuals, families, couples and groups, treating: anxiety, depression, relationship conflicts and medication management.

4421 GenSource Corporation

25572 Stanford Avenue
Valencia, CA 91355
800-949-9192
Fax: 661-294-1310
E-mail: sales@gensourcecorp.com
www.gensourcecorp.com

Greg Fisher, President/Coo
Chris Sullivan, Vp Operations

Offers a comprehensive set of fully integrated software systems for administering insurance related claims and managing risk, including workers compensation, non-occupational disability, property and casualty claims.

Year Founded: 1977

4422 Genelco Software Solutions

325 McDonnell Blvd
Hazelwood, MO 63042
800-548-2040
Fax: 314-593-3517
E-mail: info@genelco.com
www.genelco.com

Offers its flagship software systems in an ASP financial model. An ASP arrangement allows an organization to maintain control over operations without maintaining the software onsite.

4423 HCIA Response

950 Winter Street
Suite 3450
Waltham, MA 02451-1486
800-522-1440
Fax: 781-768-1811

4424 HMS Healthcare Management Systems

3102 W End Avenue
Suite 400
Nashville, TN 37203
615-383-7300
800-383-3317
Fax: 615-383-6093
www.hmstn.com

Automates processes including billing, scheduling and auditing within healthcare organizations.

4425 HMS Software

1912 Lakeview Drive
Harker Heights, TX 75240-6786
254-698-7535

Alexander Houtzeel, Co-Founder/President

4426 HSA-Mental Health

1080 Emeline Avenue
Santa Cruz, CA 95060
831-454-4000
Fax: 831-454-4770
TDD: 831-454-2123
E-mail: info@santacruzhealth.org
www.santacruzhealth.org

Exists to protect and improve the health of the people in Santa Cruz County. Provides programs in environmental health, public health, medical care, substance abuse prevention and treatment, and mental health. Clients are entitled to information on the costs of care and their options for getting health insurance coverage through a variety of programs.

4427 HZI Research Center

150 White Plains Road
Tarrytown, NY 10591
914-631-3315

Tele-Map EEG Service provides the most advanced neuroimaging technologies.

4428 Habilitation Software

204 N Sterling Street
Morganton, NC 28655
828-438-9455
Fax: 828-438-9488
E-mail: info@habsoft.com
www.habsoft.com

Personal Planning System, Windows-based computer program which assists agencies serving people with developmental disabilities with the tasks of person-centered planning; tracks outcomes, services and supports, assists with assesments and quarterly reviews, and maintains a customizable library of training programs. Also includes a census system for agencies which must maintain an exact midnight census, as well as an Accident/Incident system.

4429 Hanover Insurance

440 Lincoln Street
Worcester, MA 01653-0002
508-855-1000
800-853-0456
www.www.hanover.com

Offers hospice programs, rehabilitation groups and mental health services.

4430 Health Probe

5693 Bear Wallow Road
Suite 100
Morgantown, IN 46160
765-342-9947
E-mail: support@healthprobe.com
www.healthprobe.com

EMR created to eliminate the need for paper with electronic medical records.

4431 HealthLine Systems
17085 Camino San Bernardo
San Diego, CA 92127
858-673-1700
800-733-8737
Fax: 858-673-9866
E-mail: sales@healthlinesystems.com
www.www.healthlinesystems.com

Provide peerless information management solutions and services that maximize the quality and delivery of healthcare.

4432 HealthSoft
PO Box 536489
Orlando, FL 32853
407-648-4857
800-235-0882
Fax: 407-426-7440
E-mail: admin@healthsoftonline.com
www.www.healthsoftonline.com

CD - ROM and web based software for professionals on mental health nursing and developmental disabilities nursing.

4433 Healthcare Vision
2601 Scott Avenue
Suite 600
Fort Worth, TX 76103
817-531-8992
888-836-7428
Fax: 817-531-2360
E-mail: sales1@healthcaare-vision.com
www.www.healthcare-vision.com

HCV's innovative telemedicine software solutions and research and development capability enables HCV to deliver high-tech software solutions with features and benefits for quality healthcare, today and in the future.

Year Founded: 1992

4434 Healthline Systems
17085 Camino San Bernardo
San Diego, CA 92127
858-673-1700
800-254-7347
Fax: 858-673-9866
E-mail: sales@healthlinesystems.com
www.getproof.com

Provider of Document Management and Physician Credentialing software solutions.

4435 Healthport
120 Bluegrass Valley Parkway
Alpharetta, GA 30005
800-367-1500
www.www.healthport.com

Develops and sells Companion EMR, an electronic medical record system that eliminates paperwork, improves accuracy of information, provides instant access to patient and clinical information, and helps cuts costs while increasing revenue.

4436 Hogan Assessment Systems
2622 East 21st Street
Tulsa, OK 74114
918-749-0632
800-756-0632

Fax: 918-749-0635
www.hoganassessments.com

Robert Hogan, President/CEO

Focuses on five dimensions of personality including emotional stability, extroversion, likeability, conscientiousness and the degree to which a person needs stimulation.

4437 IBM Global Healthcare Industry
404 Wyman Street
Waltham, MA 02454
781-895-2911
Fax: 617-361-2485
E-mail: tgaffin@us.ibm.com
www.ibm.com/industries/healthcare

IBM has been strategically involved in assisting the healthcare industry in addressing numerous IT challenges. IBM provides clients and partners with the industry's broadest portfolio of technology, services, skills, and insight.

4438 IDX Systems Corporation
40 IDX Drive
South Burlington, VT 05402
802-862-1022
Fax: 802-862-6848
www.idx.com

Provides information technology solutions to maximize value in the delivery of healthcare, improve the quality of patient service, enhance medical outcomes, and reduce the costs of care.

Year Founded: 1969

4439 IMNET Systems
3015 Windward Plaza
Alpharetta, GA 30005
770-521-5600
800-329-2777

Develops, markets, installs and services electronic information and document management systems for the healthcare industry and other document intensive businesses.

4440 InfoMC
101 W Elm Street
Suite G10
Conshohocken, PA 19428
484-530-0100
Fax: 484-530-0111
E-mail: sales@infomc.com
www.infomc.com

Develops software solutions for Managed Care organizations, EAP/Work-Life organizations, and Health and Human Services agencies.

Year Founded: 1994

4441 Information Management Solutions
2422 Freedom Street
San Antonio, TX 78217
210-826-4994
800-255-3190
Fax: 210-826-2676
E-mail: john@totalims.com
www.www.totalims.com

Kelly Dowe, Sales/Corporate Information
John Reed, Sales Contact

Provides complete electronic Document Imaging Services to covert paper, microfilm, microfiche and engineering drawings to electronic images.

4442 Informix Software
IBM Corporation
1133 Westchester Avenue
White Plains, NY 10604
877-426-6006
www.ibm.com/software

IBM Informix® software includes a comprehensive array of high-performance, stand-alone and integration tools that enable efficient application and Web development, information integration , and database administration.

4443 Inforum
777 E Eisenhower Parkway
Ann Arbor, MI 48108
734-913-3000
www.medstat.com

Medstat has designed information solutions to strengthen healthcare policy and management decision-making.

Year Founded: 1981

4444 Inhealth Record Systems
5076 Winters Chapel Road
Atlanta, GA 30360
770-396-4994
800-477-7374
E-mail: sales@inhealth.us
www.inhealthrecords.com

Jeffrey Adams, EVP/COO

Provides variety of record keeping system products for health care practices and organizations.

Year Founded: 1979

4445 Innovative Data Solutions
386 Newberry Drive
Suite 100
Elk Grove Village, IL 60007
847-923-1926
E-mail: info@idsincp.com
www.idsincp.com

Mark Parianos, President/CEO

Provide effective web based and software solutions for business, small offices and fortune 500 clients.

Year Founded: 1991

4446 Innovative Health Systems/SoftMed
160 Blue Ravine Road
Suite A
Folsom, CA 95630
916-605-2050
800-695-4447
Fax: 916-605-2065
www.www.softmed.com

Don Ratcliff, Founder/President/EVP

4447 Integrated Business Services
736 N Western Ave
125
Lake Forest, IL 60045-1820
800-451-5478
Fax: 847-735-1692

E-mail: info@medbase200.com
www.medbase200.com

A medical research and information marketing firm providing access to highly selectable medical databases.

Year Founded: 1982

4448 Integrated Computer Products
125 Commerce Drive
Fayetteville, GA 30214-7336
770-719-1500

4449 InternetPhone
VocalTec
1 Executive Drive
Fort Lee, NJ 07024-3309
201-228-7000
Fax: 201-363-8986
E-mail: info@vocaltec.com
www.vocaltec.com

Elon Ganor, Chairman
Joseph Albagli, President/CEO
Laura Gavin, Manager

Telephone solution with availability on multiple platforms; one week free trial period for mental health related software is available.

4450 Keane Care
Keane Care
8383 158th Avenue NE
Suite 100
Redmond, WA 98052
800-426-2675
Fax: 425-307-2220
E-mail: kim_A_Allen@keane.com
www.www.keanecare.com

Kim Allen, Director Product Support
Jim Ingalls, Director Sales

Care Computer Systems develops, markets, and supports a range of clinical and financial software.

Year Founded: 1969

4451 LanVision Systems
5481 Creek Road
Cincinnati, OH 45242-4001
800-878-5262

JB Patsy, Chairman/President/CEO
Paul W Bridge, Jr, CFO/Treasurer
William A Geers, COO
Eric S Lombardo, Secretary

The system enables to access electronically both structured and unstructured patient data and various forms of healthcare information such as clinician's handwritten notes, lab reports, photographs and insurance cards.

4452 Lexical Technologies
151 W Atlantic Avenue
Alameda, CA 94501
501-865-8500

Provide the delivery of healthcare across enterprises through the application of integrated component solutions.

Year Founded: 1984

4453 M/MGMT Systems
2335 American River Drive
Suite 402
Sacramento, CA 95825
916-648-9010
800-664-8797
Fax: 916-648-9040
E-mail: mlab@mmgmt.com
www.mmgmt.com

Provides a comprehensive support and maintenance program to service the public health laboratories and license M/LAB.

Year Founded: 1982

4454 MEDCOM Information Systems
2117 Stonington Avenue
Hoffman Estates, IL 60195
847-885-1553
800-213-2161
Fax: 847-885-1591
E-mail: medcom@emirj.com
www.emirj.com

Provides a wide variety of products and services to the independent physician clinic as well as the hospital and private clinical laboratories.

Year Founded: 1991

4455 MEDecision
601 Lee Road
Chesterbrook Corporate Center
Wayne, PA 19087
610-254-0202
Fax: 610-254-0270
E-mail: salesinfo@medecision.com
www.MEDecision.com

Providing managed care organizations with powerful and flexible care management solutions. MEDecision's tools help managed care organizations improve care management processes and align more closely with their members and providers to improve the quality and cost outcomes of healthcare.

Year Founded: 1988

4456 McHenry County M/H Board
620 Dakota Street
Crystal Lake, IL 60012
815-455-2828
Fax: 815-455-2925
E-mail: webadmin@mc708.org
www.mc708.org

Sandy Lewis, Executive Director
Robert Lesser, Deputy Director

Our misson is to provide leadership and be accountable for the provision of prevention and treatment of mental illness, developmental disabilities, and chemical abuse by coordinative, developing and contracting services for all citizens of McHenry County.

4457 McKesson HBOC
2700 Snelling Ave N
Roseville, MN 55113
651-697-5900
Fax: 651-697-5910
www.www.mckesson.com

Our products and services are designed to meet the information needs of all participants in the integrated health system.

4458 Med Data Systems
1950 Old Cuthbert Road
Suite L
Cherry Hill, NJ 08034
856-428-1550
800-842-0011
Fax: 856-428-8172
E-mail: information@md-systems.com
www.md-systems.com

Jerold Zebrick, President/CEO

Provides an extensive suite of software programs to the healthcare and industrial markets which encompass Outcome Measurements, Baseline-Progress-Discharge Reports as well as Ergonomic and Work Hardening Analysis.

4459 MedPLus
4690 Parkway Drive
Mason, OH 45040
513-229-5500
800-444-6235
Fax: 513-229-5505
E-mail: info@medplus.com
www.www.medplus.com

Richard A Mahoney, President
Thomas R Wagner, CTO
Philip S Present, II, COO

Developer and integrator of clinical connectivity and data management solutions for health care organizations and clinicians.

Year Founded: 1991

4460 Medai
Millenia Park One
4901 Vineland Rd Suite 450
Orlando, FL 32811
321-281-4480
800-446-3324
Fax: 321-281-4499
www.www.medai.com

Steve Epstein, Ceo/Co Founder
Diane Lee, EVP/Co Founder
Swati Abbott, President

Provides solutions for the improvement of healthcare delivery. Utilizing cutting-edge technology, payers are able to predict patients at risk, identify cost drivers for their high-risk population, predict future health plan costs, evaluate patient patterns over time, and improve outcomes.

4461 Medcomp Software
PO Box 16687
Golden, CO 80402-6010
303-277-0772
Fax: 303-277-9801
E-mail: customerservice@medcompsoftware.com
www.medcompsoftware.com

Developing and designing case management systems for a wide variety of applications.

Year Founded: 1995

4462 Medi-Span
8425 Woodfield Crossing Boulevard
Suite 490
Indianapolis, IN 46240
317-735-5300
800-388-8884
E-mail: medispan-support@wolterskluwer.com
www.www.medispan.com

Medi-Span offers a complete line of drug databases, including clinical decision support and disease suite modules, application programming interfaces, and stand-alone PC products.

4463 Medical Records Institute
425 Boylston Street
Boston, MA 02116
617-964-3923
Fax: 617-964-3926
E-mail: peter@medrecinst.com
www.medrecinst.com

Peter Waegemann, CEO

Promote and enhance the journey towards electronic health records, e-health, mobile health, mental health assessment, and related applications of information technologies (IT).

4464 Medical Records Solution
Creative Solutions Unlimited
203 Gilman Street
PO Box 550
Sheffield, IA 50475
800-253-7697
E-mail: mkoch@csumail.com
www.creativesolutionsunlimited.com

Martha Koch, Vp

Reliable, comprehensive, intuitive, fully-integrated clinical software able to manage MDS 2.0 electronic submission, RUGs/PPS, triggers, Quick RAP's, survey reports, QI's, assessments, care plans, Quick Plans, physician orders, CQI, census, and hundreds of reports. Creative Solutions Unlimited provides outstanding toll-free support, training, updates, user groups, newsletters, and continuing education.

Year Founded: 1988

4465 Medipay
620 SW 5th Avenue
Suite 610
Portland, OR 97204-1421
503-227-6491
Fax: 503-299-6490

Medipay's information technology products and services monitor and control quality, manage clinical and financial risk, collaborate and integrate with external stakeholders, and empower front line staff.

4466 Medix Systems Consultants
17050 S Park Avenue
Suites C-D
S Holland, IL 60473
708-331-1271
Fax: 708-331-1272
E-mail: info@imsci.com
www.imsci.com

Systems integration and development company committed to client/server multi vendor(open systems) solutions for a diverse vertical market ranging from education and healthcare.

Year Founded: 1987

4467 Medware
2650 North Dixie Freeway
New Smyrna Beach, FL 32168
877-932-6301
E-mail: medwaresales@sage.com
www.medware.com

Integrated medical management software.

4468 Mental Health Connections
21 Blossom Street
Lexington, MA 02421
617-510-1318
www.mhc.com

Robert Patterson, MD, Founder/Principal

Developer of medical management software for physicians and research scientists. Their primary product is desigend to identify drug interactions based on the mainstream of drug metabolism research.

4469 Mental Health Outcomes
2941 S Lake Vista Drive
Lewisville, TX 75057
800-266-4440
Fax: 972-420-8215
E-mail: johan.smith@horizonhealth.com
www.www.mho-inc.net

Johan Smith, VP Operations/Development

Designs and implements custom outcome measurement systems specifically for behavioral helath programs through its CQI Outcomes Measurement System. This system provides information for a wide range of patient and treatment focused variables for child, adolesent, adult, geriatric and substance abuse programs in the inpatient, partial hospital, residential treatment and outpatient settings.

Year Founded: 1994

4470 Meritcare Health System
PO Box M.C
Fargo, ND 58122
701-234-2000
800-437-4010
www.www.meritcare.com

Roger Gilbertson, MD, President/CEO
Craig Hewitt, CIO

MeritCare is able to track your employees' health trends due to a new software program called Occusource.

4471 Micro Design International
45 Skyline Drive
Suite 1017
Lake Mary, FL 32746
407-472-6000
800-228-0891
Fax: 407-472-6100
E-mail: info@mdi.com
www.mdi.com

Provides optical (CD/DVD/MO) storage solutions through innovative achivements, easy-to-use data access, and exceptional service and support.

Year Founded: 1978

4472 Micro Office Systems
3825 Severn Road
Cleveland, OH 44118
216-297-0160
Fax: 216-297-0163
E-mail: normane@micro-officesystems.com
www.www.micro-officesystems.com

Norman Efroymson, Contact

4473 Micromedex
6200 S Syracuse Way
Suite 300
Englewood, CO 80111
800-525-9083
Fax: 303-486-6450
www.micromedex.com

A comprehensive suite of alerts, answers, protocols, and interventions directly addresses clinicians need for evidence-based information. This vital information is used to support patient care and improve outcomes.

Year Founded: 1974

4474 Misys Health Care Systems
8529 Six Forks Road
Raleigh, NC 27615
866-647-9787
www.www.misyshealthcare.com

Develops and supports software and services for physicians and caregivers.

4475 MphasiS(BPO)
5353 N 16th Street
Suite 400
Phoenix, AZ 85016
602-604-3100
Fax: 602-604-3115
E-mail: fred.thierbach@mphasis.com
www.www.mphasis.com

Fred Thierbach, Contact

Focused on financial services, logistics and technology verticals and spans across architecture, application development and integration, application management and business process outsourcing, including the operation of large scale customer contact centers.

4476 Mutual of Omaha Companies' Integrated Behavioral Services
Mutual of Omaha Plaza
S-3 Group Compliance
Omaha, NE 68175-0001
402-342-7600
Fax: 402-351-2880

Linda McDowell, BMC Software

Provider of enterprise management solutions that empower companies to manage their IT infrastructure from a business perspective.

Year Founded: 1980

4477 National Families in Action
2957 Clairmont Road Ne
Suite 150
Atlanta, GA 30329
404-248-9676
Fax: 404-248-1312

E-mail: nfia@nationalfamilies.org
www.nationalfamilies.org

An interactive database of ever-changing names of drugs that people use and abuse for illnesses.

Year Founded: 1977

4478 National Medical Health Card Systems
26 Harbor Park Drive
Port Washington, NY 11050
800-251-3883
Fax: 516-605-6981
www.nmhc.com

Software to electronically manage combined medical and Rx deductibles for the healthcare industry.

4479 NetMeeting
Microsoft Corporation
Customer Advocate Center
One Microsoft Way
Redmond, WA 98052
800-642-7676
Fax: 425-936-7329
www.microsoft.com

NetMeeting delivers a complete Internet conferencing solution for all Window users with multi-point data conferencing, text chat, whiteboard, and file transfer, as well as point-to-point audio and video.

4480 Netsmart Technologies
570 Metro Place N
Dublin, OH 43017
614-764-0143
800-434-2642
Fax: 614-799-3159
www.www.ntst.com

James Conway, CEO/Chair

Offers information systems for mental health, behavioral and public health organizations.

4481 Nightingale Vantagemed Corporation
10670 White Rock Road
Suite 300
Rancho Cordova, CA 95670
916-638-4744
E-mail: info@nightingale.md
www.www.nightingale.md

Therapist Helper, the leading practice management software program, processes patient and insurance billing transactins, accounts receivable, statements, and tracks payments. Therapist Helper will also assist in scheduling managed care tracking, and electronic claims submission. Will network at no additional charge. All you'll need is IMB or compatible Pentium with 16 MB RAM and at least 25 MB available hard drive space. Download a free, full working demo at our website.

4482 Northwest Analytical
111 SW 5th Avenue
Suite 800
Portland, OR 97204-3604
503-224-7727
888-692-7638
Fax: 503-224-5236
E-mail: info@nwasoft.com
www.nwasoft.com

Jeff Cawley, VP

Provides comprehensive SPC software tools meeting technically stringent mental health industry requirements.

4483 OPTAIO-Optimizing Practice Through Assessment, Intervention and Outcome
Harcourt Assessment/PsychCorp
19500 Bulverde Road
San Antonio, TX 78259
800-622-3231

Provides the clinical information necessary for proactive decision making.

4484 Occupational Health Software
6609 NE Tara Lane
Bainbridge Island, WA 98110
206-842-5838

Provides a wide range of consulting and training services, addressing occupational health and safety, workers compensation management, medical surveillance and industrial hygiene.

4485 Optio Software
3015 Windward Plaza
Windward Fairways II
Alpharetta, GA 30005
770-576-3500
Fax: 770-576-3699
E-mail: info@optio.com
www.optiosoftware.com

C Wayne Cape, Chairman/President/CEO
Caroline Bembry, CFO
Daryl G Hatton, CTO
Donald French, SVP Research/Development

Provides software solutions that enable organizations to achieve unprecedented speed, accuracy, functionality and quality in their document processes such as procure-to-pay, order-to-case, manufacturing and healthcare.

Year Founded: 1981

4486 Oracle Corporation
500 Oracle Parkway
Redwood Shores, CA 94065
650-506-7000
www.www.oracle.com

Charles Phillips, President
Larry Ellison, CEO

PeopleSoft provides a range of applications from traditional human resources, payroll and benefits to financials.

Year Founded: 1977

4487 Orion Healthcare Technology
1016 Leavenworth Street
Omaha, NE 68102
402-341-8880
800-324-7966
Fax: 402-341-8911
E-mail: info@orionhealthcare.com
www.www.myaccucare.com

Orion provides technology solutions to meet the ever changing needs of the healthcare industry. To accomodate the behavioral health field, Orion developed the AccuCare software system, a highly integrated and adaptive approach to the clinical practice environment. AccuCare enables cli-

nicians to quickly realize value, effiency and standardization without disrupting their primary focus to provide excellence in health care.

4488 P and W Software
5655 Lindero Canyon Road
Suite 403
Westlake Village, CA 91362
818-707-7690
Fax: 818-707-9097
E-mail: pwsoft@pwsoftware.com
www.pwsoftware.com
Bud Bockoven, Director Marketing/Sales

POWERPLUS was developed as a flexible toolkit, one which would allow each user to administer benefits according to his or her specific model. With user-defined codes and values and company level processing defaults.

Year Founded: 1984

4489 PRISMED Corporation
725 Town & Country
Suite 200
Orange, CA 92868
714-689-1544
E-mail: response@arbormed.com
www.psi-med.com

James Reitsema, President/CTO

Offers a full line of medical billing, accounting products and services to practices, clinics, and universities.

Year Founded: 1976

4490 Parrot Software
PO Box 250755
W Bloomfield, MI 48322
248-788-3223
800-727-7681
Fax: 248-788-3224
E-mail: support@parrotsoftware.com
www.parrotsoftware.com

Provide 60 different software programs for the remediation of speech, cognitive, language, attention, and memory deficits seen in individuals who have suffered aphasia from stroke or head injury.

Year Founded: 1981

4491 Patient Infosystems
46 Prince Street
Rochester, NY 14607-1023
716-242-7271
800-276-2575
Fax: 716-244-1367
E-mail: sales@ptisys.com
www.ptisys.com

Christine St. Andre, President/COO
Roger Chaufournier, Chairman/CEO
James Martin, VP Development/CTO
Nancy Cox, SVP Marketing/Sales

Offers a comprehensive portfolio of health management products and services, including a 24/7 nurse help line, chronic condition management, case management, utilization management and preventive care management.

Year Founded: 1995

4492 Perot Systems
2300 West Plano Parkway
Plano, TX 75075
972-577-0000
888-317-3768
E-mail: americas@ps.net
www.perotsystems.com

Deliveres technology based business solutions to help organizations worldwide control costs and cultivate growth.

Year Founded: 1988

4493 Primary Care Medicine on CD
Facts and Comparisons
77 West Port Plaza
Suite 450
Saint Louis, MO 63146
800-223-0554
Fax: 314-216-2100
www.factsandcomparisons.

Current, comprehensive coverage of what's happening in the discipline; quarterly updates include summary, analysis and critique of relevant studies on ambulatory care, family medicine, internal medicine, pharmacology, cardiology, therapeutic advances, plus twelve critical reviews of major new studies in the field of medical practice.

4494 Psychological Assessment Resources
16204 N Florida Avenue
Lutz, FL 33549
813-968-3003
800-331-8378
Fax: 800-727-9329
www.parinc.com

This program produces normative-based interpretive hypotheses based on your client's scores. It produces a profile of T scores, a listing of the associated raw and percentile scores, and interpretive hypotheses for each scale. Although this program is not designed to produce a finished clinical report, it allows you to integrate BRS and SRI data with other sources of information about your client. The report can be generated as a text file for editing.

Year Founded: 1978

4495 Psychological Software Services
6555 Carrollton Avenue
Indianapolis, IN 46220
317-257-9672
Fax: 317-257-9674
E-mail: nsc@netdirect.net
www.www.neuroscience.cnter.com

Comprehensive and easy-to-use multimedia cognitive rehabilitation software. Packages include 64 computerized therapy tasks with modifiable parameters that will accommodate most requirements. Exercises extend from simple attention and executive skills, through multiple modalities of visuospatial and memory skills. For clinical and educational use with head injury, stroke, LD/ADD and other brain compromises. Price range: $260-$2,500.

Year Founded: 1984

4496 Psychometric Software
2210 Front Street
Suite 208
Melbourne, FL 32901
407-729-6390
800-882-9811

Fax: 321-951-9508
E-mail: psi@digital.net
www.psipsych.com

Specializes in behavioral medicine, neuropsychological assessment, cognitive rehabilitation and biofeedback software.

Year Founded: 1978

4497 QuadraMed Corporation
12110 Sunset Hills Road
Reston, VA 20190
703-709-2300
800-393-0278
Fax: 703-709-2490
E-mail: boardofdirectors@quadramed.com
www.quadramed.com

Keith Hagen, President/Ceo
James Milligan, Svp Sales/Government Programs

4498 RCF Information Systems
4200 Colonel Glenn Highway
Suite 100
Beavercreek, OH 45431
937-427-5680
Fax: 937-427-5689
www.www.rcfinfo.com

Roger K Harris, President

Healthcare software.

4499 Raintree Systems
28765 Single Oak Drive
Suite 200
Temecula, CA 92590
951-252-9400
800-333-1033
www.raintreeinc.com

Richard Welty, President/CTO

Provides practice management software for commerical, not-for-profit, government healthcare providers, rehabilitation facilities, and social service agencies.

Year Founded: 1983

4500 Right On Programs/PRN Medical Software
778 New York Avenue
Huntington, NY 11743-4413
631-424-7777
Fax: 631-424-7207
E-mail: riteonsoft@aol.com
www.rightonprograms.com

Computer software for mental health, medical and other organizations requiring cataloging and searching a wide range of materials. Software is especially easy to learn and use. Programs include The Circulation Desk for cataloging and circulation of books, CDs, videos, photos, booklets, etc., Computer Access Catalog for cataloging without the circulation module, and Periodical Manager for periodicals including supplements.

Year Founded: 1980

4501 SHS Computer Service
759 Main Street
Stroudsburg, PA 18360
570-424-5676
Fax: 570-424-7437

E-mail: sales@shscomputer.com
www.shscomputer.com

Sheryl Hope Shay, President

Client and Fund Tracking System with HIPAA Billing, Pennsylvania CCRS/POMS State Reporting, and adhoc reports for behavioral health organizations.

Year Founded: 1986

4502 SPSS
233 S Wacker Drive
11th Floor
Chicago, IL 60606
312-651-3000
www.spss.com

Jack Noonan, President/CEO

Worldwide provider of predictive analytics software and solutions.

Year Founded: 1968

4503 Saner Software
761 N 17th Street
Unit 11
Saint Charles, IL 60174
630-513-5599
E-mail: sales@sanersoftware.com
www.sanersoftware.com

Develops health practice management software.

Year Founded: 1988

4504 Scinet
11117 Mockingbird Drive
Omaha, NE 68137
402-331-6660
E-mail: info@scinetinc.com
www.scinetinc.com

Provides all payer electronic claims transactions, electronic remittance advice, and electronic patient statements.

Year Founded: 1986

4505 Siemens Health Services Corporation
400 Lakemont Park Boulevard
Altoona, PA 16602
814-944-1651
Fax: 814-942-0125

Frank Lavelle, CEO
Jon Zimmerman, VP Health Connections

Clinical-Link is a fully integrated home care system including electronic billing, statistics, plans of treatment, individualized care plans, scheduling, financials, referal/admissions and a field automated clinical documentation.

4506 Skypek Group
2528 W Tennessee Avenue
Tampa, FL 33629-6255
813-254-3926
Fax: 813-254-3926

4507 Sls Residential
2505 Carmel Ave
Suite 210
Brewster, NY 10509
888-822-7348
www.www.slshealth.com

Fully intergrated informatics software solutions; clinical, billing/AR, administration, outcomes.

4508 Star Systems Corporation
4083 North Shiloh Drive
Suite 8
Fayetteville, AR 72703
501-587-0882
Fax: 501-587-9449
E-mail: frank@starsyscorp.com
www.starsyscorp.com

Frank W Woods, Founder

Provides healthcare software.

Year Founded: 1980

4509 Stephens Systems Services
267 5th Avenue
Suite 812
New York, NY 10016
212-545-7788
Fax: 212-545-9081

Provides healthcare software.

4510 Strategic Advantage
3353 Peachtree Road NE
Suite 400
Atlanta, GA 30326-1414
404-231-8676
800-330-8889
Fax: 404-237-1291

4511 SumTime Software®
4713 Goodrich Avenue NE
Albuquerque, NM 87110
888-821-0771
Fax: 505-888-2653
E-mail: sumtime@sumtime.com
www.sumtime.com

Is the practice management solution for health care professionals. We offer the most comprehensive means for preparing billing statements and tracking payments and maintaining records.

4512 Sun Microsystems
4150 Network Circle
Santa Clara, CA 95054
650-960-1300
800-555-9786

Provider of healthcare software.

Year Founded: 1982

4513 SunGard Pentamation
3 West Broad Street
Bethlehem, PA 18018
610-691-3616
866-905-8989
www.pentamation.com

Provides secure and reliable K-12 student information systems, special education management, financial and human resource management software to school districts.

Year Founded: 1992

4514 Sweetwater Health Enterprises
3939 Belt Line Road
Suite 600
Dallas, TX 75244
972-888-5638
Fax: 972-620-7351
E-mail: mktg@sweetwaterhealth.com
www.sweetwaterhealth.com

Cherie Holmes-Henry, VP Sales/Marketing

4515 Synergistic Office Solutions (SOS Software)
17445 E Apshawa Road
Clermont, FL 34711
352-242-9100
Fax: 352-242-9104
E-mail: sales@sosoft.com
www.sosoft.com

Seth R Krieger, PhD, President

Produce patient management software for behavioral health service providers, including billing, scheduling and clinical records.

Year Founded: 1985

4516 Tempus Software
225 Water Street
Suite 250
Jacksonville, FL 32202
Fax: 904-355-3322

Keith B Hagen, President/CEO

Provide the most comprehensive range of innovative, installable and practical healthcare information technology solutions that increase efficiencies, and empower clinicians to improve patient care through smarter healthcare technology solutions.

Year Founded: 1993

4517 Thomson ResearchSoft
2141 Palomar Airport Road
Suite 350
Carlsbad, CA 92011
760-438-5526
800-722-1227
Fax: 760-438-5573
www.risinc.com

Software for wherever research is performed worldwide including all leading academic, corporate and government institutions, healthcare.

4518 TriZetto Group
567 San Nicolas Drive
Suite 360
Newport Beach, CA 92660
800-569-1222
E-mail: salesinfo@trizetto.com
www.www.trizetto.com

Jeff Margolis, Chairman/CEO
Kathleen Earley, President/COO

Focuses on the business of healthcare and offers a broad portfolio of technology products and services.

Year Founded: 1997

4519 Turbo-Doc EMR
771 Buschmann Road
Suite G
Paradise, CA 95969

800-977-4868
Fax: 530-877-8621
E-mail: turbodoc@turbodoc.com
www.turbodoc.com

An electronic medical record system designed to assist physicians and other health care workers in completing medical record tasks.

4520 UNI/CARE Systems
540 North Tamiami Trail
Sarasota, FL 34236
941-954-3403
Fax: 941-954-2033
E-mail: sales@unicaresys.com
www.unicaresys.com

Provides fully-integrated software solutions for all facets of Behavioral Healthcare. Our software is designed for use in every setting, from Inpatient to Outpatient, from Day Treatment and Partial Hospitalization to Case Management. The Uni/Care Information System is a flexible and user-friendly network of software modules that support integrated clinical and financial data with powerful reporting capabilities. Uni/Care is an industry leader with a track record of responding to the ever-changing behavioral health environment.

Year Founded: 1981

4521 Universal Behavioral Service
3590 N Meridian Street
Indianapolis, IN 46208
317-684-0442

4522 Vann Data Services
1801 Dunn Avenue
Daytona Beach, FL 32114
386-238-1200
Fax: 386-238-1454
E-mail: sales@vanndata.com
www.vanndata.com

George Van Arnam, Founder

Healthcare practice software.

4523 Velocity Healthcare Informatics
8441 Wayzata Boulevard
Suite 105
Minneapolis, MN 55426
800-844-5648
E-mail: info@velocity.com

Ellen B White, President/CEO

Provides outcomes management system.

4524 VersaForm Systems Corporation
591 W Hamilton Avenue
Suite 230
Campbell, CA 95008
800-678-1111
www.versaform.com

Electronic medical records and practice management.

4525 Virtual Software Systems
PO Box 815
Bethel Park, PA 15102
412-835-9417
Fax: 412-835-9419
E-mail: sales@vss3.com
www.vss3.com

Thomas Palmquist, Contact

Easy to use practice management, billing, and scheduling software. *$3500.00*

4526 Wang Software

290 Concord Road
Billerica, MA 01821-3499
770-594-9473

4527 Wellness Integrated Network

3435 Ocean Park Boulevard
Suite 108
Santa Monica, CA 90405-3309
310-452-4946

4528 Woodlands

195 Union Street
Suite B1
Newark, OH 43055
740-349-7066
800-686-2756
Fax: 740-345-6028
www.www.thewoodland.org

4529 Work Group for the Computerization of Behavioral Health

4 Brattle Street
Suite 207
Cambridge, MA 02138-3714
617-864-6769
Fax: 617-492-3673
www.workgroup.org

4530 Worldwide Healthcare Solutions: IBM

404 Wyman Street
Waltham, MA 02451-1264
781-895-2486
Fax: 781-895-2235

4531 XI Tech Corporation

34 Regis Avenue
Pittsburgh, PA 15236
412-655-2120

4532 Zy-Doc Technologies

1455 Veterans Highway
Hauppauge, NY 11749
800-546-5633
Fax: 516-908-3718
E-mail: sales@zydoc.com
www.zydoc.com

Information Services

4533 3m Health Information Systems

575 Murray Boulevard
Murray, UT 84123
801-265-4400

4534 ADL Data Systems

9 Skyline Drive
Hawthorne, NY 10532
914-591-1800
Fax: 914-591-1818
E-mail: sales@mail.adldata.com
www.adldata.com

David Pollack, President

The most comprehensive software solution for MH/MRDD and the continuum of care. 38 modules to choose from. Designed to meet all financial, clinical, and administrative needs. For organizations requiring greater flexiblity and processing power. Ask about new Windows-based products utilizing the latest in technology, including bar coding, scanning, etc.

Year Founded: 1977

4535 Accumedic Computer Systems

11 Grace Avenue
Suite 401
Great Neck, NY 11021
516-466-6800
800-765-9300
Fax: 516-466-6880
E-mail: sales@accumedic.com
www.accumedic.com

Practice management solutions for mental health facilities: scheduling, billing, EMR, HIPAA.

4536 American Institute for Preventive Medicine

30445 Northwestern Highway
Suite 350
Farmington Hills, MI 48334
248-539-1800
800-345-2476
Fax: 248-539-1808
E-mail: aipm@healthylife.com
www.www.healthylife.com

4537 American Nurses Foundation: National Communications

8515 Georgia Ave
Suite 400 W
Silver Spring, MD 20910
301-628-5227
Fax: 301-628-5354
E-mail: anf@ana.org

4538 Apache Medical Systems

1650 Tysons Boulevard
Suite 300
McLean, VA 22102
703-847-1400
Fax: 703-847-1401

4539 Applied Computing Services

2764 Allen Road W
Elk, WA 99009
800-553-4055

4540 Applied Informatics (ILIAD)

295 Chipeta Way
Salt Lake City, UT 84108
801-584-6485

4541 Arbour Health System-Human Resource Institute Hospital

227 Babcock Street
Brookline, MA 02446
617-731-3200
www.arbourhealth.com

4542 Arservices, Limited
7767 Armistead Rd
Suite 160
Lorton, VA 22079
703-824-6298
Fax: 703-824-6438
www.www.arserviceslimited.com

4543 Artificial Intelligence
345 Upland Drive
Seattle, WA 98188-3802
206-575-2135

**4544 Association for Ambulatory Behavioral
Healthcare**
247 Douglas Ave
Portsmouth, VA 23707
757-673-3741
Fax: 757-966-7734
E-mail: mickey@aabh.org
www.www.aabh.org

Larry Meikel, President

Powerful forum for people engaged in providing mental
health services. Promoting the evolution of flexible models
of responsive cost-effective ambulatory behavioral
healthcare.

**4545 Behavioral Intervention Planning: Completing
a Functional Behavioral Assessment and
Developing a Behavioral Intervention Plan**
Pro-Ed Publications
8700 Shoal Creek Boulevard
Austin, TX 78757-6897
512-451-3246
800-897-3202
Fax: 800-397-7633
www.proedinc.com

Provides school personnel with all tools necessary to complete a functional behavioral assessment, determine
whether a behavior is related to the disability of the student,
and develop a behavioral intervention plan. *$22.00*

**4546 Breining Institute College for the Advanced
Study of Addictive Disorders**
8894 Greenback Lane
Orangevale, CA 95662-4019
916-987-2007
Fax: 916-987-8823
E-mail: college@breining.edu
www.breining.edu

Kathy Breining, Dean of Students

4547 Brief Therapy Institute of Denver
1333 W 120th Ave
Suite 220
Westminster, CO 80234
303-426-8757
www.btid.com

Marne Wine, Therapist

Our form of psychotherapy emphasizes goals, active participation between therapist and client, client strengths, resources, resiliencies and accountability of the therapy
process.

4548 Buckley Productions
238 E Blithedale Avenue
Mill Valley, CA 94941
877-508-3979
Fax: 415-383-5031
E-mail: buckleypro@aol.com
www.buckleyproductions.com

Richard Buckley, President

Alcohol and drug education handbooks, videos, and
web-based products for safety sensitive employers,
supervisiors and employees who are covered by the Department of Transportaion rules. We provide training materials
for Substance Abuse Professional (SAPs) and urine collec-
tors.

4549 CBI Group
100 S Prospect Avenue
Park Ridge, IL 60068
847-698-1090

4550 CMHC Systems
570 Metro Place N
Dublin, OH 43017
614-764-0143

4551 COMPSYCH Software Information Services
Peter Hornby and Margaret Anderson, SUNY
101 Broad Street
Plattsburgh, NY 12901
www.plattsburgh.edu.compsych/

Provides information about psychological software, arranged in topical categories such as statistics, cognitive,
physiological, and personality testing.

4552 CareCounsel
68 Mitchell Boulevard
Suite 200
San Rafael, CA 94903
415-472-2366
Fax: 415-472-5528
www.www.carecounsel.com

**4553 Catholic Community Services of Western
Washington**
100 23rd Avenue S
Seattle, WA 98144
206-328-5696
E-mail: info@ccsww.org
www.www.ccsww.org

4554 Center for Creative Living
2011 Crooks Road
Royal Oak, MI 48073
248-414-4050
Fax: 248-414-4053
E-mail: cclro@aol.com
www.www.centerforcreativeliving.com

4555 Central Washington Comprehensive M/H
PO Box 959
402 S 4th Ave
Yakima, WA 98907
509-575-4084
800-572-8122
Fax: 509-575-4811

4556 Child Welfare Information Gateway
1250 Maryland Avenue, SW
8th Floor
Washington, DC 20024
703-385-7565
800-394-3366
Fax: 703-385-3206
www.www.childwelfare.gov

The clearinghouse serves as a facilitator of information and knowledge exchange; the Children's Bureau and its training and technical assistant network; the child abuse and neglect, child welfare, and adoption communities; and allied agencies and professions.

4557 Choice Health
12000 Pecos Street
Suite 350
Denver, CO 80234-2079
303-252-1120
Fax: 303-252-1194

4558 Cirrus Technology
403 Chris Drive
Building 4 Suite H
Huntsville, AL 35802
E-mail: info@cirrusti.com
www.www.cirrusti.com

4559 Community Psychiatric Clinic
4319 Stone Way North
Seattle, WA 98103-7490
206-461-3614
www.www.cpcwa.org

4560 Community Sector Systems
700 5th Avenue
Suite 6100
Seattle, WA 98104-5061
206-521-2588
800-988-6392
Fax: 206-467-9237
www.cssi.com

4561 Community Solutions
PO Box 546
Morgan Hill, CA 95038
408-842-7138
Fax: 408-778-9672
E-mail: cs@communitysolutions.org
www.www.communitysolutions.org

4562 Compass Information Systems
1060 1st Avenue
Suite 410
King of Prussia, PA 19406-1336
610-992-7060
Fax: 610-992-7070
E-mail: quality@compass-is.com
www.compass-is.com

Compass Treatment Assessment System is a scientifically-based system of measuring and managing a the course of behavioral health treatment.

4563 Computer Billing and Office Managment Programs
Ed Zuckrman
www.cmch.com/guide/pro24.html

Includes a detailed review of computer billing and office management programs, where to buy or use electronic claims submission, other computer programs of interest to clinicians, resources, references and readings, and programs for writing assistance.

4564 Consultec Managed Care Systems
9040 Roswell Road
Suite 700
Atlanta, GA 30350-7530
813-784-7947
Fax: 813-789-6136

4565 Consumer Health Information Corporation
8300 Greensboro Drive
Suite 1220
McLean Va, VA 22102
703-734-0650
Fax: 703-734-1459
www.www.consumer-health.com

4566 Control-O-Fax Corporation
3070 W Airline Highway
Waterloo, IA 50704-0778
800-553-0070
E-mail: info@controlofax.com
www.www.controlofax.com

4567 DCC/The Dependent Care Connection
500 Nyla Farms
Westport, CT 06880
203-226-2680

4568 Dean Foundation for Health, Research and Education
2711 Allen Boulevard
Suite 300
Middleton, WI 53562
608-827-2300
800-844-6015
Fax: 608-827-2399
www.www.dean.senscia.com

The Dean Foundation is the non-profit research and education entity of DHS. The Foundation currently encompasses Dean's Educational Services Department, supports community service and health education projects, funds research grants, and conducts its own ancillary research including several outcomes management studies and computer-assisted, voice-activated programs for behavioral medicine.

4569 Distance Learning Network
111 Boal Ave
Boalsburg, PA 16827
814-466-7808

Eric Porterfield, Director

Broadcast and multimedia company dedicated solely to meeting the medical education and communications needs of physicians through the use of both traditional and innovative media formats. More than 150,000 physicians, nurses and pharmacists turn to DLN each year for their medical education.

Year Founded: 1996

4570 Dorland Healthcare Information
PO Box 25128
Salt Lake City, UT 84121

800-784-2332
Fax: 801-365-2300
E-mail: info@dorlandhealth.com
www.dorlandhealth.com

4571 Drug and Crime Prevention Funding News
Government Information Services
4301 Fairfax Drive
Ste 875
Arlington, VA 22203-1635
703-920-7600
800-876-0226
www.grantsandfunding.com

Provides federal and private drug and crime funding information, including congressional legislation and appropriations. Also features grant alert a weekly compilation of federal grants and contracts. Recurring features include a collection, reports of meetings, and notices of publications available. *$289.00*

10-12 pages 56 per year ISSN 1076-1519

4572 FOCUS: Family Oriented Counseling Services
PO Box 921
1435 Hauck Drive
Rolla, MO 65401
573-364-7551
800-356-5395
Fax: 573-364-4898
www.www.rollanet.org

4573 Federation of Families for Children's Mental Health
9605 Medical Center Drive
Suite 280
Rockville, MD 20850
240-403-1901
Fax: 240-403-1909
E-mail: ffcmh@ffcmh.org
www.ffcmh.org

National family-run organization dedicated exclusively to children and adolesents with mental health needs and their families. Our voice speaks through our work in policy, training and technical assistance programs. Publishes a quarterly newsletter and sponsors an annual conference and exhibits.

4574 HSA-Mental Health
1080 Emeline Avenue
Santa Cruz, CA 95060
831-454-4000
Fax: 831-454-4770
TDD: 831-454-2123
E-mail: info@santacruzhealth.org
www.santacruzhealth.org

Exists to protect and improve the health of the people in Santa Cruz County. Provides programs in environmental health, public health, medical care, substance abuse prevention and treatment, and mental health. Clients are entitled to information on the costs of care and their options for getting health insurance coverage through a variety of programs.

4575 Hagar and Associates
164 W Hospitality Lane
San Bernardino, CA 92408-3343
909-890-4050

Deborah Hagar, CEO
Provides clients with data, from national databases, of outcomes, patient demographics, and benchmark data. Can provide technology and/or automated data connection. Provides support in objective outcomes measurement.

4576 HealthOnline
PO Box 339
Brighton, CO 80601-0339
303-659-2252
Fax: 303-659-7995

4577 Healthcare Management Systems
3102 W End Avenue
Suite 400
Nashville, TN 37203
615-383-7300
Fax: 615-383-6093
www.www.hmstn.com

4578 Healthcheck
3954 Youngfield Street
Wheat Ridge, CO 80033
916-556-1880

4579 Human Resources Consulting Group
1202 Dover Drive
Provo, UT 84604
801-765-4417
Fax: 801-765-4418
www.hrconsultinggroup.com

Consultants in Human Resourses and benefits plan design. Software systems and evolutions nation wide.

4580 INMED/MotherNet America
45449 Severn Way
Suite 161
Sterling, VA 20166
703-444-4477
Fax: 703-444-4471
www.www.inmed.org

4581 InfoNation Systems
2701 University Avenue
Suite 465
Madison, WI 53705
608-209-1950
www.infonat.com

Info Nation Systems is a team of experienced health care and computer professionals offering consulting services to help healthcare providers implement solutions to their data management needs. Our team delivers fast, cost effective systems that are easy to learn, use and customize. We feature an architecture that allows maximum performance, flexibility and access to information at a significantly lower cost than other approaches.

4582 Information Access Technology
1100 E 6600 S
Suite 300
Salt Lake City, UT 84121
800-574-8801
Fax: 801-265-8880
www.www.iat-cti.com

4583 Informedics
4000 Kruse Way Place
Lake Oswego, OR 97035
503-697-3000
www.www.informedics.com

4584 Lad Lake
PO Box 158
W350 S1401 Waterville Rd
Dousman, WI 53118
414-342-0607
Fax: 414-965-4107
www.www.ladlake.org

4585 Lanstat Resources
PO Box 1388
270 Beckett Point Road
Port Townsend, WA 98368
360-379-8628
800-672-3166
Fax: 360-379-8949
www.www.lanstat.com

4586 Liberty Healthcare Management Group
75 Seminary Hill Road
Carmel, NY 10512
845-225-3400

Liberty provides individualized programs and a continuum
of services for psychiatric and substance abuse treatment at
our centers located throughout the Northeast, Oklahoma
and Florida. Liberty's commitment to medical excellence
within an environment of results-oriented care is evident in
our outstanding record of clinical success.

4587 Lifelink Corporation/Bensenville Home Society
331 S York Road
Bensenville, IL 60106-2600
630-766-3570
www.www.lifelink.org

4588 MADNESS
146-5 Chrystal Terrace
Suite 5
Santa Cruz, CA 95060
408-426-5335
Fax: 408-426-5335

4589 Managed Care Local Market Overviews
Dorland Healthcare Information
PO Box 25128
Salt Lake City, UT 84125
800-784-2332
Fax: 801-365-2300
E-mail: info@dorlandhealth.com
www.dorlandhealth.com

Delivers valuable intelligence on local health and managed
care marekts. Each of these 71 reports describes key market
participants and competitive environment in one US market, including information on: local trends in events, key
players, alliances among MCOs and providers, legislative
developments, regulatory development, statistics on Managed Penetration. *$475.00*

4590 Manisses Communication Group
Manisses Communications Group
208 Governor Street
Providence, RI 02906

401-831-6020
Fax: 401-861-6370
www.manisses.com
Fraser Lang, President/Publisher
Paul Newman, Director Of Sales

4591 Mayo HealthQuest/Mayo Clinic Health Information
200 1st Street SW
Rochester, MN 55905
507-284-2511
Fax: 507-284-0161

4592 Medical Data Research
5225 Wiley Post Way
Suite 500
Salt Lake City, UT 84116
801-536-1110
Karen Beckstead, Contact

4593 Medical Online Resources
67 Shaker Road
Suite 8
Gray, ME 04039-9640
207-729-6228

4594 Medipay
521 SW 11th Avenue
Suite 200
Portland, OR 97205
503-227-6491

Complete information technology solutions for integrated
continuum of managed behavioral health care.

4595 Meridian Resource Corporation
1401 Enclave Parkway
Suite 300
Houston, TX 77077
281-597-7000
Fax: 281-597-8880

4596 Microsoft Corporation
1 Microsoft Way
Redmond, WA 98052
800-642-7676
Fax: 425-936-7329
www.www.support.microsoft.com

4597 Multimedia Medical Systems
400 Ray C Hunt Drive
Suite 380
Charlottesville, VA 22903
804-977-8710

4598 NASW West Virginia Chapter
1608 Virginia Street E
Charleston, WV 25311
304-345-6279
Fax: 304-343-3295
E-mail: naswwv@aol.com

4599 National Child Support Network
PO Box 1018
Fayetteville, AR 72702
479-582-2300
www.childsupport.org

4600 National Council on Alcoholism and Drug Dependence
244 East 58th Street
4th Floor
New York, NY 10022
212-269-7797
Fax: 212-269-7510
E-mail: national@ncadd.org
www.ncadd.org

4601 National Families in Action
2957 Clairmont Road NE
Suite 150
Atlanta, GA 30329
404-248-9676
Fax: 404-248-1312
E-mail: nfia@nationalfamilies.org
www.www.nationalfamilies.org

4602 National Mental Health Self-Help Clearinghouse
1211 Chestnut Street
Suite 1207
Philadelphia, PA 19107
215-751-1810
800-553-4539
Fax: 215-636-6312
E-mail: info@mhselfhelp.org
www.www.mhselfhelp.org

4603 North Bay Center for Behavioral Medicine
1100 Trancas Street
Suite 244
Napa, CA 94558
707-255-7786
www.behavioralmed.org

Frank Lucchetti, Psychologist

Represents comprehensive assessment and a balanced schedule of medical and/or psychological treatments for individuals with disabilities needing relief from chronic pain, disabling conditions and stress related to depression, anxiety, and unhealthy work, community or family conditions.

4604 On-Line Information Services
202 W Firetower Road
Winterville, NC 28590
252-758-4141
800-765-8268
www.www.onlineinfoservices.com

4605 Open Minds
Behavioral Health Industry News
163 York Street
Gettysburg, PA 17325
717-334-1329
877-350-6463
Fax: 717-334-0538
E-mail: openminds@openminds.com
www.openminds.com

Provides information on marketing, financial, and legal trends in the delivery of mental health and chemical dependency benefits and services. Recurring features include interviews, news of research, a calendar of events, job listings, book reviews, notices of publications available, and industry statistics. *$185.00*

12 pages 12 per year ISSN 1043-3880

4606 Optum
Mail Route MN010-S203
6300 Olson Memorial Highway
Golden Valley, MN 55427
888-262-4614
www.www.optucare.com

A market leader in providing comprehensive information, education and support services that enhance quality of life through improved health and well-being. Through multiple access points-the telephone, audio tapes, print materials, in-person consultations and the Internet-Optum helps participants address daily living concerns, make appropriate health care decisions, and become more effective managers of their own health and well-being.

4607 Our Town Family Center
3830 E Bellevue
Street 85716
Tucson, AZ 85726
520-323-1708

A general social services agency which focuses on serving children, youth, and their families. We offer low or no cost assistance with counseling, prevention, services for homeless youth and runaways (their families too) mediation, services for at risk youth, residential programs, parent mentoring, and much more. Our Town has made a conscious decision to keep its services focused in Pima County, in order to better serve our community. We are nonprofit, and funded by United Way, private donations, and grants with the state, county and city.

4608 Ovid Online
Ovid Technologies
333 7th Avenue
New York, NY 10001
646-674-6300
800-950-2035
Fax: 646-674-6301
E-mail: sales@ovid.com
www.www.ovid.com

Online reference and database information provider.
$.50/record

4609 Patient Medical Records
901 Tahoka Road
Brownfield, TX 79316
806-637-2556
800-285-7627

4610 Penelope Price
4281 MacDuff Pl
Dublin, OH 43017
614-793-0165

4611 Physicians' ONLINE
560 White Plains Road
Tarrytown, NY 10591
914-333-5800

4612 Piedmont Community Services
24 Clay Street
Martinsville, VA 24112
276-632-7128
Fax: 276-632-9998

4613 Point of Care Technologies
6 Taft Court
Rockville, MD 20850
301-610-2400

4614 Preferred Medical Informatics
1251 W Glen Oaks Lane
Mequon, WI 53092
414-290-6749
Fax: 414-290-6780

4615 PsychAccess
700 5th Avenue
Sutie 5500
Seattle, WA 98104-5016
206-521-2588

4616 Quadramed
12110 Sunset Hills Road
Reston, VA 20190
703-709-2300
800-393-0278
Fax: 703-709-2490
www.www.quadramed.com

4617 RTI Business Systems
5622 Ox Road
Suite 220
Fairfax Station, VA 22039-1018
703-503-9600
Fax: 703-503-9696

4618 Servisource
40520 Hayes Road
Clinton Township, MI 48038
586-286-1101

4619 SilverPlatter Information
100 River Ridge Drive
Suite 200
Norwood, MA 02062-5041
781-769-2599
Fax: 781-769-8763

4620 Stress Management Research Associates
10609-B Grant Road
Houston, TX 77070
281-890-8575
E-mail: relax@stresscontrol.com
www.stresscontrol.com

Edward Charlesworth, Contact

4621 Supervised Lifestyles
2505 Carmel Ave
Suite 210
Brewster, NY 10509
888-822-7348
E-mail: sls@slshealth.com
www.slshealth.com

4622 Technical Support Systems
775 E 3300 S
1
Salt Lake City, UT 84106
801-484-1283

4623 Telepad Corporation
380 Herndon Parkway
Suite 1900
Herndon, VA 20170
703-834-9000

4624 Traumatic Incident Reduction Association
5145 Pontiac Trail
Ann Arbor, MI 48105
734-761-6268
800-499-2751
Fax: 734-663-6861
E-mail: info@tir.org
www.tir.org

4625 UNISYS Corporation
8008 Westpark Drive
McLean, VA 22102
703-847-2412

4626 Universal Behavioral Service
3590 N Meridian Street
Indianapolis, IN 46208
317-684-0442

4627 Virginia Beach Community Service Board
289 Independence Blvd
#138
Virginia Beach, VA 23462
757-437-6150

4628 Well Mind Association
1201 Western Ave
Seattle, WA 98101
206-728-9770
800-556-5829
Fax: 206-728-1500
www.speakeasy.net

Well Mind Association distributes information on current research and promotes alternative therapies for mental illness and related disorders. WMA believes that physical conditions and treatable biochemical imbalances are the causes of many mental, emotional and behavioral problems.

4629 WordPerfect Corporation
1555 N Technology Way
Orem, UT 84057-2399
801-225-5000
Fax: 801-222-5077

Pharmaceutical Companies

Manufacturers A-Z

4630 Abbott Laboratories
100 Abbott Park Road
Abbott Park, IL 60064-6400
847-937-6100
Fax: 847-937-1511
www.abbott.com

Miles White, Chairman/Chief Executive Officer

Manufactures the following psychological drugs: Cylert, Desoxyn, Depakote, Nembutal, Placidyl, Prosom, Tranxene.

4631 Akzo Nobel
525 W Van Buren Street
Chicago, IL 60606
312-544-7000
800-906-9977
Fax: 312-544-7159
E-mail: csrusa@sc.akzonobel.com
www.surface.akzonobelusa.com

Hans Wijers, CEO
Rob Frohn, CFO

Manufactures the following psychological drugs: Remeron, Tolvon.

4632 Astra Zeneca Pharmaceuticals
1800 Concord Pike
PO Box 15437
Wilmington, DE 19850
302-886-3000
Fax: 302-886-3119
www.astrazeneca-us.com

Tony Zook, President/CEO
David Elkins, Vice President/CFO

Full range of products in six therapeutic areas; gastrointestinal, oncology, anesthesia, cardiovascular, central nervous system and respiratory.

4633 Bristol-Myers Squibb
345 Park Avenue
New York, NY 10154-0037
212-546-4000
www.bms.com

James Cornelius, Chairman/CEO

Manufactures the following psychological drugs: Avapro, Enfamil, Abilify, Provachol.

4634 Cephalon
41 Moores Road
Frazer, PA 19355
610-344-0200
E-mail: humanresources@cephalon.com
www.cephalon.com

J.Kevin Buchi, Executive VP/CFO
Frank Baldino, Chairman/CEO

Manufactures the following pharmaceuticals: Provigil, Amrix, Fentora, Vivitrol, Trisenox, Nuvigil.

4635 Eisai
100 Tice Blvd
Woodcliff Lake, NJ 07677
201-692-1100
www.eisai.com

Judee Shuler, Dir. Corp. Plans/Communications
Robert Feeney, Dir. Investor & Gov. Relations

Manufactures the following psychological drug: Aricept, Aciphex, Fragmin, Zonegran.

4636 Eli Lilly and Company
Lilly Corporate Center
Indianapolis, IN 46285
317-276-2000
Fax: 317-277-6579
www.lilly.com

Sidney Taurel, Chairman/CEO
Robert Armitage, Senior VP/General Counsel

Manufactures the following psychological drugs: Prozac, Ceclor, Zyprexa, Cialis, Strattera, and Symbyax.

4637 First Horizon Pharmaceutical
6195 Shiloh Road
Alpharetta, GA 30005
770-442-9707
Fax: 770-442-9594
www.horizonpharm.com

Manufactures the following products: Triglide, Fortamet, and Altopren.

4638 Forest Laboratories
909 Third Avenue
New York, NY 10022
212-421-7850
800-947-5227
www.frx.com

Howard Solomon, CEO

Manufactures the following psychological drugs: Lexapro, Benicar, Campral, Celexa, Namenda, and Tiazac.

4639 GlaxoSmithKline
5 Moore Drive
PO Box 13398
Research Triangle Park, NC 27709
888-825-5249
Fax: 919-483-5249
www.gsk.com

JP Garnier, CEO

Manufactures the following psychological drugs: Wellbutrin, Lamictal, Paxil, Parnate.

4640 Hoffman-La Roche
340 Kingsland Street
Nutley, NJ 07110
973-235-5000
Fax: 973-235-7605
www.rocheusa.com

George Abercrombie, President/CEO

Manufactures the following psychological drugs: Boniva Valium, Klonopin, Valcyte, Zenapax.

4641 Janssen
1125 Trenton-Harbourton Road
PO Box 200
Titusville, NJ 08560-0200
609-730-2000
800-526-7736
www.www.janssen.com

Timothy Cost, Senior VP Corporate Affairs

Janssen markets prescription medications for the treatment of schizophrenia and bipolar mania.

4642 Johnson & Johnson
One Johnson & Johnson Plaza
New Brunswick, NJ 08933
732-524-0400
Fax: 732-524-3300
www.jnj.com

William Weldon, Chairman/CEO

Manufactures the following:Reminyl, Risperdal, Concerta, Daktarin, Ertaczo, Levaquin.

4643 King Pharmaceuticals
501 Fifth Street
Bristol, TN 37620
423-989-8000
800-776-7637
Fax: 866-990-0545
www.kingpharm.com

James Green, Executive VP Corporate Affairs
David Robinson, Senior Dir. Corporate Affairs

Manufactures some of the following medications: Sonata, Corgard, Cytomel, Humatin, Levoxyl, Procanbid, and Septra.

4644 Mallinckrodt
Corporate Headquarters
675 McDonnell Boulevard
Hazelwood, MO 63042
314-654-2000
Fax: 314-654-5380
www.mallinckrodt.com

Douglas McKinney, VP Of Finance/CFO
Lisa Britt, VP Of Human Resources

Manufactures the following psychological drugs: Dexedrine, Methylin.

4645 Merck
One Merck Drive
PO Box 100
Whitehouse Station, NJ 08889-0100
908-423-1000
www.merck.com

Peter Kellogg, Executive VP/CFO
Mirian Graddick-Weir, Executive VP Human Resources

Manufactures Vioxx, Zocor, Fosamax, Cozaar, Januvia, and others.

4646 Mutual Pharmaceutical Company
1100 Orthodox Street
Philadelphia, PA 19124
800-523-3684
Fax: 215-288-6559
E-mail: jsmurray@urlmutual.com
www.www.urlmutual.com

Richard H Roberts MD PhD, President/CEO/Chairman

Manufactures the following medication for treatment of depression with anxiety: Triavil.

4647 Novartis
400 Technology Square
Cambridge, MA 02139

617-871-8000
Fax: 617-871-8911
www.novartis.com

Daniel Vasella, Chairman/CEO
Raymund Breu, CFO

Manufactures the following products Diovan, Glivec, Lamisil, Zometa , Excedrin and more.

4648 Organon Schering Plough
56 Livingston Avenue
Roseland, NJ 07068
973-325-4500
Fax: 973-325-4589
www.organon-usa.com

Manufactures the following: Nuvaring, Follistia, Ganirelix, and Zemuron.

4649 Ortho-McNeil Pharmaceutical
1125 Trenton Harbourton Road
PO Box 200
Titusville, NJ 08560-200
800-526-7736
www.ortho-mcneil.com

Manufactures the following Elmiron, Modicon, Ortho-Novum, and Terazol 3.

4650 Parke-Davis Pharmaceutcials
235 E 42nd Street
New York, NY 10017
212-733-2323
www.www.pfizer.com

Manufactures the following bipolar disorder medication: Neurontin.

4651 Pfizer
235 E 42nd Street
New York, NY 10017
212-733-2323
Fax: 212-573-2273
www.pfizer.com

Jeffrey Kindler, Chairman/CEO

Manufactures the following psychological drugs: Aricept, Zoloft, Geodon.

4652 Pharmacia & Upjohn
100 Route 206
Peapack, NJ 07977
888-768-5501

F Hassan, President/CEO

Manufactures the following medication: Reboxetine.

4653 Roxane Laboratories
1809 Wilson Road
PO Box 16532
Columbus, OH 43216
614-276-4000
Fax: 614-274-0974

Manufactures detoxification medication: Dolophine.

4654 Sanofi-Aventis
55 Corporate Drive
Bridgewater, NJ 08807
800-981-2491
www.www.sanofi-aventis.us

Manufacturer of medications for cardiovascular disease, thrombosis, oncology, diabetes, central nervous system, internal medicine, and vaccines.

4655 Sanofi-Synthelabo
55 Corporate Drive
Bridgewater, NJ 08807
800-981-2491
800-207-8049
www.sanofi-aventis.us

Timothy Rothwell, Chairman

Manufactures the following: Ambien, Carac, Eligard, Klaron, Lovenox, Lantus, Penlac, Uroxatral.

4656 Sepracor Pharmaceuticals
84 Waterford Drive
Marlborough, MA 01752
508-481-6700
800-586-3782
E-mail: info@sepracor.com
www.www.sepracor.com

Adrian Adams, President/CEO
Mark Iwicki, Exeecutive Vice President/COO

Manufactures sleep disorder drug Lunesta,as well as other medications Xopenex, and Brovana.

4657 Shire Richwood
725 Chesterbrook Blvd
Wayne, PA 19087-5637
484-595-8800
Fax: 484-595-8200
www.shire.com

Matthew Emmens, CEO
Barbara Deptula, Exec. VP Bussiness Development

Manufactures the following psychological drugs: Adderall, DextroStat.

4658 Solvay Pharmaceuticals
901 Sawyer Road
Marietta, GA 30062
770-578-9000
Fax: 770-578-5597
www.solvaypharmaceuticals.com

Neil Hirsch, Contact
Jessica Mumaw, Contact

Manufactures the following psychological drugs: Klonopin, Lithobid, Lithonate.

4659 Somerset Pharmaceuticals
5415 W Laurel Street
Tampa, FL 33607
813-288-0040
www.somersetpharm.com

Manufactures the following psychological drug: Eldepryl.

4660 Synthon Pharmaceuticals
9000 Development Drive
PO Box 110487
Research Triangle, NC 27709
919-493-6006
Fax: 919-493-6104
E-mail: info@synthon.com
www.www.synthon-usa.com

Develops, produces and sells high quality alternatives to innovative medicines. Our products are marketed at the earliest possible opportunity and we sell them at competitive prices.

4661 Takeda Pharmaceuticals North America
One Takeda Parkway
Deerfield, IL 60015
224-554-6500
877-582-5332
www.tpna.com

Mark Booth, President

Manufacturer of Rozerem, Duetact, Amitiza, and Actos.

4662 Valeant Pharmaceuticals International
One Enterprise
Aliso Viejo, CA 92656
949-461-6000
800-548-5100
Fax: 949-461-6609
www.www.valeant.cm

J Michael Pearson, CEO

Develops, manufactures and markets pharmaceutical products primarily in the areas of neurology, dermatology and infectious disease.

4663 Watson Pharmaceuticals
311 Bonnie Circle
Corona, CA 92880
951-493-5300
www.www.watson.com

Paul M Bisaro, President/CEO

Manufactures the following medications: Ferrlecit, Quasense, Androderm, Nicotine Polacrilex Gum USP, Trelstar, Oxycodone and Acetaminophen Tablets USP, Oxytrol.

4664 Wyeth
5 Giralda Farms
Madison, NJ 07940
973-660-5500
Fax: 973-660-7026
www.wyeth.com

Timothy Cost, Senior VP Corporate Affairs

Manufactures the following products: Advil brands, Alavert, Anbesol ,Caltrate, Centrum brands, Dimetapp, FiberCon, Preparation H, Robitussin brands and more.

Drugs A-Z

4665 Abilify
Generic: Aripiprazole

Used in the treatment of schizophrenia and bi-polar disorder. This product is manufactured by Bristol-Myers Squibb. See manufacturers section for company information.

4666 Adderall/Adderall XR
Generic: Amphetamine/Dextroamphetamine

Used to manage anxiety disorders and some cases of attention deficit hyperactivity disorder. This product is manufactured by Shire Richwood. See Manufacturers section for company information.

4667 Ambien/Ambien CR
Generic: Zolpidem

Used in the treatment of insomnia, also sold as Tovalt. This product is manufactured by Sanofi-Synthelabo. See Manufacturers section for company information.

4668 Anafranil
Generic: Clomipramine

Used in the treatment of obsessive-compulsive disorder. This product is manufactured by Novartis Consumer Health Corporation. See Manufacturers section for company information.

4669 Antabuse
Generic: Disulfiram

Used in the treatment of alcohol and substance abuse. This product is manufactured by Wyeth-Ayers. See Manufacturers section for company information.

4670 Aricept
Generic: Donepezil

Used in the treatment of Alzheimer's disease. This product is manufactured by Pfizer and Eisai. See Manufacturers section for company information.

4671 Ativan
Generic: Lorazepam

Used in the treatment of insomnia and as a preanesthetic medication in adults. This product is manufactured by Wyeth-Ayerst Laboratories. See Manufacturers section for company information.

4672 BuSpar
Generic: Buspirone

Used in the treatment of anxiety. This product is manufactured by Bristol-Myers Squibb. See Manufacturers section for company information.

4673 Campral
Generic: Acamprosate

Used in the treatment of alcohol dependence. This product is manufactured by Merck. See Manufacturers section for company information.

4674 Celexa
Generic: Citalopram

Used in the treatment of depression. This product is manufactured by Forest Laboratories. See Manufacturers section for company information.

4675 Cialis
Generic: Tadalafil

Used in the treatment of erectile dysfunction. Manufactured by Eli Lilly. See Manufacturers section for company information.

4676 Clozaril
Generic: Clozapine

Used in the treatment of severe schizophrenia, and also sold as Clozaril and Fazaclo. This product is manufactured by Norvartis. See Manufacturers section for company information.

4677 Cognex
Generic: Tacrine

Used in the treatment of Alzheimer's disease. This product is manufactured by First Horizon Pharmaceutical. See Manufacturers section for company information.

4678 Concerta
Generic: Methylphenidate

Used in the treatment of attention deficit disorder, and also sold as Daytrana and Desoxyn. This product is manufactured by Johnson & Johnson. See Manufacturers section for company information.

4679 Cymbalta
Generic: Dulozetine

Used in the treatment of depression and anxiety. Manufactured by Eli Lilly and Company. See Manufacturers section for company information.

4680 Depakote
Generic: Valproic Acid

Used in the treatment of manic episodes associated with bi-polar disorder and mania, and also sold as Depakene. This product is manufactured by Abbott Laboratories. See Manufacturers section for company information.

4681 Desoxyn

Used in the treatment of attention deficit hyperactive disorder. This product is manufactured by Abbott Laboratories. See Manufacturers section for company information.

4682 Dexedrine
Generic: Dextroamphetamine

Used in the treatment of attention deficit hyperactive disorder, and also sold as DextroState, Focalin (by Novartis), Metadate, and Methylin. This product is manufactured by Mallinckrodt. See Manufacturers section for company information.

4683 Dolophine
Generic: Methadone

Used in the treatment of detoxifcation and temporary maintenance from narcotic addiction. This product is manufactured by Roxane Laboratories. See manufacturers section for company information.

4684 Effexor
Generic: Venlafazine

Used in the treatment of depression and generalized anxiety disorder. This product is manufactured by Wyeth-Ayerst Laboratories. See Manufacturers section for company information.

4685 Elavil
Generic: Amitryptaline

Used in the treatment of depression, also sold as Limbitrol (by Valeant). This product is manufactured by Astra Zeneca Pharmaceuticals. See Manufacturers section for company information.

4686 Emsam
Generic: Selegiline

Used in the treatment of major depressive disorder. This product is manufactured by Bristol-Myers Squibb. See manufacturers section for company information.

4687 Eskalith
Generic: Lithium

Used in the treatment of bipolar disorder. This product is manufactured by GlaxoSmithKline. See Manufacturers section for company information.

4688 Exelon
Generic: Rivastigmine

Used in the treatment of Alzheimer's disease. This product is manufactured by Novartis. See Manufacturers section for company information.

4689 Fluvoxamine
Generic: Luvox

Used in the treatment of OCD. This product is manufactured by Solvay Pharmaceuticals. See manufacturers section for company information.

4690 Geodon
Generic: Ziprasidone

Used in the treatment of psychotic episodes. This product is manufactured by Pfizer. See Manufacturers section for company information.

4691 Haldol
Generic: Haloperidol

Used in the treatment of psychosis, Tourette's disorder. This product is manufactured by Ortho-McNeil Pharmaceuticals. See manufacturers section for company information.

4692 Invega
Generic: Paliperidone

Used in the treatment of Schizophrenia. This product is manufactured by Janssen. See manufacturers section for company information.

4693 Klonopin
Generic: Clonazepam

Used in the treatment of panic disorder. This product is manufactured by Hoffman-La Roche. See Manufacturers section for company information.

4694 Lamictal
Generic: Lamotrigine

Used in the treatment of bipolar disorder. This product is manufactured by GlaxoSmithKline. See Manufacturers section for company information.

4695 Leponex
Generic: Clozapine

Used in the treatment of psychotic episodes. This product is manufactured by Novartis. See Manufacturers section for company information.

4696 Levitra
Generic: Vardenafil

Used in the treatment of erectile dysfunction. Manufactured by GlaxoSmithKline. See Manufacturers section for company information.

4697 Lexapro
Generic: Escitalopram

Used in the treatment of depression. This product is manufactured by Forest Laboratories. See Manufacturers section for company information.

4698 Lithobid
Generic: Lithium; Eskalith

Used in the treatment of bipolar disorder and depression. This product is manufactured by Solvay Pharmaceuticals. See Manufacturers section for company information.

4699 Loxitane
Generic: Loxapine

Used in the treatment of Schizophrenia. This product is manufactured by Watson Pharmaceuticals. See manufacturers section for company information.

4700 Lunesta
Generic: Eszopiclone

Used in the treatment of insomnia. This product is manufactured by Sepracor. See Manufacturers section for company information.

4701 Luvox
Generic: Fluvoxamine

Used in the treatment of obsessive compulsive disorder. This product is manufactured by Solvay Pharmaceuticals. See Manufacturers section for company information.

4702 Marplan
Generic: Isocarboxazid

Used in the treatment of manage depression, anxiety and panic disorders. Manufactured by Hoffman-La Roche. See Manufacturers section for company information.

4703 Methylin
Generic: Methylphenidate

Used in the treatment of attention deficit disorder. This product is manufactured by Mallinckrodt. See Manufacturers section for company information.

4704 Namenda
Generic: Memantine

Used in the treatment of Alzheimer's. This product is manufactured by Forest Pharmaceuticals. See Manufacturers section for company information.

4705 Nardil
Generic: Phenelzine

Used in the treatment of atypical depression. This product is manufactured by Pfizer. See Manufacturers section for company information.

4706 Nefazodone
Generic: Serzone

Used in the treatment of depression. This product is manufactured by Bristol-Myers Squibb. See Manufacturers section for company information.

4707 Neurontin
Generic: Gabapentin

Used in the treatment of bipolar disorder. This product is manufactured by Parke-Davis Pharmacutical Company. See Manufacturers section for company information.

4708 Norpramin
Generic: Desipramine

Used in the treatment of depression. This product is manufactured by Sanofi-Aventis Pharmaceuticals. See Manufacturers section for company information.

4709 Nuvigil
Generic: Amodafinil

Used in the treatment to promote wakefulness. This product is manufactured by Cephalon. See Manufacturers section for company information.

4710 Pamelor
Generic: Nortriptyline

Used in the treatment of depression. This product is manufactured by Novartis Pharmaceuticals. See Manufacturers section for company information.

4711 Parnate
Generic: Tranylcypromine

Used to help manage depression. This product is manufactured by GlaxoSmithKline. See Manufacturers section for company information.

4712 Paxil
Generic: Parozetine

Used in the treatment of depression, social anxiety, obsessive-compulsive disorder, generalized anxiety disorder and panic disorder. This product is manufactured by GlaxoSmithKline. Sold also as Pexeva by Synthon. See Manufacturers section for company information.

4713 Prolixin
Generic: Fluphenazine

Used in the treatment of schizophrenia and other psychotic disorders. This product is manufactured by Bristol-Myers Squibb. See Manufacturers section for company information.

4714 Provigil
Generic: Modafinil

Used in the treatment of sleep disorders. This product is manufactured by Cephalon. See Manufacturers section for company information.

4715 Prozac
Generic: Fluozetine

Used in the treatment of depression and obsessive-compulsive disorder. This product is manufactured by Eli Lilly and Company. See Manufacturers section for company information.

4716 Razadyne ER
Generic: Galantamine

Used in the treatment of mild to moderate Alzheimer's. This product is manufactured by Ortho-McNeil. See Manufacturers section for company information.

4717 Reboxetine
Generic: Vestra

Used in the treatment of depression. This product is manufactured by Pharmacia & Upjohn. See Manufacturers section for company information.

4718 Remeron
Generic: Mirtazapine

Used in the treatment of manage depression. This product is manufactured by Organon and Akzo Nobel. See Manufacturers section for company information.

4719 Reminyl
Generic: Razadine

Used in the treatment of Alzheimer's disease. This product is manufactured by Johnson & Johnson. See Manufacturers section for company information.

4720 Risperdal
Generic: Risperidone

Used in the treatment of schizophrenia and other mental illnesses such as psychosis. This product is manufactured by Johnson & Johnson. See Manufacturers section for company information.

4721 Ritalin
Generic: Methylphenidate

Used in the treatment of attention deficit disorders and in some forms of narcolepsy. This product is manufactured by Novartis. See Manufacturers section for company information.

4722 Rozerem
Generic: Ramelteon

Used in the treatment of insomnia. This product is manufactured by Takeda Pharmaceuticals. See Manufacturers section for company information.

4723 Seroquel
Generic: Quetiapine

Used in the treatment of psychotic disorders. This product is manufactured by Astra Zeneca Pharmaceuticals. See Manufacturers section for company information.

4724 Sonata
Generic: Zalplon

Used in the treatment of insomnia. This product is manufactured by King Pharmaceuticals. See Manufacturers section for company information.

4725 Strattera
Generic: Atomoxetine

Used in the treatment of attention deficit disorder. This product is manufactured by Eli Lilly & Company. See Manufacturers section for company information.

4726 Surmontil
Generic: Trimipramine

Used in the treatment of depression. This product is manufactured by Wyeth-Ayerst Laboratories. See Manufacturers section for company information.

4727 Symbyax
Generic: Fluoxetine

Used in the treatment of depression associated with bipolar disorder. This product is manufactured by Eli-Lilly & Company. See Manufacturers section for company information.

4728 Tofranil
Generic: Imipramine

Used in the treatment of depression. This product is manufactured by Novartis Pharmaceuticals. See Manufacturers section for company information.

4729 Tolvon
Generic: Mianserin Hydrochloride

Used in the treatment of depression. This product is manufactured by Akzo Nobel. See Manufacturers section for company information.

4730 Topamax
Generic: Topiramate

Used in the treatment of bipolar disorder. This product is manufactured by Ortho-McNeil Pharmacutical. See Manufacturers section for company information.

4731 Tranxene
Generic: Clorazepate

Used in the treatment of insomnia, or as a tranquilizer. This product is manufactured by Abbott Laboratories. See Manufacturers section for company information.

4732 Triavil
Generic: Perphenazine

Used in the treatment of depression with anxiety. This product is manufactured by Mutual Pharmaceutical Trade. See Manufacturers section for company information.

4733 Valium
Generic: Diazepam

Used in the treatment of anxiety. This product is manufactured by Hoffman-La Roche. See Manufacturers section for company information.

4734 Viagra
Generic: Sildenafil

Used in the treatment of erectile dysfunction. Manufactured by Pfizer. See Manufacturers section for company information.

4735 Vyvanse
Generic: Lixdexamfetamine

Used in the treatment of ADHD in children 6-12 years of age. This product is manufactured by Shire Richwood. See Manufacturers section for company information.

4736 Wellbutrin
Generic: Bupropion

Used in the treatment of depression. This product is manufactured by GlaxoSmithKline. See Manufacturers section for company information.

4737 Xanax
Generic: Alprazolam

Used in the treatment of anxiety, also sold as Niravam. This product is manufactured by Pharmacia & Upjohn. See Manufacturers section for company information.

4738 Zoloft
Generic: Sertraline

Used in the treatment of depression, post traumatic stress disorder, obsessive-compulsive disorder and panic disorder. This product is manufactured by Pfizer. See Manufacturers section for company information.

4739 Zyprexa
Generic: Olanzapine

Used in the treatment of psychotic disorders. This product is manufactured by Eli Lilly and Company. See Manufacturers section for company information.

ADHD

AD/HD Forms Book: Identification, Measurement, and Intervention, 402

ADD & Learning Disabilities: Reality, Myths, & Controversial Treatments, 403

ADD & Romance, 404

ADD Hyperactivity Handbook for Schools, 405

ADD Kaleidoscope: The Many Facets of Adult Attention Deficit Disorder, 406

ADD Success Stories: Guide to Fulfillment for Families with Attention Deficit Disorder, 407

ADD and Adolescence: Strategies for Success, 408

ADD in the Workplace: Choices, Changes and Challenges, 409

ADD/ADHD Checklist: an Easy Reference for Parents & Teachers, 410

ADHD Monitoring System, 411

ADHD Parenting Handbook: Practical Advise fo r Parents, 412

ADHD Report, 474

ADHD Survival Guide for Parents and Teachers, 413

ADHD and Teens: Parent's Guide to Making it Through the Tough Years, 414

ADHD and the Nature of Self-Control, 415

ADHD in Adolesents: Diagnosis and Treatment, 2952

ADHD in Adulthood: Guide to Current Theory, Diagnosis and Treatment, 2953

ADHD in the Young Child: Driven to Redirection, 416

ADHD: A Complete and Authoritative Guide, 417

ADHD: What Can We Do?, 479

ADHD: What Do We Know?, 480

Adults with Attention Deficit Disorder: ADD Isn't Just Kids Stuff, 481

Adventures in Fast Forward: Life, Love and Work for the ADD Adult, 418

Aggression Replacement Training Video: A Comprehensive Intervention for Aggressive Youth, 1633

Aggression Replacement Training: A Comprehensive Intervention for Aggressive Youth, 1596

All About ADHD: Complete Practical Guide for Classroom Teachers, 2954

All About Attention Deficit Disorder: Revised Edition, 419

All Kinds of Minds, 420

Answers to Distraction, 421

Attention Deficit Disorder ADHD and ADD Syndromes, 2955

Attention Deficit Disorder Association, 390

Attention Deficit Disorder and Learning Disabilities: Realities, Myths and Controversial Treatments, 422, 2956

Attention Deficit Hyperactivity Disorder in Children: A Medication Guide, 423

Attention Deficit/Hyperactivity Disorder, 2957

Attention Deficits and Hyperactivity in Children: Developmental Clinical Psychology and Psychiatry, 424

Attention-Deficit Hyperactivity Disorder: A Handbook for Diagnosis and Treatment, 2958

Attention-Deficit/Hyperactivity Disorder in the Classroom, 2959

Beyond Ritalin, 426

Birds-Eye View of Life with ADD and ADHD: Ad vice from Young Survivors, Second Edition, 427

CARE Child and Adolescent Risk Evaluation: A Measure of the Risk for Violent Behavior, 1600

Center For Mental Health Services, 391

Clinical Dimensions of Anticipatory Mourning, 2711

Communicating in Relationships: A Guide for Couples and Professionals, 2715

Conduct Disorders in Children and Adolesents, 428

Council for Learning Disabilities, 1726

Daredevils and Daydreamers: New Perspectives on Attention Deficit/Hyperactivity Disorder, 430

Distant Drums, Different Drummers: A Guide for Young People with ADHD, 431

Don't Give Up Kid, 432

Down and Dirty Guide to Adult Attention Deficit Disorder, 433

Driven to Distraction: Recognizing and Coping with Attention Deficit Disorder from Childhood through, 434

Eagle Eyes: A Child's View of Attention Deficit Disorder, 436

Educating Inattentive Children, 482

Eukee the Jumpy, Jumpy Elephant, 437

Facing AD/HD: A Survival Guide for Parents, 438

Family Therapy for ADHD: Treating Children, Adolescents and Adults, 2960

First Star I See, 439

Forms for Behavior Analysis with Children, 1604

Gangs in Schools: Signs, Symbols and Solutions, 1606

Gene Bomb, 440

Give Your ADD Teen a Chance: A Guide for Parents of Teenagers with Attention Deficit Disorder, 441

Grandma's Pet Wildebeest Ate My Homework, 442

Healing ADD: Simple Exercises That Will Change Your Daily Life, 443

Help 4 ADD@High School, 444

Help This Kid's Driving Me Crazy - the Young Child with Attention Deficit Disorder, 3496

Helper's Journey: Working with People Facing Grief, Loss, and Life-Threatening Illness, 2764

HomeTOVA: Attention Screening Test, 445

How to Operate an ADHD Clinic or Subspecialty Practice, 2961

Hyperactive Child, Adolescent, and Adult, 447

Hyperactive Children Grown Up: ADHD in Children, Adolescents, and Adults, 448

Is Your Child Hyperactive? Inattentive? Impulsive? Distractible?, 450

Learning Disabilities Association of America, 395

Learning to Slow Down and Pay Attention, 451

Legacy of Childhood Trauma: Not Always Who They Seem, 1637

Living with Attention Deficit Disorder: a Workbook for Adults with ADD, 452

Mallinckrodt, 4644

Medication for ADHD, 483

Medications for Attention Disorders and Related Medical Problems: A Comprehensive Handbook, 453, 2962

Meeting the ADD Challenge: A Practical Guide for Teachers, 454

Misunderstood Child: Understanding and Coping with Your Child's Learning Disabilities, 455

My Brother's a World Class Pain: a Sibling's Guide to ADHD, 456

New Look at ADHD: Inhibition, Time and Self Control, 484

Parenting a Child With Attention Deficit/Hyperactivity Disorder, 2963

Pfeiffer Treatment Center and Health Researc h Institute, 3846

Pretenders: Gifted People Who Have Difficulty Learning, 2964

A Primer on Rational Emotive Behavior Therapy, 2687

Put Yourself in Their Shoes: Understanding Teenagers with Attention Deficit Hyperactivity Disorder, 457

Rational Emotive Therapy, 3507

Shelley, The Hyperative Turtle, 459

Sometimes I Drive My Mom Crazy, But I Know She's Crazy About Me, 460

Succeeding in College with Attention Deficit Disorders: Issues and Strategies for Students, Counselo, 462

Survival Guide for College Students with ADD or LD, 463

Survival Strategies for Parenting Your ADD Child, 464

Taking Charge of ADHD: Complete, Authoritative Guide for Parents, 465

Teenagers with ADD and ADHD, 2nd Edition: A Guide for Parents and Professionals, 466

Teenagers with ADD: A Parent's Guide, 467

Treatment of Complicated Mourning, 2868

Understanding Girls with Attention Deficit Hyperactivity Disorder, 468

Understanding the Defiant Child, 487

Voices From Fatherhood: Fathers, Sons and ADHD, 469

What Makes Ryan Tick?, 470

What Works When with Children and Adolescents: A Handbook of Individual Counseling Techniques, 1615

Why Won't My Child Pay Attention?, 488

Women with Attention Deficit Disorder, 471

Writing Behavioral Contracts: A Case Simulation Practice Manual, 2878

You Mean I'm Not Lazy, Stupid or Crazy?, 472

www.LD-ADD.com, 490

www.aap.org, 491

www.add.about.com, 492

www.add.org, 493

www.additudemag.com, 494

www.addvance.com, 495

www.babycenter.com/rcindex.html, 498

www.chadd.org, 3527

www.nimh.nih.gov/publicat/adhd.cfm, 503

www.oneaddplace.com, 504

Adjustment Disorders

Adolesent in Family Therapy: Breaking the Cycle of Conflict and Control, 3094

Alive Alone, 2

Ambiguous Loss: Learning to Live with Unresolved Grief, 2880

AtHealth.Com, 4

Attachment and Interaction, 2881

Bereaved Parents of the USA, 5

Body Image: Understanding Body Dissatisfaction in Men, Women and Children, 2882

Center for Loss in Multiple Birth (CLIMB), 8

Collaborative Therapy with Multi-Stressed Families, 2714

Couples and Infertility - Moving Beyond Loss, 3492

Drug Therapy and Adjustment Disorders, 27

First Candle/SIDS Alliance, 9

Grief Recovery After Substance Passing (GRASP), 10

The M.I.S.S. Foundation, 19

Narrative Therapies with Children and Adolescents, 3140

National Organization of Parents of Murdered Children, 14

Ordinary Families, Special Children: Systems Approach to Childhood Disability, 3143

Power and Compassion: Working with Difficult Adolescents and Abused Parents, 3147

Reaching Out in Family Therapy: Home Based, School, and Community Interventions, 2840

Save Our Sons And Daughters (SOSAD), 16

Stress Response Syndromes: Personality Styles and Interventions, 29

Triplet Connection, 20

UNITE Inc Grief Support, 21

What Psychotherapists Should Know About Disability, 2872

When A Friend Dies, 32

www.DivorceNet.com, 42

www.alivealone.org, 43

www.athealth.com, 44

www.compassionatefriends.org, 48

www.counselingforloss.com, 49, 3531

www.death-dying.com, 51

www.divorceasfriends.com, 52

www.divorcecentral.com, 53

www.divorceinfo.com, 54

www.divorcemag.com, 55

www.divorcesupport.com, 56

www.griefnet.org, 59

www.misschildren.org, 61

www.psycom.net/depression.central.grief.html, 67

www.spig.clara.net/guidline.htm, 72

www.utexas.edu, 76

www.widownet.org, 77

Alcohol/Substance Abuse & Dependence

About Alcohol, 156

About Crack Cocaine, 157

About Drug Addiction, 158

Addiction Workbook: A Step by Step Guide to Quitting Alcohol and Drugs, 105

Addiction: Why Can't They Just Stop?, 106

Addictive Behaviors Across the Life Span, 2885

Adolescents, Alcohol and Drugs: A Practical Guide for Those Who Work With Young People, 2887

Adult Children of Alcoholics World Services Organization, 198

Al-Anon Family Group National Referral Hotline, 199

Alateen Talk, 159

Alateen and Al-Anon Family Groups, 1624

Alcohol & Drug Abuse Weekly, 3210

Alcohol ABC's, 160

Alcohol Issues Insights, 161

Alcohol Self-Test, 162

Alcohol and the Community, 108

Alcohol: Incredible Facts, 163

Alcohol: the Substance, the Addiction, the Solution, 214

Alcoholics Anonymous (AA): World Services, 200

Alcoholics Anonymous (AA): Worldwide, 81

Alcoholism Sourcebook, 109

Alcoholism: A Merry-Go-Round Named Denial, 164

Alcoholism: A Treatable Disease, 165

American Academy of Addiction Psychiatry (AAAP), 82

American Academy of Addiction Psychiatry: Annual Meeting, 3168

American Council on Alcoholism, 83

American Hospital Association: Section for Psychiatric and Substance Abuse, 2545

American Journal on Addictions, 166

American Psychiatric Press Textbook of Substance Abuse Treatment, 2889

American Society of Addiction Medicine, 3197

Before It's Too Late: Working with Substance Abuse in the Family, 2892

Behavioral Health Systems, 2595

Behind Bars: Substance Abuse and America's Prison Population, 2893

Binge Drinking: Am I At Risk?, 167

Blaming the Brain: The Truth About Drugs and Mental Health, 2894

Broken, 111

Brown University: Digest of Addiction Theory and Application (DATA), 3217

California Association of Social Rehabilitation Agencies, 1823

Candler General Hospital: Rehabilitation Unit, 3813

Chalice, 168

Chemical Dependency Treatment Planning Handbook, 3597

Chemically Dependent Anonymous, 201

Clinical Supervision in Alcohol and Drug Abuse Counseling, 112

Clinician's Guide to the Personality Profiles of Alcohol and Drug Abusers: Typological Descriptions, 2897

Cocaine & Crack: Back from the Abyss, 216

Cocaine Anonymous, 202

Community Anti-Drug Coalitions of America:, 2606

Concerned Intervention: When Your Loved One Won't Quit Alcohol or Drugs, 113

Concise Guide to Treatment of Alcoholism and Addictions, 114

Critical Incidents: Ethical Issues in Substance Abuse Prevention and Treatment, 2898

Cross Addiction: Back Door to Relapse, 217

Crossing the Thin Line: Between Social Drinking and Alcoholism, 170

Culture & Psychotherapy: A Guide to Clinical Practice, 2728

Dangerous Liaisons: Substance Abuse and Sex, 2899

Dauphin County Drug and Alcohol, 2418

Designer Drugs, 171

Determinants of Substance Abuse: Biological, Psychological, and Environmental Factors, 2900

Disease of Alcoholism Video, 218

Drug ABC's, 173

Drug Abuse Sourcebook, 115

Drug Dependence, Alcohol Abuse and Alcoholism, 174

Drug Facts Pamphlet, 175

Drug and Alcohol Dependence, 176

DrugLink, 177

Drugs: Talking With Your Teen, 178

Dynamics of Addiction, 116

Eye Opener, 117

Fetal Alcohol Syndrome & Fetal Alcohol Effect, 118, 179, 219

Fetal Alcohol Syndrome and Effect, Stories of Help and Hope, 220

Five Smart Steps to Safer Drinking, 180

Florida Alcohol and Drug Abuse Association, 1866

Geauga Board of Mental Health, Alcohol and Drug Addiction Services, 4202

Getting Beyond Sobriety, 119

Getting Hooked: Rationality and Addiction, 120

Getting Involved in AA, 181

Getting Started in AA, 182

Getting What You Want From Drinking, 183

Handbook of the Medical Consequences of Alco hol and Drug Abuse, 121

Hazelden Voice, 184

Helping Women Recover: Special Edition for Use in the Criminal Justice System, 122

Heroin: What Am I Going To Do?, 221

Hispanic Substance Abuse, 2904

I Can't Be an Alcoholic Because..., 185

I'll Quit Tomorrow, 222

ICPA Reporter, 186

Infoline, 203

Inside a Support Group, 124

Integrated Treatment of Psychiatric Disorders, 2778

Join Together Online, 204

Journal of Substance Abuse Treatment, 187

Kicking Addictive Habits Once & For All, 125

LSD: Still With Us After All These Years, 126

Let's Talk Facts About Substance Abuse & Addiction, 127

Living Sober I, 129

Living Sober II, 130

MADD-Mothers Against Drunk Drivers, 205

Making the Grade: Guide to School Drug Prevention Programs, 3136

Malignant Neglect: Substance Abuse and America's Schools, 2907

Marijuana ABC's, 188

Marijuana Anonymous, 206

Marijuana: Escape to Nowhere, 223

Meaning of Addiction, 131
Medical Aspects of Chemical Dependency
The Neurobiology of Addiction, 132, 224,
3503
Methamphetamine: Decide to Live
Prevention Video, 225
Missed Opportunity: National Survey of
Primary Care Physicians and Patients on
Substance Abuse, 2908
Mother's Survival Guide to Recovery: All
About Alcohol, Drugs & Babies, 133
Motivating Behavior Changes Among
Illicit-Drug Abusers, 134
Motivational Interviewing: Prepare People to
Change Addictive Behavior, 3020
Motivational Interviewing: Preparing People
to Change Addictive Behavior, 189
Nar-Anon Family Group, 207
Narcotics Anonymous, 208
Narrative Means to Sober Ends: Treating
Addiction and Its Aftermath, 2909
National Association of Addiction Treatment
Providers, 2635
National Association of Alcohol and Drug
Abuse Counselors (NAADAC), 90
National Association of State Alcohol and
Drug Abuse Directors, 91
National Directory of Drug and Alcohol
Abuse Treatment Programs, 135
National Institute of Drug Abuse (NIDA),
190, 1764
National Institute on Alcohol Abuse and
Alcoholism, 96
National Organization on Fetal Alcohol
Syndrome, 100
National Rehabilitation Association, 1770
National Survey of American Attitudes on
Substance Abuse VI: Teens, 3141
New Treaments for Chemical Addictions,
136
No Place to Hide: Substance Abuse in
Mid-Size Cities and Rural America, 2910
No Safe Haven: Children of
Substance-Abusing Parents, 2911
PTSD in Children and Adolesents, 3054
Pathways to Promise, 209
Points for Parents Perplexed about Drugs,
137
Prescription Drugs: Recovery from the
Hidden Addiction, 226
The Prevention Researcher, 194
Principles of Addiction Medicine, 2914
Psychological Theories of Drinking and
Alcoholism, 2916
Rational Recovery, 210
Real World Drinking, 191
Reality Check: Marijuana Prevention Video,
227
Recovery, 356, 928, 1414, 1783
Relapse Prevention Maintenance: Strategies
in the Treatment of Addictive Behaviors,
2917
Relapse Prevention Maintenance: Strategies
in the Treatment of Addictive Behaviors,
2918
Roster: Substance Abuse Treatment Centers,
3664
SMART-Self Management and Recovery
Training, 212
Samhsa's National Clearinghouse For
Alcohol And Drug Information, 102
Save Our Sons and Daughters Newsletter
(SOSAD), 192

The Science of Addiction: From
Neurobiology to Treatment, 148
Science of Prevention: Methodological
Advances from Alcohol and Substance
Research, 140
Section for Psychiatric and Substance Abuse
Services (SPSPAS), 103
Selfish Brain: Learning from Addiction, 141
Seven Points of Alcoholics Anonymous, 142
Sex, Drugs, Gambling and Chocolate:
Workbook for Overcoming Addictions,
143
SmokeFree TV: A Nicotine Prevention
Video, 228
So Help Me God: Substance Abuse, Religion
and Spirituality, 2919
Solutions Step by Step - Substance Abuse
Treatment Videotape, 3508
Solutions Step by Step: Substance Abuse
Treatment Manual, 2920
Somatoform and Factitious Disorders, 3077
Southwest Behavorial Health Services, 3743
Step Workbook for Adolescent Chemical
Dependency Recovery, 3615
Straight Talk About Substance Use and
Violence, 229
Substance Abuse and Learning Disabilities:
Peas in a Pod or Apples and Oranges?,
2921
Substance Abuse: A Comprehensive
Textbook, 2922
Teens and Drinking, 193
Therapeutic Communities of America, 2679
Treating Alcohol Dependence: a Coping
Skills Training Guide, 3619
Treating Alcoholism, 149
Treating Substance Abuse: Part 1, 2925
Treating Substance Abuse: Part 2, 2926
Treating the Alcoholic: Developmental
Model of Recovery, 2927
Troubled Teens: Multidimensional Family
Therapy, 3160
Twelve-Step Facilitation Handbook, 150
Twenty-Four Hours a Day, 151
Under the Rug: Substance Abuse and the
Mature Woman, 2928
Understanding Psychiatric Medications in
the Treatment of Chemical Dependency
and Dual Diagnoses, 2929
When Someone You Care About Abuses
Drugs and Alcohol: When to Act, What to
Say, 196
Why Haven't I Been Able to Help?, 197
Williamson County Council on Alcohol and
Drug Prevention, 2447
Woman's Journal, Special Edition for Use in
the Criminal Justice System, 153
You Can Free Yourself From Alcohol &
Drugs: Work a Program That Keeps You
in Charge, 154
Your Brain on Drugs, 155
Your Drug May Be Your Problem: How and
Why to Stop Taking Pyschiatric
Medications, 2930
www.Ncadi.Samhsa.Gov, 231
www.aca-usa.org, 233
www.addictionresourceguide.com, 234
www.adultchildren.org, 235
www.al-anon.alateen.org, 236
www.alcoholism.about.com/library, 237
www.doitnow.org/pages/pubhub.hmtl, 239
www.jacsweb.org, 240
www.jointogether.org, 241

www.madd.org, 242
www.mentalhealth.samhsa.gov, 244
www.naadac.org, 246
www.nccbh.org, 247
www.niaaa.nih.gov, 248
www.nida.nih.gov, 249
www.nida.nih.gov/drugpages, 250
www.nofas.org, 251
www.sadd.org, 253
www.samhsa.gov, 254
www.smartrecovery.org, 255
www.soulselfhelp.on.ca/coda.html, 256
www.unhooked.com, 257
www.well.com, 258

Anxiety Disorders

Agoraphobics Building Independent Lives,
353
Agoraphobics in Motion, 260
Aleppos Foundation, 1693
An End to Panic: Breakthrough Techniques
for Overcoming Panic Disorder, 279
Anxiety & Phobia Workbook, 280
Anxiety Cure: Eight Step-Program for
Getting Well, 281
Anxiety Disorders Association of America,
261
Anxiety Disorders Fact Sheet, 336
Anxiety Disorders: A Scientific Approach
for Selecting the Most Effective
Treatment, 2931
Anxiety and Its Disorders, 283
Anxiety and Phobia Treatment Center, 262
Anxiety, Phobias, and Panic: a Step-By-Step
Program for Regaining Control of Your
Life, 285
Applied Relaxation Training in the
Treatment of PTSD and Other Anxiety
Disorders, 2932
Assimilation, Rational Thinking, and
Suppression in the Treatment of PTSD and
Other Anxiety Disorder, 2933
Association for Research in Nervous and
Ment al Disease, 2587
Bristol-Myers Squibb, 4633
Client's Manual for the Cognitive Behavioral
Treatment of Anxiety Disorders, 2934
Cognitive Therapy for Delusions, Voices,
and Paranoia, 3079
Cognitive Therapy of Personality Disorders,
3031
Comorbidity of Mood and Anxiety
Disorders, 289
Concise Guide to Anxiety Disorders, 290
Coping with Trauma: A Guide to Self
Understanding, 294
Delusional Beliefs, 3080
Don't Panic: Taking Control of Anxiety
Attacks, 295
Driving Far from Home, 359
Dying of Embarrassment: Help for Social
Anxiety and Social Phobia, 297
Encyclopedia of Phobias, Fears, and
Anxieties, 298
Facts About Anxiety Disorders, 337
Five Smart Steps to Less Stress, 339
Five Weeks to Healing Stress: the Wellness
Option, 299
Flying Without Fear, 300

Free from Fears: New Help for Anxiety, Panic and Agoraphobia, 301

Gender Differences in Mood and Anxiety Disorders: From Bench to Bedside, 2936

Generalized Anxiety Disorder: Diagnosis, Treatment and Its Relationship to Other Anxiety Disorders, 2937

Getting What You Want From Stress, 341

Healing Fear: New Approaches to Overcoming Anxiety, 303

How to Help Your Loved One Recover from Agoraphobia, 304

Impulsivity and Compulsivity, 1139

Institute of Living Anxiety Disorders Center, 1740

Integrative Treatment of Anxiety Disorders, 2938

International Critical Incident Stress Foundation, 267

It's Not All In Your Head: Now Women Can Discover the Real Causes of their Most Misdiagnosed Health, 306

Journal of Anxiety Disorders, 342

Let's Talk Facts About Panic Disorder, 343

Life Is Hard: Audio Guide to Healing Emotional Pain, 3500

Long-Term Treatments of Anxiety Disorders, 2939

Manual of Panic: Focused Psychodynamic Psychotherapy, 3073

Master Your Panic and Take Back Your Life, 308

Master Your Panic and Take Back Your Life: Twelve Treatment Sessions to Overcome High Anxiety, 309

National Anxiety Foundation, 269

No More Butterflies: Overcoming Shyness, Stagefright, Interview Anxiety, and Fear of Public Speaking, 312

One Hundred One Stress Busters, 344

Overcoming Specific Phobia, 3074

Panic Attacks, 345

Panic Disorder: Clinical Diagnosis, Management and Mechanisms, 2941

Panic Disorder: Critical Analysis, 314

Panic Disorder: Theory, Research and Therapy, 2942

Pass-Group, 354

Perturbing the Organism: The Biology of Stressful Experience, 3055

Phobias: Handbook of Theory, Reseach and Treatment, 2943

Phobics Anonymous, 355

Post Traumatic Stress Disorder, 3056

Real Illness: Generalized Anxiety Disorder, 346

Real Illness: Panic Disorder, 347

Real Illness: Social Phobia Disorder, 348

Relaxation & Stress Reduction Workbook, 317, 3613

Selective Mutism Foundation, 274

Shy Children, Phobic Adults: Nature and Trea tment of Social Phobia, 2945

Social Phobia: Clinical and Research Perspectives, 2946

Social Phobia: From Shyness to Stage Fright, 320

Somatization, Physical Symptoms and Psychological Illness, 3075

Stop Obsessing: How to Overcome Your Obsessions and Compulsions, 321

Stress, 349

Stress Management Training: Group Leader's Guide, 3616

Stress Owner's Manual: Meaning, Balance and Health in Your Life, 3617

Stress-Related Disorders Sourcebook, 322

Territorial Apprehensiveness (TERRAP) Programs, 276

Textbook of Anxiety Disorders, 324

Treating Anxiety Disorders, 2947

Treating Anxiety Disorders with a Cognitive, 2948

Treating Panic Disorder and Agoraphobia: A Step by Step Clinical Guide, 2949

Triumph Over Fear: a Book of Help and Hope for People with Anxiety, Panic Attacks, and Phobias, 331

Worry Control Workbook, 334

www.adaa.org, 361

www.aim-hq.org, 362

www.algy.com/anxiety/files/barlow.html, 363

www.apa.org, 364

www.cyberpsych.org, 50, 366, 500, 685, 759, 810, 850, 940, 973, 1073, 1211, 1272, 1320, 1418, 1480, 1522, 3532

www.dstress.com/guided.htm, 367

www.freedomfromfear.org, 369

www.guidetopsychology.com, 371

www.healthanxiety.org, 372

www.healthyminds.org, 373

www.intelihealth.com, 375

www.jobstresshelp.com, 376

www.lexington-on-line.com, 377

www.npadnews.com, 380

www.panicattacks.com.au, 381

www.panicdisorder.about.com, 382

www.selectivemutismfoundation.org, 385

www.selfhelpmagazine.com/articles/stress, 386

www.terraphouston.com, 387

Asperger's Syndrome

Apserger Syndrome Education Network of America (ASPEN), 509

Asperger's Association of New England (AANE), 510

Autism Network International, 511

Autism Treatment Center of America: The Son -Rise Program, 514

Families of Adults Afflicted with Asperger's Syndrome (FAAAS), 515

More Advanced Persons with Autism and Asperger's Syndrome (MAAP), 516

National Institute of Neurological Disorders and Stroke Brain Information Network (BRAIN), 518

National Institute on Deafness and Other Communication Disorders Information Clearinghouse, 519

www.aspergerinfo.com, 532

www.aspergers.com, 533

www.aspergersyndrome.org, 534

www.aspiesforfreedom.com, 535

www.wrongplanet.net, 536

Associations & Organizations

National Alliance on Mental Illness: South Carolina, 2083, 2094

National Alliance on Mental Illness: Alabama, 1805

National Alliance on Mental Illness: Iowa, 1907

National Alliance on Mental Illness: Kentuck y, 1918

National Alliance on Mental Illness: Louisia na, 1925

National Alliance on Mental Illness: Maine, 1928

National Alliance on Mental Illness: Marylan d, 1936

National Alliance on Mental Illness: Massach usetts, 1948

National Alliance on Mental Illness: Michiga n, 1961

National Alliance on Mental Illness: Mississ ippi, 1975

National Alliance on Mental Illness: Missour i, 1981

National Alliance on Mental Illness: Montana, 1985

National Alliance on Mental Illness: Nebrask a, 1988

National Alliance on Mental Illness: Nevada, 1994

National Alliance on Mental Illness: New Ham pshire, 1998

National Alliance on Mental Illness: New Jer sey, 2005

National Alliance on Mental Illness: New Mex ico, 2011

National Alliance on Mental Illness: New Yor k, 2024

National Alliance on Mental Illness: North C arolina, 2038

National Alliance on Mental Illness: North D akota, 2043

National Alliance on Mental Illness: Ohio, 2053

National Alliance on Mental Illness: Oklahom a, 2062

National Alliance on Mental Illness: Oregon, 2067

National Alliance on Mental Illness: Pennsyl vania, 2074

National Alliance on Mental Illness: South D akota, 2101

National Alliance on Mental Illness: Tenness ee, 2104

National Alliance on Mental Illness: Texas, 2117

National Alliance on Mental Illness: Utah, 2128

National Alliance on Mental Illness: Vermont, 2132

National Alliance on Mental Illness: Virgini a, 2141

National Alliance on Mental Illness: Washing ton, 2152

National Alliance on Mental Illness: West Vi rginia, 2166

National Alliance on Mental Illness: Wiscons in, 2171

National Alliance on Mental Illness: Wyoming, 2177

National Association for the Dually Diagnose d (NADD), 270, 989, 1104, 1128, 1167, 1225, 1239, 1286, 1339, 1471, 1537, 1754

Autistic Disorder

Activities for Developing Pre-Skill Concepts in Children with Autism, 562
Adults with Autism, 563
Advocate: Autism Society of America, 3209
Are You Alone on Purpose?, 564
Aspects of Autism: Biological Research, 565
Asperger Syndrome, 566
Asperger Syndrome Education Network (ASPEN), 540
Asperger Syndrome: A Practical Guide for Teachers, 567
Asperger's Association of New England, 541
Asperger's Syndrome: A Guide for Parents and Professionals, 568
Aspergers Syndrome: A Guide for Educators and Parents, Second Edition, 569
Autism, 570
Autism & Asperger Syndrome, 571
Autism & Sensing: The Unlost Instinct, 572
Autism Bibliography, 573
Autism Newslink, 641
Autism Research Foundation, 542
Autism Research Institute, 512, 543
Autism Research Review International, 642
Autism Services Center, 544, 652
Autism Society News, 643
Autism Society of America, 513, 545, 653
Autism Spectrum, 574
Autism Spectrum Disorders: The Complete Guid to Understanding Autism, Asperger's Syndrome, Pervasiv, 575
Autism Treatment Center of America Son-Rise Program, 654
Autism Treatment Guide, 576
Autism and Pervasive Developmental Disorders, 577
Autism in Children and Adolescents, 644
Autism: A Strange, Silent World, 660
Autism: A World Apart, 661
Autism: An Inside-Out Approach An Innovative Look at the Mechanics of Autism and its Developmental, 578
Autism: An Introduction to Psychological Theory, 579
Autism: Being Friends, 662
Autism: Explaining the Enigma, 580
Autism: From Tragedy to Triumph, 581
Autism: Identification, Education and Treatment, 582
Autism: Nature, Diagnosis and Treatment, 583
Autism: Strategies for Change, 584
Autistic Adults at Bittersweet Farms, 585
Avoiding Unfortunate Situations, 586
Beyond Gentle Teaching, 587
Biology of the Autistic Syndromes, 588
A Book: A Collection of Writings from the Advocate, 561
Breakthroughs: How to Reach Students with Autism, 664
Children with Autism: A Developmental Perspective, 589
Children with Autism: Parents' Guide, 590
Communication Unbound: How Facilitated Communication Is Challenging Views, 591
Community Services for Autistic Adults and Children, 549
Diagnosis and Treatment of Autism, 592
Edgewood Children's Center, 3937

Facilitated Communication and Technology Guide, 593
Facilitated Learning at Syracuse University, 650
Facts About Autism, 645
Families for Early Autism Treatment, 550
Fighting for Darla: Challenges for Family Care & Professional Responsibility, 594
Fragile Success - Ten Autistic Children, Childhood to Adulthood, 595
Getting Started with Facilitated Communication, 596
Going to School with Facilitated Communication, 666
Handbook for the Study of Mental Health, 3602
Handbook of Autism and Pervasive Developmental Disorders, 597
Health Care Desensitization, 667
Helping People with Autism Manage Their Behavior, 598
Hidden Child: The Linwood Method for Reaching the Autistic Child, 599
How to Teach Autistic & Severely Handicapped Children, 600
I'm Not Autistic on the Typewriter, 601, 668
Inner Life of Children with Special Needs, 602
Joey and Sam, 603
Journal of Autism and Developmental Disorders, 646
Keys to Parenting the Child with Autism, 604
Kristy and the Secret of Susan, 605
Learning and Cognition in Autism, 606
Let Community Employment Be the Goal For Individuals with Autism, 607
Let Me Hear Your Voice, 608
Letting Go, 609
MAAP, 647
Management of Autistic Behavior, 610
Mental Health Resources Catalog, 2796
Mindblindness: An Essay on Autism and Theory of Mind, 611
Mixed Blessings, 612
More Advanced Autistic People Services (MAAPS), 551
More Laughing and Loving with Autism, 613
Neurobiology of Autism 2nd Edition, 614
New England Center for Children, 556
News from the Border: a Mother's Memoir of Her Autistic Son, 615
Nobody Nowhere, 616
1001 Great Ideas for Teaching or Raising Chi ldren with Autism Spectrum Disorders, 560
Parent Survival Manual, 617
Parent's Guide to Autism, 618
Please Don't Say Hello, 619
Preschool Issues in Autism, 620
Psychoeducational Profile, 621
Reaching the Autistic Child: a Parent Training Program, 622
Record Books for Individuals with Autism, 623
Russell Is Extra Special, 624
Samhsa's National Mental Health Information Center, 558
Schools for Children With Autism Spectrum Disorders, 625
Sense of Belonging: Including Students with Autism in Their School Community, 672
Sex Education: Issues for the Person with Autism, 626, 648

Siblings of Children with Autism: A Guide for Families, 627
Somebody Somewhere, 628
Son-Rise Program at the Option Institute Autism Treatment Center of America, 559
Soon Will Come the Light, 629
Straight Talk About Autism with Parents and Kids, 673
TEACCH, 651
Teaching Children with Autism: Strategies to Enhance Communication, 630
Teaching and Mainstreaming Autistic Children, 631
Then Things Every Child with Autism Wishes Y ou Knew, 633
Thinking In Pictures, Expanded Edition: My L Life with Autism, 634
Ultimate Stranger: The Autistic Child, 635
Understanding Autism, 636
Until Tomorrow: A Family Lives with Autism, 637
When Snow Turns to Rain, 638
Winter's Flower, 639
Without Reason, 640
www.aane.org, 674
www.ani.ac, 675
www.aspennj.org, 676
www.autism-society.org, 677
www.autism.org, 678
www.autismresearchinstitute.org, 679
www.autismservicescenter.org, 680
www.autismspeaks.org, 681
www.autisticservices.com, 682
www.csaac.org, 684
www.feat.org, 686
www.iidc.indiana.edu, 687
www.ladders.org, 688
www.maapservices.org, 689
www.necc.org, 693
www.resourcesnyc.org, 695
www.son-rise.org, 696

Bipolar Disorders

Bipolar Clinic and Research Program, 746
Bipolar Disorders Clinic, 747
Bipolar Disorders Treatment Information Center, 704
Bipolar Disorders: A Guide to Helping Children and Adolescents, 720
Bipolar Disorders: Clinical Course and Outcome, 721
Bipolar Puzzle Solution, 722
Bipolar Research at University of Pennsylvan ia, 748
Child and Adolescent Bipolar Disorder: An Update from the National Institute of Mental Health, 735
Concise Guide to Mood Disorders, 2720
Epidemiology-Genetics Program in Psychiatry, 749
Guildeline for Treatment of Patients with Bipolar Disorder, 726
Lithium Information Center, 709
Management of Bipolar Disorder: Pocketbook, 729
Mood Disorders, 743
Novartis, 4647
UT Southwestern Medical Center, 750
Yale Mood Disorders Research Program, 751
www.bpso.org, 756, 3524

www.bpso.org/nomania.htm, 757, 3525
www.cfsny.org, 46, 238, 365, 499, 683, 758
www.dbsalliance.org, 760
www.goodwill-suncoast.org, 370, 762
www.manicdepressive.org, 763
www.med.yale.edu, 764
www.mentalhealth.Samhsa.Gov, 378, 690,
  765
www.mentalhealth.com/p20-grp.html, 3556
www.mhselfhelp.org, 60, 245, 691, 766
www.miminc.org, 767
www.moodswing.org/bdfaq.html, 768, 3563
www.nami.org, 379, 501, 692, 769
www.thenadd.org, 388, 507, 697, 772
www.utsouthwestern.edu, 773

Clinical Management

ACS Healthcare Solutions, 4353
ADL Data Systems, 4534
AHMAC, 4354
AIMS, 4355
AMCO Computers, 4356
Accumedic Computer Systems, 4359, 4535
Adam Software, 4360
Advanced Data Systems, 4361
Agilent Technologies, 4362
American Institute for Preventive Medicine,
  4536
American Medical Software, 4363
American Nurses Foundation: National
  Communications, 4537
American Psychiatric Press Reference
  Library CD-ROM, 4364
Anasazi Software, 4365
Andrew and Associates, 4366
Apache Medical Systems, 4538
Applied Computing Services, 4539
Applied Informatics (ILIAD), 4540
Arbour Health System-Human Resource
  Institute Hospital, 4541
Aries Systems Corporation, 4367
Arservices, Limited, 4542
Ascent, 4368
Askesis Development Group, 4369
Assist Technologies, 4370
Association for Ambulatory Behavioral
  Healthcare, 4544
Austin Travis County Mental Health Mental
  Retardation Center, 4371
Aware Resources, 4372
BOSS Inc, 4373
Beaver Creek Software, 4374
Behavioral Health Advisor, 4375
Behavioral Intervention Planning:
  Completing a Functional Behavioral
  Assessment and Developing a Beh, 4545
Behaviordata, 4376
Bellefaire Jewish Children's Bureau, 4377
BetaData Systems, 4378
Body Logic, 4379
Breining Institute College for the Advanced
  Study of Addictive Disorders, 3355, 4546
Brief Therapy Institute of Denver, 4547
Buckley Productions, 4548
Bull HN Information Systems, 4380
Business Objects, 4381
CASCAP, 4382
CBI Group, 4549
CLARC Services, 4383
CMHC Systems, 4550

CSI Software, 4384
Cardiff Software: Vista, 4385
CareCounsel, 4552
Catholic Community Services of Western
  Washington, 4553
Center for Clinical Computing, 4386
Center for Creative Living, 4554
Center for Health Policy Studies, 3359, 4387
Central Washington Comprehensive M/H,
  4555
Ceridian Corporation, 4388
Chartman Software, 4389
Child Welfare Information Gateway, 4556
Cincom Systems, 4390
Cirrus Technology, 4558
Client Management Information System,
  4391
CliniSphere version 2.0, 4392
Clinical Nutrition Center, 4393
Community Psychiatric Clinic, 4559
Community Solutions, 4561
Compu-Care Management and Systems, 4394
CompuLab Healthcare Systems Corporation,
  4395
Computer Transition Services, 4396
Consumer Health Information Corporation,
  4565
Control-0-Fax Corporation, 4397
Control-O-Fax Corporation, 4566
Cornucopia Software, 4399
Creative Socio-Medics Corporation, 4401
DB Consultants, 4402
DCC/The Dependent Care Connection, 4567
DST Output, 4403
DataMark, 4404
Dean Foundation for Health, Research and
  Education, 4568
Distance Learning Network, 3371, 4406,
  4569
Docu Trac, 4407
DocuMed, 4408
Dorland Healthcare Information, 4570
E Services Group, 4409
EAP Technology Systems, 4410
Echo Group, 4411
Eclipsys Corporation, 4412
Electronic Healthcare Systems, 4413
Emedeon Practice Services, 4414
Entre Technology Services, 4415
Experior Corporation, 4416
FOCUS: Family Oriented Counseling
  Services, 4572
Facts Services, 4417
Family Services of Delaware County, 4418
Federation of Families for Children's
  Mental Health, 1579, 1733, 4573
First Data Bank, 4419
Gelbart and Associates, 4420
GenSource Corporation, 4421
Genelco Software Solutions, 4422
HMS Healthcare Management Systems, 4424
HSA-Mental Health, 4426, 4574
HZI Research Center, 4427
Habilitation Software, 4428
Hagar and Associates, 4575
Hanover Insurance, 4429
Health Probe, 4430
HealthLine Systems, 4431
HealthSoft, 4432
Healthcare Management Systems, 4577
Healthcare Vision, 4433
Healthcheck, 4578
Healthline Systems, 4434

Healthport, 4435
Hogan Assessment Systems, 4436
Human Resources Consulting Group, 4579
IBM Global Healthcare Industry, 4437
IDX Systems Corporation, 4438
IMNET Systems, 4439
INMED/MotherNet America, 4580
InfoMC, 4440
Information Access Technology, 4582
Information Management Solutions, 4441
Informedics, 4583
Informix Software, 4442
Inforum, 4443
Inhealth Record Systems, 4444
Innovative Data Solutions, 4445
Innovative Health Systems/SoftMed, 4446
Integrated Business Services, 4447
Keane Care, 4450
Lad Lake, 4584
Lanstat Resources, 4585
Lexical Technologies, 4452
Liberty Healthcare Management Group, 4586
Lifelink Corporation/Bensenville Home
  Society, 4587
M/MGMT Systems, 4453
MEDCOM Information Systems, 4454
MEDecision, 4455
Managed Care Local Market Overviews,
  4589
Manisses Communication Group, 4590
Mayo HealthQuest/Mayo Clinic Health
  Information, 4591
McHenry County M/H Board, 4456
McKesson HBOC, 4457
Med Data Systems, 4458
MedPLus, 4459
Medai, 4460
Medcomp Software, 4461
Medi-Span, 4462
Medical Data Research, 4592
Medical Records Institute, 4463
Medical Records Solution, 4464
Medipay, 4465, 4594
Medix Systems Consultants, 4466
Medware, 4467
Mental Health Connections, 4468
Mental Health Outcomes, 4469
Meridian Resource Corporation, 4595
Meritcare Health System, 4470
Micro Design International, 4471
Micro Office Systems, 4472
Micromedex, 4473
Microsoft Corporation, 4596
Misys Health Care Systems, 4474
MphasiS(BPO), 4475
NASW West Virginia Chapter, 4598
National Child Support Network, 1583, 4599
National Council on Alcoholism and Drug
  Dependence, 95, 2348, 4600
National Families in Action, 4477, 4601
National Medical Health Card Systems, 4478
National Mental Health Self-Help
  Clearinghouse, 4602
NetMeeting, 4479
Netsmart Technologies, 4480
Nightingale Vantagemed Corporation, 4481
North Bay Center for Behavioral Medicine,
  4603
Northwest Analytical, 4482
OPTAIO-Optimizing Practice Through
  Assessment, Intervention and Outcome,
  4483
Occupational Health Software, 4484

On-Line Information Services, 4604
Open Minds, 4605
Optio Software, 4485
Optum, 4606
Oracle Corporation, 4486
Orion Healthcare Technology, 4487
Our Town Family Center, 4607
Ovid Online, 4608
P and W Software, 4488
Parrot Software, 4490
Patient Medical Records, 4609
Penelope Price, 3417, 4610
Perot Systems, 4492
Physicians' ONLINE, 4611
Piedmont Community Services, 4612
Point of Care Technologies, 4613
Preferred Medical Informatics, 4614
Primary Care Medicine on CD, 4493
Psychological Assessment Resources, 4494
Psychological Software Services, 4495
Psychometric Software, 4496
QuadraMed Corporation, 3431, 4497
Quadramed, 4616
RCF Information Systems, 4498
Raintree Systems, 4499
Right On Programs/PRN Medical Software,
    4500
SHS Computer Service, 4501
SPSS, 4502
Saner Software, 4503
Scinet, 4504
Servisource, 4618
SilverPlatter Information, 4619
Sls Residential, 4507
Star Systems Corporation, 4508
Stephens Systems Services, 4509
Strategic Advantage, 4510
Stress Management Research Associates,
    4620
SumTime Software®, 4511
Sun Microsystems, 4512
SunGard Pentamation, 4513
Supervised Lifestyles, 4621
Synergistic Office Solutions (SOS Software),
    4515
Technical Support Systems, 4622
Telepad Corporation, 4623
Tempus Software, 4516
Thomson ResearchSoft, 4517
3m Health Information Systems, 4533
Traumatic Incident Reduction Association,
    4624
TriZetto Group, 4518
Turbo-Doc EMR, 4519
UNI/CARE Systems, 4520
UNISYS Corporation, 4625
Universal Behavioral Service, 4521, 4626
Vann Data Services, 4522
Velocity Healthcare Informatics, 4523
VersaForm Systems Corporation, 4524
Virginia Beach Community Service Board,
    4627
Virtual Software Systems, 4525
Well Mind Association, 4628
Woodlands, 4528
WordPerfect Corporation, 4629
Zy-Doc Technologies, 4532

Cognitive Disorders

Agitation in Patients with Dementia: a
    Practical Guide to Diagnosis and
    Management, 788
Alzheimer's Association National Office, 775
Alzheimer's Disease Education and Referral
    Center, 776
Alzheimer's Disease Research and the
    American Health Assistance Foundation,
    799
Alzheimer's Disease Sourcebook, 789
Alzheimer's Disease: Activity-Focused Care,
    Second Edition, 790
American Health Assistance Foundation, 777
American Psychiatric Association Practice
    Guideline for the Treatment of Patients
    with Delirium, 110, 791
Behavioral Complications in Alzheimer's
    Disease, 792
Care That Works: A Relationship Approach
    to Persons With Dementia, 793
Cognitive Behavioral Assessment, 3491
Cognitive Therapy, 2935
Cognitive Therapy in Practice, 2713
Covert Modeling & Covert Reinforcement,
    752
Dementia: A Clinical Approach, 794
Developing Mind: Toward a Neurobiology
    of Interpersonal Experience, 2735
Disorders of Brain and Mind: Volume 1, 795
Educating Clients about the Cognitive
    Model, 3493
Guidelines for the Treatment of Patients
    with Alzheimer's Disease and Other
    Dementias of Late Life, 1378, 2967
Living Skills Recovery Workbook, 3611
Loss of Self: Family Resource for the Care
    of Alzheimer's Disease and Related
    Disorders, 2968
National Association Councils on
    Developmental Disabilities, 780
National Family Caregivers Association, 782
National Institute of Neurological Disorders
    and Stroke, 783
National Niemann-Pick Disease Foundation,
    786
Neurobiology of Primary Dementia, 2969
Practical Guide to Cognitive Therapy, 2818
Progress in Alzheimer's Disease and Similar
    Conditions, 797
Victims of Dementia: Service, Support, and
    Care, 798
Virginia Federation of Families for
    Children's Mental Health, 2146
www.Nia.Nih.Gov/Alzheimers, 801
www.aan.com, 802, 3511
www.agelessdesign.com, 803
www.ahaf.org/alzdis/about/adabout.htm, 804
www.alz.co.uk, 805
www.alzforum.org, 806
www.alzheimersbooks.com/, 807
www.alzheimersupport.Com, 808
www.biostat.wustl.edu, 809
www.elderlyplace.com, 811
www.habitsmart.com/cogtitle.html, 812
www.mayohealth.org/mayo/common/htm/,
    813
www.mentalhealth.smahsa.gov, 815
www.mindstreet.com/training.html, 816
www.ninds.nih.gov, 817
www.noah-health.org/en/bns/disorders/
    alzheimer.html, 818
www.ohioalzcenter.org/facts.html, 819
www.psych.org/clin_res/pg_dementia.cfm,
    821
www.rcpsych.ac.uk/info/help/memory, 823
www.zarcrom.com/users/alzheimers, 824
www.zarcrom.com/users/yeartorem, 825

Conduct Disorder

Active Parenting Now, 847
Antisocial Behavior by Young People, 834
Association for Behavioral and Cognitive
    Therapies, 827
Bad Men Do What Good Men Dream: a
    Forensic Psychiatrist Illuminates the
    Darker Side of Human Behavi, 835
Behavior Rating Profile, 3099
Child & Family Center, 846
Cognitive Therapy for Depression and
    Anxiety, 288
Conduct Disorders in Childhood and
    Adolescence, Developmental Clinical
    Psychology and Psychiatry, 836
Creative Therapy 2: Working with Parents,
    837
Defiant Teens, 3119
Difficult Child, 838
Inclusion Strategies for Students with
    Learning and Behavior Problems, 2976
Neurobiology of Violence, 2802
Outrageous Behavior Mood: Handbook of
    Strategic Interventions for Managing
    Impossible Students, 2977
Preventing Antisocial Behavior Interventions
    from Birth through Adolescence, 841
Skills Training for Children with Behavior
    Disorders, 842
Society of Behavioral Medicine, 2676
Treatment of Children with Mental
    Disorders, 34, 476, 649, 845
Treatment of Suicidal Patients in Managed
    Care, 3092
Understanding & Managing the Defiant
    Child, 848
www.members.aol.com/AngriesOut, 1157
www.mentalhelp.net/psyhelp/chap7, 1159

Depression

Active Treatment of Depression, 2979
Against Depression, 871
Akzo Nobel, 4631
Antidepressant Fact Book: What Your
    Doctor Won't Tell You About Prozac,
    Zoloft, Paxil, Celexa and Lu, 2980
Antipsychotic Medications: A Guide, 2981
Anxiety and Depression in Adults and
    Children, Banff International Behavioral
    Science Series, 872
Attention-Deficit Hyperactivity Disorder in
    Adults: A Guide, 425
Bipolar Disorder, 734
Breaking the Patterns of Depression, 873
Brief Therapy for Adolescent Depression,
    2982
Broken Connection: On Death and the
    Continuity of Life, 874

Carbamazepine and Manic Depression: A Guide, 723
Clinical Guide to Depression in Children and Adolescents, 875
The Cognitive Behavorial Workbook for Depression: A Step-by-Step Program, 904
Cognitive Therapy of Depression, 2983
Coping With Unexpected Events: Depression & Trauma, 736
Coping with Depression, 930
Day for Night: Recognizing Teenage Depression, 931
Depressed Anonymous, 927
Depression, 911
Depression & Antidepressants, 2985
Depression & Anxiety Management, 876
Depression & Bi-Polar Support Alliance, 855
Depression & BiPolar Support Alliance, 708
Depression & Related Affective Disorders Association (DRADA), 856
Depression After Delivery, 857
Depression Workbook: a Guide for Living with Depression, 877
Depression and Bi-Polar Alliance, 858
Depression and Its Treatment, 878
Depression and Manic Depression, 932
Depression in Children and Adolescents: A Fact Sheet for Physicians, 912
Depression in Context: Strategies for Guided Action, 2986
Depression, the Mood Disease, 879
Depression: Help On the Way, 913
Depression: What Every Woman Should Know, 914
Depressive and Manic-Depressive Association of St. Louis, 1976
Diagnosis and Treatment of Depression in Lat e Life: Results of the NIH Consensus Development Confer, 880
Divalproex and Bipolar Disorder: A Guide, 725
Eating Disorders: Facts About Eating Disorders and the Search for Solutions, 1052
Electroconvulsive Therapy: A Guide, 2741
Eli Lilly and Company, 4636
Emotions Anonymous International Service Center, 859
Encyclopedia of Depression, 882
Evaluation and Treatment of Postpartum Emotional Disorders, 2987
Forest Laboratories, 4638
Freedom From Fear, 266, 860
Gender Differences in Depression: Marital Therapy Approach, 3494
Growing Up Sad: Childhood Depression and Its Treatment, 883
Handbook of Depression, 2988
Help Me, I'm Sad: Recognizing, Treating, and Preventing Childhood and Adolescent Depression, 884
Helping Your Depressed Teenager: a Guide for Parents and Caregivers, 885
Let's Talk About Depression, 915
Lithium and Manic Depression: A Guide, 727
Living Without Depression & Manic Depression: a Workbook for Maintaining Mood Stability, 728
Living with Depression and Manic Depression, 933
Lonely, Sad, and Angry: a Parent's Guide to Depression in Children and Adolescents, 886

Management of Depression, 887
Mania: Clinical and Research Perspectives, 730
Mayo Clinic on Depression, 889
Medications, 3272
Men and Depression, 917
Mood Apart, 890
Mood Apart: Thinker's Guide to Emotion & It's Disorders, 891
New Message, 918
New York City Depressive & Manic Depressive Group, 2028
Organon Schering Plough, 4648
Overcoming Depression, 893
Oxcarbazepine and Bipolar Disorder: A Guide, 731
Pain Behind the Mask: Overcoming Masculine Depression, 894
Panic Disorder and Agoraphobia: A Guide, 313
Pastoral Care of Depression, 895
Physicians Living with Depression, 3506
Post-Natal Depression: Psychology, Science and the Transition to Motherhood, 896
Postpartum Mood Disorders, 897, 2990
Postpartum Support International, 868
Practice Guideline for Major Depressive Disorders in Adults, 898
Predictors of Treatment Response in Mood Disorders, 899
Premenstrual Dysphoric Disorder: A Guide, 2991
Prozac Nation: Young & Depressed in America, a Memoir, 900
Questions & Answers About Depression & Its Treatment, 901
Recovering Your Mental Health: a Self-Help Guide, 919
Scientific Foundations of Cognitive Theory and Therapy of Depression, 2992
Seasonal Affective Disorder and Beyond: Light Treatment for SAD and Non-SAD Conditions, 902
Sid W Richardson Institute for Preventive Medicine of the Methodist Hospital, 924
Social Anxiety Disorder: A Guide, 319
Stories of Depression: Does this Sound Like You?, 903
Storm In My Brain, 920
Symptoms of Depression, 2993
Testing Automatic Thoughts with Thought Records, 3509
Treating Depression, 2995
Treatment Plans and Interventions for Depression and Anxiety Disorders, 329, 905
Treatment for Chronic Depression: Cognitive Behavioral Analysis System of Psychotherapy (CBASP), 906
Treatment of Recurrent Depression, 2996
Trichotillomania: A Guide, 330
University of Texas: Mental Health Clinical Research Center, 925
What Do These Students Have in Common?, 921
What to do When a Friend is Depressed: Guide for Students, 922
When Nothing Matters Anymore: A Survival Guide for Depressed Teens, 907
Why Isn't My Child Happy? Video Guide About Childhood Depression, 934
Winter Blues, 908

A Woman Doctor's Guide to Depression, 2978
Women and Depression, 935
Yale University: Depression Research Program, 926
Yesterday's Tomorrow, 909
You Can Beat Depression: Guide to Prevention and Recovery, 910
www.Depressedteens.Com, 936
www.Ifred.Org, 937
www.befrienders.org, 938
www.blarg.net/~charlatn/voices, 939, 3523
www.geocities.com, 3534
www.klis.com/chandler/pamphlet/dep/, 942
www.med.jhu.edu/drada/creativity.html, 3549
www.mentalhealth.com/story, 3557
www.ndmda.org/justmood.htm, 3566
www.nimh.nih.gov/publicat/depressionmenu.c fm, 943
www.nimh.nih.gov/publist/964033.htm, 944
www.psychologyinfo.com/depression, 947
www.psycom.net/depression.central.html, 948, 3580
www.queendom.com/selfhelp/depression/ depression.html, 949
www.shpm.com, 950
www.shpm.com/articles/depress, 3588
www.wingofmadness.com, 951, 3594

Dissociative Disorders

Amongst Ourselves: A Self-Help Guide to Living with Dissociative Identity Disorder, 960
Dissociation, 961
Dissociation and the Dissociative Disorders: DSM-V and Beyond, 962
Dissociative Child: Diagnosis, Treatment and Management, 963
Dissociative Identity Disorder: Diagnosis, Clinical Features, and Treatment of Multiple Personality, 2997
Eisai, 4635
First Horizon Pharmaceutical, 4637
Got Parts? An Insider's Guide to Managing Li fe Successfully with Dissociative Identity Disorder (Ne, 965
Handbook for the Assessment of Dissociation: a Clinical Guide, 966
Handbook of Dissociation: Theoretical, Empirical, and Clinical Perspectives, 2998
International Society for the Study of Dissociation, 954
Rebuilding Shattered Lives: Responsible Treatment of Complex Post-Traumatic and Dissociative Disorde, 968, 1306, 3059
Standing in the Spaces: Essays on Clinical Process, Trauma, and Dissociation, 3061
Treatment of Multiple Personality Disorder, 969
Understanding Dissociative Disorders and Addiction, 195, 970
Understanding Dissociative Disorders: A Guid e for Family Physicians and Healthcare Workers, 971
www.fmsf.com, 974
www.isst-D.Org, 975

Eating Disorders

American Anorexia/Bulimia Association, 980
American Anorexia/Bulimia Association News, 1045
Anorexia Bulimia Treatment and Education Center, 981
Anorexia Nervosa & Recovery: a Hunger for Meaning, 1000
Anorexia Nervosa and Related Eating Disorders, 982
Anorexia: Am I at Risk?, 1046
Assessment of Eating Disorders, 1001
Beyond Anorexia, 1002
Binge Eating: Nature, Assessment and Treatment, 1003
Body Image, 1047
Body Image Workbook: An 8 Step Program for Learning to Like Your Looks, 1004
Body Image, Eating Disorders, and Obesity in Youth, 1005
Brief Therapy and Eating Disorders, 1006
Bulimia, 1007, 1048
Bulimia Nervosa, 1008
Bulimia Nervosa & Binge Eating: A Guide To Recovery, 1009
Bulimia: a Guide to Recovery, 1010
Center for the Study of Adolescence, 1059
Center for the Study of Anorexia and Bulimia, 1060
Change for Good Coaching and Counseling, 984
Clinical Handbook of Eating Disorders: An In tegrated Approach (Medical Psychiatry, 26), 1011
Controlling Eating Disorders with Facts, Advice and Resources, 1012
Conversations with Anorexics: A Compassionate & Hopeful Journey, 1013
Coping with Eating Disorders, 1014
Council on Size and Weight Discrimination (CSWD), 985
Cult of Thinness, 1015
Developmental Psychopathology of Eating Disorders: Implications for Research, Prevention and Treatme, 1016
Eating Disorder Council of Long Island, 2017
Eating Disorder Sourcebook, 1049
Eating Disorder Video, 1068
Eating Disorders, 1050
Eating Disorders & Obesity: a Comprehensive Handbook, 1017
Eating Disorders Association of New Jersey, 2002
Eating Disorders Factsheet, 1051
Eating Disorders Research and Treatment Program, 1061
Eating Disorders Sourcebook, 1018
Eating Disorders and Obesity, Second Edition : A Comprehensive Handbook, 1019
Eating Disorders: Reference Sourcebook, 1020
Eating Disorders: When Food Hurts, 1069
Eating Disorders: When Food Turns Against You, 1021
Emotional Eating: A Practical Guide to Taking Control, 1022
Encyclopedia of Obesity and Eating Disorders, 1023
Etiology and Treatment of Bulimia Nervosa, 1024

Fats of Life, 1053
Feminist Perspectives on Eating Disorders, 1025
Food Addicts Anonymous, 1064
Food and Feelings, 1054
Food for Recovery: The Next Step, 1026
Getting What You Want from Your Body Image, 1055
Golden Cage, The Enigma of Anorexia Nervosa, 1027
Group Psychotherapy for Eating Disorders, 1028
Group Work for Eating Disorders and Food Issues, 3495
Handbook of Treatment for Eating Disorders, 3001
Helping Athletes with Eating Disorders, 1029
Hunger So Wide and Deep, 1030
Hungry Self; Women, Eating and Identity, 1031
Insights in the Dynamic Psychotherapy of Anorexia and Bulimia, 1032
International Association of Eating Disorders Professionals, 986
Interpersonal Psychotherapy, 2989, 3002
Largesse, The Network for Size Esteem, 987
Lifetime Weight Control, 1033
MEDA, 1065
Making Peace with Food, 1034
Metro Intergroup of Overeaters Anonymous, 2023
National Association of Anorexia Nervosa and Associated Disorders (ANAD), 990
National Association to Advance Fat Acceptance (NAAFA), 991
National Center for Overcoming Overeating, 1066
National Eating Disorders Association, 992
New Jersey Support Groups, 2010
O-Anon General Service Office (OGSO), 996
Obesity Research Center, 1062
Obesity: Theory and Therapy, 1035
Overeaters Anonymous, 1036, 1067
Pennsylvania Chapter of the American Anorexia Bulimia Association, 2077
Psychobiology and Treatment of Anorexia Nervosa and Bulimia Nervosa, 1037
Psychodynamic Technique in the Treatment of the Eating Disorders, 1038
Psychosomatic Families: Anorexia Nervosa in Context, 1039
Restrictive Eating, 1056
Richmond Support Group, 2143
Self-Starvation, 1040
Sexual Abuse and Eating Disorders, 3003
Starving to Death in a Sea of Objects, 1041
Surviving an Eating Disorder: Perspectives and Strategies, 1042
TOPS Club, 998
Teen Image, 1057
Treating Eating Disorders, 1043
University of Pennsylvania Weight and Eating Disorders Program, 1063
We Insist on Natural Shapes, 999
Westchester Task Force on Eating Disorders, 2035
When Food Is Love, 1044
Working Together, 1058
www.alt.support.eating.disord, 1070
www.anred.com, 1071
www.closetoyou.org/eatingdisorders, 1072
www.edap.org, 1074
www.gurze.com, 1075

www.healthyplace.com/Communities/, 1076
www.kidsource.com/nedo/, 1077
www.mentalhelp.net, 1078
www.mirror-mirror.org/eatdis.htm, 1079, 3562
www.something-fishy.com, 1082

Factitious Disorder

Disorders of Simulation: Malingering, Factit ious Disorders, and Compensation Neurosis, 1090
Munchausen by Proxy: Identification, Interve ntion, and Case Management, 1092
National Association for the Dually Diagnosed (NADD), 11, 33, 397, 553, 712, 781, 830, 864, 955, 1086
Playing Sick?: Untangling the Web of Munchau sen Syndrome, Munchausen by Proxy, Malingering, and Fac, 1095

Gender Identity Disorder

Gender Identity Disorder: A Medical Dictiona ry, Bibliography, and Annotated Research Guide to Inter, 1111
Gender Loving Care, 3007
Handbook of Sexual and Gender Identity Disor der, 1112
Identity Without Selfhood, 1113
National Gay and Lesbian Task Force, 1105
National Institute of Mental Health, 517, 865, 993, 1106
Parents, Families and Friends of Lesbians and Gays, 1109
Psychoanalytic Therapy & the Gay Man, 3011
Transvestites and Transsexuals: Toward a Theory of Cross-Gender Behavior, 3012
www.kidspeace.org, 1118

Government Agencies

Administration on Aging, 2182
Administration on Developmental Disabilities US Department of Health & Human Services, 2183
Agency for Healthcare Research and Quality: Office of Communications and Knowledge Transfer, 2184
Alabama Department of Human Resources, 2231
Alabama Department of Mental Health and Mental Retardation, 2232
Alabama Department of Public Health, 2233
Alabama Disabilities Advocacy Program, 2234
Alaska Council on Emergency Medical Services, 2235
Alaska Department of Health & Social Services, 2236
Alaska Division of Mental Health and Developmental Disabilities, 2237
Alaska Health and Social Services Division of Behavioral Health, 2238

Alaska Mental Health Board, 2239
Alcohol and Drug Council of Middle Tennessee, 2437
Arizona Department of Health Services, 2241
Arizona Department of Health Services: Behavioral Services, 2242
Arizona Department of Health Services: Child Fatality Review, 2243
Arizona Department of Health: Substance Abuse, 2244
Arkansas Department Health & Human Services, 2246
Arkansas Division of Children & Family Service, 2247
Arkansas Division on Youth Services, 2248
Arkansas State Mental Hospital, 2249
Association of Maternal and Child Health Programs (AMCHP), 2185
Austin Travis County Mental Health: Mental Retardation Center, 2448
Bureau of Mental Health and Substance Abuse Services, 2476
Bureau of TennCare: State of Tennessee, 2438
California Department of Alcohol and Drug Programs, 2228
California Department of Alcohol and Drug Programs: Resource Center, 2251
California Department of Corrections and Reh abilitation, 2252
California Department of Education: Healthy Kids, Healthy California, 2253
California Department of Health Services: Medicaid, 2254
California Department of Health Services: Medi-Cal Drug Discount, 2255
California Department of Health and Human Services, 2274
California Department of Mental Health, 2256
California Hispanic Commission on Alcohol Drug Abuse, 2257
California Institute for Mental Health, 2258
California Mental Health Directors Association, 2259
California Women's Commission on Addictions, 2260
Center for Mental Health Services Homeless Programs Branch, 2186
Center for Substance Abuse Treatment, 2187
Centers for Disease Control & Prevention, 2188
Centers for Medicare & Medicaid Services/CMS: Office of Research, Statisctics, Data and Systems, 2330
Centers for Medicare & Medicaid Services, 2331
Centers for Medicare & Medicaid Services: Office of Policy, 2189, 2332
Centers for Medicare and Medicaid Services: Office of Financial Management/OFM, 2333
Chattanooga/Plateau Council for Alcohol and Drug Abuse, 2439
Colorado Department of Health Care Policy and Financing, 2261
Colorado Department of Human Services (CDHS), 2262
Colorado Department of Human Services: Alcohol and Drug Abuse Division, 2263
Colorado Division of Mental Health, 2264
Colorado Medical Assistance Program Information Center, 2265

Colorado Traumatic Brain Injury Trust Fund Program, 2266
Comcare of Sedgwick County, 2315
Connecticut Department of Mental Health and Addiction Services, 2269
Connecticut Department of Children and Families, 2270
DC Commission on Mental Health Services, 2275
DC Department of Human Services, 2276
DC Department of Mental Health, 2191
Dane County Mental Health Center, 2477
Delaware Department of Health & Social Services, 2271
Delaware Division of Child Mental Health Services, 2272
Delaware Division of Family Services, 2273
Denver County Department of Social Services, 2267
Department of Health and Family Services: Southern Region, 2478
Department of Health and Welfare: Medicaid Division, 2288
Department of Health and Welfare: Community Rehab, 2289
Department of Human Services: Chemical Health Division, 2349
Division of Health Care Policy, 2316
El Paso County Human Services, 2268
Equal Employment Opportunity Commission, 2192
Florida Department Health and Human Services: Substance Abuse Program, 2278
Florida Department of Children and Families, 2279
Florida Department of Health and Human Services, 2280
Florida Department of Mental Health and Rehabilitative Services, 2281
Florida Medicaid State Plan, 2282
Georgia Department of Human Resources, 2283
Georgia Department of Human Resources: Division of Public Health, 2284
Georgia Division of Mental Health Developmental Disabilities and Addictive Diseases (MHDDAD), 2285
Harris County Mental Health: Mental Retardation Authority, 2449
Hawaii Department of Adult Mental Health, 2286
Hawaii Department of Health, 2287
Health & Medicine Counsel of Washington DDNC Digestive Disease National Coalition, 2277
Health Care For All(HCFA), 2193
Health Systems and Financing Group, 2194
Health and Human Services Office of Assistant Secretary for Planning & Evaluation, 2195
Idaho Bureau of Maternal and Child Health, 2290
Idaho Bureau of Mental Health and Substance Abuse, Division of Family & Community Service, 2291
Idaho Department of Health & Welfare, 2292
Idaho Department of Health and Welfare: Family and Child Services, 2293
Idaho Mental Health Center, 2294
Illinois Alcoholism and Drug Dependency Association, 1893, 2295
Illinois Department of Alcoholism and Substance Abuse, 2296

Illinois Department of Children and Family Services, 2297
Illinois Department of Health and Human Services, 2298
Illinois Department of Human Services: Office of Mental Health, 2299
Illinois Department of Mental Health and Drug Dependence, 2300
Illinois Department of Mental Health and Developmental Disabilities, 2301
Illinois Department of Public Aid, 2302
Illinois Department of Public Health: Division of Food, Drugs and Dairies/FDD, 2303
The Indiana Consortium for Mental Health Services Research (ICMHSR), 2310
Indiana Department of Public Welfare Division of Family Independence: Food Stamps/Medicaid/Training, 2305
Indiana Family & Social Services Administration, 2306
Indiana Family And Social Services Administration, 2307
Indiana Family and Social Services Administration: Division of Mental Health, 2308
Information Resources and Inquiries Branch, 2196
Iowa Department Human Services, 2311
Iowa Department of Public Health, 2312
Iowa Department of Public Health: Division of Substance Abuse, 2313
Iowa Division of Mental Health & Developmental Disabilities: Department of Human Services, 2314
Juvenile Justice Commission, 2383
Kansas Council on Developmental Disabilities Kansas Department of Social and Rehabilitation Services, 2317
Kansas Department of Mental Health and Retardation and Social Services, 2318
Kentucky Cabinet for Health and Human Services, 2319
Kentucky Department for Human Support Services, 2320
Kentucky Department for Medicaid Services, 2321
Kentucky Department of Mental Health and Mental Retardation, 2322
Kentucky Justice Cabinet: Department of Juvenile Justice, 2323
LRADAC The Behavioral Health Center of the Midlands, 2429
Louisiana Commission on Law Enforcement and Administration (LCLE), 2324
Louisiana Department of Health and Hospitals: Office of Mental Health, 2325
Louisiana Department of Health and Hospitals: Louisiana Office for Addictive Disorders, 2326
Maine Department Health and Human Services Children's Behavioral Health Services, 2327
Maine Department of Behavioral and Developmental Services, 2328
Maine Office of Substance Abuse: Information and Resource Center, 2329
Marion County Health Department, 2411
Maryland Alcohol and Drug Abuse Administration, 2334
Maryland Department of Health and Mental Hygiene, 2335
Maryland Department of Human Resources, 2336

Maryland Division of Mental Health, 2337

Massachusetts Department of Mental Health, 2338

Massachusetts Department of Public Health, 2339

Massachusetts Department of Public Health: Bureau of Substance Abuse Services, 2340

Massachusetts Department of Social Services, 2341

Massachusetts Department of Transitional Assistance, 2342

Massachusetts Division of Medical Assistance MassHealth Program, 2343

Massachusetts Executive Office of Public Safety, 2344

Memphis Alcohol and Drug Council, 2440

Mental Health Association in Alaska, 2240

Mental Health Association in Illinois, 2304

Mental Health Association in South Carolina, 2430

Mental Health Association of Greater Dallas, 2450

Mental Health Council of Arkansas, 2250

Michigan Department of Community Health, 2345

Michigan Department of Human Services, 2346

Michigan State Representative: Co-Chair Public Health, 2347

Middle Tennessee Mental Health Institute, 2441

Minnesota Department of Human Services, 2350

Minnesota Youth Services Bureau, 2351

Mississippi Alcohol Safety Education Program, 2352

Mississippi Department Mental Health Mental Retardation Services, 2353

Mississippi Department of Human Services, 2354

Mississippi Department of Mental Health: Division of Alcohol and Drug Abuse, 2355

Mississippi Department of Mental Health: Division of Medicaid, 2356

Mississippi Department of Rehabilitation Services: Office of Vocational Rehabilitation (OVR), 2357

Missouri Department Health & Senior Services, 2358

Missouri Department of Mental Health, 2359

Missouri Department of Public Safety, 2360

Missouri Department of Social Services, 2361

Missouri Department of Social Services: Medical Services Division, 2362

Missouri Division of Alcohol and Drug Abuse, 2363

Missouri Division of Comprehensive Psychiatric Service, 2364

Missouri Division of Mental Retardation and Developmental Disabilities, 2365

Monatana Department of Human & Community Services, 2229

Montana Department of Health and Human Services: Child & Family Services Division, 2366

Montana Department of Public Health & Human Services: Addictive and Mental Disorders, 2367

Montana Department of Public Health and Human Services: Montana Vocational Rehabilitation Programs, 2368

National Institutes of Mental Health Division of Intramural Research Programs (DIRP), 2197

National Center for HIV, STD and TB Prevention, 2198

National Clearinghouse for Drug & Alcohol, 2199

National Institute of Alcohol Abuse and Alcoholism: Treatment Research Branch, 2200

National Institute of Alcohol Abuse and Alcoholism: Homeless Demonstration and Evaluation Branch, 2201

National Institute of Alcohol Abuse and Alcoholism: Office of Policy Analysis, 2202

National Institute of Drug Abuse: NIDA, 2203

National Institute of Mental Health: Schizophrenia Research Branch, 2204

National Institute of Mental Health: Mental Disorders of the Aging, 2205

National Institute of Mental Health: Office of Science Policy, Planning, and Communications, 2206

National Institute on Drug Abuse: Office of Science Policy and Communications, 2207

National Institute on Drug Abuse: Division of Clinical Neurosciences and Behavioral Research, 2208

National Institutes of Health: National Center for Research Resources (NCCR), 2209

National Institutes of Mental Health: Office on AIDS, 2210

National Library of Medicine, 2211

Nebraska Department of Health and Human Services (NHHS), 2369

Nebraska Health & Human Services: Medicaid and Managed Care Division, 2370

Nebraska Health and Human Services Division: Department of Mental Health, 2371

Nebraska Mental Health Centers, 2372

Nevada Department of Health & Human Services Health Care Financing and Policy, 2373

Nevada Department of Health and Human Services, 2374

Nevada Division of Mental Health & Developmental Services, 2375

Nevada Employment Training & Rehabilitation Department, 2376

Nevada State Health Division: Bureau of Alcohol & Drug Abuse, 2377

New Hampshire Department of Health & Human Services: Bureau of Community Health Services, 2380

New Hampshire Department of Health and Human Services: Bureau of Developmental Services, 2381

New Hampshire Department of Health and Human Services: Bureau of Behavioral Health, 2382

New Jersey Department of Human Services, 2384

New Jersey Division of Mental Health Services, 2385

New Jersey Division of Youth & Family Services, 2386

New Jersey Office of Managed Care, 2387

New Mexico Behavioral Health Collaborative, 2388

New Mexico Department of Health, 2389

New Mexico Department of Human Services, 2390

New Mexico Department of Human Services: Medical Assistance Division, 2391

New Mexico Health & Environment Department, 2392

New Mexico Kids, Parents and Families Office of Child Development: Children, Youth and Families Dep, 2393

New York Office of Alcohol & Substance Abuse Services, 2394

New York State Department of Health Individual County Listings of Social Services Departments, 2395

New York State Office of Mental Health, 2396

North Carolina Department of Human Resources, 2397

North Carolina Division of Mental Health, 2398

North Carolina Division of Social Services, 2399

North Carolina Substance Abuse Professional Certification Board (NCSAPCB), 2400

North Dakota Department of Human Services: Medicaid Program, 2401

North Dakota Department of Human Services: Mental Health Services Division, 2402

North Dakota Department of Human Services Division of Mental Health and Substance Abuse Services, 2403

Northern Arizona Regional Behavioral Health Authority, 2245

Northern Nevada Adult Mental Health Services, 2378

Office of Applied Studies, SA & Mental Health Services, 2212

Office of Disease Prevention & Health Promotion, 2213

Office of Medicaid Policy & Planning (OMPP), 2309

Office of Mental Health and Addiction Services Training & Resource Center, 2412

Office of National Drug Control Policy, 2214

Office of Program and Policy Development, 2215

Office of Science Policy OD/NIH, 2216

Ohio Community Drug Board, 2404

Ohio Department of Mental Health, 2405

Oklahoma Department of Human Services, 2406

Oklahoma Department of Mental Health and Substance Abuse Service (ODMHSAS), 2407

Oklahoma Healthcare Authority, 2408

Oklahoma Mental Health Consumer Council, 2409

Oklahoma Office of Juvenile Affairs, 2410

Oregon Commission on Children and Families, 2413

Oregon Department of Human Resources: Division of Health Services, 2414

Oregon Department of Human Services: Mental Health Services, 2415

Oregon Department of Human Services: Office of Developmental Disabilities, 2416

Oregon Health Policy and Research: Policy and Analysis Unit, 2417

Pennsylvania Bureau Drug and Alcohol Programs: Monitoring, 2419

Pennsylvania Bureau of Community Program Standards: Licensure and Certification, 2420

Pennsylvania Bureau of Drug and Alcohol Programs: Information Bulletins, 2421

Pennsylvania Department of Health: Bureau of Drug and Alcohol Programs, 2422

Pennsylvania Department of Public Welfare and Mental Health Services, 2423

Pennsylvania Division of Drug and Alcohol Prevention: Treatment, 2424

Pennsylvania Medical Assistance Programs, 2425

President's Committee on Mental Retardation, 2217

Presidential Commission on Employment of the Disabled, 2218

Protection and Advocacy Program for the Mentally Ill, 2219

Public Health Foundation, 2220

Rhode Island Council on Alcoholism and Other Drug Dependence, 2230

Rhode Island Department of Human Services, 2426

Rhode Island Division of Substance Abuse, 2427

South Carolina Department of Alcohol and Other Drug Abuse Services, 2431

South Carolina Department of Mental Health, 2432

South Carolina Department of Social Services, 2433

South Dakota Department of Human Services: Division of Mental Health, 2434

South Dakota Department of Social Services Office of Medical Services, 2435

South Dakota Human Services Center, 2436

Southern Nevada Adult Mental Health Services, 2379

State of Rhode Island Department of Mental Health, Retardation and Hospitals, 2428

State of Vermont Developmental Disabilities Services, 2462

Substance Abuse & Mental Health Services Adminstration (SAMHSA), 2221

Substance Abuse and Mental Health Services Administration: Center for Mental Health Services, 2222

Tarrant County Mental Health: Mental Retardation Services, 2451

Tennessee Commission on Children and Youth, 2442

Tennessee Department of Health, 2443

Tennessee Department of Health: Alcohol and Drug Abuse, 2444

Tennessee Department of Human Services, 2445

Tennessee Department of Mental Health and Developmental Disabilities, 2446

Texas Commission on Alcohol and Drug Abuse, 2452

Texas Department of Aging and Disability Services: Mental Retardation Services, 2453

Texas Department of Family and Protective Services, 2454

Texas Health & Human Services Commission, 2455

US Department of Health & Human Services: Indian Health Service, 2223

US Department of Health and Human Services Planning and Evaluation, 2224

US Department of Health and Human Services Bureau of Primary Health, 2225

US Department of Health and Human Services: Office of Women's Health, 2226

US Veterans Administration: Mental Health and Behavioral Sciences Services, 2227

University of Wisconsin Center for Health Policy and Program Evaluation, 2479

Utah Commission on Criminal and Juvenile Justice, 2456

Utah Department of Health, 2457

Utah Department of Health: Health Care Financing, 2458

Utah Department of Human Services, 2459

Utah Department of Human Services: Division of Substance Abuse And Mental Health, 2460

Utah Department of Mental Health, 2461

Vermont Department for Children and Families Economic Services Division (ESD), 2463

Vermont Department of Health: Division of Mental Health Services, 2464

Virginia Department of Medical Assistance Services, 2465

Virginia Department of Mental Health, Mental Retardation and Substance Abuse Services (DMHMRSAS), 2466

Virginia Department of Social Services, 2467

Virginia Office of the Secretary of Health and Human Resources, 2468

Washington Department of Alcohol and Substance Abuse: Department of Social and Health Service, 2469

Washington Department of Social & Health Services, 2470

Washington Department of Social and Health Services: Mental Health Division, 2471

West Virginia Bureau for Behavioral Health and Health Facilities, 2472

West Virginia Department of Health & Human Resources (DHHR), 2473

West Virginia Department of Welfare Bureau for Children and Families, 2474

West Virginia Division of Criminal Justice Services (DCJS), 2475

Wisconsin Bureau of Health Care Financing, 2480

Wisconsin Department of Health and Family Services, 2481

Wyoming Department of Family Services, 2482

Wyoming Department of Health: Division of Health Care Finance, 2483

Wyoming Mental Health Division, 2484

Impulse Control Disorders

Abusive Personality: Violence and Control in Intimate Relationships, 3013

Clinical Manual of Impulse-Control Disorders, 1135

Coping With Self-Mutilation: a Helping Book for Teens Who Hurt Themselves, 3014

Dealing with Anger Problems: Rational-Emotive Therapeutic Interventions, 3015

Domestic Violence 2000: Integrated Skills Program for Men, 3016

Dysinhibition Syndrome How to Handle Anger and Rage in Your Child or Spouse, 839, 1137

Gam-Anon Family Groups, 1147

Gamblers Anonymous, 1148

Impulse Control Disorders: A Clinician's Gui de to Understanding and Treating Behavioral Addictions, 1138

Mental Health Matters, 1127

Play Therapy with Children in Crisis: Individual, Group and Family Treatment, 3146

Sex Murder and Sex Aggression: Phenomenology Psychopathology, Psychodynamics and Prognosis, 3017

Stop Me Because I Can't Stop Myself: Taking Control of Impulsive Behavior, 1143

Strange Behavior Tales of Evolutionary Neurolgy, 2970

Teaching Behavioral Self Control to Students, 3018

Youth with Impulse-Control Disorders: On the Spur of the Moment (Helping Youth with Mental, Physica, 1146

www.apa.org/pubinfo/anger.html, 1153

Obsessive Compulsive Disorder

Boy Who Couldn't Stop Washing, 1175

Brain Lock: Free Yourself from Obsessive Compulsive Behavior, 1176

Childhood Obsessive Compulsive Disorder, 1177

Current Treatments of Obsessive-Compulsive Disorder, 3019

Freeing Your Child from Obsessive-Compulsive Disorder: A Powerful, Practical Program for Parents of, 1179

Funny, You Don't Look Crazy: Life With Obsessive Compulsive Disorder, 1180

Getting Control: Overcoming Your Obsessions and Compulsions, 1181

Hope & Solutions for Obsessive Compulsive Disorder: Part III, 1207

Hope and Solutions for OCD, 1208

Imp of the Mind: Exploring the Silent Epidemic of Obsessive Bad Thoughts, 1182

Let's Talk Facts About Obsessive Compulsive Disorder, 1183

North American Training Institute: Division of the Minnesota Council on Compulsive Gambling, 1971

OCD Newsletter, 1204

OCD Workbook: Your Guide to Breaking Free From Obsessive-Compulsive Disorder, 1184

OCD in Children and Adolescents: A Cognitive-Behavioral Treatment Manual, 1185

Obsessive Compulsive Anonymous, 1170

Obsessive Compulsive Foundation, 1171

Obsessive Compulsive Information Center, 1172

Obsessive-Compulsive Anonymous, 1205

Obsessive-Compulsive Disorder Casebook, 1186

Obsessive-Compulsive Disorder Spectrum, 1187

Obsessive-Compulsive Disorder in Children and Adolescents: A Guide, 1188

Obsessive-Compulsive Disorder in Children and Adolescents, 1189

Obsessive-Compulsive Disorder: Contemporary Issues in Treatment, 3021

Obsessive-Compulsive Disorder: Theory, Research and Treatment, 1190

Obsessive-Compulsive Disorders: A Complete Guide to Getting Well and Staying Well, 1191

Obsessive-Compulsive Disorders: A Complete G uide to Getting Well and Staying Well, 1192

Obsessive-Compulsive Disorders: Practical Management, 1193

Obsessive-Compulsive Disorders: The Latest Assessment and Treatment Strategies, 1194

Obsessive-Compulsive Foundation, 1206

Obsessive-Compulsive Related Disorders, 1195

Obsessive-Compulsive and Related Disorders in Adults: a Comprehensive Clinical Guide, 3022

Over and Over Again: Understanding Obsessive-Compulsive Disorder, 1196

Overcoming Agoraphobia and Panic Disorder, 2940

Overcoming Obsessive-Compulsive Disorder, 3023

Phobic and Obsessive-Compulsive Disorders: Theory, Research, and Practice, 1197

Real Illness: Obsessive-Compulsive Disorder, 1198

Relapse Prevention for Addictive Behaviors: a Manual for Therapists, 138

Rewind, Replay, Repeat: A Memoir of Obsessive-Compulsive Disorder, 1199

School Personnel, 1200

Solvay Pharmaceuticals, 4658

A Story of Bipolar Disorder (Manic-Depressive Illness) Does this Sound Like You?, 717

Suncoast Residential Training Center/Developmental Services Program, 275, 833, 870, 1244, 1290, 1367, 3808

Tormenting Thoughts and Secret Rituals: The Hidden Epidemic of Obsessive-Compulsive Disorder, 1201

Touching Tree, 1209

Treatment of Obsessive Compulsive Disorder, 3024

When Once Is Not Enough: Help for Obsessive Compulsives, 1202

When Perfect Isn't Good Enough: Strategies for Coping with Perfectionism, 1203

www.fairlite.com/ocd/, 1212

www.interlog.com/~calex/ocd, 1213

www.lexington-on-line.com/, 1214

www.mayoclinic.com, 1215

www.nimh.nih.gov/anxiety/anxiety/ocd, 1216

www.nursece.com/OCD.htm, 1218

www.ocfoundation.org, 1220

Paraphilias (Perversions)

Perversion (Ideas in Psychoanalysis), 1230

The World of Perversion: Psychoanalysis and the Impossible Absolute of Desire, 1231

Pediatric & Adolescent Issues

AACAP News, 3202

ASAP Newsletter, 3208

Activities for Adolescents in Therapy, 3595

Activities for Children in Therapy: Guide for Planning and Facilitating Therapy with Troubled Childr, 3596

Administration for Children and Families, 2180

Administration for Children, Youth and Families, 2181

Adolescents in Psychiatric Hospitals: A Psychodynamic Approach to Evaluation and Treatment, 3093

After School And More, 78

Alliance for Children and Families, 2508

American Academy of Child and Adolescent Psychiatry (AACAP): Annual Meeting, 3167

American Academy of Child & Adolescent Psychiatry, 2509

American Academy of Child and Adolescent Psychiatry - Membership Directory, 1573, 1695, 3347, 3622

American Academy of Pediatrics, 1574, 1696

American Association for Protecting Children, 2515

American Association of Children's Residential Center Annual Conference, 2518, 3171

American Association of Psychiatric Services for Children (AAPSC), 1698

American Pediatrics Society, 1575, 1702

American Society for Adolescent Psychiatry (ASAP), 2565

American Society for Adolescent Psychiatry: Annual Meeting, 3183

An Elephant in the Living Room: Leader's Guide for Helping Children of Alcoholics, 2890

Annie E Casey Foundation, 2573

Anxiety Disorders in Children and Adolescents, 1616

Association for Child Psychoanalysis Newsletter, 3213

Association for Child Psychoanalysts, 2581

Association for Children of New Jersey, 2001

Association for the Care of Children's Health, 1705

Association for the Help of Retarded Children, 1576, 1706

At-Risk Youth in Crises, 3095

Attachment, Trauma and Healing: Understanding and Treating Attachment Disorder in Children and Famil, 3096

Autism Spectrum Disorders in Children and Adolescents, 1618

Baby Fold, 1886

Basic Child Psychiatry, 3097

Behavior Modification for Exceptional Children and Youth, 3098

Behavioral Approach to Assessment of Youth with Emotional/Behavioral Disorders, 3100

Behavioral Approaches: Problem Child, 3101

Berkshire Farm Center and Services for Youth, 3958

Beyond Behavior Modification: Cognitive-Behavioral Approach to Behavior Management in the School, 2973

Bibliotherapy Starter Set, 1597

Book of Psychotherapeutic Homework, 1598

Boysville of Michigan, 1952

Brown University: Child & Adolescent Psychopharmacology Update, 3216

CHINS UP Youth and Family Services, 1842

Camps 2008, 79

Candor, Connection and Enterprise in Adolesent Therapy, 3102

Center for Family Support (CFS), 7, 264, 392, 547, 706, 778, 829, 854, 953, 983, 1102, 1125, 1166, 1224, 1237, 1282, 1334, 1357, 1440, 1469, 1535

Chicago Child Care Society, 1888

Child Friendly Therapy: Biophysical Innovations for Children and Families, 3103

Child Psychiatry, 3104

Child Psychopharmacology, 3105

Child Welfare League of America, 1721

Child and Adolescent Mental Health Consultation in Hospitals, Schools and Courts, 3106

Child and Adolescent Psychiatry, 3223

Child and Adolescent Psychiatry: Modern Approaches, 3107

Child and Adolescent Psychopharmacology Information, 2169

Child-Centered Counseling and Psychotherapy, 3108

Childhood Behavior Disorders: Applied Research and Educational Practice, 3109

Childhood Disorders, 3110

Children and Adolescents with Emotional and Behavioral Disorders, 3360

Children and Adults with AD/HD (CHADD), 394, 1625

Children and Trauma: Guide for Parents and Professionals, 1293, 1601

Children and Youth Funding Report, 169

Children's Alliance, 1912, 2147

Children's Health Council, 2600

Children's Home of the Wyoming Conference, Quality Improvement, 4156

Children: Experts on Divorce, 1635

Childs Work/Childs Play, 1602, 3111

Chill: Straight Talk About Stress, 1636

Chronicle, 3224

Clinical & Forensic Interviewing of Children & Families, 3112

Clinical Application of Projective Drawings, 3113

Clinical Child Documentation Sourcebook, 3114

Cognitive Behavior Therapy Child, 3115

Comprehensive Directory: Programs and Services for Children with Disabilities and Their Families, 3599

Concerned Advocates Serving Children & Families, 2050

Concise Guide to Child and Adolescent Psychiatry, 3116

Concord Family and Adolescent Services, 3909

Conduct Disorder in Children and Adolescents, 843, 1619

Council on Accreditation (COA) of Services for Families and Children, 2492

Counseling Children with Special Needs, 3117

Covenant House Nineline, 1626

Creative Therapy with Children and Adolescents, 1603, 3118

Crossroad: Fort Wayne's Children's Home, 3856

Delaware Guidance Services for Children and Youth, 1856

Department of Human Services For Youth & Families, 1864

Developmental Therapy/Developmental Teaching, 3120

Don't Feed the Monster on Tuesdays: The Children's Self-Esteem Book, 24

Don't Rant and Rave on Wednesdays: The Children's Anger-Control Book, 26

Effective Discipline, 2974

Elon Homes for Children, 4182

Empowering Adolesent Girls, 2902

Enhancing Social Competence in Young Students, 3121

Exceptional Parent, 3234

FAT City: How Difficult Can This Be?, 360

Families Can Help Children Cope with Fear, Anxiety, 338, 1620

Families United of Milwaukee, 2170

Federation for Children with Special Needs (FCSN), 1578, 1732

Federation of Families for Children's Mental Health, 1845

First Connections and Healthy Families, 3910

Five Acres: Boys and Girls Aid Society of Los Angeles County, 1830

Florida Federation of Families for Children's Mental Health, 1867

Focal Point: Research, Policy and Practice in Children's Mental Health, 3235

Forms-5 Book Set, 1605

Gender Respect Workbook, 1607

Georgia Association of Homes and Services for Children, 1874

Girls and Boys Town of New York, 1627

Good Will-Hinckley Homes for Boys and Girls, 3888

Graham-Windham Services for Children and Families: Manhattan Mental Health Center, 3973

Grip Project, 3911

Groden Center, 4044

Group Therapy With Children and Adolescents, 3122

Handbook of Child Behavior in Therapy and in the Psychiatric Setting, 3123

Handbook of Infant Mental Health, 3124

Handbook of Parent Training: Parents as Co-Therapists for Children's Behavior Problems, 3125

Handbook of Psychiatric Practice in the Juvenile Court, 3126

Hannah Neil Center for Children, 4009

Helping Parents, Youth, and Teachers Understand Medications for Behavioral and Emotional Problems, 840, 2975, 3127

How to Do Homework without Throwing Up, 446

I Love You Like Crazy: Being a Parent with Mental Illness, 3497

I Wish Daddy Didn't Drink So Much, 1608

I'm Somebody, Too!, 449

Illinois Federation of Families for Children's Mental Health, 1895

In the Long Run... Longitudinal Studies of Psychopathology in Children, 3129

Infants, Toddlers and Families: Framework for Support and Intervention, 3130

Insider, 3248

Interventions for Students with Emotional Disorders, 3131

Interviewing Children and Adolescents: Skills and Strategies for Effective DSM-IV Diagnosis, 3132

Iowa Federation of Families for Children's Mental Health, 1906

Judge Baker Children's Center, 1743

Just Say No International, 1628

Keys for Networking: Kansas Parent Informati on & Resource Center, 1910

Kid Power Tactics for Dealing with Depression & Parent's Survival Guide to Childhood Depression, 1609

Kidspeace National Centers, 1629

Learning Disorders and Disorders of the Self in Children and Adolesents, 3134

Lifespire, 1580, 1746

Littleton Group Home, 3912

Living on the Razor's Edge: Solution-Oriented Brief Family Therapy with Self-Harming Adolescents, 3135

Louisiana Federation of Families for Children's Mental Health, 1924

Major Depression in Children and Adolescents, 916, 1622

Manual of Clinical Child and Adolescent Psychiatry, 3137

Meadowridge Pelham Academy, 3913

Meadowridge Walden Street School, 3914

Mental Affections Childhood, 3138

Mental, Emotional, and Behavior Disorders in Children and Adolescents, 844, 1623

Mentally Ill Kids in Distress, 1581, 1750

Metropolitan Area Chapter of Federation of Families for Children's Mental Health, 1957

Michigan Association for Children with Emotional Disorders: MACED, 1959

Michigan Association for Children's Mental Health, 1582, 1960

Minnesota Association for Children's Mental Health, 1966

My Body is Mine, My Feelings are Mine, 1610

My Listening Friend: A Story About the Benefits of Counseling, 1611

Myth of Maturity: What Teenagers Need from Parents to Become Adults, 3139

NAMI Beginnings, 3282

National Association For Childrens Behavioral Health, 2632

National Council of Juvenile and Family Court Judges, 2645

National Dissemination Center for Children with Disabilities, 398, 1584

National Federation of Families for Children 's Mental Health, 1938

National Technical Assistance Center for Children's Mental Health, 1585, 1773

National Youth Crisis Hotline, 1630

Navajo Nation K'E Project, 1814

Navajo Nation K'E Project-Shiprock, 2012

Navajo Nation K'E Project: Chinle, 1815

Navajo Nation K'E Project: Tuba City, 1816

Navajo Nation K'E Project: Winslow, 1817

New England Home for Little Wanderers, 3915

No-Talk Therapy for Children and Adolescents, 3142

Non Medical Marijuana: Rite of Passage or Russian Roulette?, 2912

North Dakota Federation of Families for Children's Mental Health: Region II, 2045

North Dakota Federation of Families for Children's Mental Health: Region V, 2047

North Dakota Federation of Families for Children's Mental Health: Region VII, 2048

North Dakota Federation of Families for Children's Mental Health, 2049

OK Parents as Partners, 2063

Outcomes for Children and Youth with Emotional and Behavioral Disorders and their Families, 3144

Parents Helping Parents, 1586

Parents Information Network, 1587

Parents United Network: Parsons Child Family Center, 2031

Pennsylvania Society for Services to Children, 2078

Pilot Parents: PP, 1588

Preventing Maladjustment from Infancy Through Adolescence, 28

Proven Youth Development Model that Prevents Substance Abuse and Builds Communities, 2915

Psychological Examination of the Child, 3149

Psychotherapies with Children and Adolescents, 3150

Rainbows, 39, 1631

Research and Training Center for Children's Mental Health, 1589

Research and Training Center on Family Support and Children's Mental Health, 1590, 1786

Research and Training for Children's Mental Health-Update, 3308

Resources for Children with Special Needs, 1591, 1787

SADD: Students Against Destructive Decisions, 211, 1632

SPOKES Federation of Families for Children's Mental Health, 1921

Saddest Time, 1612

Salem Children's Home, 3847

Seelig and Company: Child Welfare and Behavioral Healthcare, 4322

Severe Stress and Mental Disturbance in Children, 3152

Society for Adolescent Psychiatry Newsletter, 3314

Society for Pediatric Psychology (SPP), 2670

Specialized Alternatives for Families & Youth of America (SAFY), 4326

St. Mary's Home for Boys, 4027

Structured Adolescent Pscyhotherapy Groups, 3153

Teen Relationship Workbook, 1613

Texas Federation of Families for Children's Mental Health, 2121

Textbook of Child and Adolescent Psychiatry, 3154

Textbook of Pediatric Neuropsychiatry, 3155

Thirteen Steps to Help Families Stop Fightin Solve Problems Peacefully, 1614

Three Springs LEAPS, 4058

Transition Matters-From School to Independence, 2866

Treating Depressed Children: A Therapeutic Manual of Proven Cognitive Behavior Techniques, 2994, 3157

Treating the Tough Adolesent: Family Based Step by Step Guide, 3159
Understanding and Teaching Emotionally Disturbed Children and Adolescents, 3161
United Advocates for Children of California, 1840
United Families for Children's Mental Health, 1592, 1791
United Families for Children's Mental Health, 1929
Ups & Downs: How to Beat the Blues and Teen Depression, 3162
Vermont Federation of Families for Children's Mental Health, 2136
Victor School, 3918
Virginia Federation of Families, 2145
Western North Carolina Families (CAN), 2042
Westlund Child Guidance Clinic, 3928
Wisconsin Association of Family and Child Agency, 2174
Young Adult Institute and Workshop (YAI), 1593
Youth Services International, 1594, 1798
Youth Violence: Prevention, Intervention, and Social Policy, 3164
Zero to Three, 1595, 1799
www.Al-Anon-Alateen.org, 1638
www.CHADD.org, 489, 1639
www.aacap.org, 3510
www.abcparenting.com, 1640
www.aboutteensnow.com/dramas, 1641
www.adhdnews.com.ssi.htm, 1642
www.adhdnews.com/Advocate.htm, 496, 1643
www.adhdnews.com/sped.htm, 497, 1644
www.cfc-efc.ca/docs/00000095.htm, 1645
www.couns.uiuc.edu, 1646
www.divorcedfather.com, 1647
www.duanev/family/dads.html, 1648
www.education.indiana.edu/cas/adol/adol.html, 1649
www.ericps.crc.uiuc.edu/npin/index.html, 1650
www.ericps.crc.uiuc.edu/npin/library/texts.html, 1651
www.fathermag.com, 1652
www.fathers.com, 1653
www.flyingsolo.com, 1654
www.fsbassociates.com/fsg/whydivorce.html, 1656
www.geocities.com/enchantedforest/1068, 761, 1657, 3535
www.home.clara.net/spig/guidline.htm, 1658
www.hometown.aol.com/DrgnKprl/BPCAT.html, 1659
www.ianrpubs.unl.edu/family/nf223.htm, 1660
www.kidshealth.org/kid/feeling/index.html, 1661
www.kidsource.com/kidsource/pages/parenting, 1662
www.klis.com/chandler/pamphlet/bipolar/bipolarpamphlet.html, 1663
www.klis.com/chandler/pamphlet/bipolar/bipol arpamphlet.htm, 1664
www.magicnet.net/~hedyyumi/child.html, 1666
www.mentalhealth.org/publications/allpubs/, 1667
www.muextension.missouri.edu/xpor/hesguide/, 1668
www.naturalchild.com/home, 1669

www.nichcy.org, 502, 1670
www.nnfr.org/curriculum/topics/sep_div.html, 1671
www.nospank.org/toc.htm, 1672
www.npin.org/pnews/pnews997/, 1673
www.oznet.ksu.edu/library/famlf2/, 1674, 3570
www.parentcity.com/read/library, 1675
www.parenthoodweb.com, 1676, 3573
www.parenthoodweb.com, 1677
www.personal.psu.edu/faculty, 1678
www.positive-way.com/step.htm, 1679, 3575
www.pta.org/commonsense, 1680
www.safecrossingsfoundation.org, 70
www.stepfamily.org/tensteps.htm, 1681, 3590
www.stepfamilyinfo.org/sitemap.htm, 1682, 3591
www.teenwire.com/index.asp, 1683
www.todaysparent.com, 1684
www.users.aol.com:80/jimams/, 1685
www.users.aol.com:80/jimams/answers1, 1686
www.wholefamily.com/kidteencenter/, 1687
www.worldcollegehealth.org, 1688
www2.mc.duke.edu/pcaad, 1689

Personality Disorders

Angry Heart: Overcoming Borderline and Addictive Disorders, 1245
Assess Dialogue Personality Disorders, 1246
Bad Boys, Bad Men: Confronting Antisocial Personality Disorder, 3025
Biological Basis of Personality, 3026
Biology of Personality Disorders, 3027
Biology of Personality Disorders, Review of Psychiatry, 1247
Borderline Personality Disorder, 1248
The Borderline Personality Disorder Survival Guide, 1270
Borderline Personality Disorder: Multidimensional Approach, 1249
Borderline Personality Disorder: A Therapist Guide to Taking Control, 3028
Borderline Personality Disorder: Etilogy and Treatment, 1251
Borderline Personality Disorder: Tailoring the Psychotherapy to the Patient, 1252, 3029
Center for Attitudinal Healing (CAH), 1715
Challenging Behavior, 1253
Clinical Assessment and Management of Severe Personality Disorders, 1254
Cognitive Analytic Therapy & Borderline Personality Disorder: Model and the Method, 1255
Cognitive Therapy for Personality Disorders: a Schema-Focused Approach, 3030
Cognitive Therapy of Personality Disorders, Second Edition, 1256
Dealing With the Problem of Low Self-Esteem: Common Characteristics and Treatment, 3032
Developmental Model of Borderline Personality Disorder: Understanding Variations in Course and Outco, 1257
Disordered Personalities, 1258
Disorders of Narcissism: Diagnostic, Clinical, and Empirical Implications, 1259

Disorders of Personality: DSM-IV and Beyond, 3033
Fatal Flaws: Navigating Destructive Relation ships with People with Disorders, 1261
Field Guide to Personality Disorders, 1262
Forty Two Lives in Treatment: a Study of Psychoanalysis and Psychotherapy, 3236
Group Exercises for Enhancing Social Skills & Self-Esteem, 3034
Life After Trauma: Workbook for Healing, 3051
Lost in the Mirror: An Inside Look at Borderline Personality Disorder, 967, 1263
Management of Countertransference with Borderline Patients, 1264
Personality Characteristics of the Personality Disordered, 3035
Personality Disorders and Culture: Clinical and Conceptual Interactions, 3036
Personality Disorders in Modern Life, 1265
Personality and Psychopathology, 1266
Personality and Stress Center for Applications of Psychological Type, 3505
Personality and Stress: Individual Differences in the Stress Process, 3037
Psychotherapy for Borderline Personality, 3038
Role of Sexual Abuse in the Etiology of Borderline Personality Disorder, 1267, 3039
SAFE Alternatives, 1271
SAMHSA's National Mental Health Information Center, 15, 273, 715, 787, 959, 997, 1089, 1110, 1131, 1174, 1229, 1243
Shorter Term Treatments for Borderline Personality Disorders, 3040
Skills Training Manual for Treating Borderline Personality Disorder, Companion Workbook, 3614
Stop Walking on Eggshells, 1268
Structured Interview for DSM-IV Personality (SIDP-IV), 1269
Treating Difficult Personality Disorders, 3041
www.mhsanctuary.com/borderline, 1274
www.nimh.nih.gov/publicat/ocdmenu.cfm, 1217, 1275
www.ocdhope.com/gdlines.htm, 1219, 1276

Post Traumatic Stress Disorder

Academy of Psychosomatic Medicine, 2505
Advanced Psychotherapy Association, 2506
After the Crash: Assessment and Treatment of Motor Vehicle Accident Survivors, 1291
Aging and Post Traumatic Stress Disorder, 1292
American Psychosomatic Society, 2564
American Society of Group Psychotherapy & Psychodrama, 2568
Anxiety Disorders, 282, 335, 357, 1313
Association of Traumatic Stress Specialists, 1280
Body Remembers: Psychophysiology of Trauma and Trauma Treatment, 3042
Concise Guide to Brief Dynamic Psychotherapy, 3045
Coping with Post-Traumatic Stress Disorder, 1294

Coping with Trauma: A Guide to Self Understanding, 1295

Don't Despair on Thursdays: the Children's Grief-Management Book, 23

Don't Pop Your Cork on Mondays: The Children's Anti-Stress Book, 25

E-Productivity-Services.Net, 1283

Effecive Treatments for PTSD: Practice Guide lines from the International Society for Traumatic Stre, 1296

Effective Treatments for PTSD, 1297

Effective Treatments for PTSD: Practice Guidelines from the International Society for Traumatic Stre, 3047

Even from a Broken Web: Brief, Respectful Solution Oriented Therapy for Sexual Abuse and Trauma, 3048

Functional Somatic Syndromes, 3072

Group Treatments for Post-Traumatic Stress Disorder, 3050

Handbook of PTSD: Science and Practice, 1298

Haunted by Combat: Understanding PTSD in War Veterans, 1299

Helping Children and Adolescents Cope with Violence and Disasters, 1314

Hoffman-La Roche, 4640

I Can't Get Over It: Handbook for Trauma Survivors, 1300

International Society for Traumatic Stress Studies, 1284

Let's Talk Facts About Post-Traumatic Stress Disorder, 1315

Life Passage in the Face of Death, Volume I: A Brief Psychotherapy, 3501

Memory, Trauma and the Law, 3052

National SHARE Office, 37

Parents of Murdered Children, 38

Post Traumatic Stress Disorder: Complete Treatment Guide, 3057

Post-Traumatic Stress Disorder: Assessment, Differential Diagnosis, and Forensic Evaluation, 1302

Posttraumatic Stress Disorder in Litigation: Guidelines for Forensic Assessment, 1303

Posttraumatic Stress Disorder: A Guide, 1304

Psychological Trauma, 1305

Psychosomatic Medicine, 3305

Real Illness: Post-Traumatic Stress Disorder, 1316

Remembering Trauma: Psychotherapist's Guide to Memory & Illusion, 3060

Risk Factors for Posttraumatic Stress Disorder, 1307

Sidran Traumatic Stress Institute, 1788

Take Charge: Handling a Crisis and Moving Forward, 1308

Through the Eyes of a Child, 3156

Transforming Trauma: EMDR, 3066

Trauma Response, 3067

Traumatic Events & Mental Health, 3068

Traumatic Stress: Effects of Overwhelming Experience on Mind, Body and Society, 1309

Treating Trauma Disorders Effectively, 1317

Treatment of Stress Response Syndromes, 31

Trust After Trauma: A Guide to Relationships for Survivors and Those Who Love Them, 1310

Understanding Post Traumatic Stress Disorder and Addiction, 1311

www.apa.org/practice/traumaticstress.html, 1318

www.bcm.tmc.edu/civitas/caregivers.htm, 1319

www.factsforhealth.org, 368, 1321, 3533

www.grieftalk.com/help1.html, 3537

www.icisf.org, 374, 1322

www.ncptsd.org, 1324

www.ptsdalliance.org, 1327

www.sidran.org, 978, 1328

www.sidran.org/trauma.html, 1329

www.sni.net/trips/links.html, 1330

www.trauma-pages.com, 1331

Professional

Ackerman Institute for the Family, 3342

Active Intervention, 3343

Alfred Adler Institute (AAI), 3344

Alliance Behavioral Care: University of Cincinnati Psychiatric Services, 3345

Alton Ochsner Medical Foundation, Psychiatry Residency, 3346

American College of Women's Health Physicians, 3349

Andrus Children's Center, 3350

Asian Pacific Development Center for Human Development, 3351

Assessment and Treatment of Anxiety Disorders in Persons with Mental Retardation, 3316

Assessment of Neuropsychiatry and Mental Health Services, 3317

Attention-Deficit/Hyperactivity Disorder Test: a Method for Identifying Individuals with ADHD, 1617, 3318

Behavioral Medicine and Biofeedback Consultants, 3353

Behavioral and Emotional Rating Scale, 3319

Brandeis University/Heller School, 3354

Brown Schools Behavioral Health System, 3356

CPP Incorporated, 3320

California Institute of Behavioral Sciences, 3357

Cambridge Hospital: Department of Psychiatry, 3358

Childhood History Form for Attention Disorders, 3321

Children's Depression Inventory, 3322

Clinical Evaluations of School Aged Children, 3323

Clinical Interview of the Adolescent: From Assessment and Formulation to Treatment Planning, 3324

College of Health and Human Services: SE Missouri State, 3361

Colonial Services Board, 3363

Columbia Counseling Center, 3364

Concise Guide to Assessment and Management of Violent Patients, 3325

Conducting Insanity Evaluations, 3326

Conners' Rating Scales, 3327

Copper Hills Youth Center, 3365

Daniel and Yeager Healthcare Staffing Solutions, 3369

Department of Psychiatry: Dartmouth University, 3370

Depression and Anxiety in Youth Scale, 3328

Diagnosis and Treatment of Multiple Personality Disorder, 3329

Diagnosis and Treatment of Sociopaths and Clients with Sociopathic Traits, 3330

Diagnostic Interview Schedule for Children: CDISC, 3331

Downstate Mental Hygiene Association, 3372

Draw a Person: Screening Procedure for Emotional Disturbance, 3332

East Carolina University Department of Psychiatric Medicine, 3373

Eastern County Mental Health Center, 3374

Emory University School of Medicine, Psychology and Behavior, 3375

Emory University: Psychological Center, 3376

Functional Assessment and Intervention: Guide to Understanding Problem Behavior, 3333

Genesis Learning Center (Devereux), 3378

George Washington University, 3379

Handbook of Psychological Assessment, 3334

Harper House: Change Alternative Living, 3380

Harvard Medical School Guide to Suicide Assessment and Intervention, 1505, 3335

Haymarket Center, Professional Development, 3381

Health Watch, 3336

Heartshare Human Services, 3382

Hillcrest Utica Psychiatric Services, 3383

Jacobs Institute of Women's Health, 3385

Jefferson Drug/Alcohol, 3386

John A Burns School of Medicine Department of Psychiatry, 3387

Langley Porter Psych Institute at UCSF Parnassus Campus, 3388

Laurelwood Hospital and Counseling Centers, 3389

Life Science Associates, 3390

Locumtenens.com, 3391

MCG Telemedicine Center, 3392

MCW Department of Psychiatry and Behavioral Medicine, 3393

Management Recruiters of Washington, DC, 3394

Marsh Foundation, 3395

Masters of Behavioral Healthcare Management, 3396

Medical College of Georgia, 3397

Medical College of Ohio, Psychiatry, 3398

Medical College of Pennsylvania, 3399

Medical College of Wisconsin, 3401

Medical Doctor Associates, 3402

Medical University of South Carolina Institute of Psychiatry, Psychiatry Access Center, 3403

Meharry Medical College, 3404

Menninger Division of Continuing Education, 3405

NEOUCOM-Northeastern Ohio Universities College of Medicine, 3406

Nathan S Kline Institute for Psychiatric Research, 3407

National Association of Alcholism and Drug Abuse Counselors, 3408

National Association of School Psychologists, 2639, 3409

New York University Behavioral Health Programs, 3410

Nickerson Center, 3411

Northwestern University Medical School Feinberg School of Medicine, 3412

Ochester Psychological Service, 3413

Onslow County Behavioral Health, 3414

PRIMA A D D Corp., 3415

Parent Child Center, 3416
Penn State Hershey Medical Center, 3418
Pepperdine University, Graduate School of
    Education and Psychology, 3419
Postgraduate Center for Mental Health, 3421
Pressley Ridge Schools, 3422
Psych-Med Association, St. Francis Medical,
    3424
PsychTemps, 3425
Psychiatric Associates, 3426
Psychological Center, 3428
Psychology Department, 3430
Regional Research Institute for Human
    Services of Portland University, 3432
Research Center for Children's Mental
    Health, Department of Children and
    Family, 3433
River City Mental Health Clinic, 3434
Riveredge Hospital, 3435
Riverside Center, 3436
Rockland Children's Psychiatric Center, 3437
Rosemont Center, 3438
Scale for Assessing Emotional Disturbance,
    3337
Schneider Institute for Health Policy, 3440
School of Nursing, UCLA, 3441
Screening for Brain Dysfunction in
    Psychiatric Patients, 3338
Sexual Dysfunction: Guide for Assessment
    and Treatment, 3339
Social-Emotional Dimension Scale, 3340
Southern Illinois University School of
    Medicine: Department of Psychiatry, 3442
Southern Illinois University School of
    Medicine, 3443
St. Francis Medical Center, 3444
St. Joseph Behavioral Medicine Network,
    3445
St. Louis Behavioral Medicine Institute, 3446
Stonington Institute, 3447
Success Day Training Program, 3448
Test Collection at ETS, 3341
Topeka Institute for Psychoanalysis, 3449
Training Behavioral Healthcare
    Professionals, 3451
UCLA Neuropsychiatric Institute and
    Hospital, 3452
UCSF-Department of Psychiatry, Cultural
    Competence, 3453
USC Psychiatry and Psychology Associates,
    3454
USC School of Medicine, 3455
Ulster County Mental Health Department,
    3456
Union County Psychiatric Clinic, 3457
University Behavioral Healthcare, 3458
University of California at Davis Psychiatry
    and Behavioral Sciences Department, 3459
University of Cincinnati College of Medical
    Department of Psychiatry, 3460
University of Colorado Health Sciences
    Center, 3461
University of Connecticut Health Center,
    3462
University of Iowa Hospital, 3463
University of Kansas Medical Center, 3464
University of Kansas School of Medicine,
    3465
University of Louisville School of Medicine,
    3466
University of Maryland Medical Systems,
    3467

University of Maryland School of Medicine,
    3468
University of Massachusetts Medical Center,
    3469
University of Miami - Department of
    Psychology, 3470
University of Michigan, 3471
University of Minnesota Fairview Health
    Systems, 3472
University of Minnesota, Family Social
    Science, 3473
University of New Mexico, School of
    Medicine Health Sciences Center, 3474
University of North Carolina School of Socia
    l Work, 3475
University of North Carolina, School of
    Medicine, 3476
University of Pennsylvania Health System,
    3477
University of Pennsylvania, Department of
    Psychiatry, 3478
University of Tennessee Medical Group:
    Department of Medicine and Psychiatry,
    3479
University of Texas Medical Branch
    Managed Care, 3480
University of Texas, Southwestern Medical
    Center, 3481
University of Texas-Houston Health Science
    Center, 3482
University of Utah Neuropsychiatric, 3483
Wake Forest University, 3484
Wayne University-University of Psychiatric
    Center-Jefferson: Outpatient Mental
    Health for Children,, 3485
West Jefferson Medical Center, 3486
Western Psychiatric Institute and Clinic, 3487
Wordsworth, 3488
Yale University School of Medicine: Child
    Study Center, 3489

Psychosomatic (Somatizing) Disorders

Astra Zeneca Pharmaceuticals, 4632
Brief Therapy for Post Traumatic Stress
    Disorder, 3043
Cognitive Processing Therapy for Rape
    Victims, 3044
Deborah MacWilliams, 1336
The Divided Mind: The Epidemic of
    Mindbody D isorders, 1349
Effective Learning Systems, 1350
Essentials of Psychosomatic Medicine, 1344
Eye Movement Desensitization and
    Reprocessing: Basic Principles, Protocols,
    and Procedures, 3049
Family Stress, Coping, and Social Support,
    2751
Hypochondria: Woeful Imaginings, 1345
Institute for Contemporary Psychotherapy,
    1337
Mind-Body Problems: Psychotherapy with
    Psychosomatic Disorders, 1346
Overcoming Post-Traumatic Stress Disorder,
    3053
Phantom Illness: Recognizing,
    Understanding, and Overcoming
    Hypochondria, 1347
Somatoform and Factitious Disorders
    (Review of Psychiatry), 1348

www.users.lanminds.com/~eds/, 1354

Schizophrenia

Behavioral High-Risk Paradigm in
    Psychopathology, 3078
Biology of Schizophrenia and Affective
    Disease, 1368
Bonnie Tapes, 1416
The Bonnie Tapes Mental Illness in the
    Family; Recovering from Mental Illness;
    My Sister is Mentally, 755
Breakthroughs in Antipsychotic Medications:
    A Guide for Consumers, Families, and
    Clinicians, 1369
Career Assessment & Planning Services,
    263, 828, 1165, 1236, 1281, 1333, 1356
The Center Cannot Hold: My Journey
    Through M adness, 1401
Center for Mental Health Services, 1335,
    1358
The Complete Family Guide to
    Schizophrenia: Helping Your Loved One
    Get the Most Out of Life, 1402
Concept of Schizophrenia: Historical
    Perspectives, 1370
Contemporary Issues in the Treatment of
    Schizophrenia, 1371
Encyclopedia of Schizophrenia and the
    Psychotic Disorders, 1373
Families Coping with Mental Illness, 754,
    1417
Families Coping with Schizophrenia:
    Practitioner's Guide to Family Groups,
    3081
Family Care of Schizophrenia: a
    Problem-Solving Approach..., 1374
Family Work for Schizophrenia: a Practical
    Guide, 1375
Family-to-Family: National Alliance on
    Mental Illness, 1413
First Episode Psychosis, 1376
Group Therapy for Schizophrenic Patients,
    1377
How to Cope with Mental Illness In Your
    Family: A Guide for Siblings and
    Offspring, 1379
Innovative Approaches for Difficult to Treat
    Populations, 1380, 2775
Janssen, 4641
Johnson & Johnson, 4642
Me, Myself, and Them: A Firsthand Account
    of One Young Person's Experience with
    Schizophrenia (Adol, 1381
NARSA: The Mental Health Research
    Associatio n, 1410
NARSAD: The Mental Health Research
    Associati on, 862, 1359
National Alliance for Research on
    Schizophrenia and Depression, 923, 1360
National Association for The Dually
    Diagnose d (NADD), 1362
National Mental Health Association, 97, 1363
Natural History of Mania, Depression and
    Schizophrenia, 892, 1382
New Pharmacotherapy of Schizophrenia,
    1383
Office Treatment of Schizophrenia, 1384
Practice Guideline for the Treatment of
    Patients with Schizophrenia, 2944, 3082

Practicing Psychiatry in the Community: a Manual, 1385
Prenatal Exposures in Schizophrenia, 1386
Psychiatric Rehabilitation of Chronic Mental Patients, 1387
Psychoses and Pervasive Development Disorders in Childhood and Adolescence, 1388
Return From Madness, 1389
Schizophrenia, 1390, 1406
Schizophrenia Bulletin: Superintendent of Documents, 1407
Schizophrenia Fact Sheet, 1408
Schizophrenia Research, 1409
Schizophrenia Research Branch: Division of Clinical and Treatment Research, 1411
Schizophrenia Revealed: From Neurons to Soci al Interactions, 1391
Schizophrenia Revealed: From Nuerons to Social Interactions, 1392, 3083
Schizophrenia and Genetic Risks, 1393
Schizophrenia and Manic Depressive Disorder, 1394
Schizophrenia and Primitive Mental States, 1395
Schizophrenia in a Molecular Age, 1396
Schizophrenia: From Mind to Molecule, 1397
Schizophrenia: Straight Talk for Family and Friends, 1398
Schizophrenic Biologic Research Center, 1412
Schizophrenics Anonymous Forum, 1415
Stigma and Mental Illness, 1399
Surviving Schizophrenia: A Manual for Families, Consumers and Providers, 1400
Treating Schizophrenia, 1403
Understanding Schizophrenia: Guide to the New Research on Causes & Treatment, 1404
Water Balance in Schizophrenia, 1405
www.health-center.com/mentalhealth/ schizophrenia/default.htm, 1419
www.hopkinsmedicine.org/epigen, 1420
www.members.aol.com/leonardjk/USA.htm, 1421
www.mentalhealth.com/book, 3555
www.mentalhelp.net/guide/schizo.htm, 1423
www.mgl.ca/~chovil, 1424
www.mhsource.com/ advocacy/narsad/order.html, 1425
www.mhsource.com/advocacy/ narsad/newsletter.html, 1426
www.mhsource.com/advocacy/narsad /narsadfaqs.html, 1427
www.mhsource.com/advocacy/narsad/ studyops.html, 1428
www.mhsource.com/narsad.html, 1429
www.naminys.org, 1430
www.nimh.nih.gov/publicat/schizoph.htm, 1431
www.recovery-inc.com, 1434
www.schizophrenia.com, 1435, 3584
www.schizophrenia.com/ami, 3585
www.schizophrenia.com/discuss/, 1436
www.schizophrenia.com/newsletter, 1437, 3586
www.schizophrenia.com/newsletter/buckets/ success.html, 1438

Sexual Disorders

Back on Track: Boys Dealing with Sexual Abuse, 1445
Dangerous Sex Offenders: a Task Force Report of the American Psychiatric Association, 1446
Erectile Dysfunction: Integrating Couple Therapy, Sex Therapy and Medical Treatment, 3085
Family Violence & Sexual Assault Bulletin, 1457
Family Violence & Sexual Assault Institute, 1731
Handbook of Sexual and Gender Identity Disorder, 1447
Homosexuality and American Psychiatry: The Politics of Diagnosis, 3008
Hypoactive Sexual Desire: Integrating Sex and Couple Therapy, 3086
Interviewing the Sexually Abused Child, 1448, 3133
Masculinity and Sexuality: Selected Topics in the Psychology of Men, 1449
National Assocaition for the Dually Diagnose d (NADD), 1441
Principles and Practice of Sex Therapy, 1450, 3010
Quickies: The Handbook of Brief Sex Therapy, 1452
Sexual Aggression, 1453
Sexuality and People with Disabilities, 1454
Therapy for Adults Molested as Children: Beyond Survival, 1455
Treating Intellectually Disabled Sex Offenders: A Model Residential Program, 1456
Treating the Aftermath of Sexual Abuse: a Handbook for Working with Children in Care, 3158
www.cs.uu.nl/wais/html/na-bng/alt.support.ab use-partners.html, 1458
www.emdr.com, 941, 1459
www.firelily.com/gender/sstgfaq, 1460
www.priory.com/sex.htm, 1463
www.shrinktank.com, 1465
www.xs4all.nl/~rosalind/cha-assr.html, 1466

Sleep Disorders

Abbott Laboratories, 4630
American Academy of Sleep Medicine, 1468
Cephalon, 4634
Concise Guide to Evaluation and Management of Sleep Disorders, 1475
Principles and Practice of Sleep Medicine, 1477
Sleep Disorders Sourcebook, Second Edition, 1478
Sleep Disorders Unit of Beth Israel Hospital, 3916
Synthon Pharmaceuticals, 4660
Valeant Pharmaceuticals International, 4662
Wyeth, 4664
www.aasmnet.org, 1479
www.nhlbi.nih.gov/about/ncsdr, 1482
www.nlm.nih.gov/medlineplus/sleepdisorders. html, 1483
www.sleepdisorders.about.com, 1486
www.sleepdisorders.com, 1487
www.sleepfoundation.org, 1488
www.sleepnet.com, 1489
www.talhost.net/sleep/links.htm, 1490

Suicide

Adolescent Suicide, 1499
Adolescent Suicide: A School-Based Approach to Assessment and Intervention, 1500
American Association of Suicidology, 1492
American Foundation for Suicide Prevention, 1493
An Unquiet Mind: A Memoir of Moods and Madne ss, 1501
Anatomy of Suicide: Silence of the Heart, 1502
Assessment and Prediction of Suicide, 3087
Brilliant Madness: Living with Manic-Depressive Illness, 1503
Compassionate Friends, 35
Comprehensive Textbook of Suicidology, 3088
Exubernace: The Passion for Life, 1504
Friends for Survival, 36, 1519
In the Wake of Suicide, 1506
Left Alive: After a Suicide Death in the Family, 1507
Manic-Depressive Illness: Bipolar Disorders and Recurrent Depression, 888, 1508
My Son...My Son: A Guide to Healing After De ath, Loss, or Suicide, 1509
Night Falls Fast: Understanding Suicide, 1510
NineLine, 1520
No Time to Say Goodbye: Surviving the Suicid e of a Loved One, 1511
Suicidal Patient: Principles of Assesment, Treatment, and Case Management, 1512
Suicide From a Psychological Prespective, 3090
Suicide Over the Life Cycle, 1513
Suicide Prevention Action Network USA (SPANUSA), 1498
Suicide Talk: What To Do If You Hear It, 1516
Suicide: Fast Fact 3, 1517
Suicide: Who Is at Risk?, 1518
Survivors of Loved Ones' Suicides (SOLOS), 17, 40, 1521
Touched with Fire: Manic-Depressive Illness and The Artistic Temperament, 1514
Understanding and Preventing Suicide: New Perspectives, 1515
www.1000deaths.com, 41
www.friendsforsurvival.org, 57
www.lollie.com/about/suicide.html, 1523
www.lollie.com/blue/suicide.html, 3547
www.members.aol.com/dswgriff, 3554
www.members.aol.com/dswgriff/suicide.html, 1524
www.members.tripod.com/~suicideprevention / index, 1525
www.metanoia.org/suicide/, 1527, 3558
www.psycom.net/depression.central.suicide. html, 1530
www.save.org, 1531, 3583
www.vcc.mit.edu/comm/samaritans/brochure. html, 1532
www.vvc.mit.edu/comm/samaritans/warning. html, 1533

Tic Disorders

Adam and the Magic Marble, 1542
After the Diagnosis...The Next Steps, 1561
Children with Tourette Syndrome: A
  Parent's Guide, 1543
Children with Tourette Syndrome: A
  Parents' Guide, 1544
Clinical Counseling: Toward a Better
  Understanding of TS, 1562
Complexities of TS Treatment: Physician's
  Roundtable, 1563
Don't Think About Monkeys: Extraordinary
  Stories Written by People with Tourette
  Syndrome, 1545
Echolalia: an Adult's Story of Tourette
  Syndrome, 1546
Family Life with Tourette Syndrome...
  Personal Stories, 1564
Hi, I'm Adam: a Child's Story of Tourette
  Syndrome, 1547
I Can't Stop!: A Story About Tourette
  Syndrome, 1548
Mind of its Own, Tourette's Syndrome:
  Story and a Guide, 1549
National Alliance on Mental Illness, 268,
  396, 552, 710, 863, 988, 1238, 1285, 1361,
  1470, 1494, 1536
National Mental Health Consumers'
  Self-Help Clearinghouse, 13, 99, 272,
  400, 555, 714, 785, 832, 867, 957, 995,
  1088, 1107, 1130, 1169, 1227, 1241, 1288,
  1341, 1365, 1443
RYAN: A Mother's Story of Her
  Hyperactive/ Tourette Syndrome Child,
  458
RYAN: a Mother's Story of Her
  Hyperactive/Tourette Syndrome Child,
  1550
Raising Joshua, 1551
SAMHSA'S National Mental Health
  Information Center, 869, 1289, 1342,
  1366, 1444, 1474, 1497, 1540
Tics and Tourette Syndrome: A Handbook
  for Parents and Professionals, 1552
Tourette Syndrome, 1553
Tourette Syndrome Association, 1541, 1560
Tourette Syndrome and Human Behavior,
  1554
Tourette's Syndrome, Tics, Obsession,
  Compulsions: Developmental
  Psychopathology & Clinical Care, 1555
Tourette's Syndrome: The Facts, Second
  Edition, 1556
Tourette's Syndrome: Tics, Obsessions,
  Compulsions, 1557
Treating Tourette Syndrome and Tic
  Disorders : A Guide for Practitioners, 1558
Understanding and Treating the Hereditary
  Psychiatric Spectrum Disorders, 849,
  1210, 1565
What Makes Ryan Tic?, 1559
www.mentalhealth.com, 243, 814, 1232,
  1273, 1323, 1351, 1422, 1461, 1481, 1526,
  1566
www.planetpsych.com, 383, 505, 694, 770,
  820, 851, 945, 976, 1080, 1221, 1233,
  1277, 1325, 1352, 1432, 1462, 1484, 1528,
  1567
www.psychcentral.com, 252, 384, 506, 771,
  822, 852, 946, 977, 1081, 1222, 1234,
  1278, 1326, 1353, 1433, 1464, 1485, 1529,
  1568
www.tourette-syndrome.com, 1569
www.tourettesyndrome.net, 1570
www.tsa-usa.com, 1571
www.tsa-usa.org, 1572

A

AA-Alcoholics Anonymous, 232
AACAP, 3202
AACAP News, 3202
AACP, 3226
AAHP/Dorland Directory of Health Plans, 3621
AAMA Annual Conference, 3165
AAMI Newsletter, 3203
AAMR: American Association on Mental Retardation, 1690
AAPL Newsletter, 3204
ABCs of Parenting, 1640
ABE American Board of Examiners in Clinical Social Work, 4112
ACC, 4352
ACORN Behavioral Care Management Corporation, 4113
ACS Healthcare Solutions, 4353
AD/HD Forms Book: Identification, Measurement, and Intervention, 402
ADD & Learning Disabilities: Reality, Myths, & Controversial Treatments, 403
ADD & Romance, 404
ADD Hyperactivity Handbook for Schools, 405
ADD Kaleidoscope: The Many Facets of Adult Attention Deficit Disorder, 406
ADD Success Stories: Guide to Fulfillment for Families with Attention Deficit Disorder, 407
ADD Warehouse, 473, 477, 478, 485, 886
ADD and Adolescence: Strategies for Success, 408
ADD in the Workplace: Choices, Changes and Challenges, 409
ADD/ADHD Checklist: an Easy Reference for Parents & Teachers, 410
ADDitude Magazine, 473
ADHD & LD: Powerful Teaching Strategies & Ac comodations, 477
ADHD Monitoring System, 411
ADHD Parenting Handbook: Practical Advise fo r Parents, 412
ADHD Report, 474
ADHD Survival Guide for Parents and Teachers, 413
ADHD and Teens: Parent's Guide to Making it Through the Tough Years, 414
ADHD and the Nature of Self-Control, 415
ADHD in Adolesents: Diagnosis and Treatment, 2952
ADHD in Adulthood: Guide to Current Theory, Diagnosis and Treatment, 2953
ADHD in the Young Child: Driven to Redirection, 416
ADHD-Inclusive Instruction & Collaborative Practices, 478
ADHD: A Complete and Authoritative Guide, 417
ADHD: What Can We Do?, 479
ADHD: What Do We Know?, 480
ADL Data Systems, 4534
AHMAC, 4354
AIMS, 4355
AJMR-American Journal on Mental Retardation, 3205
AMA's Annual Medical Communications Conferen ce, 3166
AMCO Computers, 4356
ANCOR, 3624

ANKA Behavioral Health, 3746
AP-LS Central Office, 2563
APA Books, 1005
APA Monitor, 3206
ARC News, 3207
ARH Psychiatric Center, 3872
ASAP Newsletter, 3208
ASD: Heads Up for the Low Down, 655
ASP Software, 4357
Abbott Laboratories, 4630
Abilify, 4665
About Alcohol, 156
About Crack Cocaine, 157
About Drug Addiction, 158
About Teens Now, 1687
About.Com, 3514
About.com on Sleep Disorders, 1486
Abusive Personality: Violence and Control in Intimate Relationships, 3013
Academy for International Health Studies, 3187
Academy of Managed Care Providers, 4115
Academy of Psychosomatic Medicine, 2505
Acceptance and Commitment Therapy for Anxiet y Disorders, 278
Access Behavioral Care, 4116
Accreditation Services, 4358
Accumedic Computer Systems, 4359, 4535
Ackerman Institute for the Family, 3342
Action Autonomie, 1691
Action Healthcare Management, 4117
Active Intervention, 3343
Active Parenting Now, 847
Active Parenting Publishers, 3665, 847, 1068
Active Treatment of Depression, 2979
Activities for Adolescents in Therapy, 3595
Activities for Children in Therapy: Guide for Planning and Facilitating Therapy with Troubled Children, 3596
Activities for Developing Pre-Skill Concepts in Children with Autism, 562
Adam Software, 4360
Adam and the Magic Marble, 1542
Adanta Group-Behavioral Health Services, 4118
Adaptive Behavior and Its Measurement Implications for the Field of Mental Retardation, 2689
Adderall/Adderall XR, 4666
Addiction Resource Guide, 234
Addiction Treatment Homework Planner, 2883
Addiction Treatment Planner, 2884
Addiction Workbook: A Step by Step Guide to Quitting Alcohol and Drugs, 105
Addiction: Why Can't They Just Stop?, 106
Addictive Behaviors Across the Life Span, 2885
Addictive Thinking: Understanding Self-Deception, 2886
Addressing the Specific needs of Women with Co-Occuring Disorders in the Criminal Justice System, 2690
Administration for Children and Families, 2180
Administration for Children, Youth and Families, 2181
Administration on Aging, 2182
Administration on Developmental Disabilities US Department of Health & Human Services, 2183
Adolescence Directory On-Line, 1649

Adolescent Suicide, 1499
Adolescent Suicide: A School-Based Approach to Assessment and Intervention, 1500
Adolescent and Family Institute of Colorado, 1841
Adolescents in Psychiatric Hospitals: A Psychodynamic Approach to Evaluation and Treatment, 3093
Adolescents, Alcohol and Drugs: A Practical Guide for Those Who Work With Young People, 2887
Adolescents, Alcohol and Substance Abuse: Reaching Teens through Brief Interventions, 2888
Adolesent in Family Therapy: Breaking the Cycle of Conflict and Control, 3094
Adult Children of Alcoholics World Services Organization, 198, 235
Adult Learning Systems, 4119
Adults with Attention Deficit Disorder: ADD Isn't Just Kids Stuff, 481
Adults with Autism, 563
Advanced Data Systems, 4361
Advanced Psychotherapy Association, 2506
Advances in Projective Drawing Interpetation, 2691
Advancing DSM: Dilemmas in Psychiatric Diagnosis, 2692
Advanstar Communications, 3240
Adventures in Fast Forward: Life, Love and Work for the ADD Adult, 418
Adverse Effects of Psychotropic Drugs, 2693
Advocate Ravenswood Hospital Medical Center, 3825
Advocate: Autism Society of America, 3209
Advocates for Human Potential, 1692
Advocating for Your Child, 496, 1643
Aetna InteliHealth, 1117
Aetna-US HealthCare, 4120
After School And More, 78
After School and More, 698
After the Crash: Assessment and Treatment of Motor Vehicle Accident Survivors, 1291
After the Diagnosis...The Next Steps, 1561
Against Depression, 871
Ageless Design, 803
Agency for Healthcare Research & Quality, 2507
Agency for Healthcare Research and Quality: Office of Communications and Knowledge Transfer, 2184
Aggression Replacement Training Video: A Comprehensive Intervention for Aggressive Youth, 1633
Aggression Replacement Training: A Comprehensive Intervention for Aggressive Youth, 1596
Agilent Technologies, 4362
Agility in Health Care, 2694
Aging and Post Traumatic Stress Disorder, 1292
Agitation in Patients with Dementia: a Practical Guide to Diagnosis and Management, 788
The Agoraphobia Workbook, 325
Agoraphobia: For Friends/Family, 382
Agoraphobics Building Independent Lives, 353
Agoraphobics in Motion, 260, 362
Akzo Nobel, 4631
Al-Anon Family Group Headquarters, 159

Al-Anon Family Group National Referral Hotline, 199
Al-Anon and Alateen, 1638
Al-Anon/Alateen, 236
Alabama Alliance for the Mentally Ill, 1800
Alabama Department of Human Resources, 2231
Alabama Department of Mental Health and Mental Retardation, 2232
Alabama Department of Public Health, 2233
Alabama Disabilities Advocacy Program, 2234
Alaska Alliance for the Mentally Ill, 1806
Alaska Council on Emergency Medical Services, 2235
Alaska Department of Health & Social Services, 2236
Alaska Division of Mental Health and Developmental Disabilities, 2237
Alaska Health and Social Services Division of Behavioral Health, 2238
Alaska Mental Health Board, 2239
Alaska Psychiatric Institute, 3741
Alateen Talk, 159
Alateen and Al-Anon Family Groups, 1624
Albert Whitman & Company, 1548
Alcohol & Drug Abuse Weekly, 3210
Alcohol & Other Drugs: Health Facts, 107
Alcohol ABC's, 160
Alcohol Issues Insights, 161
The Alcohol Policy Information System (APIS), 2202
Alcohol Self-Test, 162
Alcohol and Drug Council of Middle Tennessee, 2437
Alcohol and Sex: Prescription for Poor Decision Making, 213
Alcohol and the Community, 108
Alcohol and the Elderly, 237
Alcohol: Incredible Facts, 163
Alcohol: the Substance, the Addiction, the Solution, 214
Alcoholics Anonymous (AA): World Services, 200
Alcoholics Anonymous (AA): Worldwide, 81
Alcoholism Sourcebook, 109
Alcoholism: A Merry-Go-Round Named Denial, 164
Alcoholism: A Treatable Disease, 165
Aldrich and Cox, 4121
Aleppos Foundation, 1693
Alexian Brothers Bonaventure House, 3826
Alfred Adler Institute (AAI), 3344
Alive Alone, 2, 43
All About ADHD: Complete Practical Guide for Classroom Teachers, 2954
All About Attention Deficit Disorder: Revised Edition, 419
All Kinds of Minds, 420
Allendale Association, 1885
Allentown State Hospital, 4028
Alliance Behavioral Care, 4122
Alliance Behavioral Care: University of Cincinnati Psychiatric Services, 3345
Alliance For Community Care, 4123
Alliance for Children and Families, 2508, 3248
Alliance for the Mentally Ill, 3585
Alliance for the Mentally Ill: Friends & Advocates of the Mentally Ill, 2014
Alliance of Genetic Support Groups, 1694
Allies for Youth & Families, 2125

Allina Hospitals & Clinics Behavioral Health Services, 4124
Allyn & Bacon, 145
Alpha, 733
Alternative Support for Eating Disorder, 1070
Alton Mental Health Center, 3827
Alton Ochsner Medical Foundation, Psychiatry Residency, 3346
Alzheimer Research Forum, 806
Alzheimer's Association National Office, 775
Alzheimer's Disease Bookstore, 807
Alzheimer's Disease Education and Referral, 801
Alzheimer's Disease Education and Referral Center, 776
Alzheimer's Disease International, 805
Alzheimer's Disease Research and the American Health Assistance Foundation, 799
Alzheimer's Disease Sourcebook, 789
Alzheimer's Disease: Activity-Focused Care, Second Edition, 790
Alzheimer's Outreach, 824
AlzheimerSupport.com, 808
Ambien/Ambien CR, 4667
Ambiguous Loss: Learning to Live with Unresolved Grief, 2880
Ameican Society on Aging, 1748
AmeriChoice, 4125
Amerian Medical Group Association, 3241
Americal Board of Medical Psychotherapists & Psychodiagnosticians, 3271
American Academy of Child and Adolescent Psychiatry (AACAP): Annual Meeting, 3167
American Academy Of Pediatrics, 417
American Academy of Addiction Psychiatry, 166
American Academy of Addiction Psychiatry (AAAP), 82
American Academy of Addiction Psychiatry: Annual Meeting, 3168
American Academy of Child & Adolescent Psychiatry, 2509
American Academy of Child and Adolescent Psychiatry, 1573, 1695, 3347, 3622, 3223, 3510
American Academy of Clinical Psychiatrists, 2510
American Academy of Medical Administrators, 2511, 3165
American Academy of Neurology, 802, 3511
American Academy of Pediatrics, 1574, 1696
American Academy of Pediatrics Practice Guidelines on ADHD, 491
American Academy of Psychiatry & Law, 3169
American Academy of Psychiatry & Law Annual Conference, 3169
American Academy of Psychiatry and the Law, 3204
American Academy of Psychiatry and the Law (AAPL), 2512
American Academy of Psychoanalysis Preliminary Meeting, 3170
American Academy of Psychoanalysis and Dynam ic Psychiatry, 2513, 3623
American Academy of Psychoanalysis and Dynamic Psychiatry, 3170, 3623
American Academy of Sleep Medicine, 1468, 1479
American Anorexia/Bulimia Association, 980

American Anorexia/Bulimia Association News, 1045
American Association for Geriatric Psychiatry, 1697
American Association for Marriage and Family Therapy, 2514
American Association for Protecting Children, 2515
American Association of Black Psychologists, 3515
American Association of Chairs of Department s of Psychiatry, 2517
American Association of Children's Residential Centers, 2518, 3171
American Association of Community Psychiatrists (AACP), 2516, 3211
American Association of Directors of Psychiatric Residency Training, 2519
American Association of Geriatric Psychiatry (AAGP), 2520
American Association of Geriatric Psychiatry Annual Meetings, 3172
American Association of Health Care Consultants, 3173
American Association of Health Plans, 2521
American Association of Healthcare Consultants, 2522
American Association of Homes & Services for the Aging, 3174
American Association of Homes and Services for the Aging, 2523
American Association of Mental Health Professionals in Corrections (AAMHPC), 2524
American Association of Pastoral Counselors, 2525
American Association of Pharmaceutical Scientists, 2526
American Association of Psychiatric Services for Children (AAPSC), 1698
American Association of Retired Persons, 2527
American Association of Suicidology, 1492
American Association on Intellectual and Dev elopmental Disabilities Annual Meeting, 3175
American Association on Mental Retardation (AAR), 2528
American Bar Association, 3273
American Board of Disability Analysts Annual Conference, 3176
American Board of Examiners in Clinical Social Work, 2485, 2529, 3513
American Board of Examiners of Clinical Social Work Regional Offices, 2486
American Board of Professional Psychology (ABPP), 2530
American Board of Psychiatry and Neurology (ABPN), 2531
American College Health Association, 2532
American College of Health Care Administrators: ACHCA Annual Meeting, 3177
American College of Health Care Administrators (ACHCA), 2533
American College of Healthcare Executives, 2534, 3348, 3178, 3238
American College of Healthcare Executives Educational Events, 3178
American College of Mental Health Administration (ACMHA), 2535
American College of Osteopathic Neurologists & Psychiatrists, 2536
American College of Psychiatrists, 2537

American College of Psychiatrists Annual Meeting, 3179

American College of Psychoanalysts (ACPA), 2538

American College of Women's Health Physicians, 3349

American Council on Alcoholism, 83, 233

American Counseling Association, 2539, 357, 2925, 2926, 3495, 3499, 3530

American Counseling Association (ACA), 2540

American Foundation for Suicide Prevention, 1493

American Geriatrics Society, 2541

American Group Psychotherapy Association, 2542, 3180

American Group Psychotherapy Association Annual Conference, 3180

American Health Assistance Foundation, 777, 799, 804

American Health Care Association, 2543, 3290

American Health Care Association Annual Convention, 3181

American Health Information Management Association Annual Exhibition and Conference, 2544, 3182

American Health Information Management Association, 3254, 3255

American Holistic Health Association, 1699

American Hospital Association: Section for Psychiatric and Substance Abuse, 2545

American Institute for Preventive Medicine, 3212, 4536, 1308

American Institute for Preventive Medicine Press, 3212

American Journal on Addictions, 166

American Managed Behavioral Healthcare Association, 1700, 2546, 4126

American Medical Association, 2547, 3166, 3516

American Medical Directors Association, 2548

American Medical Group Association, 2549

American Medical Informatics Association, 2550, 3264

American Medical Software, 4363

American Mental Health Counselors Association (AMHCA), 2551

American Network of Community Options and Resources-Directory of Members, 1701, 3624

American Neuropsychiatric Association, 2552, 3261

American Nurses Association, 2553

American Nurses Foundation: National Communications, 4537

American Orthopsychiatric Association, 3287

American Pediatrics Society, 1575, 1702

American Pharmacists Association, 2554

American Psychiatric Association, 1703, 821, 3576

American Psychiatric Association (APA), 2555

American Psychiatric Association Practice Guideline for the Treatment of Patients With Substance Use Disorders, 110

American Psychiatric Association Practice Guideline for the Treatment of Patients with Delirium, 791

American Psychiatric Association-Membership Directory, 3625

American Psychiatric Glossary, 2695

American Psychiatric Nurses Association, 2556, 3519

American Psychiatric Press, 2729, 2827, 2975, 3126

American Psychiatric Press Reference Library CD-ROM, 4364

American Psychiatric Press Textbook of Substance Abuse Treatment, 2889

American Psychiatric Publishing Textbook of Clinical Psychiatry, 2696

American Psychiatric Publishing (APPI), 3666

American Psychiatric Publishing Inc, 3520

The American Psychiatric Publishing Textbook of Anxiety Disorders, 326

American Psychoanalytic Association (APsaA), 2558

American Psychoanalytic Association - Roster, 3626

American Psychoanalytic Asssociation, 3521

American Psychologial Association: Division of Family Psychology, 2559

American Psychological Association, 1704, 2560, 134, 140, 318, 332, 1318, 2825, 3206, 3258, 3306, 3518, 3578, 3626

American Psychological Association Database Department/PsycINFO, 2860, 3291

American Psychological Association Division of Independent Practice (APADIP), 2561

American Psychological Association: Applied Experimental and Engineering Psychology, 2562

American Psychological Publishing, 1291, 2819

American Psychology- Law Society (AP-LS), 2563

American Psychosomatic Society, 2564, 3305

American Public Human Services Association, 84

American Society for Adolescent Psychiatry, 3208

American Society for Adolescent Psychiatry (ASAP), 2565

American Society for Adolescent Psychiatry: Annual Meeting, 3183

American Society for Clinical Pharmacology & Therapeutics, 2566

American Society of Addiction Medicine, 3197, 2914, 3185

American Society of Consultant Pharmacists, 2567

American Society of Group Psychotherapy & Psychodrama, 2568

American Society of Health System Pharmacists, 2569

American Society of Psychoanalytic Physicians (ASPP), 2570

American Society of Psychoanalytic Physicians: Membership Directory, 3627

American Society of Psychopathology of Expression (ASPE), 2571

American Society on Aging, 2572

Americans with Disabilities Act and the Emerging Workforce, 2697

AmericasDoctor.com, 3517

Amongst Ourselves: A Self-Help Guide to Living with Dissociative Identity Disorder, 960

An Elephant in the Living Room: Leader's Guide for Helping Children of Alcoholics, 2890

An End to Panic: Breakthrough Techniques for Overcoming Panic Disorder, 279

An Unquiet Mind: A Memoir of Moods and Madne ss, 1501

Anafranil, 4668

Analysis Group Economics, 4127

Analytic Press, 3667, 2785, 2822, 2826, 3011, 3061, 3266, 3285

Anasazi Software, 4365

Anatomy of Suicide: Silence of the Heart, 1502

Anatomy of a Psychiatric Illness: Healing the Mind and the Brain, 3069

Ancora Psychiatric Hospital, 3733

Andrew McFarland Mental Health Center, 3828

Andrew and Associates, 4366

Andrus Children's Center, 3350

The Anger Control Workbook, 1144

Anger and Aggression, 1159

Angry All the Time, 1134

Angry Heart: Overcoming Borderline and Addictive Disorders, 1245

Ann Arbor Consultation Services Performance & Health Solutions, 1950

Ann Klein Forensic Center, 3948

Annie E Casey Foundation, 2573

Annual Early Childhood Conference: Effective Relationship-Based Practices in Promoting Positive Child Outcomes, 3184

Annual Meeting & Medical-Scientific Conference, 3185

Annual Santa Fe Psychiatric Symposium, 3186

Annual Summit on International Managed Care Trends, 3187

Anorexia Bulimia Treatment and Education Center, 981

Anorexia Nervosa & Recovery: a Hunger for Meaning, 1000

Anorexia Nervosa General Information, 1078

Anorexia Nervosa and Related Eating Disorders, 982, 1071

Anorexia/Bulimia Association of New Jersey, 2010

Anorexia: Am I at Risk?, 1046

Answers to Distraction, 421

Answers to Your Questions About ADD, 495

Answers to Your Questions about Panic Disorder, 364

Antabuse, 4669

Anthem BC/BS of Virginia, 2137

Antidepressant Fact Book: What Your Doctor Won't Tell You About Prozac, Zoloft, Paxil, Celexa and Luvox, 2980

Antipsychotic Medications: A Guide, 2981

Antisocial Behavior by Young People, 834

Anxiety & Phobia Workbook, 280

The Anxiety & Phobia Workbook, Fourth Editio n, 327

The Anxiety Cure for Kids: A Guide for Paren ts, 328

Anxiety Cure: Eight Step-Program for Getting Well, 281

Anxiety Disorders, 282, 335, 357, 1313, 373

Anxiety Disorders Association of America, 261, 294, 295, 301, 304, 306, 308, 320, 321, 331, 361

Anxiety Disorders Fact Sheet, 336

Anxiety Disorders in Children and Adolescents, 1616

Anxiety Disorders: A Scientific Approach for Selecting the Most Effective Treatment, 2931
Anxiety Panic Hub, 381
Anxiety and Depression in Adults and Children, Banff International Behavioral Science Series, 872
Anxiety and Its Disorders, 283
Anxiety and Phobia Treatment Center, 262, 372
Anxiety, Phobias, and Panic, 284
Anxiety, Phobias, and Panic: a Step-By-Step Program for Regaining Control of Your Life, 285
Aon Consulting Group, 4128
Apache Medical Systems, 4538
Appalachian Behavioral Healthcare System, 4006
Applied Computing Services, 4539
Applied Informatics (ILIAD), 4540
Applied Relaxation Training in the Treatment of PTSD and Other Anxiety Disorders, 2932
Apserger Syndrome Education Network of America (ASPEN), 509
Arbour Health System-Human Resource Institute Hospital, 4541
Arbour-Fuller Hospital, 3905
Archways-A Bridge To A Brighter Future, 3790
Are You Alone on Purpose?, 564
Are the Kids Alright?, 1634
Aricept, 4670
Aries Systems Corporation, 4367
Arizona Alliance for the Mentally Ill, 1809
Arizona Alliance for the Mentally Ill (NAMI Arizona), 3203
Arizona Center For Mental Health PHD, 4129
Arizona Department of Health Services, 2241
Arizona Department of Health Services: Behavioral Services, 2242
Arizona Department of Health Services: Child Fatality Review, 2243
Arizona Department of Health: Substance Abuse, 2244
Arizona State Hospital, 3742
Arkansas Alliance for the Mentally Ill, 1818
Arkansas Department Health & Human Services, 2246
Arkansas Division of Children & Family Service, 2247
Arkansas Division on Youth Services, 2248
Arkansas State Hospital, 3744
Arkansas State Mental Hospital, 2249
Arms Acres, 3957
Arservices, Limited, 4542
Arthur Brisbane Child Treatment Center, 3949
Arthur S Shorr and Associates, 4130
Artificial Intelligence, 4543
Ascent, 4368
Asher Meadow, 1097
Asher Meadow Newsletter, 1096
Asian Pacific Development Center for Human Development, 3351
Ask NOAH About: Aging and Alzheimer's Disease, 818
Askesis Development Group, 4369
Aspects of Autism: Biological Research, 565
The Asperger Parent: How to Raise a Child with Asperger Syndrome and Maintain Your Sense of Humor, 531

Asperger Syndrome, 566
Asperger Syndrome Diagnostic Scale (ASDS), 2950
Asperger Syndrome Education Network (ASPEN), 540, 676
Asperger Syndrome Education Network (ASPEN) Conference, 537
Asperger Syndrome: A Practical Guide for Teachers, 567
Asperger Syndrome: Living Outside the Bell Curve, 522
Asperger Syndrome: a Practical Guide for Teachers, 2965
Asperger's Association of New England, 541, 674
Asperger's Association of New England (AANE), 510
Asperger's Diagnostic Assessment with Dr. Tony Attwood, 3490
Asperger's Syndrome: A Guide for Parents and Professionals, 568
Asperger's Syndrome: A Video Guide for Parents and Professionals, 523
Asperger's Syndrome: An Interview with Lars Perner and Philip Brousseau, 524
Asperger's Syndrome: Autism and Obsessive Behavior, 525
Asperger's Unplugged, an Interview with Jerry Newport, 526
Aspergers Resource Links, 532, 533, 534
Aspergers Syndrome: A Guide for Educators and Parents, Second Edition, 569
Aspies for Freedom, 535
Assesing Problem Behaviors, 2698
Assess Dialogue Personality Disorders, 1246
Assessing Sex Offenders: Problems and Pitfalls, 3084
Assessing Substance Abusers with the Million Clinical Multiaxial Inventory, 2891
Assessment and Prediction of Suicide, 3087
Assessment and Treatment of Anxiety Disorders in Persons with Mental Retardation, 3316
Assessment of Eating Disorders, 1001
Assessment of Neuropsychiatry and Mental Health Services, 3317
Assimilation, Rational Thinking, and Suppression in the Treatment of PTSD and Other Anxiety Disorders, 2933
Assist Technologies, 4370
Assistance League of Southern California, 1820
Associated Counseling Services, 4131
Association for Academic Psychiatry (AAP), 2574
Association for Advancement of Behavior Therapy: Membership Directory, 3628
Association for Advancement of Mental Health, 2000
Association for Advancement of Psychoanalysis: Karen Horney Psychoanalytic Institute and Center, 2575
Association for Ambulatory Behavioral Healthcare, 2576, 3188, 4544
Association for Applied Psychophysiology & Biofeedback, 2577
Association for Applied Psychophysiology and Biofeedback, 3512
Association for Behavior Analysis, 2578
Association for Behavioral and Cognitive Therapies, 827
Association for Behavioral and Cognitive Therapies, 2579
Association for Birth Psychology, 2580

Association for Child Psychoanalysis, 3213
Association for Child Psychoanalysis Newsletter, 3213
Association for Child Psychoanalysts, 2581
Association for Children of New Jersey, 2001
Association for Hospital Medical Education, 2582
Association for Humanistic Psychology, 2583
Association for Pre- & Perinatal Psychology and Health, 2584
Association for Psychoanalytic Medicine (APM), 2585
Association for Psychological Science, 2586
Association for Psychological Type, 3221
Association for Research in Nervous and Ment al Disease, 2587
Association for Retarded Citizens-Pennsylvania, 3207
Association for Women in Psychology, 2588
Association for the Advancement of Psycholog y, 2589
Association for the Care of Children's Health, 1705
Association for the Help of Retarded Children, 1576
Association for the Help of Retarded Children, 1706
Association for the Help of Retarded Children (AHRC), 3224
Association for the Scientific Study of Consciousness, 3522
Association of Black Psychologists, 2590, 3293
Association of Black Psychologists Annual Convention, 3189
Association of Maternal and Child Health Programs (AMCHP), 2185
Association of Mental Health Librarians (AMHL), 1707
Association of State and Provincial Psychology Boards, 2591
Association of Traumatic Stress Specialists, 1280
Association of University Centers on Disabilities (UACD), 2592
Association of the Advancement of Gestalt Therapy, 2593
Astra Zeneca Pharmaceuticals, 4632
At Health, 3, 44
At Health Incorporated, 3629
At-Risk Youth in Crises, 3095
AtHealth.Com, 4
Atascadero State Hospital, 3747
Ativan, 4671
Attachment and Interaction, 2881
Attachment, Trauma and Healing: Understanding and Treating Attachment Disorder in Children and Families, 3096
Attention Deficit Disorder, 492
Attention Deficit Disorder ADHD and ADD Syndromes, 2955
Attention Deficit Disorder Association, 390, 493
Attention Deficit Disorder and Learning Disabilities: Realities, Myths and Controversial Treatments, 422, 2956
Attention Deficit Disorder and Parenting Site, 490
Attention Deficit Hyperactivity Disorder, 503
Attention Deficit Hyperactivity Disorder in Children: A Medication Guide, 423
Attention Deficit/Hyperactivity Disorder, 2957

Attention Deficits and Hyperactivity in Children: Developmental Clinical Psychology and Psychiatry, 424
Attention-Deficit Hyperactivity Disorder in Adults: A Guide, 425
Attention-Deficit Hyperactivity Disorder: A Handbook for Diagnosis and Treatment, 2958
Attention-Deficit/Hyperactivity Disorder Test: a Method for Identifying Individuals with ADHD, 3318
Attention-Deficit/Hyperactivity Disorder in Children and Adolescents, 1617
Attention-Deficit/Hyperactivity Disorder in the Classroom, 2959
Attention-Deficit/Hyperactiviy Disorder in Children and Adolescents, 1667
Augustus F Hawkins Community Mental Health Center, 3748
Austin State Hospital, 4061
Austin Travis County Mental Health Mental Retardation Center, 4371
Austin Travis County Mental Health: Mental Retardation Center, 2448
Autism, 570
Autism & Asperger Syndrome, 571
Autism & Sensing: The Unlost Instinct, 572
Autism Asperger Publishing, 530
Autism Asperger Publishing Company, 531
Autism Bibliography, 573
Autism DVD Package, 656
Autism Network International, 511, 675
Autism Newslink, 641
Autism Research Foundation, 542
The Autism Research Foundation, 688
Autism Research Institute, 512, 543, 642, 679
Autism Research Review International, 642
Autism Services Center, 544, 652, 680
Autism Society News, 643
Autism Society Ontario, 641
Autism Society of America, 513, 545, 653, 677, 3209
Autism Society of North Carolina, 2037
Autism Spectrum, 574
Autism Spectrum Disorders and the SCERTS, 657
Autism Spectrum Disorders in Children and Adolescents, 1618
Autism Spectrum Disorders: The Complete Guid to Understanding Autism, Asperger's Syndrome, Pervasive Developmental Disorder, and, 575
Autism Treatment Center of America Son-Rise Program, 654
Autism Treatment Center of America: The Son -Rise Program, 514
Autism Treatment Guide, 576
Autism and Pervasive Developmental Disorders, 577
Autism in Children and Adolescents, 644
Autism in the Classroom, 658
Autism is a World, 659
Autism: A Strange, Silent World, 660
Autism: A World Apart, 661
Autism: An Inside-Out Approach An Innovative Look at the Mechanics of Autism and its Developmental Cousins, 578
Autism: An Introduction to Psychological Theory, 579
Autism: Being Friends, 662
Autism: Explaining the Enigma, 580
Autism: From Tragedy to Triumph, 581

Autism: Identification, Education and Treatment, 582
Autism: Nature, Diagnosis and Treatment, 583
Autism: Strategies for Change, 584
Autistic Adults at Bittersweet Farms, 585
Autistic Services, 546, 682
Avoiding The Turbulance: Guiding Families of Children Diagnosed with Autism, 663
Avoiding Unfortunate Situations, 586
Aware Resources, 4372
Awareness Foundation for OCD, 1207

B

BOSS Inc, 4373
BPSO-Bipolar Significant Others, 756, 3524
Baby Fold, 1886
BabyCenter, 498
Babylon Consultation Center, 2015
Back on Track: Boys Dealing with Sexual Abuse, 1445
Bad Boys, Bad Men: Confronting Antisocial Personality Disorder, 3025
Bad Men Do What Good Men Dream: a Forensic Psychiatrist Illuminates the Darker Side of Human Behavior, 835
Baker & Taylor International, 591, 594
Baker and Taylor, 3668
Baldpate Hospital, 3906
Bantam Books, 1503
Bantam Doubleday Dell Publishing, 403, 422, 838, 2755
Barbanell Associates, 4132
Barry Associates, 4133
Basic Books, 890
Basic Child Psychiatry, 3097
Basic Guided Relaxation: Advanced Technique, 367
Basic Personal Counseling: Training Manual for Counslers, 2699
Baywood Publishing Company, 3251, 3252, 3253, 3257
Bazelon Center for Mental Health Law, 1708, 2594
Beaver Creek Software, 4374
Beer Marketer's Insights, 161
Before It's Too Late: Working with Substance Abuse in the Family, 2892
Behavior Modification for Exceptional Children and Youth, 3098
Behavior Rating Profile, 3099
Behavioral Approach to Assessment of Youth with Emotional/Behavioral Disorders, 3100
Behavioral Approaches: Problem Child, 3101
Behavioral Complications in Alzheimer's Disease, 792
Behavioral Health Advisor, 4375
Behavioral Health Care, 4134
Behavioral Health Care Consultants, 4135
Behavioral Health Industry News, 3214, 3288, 4605
Behavioral Health Management, 3215
Behavioral Health Management Group, 4136
Behavioral Health Options: Sierra Health Services, 3943
Behavioral Health Partners, 4137
Behavioral Health Record Section-AMRA, 3237
Behavioral Health Services, 4138

Behavioral Health Systems, 2595, 4139
Behavioral Healthcare Center, 3352
Behavioral Healthcare Resource Institute, 3475
Behavioral High-Risk Paradigm in Psychopathology, 3078
Behavioral Intervention Planning: Completing a Functional Behavioral Assessment and Developing a Behavioral Intervention Plan, 4545
Behavioral Measurement Database Services, 3630
Behavioral Medicine and Biofeedback Consultants, 3353
Behavioral Risk Management, 2972
Behavioral and Emotional Rating Scale, 3319
Behaviordata, 4376
Behind Bars: Substance Abuse and America's Prison Population, 2893
Bellefaire Jewish Children's Bureau, 4377
Bellin Psychiatric Center, 4107
Bereaved Parents of the USA, 5
Bereaved Parents' Network, 45
Berkowitz Chassion and Sklar, 4140
Berkshire Center, 3907
Berkshire Farm Center and Services for Youth, 3958
Best Buddies International (BBI), 1709
Best of AAMR: Families and Mental Retardation, 2700
BetaData Systems, 4378
Bethesda Lutheran Homes and Services, 1710
Beyond Anorexia, 1002
Beyond Anxiety and Phobia, 286
Beyond Behavior Modification: Cognitive-Behavioral Approach to Behavior Management in the School, 2973
Beyond Gentle Teaching, 587
Beyond Ritalin, 426
Bibliotherapy Starter Set, 1597
Big Spring State Hospital, 4062
Bill Ferguson's How to Divorce as Friends, 52
Binge Drinking, 215
Binge Drinking: Am I At Risk?, 167
Binge Eating: Nature, Assessment and Treatment, 1003
Biological Basis of Personality, 3026
Biology of Anxiety Disorders, 287
Biology of Personality Disorders, 3027
Biology of Personality Disorders, Review of Psychiatry, 1247
Biology of Schizophrenia and Affective Disease, 1368
Biology of the Autistic Syndromes, 588
Bipolar Affective Disorder in Children and Adolescents, 1663
Bipolar Children and Teens Homepage, 1659
Bipolar Clinic and Research Program, 746
Bipolar Disorder, 734
Bipolar Disorder Frequently Asked Questions, 768, 3563
Bipolar Disorder Survival Guide: What You and Your Family Need to Know, 718
Bipolar Disorder for Dummies, 719
Bipolar Disorders Clinic, 747
Bipolar Disorders Treatment Information Center, 704, 767
Bipolar Disorders: A Guide to Helping Children and Adolescents, 720
Bipolar Disorders: Clinical Course and Outcome, 721
Bipolar Kids Homepage, 761, 1657, 3535

Bipolar Puzzle Solution, 722
Bipolar Research at University of
   Pennsylvan ia, 748
Birds-Eye View of Life with ADD and
   ADHD: Ad vice from Young Survivors,
   Second Edition, 427
Birmingham Psychiatry, 1801
Biting The Hand That Starves You: Inspiring
   Resistance to Anorexia/Bulimia, 2999
Black Mental Health Alliance (BMHA), 1711
Blackwell Publishing, 138
Blaming the Brain: The Truth About Drugs
   and Mental Health, 2894
Blended Families, 1677, 3573
Blue Mountain Recovery Center, 4024
Body Image, 1047
Body Image Workbook: An 8 Step Program
   for Learning to Like Your Looks, 1004
Body Image, Eating Disorders, and Obesity
   in Youth, 1005
Body Image: Understanding Body
   Dissatisfaction in Men, Women and
   Children, 2882
Body Logic, 4379
The Body Remembers Casebook: Unifying
   Methods and Models in the Treatment of
   Trauma and PTSD, 3062
Body Remembers: Psychophysiology of
   Trauma and Trauma Treatment, 3042
The Body Remembers: The Psychphysiology
   of Trauma and Trauma Treatment, 3063
Bolton Press Atlanta, 1509
Bonnie Tapes, 1416
The Bonnie Tapes Mental Illness in the
   Family; Recovering from Mental Illness;
   My Sister is Mentally Ill, 755
Bonny Foundation, 2596
Book of Psychotherapeutic Homework, 1598
A Book: A Collection of Writings from the
   Advocate, 561
Borderline Personality Disorder, 1248
Borderline Personality Disorder Sanctuary,
   1274
The Borderline Personality Disorder Survival
   Guide, 1270
Borderline Personality Disorder:
   Multidimensional Approach, 1249
Borderline Personality Disorder: A Patient's
   Guide to Taking Control, 1250
Borderline Personality Disorder: A Therapist
   Guide to Taking Control, 3028
Borderline Personality Disorder: Etiology and
   Treatment, 1251
Borderline Personality Disorder: Tailoring
   the Psychotherapy to the Patient, 1252
Borderline Personality Disorder: Tailoring
   the Psychotherapy to the Patient, 3029
Borgess Behavioral Medicine Services, 1951
Boundaries and Boundary Violations in
   Psychoanalysis, 2701
Boy Who Couldn't Stop Washing, 1175
Boysville of Michigan, 1952
Brain Calipers: Descriptive Psychopathology
   and the Mental Status Examination,
   Second Edition, 2702
Brain Imaging Handbook, 2487
Brain Lock: Free Yourself from Obsessive
   Compulsive Behavior, 1176
Brainerd Regional Human Services Center,
   3734
Brandeis University/Heller School, 3354
Branden Publishing Company, 581
Brattleboro Retreat, 4085

Breaking the News, 1656
Breaking the Patterns of Depression, 873
Breaking the Silence: Teaching the Next
   Generation About Mental Illness, 1599
Breakthroughs in Antipsychotic Medications:
   A Guide for Consumers, Families, and
   Clinicians, 1369, 2703
Breakthroughs: How to Reach Students with
   Autism, 664
Breining Institute College for the Advanced
   Study of Addictive Disorders, 3355, 4546
Bridges: Building Recovery & Individual
   Dre ams & Goals Through Education &
   Support, 2102
Bridgewell, 1941
Brief Coaching for Lasting Solutions, 2704
Brief Therapy Institute of Denver, 4547
Brief Therapy and Eating Disorders, 1006
Brief Therapy and Managed Care, 2705
Brief Therapy for Adolescent Depression,
   2982
Brief Therapy for Post Traumatic Stress
   Disorder, 3043
Brief Therapy with Intimidating Cases, 2706
Brilliant Madness: Living with
   Manic-Depressive Illness, 1503
Bristol-Myers Squibb, 4633
Broadway Books, 302
Broadway Books a Division of Random
   House, 1511
Broken, 111
Broken Connection: On Death and the
   Continuity of Life, 874
Bronx Children's Psychiatric Center, 3959
Bronx Psychiatric Center, 3960
Brookes Publishing, 3669
Brookings Alliance for the Mentally Ill, 2099
Brookline Books/Lumen Editions, 3670, 622
Brooklyn Children's Center, 3961
Broughton Hospital, 4001
Broward County Healthcare Management,
   4141
Brown Consulting, 4142
Brown Schools Behavioral Health System,
   3356
Brown University: Child & Adolescent
   Psychopharmacology Update, 3216
Brown University: Digest of Addiction
   Theory and Application (DATA), 3217
Brown University: Geriatric
   Psychopharmacology Update, 3218
Brown University: Psychopharmacology
   Update, 3219
Brunner-Routledge Mental Health, 3671
Brunner/Routledge, 2773, 2789, 3050, 3110
BryLin Hospitals, 3962
Bryce Hospital, 3735
BuSpar, 4672
Buckley Productions, 4548
Buffalo Psychiatric Center, 3963
Building Bridges: States Respond to
   Substance Abuse and Welfare Reform,
   2895
Bulimia, 1007, 1048
Bulimia Nervosa, 1008
Bulimia Nervosa & Binge Eating: A Guide
   To Recovery, 1009
Bulimia: a Guide to Recovery, 1010
Bull HN Information Systems, 4380
Bull Publishing Company, 3672
Bulletin of Menninger Clinic, 3220
Bulletin of Psychological Type, 3221
Bundle of Blues, 929

Bureau of Mental Health and Substance
   Abuse Services, 2476
Bureau of TennCare: State of Tennessee,
   2438
Business Objects, 4381
Business Publishers, 3275, 3276
Butler Hospital, 4042

C

CAFCA, 4143
CAMC Family Medicine Center of
   Charleston, 2164
CARE Child and Adolescent Risk
   Evaluation: A Measure of the Risk for
   Violent Behavior, 1600
CARF Directory of Organizations with
   Accredited Programs, 3631
CARF: Commission on Accreditation of
   Rehabil itation Facilities, 2488
CASAWORKS for Families: Promising
   Approach to Welfare Reform and
   Substance-Abusing Women, 2896
CASCAP, 4382
CBCA, 4144
CBI Group, 4145, 4549
CD Publications, 169, 3230, 3277
CG Jung Foundation for Analytical
   Psychology, 2597
CHADD, 408, 3527
CHADD: Children/Adults with Attention
   Deficit/Hyperactivity Disorder, 1639
CHINS UP Youth and Family Services, 1842
CIGNA Behavioral Care, 4146
CIGNA Corporation, 4147
CLARC Services, 4383
CM Tucker Jr Nursing Care Center, 4045
CME Mental Health InfoSource, 3559
CME Psychiatric Time, 3560
CME, Medical Information Source, 3551
CMHC Systems, 4550
CNN Health Section, 3528
COMPSYCH Software Information
   Services, 4551
CPP Incorporated, 3320
CSI Software, 4384
Cabrini Medical Center, 3964
California Alliance for the Mentally Ill, 1821
California Association of Marriage and
   Family Therapists, 1822
California Association of Social
   Rehabilitation Agencies, 1823
California Department of Alcohol and Drug
   Programs: Resource Center, 2228, 2251
California Department of Corrections and
   Reh abilitation, 2252
California Department of Education: Healthy
   Kids, Healthy California, 2253
California Department of Health Services:
   Medi-Cal Drug Discount, 2255
California Department of Health Services:
   Medicaid, 2254
California Department of Health and Human
   Services, 2274
California Department of Managed Health
   Care, 3760
California Department of Mental Health,
   2256, 3763, 3768
California Health Information Association,
   1824

California Hispanic Commission on Alcohol Drug Abuse, 2257
California Institute for Mental Health, 1825, 2258
California Institute of Behavioral Sciences, 3357
California Mental Health Directors Association, 2259
California Psychiatric Association (CPA), 1826
California Psychological Association, 1827
California School of Professional Psychology, 3396
California Women's Commission on Addictions, 2260
Calix Society, 168
Calland and Company, 4148
Calnet, 1828
Cambridge Handbook of Psychology, Health and Medicine, 2707
Cambridge Hospital: Department of Psychiatry, 3358
Cameron and Associates, 4149
Campobello Chemical Dependency Treatment Services, 3749
Campral, 4673
Camps 2008, 79, 699
Canadian Art Therapy Association, 1712
Canadian Federation of Mental Health Nurses, 1713
Canadian Mental Health Association, 1714
Candler General Hospital: Rehabilitation Unit, 3813
Candor, Connection and Enterprise in Adolesent Therapy, 3102
Cape Cod Institute, 3526
Capital District Psychiatric Center, 3965
Capitation Report, 3222
Capitol Publications, 3246
Carbamazepine and Manic Depression: A Guide, 723
Cardiff Software: Vista, 4385
Care That Works: A Relationship Approach to Persons With Dementia, 793
CareCounsel, 4552
Career Assessment & Planning Services, 85, 263, 705, 828, 1124, 1165, 1236, 1281, 1333, 1356, 370
Caregivers Series, 1319
Carewise, 4150
Caro Center, 3920
Carson City Alliance for the Mentally Ill Share & Care Group, 1993
Case Management Resource Guide, 3632
Case Management Resource Guide (Health Care), 3633
Case Manager Database, 3634
Casey Family Services, 4151
Catawba Hospital, 4088
Catholic Community Services of Western Washington, 4553
Causes of Anxiety and Panic Attacks, 363
Cedarcrest Hospital, 3778
Celexa, 4674
Cenaps Corporation, 2489
Centennial Mental Health Center, 3774
The Center Cannot Hold: My Journey Through M adness, 1401
Center For Communications, 2231
Center For Mental Health Services, 6, 391
Center For Prevention and Rehabilitation, 4029

Center for Applications of Psychological Type, 2598
Center for Attitudinal Healing (CAH), 1715
Center for Clinical Computing, 4386
Center for Creative Living, 4554
Center for Family Services, 758
Center for Family Support, 46, 238, 499, 1154
Center for Health Policy Studies, 3359, 4152, 4387
Center for Loss in Multiple Birth, 47
Center for Loss in Multiple Birth (CLIMB), 8
Center for Mental Health Services, 1335, 1358, 1717
Center for Mental Health Services Homeless Programs Branch, 2186
Center for Mental Health Services Knowledge, 87, 265, 393, 548, 707, 779, 1085, 1103, 1126
Center for Mental Health Services Knowledge Exchange Network, 378, 690, 765, 1158
Center for Mental Health Services: Knowledge Exchange Network, 336, 338, 644, 743, 1616, 1617, 1618, 1619, 1620, 1622, 1623
Center for Outcomes Research and Effectiveness, 3745
Center for Substance Abuse Treatment, 2187
Center for the Advancement of Health, 4153
Center for the Study of Adolescence, 1059
Center for the Study of Anorexia and Bulimia, 1060
Center for the Study of Autism (CSA), 678
Center for the Study of Issues in Public Mental Health, 1718
Center on Addiction at Columbia University, 2893, 2895, 2896, 2899, 2907, 2908, 2910, 2911, 2912, 2915, 2919, 2921, 2928, 3141
Centers For Disease Control and Prevention, 2198
Centers for Disease Control & Prevention, 2188
Centers for Medicare & Medicaid Services, 2331
Centers for Medicare & Medicaid Services/CMS: Office of Research, Statisctics, Data and Systems, 2330
Centers for Medicare & Medicaid Services: Health Policy, 2189
Centers for Medicare & Medicaid Services: Office of Policy, 2332
Centers for Medicare and Medicaid Services: Office of Financial Management/OFM, 2333
Centers for Mental Healthcare Research, 4154
Central Behavioral Healthcare, 4007
Central Louisiana State Hospital, 3879
Central New York Psychiatric Center, 3966
Central Regional Hospital, 4002
Central State Hospital, 3814, 3873, 4089
Central Washington Comprehensive M/H, 4555
Central Wyoming Behavioral Health at Lander Valley, 2176
Centre for Addiction & Mental Health, 1719
Centre for Mental Health Solutions: Minnesota Bio Brain Association, 1965
Century Financial Services, 4155
Cephalon, 4634
Ceridian Corporation, 4388
Chaddock, 1887

Chalice, 168
Challenging Behavior, 1253
Challenging Behavior of Persons with Mental Health Disorders and Severe Developmental Disabilities, 2708
Change for Good Coaching and Counseling, 984
A Change of Character, 800
Changing Echoes, 3750
Changing Health Care Marketplace, 2709
Charles C Thomas Publishers, 3674, 152, 1301, 1312, 1451, 2768, 2832, 2858, 2863, 2870, 2891, 3064, 3084
Charles Press Publishers, 901
Charter BHS of Wisconsin/Brown Deer, 2168
Chartman Software, 4389
Chattanooga/Plateau Council for Alcohol and Drug Abuse, 2439
Chelsea House Publications, 1141
Chemical Dependency Treatment Planning Handbook, 3597
Chemically Dependent Anonymous, 201
Cherish the Children, 427
Cherokee Health Systems, 4053
Cherokee Mental Health Institute, 3862
Cherry Hospital, 4003
Chester Mental Health Center, 3829
Chicago Child Care Society, 1888
Child & Family Center, 846
Child & Parent Resource Institute, 1720
Child Friendly Therapy: Biophysical Innovations for Children and Families, 3103
Child Psychiatry, 3104
Child Psychopharmacology, 3105
Child Study & Treatment Center, 4099
Child Welfare Information Gateway, 4556
Child Welfare League of America, 1721, 3158
Child Welfare League of America: Washington, 2599
Child and Adolescent Bipolar Disorder: An Update from the National Institute of Mental Health, 735
Child and Adolescent Mental Health Consultation in Hospitals, Schools and Courts, 3106
Child and Adolescent Psychiatry, 3223
Child and Adolescent Psychiatry: Modern Approaches, 3107
Child and Adolescent Psychopharmacology Information, 2169
Child-Centered Counseling and Psychotherapy, 3108
Childhood Behavior Disorders: Applied Research and Educational Practice, 3109
Childhood Disorders, 3110
Childhood History Form for Attention Disorders, 3321
Childhood Obsessive Compulsive Disorder, 1177
Children and Adolescents with Emotional and Behavioral Disorders, 3360
Children and Adults with AD/HD (CHADD), 394, 1625
Children and Autism: Time is Brain, 665
Children and Trauma: Guide for Parents and Professionals, 1293, 1601
Children and Youth Funding Report, 169
Children and Youth with Asperger Syndrome, 2951
Children in Therapy: Using the Family as a Resource, 2710

Children of Hope Family Hospital, 3822
Children with Autism: A Developmental Perspective, 589
Children with Autism: Parents' Guide, 590
Children with Tourette Syndrome: A Parent's Guide, 1543
Children with Tourette Syndrome: A Parents' Guide, 1544
Children's Alliance, 1912, 2147
Children's Depression Inventory, 3322
Children's Health Council, 2600
Children's Home Association of Illinois, 1889
Children's Home of the Wyoming Conference, Quality Improvement, 4156
Children's Mental Health Partnership, 2110
Children/Adults with Attention Deficit/Hyperactivity Disorder, 489
Children: Experts on Divorce, 1635
Childs Work/Childs Play, 1602, 3111, 1597, 1598, 1605, 1607, 1608, 1609, 1610, 1611, 1612, 1613, 1614, 1636
Chill: Straight Talk About Stress, 1636
Choate Health Management, 3908
Choate Mental Health and Development Center, 3830
Choice Health, 4557
ChoiceCare, 4157
Choices Adolescent Treatment Center, 4063
Christian Association for Psychological Studies, 2601
Christian Horizons, 1722
Christopher Alsten, PhD, 3498
Chronicle, 3224
Cialis, 4675
Cincom Systems, 4390
Cindy Hide, 3417
Cirrus Technology, 4558
Citadel, 2670
Clarinda Mental Health Treatment Complex, 3863
Clarks Summit State Hospital, 4030
Clermont Counseling Center, 4008
Client Management Information System, 4391
Client's Manual for the Cognitive Behavioral Treatment of Anxiety Disorders, 2934
Clifton T Perkins Hospital Center, 3891
CliniSphere version 2.0, 4392
Clinical & Forensic Interviewing of Children & Families, 3112
Clinical Application of Projective Drawings, 3113
Clinical Assessment and Management of Severe Personality Disorders, 1254
Clinical Child Documentation Sourcebook, 3114
Clinical Counseling: Toward a Better Understanding of TS, 1562
Clinical Dimensions of Anticipatory Mourning, 2711
Clinical Evaluations of School Aged Children, 3323
Clinical Guide to Depression in Children and Adolescents, 875
Clinical Handbook of Eating Disorders: An Integrated Approach (Medical Psychiatry, 26), 1011
Clinical Integration, 2712
Clinical Interview of the Adolescent: From Assessment and Formulation to Treatment Planning, 3324

Clinical Manual of Impulse-Control Disorders, 1135
Clinical Manual of Supportive Psychotherapy, 3598
Clinical Nutrition Center, 4393
Clinical Psychiatry News, 3225
Clinical Psychiatry Quarterly, 3226
Clinical Social Work Federation, 2602
Clinical Supervision in Alcohol and Drug Abuse Counseling, 112
Clinician's Guide to the Personality Profiles of Alcohol and Drug Abusers: Typological Descriptions Using the MMPI, 2897
Close to You, 1072
Clozaril, 4676
Coalition of Illinois Counselors Organization, 1890
Coalition of Voluntary Mental Health Agencies, 1723
Cocaine & Crack: Back from the Abyss, 216
Cocaine Anonymous, 202
Cognex, 4677
Cognitive Analytic Therapy & Borderline Personality Disorder: Model and the Method, 1255
Cognitive Behavior Therapy Child, 3115
Cognitive Behavioral Assessment, 3491
The Cognitive Behavorial Workbook for Depression: A Step-by-Step Program, 904
Cognitive Processing Therapy for Rape Victims, 3044
Cognitive Therapy, 2935
Cognitive Therapy Pages, 812, 3538
Cognitive Therapy for Delusions, Voices, and Paranoia, 3079
Cognitive Therapy for Depression and Anxiety, 288
Cognitive Therapy for Personality Disorders: a Schema-Focused Approach, 3030
Cognitive Therapy in Practice, 2713
Cognitive Therapy of Depression, 2983
Cognitive Therapy of Personality Disorders, 3031
Cognitive Therapy of Personality Disorders, Second Edition, 1256
Cognitive Therapy: A Multimedia Learning Program, 816
Colin A Ross Institute for Psychological Trauma, 1317
Collaborative Therapy with Multi-Stressed Families, 2714
College Health IPA, 4158
College of Dupage, 4159
College of Health and Human Services: SE Missouri State, 3361
College of Southern Idaho, 3362, 4160
Colonial Services Board, 3363
Colorado Chapter, 1845
Colorado Department of Health Care Policy and Financing, 2261
Colorado Department of Human Services, 2264
Colorado Department of Human Services (CDHS), 2262
Colorado Department of Human Services: Alcohol and Drug Abuse Division, 2263
Colorado Division of Mental Health, 2264
Colorado Health Networks-Value Options, 1843
Colorado Medical Assistance Program Information Center, 2265
Colorado Mental Health Institute at Fort Logan, 3775

Colorado Mental Health Institute at Pueblo, 3776
Colorado Traumatic Brain Injury Trust Fund Program, 2266
Columbia Counseling Center, 3364
Columbia DISC Development Group, 3331
Columbia Hospital M/H Services, 4161
ComPsych, 4162
Combined Addicts and Professionals Services CAPS/Residential Unit, 3751
Comcare of Sedgwick County, 2315
Comeback Treatment Centers, 3752
Commission on Accreditation of Rehabilitation Facilities, 2603
Commission on the Mentally Disabled, 2794
Committee for Truth in Psychiatry: CTIP, 2190
Common Sense: Strategies for Raising Alcoholic/Drug-/Free Children, 1680
Common Voice for Pierce County Parents, 2148
Commonly Abused Drugs: Street Names for Drugs of Abuse, 250
Commonwealth Center for Children and Adolescents, 4090
Commonwealth Fund, 2604
Communicating in Relationships: A Guide for Couples and Professionals, 2715
Communication Unbound: How Facilitated Communication Is Challenging Views, 591
Community Access, 1724
Community Action Partnership, 2605
Community Anti-Drug Coalitions of America:, 2606
Community Behavioral Health Association of Maryland: CBH, 1930
Community Hospital Anderson, 3855
Community Mental Health Directory, 3635
Community Partnership of Southern Arizona, 1810
Community Psychiatric Clinic, 4559
Community Resource Council, 1829
Community Sector Systems, 4560
Community Service Options, 1725
Community Services for Autistic Adults & Children, 684
Community Services for Autistic Adults and Children, 549
Community Solutions, 4561
Community-Based Instructional Support, 2716
Comorbidity of Mood and Anxiety Disorders, 289
CompHealth Credentialing, 2490
Compact Clinicals, 1194
Compass Information Systems, 4562
Compassionate Friends, 35, 48
Compeer, 2016
Compilation of Writings by People Suffering from Depression, 3523
Complete Directory for People with Disabilities, 3636
The Complete Family Guide to Schizophrenia: Helping Your Loved One Get the Most Out of Life, 1402
Complete Learning Disabilities Directory, 3637
Complete Mental Health Directory, 3638
Complexities of TS Treatment: Physician's Roundtable, 1563
Comprehensive Approach to Suicide Prevention, 1523, 3547
Comprehensive Care Corporation, 4163

Comprehensive Center For Pain Management, 4164
The Comprehensive Directory, 701
Comprehensive Directory: Programs and Services for Children with Disabilities and Their Families, 3599
Comprehensive Textbook of Geriatric Psychi- try, 2717
Comprehensive Textbook of Suicidology, 3088
Compu-Care Management and Systems, 4394
CompuLab Healthcare Systems Corporation, 4395
Computer Billing and Office Managment Programs, 4563
Computer Transition Services, 4396
Computerization of Behavioral Healthcare, 2718
Concept of Schizophrenia: Historical Perspectives, 1370
Concerned Advocates Serving Children & Families, 2050
Concerned Intervention: When Your Loved One Won't Quit Alcohol or Drugs, 113
Concerta, 4678
Concise Guide to Anxiety Disorders, 290
Concise Guide to Assessment and Management of Violent Patients, 3325
Concise Guide to Brief Dynamic Psychotherapy, 3045
Concise Guide to Child and Adolescent Psychiatry, 3116
Concise Guide to Evaluation and Management of Sleep Disorders, 1475
Concise Guide to Laboratory and Diagnostic Testing in Psychiatry, 3600
Concise Guide to Marriage and Family Therapy, 2719
Concise Guide to Mood Disorders, 2720
Concise Guide to Neuropsychiatry and Behavioral Neurology, 3070
Concise Guide to Psychiatry and Law for Clinicians, 2721
Concise Guide to Psychodynamic Psychotherapy: Principles and Techniques in the Era of Managed Care, 3071
Concise Guide to Psychopharmacology, 2722
Concise Guide to Treatment of Alcoholism and Addictions, 114
Concise Guide to Women's Mental Health, 2984
Concord Family and Adolescent Services, 3909
Concord Family and Youth Services A Division of Justice Resource Institute, 1942
Conduct Disorder in Children and Adolescents, 843, 1619
Conduct Disorders in Childhood and Adolescence, Developmental Clinical Psychology and Psychiatry, 836
Conduct Disorders in Children and Adolesents, 428
Conducting Insanity Evaluations, 3326
Connecticut Department of Children and Families, 2270
Connecticut Department of Mental Health and Addiction Services, 2269
Connecticut Families United for Children's Mental Health, 1848
Connecticut National Association of Mentally Ill, 1849
Connecticut Valley Hospital General Psychiatric Division, 3779

Conners' Rating Scales, 3327
Consent Handbook for Self-Advocates and Support Staff, 2723
Consultec Managed Care Systems, 4564
Consumer Health Information Corporation, 4565
Consumer Satisfaction Team, 2491
Consumer's Guide to Psychiatric Drugs, 22, 291, 429, 724
Contact Behavioral Health Services, 4165
Contemporary Issues in the Treatment of Schizophrenia, 1371
Continuing Medical Education, 3296
Control-0-Fax Corporation, 4397
Control-O-Fax Corporation, 4566
Controlling Anger-Before It Controls You, 1153
Controlling Eating Disorders with Facts, Advice and Resources, 1012
Conversations with Anorexics: A Compassionate & Hopeful Journey, 1013
CoolTalk, 4398
Coping With Self-Mutilation: a Helping Book for Teens Who Hurt Themselves, 3014
Coping With Unexpected Events: Depression & Trauma, 736
Coping with Anxiety, 292
Coping with Depression, 930
Coping with Eating Disorders, 1014
Coping with Mood Changes Later in Life, 737
Coping with Post-Traumatic Stress Disorder, 1294
Coping with Separation and Divorce: A Parenting Seminar, 1671
Coping with Social Anxiety: The Definitive G uide to Effective Treatment Options, 293
Coping with Trauma: A Guide to Self Understanding, 294, 1295
Copper Hills Youth Center, 3365
Cornell Interventions Lifeworks, 3831
Cornerstone of Rhinebeck, 3967
Cornucopia Software, 4399
Corphealth, 3366, 4166
Corporate Counseling Associates, 2607
Corporate Health Systems, 4167
Council for Learning Disabilities, 1726
Council of Behavioral Group Practice, 2608
Council on Accreditation (COA) of Services for Families and Children, 2492
Council on Quality and Leadership, 1727
Council on Size and Weight Discrimination (CSWD), 985
Council on Social Work Education, 2493, 2609
Counseling Associates, 4168
Counseling Children with Special Needs, 3117
Counseling Services, 3367
Counseling for Loss and Life Changes, 49, 3531
Countertransference Issues in Psychiatric Treatment, 2724
Couples Therapy in Managed Care, 3227
Couples and Infertility - Moving Beyond Loss, 3492
Courage to Change, 842, 848, 1601, 1635
Covenant Home Healthcare, 4169
Covenant House Nineline, 1626
Coventry Health Care of Iowa, 4170
Covert Modeling & Covert Reinforcement, 752

Craig Academy, 4031
Craig Counseling & Biofeedback Services, 1844
Creating and Implementing Your Strategic Plan: Workbook for Public and Nonprofit Organizations, 3601
Creative Computer Applications, 4400
Creative Health Concepts, 4171
Creative Socio-Medics Corporation, 4401
Creative Solutions Unlimited, 4464
Creative Therapy 2: Working with Parents, 837
Creative Therapy with Children and Adolescents, 3118
Creative Therapy with Children and Adolescents, 1603
Creativity and Depression and Manic-Depression, 3549
Creedmoor Psychiatric Center, 3968
Crisis: Prevention and Response in the Community, 2725
Critical Incidents: Ethical Issues in Substance Abuse Prevention and Treatment, 2898
Cross Addiction: Back Door to Relapse, 217
Cross-Cultural Perspectives on Quality of Life, 2726
Crossing the Thin Line: Between Social Drinking and Alcoholism, 170
Crossroad Publishing, 3675
Crossroad: Fort Wayne's Children's Home, 3856
Crown House Publishing, 971
Crown Publishing Group, 1026, 1179
Crownsville Hospital Center, 3892
Cruel Compassion: Psychiatric Control of Society's Unwanted, 2727
Cult of Thinness, 1015
Culture & Psychotherapy: A Guide to Clinical Practice, 2728
Cumberland River Regional Board, 3874
Current Treatments of Obsessive-Compulsive Disorder, 3019
Customer Support Department, 3229, 3298
Customer Support Services, 176
Cutting-Edge Medicine: What Psychiatrists Need to Know, 2729
CyberPsych, 50, 366, 500, 685, 759, 810, 850, 940, 973, 1073, 1114, 1155, 1211, 1272, 1320, 1418, 1480, 1522, 3532
Cybermedicine, 2730
Cymbalta, 4679
Cypruss Communications, 4172

D

DB Consultants, 4402
DBSA Support Groups: An Important Step on the Road to Wellness, 738
DC Alliance for the Mentally Ill, 1860
DC Commission on Mental Health Services, 2275
DC Department of Human Services, 2276
DC Department of Mental Health, 2191
DCC/The Dependent Care Connection, 4567
DD Fischer Consulting, 4173
DMDA/DBSA: Uplift, 2126
DML Training and Consulting, 4174
DRADA-Depression and Related Affective Disorders Association, 931
DRG Handbook, 2731

DSM-IV Anxiety Disorders New Diagnostic Issues, 358

DSM-IV Psychotic Disorders: New Diagnostic Issue, 3639

DSM: IV Diagnostic & Statistical Manual of Mental Disorders, 2732

DSM: IV Personality Disorders, 2733

DST Output, 4403

Dallas Federation of Families for Children's Mental Health, 2111

Dallas Metrocare Services, 4064

Dane County Mental Health Center, 2477

Dangerous Liaisons: Substance Abuse and Sex, 2899

Dangerous Sex Offenders: a Task Force Report of the American Psychiatric Association, 1446

Daniel Memorial Institute, 3368

Daniel and Yeager Healthcare Staffing Solutions, 3369

Daredevils and Daydreamers: New Perspectives on Attention Deficit/Hyperactivity Disorder, 430

Dark Glasses and Kaleidoscopes: Living with Manic Depression, 753

DataMark, 4404

DataStar/Dialog, 3546

Dauphin County Drug and Alcohol, 2418

David Baldwin's Trauma Information Pages, 1331

Day for Night: Recognizing Teenage Depression, 931

Daytop Residential Services Division, 3780

Dealing With the Problem of Low Self-Esteem: Common Characteristics and Treatment, 3032

Dealing with Anger Problems: Rational-Emotive Therapeutic Interventions, 3015

Dealing with Feelings, 1661

Dean Foundation for Health, Research and Education, 4568

Death and Dying Grief Support, 51

Deborah MacWilliams, 1336

Defiant Teens, 3119

Delaware Alliance for the Mentally Ill, 1855

Delaware Department of Health & Social Services, 2271

Delaware Division of Child Mental Health Services, 2272

Delaware Division of Family Services, 2273

Delaware Guidance Services for Children and Youth, 1856

Delaware State Hospital, 3788

Deloitte and Touche LLP Management Consulting, 4175

Delta Center, 3832

DeltaMetrics, 4176, 4405

Delusional Beliefs, 3080

Dementia: A Clinical Approach, 794

Denver County Department of Social Services, 2267

Depakote, 4680

Department Of Psychology, 2625

Department of Children and Families, 2278, 2281

Department of Community Health, 3635

Department of Health Care Policy and Financing, 2265

Department of Health and Family Services, 2476

Department of Health and Family Services: Southern Region, 2478

Department of Health and Human Services Regulation and Licensure, 1986

Department of Health and Human Services/OAS, 1861

Department of Health and Welfare: Community Rehab, 2289

Department of Health and Welfare: Medicaid Division, 2288

Department of Human Services For Youth & Families, 1864

Department of Human Services: Chemical Health Division, 2349

Department of Mental Health, 2345

Department of Mental Health Vacaville Psychiatric Program, 3753

Department of Psychiatry, 751

Department of Psychiatry and Behavioral Science, 2033

Department of Psychiatry: Dartmouth University, 3370

Depressed Anonymous, 927

Depression, 911

Depression & Antidepressants, 2985

Depression & Anxiety Management, 876

Depression & Bi-Polar Support Alliance, 855, 760, 920

Depression & BiPolar Support Alliance, 708, 736

Depression & Related Affective Disorders Association (DRADA), 856

Depression After Delivery, 857

Depression Workbook: a Guide for Living with Depression, 877

Depression and Anxiety in Youth Scale, 3328

Depression and Bi-Polar Alliance, 858

Depression and Bipolar Support Alliance, 737, 738, 739, 740, 741, 744, 745, 753

Depression and Bipolar Support Alliance of Houston and Harris County, 2112

Depression and Its Treatment, 878

Depression and Manic Depression, 932

Depression and Related Affective Disorders Association, 936, 3309

Depression in Children and Adolescents, 1664

Depression in Children and Adolescents: A Fact Sheet for Physicians, 912

Depression in Context: Strategies for Guided Action, 2986

Depression, the Mood Disease, 879

Depression: Help On the Way, 913

Depression: What Every Woman Should Know, 914

Depressive and Manic-Depressive Association of Boston, 1943

Depressive and Manic-Depressive Association of St. Louis, 1976

Designer Drugs, 171

Designing Positive Behavior Support Plans, 2734

Desoxyn, 4681

A Desperate Act, 1150

Determinants of Substance Abuse: Biological, Psychological, and Environmental Factors, 2900

Detwiler's Directory of Health and Medical Resources, 3640

Developing Mind: Toward a Neurobiology of Interpersonal Experience, 2735

Development & Psychopathology, 3228

Developmental Brain Research, 3229

Developmental Disabilities Nurses Association, 2610

Developmental Model of Borderline Personality Disorder: Understanding Variations in Course and Outcome, 1257

Developmental Psychopathology of Eating Disorders: Implications for Research, Prevention and Treatment, 1016

Developmental Therapy/Developmental Teaching, 3120

Devereux Arizona Treatment Network, 1811

Dexedrine, 4682

Dhs-Division of Alcoholism and Substance Abuse, 2300

Diagnosis and Treatment of Autism, 592

Diagnosis and Treatment of Depression in Lat e Life: Results of the NIH Consensus Development Conference, 880

Diagnosis and Treatment of Multiple Personality Disorder, 3329

Diagnosis and Treatment of Sociopaths and Clients with Sociopathic Traits, 3330

Diagnostic Interview Schedule for Children: CDISC, 3331

Different From You, 972

Difficult Child, 838

Dilligaf Publishing, 1180

Dilligaf Publishing for Awareness Project, 1553

Directory for People with Chronic Illness, 3641

Directory of Developmental Disabilities Services, 3642

Directory of Health Care Professionals, 3643

Directory of Hospital Personnel, 3644

Directory of Physician Groups & Networks, 3645

Directory of Physician Groups and Networks, 3646

Disability Funding Week, 3230

Disability Services Division, 2368

Disability at the Dawn of the 21st Century and the State of the States, 2736

Disease of Alcoholism Video, 218

Disordered Personalities, 1258

Disorders of Brain and Mind: Volume 1, 795

Disorders of Narcissism: Diagnostic, Clinical, and Empirical Implications, 1259

Disorders of Personality: DSM-IV and Beyond, 3033

Disorders of Simulation: Malingering, Factit ious Disorders, and Compensation Neurosis, 1090

Dissociation, 961

Dissociation and the Dissociative Disorders: DSM-V and Beyond, 962

Dissociative Child: Diagnosis, Treatment and Management, 963

Dissociative Identity Disorder: Diagnosis, Clinical Features, and Treatment of Multiple Personality, 2997

Distance Learning Network, 3371, 4406, 4569

Distant Drums, Different Drummers: A Guide for Young People with ADHD, 431

Divalproex and Bipolar Disorder: A Guide, 725

Diversified Group Administrators, 4177

Diversity in Psychotherapy: The Politics of Race, Ethnicity, and Gender, 2737

The Divided Mind: The Epidemic of Mindbody D isorders, 1349

Division of Behavioral Healthcare Services, 2428

Division of Health Care Policy, 2316

A Division of Justice Resource Institute, Inc, 3909, 3910, 3911, 3912, 3913, 3914, 3918

Division of Special Education And Student Services, 2142

Divorce Information, 54

Divorce Magazine, 55

Divorce Support, 56

DivorceNet, 42

The Do It Now Foundation, 239

Do No Harm?, 1091

Doctoral Program in Clinical Psychology, 2663

Docu Trac, 4407

DocuMed, 4408

Does Stress Damage the Brain? Understanding Trauma-Related Disorders from a Mind-Body Perspective, 3046

Doing What Comes Naturally: Dispelling Myths and Fallacies About Sexuality and People with Developmental Disabilities, 2738

Dolophine, 4683

Domestic Violence 2000: Integrated Skills Program for Men, 3016

Dominion Hospital, 4091

Don't Despair on Thursdays: the Children's Grief-Management Book, 23

Don't Feed the Monster on Tuesdays: The Children's Self-Esteem Book, 24

Don't Give Up Kid, 432

Don't Panic: Taking Control of Anxiety Attacks, 295

Don't Pop Your Cork on Mondays: The Children's Anti-Stress Book, 25

Don't Rant and Rave on Wednesdays: The Children's Anger-Control Book, 26

Don't Think About Monkeys: Extraordinary Stories Written by People with Tourette Syndrome, 1545

Dorenfest Group, 4178

Dorland Healthcare Information, 4570, 2731, 3621, 3632, 3633, 3634, 3640, 3643, 3645, 3646, 3647, 3649, 3653, 4281, 4589

Dorland's Medical Directory, 3647

Dorthea Dix Hospital, 4004

Dorthea Dix Psychiatric Center, 3887

Dougherty Management Associates Health Strategies, 4179

Down and Dirty Guide to Adult Attention Deficit Disorder, 433

Downstate Mental Hygiene Association, 3372

Dr. Ivan's Depression Central, 948, 3580

Dr. Tony Attwood: Asperger's Syndrome Volume 2 DVD, 527

Draw a Person: Screening Procedure for Emotional Disturbance, 3332

Drinking Facts, 172

Driven to Distraction: Recognizing and Coping with Attention Deficit Disorder from Childhood through Adulthood, 434

Driving Far from Home, 359

Drug ABC's, 173

Drug Abuse Sourcebook, 115

Drug Dependence, Alcohol Abuse and Alcoholism, 174

Drug Facts Pamphlet, 175

Drug Information Handbook for Psychiatry, 3648

Drug Information for Teens: Health Tips about the Physical and Mental Effects of Substance Abuse, 2901

Drug Policy Information Clearinghouse, 2214

Drug Strategies, 3136, 3151

Drug Therapy and Adjustment Disorders, 27

Drug Therapy and Anxiety Disorders, 296

Drug Therapy and Childhood & Adolescent Diso rders, 435

Drug Therapy and Cognitive Disorders, 796

Drug Therapy and Dissociative Disorders, 964

Drug Therapy and Impulse Control Disorders, 1136

Drug Therapy and Obsessive-Compulsive Disord er, 1178

Drug Therapy and Personality Disorders, 1260

Drug Therapy and Postpartum Disorders, 881

Drug Therapy and Psychosomatic Disorders, 1343

Drug Therapy and Schizophrenia, 1372

Drug Therapy and Sleep Disorders, 1476

Drug Therpay and Eating Disorders, 3000

Drug and Alcohol Dependence, 176

Drug and Crime Prevention Funding News, 4571

DrugLink, 177

Drugs: Talking With Your Teen, 178

Duke University's Program in Child and Adolescent Anxiety Disorder, 1689

Dupage County Health Department, 4180

Dying of Embarrassment: Help for Social Anxiety and Social Phobia, 297

Dynamic Psychotherapy: An Introductory Approach, 2739

Dynamics of Addiction, 116

Dysinhibition Syndrome How to Handle Anger and Rage in Your Child or Spouse, 839, 1137

E

E Lansing Center for Family, 3921

E Services Group, 4409

E-Productivity-Services.Net, 1283, 3195

EAP Technology Systems, 4410

EAPA Exchange, 3231

EBSCO Publishing, 3676

EMDR Institute, 941, 1459

EPIC, 3569

Eagle Eyes: A Child's View of Attention Deficit Disorder, 436

Earle E Morris Jr Alcohol & Drug Treatment Center, 4046

East Bay Alliance for the Mentally Ill, 2081

East Carolina University Department of Psychiatric Medicine, 3373

East Division Greenwell Springs Campus, 3880

East Mississippi State Hospital, 3933

Eastern County Mental Health Center, 3374

Eastern Louisiana Mental Health System, 3881

Eastern Shore Hospital Center, 3893

Eastern State Hospital, 3875, 4092, 4100

Eating Disorder Council of Long Island, 2017

Eating Disorder Sourcebook, 1049

Eating Disorder Video, 1068

Eating Disorders, 1050

Eating Disorders & Obesity: a Comprehensive Handbook, 1017

Eating Disorders Association of New Jersey, 2002

Eating Disorders Awareness and Prevention, 1074

Eating Disorders Factsheet, 1051

Eating Disorders Research and Treatment Program, 1061

Eating Disorders Sourcebook, 1018

Eating Disorders and Obesity, Second Edition : A Comprehensive Handbook, 1019

Eating Disorders: Facts About Eating Disorders and the Search for Solutions, 1052

Eating Disorders: Reference Sourcebook, 1020

Eating Disorders: When Food Hurts, 1069

Eating Disorders: When Food Turns Against You, 1021

Echo Group, 4411

Echo Management Group, 4181

Echolalia: an Adult's Story of Tourette Syndrome, 1546

Eclipsys Corporation, 4412

Ed Zuckrman, 4563

Edgewood Children's Center, 3937

Educating Clients about the Cognitive Model, 3493

Educating Inattentive Children, 482

Educational Testing Service, 3341

Effecive Treatments for PTSD: Practice Guide lines from the International Society for Traumatic Stress Studies, 1296

Effective Discipline, 2974

Effective Learning Systems, 1350

Effective Treatments for PTSD, 1297

Effective Treatments for PTSD: Practice Guidelines from the International Society for Traumatic Stress Studies, 3047

Effexor, 4684

Efficacy of Special Education and Related Services, 2740

Eisai, 4635

El Paso County Human Services, 2268

El Paso Psychiatric Center, 4065

Elavil, 4685

Elderly Place, 811

Electroconvulsive Therapy: A Guide, 2741

Electronic Healthcare Systems, 4413

Elgin Mental Health Center, 3833

Eli Lilly and Company, 4636

Elmira Psychiatric Center, 3969

Elon Homes for Children, 4182

Elsevier, 1193

Elsevier Health Sciences, 794

Elsevier Publishing, 174, 187, 342

Elsevier Science, 128, 3239, 3611

Elsevier/WB Saunders Company, 1477

Embarking on a New Century: Mental Retardation at the end of the Twentieth Century, 2742

Emedeon Practice Services, 4414

Emergencies in Mental Health Practice, 2743

Emily Griffith Center, 3777

Emory University School of Medicine, Psychology and Behavior, 3375

Emory University: Psychological Center, 3376

Emotional Eating: A Practical Guide to Taking Control, 1022

Emotions Anonymous, 918

Emotions Anonymous International Service Center, 859

Employee Assistance Professionals, 4183

Employee Assistance Professionals Association, 2611

Employee Assistance Professionals Association, 3231
Employee Assistance Society of North America, 2612
Employee Benefit Specialists, 4184
Employee Benefits Journal, 3233
Employee Network, 4185
Empowering Adolesent Girls, 2902
Emsam, 4686
Encyclopedia of Depression, 882
Encyclopedia of Obesity and Eating Disorders, 1023
Encyclopedia of Phobias, Fears, and Anxieties, 298
Encyclopedia of Schizophrenia and the Psychotic Disorders, 1373
Enhancing Social Competence in Young Students, 3121
Enslow Publishers, 1142
Entre Technology Services, 4415
Entropy Limited, 4186
Epidemiology-Genetics Program in Psychiatry, 749
Epidemology-Genetics Program in Psychiatry, 1420
Equal Employment Opportunity Commission, 2192
Erectile Dysfunction: Integrating Couple Therapy, Sex Therapy and Medical Treatment, 3085
Eskalith, 4687
Essential Guide to Psychiatric Drugs, 2744
Essentials of Clinical Psychiatry: Based on the American Psychiatric Press Textbook of Psychiatry, 2745
Essentials of Psychosomatic Medicine, 1344
Essi Systems, 4187
Ethical Way, 2746
Ethics for Addiction Professionals, 2903
Ethos Consulting, 4188
Etiology and Treatment of Bulimia Nervosa, 1024
Eukee the Jumpy, Jumpy Elephant, 437
Evaluation Center at HSRI, 4189
Evaluation and Treatment of Postpartum Emotional Disorders, 2987
Even from a Broken Web: Brief, Respectful Solution Oriented Therapy for Sexual Abuse and Trauma, 3048
Evidence-Based Mental Health Practice: A Textbook, 2747
Exceptional Parent, 3234
Executive Guide to Case Management Strategies, 2748
Exelon, 4688
Exemplar Employee: Rewarding & Recognizing Direct Contact Employees, 2749
Exodus Recovery Center, 3754
Experience of Schizophrenia, 1424
Experior Corporation, 4416
Exubernace: The Passion for Life, 1504
Eye Movement Desensitization and Reprocessing International Association (EMDRIA), 1728
Eye Movement Desensitization and Reprocessing: Basic Principles, Protocols, and Procedures, 3049
Eye Opener, 117

F

FACES of the Blue Grass, 1913
FAT City: How Difficult Can This Be?, 360
FCS, 4190
FHN Family Counseling Center, 3834
FOCUS: Family Oriented Counseling Services, 4572
FPM Behavioral Health: Corporate Marketing, 4191
Facilitated Communication and Technology Guide, 593
Facilitated Learning at Syracuse University, 650
Facing AD/HD: A Survival Guide for Parents, 438
Facts About Anxiety Disorders, 337
Facts About Autism, 645
Facts Services, 4417
Facts and Comparisons, 177, 4392, 4493
Facts on File, 298, 882, 1023, 1373
Fairwinds Treatment Center, 3791
False Memory Syndrome Facts, 974
Families Anonymous, 1729
Families Can Help Children Cope with Fear, Anxiety, 338, 1620
Families Coping with Mental Illness, 754, 1417
Families Coping with Schizophrenia: Practitioner's Guide to Family Groups, 3081
Families Involved Together, 1931
Families Together in New York State, 2018
Families United of Milwaukee, 2170
Families for Early Autism Treatment, 550, 686
Families of Adults Afflicted with Asperger's Syndrome (FAAAS), 515
Family & Community Alliance Project, 1850
Family Advocacy & Support Association, 1730, 1862
Family Approach to Psychiatric Disorders, 2750
Family Care of Schizophrenia: a Problem-Solving Approach..., 1374
Family Experiences Productions, 3677
Family Life Library, 1674, 3570
Family Life with Tourette Syndrome... Personal Stories, 1564
Family Managed Care, 4192
Family Network on Disabilities of Florida, 1865
Family Relations, 1678
Family Service Agency, 3755
Family Service Association of Greater Elgin Area, 1891
Family Services of Delaware County, 4418
Family Stress, Coping, and Social Support, 2751
Family Support Network, 1982
Family Therapy Progress Notes Planner, 2752
Family Therapy for ADHD: Treating Children, Adolesents and Adults, 2960
Family Violence & Sexual Assault Bulletin, 1457
Family Violence & Sexual Assault Institute, 1731, 1457
Family Work for Schizophrenia: a Practical Guide, 1375
Family and Social Services Administration, 2305

A Family-Centered Approach to People with Mental Retardation, 2684
Family-to-Family: National Alliance on Mental Illness, 1413
Fanlight Productions, 3678, 636, 661, 800, 929, 932, 935, 1069, 1634
Fanlight Publications, 972
Fatal Flaws: Navigating Destructive Relation ships with People with Disorders, 1261
Fatherhood Project, 1653
Fathering Magazine, 1652
Fats of Life, 1053
Faulkner & Gray, 3245
Federation for Children with Special Needs (FCSN), 1578, 1732
Federation of Families for Children's Mental Health, 1733
Federation of Families for Children's Mental Health, 1579, 4573
Federation of Families for Children's Mental Health, 1845
Federation of Families of South Carolina, 2093
Feminist Perspectives on Eating Disorders, 1025
Fergus Falls Regional Treatment Center, 3929
Fetal Alcohol Syndrome & Fetal Alcohol Effect, 118, 179, 219
Fetal Alcohol Syndrome and Effect, Stories of Help and Hope, 220
Field Guide to Personality Disorders, 1262
Fifty Ways to Avoid Malpractice: A Guidebook for Mental Health Professionals, 2753
Fighting for Darla: Challenges for Family Care & Professional Responsibility, 594
Filipino American Service Group, 3756
Filmakers Library, 660
Finding Peacce of Mind: Treatment Strategies for Depression and Bipolar Disorder, 739
Findley, Davies and Company, 4193
Finger Lakes Parent Network, 2019
First Candle/SIDS Alliance, 9, 71
First Connections and Healthy Families, 3910
First Consulting Group, 4194
First Corp-Health Consulting, 4195
First Data Bank, 4419
First Episode Psychosis, 1376
First Horizon Pharmaceutical, 4637
First Hospital Corporation, 2138
First Star I See, 439
First Step of Sarasota, 3792
First Therapy Session, 2754
Five Acres: Boys and Girls Aid Society of Los Angeles County, 1830
Five Smart Steps to Less Stress, 339
Five Smart Steps to Safer Drinking, 180
Five Ways to Stop Stress, 340
Five Weeks to Healing Stress: the Wellness Option, 299
Five-HTP: The Natural Way to Overcome Depression, Obesity, and Insomnia, 2755
Flawless Consulting, 2756
Fletcher Allen Health Care, 2131, 3377
Florida Alcohol and Drug Abuse Association, 1866
Florida Department Health and Human Services: Substance Abuse Program, 2278
Florida Department of Children and Families, 2279

Florida Department of Health and Human Services, 2280
Florida Department of Mental Health and Rehabilitative Services, 2281
Florida Federation of Families for Children's Mental Health, 1867
Florida Health Care Association, 1868
Florida Health Information Management Association, 1869
Florida International University, 2588
Florida Medicaid State Plan, 2282
Florida National Alliance for the Mentally Ill, 1870
Florida State Hospital, 3793
Fluvoxamine, 4689
Flying Solo, 1654
Flying Without Fear, 300
Focal Point: Research, Policy and Practice in Children's Mental Health, 3235
Focus on Kids: The Effects of Divorce on Children, 1668
Food Addicts Anonymous, 1064
Food and Feelings, 1054
Food for Recovery: The Next Step, 1026
Forensic Division, 3882
Forensic Treatment Center, 4038
Forest Laboratories, 4638
Forgiveness: Theory, Research and Practice, 2757
Forms for Behavior Analysis with Children, 1604
Forms-5 Book Set, 1605
Forty Two Lives in Treatment: a Study of Psychoanalysis and Psychotherapy, 3236
Foundations of Mental Health Counseling, 2758
Four Seasons Counseling Clinic, 3864
Fowler Healthcare Affiliates, 4196
Fox Counseling Service, 2113
Fragile Success - Ten Autistic Children, Childhood to Adulthood, 595
Franklin Electronic Publishers, 3679
Franklin Watts, 1021
Franklin-Williamson Human Services, 3835
Frankling Electronic Publishers, 3679
Free Press, 1404, 1514, 2894
Free Spirit Publishing, 3680, 32, 333, 907
Free from Fears: New Help for Anxiety, Panic and Agoraphobia, 301
Freedom From Fear, 266, 860, 369
Freedom Ranch, 3970
Freedom To Fly, 4197
Freedom Village USA, 3971, 1655
Freeing Your Child from Anxiety: Powerful, Practical Solutions to Overcome Your Child's Fears, Worries, and Phobias, 302
Freeing Your Child from Obsessive-Compulsive Disorder: A Powerful, Practical Program for Parents of Children and Adolescents, 1179
Fremont Hospital, 3757
Friends for Survival, 36, 1519, 57
From the Couch, 3237
Frontiers of Health Services Management, 3238
Full Circle Programs, 4198
Functional Assessment and Intervention: Guide to Understanding Problem Behavior, 3333
Functional Somatic Syndromes, 3072
Fundamentals of Psychiatric Treatment Planning, 2759

Funny, You Don't Look Crazy: Life With Obsessive Compulsive Disorder, 1180
Future Horizons, 560, 633

G

G Pierce Wood Memorial Hospital, 3794
G Werber Bryan Psychiatric Hospital, 4047
GMR Group, 4199
GPS Proposals, 3190
Gam-Anon Family Groups, 1147
Gamblers Anonymous, 1148
Gangs in Schools: Signs, Symbols and Solutions, 1606
Garner Consulting, 4200
Garnett Day Treatment Center, 2139
Gateway Community Services, 3795
Gateway Healthcare, 4043
Gaynor and Associates, 4201
Geauga Board of Mental Health, Alcohol and Drug Addiction Services, 4202
Gelbart and Associates, 4420
GenSource Corporation, 4421
Gender Differences in Depression: Marital Therapy Approach, 3494
Gender Differences in Mood and Anxiety Disorders: From Bench to Bedside, 2936
Gender Identity Disorder: A Medical Dictionary, Bibliography, and Annotated Research Guide to Internet References, 1111
Gender Loving Care, 3007
Gender Respect Workbook, 1607
Gene Bomb, 440
Geneen Roth and Associates, 1044
Genelco Software Solutions, 4422
General Hospital Psychiatry: Psychiatry, Medicine and Primary Care, 3239
Generalized Anxiety Disorder: Diagnosis, Treatment and Its Relationship to Other Anxiety Disorders, 2937
Generic: Acamprosate, 4673
Generic: Alprazolam, 4737
Generic: Amitryptaline, 4685
Generic: Amodafinil, 4709
Generic: Amphetamine/Dextroamphetamine, 4666
Generic: Aripiprazole, 4665
Generic: Atomoxetine, 4725
Generic: Bupropion, 4736
Generic: Buspirone, 4672
Generic: Citalopram, 4674
Generic: Clomipramine, 4668
Generic: Clonazepam, 4693
Generic: Clorazepate, 4731
Generic: Clozapine, 4676, 4695
Generic: Desipramine, 4708
Generic: Dextroamphetamine, 4682
Generic: Diazepam, 4733
Generic: Disulfiram, 4669
Generic: Donepezil, 4670
Generic: Dulozetine, 4679
Generic: Escitalopram, 4697
Generic: Eszopiclone, 4700
Generic: Fluoxine, 4727
Generic: Fluozetine, 4715
Generic: Fluphenazine, 4713
Generic: Fluvoxamine, 4701
Generic: Gabapentin, 4707
Generic: Galantamine, 4716
Generic: Haloperidol, 4691

Generic: Imipramine, 4728
Generic: Isocarboxazid, 4702
Generic: Lamotrigine, 4694
Generic: Lithium, 4687
Generic: Lithium; Eskalith, 4698
Generic: Lixdexamfetamine, 4735
Generic: Lorazepam, 4671
Generic: Loxapine, 4699
Generic: Luvox, 4689
Generic: Memantine, 4704
Generic: Methadone, 4683
Generic: Methylphenidate, 4678, 4703, 4721
Generic: Mianserin Hydrochloride, 4729
Generic: Mirtazapine, 4718
Generic: Modafinil, 4714
Generic: Nortriptyline, 4710
Generic: Olanzapine, 4739
Generic: Paliperidone, 4692
Generic: Parozetine, 4712
Generic: Perphenazine, 4732
Generic: Phenelzine, 4705
Generic: Quetiapine, 4723
Generic: Ramelteon, 4722
Generic: Razadine, 4719
Generic: Risperidone, 4720
Generic: Rivastigmine, 4688
Generic: Selegiline, 4686
Generic: Sertraline, 4738
Generic: Serzone, 4706
Generic: Sildenafil, 4734
Generic: Tacrine, 4677
Generic: Tadalafil, 4675
Generic: Topiramate, 4730
Generic: Tranylcypromine, 4711
Generic: Trimipramine, 4726
Generic: Valproic Acid, 4680
Generic: Vardenafil, 4696
Generic: Venlafazine, 4684
Generic: Vestra, 4717
Generic: Zalplon, 4724
Generic: Ziprasidone, 4690
Generic: Zolpidem, 4667
Genesis House Recovery Residence, 3796
Genesis Learning Center (Devereux), 3378
Geodon, 4690
George Washington University, 3379
Georgetown University Child Development Center, 1585, 1773
Georgia Association of Homes and Services for Children, 1874
Georgia Department of Human Resources, 2283
Georgia Department of Human Resources: Division of Public Health, 2284
Georgia Division of Mental Health Developmental Disabilities and Addictive Diseases (MHDDAD), 2285
Georgia National Alliance for the Mentally Ill, 1875
Georgia Parent Support Network, 1876
Georgia Psychological Society First Annual Conference, 3190
Georgia Regional Hospital at Atlanta, 3815
Georgia Regional Hospital at Augusta, 3816
Georgia Regional Hospital at Savannah, 3817
Geriatric Mental Health Care: A Treatment Guide for Health Professionals, 2966
Geriatrics, 3240
Gerontoligical Society of America, 2613
Get Your Angries Out, 1157
Getting Better Sleep: What You Need to Know, 740
Getting Beyond Sobriety, 119

Getting Control: Overcoming Your Obsessions and Compulsions, 1181
Getting Hooked: Rationality and Addiction, 120
Getting Involved in AA, 181
Getting Started in AA, 182
Getting Started with Facilitated Communication, 596
Getting What You Want From Drinking, 183
Getting What You Want From Stress, 341
Getting What You Want from Your Body Image, 1055
Gift of Life Home, 3972
Gilford Press, 2693
Girls and Boys Town of New York, 1627
Give Your ADD Teen a Chance: A Guide for Parents of Teenagers with Attention Deficit Disorder, 441
GlaxoSmithKline, 4639
Glazer Medical Solutions, 4203
GoAskAlice/Healthwise Columbia University, 3536
Going to School with Facilitated Communication, 666
Gold Coast Alliance for the Mentally Ill, 1831
Golden Cage, The Enigma of Anorexia Nervosa, 1027
Good Sam-W/Alliance for the Mentally Ill Family Support Group, 2149
Good Will-Hinckley Homes for Boys and Girls, 3888
Goodwill Industries-Suncoast, 85, 104, 263, 275, 705, 716, 828, 833, 870, 1124, 1132, 1165, 1236, 1244, 1281, 1290, 1333, 1356, 1367, 3808
Gorski-Cenaps Corporation Training & Consultation, 2614
Got Parts? An Insider's Guide to Managing Li fe Successfully with Dissociative Identity Disorder (New Horizons in Therapy), 965
Government Information Services, 4571
Government Printing Office, 1407
Grady Health Systems: Central Fulton CMHC, 1877
Graham-Windham Services for Children and Families: Manhattan Mental Health Center, 3973
Grand Central Publishing, 284
Grandma's Pet Wildebeest Ate My Homework, 442
Greater Binghamton Health Center, 3974
Greater Bridgeport Community Mental Health Center, 3781
Green Oaks Behavioral Healthcare Service, 4066
Greenwood Publishing Group, 3681, 2781
Greil Memorial Psychiatric Hospital, 3736
Grey House Publishing, 3636, 3637, 3638, 3641, 3644, 3650
Greystone Park Psychiatric Hospital, 3950
Grief Journey, 3537
Grief Recovery After A Substance Passing, 58
Grief Recovery After Substance Passing (GRASP), 10, 88
Grief and Bereavement, 67
GriefNet, 59
Griffin Memorial Hospital, 4019
Grip Project, 3911
Groden Center, 4044, 584

Group Exercises for Enhancing Social Skills & Self-Esteem, 3034
Group Involvement Training, 2760
Group Practice Journal, 3241
Group Psychotherapy for Eating Disorders, 1028
Group Therapy With Children and Adolescents, 3122
Group Therapy for Schizophrenic Patients, 1377
Group Treatments for Post-Traumatic Stress Disorder, 3050
Group Work for Eating Disorders and Food Issues, 3495
Group for the Advancement of Psychiatry, 2615
Growing Up Sad: Childhood Depression and Its Treatment, 883
A Guide To Psychlogy & Its Practice, 371
A Guide to Consent, 2685
Guide to Possibility Land: Fifty One Methods for Doing Brief, Respectful Therapy, 2761
Guide to Treatments That Work, 2762
Guidelines for Families Coping with OCD, 1219, 1276
Guidelines for Separating Parents, 72, 1658
Guidelines for the Treatment of Patients with Alzheimer's Disease and Other Dementias of Late Life, 2967
Guidelines for the Treatment of Patients with Schizophrenia, 1378
Guildeline for Treatment of Patients with Bipolar Disorder, 726
Guilford Press, 520, 2888
The Guilford Press, 139, 144, 718, 1001, 1019, 1256, 1296, 1298, 1402, 1450, 1558
Gurze Books, 3683, 1010, 1049
Gurze Bookstore, 1075

H

H Douglas Singer Mental Health Center, 3836
HCA Healthcare, 4204
HCIA Response, 4423
HMO & PPO Database & Directory, 3649
HMO/PPO Directory, 3650
HMS Healthcare Management Systems, 4424
HMS Software, 4425
HPN Worldwide, 4205
HSA-Mental Health, 4426, 4574
HSP Verified, 4206
HZI Research Center, 4427
Habilitation Software, 4428
Habilitative Systems, 3837
Hagar and Associates, 4575
Haldol, 4691
Hamilton Center, 3857
Hampstead Hospital, 3946
Handbook for the Assessment of Dissociation: a Clinical Guide, 966
Handbook for the Study of Mental Health, 3602
Handbook of Autism and Pervasive Developmental Disorders, 597
Handbook of Child Behavior in Therapy and in the Psychiatric Setting, 3123
Handbook of Clinical Psychopharmacology for Therapists, 3603
Handbook of Constructive Therapies, 3604

Handbook of Counseling Psychology, 3605
Handbook of Depression, 2988
Handbook of Dissociation: Theoretical, Empirical, and Clinical Perspectives, 2998
Handbook of Infant Mental Health, 3124
Handbook of Managed Behavioral Healthcare, 3606
Handbook of Medical Psychiatry, 3607
Handbook of Mental Retardation and Development, 3608
Handbook of PTSD: Science and Practice, 1298
Handbook of Parent Training: Parents as Co-Therapists for Children's Behavior Problems, 3125
Handbook of Psychiatric Education and Faculty Development, 3609
Handbook of Psychiatric Practice in the Juvenile Court, 3610
Handbook of Psychiatric Practice in the Juvenile Court, 3126
Handbook of Psychological Assessment, 3334
Handbook of Sexual and Gender Identity Disor der, 1112
Handbook of Sexual and Gender Identity Disorder, 1447
Handbook of Treatment for Eating Disorders, 3001
Handbook of the Medical Consequences of Alco hol and Drug Abuse, 121
Handbook on Quality of Life for Human Service Practitioners, 2763
Hanley & Befus, 3256
Hannah Neil Center for Children, 4009
Hanover Insurance, 4429
Happy Healthy Lifestyle Magazine for People with ADD, 494
Harcourt Assessment/PsychCorp, 4483
Harper Collins, 891, 893, 1031, 1034, 1042, 1176, 1400
Harper Collins Publishers, 3684
Harper House: Change Alternative Living, 3380
HarperCollins Publishers, 1349
Harriet Tubman Women and Children Treatment Facility Residential Program, 3838
Harris County Mental Health: Mental Retardation Authority, 2449
Harris Publishing, 3625
Hartford Hospital, 1740
Harvard Health Publications, 3242
Harvard Medical School Guide to Suicide Assessment and Intervention, 1505, 3335
Harvard Mental Health Letter, 3242
Harvard Review of Psychiatry, 3243
Harvard University Press, 3685, 579, 589, 1039, 2880
Haunted by Combat: Understanding PTSD in War Veterans, 1299
Have a Heart's Depression Home, 3534
Hawaii Alliance for the Mentally Ill, 1879
Hawaii Department of Adult Mental Health, 2286
Hawaii Department of Health, 2287
Hawaii Families As Allies, 1880
Hawaii State Hospital, 3821
Haworth Press, 3686, 585, 798, 894, 895, 1000, 3006, 3227
Hawthorn Center, 3922
Haymarket Center, Professional Development, 3381

Hays Group, 4207
Hazelden Foundation, 184
Hazelden Publishing, 150, 195
Hazelden Publishing & Educational Services, 1199
Hazelden Voice, 184
Healing ADD: Simple Exercises That Will Change Your Daily Life, 443
Healing Fear: New Approaches to Overcoming Anxiety, 303
Healing for Survivors, 1734
Health & Medicine Counsel of Washington DDNC Digestive Disease National Coalition, 2277
Health & Social Work, 3244
Health Alliance Plan, 4208
Health Capital Consultants, 4209
Health Care Desensitization, 667
Health Care For All(HCFA), 2193
Health Communications, 3688, 2886, 2913
Health Data Management, 3245
Health Decisions, 4210
Health Education, Research, Training Curriculum, 3232
Health Federation of Philadelphia, 2072
Health Grants & Contracts Weekly, 3246
Health Management Associates, 4211
Health Probe, 4430
Health Resources and Services Administration, 1932, 2194, 2225
Health Service Providers Verified, 2616
Health Services Agency: Mental Health, 1832
Health Source, 1379
Health Systems Research, 4212
Health Systems and Financing Group, 2194
Health Watch, 3336
Health and Human Services Office of Assistant Secretary for Planning & Evaluation, 2195
HealthGate, 3539
HealthLine Systems, 4431
HealthOnline, 4576
HealthPartners, 4213
HealthSoft, 4432
HealthWorld Online, 3541
Healthcare America, 4214
Healthcare Association of New York State, 2020
Healthcare Management Systems, 4577
Healthcare Value Management Group, 4215
Healthcare Vision, 4433
Healthcare in Partnership, 4216
Healthcheck, 4578
Healtheast Behavioral Care, 2494
Healthfinder, 1116
Healthline Systems, 4434
Healthport, 4435
Healthtouch Online, 3540
Healthwise, 4217
Healthwise of Utah, 2127
Healthy Companies, 4218
HeartMath, 4219
Heartland Behavioral Healthcare, 4010, 4011
Heartshare Human Services, 3382
Helix MEDLINE: GlaxoSmithKline, 3542
The Heller School for Social Policy & Management, 3440
Helms & Company, 4220
Help 4 ADD@High School, 444
Help Me, I'm Sad: Recognizing, Treating, and Preventing Childhood and Adolescent Depression, 884

Help This Kid's Driving Me Crazy - the Young Child with Attention Deficit Disorder, 3496
Helper's Journey: Working with People Facing Grief, Loss, and Life-Threatening Illness, 2764
Helping Athletes with Eating Disorders, 1029
Helping Children and Adolescents Cope with Violence and Disasters, 1314
Helping Hand, 1621
Helping Parents, Youth, and Teachers Understand Medications for Behavioral and Emotional Problems, 840, 2975, 3127
Helping People with Autism Manage Their Behavior, 598
Helping Women Recover: Special Edition for Use in the Criminal Justice System, 122
Helping Your Child Cope with Separation and Divorce, 1645
Helping Your Depressed Teenager: a Guide for Parents and Caregivers, 885
Heroin: What Am I Going To Do?, 221
Hi, I'm Adam: a Child's Story of Tourette Syndrome, 1547
Hidden Child: The Linwood Method for Reaching the Autistic Child, 599
The Hidden Child: Youth with Autism, 632
High Impact Consulting, 2765
High Tide Press, 3689, 2738, 2749, 2766, 2788, 2850, 2964, 3333
High Watch Farm, 3782
Highland Hospital, 4103
Hillcrest Utica Psychiatric Services, 3383
Hincks-Dellcrest Centre, 1735
Hiram W Davis Medical Center, 4093
Hispanic Substance Abuse, 2904
A History of Nursing in the Field of Mental Retardation, 2686
Hoffman-La Roche, 4640
Hogan Assessment Systems, 4436
Hogrefe & Huber Publishers, 3690
Holt Paperbacks, 293
Home Maintenance for Residential Service Providers, 2766
HomeTOVA: Attention Screening Test, 445
Homeward Bound, 4067
Homosexuality and American Psychiatry: The Politics of Diagnosis, 3008
Hong Fook Mental Health Association, 1736
Hope & Solutions for Obsessive Compulsive Disorder: Part III, 1207
Hope House, 3975
Hope Press, 3691, 406, 413, 440, 458, 470, 486, 839, 849, 1137, 1210, 1542, 1545, 1546, 1547, 1550, 1551, 1554, 1559, 1565
Hope and Solutions for OCD, 1208
Horizon Behavioral Services, 4221
Horizon Management Services, 4222
Horizon Mental Health Management, 4223
Horizons School, 1802
Hospital Association of Southern California, 1836
Houghton Mifflin Company, 615, 900, 1347
How to Avoid a Manic Episode, 757, 3525
How to Cope with Mental Illness In Your Family: A Guide for Siblings and Offspring, 1379
How to Do Homework without Throwing Up, 446
How to Help Someone You Care About, 1532
How to Help Your Loved One Recover from Agoraphobia, 304
How to Help a Person with Depression, 3557

How to Operate an ADHD Clinic or Subspecialty Practice, 2961
How to Partner with Managed Care, 2767
How to Teach Autistic & Severely Handicapped Children, 600
How to Teach Social Skills, 3128
Hudson River Psychiatric Center, 3976
Human Affairs International, 4224
Human Behavior Associates, 4225
Human Kinetics Publishers, 1029
Human Resources Consulting Group, 4579
Human Resources Development Institute, 1892
Human Sciences Press, 619
Human Services Research Institute, 1737, 4226
Hunger So Wide and Deep, 1030
Hungry Self; Women, Eating and Identity, 1031
Huron Alliance for the Mentally Ill, 2100
Hutchings Psychiatric Center, 3977
Hyde Park Associates, 4227
Hyland Behavioral Health System, 3938
Hyperactive Child, Adolescent, and Adult, 447
Hyperactive Children Grown Up: ADHD in Children, Adolescents, and Adults, 448
Hyperion, 1401, 2978
Hyperion Books, 3692
Hypoactive Sexual Desire: Integrating Sex and Couple Therapy, 3086
Hypochondria: Woeful Imaginings, 1345

I

I Can't Be an Alcoholic Because..., 185
I Can't Get Over It: Handbook for Trauma Survivors, 1300
I Can't Stop!: A Story About Tourette Syndrome, 1548
I Love You Like Crazy: Being a Parent with Mental Illness, 3497
I Wish Daddy Didn't Drink So Much, 1608
I'll Quit Tomorrow, 222
I'm Not Autistic on the Typewriter, 601, 668
I'm Somebody, Too!, 449
IABMCP, 3247
IABMCP Newsletter, 3247
IBM Corporation, 4442
IBM Global Healthcare Industry, 4437
ICON Health Publications, 1111
ICPA Reporter, 186
ICPADD, 186
IDX Systems Corporation, 4438
IEP-2005: Writing and Implementing Individua lized Education Programs, 2768
IHC Behavioral Health Network, 4228
IMNET Systems, 4439
INMED/MotherNet America, 4580
IQuest/Knowledge Index, 3529
Ibero-American Action League, 2032
Idaho Alliance for the Mentally Ill, 1883
Idaho Bureau of Maternal and Child Health, 2290
Idaho Bureau of Mental Health and Substance Abuse, Division of Family & Community Service, 2291
Idaho Department of Health & Welfare, 2292
Idaho Department of Health and Welfare: Family and Child Services, 2293
Idaho Mental Health Center, 2294

Identity Without Selfhood, 1113, 3009
If You Are Thinking about Suicide...Read This First, 1527, 3558
Illinois Alcoholism and Drug Dependency Association, 1893, 2295
Illinois Alliance for the Mentally Ill, 1894
Illinois Department of Alcoholism and Substance Abuse, 2296
Illinois Department of Children and Family Services, 2297
Illinois Department of Health and Human Services, 2298
Illinois Department of Human Services: Office of Mental Health, 2299
Illinois Department of Mental Health and Developmental Disabilities, 2301
Illinois Department of Mental Health and Drug Dependence, 2300
Illinois Department of Public Aid, 2302
Illinois Department of Public Health: Division of Food, Drugs and Dairies/FDD, 2303
Illinois Federation of Families for Children's Mental Health, 1895
Imp of the Mind: Exploring the Silent Epidemic of Obsessive Bad Thoughts, 1182
Impact Publishers, 3693, 143, 309, 837, 910, 1603, 2780, 2793, 2798, 3118, 3500, 3617
Improving Clinical Practice, 2769
Improving Therapeutic Communication, 2770
Impulse Control Disorders: A Clinician's Gui de to Understanding and Treating Behavioral Addictions, 1138
Impulsivity and Compulsivity, 1139
In Search of Solutions: A New Direction in Psychotherapy, 2771
In the Long Run... Longitudinal Studies of Psychopathology in Children, 3129
In the Wake of Suicide, 1506
Inclusion Strategies for Students with Learning and Behavior Problems, 2976
Increasing Variety in Adult Life, 2772
Independence Mental Health Institute, 3865
Independent Practice for the Mental Health Professional, 2773
Independent Publishing Group, 1091
Indiana Alliance for the Mentally Ill, 1900
The Indiana Consortium for Mental Health Services Research (ICMHSR), 2310
Indiana Department of Public Welfare Division of Family Independence: Food Stamps/Medicaid/Training, 2305
Indiana Family & Social Services Administration, 2306
Indiana Family And Social Services Administration, 2307
Indiana Family Support Network, MHA Indiana, 3858
Indiana Family and Social Services Administration, 2308, 2309
Indiana Institute on Disability and Community, 623, 626, 645, 662, 667, 672, 1454
Indiana Resource Center for Autism (IRCA), 1901, 687
Indiana University Psychiatric Management, 1902
Infanticide: Psychosocial and Legal Perspectives on Mothers Who Kill, 2774
Infants, Toddlers and Families: Framework for Support and Intervention, 3130
Info Management Associates, 3198
InfoMC, 4440

InfoNation Systems, 4581
Infoline, 203
Informa Healthcare, 1011
Information Access Technology, 4582
Information Centers for Lithium, Bipolar Disorders Treatment & Obsessive Compulsive Disorder, 1738
Information Management Solutions, 4441
Information Resources and Inquiries Branch, 2196
Informedics, 4583
Informix Software, 4442
Inforum, 4443
Infotrieve Medline Services Provider, 3544
Inhealth Record Systems, 4444
Inner Health Incorporated, 3498
Inner Life of Children with Special Needs, 602
Inner Peace Movement of Canada, 1739
Innovations in Clinical Practice: Source Book - Volumes 4-20, 3651
Innovative Approaches for Difficult to Treat Populations, 1380, 2775
Innovative Data Solutions, 4445
Innovative Health Systems/SoftMed, 4446
Inside Recovery How the Twelve Step Program Can Work for You, 123
Inside a Support Group, 124
Insider, 3248
Insider's Guide to Mental Health Resources Online, 2776
Insights in the Dynamic Psychotherapy of Anorexia and Bulimia, 1032
Instant Psychopharmacology, 2777
Institute for Advancement of Human Behavior, 3191
Institute for Behavioral Healthcare, 3384
Institute for Contemporary Psychotherapy, 1337
Institute for Contemproary Psychotherapy, 1338
Institute for Social Research Indiana University, 2310
Institute for the Advancement of Human Behavior (IAHB), 2617
Institute of HeartMath, 2618
Institute of Living Anxiety Disorders Center, 1740
Institute on Psychiatric Services: American Psychiatric Association, 2619
Insurance Management Institute, 4229
Integrated Behavioral Health Consultants, 2620
Integrated Business Services, 4447
Integrated Computer Products, 4448
Integrated Research Services, 194
Integrated Treatment of Psychiatric Disorders, 2778
Integrating Psychotherapy and Pharmaco-therapy: Disolving the Mind-Brain Barrier, 2779
Integrative Brief Therapy: Cognitive, Psychodynamic, Humanistic & Neurobehavioral Approaches, 2780
Integrative Treatment of Anxiety Disorders, 305, 2938
InteliHealth, 3545
Interface EAP, 4230
Interim Physicians, 4231
Interlink Health Services, 4232
International Association of Eating Disorders Professionals, 986

International Association of Psychosocialogy, 3295
International Center for the Study of Psychiatry And Psychology (ISCPP), 2621
International Critical Incident Stress Foundation, 267, 374, 1322
International Drug Therapy Newsletter, 3249
International Foundation of Employee Benefit Plans, 3233
International Handbook on Mental Health Policy, 2781
International Journal of Aging and Human Developments, 3251
International Journal of Health Services, 3252
International Journal of Neuropsychopharmacology, 3250
International Journal of Psychiatry in Medicine, 3253
International Medical News Group, 3225
International Photo Therapy Association, 1741
International Psychohistorical Assocation (IPA), 3299
International Society for Developmental Psychobiology, 2622
International Society for Traumatic Stress Studies, 1284
International Society for the Study of Dissociation, 954, 975
International Society of Political Psychology, 2623
International Society of Psychiatric-Mental Health Nurses, 1742
International Transactional Analysis Association (ITAA), 2624
Internet Mental Health, 243, 814, 1232, 1273, 1323, 1351, 1422, 1461, 1481, 1526, 1566
InternetPhone, 4449
Interpersonal Psychotherapy, 2782, 2989, 3002
Interventions for Students with Emotional Disorders, 3131
Interview with Dr. Pauline Filipek, 669
Interviewing Children and Adolesents: Skills and Strategies for Effective DSM-IV Diagnosis, 3132
Interviewing the Sexually Abused Child, 1448, 3133
Introduction to Depression and Bipolar Disor der, 741
Introduction to Time: Limited Group Psychotherapy, 2783
Introduction to the Technique of Psychotherapy: Practice Guidelines for Psychotherapists, 2784
Invega, 4692
Iowa Alliance for the Mentally Ill, 1905
Iowa Department Human Services, 2311
Iowa Department of Public Health, 2312
Iowa Department of Public Health: Division of Substance Abuse, 2313
Iowa Division of Mental Health & Developmental Disabilities: Department of Human Services, 2314
Iowa Federation of Families for Children's Mental Health, 1906
Is Your Child Hyperactive? Inattentive? Impulsive? Distractible?, 450
It's Not All In Your Head: Now Women Can Discover the Real Causes of their Most Misdiagnosed Health Problems, 306

J

JM Oher and Associates, 4233
JS Medical Group, 4234
Jacobs Institute of Women's Health, 3385
Jail Detainees with Co-Occurring Mental Health and Substance Use Disorders, 2905
James F Byrnes Medical Center, 4048
James J Peters VA Medical Center, 1412
Janssen, 4641
Jason Aronson, 1013, 1024, 1032, 1038, 1040, 1041, 1346, 1389
Jason Aronson Publishers, 3694
Jason Aronson Publishing, 1395
Jason Aronson-Rowman & Littlefield Publishers, 29
Jean Piaget Society: Society for the Study of Knowledge and Development (JPSSSKD), 2625
Jefferson Drug/Alcohol, 3386
Jeri Davis Marketing Consultants, 4235
Jerome M Sattler, 3112
Jerome M Sattler Publisher, 3695
Jersey City Medical Center Behavioral Health Center, 3951
Jessica Kingsley, 2881
Jessica Kingsley Publishers, 3696, 572, 578, 1552
Jewish Alcoholics Chemically Dependent Persons, 240
Jewish Family Service, 3783
Jewish Family Service of Atlantic County and Cape, 2003
Jewish Family Service of Dallas, 2114
Jewish Family Service of San Antonio, 2115
Jewish Family and Children's Services, 1944, 4068
Jim Chandler MD, 942
Job Stress Help, 376
Joey and Sam, 603
John A Burns School of Medicine Department of Psychiatry, 3387
John Hopkins University School of Medicine, 749
John J Madden Mental Health Center, 3839
John L. Gildner Regional Institute for Children and Adolescents, 3894
John Maynard and Associates, 4236
John R Day and Associates, 3840
John Wiley and Sons, 719
Johns Hopkins University Press, 3698, 614, 793, 879, 2953
Johnson & Johnson, 4642
Johnson, Bassin and Shaw, 4237
Join Together, 241
Join Together Online, 204
Joint Commission on Accreditation of Healthcare Organizations, 2495
Jones and Bartlett Publishers, 277
Jossey-Bass, 3699
Jossey-Bass / John Wiley & Sons, 1403
Jossey-Bass / Wiley & Sons, 112, 119, 122, 125, 126, 129, 130, 131, 153, 1505, 1506
Jossey-Bass/Wiley, 1196
Journal of AHIMA, 3254
Journal of American Health Information Management Association, 3255
Journal of American Medical Information Association, 3256
Journal of Anxiety Disorders, 342
Journal of Autism and Developmental Disorders, 646

Journal of Drug Education, 3257
Journal of Education Psychology, 3258
Journal of Emotional and Behavioral Disorders, 3259
Journal of Intellectual & Development Disability, 3260
Journal of Neuropsychiatry and Clinical Neurosciences, 3261
Journal of Positive Behavior Interventions, 3262
Journal of Practical Psychiatry, 3263
Journal of Substance Abuse Treatment, 187
Journal of the American Medical Informatics Association, 3264
Journal of the American Psychiatric Nurses Association, 3265
Journal of the American Psychoanalytic Association, 3266
Journal of the International Neuropsychological Society, 3267
Judge Baker Children's Center, 1743
Julia Dyckman Andrus Memorial, 3350
Juniper Healthcare Containment Systems, 4238
Just Say No International, 1628
Just a Mood...or Something Else, 3566
Justice in Mental Health Organizations, 1953
Juvenile Justice Commission, 2383

K

KAI Associates, 4239
KY-SPIN, 1914
Kalamazoo Psychiatric Hospital, 3923
Kansas Council on Developmental Disabilities Kansas Department of Social and Rehabilitation Services, 2317
Kansas Department of Mental Health and Retardation and Social Services, 2318
Kansas Department of Social and Rehabilitation Services, 2316
Kansas Schizophrenia Anonymous, 1909
Keane Care, 4450
Kennedy Krieger Institute, 3895
The Kennion Group Inc, 4333
Kent County Alliance for the Mentally Ill, 2082
Kentucky Alliance for the Mentally Ill, 1915
Kentucky Cabinet for Health and Family Services, 2321
Kentucky Cabinet for Health and Human Services, 2319
Kentucky Correctional Psychiatric Center, 3876
Kentucky Department for Health and Family Services, 2320
Kentucky Department for Human Support Services, 2320
Kentucky Department for Medicaid Services, 2321
Kentucky Department of Mental Health and Mental Retardation, 2322
Kentucky IMPACT, 1916
Kentucky Justice Cabinet: Department of Juvenile Justice, 2323
Kentucky Psychiatric Association, 1917
Kerrville State Hospital, 4069
Key, 3268
Keys To Recovery, 3841
Keys for Networking: Kansas Parent Informati on & Resource Center, 1910

Keys to Parenting the Child with Autism, 604
Kicking Addictive Habits Once & For All, 125
Kid Power Tactics for Dealing with Depression & Parent's Survival Guide to Childhood Depression, 1609
KidsPeace, 1118
Kidspeace National Centers, 1629
King Pharmaceuticals, 4643
Kingsboro Psychiatric Center, 3978
Kirby Forensic Psychiatric Center, 3979
Kitsap County Alliance for the Mentally Ill, 2150
Klingberg Family Centers, 3784
Klonopin, 4693
Kluwer Academic/Plenum Publishers, 606, 620, 1197, 2900, 2998, 3012
Knopf Publishing Group, 1501, 1504
Know Your Rights: Mental Health Private Practice & the Law, 3499
Kristy and the Secret of Susan, 605
Kushner and Company, 4240

L

LRADAC The Behavioral Health Center of the Midlands, 2429
LSD: Still With Us After All These Years, 126
La Hacienda Treatment Center, 4070
Lad Lake, 4584
Lake Mental Health Consultants, 4241
Lakeshore Mental Health Institute, 4054
Lamictal, 4694
LanVision Systems, 4451
Langley Porter Psych Institute at UCSF Parnassus Campus, 3388
Langley Porter Psychiatric Institute at UCSF Parnassus Campus, 1833
Languages of Psychoanalysis, 2785
Lanstat Incorporated, 2496
Lanstat Resources, 4585
Lapeer County Community Mental Health Center, 1954
Largesse, The Network for Size Esteem, 987
Larkin Center, 1896
Larned State Hospital, 3867
Las Vegas Medical Center, 3955
Laurel Regional Hospital, 3896
Laurel Ridge Treatment Center, 4071
Laurelwood Hospital and Counseling Centers, 3389
Lawrence Erlbaum Associates, 3700, 1016, 3021
Leadership and Organizational Excellence, 2786
Learning Disabilities Association of America, 395, 475
Learning Disabilities: A Multidisciplinary Journal, 475
Learning Disability Association of America, 1744
Learning Disorders and Disorders of the Self in Children and Adolesents, 3134
Learning and Cognition in Autism, 606
Learning to Get Along for the Best Interest of the Child, 1666
Learning to Slow Down and Pay Attention, 451
Left Alive: After a Suicide Death in the Family, 1507

Legacy Consulting Insurance Services, 4242
Legacy of Childhood Trauma: Not Always
　Who They Seem, 1637
Leponex, 4695
Let Community Employment Be the Goal
　For Individuals with Autism, 607
Let Me Hear Your Voice, 608
Let's Talk About Depression, 915
Let's Talk Facts About Obsessive
　Compulsive Disorder, 1183
Let's Talk Facts About Panic Disorder, 343
Let's Talk Facts About Post-Traumatic
　Stress Disorder, 1315
Let's Talk Facts About Substance Abuse &
　Addiction, 127
Letting Go, 609
Levitra, 4696
Lewin Group, 4243
Lexapro, 4697
Lexi-Comp, 2836, 3648, 3659, 3661
Lexical Technologies, 4452
Lexington Books, 3701, 1022, 3004
Liberty Healthcare Management Group, 4586
Liberty Resources, 3980
Life After Trauma: Workbook for Healing,
　3051
Life Course Perspective on Adulthood and
　Old Age, 2787
Life Development Institute, 1745
Life Is Hard: Audio Guide to Healing
　Emotional Pain, 3500
Life Passage in the Face of Death, Volume I:
　A Brief Psychotherapy, 3501
Life Passage in the Face of Death, Volume II
　: Psychological Engagement of the
　Physically Ill Patient, 3502
Life Science Associates, 3390
Life Steps Pasos de Vida, 3758
Life Transition Therapy, 3953
Life after Loss: Dealing with Grief, 76
LifeRing, 257
Lifelink Bensenville, 3842
Lifelink Corporation, 4244
Lifelink Corporation/Bensenville Home
　Society, 4587
Lifespan Care Management Agency, 4245
Lifespire, 1580, 1746
Lifetime Weight Control, 1033
Lincoln Center Campus, 3184
Lincoln Child Center, 3759
Lippincott Williams & Wilkins, 3702, 2922,
　3249
Lithium Information Center, 709
Lithium and Manic Depression: A Guide, 727
Lithobid, 4698
Little City Foundation (LCF), 1897
Littleton Group Home, 3912
Living Skills Recovery Workbook, 128, 3611
Living Sober I, 129
Living Sober II, 130
Living Without Depression & Manic
　Depression: a Workbook for Maintaining
　Mood Stability, 728
Living on the Razor's Edge:
　Solution-Oriented Brief Family Therapy
　with Self-Harming Adolesents, 3135
Living with Attention Deficit Disorder: a
　Workbook for Adults with ADD, 452
Living with Depression and Manic
　Depression, 933
Locumtenens.com, 3391

Lonely, Sad, and Angry: a Parent's Guide to
　Depression in Children and Adolescents,
　886
Long-Term Treatments of Anxiety
　Disorders, 2939
Los Angeles County Department of Mental
　Health, 3748
Loss of Self: Family Resource for the Care
　of Alzheimer's Disease and Related
　Disorders, 2968
Lost in the Mirror: An Inside Look at
　Borderline Personality Disorder, 967, 1263
Louisiana Alliance for the Mentally Ill, 1923
Louisiana Commission on Law Enforcement
　and Administration (LCLE), 2324
Louisiana Department of Health and
　Hospitals: Louisiana Office for Addictive
　Disorders, 2326
Louisiana Department of Health and
　Hospitals: Office of Mental Health, 2325
Louisiana Federation of Families for
　Children's Mental Health, 1924
Love First: A New Approach to Intervention
　for Alcoholism and Drug Addiction, 2906
Love Publishing, 3703
Love Publishing Company, 631
Loving Healing Press, 965
Loxitane, 4699
Lunesta, 4700
Luvox, 4701

M

MAAP, 647, 521
MAAP Services, 538, 647, 689
MADD-Mothers Against Drunk Drivers, 205
MADD-Mothers Against Drunk Driving, 242
MADNESS, 4588
MBP Expert Services, 1098
MCF Consulting, 4246
MCG Telemedicine Center, 3392, 4247
MCW Department of Psychiatry and
　Behavioral Medicine, 3393, 4248
MEDA, 1065
MEDCOM Information Systems, 4454
MEDLINEplus on Sleep Disorders, 1483
MEDecision, 4455
MHM Services, 3199
MHNet, 4032
MISS Foundation, 62
MJ Powers & Company, 3297
MMHR, 4249
MSI International, 4250
MacNeal Hospital, 3843
Macomb County Community Mental Health,
　1955
Macon W Freeman Center, 4072
Magellan Health Service, 4251
Magellan Public Solutions, 4252
Maine Alliance for the Mentally Ill, 1926
Maine Department Health and Human
　Services Children's Behavioral Health
　Services, 2327
Maine Department of Behavioral and
　Developmental Services, 2328
Maine Office of Substance Abuse:
　Information and Resource Center, 2329
Maine Psychiatric Association, 1927
Major Depression in Children and
　Adolescents, 916, 1622

Making Money While Making a Difference:
　Achieving Outcomes for People with
　Disabilities, 2788
Making Peace with Food, 1034
Making the Grade: Guide to School Drug
　Prevention Programs, 3136
Malignant Neglect: Substance Abuse and
　America's Schools, 2907
Mallinckrodt, 4644
Managed Care Concepts, 4253
Managed Care Consultants, 4254
Managed Care Local Market Overviews,
　4589
Managed Care Strategies, 3269
Managed Care Strategies & Psychotherapy
　Finances, 3269, 3307
Managed Health Care Association, 2626
Managed Health Network, 4255
Managed Healthcare Consultants, 4256
Managed Mental Health Care in the Public
　Sector: a Survival Manual, 2789
Managed Networks of America, 4257
Management Recruiters of Washington, DC,
　3394
Management of Autistic Behavior, 610
Management of Bipolar Disorder:
　Pocketbook, 729
Management of Countertransference with
　Borderline Patients, 1264
Management of Depression, 887
Managing Client Anger: What to Do When a
　Client is Angry with You, 2790
Managing Social Anxiety: A
　Cognitive-Behavio ral Therapy Approach
　Client Workbook (Treatments That
　Work), 307
Managing Traumatic Stress Risk: A
　Proactive Approach, 1301
Manatee Glens, 3797
Manatee Palms Youth Services, 3798
Manhattan Psychiatric Center, 3981
Mania: Clinical and Research Perspectives,
　730
Maniaci Insurance Services, 4258
Manic Depressive and Depressive
　Association of Metropolitan Detroit, 1956
Manic-Depressive Illness, 3556
Manic-Depressive Illness: Bipolar Disorders
　and Recurrent Depression, 888, 1508
Manisses Communication Group, 4590
Manisses Communications Group, 2830,
　2831, 3278, 4590
Manual of Clinical Child and Adolescent
　Psychiatry, 3137
Manual of Clinical Psychopharmacology,
　2791
Manual of Panic: Focused Psychodynamic
　Psychotherapy, 3073
Marijuana ABC's, 188
Marijuana Anonymous, 206
Marijuana: Escape to Nowhere, 223
Marin Institute, 4259
Marion County Health Department, 2411
Marplan, 4702
Marsh Foundation, 3395
Mary Starke Harper Geriatric Psychiatry
　Center, 3737
Maryland Alcohol and Drug Abuse
　Administration, 2334
Maryland Alliance for the Mentally Ill, 1933

Maryland Department of Health and Mental Hygiene, 2335
Maryland Department of Human Resources, 2336
Maryland Division of Mental Health, 2337
Maryland Psychiatric Research Center, 1934
Masculinity and Sexuality: Selected Topics in the Psychology of Men, 1449
Masn Crest Publishers, 1343
Mason Crest Publishers, 3704, 27, 296, 435, 461, 632, 796, 881, 889, 964, 1136, 1146, 1178, 1260, 1372, 1476, 2923, 3000, 3091
Massachusetts Alliance for the Mentally Ill, 1945
Massachusetts Behavioral Health Partnership, 1946
Massachusetts Department of Health and Human Services, 2342
Massachusetts Department of Mental Health, 2338
Massachusetts Department of Public Health, 2339
Massachusetts Department of Public Health: Bureau of Substance Abuse Services, 2340
Massachusetts Department of Social Services, 2341
Massachusetts Department of Transitional Assistance, 2342
Massachusetts Division of Medical Assistance MassHealth Program, 2343
Massachusetts Executive Office of Public Safety, 2344
The Massachusetts General Hospital Bipolar Clinic/Research Program, 746, 763
Master Your Panic and Take Back Your Life, 308
Master Your Panic and Take Back Your Life: Twelve Treatment Sessions to Overcome High Anxiety, 309
Mastering Your Stress Demons, 375
Mastering the Kennedy Axis V: New Psychiatric Assessment of Patient Functioning, 2792
Masters of Behavioral Healthcare Management, 3396
Mastery of Your Anxiety and Panic: Workbook, 310
Matthew: Guidance for Parents with Autistic Children, 670
Mayes Group, 4260
Mayo Clinic, 1215, 3270
Mayo Clinic Health Letter, 3270
Mayo Clinic Health Oasis, 1119
Mayo Clinic Health Oasis Library, 3548
Mayo Clinic on Depression, 889
Mayo HealthQuest/Mayo Clinic Health Information, 4591
MayoClinic.com, 813
Mayview State Hospital, 4033
McCall Foundation, 3785
McGladery and Pullen CPAs, 4261
McGraw Hill Healthcare Management, 4262
McGraw-Hill Companies, 732, 1143
McHenry County M/H Board, 4456
McHenry County Mental Health Board, 3844
McKesson Clinical Reference Systems, 4375
McKesson HBO and Company, 4263
McKesson HBOC, 4457
McMan's Depression and Bipolar Web, 742
McMan's Depression and Bipolar Weekly, 742

Me, Myself, and Them: A Firsthand Account of One Young Person's Experience with Schizophrenia (Adolescent Mental Health Initiativ, 1381
Meadowridge Pelham Academy, 3913
Meadowridge Walden Street School, 3914
Meaning of Addiction, 131
Med Advantage, 2497, 2627
Med Data Systems, 4458
MedPLus, 4459
MedWeb Emory University Health Sciences Center Library, 3553
Medai, 4460
Medcomp Software, 4461
Medi-Pages, 3652
Medi-Pages On-Line Directory, 3652
Medi-Span, 4462
Medical & Healthcare Marketplace Guide Directory, 3653
Medical Aspects of Chemical Dependency Active Parenting Publishers, 132, 224
Medical Aspects of Chemical Dependency The Neurobiology of Addiction, 3503
Medical Center of LA: Mental Health Services, 3883
Medical College of Georgia, 3397
Medical College of Ohio, Psychiatry, 3398
Medical College of Pennsylvania, 3399
Medical College of Virginia, 3400
Medical College of Wisconsin, 3401
Medical Data Research, 4592
Medical Doctor Associates, 3402
Medical Group Management Association, 2628
Medical Online Resources, 4593
Medical Psychotherapist, 3271
Medical Records Institute, 4463
Medical Records Solution, 4464
Medical University of South Carolina Institute of Psychiatry, Psychiatry Access Center, 3403
Medication for ADHD, 483
Medications, 3272
Medications for Attention Disorders and Related Medical Problems: A Comprehensive Handbook, 453, 2962
Medina CFIT, 4011
Medipay, 4465, 4594
Meditation, Guided Fantasies, and Other Stress Reducers, 386
Meditative Therapy Facilitating Inner-Directed Healing, 2793
Medix Systems Consultants, 4466
Medscape, 3552
Medware, 4467
Meeting the ADD Challenge: A Practical Guide for Teachers, 454
Meharry Medical College, 3404
Mellon HR Solutions, 4264
Memory, Trauma and the Law, 3052
Memphis Alcohol and Drug Council, 2440
Memphis Business Group on Health, 2103
Memphis Mental Health Institute, 4055
Men and Depression, 917
Mendota Mental Health Institute, 4108
Menninger Care Systems, 4265
Menninger Clinic, 1747, 846
Menninger Clinic Department of Research, 3405
Menninger Division of Continuing Education, 3405
Mental & Physical Disability Law Reporter, 3273

Mental Affections Childhood, 3138
Mental Disability Law: Primer, a Comprehensive Introduction, 2794
Mental Health & Spirituality Support Group, 2151
Mental Health Aspects of Developmental Disabilities, 3274
Mental Health Association, 2116
Mental Health Association in Alaska, 1807, 2240
Mental Health Association in Albany County, 2021
Mental Health Association in Dutchess County, 2022
Mental Health Association in Illinois, 2304
Mental Health Association in Marion County Consumer Services, 1903
Mental Health Association in Michigan, 1415
Mental Health Association in South Carolina, 2430
Mental Health Association of Arizona, 1812
Mental Health Association of Colorado, 1846
Mental Health Association of Delaware, 1857
Mental Health Association of Greater Dallas, 2450
Mental Health Association of Greater St. Louis, 1977
Mental Health Association of Maryland, 1935
Mental Health Association of Montana, 1983
Mental Health Association of New Jersey, 2004
Mental Health Association of Southeastern Pe nnsylvania (MHASP), 2073
Mental Health Association of Summit, 2051
Mental Health Association of West Florida, 1871
Mental Health Association: Connecticut, 1851
Mental Health Board of North Central Alabama, 1803
Mental Health Center of North Central Alabama, 1804
Mental Health Connections, 4468
Mental Health Consultants, 3200
Mental Health Corporations of America, 2629
Mental Health Council of Arkansas, 2250
Mental Health Directory, 3654
Mental Health Law Reporter, 3275
Mental Health Materials Center (MHMC), 2630
Mental Health Matters, 1127
Mental Health Network, 4266
Mental Health Outcomes, 4469
Mental Health Rehabilitation: Disputing Irrational Beliefs, 2795
Mental Health Report, 3276
Mental Health Research Association (NARSAD), 861
Mental Health Resources Catalog, 2796
Mental Health Views, 3277
Mental Health Weekly, 3278
Mental Health and Aging Network (MHAN) of the American Society on Aging (ASA), 1748
Mental Health and Substance Abuse Corporations of Massachusetts, 1947
Mental Illness Education Project, 1749, 3504, 754, 1416, 1417, 3497
The Mental Illness Education Project, 755
Mental Retardation, 3279
Mental Retardation: Definition, Classification, and Systems of Supports, 2797

Mental, Emotional, and Behavior Disorders in Children and Adolescents, 844, 1623
Mentalhelp, 1423
Mentally Disabled and the Law, 3280
Mentally Ill Kids in Distress, 1581, 1750
Mercer Consulting, 4267
Merck, 4645
Meridian Resource Corporation, 4268, 4595
Merit Behavioral Care of California, 3760
Meritcare Health System, 4470
Mertech, 2498
Mesa Mental Health, 4269
Metaphor in Psychotherapy: Clinical Applications of Stories and Allegories, 2798
Methamphetamine: Decide to Live Prevention Video, 225
Methylin, 4703
Metro Child and Adolescent Network, 3845
Metro Intergroup of Overeaters Anonymous, 2023, 1036
Metro Regional Treatment Center: Anoka, 3930
Metropolitan Area Chapter of Federation of Families for Children's Mental Health, 1957
Metropolitan Family Services, 1898
Metropolitan State Hospital, 3761
Michael Reese Hospital and Medical Center, 1059, 1061
Michigan Alliance for the Mentally Ill, 1958
Michigan Association for Children with Emotional Disorders: MACED, 1959
Michigan Association for Children's Mental Health, 1582
Michigan Association for Children's Mental Health, 1960
Michigan Department of Community Health, 2345
Michigan Department of Human Services, 2346
Michigan State Representative: Co-Chair Public Health, 2347
Micro Design International, 4471
Micro Office Systems, 4472
Microcounseling, 2799
Micromedex, 4473
Microsoft Corporation, 4596, 4479
Mid-Hudson Forensic Psychiatric Center, 3982
Middle Tennessee Mental Health Institute, 2441, 4056
Middletown Psychiatric Center, 3983
Mihalik Group, 4270
Mildred Mitchell-Bateman Hospital, 4104
Millcreek Children's Services, 4012
Milliman, Inc, 4271
Mills-Peninsula Hospital: Behavioral Health, 3762
Mind of its Own, Tourette's Syndrome: Story and a Guide, 1549
Mind-Body Problems: Psychotherapy with Psychosomatic Disorders, 1346
Mindblindness: An Essay on Autism and Theory of Mind, 611
Minnesota Association for Children's Mental Health, 1966
Minnesota Department of Human Services, 2350
Minnesota Psychiatric Society, 1967
Minnesota Psychological Association, 1968
Minnesota Youth Services Bureau, 2351
Mirror, Mirror, 1079, 3562

Missed Opportunity: National Survey of Primary Care Physicians and Patients on Substance Abuse, 2908
Mississippi Alcohol Safety Education Program, 2352
Mississippi Alliance for the Mentally Ill, 1973
Mississippi Department Mental Health Mental Retardation Services, 2353
Mississippi Department of Human Services, 2354
Mississippi Department of Mental Health: Division of Medicaid, 2355, 2356
Mississippi Department of Rehabilitation Services: Office of Vocational Rehabilitation (OVR), 2357
Mississippi Families as Allies, 1974
Mississippi State Hospital, 3934
Missouri Alliance for the Mentally Ill, 1978
Missouri Department Health & Senior Services, 2358
Missouri Department of Mental Health, 2359
Missouri Department of Public Safety, 2360
Missouri Department of Social Services, 2361
Missouri Department of Social Services: Medical Services Division, 2362
Missouri Division of Alcohol and Drug Abuse, 2363
Missouri Division of Comprehensive Psychiatric Service, 2364
Missouri Division of Mental Retardation and Developmental Disabilities, 2365
Missouri Institute of Mental Health, 1979
Missouri Statewide Parent Advisory Network: MO-SPAN, 1980
Misunderstood Child: Understanding and Coping with Your Child's Learning Disabilities, 455
Misys Health Care Systems, 4474
Mixed Blessings, 612
Moccasin Bend Mental Health Institute, 4057
Mohawk Valley Psychiatric Center, 3984
Monadnock Family Services, 1997
Monatana Department of Human & Community Services, 2229
Montana Alliance for the Mentally Ill, 1984
Montana Department of Health and Human Services: Child & Family Services Division, 2366
Montana Department of Public Health & Human Services: Addictive and Mental Disorders, 2367
Montana Department of Public Health and Human Services: Montana Vocational Rehabilitation Programs, 2368
Montgomery County Project SHARE, 4034
Mood Apart, 890
Mood Apart: Thinker's Guide to Emotion & It's Disorders, 891
Mood Disorders, 743
More Advanced Autistic People Services (MAAPS), 551
More Advanced Persons with Autism and Asperger's Syndrome (MAAP), 516
More Laughing and Loving with Autism, 613
Mosby, 3607
Mother's Survival Guide to Recovery: All About Alcohol, Drugs & Babies, 133
Mothers Against Munchausen Syndrome by Proxy Allegations, 1099
Mothers in Sympathy and Support, 61
Motivating Behavior Changes Among Illicit-Drug Abusers, 134

Motivational Interviewing: Prepare People to Change Addictive Behavior, 3020
Motivational Interviewing: Preparing People to Change Addictive Behavior, 189
Mount Carmel Behavioral Healthcare, 2052
Mount Pleasant Center, 3924
Mount Pleasant Mental Health Institute, 3866
Mountain State Parents Children Adolescent Network, 2165
Mountainside Treatment Center, 3786
Moynihan Institute of Global Affairs, 2623
MphasiS(BPO), 4475
Multimedia Medical Systems, 4597
Munchause Syndrome, 1100
Munchausen Syndrome by Proxy: Issues in Diagnosis and Treatment, 3004
Munchausen by Proxy Syndrome: Misunderstood Child Abuse, 3005
Munchausen by Proxy: Identification, Intervention, and Case Management, 3006
Munchausen by Proxy: Identification, Intervention, and Case Management, 1092
Munchausen's Syndrome by Proxy, 1093
Murphy-Harpst-Vashti, 4272
Mutual Pharmaceutical Company, 4646
Mutual of Omaha Companies' Integrated Behavioral Services, 4476
Mutual of Omaha's Health and Wellness Programs, 1987
My Body is Mine, My Feelings are Mine, 1610
My Brother's a World Class Pain: a Sibling's Guide to ADHD, 456
My Listening Friend: A Story About the Benefits of Counseling, 1611
My Quarter-Life Crisis: How an Anxiety Disorder Knocked Me Down, and How I Got Back Up, 311
My Son...My Son: A Guide to Healing After Death, Loss, or Suicide, 1509
Myth of Maturity: What Teenagers Need from Parents to Become Adults, 3139
Myths and Facts about Depression and Bipolar Disorders, 744

N

NADD, 3316
NADD Annual Conference & Exhibit Show, 3192
NADD Press, 11, 33
NADD-National Association for the Dually Diagnosed, 697
NADD-National Council on Alcoholism and Drug Dependence, 230
NADD: National Association for the Dually Diagnosed, 388, 772
NAMI, 2140
NAMI Advocate, 3281
NAMI Beginnings, 3282
NAMI Eastside Family Resource Center, 2160
NAMI Hawaii, 1881
NAMI National Convention, 3193
NAMI Queens/Nassau, 1599
NAMI Whidbey Island, 2163
NAMI Wyoming, 2179
NAMI-Eastside, 2158
NAMI-Eastside Family Resource Center, 2156

NAMI-New York State: National Alliance on Mental Illness, 1430

NAMI-Wisconsin, 2173

NARSA: The Mental Health Research Associatio n, 1410

NARSAD: The Mental Health Research Associati on, 862, 1359

NASAP, 2656, 3286

NASW JobLink, 4273

NASW Minnesota Chapter, 1969

NASW News, 3283

NASW West Virginia Chapter, 4598

NEOUCOM-Northeastern Ohio Universities College of Medicine, 3406

NIH Neurological Institute, 783

NPIN Resources for Parents: Full Texts of Parenting-Related Material, 1651

NPIN: National Parent Information Network, 1650

NYU Department of Psychiatry, 3550

Namenda, 4704

Nami Eastside-Family Resource Center, 2151

Napa State Hospital, 3763

Nar-Anon Family Group, 207

Narcotics Anonymous, 208

Nardil, 4705

Narrative Means to Sober Ends: Treating Addiction and Its Aftermath, 2909

Narrative Therapies with Children and Adolescents, 3140

Nathan S Kline Institute, 3985

Nathan S Kline Institute for Psychiatric Research, 3407

Nathan S Kline Institute for Psychiatric Research, 1751, 1718

Nation Alliance on Mental Illness: Californi a, 1834

National Institutes of Mental Health Division of Intramural Research Programs (DIRP), 2197

National Academy of Neuropsychology (NAN), 2631

National Aliance for the Mentally Ill, 501

National Alliance for Autism Research (NAAR), 681

National Alliance for Research on Schizophrenia and Depression, 923

National Alliance for Research on Schizophrenia and Depression, 1360, 1429

National Alliance for the Mentally Ill, 379, 692, 769, 1394, 1821, 3281

National Alliance on Mental Illness, 89, 268, 396, 552, 710, 863, 988, 1238, 1285, 1361, 1470, 1494, 1536, 1752, 722, 1369, 1393, 3193, 3282

National Alliance on Mental Illness: Alabama, 1805

National Alliance on Mental Illness: Alaska, 1808

National Alliance on Mental Illness: Arizona, 1813

National Alliance on Mental Illness: Arkansa s, 1819

National Alliance on Mental Illness: Colorad o, 1847

National Alliance on Mental Illness: Connect icut, 1852

National Alliance on Mental Illness: Davis Park, 2084

National Alliance on Mental Illness: Delawar e, 1858

National Alliance on Mental Illness: Distric t of Columbia, 1863

National Alliance on Mental Illness: Florida, 1872

National Alliance on Mental Illness: Georgia, 1878

National Alliance on Mental Illness: Hawaii, 1882

National Alliance on Mental Illness: Idaho, 1884

National Alliance on Mental Illness: Illinoi s, 1899

National Alliance on Mental Illness: Indiana, 1904

National Alliance on Mental Illness: Iowa, 1907

National Alliance on Mental Illness: Kansas, 1911

National Alliance on Mental Illness: Kentuck y, 1918

National Alliance on Mental Illness: Louisia na, 1925

National Alliance on Mental Illness: Maine, 1928

National Alliance on Mental Illness: Marylan d, 1936

National Alliance on Mental Illness: Massach usetts, 1948

National Alliance on Mental Illness: Michiga n, 1961

National Alliance on Mental Illness: Minneso ta, 1970

National Alliance on Mental Illness: Mississ ippi, 1975

National Alliance on Mental Illness: Missour i, 1981

National Alliance on Mental Illness: Montana, 1985

National Alliance on Mental Illness: Nebrask a, 1988

National Alliance on Mental Illness: Nevada, 1994

National Alliance on Mental Illness: New Ham pshire, 1998

National Alliance on Mental Illness: New Jer sey, 2005

National Alliance on Mental Illness: New Mex ico, 2011

National Alliance on Mental Illness: New Yor k, 2024

National Alliance on Mental Illness: North C arolina, 2038

National Alliance on Mental Illness: North D akota, 2043

National Alliance on Mental Illness: Ohio, 2053

National Alliance on Mental Illness: Oklahom a, 2062

National Alliance on Mental Illness: Oregon, 2067

National Alliance on Mental Illness: Pennsyl vania, 2074

National Alliance on Mental Illness: Rhode Island, 2083, 2085

National Alliance on Mental Illness: South Carolina, 2094

National Alliance on Mental Illness: South D akota, 2101

National Alliance on Mental Illness: Tenness ee, 2104

National Alliance on Mental Illness: Texas, 2117

National Alliance on Mental Illness: Utah, 2128

National Alliance on Mental Illness: Vermont, 2132

National Alliance on Mental Illness: Virgini a, 2141

National Alliance on Mental Illness: Washing ton, 2152

National Alliance on Mental Illness: West Vi rginia, 2166

National Alliance on Mental Illness: Wiscons in, 2171

National Alliance on Mental Illness: Wyoming, 2177

National Anxiety Foundation, 269

National Assocaition for the Dually, 711

National Assocaition for the Dually Diagnose d (NADD), 1441

National Association Councils on Developmental Disabilities, 780

National Association For Childrens Behavioral Health, 2632

National Association for Rural Mental Health, 1753

National Association for The Dually Diagnose d (NADD), 1362

National Association for The Dually Diagnosed: NADD, 73

National Association for the Advancement of Psychoanalysis, 2633, 3658

National Association for the Dually Diagnose d (NADD), 270, 989, 1104, 1128, 1167, 1225, 1239, 1286, 1339, 1471, 1537, 1754

National Association for the Dually Diagnosed, 507, 1163, 3192

National Association for the Dually Diagnosed (NADD), 11, 397, 553, 712, 781, 830, 864, 955, 1086

National Association for the Dually Diagnosed: NADD Newsletter, 33

National Association for the Mentally Ill of New Jersey, 2006

National Association in Women's Health Professionals, 2634

National Association of Addiction Treatment Providers, 2635

National Association of Alcholism and Drug Abuse Counselors, 3408

National Association of Alcohol and Drug Abuse Counselors, 90, 246

National Association of Anorexia Nervosa and Associated Disorders (ANAD), 990

National Association of Anorexia Nervosa and Associated Disorders, 1058

National Association of Community Health Centers, 2636, 2215

National Association of Mental Illness: California, 1835

National Association of Nouthetic Counselors, 2637

National Association of Protection and Advocacy Systems, 1755

National Association of Psychiatric Health Systems: Membership Directory, 2638, 3655

National Association of Psychiatric Health Systems, 3564

National Association of School Psychologists, 3409

National Association of School Psychologists (NASP), 2639

National Association of Social Workers, 2640, 2846, 3244

National Association of Social Workers Florida Chapter, 1873

National Association of Social Workers New York State Chapter, 2025

National Association of Social Workers: Delaware Chapter, 1859
National Association of Social Workers: Kentucky Chapter, 1919
National Association of Social Workers: Maryland Chapter, 1937
National Association of Social Workers: Nebraska Chapter, 1989
National Association of Social Workers: North Carolina Chapter, 2039
National Association of Social Workers: North Dakota Chapter, 2044
National Association of Social Workers: Ohio Chapter, 2054
National Association of Social Works, 3283, 3310, 3311, 3312, 3313
National Association of State Alcohol and Drug Abuse Directors, 91
National Association of State Mental Health Program Directors (NASMHPD), 1756, 2641
National Association of Therapeutic Wilderness Camps, 1757
National Association to Advance Fat Acceptance (NAAFA), 991
National Associaton of Social Workers, 3565
National Board for Certified Counselors, 2499
National Book Network, 1230
National Business Coalition Forum on Health (NBCH), 2642
National Center for HIV, STD and TB Prevention, 2198
National Center for Learning Disabilities, 1758
National Center for Overcoming Overeating, 1066
National Center for PTSD, 1324
National Center on Addiction and Substance Abuse at Columbia University, 1759
National Child Support Network, 1583, 1760, 4599
National Clearinghouse for Alcohol & Drug Information, 231
National Clearinghouse for Alcohol and, 92
National Clearinghouse for Alcohol and Drug, 93
National Clearinghouse for Drug & Alcohol, 2199
National Coalition for the Homeless, 2643
National Committee for Quality Assurance, 2644
National Council for Commuity Behavioral Healthcare, 247
National Council for Community Behavioral Healthcare, 1761
National Council for Community Behavioral Healthcare, 94
National Council of Juvenile and Family Court Judges, 2645
National Council on Aging, 2646
National Council on Alcoholism and Drug Dependence, 4600
National Council on Alcoholism and Drug Dependence: Greater Detriot Area, 95, 2348
National Criminal Justice Association, 2647
National Directory of Drug and Alcohol Abuse Treatment Programs, 135
National Directory of Medical Psychotherapists and Psychodiagnosticians, 3656
National Dissemination Center for Children with Disabilities, 398, 1584

National Eating Disorders Association, 992
National Eating Disorders Organization, 1077
National Eldercare Services Company, 2648
National Empowerment Center, 1762, 4274
National Families in Action, 4477, 4601
National Family Caregivers Association, 782
National Federation of Families for Children 's Mental Health, 1938
National Foundation for Depressive Illness, 937
National GAINS Center for People with Co-Occurring Disorders in the Justice System, 1763
National Gay and Lesbian Task Force, 1105
National Health Foundation, 1836
National Health Information, 3222
National Information Center for Children and Youth with Disabilities, 502, 1670
National Instiues of Health, 2211
National Institute of Alcohol Abuse and Alcoholism: Treatment Research Branch, 2200
National Institute of Alcohol Abuse and Alcoholism: Office of Policy Analysis, 2201, 2202
National Institute of Drug Abuse (NIDA), 190, 1764
National Institute of Drug Abuse: NIDA, 2203
National Institute of Health, 1216
National Institute of Health National Center on Sleep Disorders, 1482
National Institute of Mental Health (NIMH), 3567
National Institute of Mental Health Eating Disorders Program, 993
National Institute of Mental Health Information Resources and Inquiries Branch, 1765
National Institute of Mental Health: Mental Disorders of the Aging, 2205
National Institute of Mental Health: Office of Science Policy, Planning, and Communications, 2206
National Institute of Mental Health: Schizophrenia Research Branch, 2204
National Institute of Neurological Disorders and Stroke, 783
National Institute of Neurological Disorders and Stroke Brain Information Network (BRAIN), 518
National Institute of Neurological Disorders & Stroke, 817
National Institute on Alcohol Abuse & Alcoholism, 248
National Institute on Alcohol Abuse and Alcoholism, 96
National Institute on Deafness and Other Communication Disorders Information Clearinghouse, 519
National Institute on Drug Abuse, 249
National Institute on Drug Abuse: Office of Science Policy and Communications, 2207
National Institute on Drug Abuse: Division of Clinical Neurosciences and Behavioral Research, 2208
National Institutes of Health, 1115, 2205, 2206, 2210
National Institutes of Health DHHS, 517
National Institutes of Health: National Center for Research Resources (NCCR), 2209
National Institutes of Mental Health: Office on AIDS, 2210
National Library of Medicine, 2211, 1120

National Managed Health Care Congress, 2649
National Medical Health Card Systems, 4478
National Mental Health Association, 97, 1363, 1766, 2650, 3568
National Mental Health Association: Georgetown County, 2095
National Mental Health Consumer's, 98, 271, 399, 554, 1340
National Mental Health Consumer's Self-Help, 12, 713, 784, 831, 866, 956, 994, 1087, 1129, 1168, 1226, 1240, 1287, 1364, 1442, 1472, 1495, 1538
National Mental Health Consumer's Self-Help Clearinghouse, 691, 766, 1160
National Mental Health Consumers Self-Help, 3268
National Mental Health Consumers Self-Help Clearinghouse, 245
National Mental Health Consumers' Self-Help Clearinghouse, 714, 785, 832, 867, 957, 995, 1107, 1169, 1227, 1241, 1288, 1365, 1443, 1473, 1496, 1539, 1767
National Mental Health Consumers' Self-Help Clearinghouse, 13, 99, 272, 400, 555, 1088, 1130, 1341, 1789
National Mental Health Self-Help Clearinghouse, 4035, 4602
National Multicultural Conference and Summit, 3194
National Network for Mental Health, 1768
National Niemann-Pick Disease Foundation, 786
National Nurses Association, 2651
National Organization of Parents of Murdered Children, 14
National Organization on Disability, 1769
National Organization on Fetal Alcohol Syndrome, 100, 251
National Panic/Anxiety Disorder Newsletter, 380
National Pharmaceutical Council, 2652
National Psychological Association for Psychoanalysis (NPAP), 2653
National Register of Health Service Providers in Psychology, 2500, 3657
National Register of Health Service Provider s in Psychology, 2654
National Registry of Psychoanalysts, 3658
National Rehabilitation Association, 1770
National Resource Center on Homelessness & Mental Illness, 1771
National SHARE Office, 37, 63
National Self-Help Clearinghouse, 60
National Self-Help Clearinghouse Graduate School and University Center, 1772
National Sleep Foundation, 1488
National Survey of American Attitudes on Substance Abuse VI: Teens, 3141
National Technical Assistance Center for Children's Mental Health, 1585, 1773
National Treatment Alternative for Safe Communities, 2655
National Youth Crisis Hotline, 1630
National-Louis University, 1780
Natural Child Project, 1669
Natural History of Mania, Depression and Schizophrenia, 1382
Natural History of Mania, Depression and Schizophrenia, 892
Natural Supports: A Foundation for Employment, 2800
Navajo Nation K'E Project, 1814
Navajo Nation K'E Project-Shiprock, 2012

Navajo Nation K'E Project: Chinle, 1815
Navajo Nation K'E Project: Tuba City, 1816
Navajo Nation K'E Project: Winslow, 1817
Nebraska Alliance for the Mentally Ill, 1990
Nebraska Department of Health and Human
    Services (NHHS), 2369
Nebraska Family Support Network, 1991
Nebraska Health & Human Services:
    Medicaid and Managed Care Division,
    2370
Nebraska Health and Human Services, 3662,
    3663, 3664
Nebraska Health and Human Services
    Division: Department of Mental Health,
    2371
Nebraska Health and Human Services
    System, 3642
Nebraska Mental Health Centers, 2372
Nefazodone, 4706
Negotiating Managed Care: Manual for
    Clinicians, 2801
Nelson Thornes, 3705
NetMeeting, 4479
Netscape Communicatons, 4398
Netsmart Technologies, 4480
Network Behavioral Health, 4275
Neurobiology of Autism 2nd Edition, 614
Neurobiology of Primary Dementia, 2969
Neurobiology of Violence, 2802
Neurodevelopment & Adult
    Psychopathology, 2803
Neurology for Clinical Social Work: Theory
    and Practice, 2804
Neurontin, 4707
Neuropsychiatry and Mental Health Services,
    2805
Neuropsychology of Mental Disorders:
    Practical Guide, 2806
Nevada Alliance for the Mentally Ill, 1995
Nevada Department of Health & Human
    Services Health Care Financing and
    Policy, 2373
Nevada Department of Health and Human
    Services, 2374
Nevada Division of Mental Health &
    Developmental Services, 2375
Nevada Employment Training &
    Rehabilitation Department, 2376
Nevada Principals' Executive Program, 1996
Nevada State Health Division: Bureau of
    Alcohol & Drug Abuse, 2377
New Avenues Alliance for the Mentally Ill,
    2086
New Day, 4276
New England Center for Children, 556, 693
New England Home for Little Wanderers,
    3915
New England Psych Group, 4277
New Hampshire Alliance for the Mentally
    Ill, 1999
New Hampshire Department of Health &
    Human Services: Bureau of Community
    Health Services, 2380
New Hampshire Department of Health and
    Human Services: Bureau of Behavioral
    Health, 2381, 2382
New Hampshire State Hospital, 3947
The New Handbook of Cognitive Therapy
    Techniques, 2971
New Hope Foundation, 1774
New Horizons Ranch and Center, 4073
New Horizons of the Treasure Coast, 3799

New Jersey Association of Mental Health
    Agencies, 2007
New Jersey Department of Banking &
    Insurance, 2387
New Jersey Department of Human Services,
    2384
New Jersey Division of Mental Health
    Services, 2385
New Jersey Division of Youth & Family
    Services, 2386
New Jersey Office of Managed Care, 2387
New Jersey Protection and Advocacy, 2008
New Jersey Psychiatric Association, 2009
New Jersey Support Groups, 2010
New Life Recovery Centers, 3764
New Look at ADHD: Inhibition, Time and
    Self Control, 484
New Message, 918
New Mexico Alliance for the Mentally Ill,
    2013
New Mexico Behavioral Health
    Collaborative, 2388
New Mexico Department of Health, 2389
New Mexico Department of Human
    Services, 2390
New Mexico Department of Human
    Services: Medical Assistance Division,
    2391
New Mexico Health & Environment
    Department, 2392
New Mexico Kids, Parents and Families
    Office of Child Development: Children,
    Youth and Families Department, 2393
New Mexico State Hospital, 3954
New Orleans Adolescent Hospital, 3884
New Page Books, 316
New Pharmacotherapy of Schizophrenia,
    1383
New Roles for Psychiatrists in Organized
    Systems of Care, 2807
New Treatments for Chemical Addictions,
    136
New World Library, 3707
New York Association of Psychiatric
    Rehabilitation Services, 2026
New York Business Group on Health, 2027
New York City Depressive & Manic
    Depressive Group, 2028
New York Office of Alcohol & Substance
    Abuse Services, 2394
New York Psychiatric Institute, 3986
New York State Alliance for the Mentally Ill,
    2029
New York State Department of Health
    Individual County Listings of Social
    Services Departments, 2395
New York State Office of Mental Health,
    2396
New York University Behavioral Health
    Programs, 3410
New York University Press, 3708, 1009
Newbride Consultation, 4278
Newport County Alliance for the Mentally
    Ill, 2087
News & Notes, 3284
News from the Border: a Mother's Memoir
    of Her Autistic Son, 615
Newsletter of the American Psychoanalytic
    Association, 3285
Nickerson Center, 3411
Night Falls Fast: Understanding Suicide,
    1510
Nightingale Vantagemed Corporation, 4481

NineLine, 1520
No More Butterflies: Overcoming Shyness,
    Stagefright, Interview Anxiety, and Fear
    of Public Speaking, 312
No Place to Hide: Substance Abuse in
    Mid-Size Cities and Rural America, 2910
No Safe Haven: Children of
    Substance-Abusing Parents, 2911
No Time to Say Goodbye: Surviving the
    Suicid e of a Loved One, 1511
No-Talk Therapy for Children and
    Adolescents, 3142
Nobody Nowhere, 616
Non Medical Marijuana: Rite of Passage or
    Russian Roulette?, 2912
Norfolk Regional Center, 3942
Norpramin, 4708
Norristown State Hospital, 4036
North Alabama Regional Hospital, 3738
North American Society of Adlerian
    Psychology (NASAP), 2656
North American Society of Adlerian
    Psychology Newsletter, 3286
North American Training Institute: Division
    of the Minnesota Council on Compulsive
    Gambling, 1971
North Bay Center for Behavioral Medicine,
    4603
North Carolina Alliance for the Mentally Ill,
    2040
North Carolina Department of Human
    Resources, 2397
North Carolina Division of Mental Health,
    2398
North Carolina Division of Social Services,
    2399
North Carolina Mental Health Consumers
    Organization, 2041
North Carolina Substance Abuse
    Professional Certification Board
    (NCSAPCB), 2400
North Dakota Alliance for the Mentally Ill,
    2046
North Dakota Department of Human
    Services Division of Mental Health and
    Substance Abuse Services, 2403
North Dakota Department of Human
    Services: Medicaid Program, 2401
North Dakota Department of Human
    Services: Mental Health Services
    Division, 2402
North Dakota Federation of Families for
    Children's Mental Health, 2045, 2047,
    2048, 2049
North Dakota State Hospital, 4005
North Florida Evaluation and Treatment
    Center, 3800
North Mississippi State Hospital, 3935
North Sound Regional Support Network,
    2153
North Star Centre, 3801
North Texas State Hospital: Vernon Campus,
    4074
North Texas State Hospital: Wichita Falls
    Campus, 4075
Northcoast Behavioral Healthcare System,
    4013, 4014
Northeast Florida State Hospital, 3802
Northern Arizona Regional Behavioral
    Health Authority, 2245
Northern California Psychiatric Society, 1837
Northern Nevada Adult Mental Health
    Services, 2378, 3944

Northern New Mexico Rehabilitation Center, 3955
Northern Rhode Island Alliance for the Mentally Ill, 2088
Northern Virginia Mental Health Institute, 4094
Northpointe Behavioral Healthcare Systems, 1962, 3925, 4279
Northridge Hospital Medical Center, 3765
Northwest Analytical, 4482
Northwest Center for Behavioral Health, 4020
Northwest Georgia Regional Hospital, 3818
Northwest Missouri Psychiatric Rehabilitation Center, 3939
Northwest Psychiatric Hospital, 4015
Northwestern University Medical School Feinberg School of Medicine, 3412
Novartis, 4647
Now Is Not Forever: A Survival Guide, 1524, 3554
Nueva Esperanza Counseling Center, 2154
Nuvigil, 4709

O

O-Anon General Service Office (OGSO), 996
OCD Newsletter, 1204
OCD Web Server, 1212
OCD Workbook: Your Guide to Breaking Free From Obsessive-Compulsive Disorder, 1184
OCD in Children and Adolescents: A Cognitive-Behavioral Treatment Manual, 1185
OK Parents as Partners, 2063
OPTAIO-Optimizing Practice Through Assessment, Intervention and Outcome, 4483
ORTHO Update, 3287
Obesity Research Center, 1062
Obesity: Theory and Therapy, 1035
Obsessive Compulsive Anonymous, 1170
Obsessive Compulsive Disorder, 1218
Obsessive Compulsive Foundation, 1171
Obsessive Compulsive Information Center, 1172
Obsessive-Compulsive Anonymous, 1205
Obsessive-Compulsive Disorder, 1214, 1217, 1275
Obsessive-Compulsive Disorder Casebook, 1186
Obsessive-Compulsive Disorder Spectrum, 1187
Obsessive-Compulsive Disorder Web Sites, 1213
Obsessive-Compulsive Disorder in Children and Adolescents, 1189
Obsessive-Compulsive Disorder in Children and Adolescents: A Guide, 1188
Obsessive-Compulsive Disorder: Contemporary Issues in Treatment, 3021
Obsessive-Compulsive Disorder: Theory, Research and Treatment, 1190
Obsessive-Compulsive Disorders: A Complete G uide to Getting Well and Staying Well, 1192
Obsessive-Compulsive Disorders: A Complete Guide to Getting Well and Staying Well, 1191

Obsessive-Compulsive Disorders: Practical Management, 1193
Obsessive-Compulsive Disorders: The Latest Assessment and Treatment Strategies, 1194
Obsessive-Compulsive Foundation, 1206, 1200, 1209, 1220
Obsessive-Compulsive Related Disorders, 1195
Obsessive-Compulsive and Related Disorders in Adults: a Comprehensive Clinical Guide, 3022
Occupational Health Software, 4484
Ochester Psychological Service, 3413
Odyssey House, 3987
Of One Mind: The Logic of Hypnosis, the Practice of Therapy, 2808
Office Treatment of Schizophrenia, 1384
Office of Applied Studies, SA & Mental Health Services, 2212
Office of Consumer, Family & Public Information, 3654
Office of Disease Prevention & Health Promotion, 2213
Office of Medicaid Policy & Planning (OMPP), 2309
Office of Mental Health and Addiction Services Training & Resource Center, 2412
Office of National Drug Control Policy, 2214
Office of Program and Policy Development, 2215
Office of Science Policy OD/NIH, 2216
Office of Women's and Children's Health, 2243
Ohio Alliance for the Mentally Ill, 2055
Ohio Association of Child Caring Agencies, 2056
Ohio Community Drug Board, 2404
Ohio Council of Behavioral Healthcare Providers, 2057
Ohio Department of Mental Health, 2058, 2405
Oklahoma Alliance for the Mentally Ill, 2064
Oklahoma Department of Human Services, 2406
Oklahoma Department of Mental Health and Substance Abuse Service (ODMHSAS), 2407
Oklahoma Forensic Center, 4021
Oklahoma Healthcare Authority, 2408
Oklahoma Mental Health Consumer Council, 2065, 2409, 4280
Oklahoma Office of Juvenile Affairs, 2410
Oklahoma Psychiatric Physicians Association, 2066
Oklahoma Youth Center, 4022
Ollie Webb Center, 1588, 1992
Omnigraphics, 3709, 109, 115, 322, 789, 1018, 1478, 2901
On Being a Therapist, 2809
On the Client's Path: A Manual for the Practice of Brief Solution - Focused Therapy, 3612
On the Counselor's Path: A Guide to Teaching Brief Solution Focused Therapy, 2810
On-Line Information Services, 4604
On-line Dictonary of Mental Health, 3543
One ADD Place, 504
One Hundred Four Activities That Build, 1140
One Hundred One Stress Busters, 344
One Hundred Top Series, 4281

100 Q&A About Panic Disorder, 277
1001 Great Ideas for Teaching or Raising Chi ldren with Autism Spectrum Disorders, 560
Onslow County Behavioral Health, 3414
Open Minds, 3288, 4605, 3214
Opportunities for Daily Choice Making, 2811
Optimum Care Corporation, 4282
Optio Software, 4485
The Option Institute, 514
Options Health Care, 4283
Optum, 4606
Oracle Corporation, 4486
Orange County Mental Health, 3766
Orange County Mental Health Association, 2030
Orange County Psychiatric Society, 1838
Ordinary Families, Special Children: Systems Approach to Childhood Disability, 3143
Oregon Alliance for the Mentally Ill, 2068
Oregon Commission on Children and Families, 2413
Oregon Department of Human Resources: Division of Health Services, 2414
Oregon Department of Human Services: Mental Health Services, 2415
Oregon Department of Human Services: Office of Developmental Disabilities, 2416
Oregon Family Support Network, 2069
Oregon Health Policy and Research: Policy and Analysis Unit, 2417
Oregon Psychiatric Association, 2070
Oregon State Hospital: Portland, 4025
Oregon State Hospital: Salem, 4026
Organon Schering Plough, 4648
Orion Healthcare Technology, 4487
Ortho-McNeil Pharmaceutical, 4649
Oryx Press, 1012, 1020
Osawatomie State Hospital, 3868
Our Lady of Bellefonte Hospital, 3877
Our Personal Stories, 1151
Our Town Family Center, 4607
Out of Control: Gambling and Other Impulse- Control Disorders, 1141
Out of Darkness and Into the Light: Nebraska's Experience In Mental Retardation, 2812
Outcomes for Children and Youth with Emotional and Behavioral Disorders and their Families, 3144
Outrageous Behavior Mood: Handbook of Strategic Interventions for Managing Impossible Students, 2977
Outside In: A Look at Adults with Attention Deficit Disorder, 485
Over and Over Again: Understanding Obsessive-Compulsive Disorder, 1196
Overcoming Agoraphobia and Panic Disorder, 2940
Overcoming Depression, 893
Overcoming Obsessive-Compulsive Disorder, 3023
Overcoming Post-Traumatic Stress Disorder, 3053
Overcoming Specific Phobia, 3074
Overeaters Anonymous, 1036, 1067
Ovid Online, 4608
Ovid Technologies, 4608
Oxcarbazepine and Bipolar Disorder: A Guide, 731
Oxford Univeristy Press, 888

Oxford University Press, 3710, 307, 310, 447, 1015, 1191, 1192, 1381, 1508, 1549, 1556, 3025
Oxford University Press/Oxford Reference, 2762
Oxford University Press/Oxford Reference Book Society, 2828

P

P and W Software, 4488
PENN Behavioral Health, 3478
PMHCC, 4284
PRIMA A D D Corp., 3415
PRISMED Corporation, 4489
PRO Behavioral Health, 1775, 4285
PSC, 4286
PSIMED Corporation, 4287
PTSD in Children and Adolesents, 3054
Pacer Center, 1972
PacifiCare Behavioral Health, 3767
Pahl Transitional Apartments, 3988
Pain Behind the Mask: Overcoming Masculine Depression, 894
Pamelor, 4710
Panic Attacks, 345
Panic Disorder, 377
Panic Disorder and Agoraphobia: A Guide, 313
Panic Disorder, Separation, Anxiety Disorder, and Agoraphobia, 1665
Panic Disorder: Clinical Diagnosis, Management and Mechanisms, 2941
Panic Disorder: Critical Analysis, 314
Panic Disorder: Theory, Research and Therapy, 2942
PaperChase, 3572
Parent Child Center, 3416
Parent City Library, 1675
Parent Connection, 2118
Parent Professional Advocacy League, 1949
Parent Resource Center, 2142
Parent Support Network of Rhode Island, 2089
Parent Survival Manual, 617
A Parent's Guide to Asperger Syndrome and High-Functioning Autism, 520
Parent's Guide to Autism, 618
ParenthoodWeb, 1676
Parenting a Child With Attention Deficit/Hyperactivity Disorder, 2963
Parenting: General Parenting Articles, 1662
Parents Helping Parents, 1586, 1776
Parents Information Network, 1587, 1777
Parents Involved Network, 2075
Parents United Network: Parsons Child Family Center, 2031
Parents and Friends of Lesbians and Gays, 1108
Parents for Children's Mental Health, 1778
Parents of Murdered Children, 38, 65
Parents, Families and Friends of Lesbians and Gays, 1109
Paris International Corporation, 4288
Parke-Davis Pharmaceutcials, 4650
Parkview Hospital Rehabilitation Center, 3859
Parnate, 4711
Parrot Software, 4490
Participatory Evaluation for Special Education and Rehabilitation, 2813

Pass-Group, 354
Pastoral Care of Depression, 895
The Pathology of Man: A Study of Human Evil, 3064
Pathways to Promise, 209
Patient Guide to Mental Health Issues: Desk Chart, 3659
Patient Infosystems, 4491
Patient Medical Records, 4609
Patrick B Harris Psychiatric Hospital, 4049
Patton State Hospital, 3768
Paul H Brookes Company, 2796
Paxil, 4712
Peace, Love, and Hope, 1076
Pearson, 4289
Pediatric Psychopharmacology: Fast Facts, 3145
Penelope Price, 3417, 4610
Penguin, 111
Penguin Group, 3711, 1175
Penguin Group (USA), 575
Penguin Putnam, 884, 1181, 1182
Penn State Hershey Medical Center, 3418
Pennsylvania Alliance for the Mentally Ill, 2076
Pennsylvania Bureau Drug and Alcohol Programs: Monitoring, 2419
Pennsylvania Bureau of Community Program Standards: Licensure and Certification, 2420
Pennsylvania Bureau of Drug and Alcohol Programs: Information Bulletins, 2421
Pennsylvania Chapter of the American Anorexia Bulimia Association, 2077
Pennsylvania Department of Health, 2420
Pennsylvania Department of Health: Bureau of Drug and Alcohol Programs, 2422
Pennsylvania Department of Public Welfare and Mental Health Services, 2423
Pennsylvania Division of Drug and Alcohol Prevention: Treatment, 2424
Pennsylvania Medical Assistance Programs, 2425
Pennsylvania Society for Services to Children, 2078
Pensions, Benefits & Compensators Employer, 4351
People First of Oregon, 2071
Pepperdine University, Graduate School of Education and Psychology, 3419
Perfect Daughters, 2913
Performance Resource Press, 1621
Perot Systems, 4492
Perseus Books Group, 3712, 2930, 2980
Persoma Management, 4290
Person-Centered Foundation for Counseling and Psychotherapy, 2814
Personality Characteristics of the Personality Disordered, 3035
Personality Disorders and Culture: Clinical and Conceptual Interactions, 3036
Personality Disorders in Modern Life, 1265
Personality and Psychopathology, 1266
Personality and Stress Center for Applications of Psychological Type, 3505
Personality and Stress: Individual Differences in the Stress Process, 3037
Perspectives, 4291
Perturbing the Organism: The Biology of Stressful Experience, 3055
Perversion (Ideas in Psychoanalysis), 1230
Peter Hornby and Margaret Anderson, SUNY, 4551

Pfeiffer Treatment Center and Health Researc h Institute, 3846
Pfizer, 4651
Phantom Illness: Recognizing, Understanding, and Overcoming Hypochondria, 1347
PharmaCoKinetics and Therapeutic Monitering of Psychiatric Drugs, 2815
Pharmaceutical Care Management Association, 2657
Pharmacia & Upjohn, 4652
Pharmacotherapy for Mood, Anxiety and Cognit ive Disorders, 315
Philadelphia Health Management, 4292
Phobias And How to Overcome Them: Understand ing and Beating Your Fears, 316
Phobias: Handbook of Theory, Reseach and Treatment, 2943
Phobic and Obsessive-Compulsive Disorders: Theory, Research, and Practice, 1197
Phobics Anonymous, 355
Phoenix Care Systems, Inc: Willowglen Academ y, 1779
Phoenix House, 3989
Phoenix Programs Inc, 3769
Physician's Guide to Depression and Bipolar Disorders, 732
Physicians Living with Depression, 3506
Physicians for a National Health Program, 2658
Physicians' ONLINE, 4611
Piedmont Community Services, 4612
Piedmont Geriatric Hospital, 4095
Pierce County Alliance for the Mentally Ill, 2155
Pilgrim Psychiatric Center, 3990
Pilot Parents: PP, 1588, 1992
Pinal Gila Behavioral Health Association, 4293
Pittsburgh Health Research Institute, 3420
Placebo Effect Accounts for Fifty Percent of Improvement, 3588
Planet Psych, 1121
PlanetPsych.com, 64, 851
Planetpsych.com, 383, 505, 694, 770, 820, 945, 976, 1080, 1221, 1233, 1277, 1325, 1352, 1432, 1462, 1484, 1528, 1567, 3574
Planned Lifetime Assistance Network of Northeast Ohio, 2059
Play Therapy with Children in Crisis: Individual, Group and Family Treatment, 3146
Playing Sick, 1094
Playing Sick?: Untangling the Web of Munchau sen Syndrome, Munchausen by Proxy, Malingering, and Factitious Disorder, 1095
Please Don't Say Hello, 619
Point of Care Technologies, 4613
Points for Parents Perplexed about Drugs, 137
Policy Research Associates, 2690, 2905
Porter Novelli, 4294
Portland State University/Regional Research Institute, 1590, 1786
Posen Consulting Group, 4295
Positive Bahavior Support for People with Developmental Disabilities: A Research Synthesis, 2816
Positive Behavior Support Training Curriculum, 2817

Positive Education Program, 2060
Post Traumatic Stress Disorder, 3056
Post Traumatic Stress Disorder Alliance, 1327
Post Traumatic Stress Disorder: Complete Treatment Guide, 3057
Post Traumatic Stress Resources, 1330
Post-Natal Depression: Psychology, Science and the Transition to Motherhood, 896
Post-Traumatic Stress Disorder: Assessment, Differential Diagnosis, and Forensic Evaluation, 1302
Postgraduate Center for Mental Health, 3421
Postpartum Mood Disorders, 897, 2990
Postpartum Support International, 868
Posttraumatic Stress Disorder in Litigation: Guidelines for Forensic Assessment, 1303
Posttraumatic Stress Disorder: A Guide, 1304
Posttraumatic Stress Disorders in Children and Adolescents Handbook, 3058
Power and Compassion: Working with Difficult Adolesents and Abused Parents, 3147
Practical Art of Suicide Assessment: A Guide for Mental Health Professionals and Substance Abuse Counselors, 3089
Practical Charts for Managing Behavior, 3148
Practical Guide to Cognitive Therapy, 2818
Practical Psychiatric Practice Forms and Protocols for Clinical Use, 2819
Practice Guideline for Major Depressive Disorders in Adults, 898
Practice Guideline for the Treatment of Patients with Panic Disorder, 2944
Practice Guideline for the Treatment of Patients with Schizophrenia, 3082
Practice Guidelines for Extended Psychiatric Residential Care: From Chaos to Collaboration, 2820
Practice Management Resource Group, 4296
Practicing Psychiatry in the Community: a Manual, 1385
Praeger, 2737
Praeger Security International General Interest-Cloth, 1299
Pragmatix, 4297
Prairie View, 3869
Predictors of Treatment Response in Mood Disorders, 899
Preferred Medical Informatics, 4614
Preferred Mental Health Management, 4298
Premenstrual Dysphoric Disorder: A Guide, 2991
Prenatal Exposures in Schizophrenia, 1386
Presbyterian Intercommunity Hospital Mental Health Center, 3770
Preschool Issues in Autism, 620
Prescription Drugs: Recovery from the Hidden Addiction, 226
President's Committee on Mental Retardation, 2217
Presidential Commission on Employment of the Disabled, 2218
Pressley Ridge Schools, 3422
Pretenders: Gifted People Who Have Difficulty Learning, 2964
Preventing Antisocial Behavior Interventions from Birth through Adolescence, 841
Preventing Maladjustment from Infancy Through Adolescence, 28
The Prevention Researcher, 194
Price Stern Sloan Publishing, 3162
Primary Care Medicine on CD, 4493

Prime Care Consultants, 4299
Primer of Brief Psychotherapy, 2821
Primer of Supportive Psychotherapy, 2822
A Primer on Rational Emotive Behavior Therapy, 2687
Princeton University Press, 3713, 3008
Principles and Practice of Sex Therapy, 1450, 3010
Principles and Practice of Sleep Medicine, 1477
Principles of Addiction Medicine, 2914
Pro-Ed, 2950
ProAmerica Managed Care, 4300
ProMetrics CAREeval, 4301
ProMetrics Consulting & Susquehanna PathFinders, 4302
Process Strategies Institute, 4303
Professional Academy of Custody Evaluators, 3571
Professional Assistance Center for Education (PACE), 1780
Professional Counselor, 3289
Professional Horizons, Mental Health Service, 3423
Professional Resource Press, 3715, 1302, 2753, 2847, 2849, 2879, 2931, 2982, 2987, 3015, 3030, 3034, 3153, 3323, 3616, 3651
Professional Risk Management Services, 2659, 4304
Professional Services Consultants, 4305
Program Development Associates, 522, 523, 524, 525, 526, 527, 528, 529, 655, 656, 657, 658, 659, 663, 665, 669, 670, 671, 2951, 3490
Progress in Alzheimer's Disease and Similar Conditions, 797
Project LINK, 2032
Project NoSpank, 1672
Project Vision, 1920
Prolixin, 4713
Protection and Advocacy Program for the Mentally Ill, 2219
Proven Youth Development Model that Prevents Substance Abuse and Builds Communities, 2915
Providence Behavioral Health Connections, 4306
Provider Magazine, 3290
Provigil, 4714
Prozac, 4715
Prozac Nation: Young & Depressed in America, a Memoir, 900
Psy Care, 4307
PsycHealth, 4308
PsycINFO Database, 3660
PsycINFO News, 3291
PsycINFO, American Psychological Association, 3660
PsycINFO/American Psychological Association, 3292, 3300
PsycSCAN Series, 3292
Psych Discourse, 3293
Psych-Med Association, St. Francis Medical, 3424
Psych-Media, 3274
PsychAccess, 4615
PsychTemps, 3425
Psychiatric Associates, 3426, 4309
Psychiatric Clinical Research Center, 1781
Psychiatric Disorders In Current Medical Diagnosis and Treatment, 2823
Psychiatric News, 3294
Psychiatric Rehabilitation Journal, 3295

Psychiatric Rehabilitation of Chronic Mental Patients, 1387
Psychiatric Society Of Informatics American Association For Technology In Psychiatry, 2660
Psychiatric Solutions, 3757
Psychiatric Times, 3296
Psychiatric Treatment of Victims and Survivors of Sexual Trauma: A Neuro-Bio-Psychological Approach, 1451
The Psychiatrists' Program, 2659
Psychiatry Department, 3186
Psychiatry Drug Alerts, 3297
Psychiatry Research, 3298
Psychiatry in the New Millennium, 2824
Psycho Medical Chirologists, 4310
Psychoanalysis, Behavior Therapy & the Relational World, 2825
Psychoanalytic Therapy & the Gay Man, 3011
Psychoanalytic Therapy as Health Care Effectiveness and Economics in the 21st Century, 2826
Psychobiology and Treatment of Anorexia Nervosa and Bulimia Nervosa, 1037
Psychodynamic Technique in the Treatment of the Eating Disorders, 1038
Psychoeducational Profile, 621
Psychohistory Forum, 2661
Psychohistory News, 3299
Psychological Abstracts, 3300
Psychological Aspects of Women's Health Care, 2827
Psychological Assessment Resources, 3301, 4494
Psychological Associates-Texas, 3427
Psychological Center, 3428
Psychological Diagnostic Services, 3429
Psychological Examination of the Child, 3149
Psychological Science Agenda, 3302
Psychological Software Services, 4495
Psychological Theories of Drinking and Alcoholism, 2916
Psychological Trauma, 1305
Psychologists' Desk Reference, 2828
Psychology Department, 3430
Psychology Information On-line: Depression, 947
Psychology Society (PS), 2662
Psychology Teacher Network Education Directorate, 3303
Psychology of Religion, 2663
Psychometric Software, 4496
Psychoneuroendocrinology: The Scientific Basis of Clinical Practice, 2829
Psychonomic Society, 2664
Psychopharmacology Desktop Reference, 2830
Psychopharmacology Update, 2831
Psychophysiology, 3304
Psychoses and Pervasive Development Disorders in Childhood and Adolescence, 1388
Psychosocial Aspects of Disability, 2832
Psychosocial Press, 1090
Psychosomatic Families: Anorexia Nervosa in Context, 1039
Psychosomatic Medicine, 3305
Psychotherapies with Children and Adolescents, 3150
Psychotherapist's Duty to Warn or Protect, 2833

Psychotherapist's Guide to Cost Containment: How to Survive and Thrive in an Age of Managed Care, 2834
Psychotherapy Bulletin, 3306
Psychotherapy Finances, 3307
Psychotherapy Indications and Outcomes, 2835
Psychotherapy for Borderline Personality, 3038
Psychotropic Drug Information Handbook, 2836
Psychotropic Drugs: Fast Facts, 2837
Public Consulting Group, 4311
Public Health Foundation, 2220
Put Yourself in Their Shoes: Understanding Teenagers with Attention Deficit Hyperactivity Disorder, 457
Pyrce Healthcare Group, 4312
Pyromania, Kleptomania, and Other Impulse- Control Disorder, 1142

Q

QuadraMed Corporation, 3431, 4497
Quadramed, 4616
QualChoice Health Plan, 4313
Quality of Life: Volume II, 2838
Queendom, 949
Queens Children's Psychiatric Center, 3991
Questions & Answers About Depression & Its Treatment, 901
Questions from Adolescents about ADD, 1685
Questions from Younger Children about ADD, 1686
Questions of Competence, 2839
Quickies: The Handbook of Brief Sex Therapy, 1452
Quinco Behavioral Health Systems, 4314

R

RCF Information Systems, 4498
REC Management, 4315
RICA: Baltimore, 3897
RICA: Southern Maryland, 3898
RTI Business Systems, 4617
RYAN: A Mother's Story of Her Hyperactive/ Tourette Syndrome Child, 458
RYAN: a Mother's Story of Her Hyperactive/Tourette Syndrome Child, 1550
Rainbow Mental Health Facility, 3870
Rainbows, 39, 1631, 68
Raintree Systems, 4499
Raising Joshua, 1551
Random House, 873, 1027, 1201
Rapid Psychler Press, 2665, 3716, 1258, 1262, 2702, 2733, 2861
Rating Scales in Mental Health, 3661
Rational Emotive Therapy, 3507
Rational Recovery, 210
Raven Press, 1035
Razadyne ER, 4716
Reaching Out in Family Therapy: Home Based, School, and Community Interventions, 2840

Reaching the Autistic Child: a Parent Training Program, 622
Real Illness: Generalized Anxiety Disorder, 346
Real Illness: Obsessive-Compulsive Disorder, 1198
Real Illness: Panic Disorder, 347
Real Illness: Post-Traumatic Stress Disorder, 1316
Real Illness: Social Phobia Disorder, 348
Real World Drinking, 191
Reality Check: Marijuana Prevention Video, 227
Reboxetine, 4717
Rebuilding Shattered Lives: Responsible Treatment of Complex Post-Traumatic and Dissociative Disorders, 968, 1306, 3059
Reclamation, 1782
Recognition and Treatment of Psychiatric Disorders: Psychopharmacology Handbook for Primary Care, 2841
Recognition of Early Psychosis, 2842
Record Books for Individuals with Autism, 623
Recovering Your Mental Health: a Self-Help Guide, 919
Recovery, 356, 928, 1414, 1783, 1434, 3581
Refuah, 1784
Regional Research Institue-Portland State University, 3235
Regional Research Institute for Human Services of Portland University, 3432
Rehabilitation Accreditation Commission, 3631
Relapse Prevention Maintenance: Strategies in the Treatment of Addictive Behaviors, 2917, 2918
Relapse Prevention for Addictive Behaviors: a Manual for Therapists, 138
Relationship and Learning Center, 69
Relaxation & Stress Reduction Workbook, 317, 3613
Remembering Trauma: Psychotherapist's Guide to Memory & Illusion, 3060
Remeron, 4718
Reminyl, 4719
Renaissance Manor, 3803
Renfrew Center Foundation, 4037
A Research Agenda for DSM-V, 2688
Research Center for Children's Mental Health, Department of Children and Family, 3433
Research Center for Severe Mental Illnesses, 1785
Research Press, 402, 438, 454, 1500, 1596, 1600, 1604, 1606, 1615, 1633, 1637, 2687, 2711, 2715, 2764, 2868, 2878, 3507
Research Press Publishers, 3717
Research and Training Center for Children's Mental Health, 1589
Research and Training Center on Family Support and Children's Mental Health, 1590, 1786
Research and Training for Children's Mental Health-Update, 3308
Resources For Children with Special Needs, 700, 701
Resources for Children with Special Needs, 1591, 1787, 78, 79, 625, 695, 698, 699, 702, 2866, 3599
Restrictive Eating, 1056
Rethinking Substance Abuse: What the Science Shows, and What We Should Do about It, 139

Retreat Healthcare, 2133
Return From Madness, 1389
Reuters Health, 3582
Review of Psychiatry, 2843
Rewind, Replay, Repeat: A Memoir of Obsessive-Compulsive Disorder, 1199
Rhode Island Council on Alcoholism and Other Drug Dependence, 2230
Rhode Island Department of Human Services, 2426
Rhode Island Division of Substance Abuse, 2427
Richmond State Hospital, 3860
Richmond Support Group, 2143
Right On Programs/PRN Medical Software, 4500
Rio Grande State Center, 4076
Rising Above a Diagnosis of Autism, 671
Risk Factors for Posttraumatic Stress Disorder, 1307
Risk and Insurance Management Society, 2666
Risperdal, 4720
Ritalin, 4721
River City Mental Health Clinic, 3434
River Oaks Hospital, 3885
River Valley Behavioral Health, 3201
Riveredge Hospital, 3435
Riverside Center, 3436
Riverside Publishing, 3718
Riverview Psychiatric Center, 3889
Rochester Psychiatric Center, 3992
Rockland Children's Psychiatric Center, 3437, 3993
Rockland Psychiatric Center, 3994
Rodale Books, 106
Role of Sexual Abuse in the Etiology of Borderline Personality Disorder, 1267, 3039
Rosemont Center, 3438
Rosen Publishing, 147
Rosen Publishing Group, 124, 1014, 1294, 3014
The Rosen Publishing Group, 123
Roster: Centers for the Developmentally Disabled, 3662
Roster: Health Clinics, 3663
Roster: Substance Abuse Treatment Centers, 3664
Routledge, 896, 962, 1092, 1095, 2882
Routledge Publishing, 1094
Roxane Laboratories, 4653
Royal College of Psychiatrists, 823
Rozerem, 4722
Rusk State Hospital, 4077
Russell Is Extra Special, 624
Rylee's Gift - Asperger Syndrome, 528
Ryther Child Center, 4101

S

SA/VE - Suicide Awareness/Voices of Education, 1531, 3583
SADD-Students Against Destructive Decisions, 253
SADD: Students Against Destructive Decisions, 211, 1632
SAFE Alternatives, 1271
SAFY of America, 3439
SAFY of America: Specialized Alternatives for Families and Youth, 2501

SAMHSA, 2222

SAMHSA'S National Mental Health Informantion Center, 919

SAMHSA'S National Mental Health Information, 958, 1173, 1228, 1242

SAMHSA'S National Mental Health Information Center, 869, 1289, 1342, 1366, 1444, 1474, 1497, 1540, 843, 844, 1051, 1313, 1408, 1517

SAMHSA's National Mental Health Info Center, 244

SAMHSA's National Mental Health Information Center, 15, 101, 273, 401, 557, 715, 787, 959, 997, 1089, 1110, 1131, 1174, 1229, 1243, 916

SAMSHA, 1335, 1358, 1717

SHS Computer Service, 4501

SIU School of Medicine, 3443

SMAHSA'S National Mental Health Information Center, 815

SMART-Self Management and Recovery Training, 212

SMART: Self-Management and Recovery Training, 255

SPOKES Federation of Families for Children's Mental Health, 1921

SPSS, 4502

SUPRA Management, 2502

Saddest Time, 1612

Safe Crossings Foundation, 70

Safe Schools/Safe Students: Guide to Violence Prevention Stategies, 3151

Safer Society Foundation, 1456

Sagamore Children's Psychiatric Center, 3995

Sagamore Children's Services: Woodside CSN, 4016

Sage Publications, 3719, 28, 424, 836, 872, 1177, 2834, 2875, 2885, 3005, 3044

Sage Publishing, 3265

Salem Children's Home, 3847

Salud Management Associates, 4316

Samaritan Counseling Center, 3926

Samaritan Village, 3996

Samaritans International, 938

Samhsa's National Clearinghouse For Alcohol And Drug Information, 102

Samhsa's National Mental Health Information Center, 558

San Antonio State Hospital, 4078

Sandplay Therapy: Step By Step Manual for Physchotherapists of Diverse Orientations, 2844

Sandra Fields-Neal and Associates, 4317

Saner Software, 4503

Sanofi-Aventis, 4654

Sanofi-Synthelabo, 4655

Sarmul Consultants, 4318

Save Our Sons And Daughters (SOSAD), 16

Save Our Sons and Daughters Newsletter (SOSAD), 192

Scale for Assessing Emotional Disturbance, 3337

Schafer Consulting, 4319

Scheur and Associates, 4320

Schizophrenia, 1390, 1406, 1419, 1425, 1426, 1427, 1428, 1431, 1435, 1436, 1437, 1438

Schizophrenia Bulletin: Superintendent of Documents, 1407

Schizophrenia Fact Sheet, 1408

Schizophrenia Research, 1409

Schizophrenia Research Branch: Division of Clinical and Treatment Research, 1411

Schizophrenia Revealed: From Neurons to Soci al Interactions, 1391

Schizophrenia Revealed: From Nuerons to Social Interactions, 1392, 3083

Schizophrenia Support Organizations, 1421

Schizophrenia and Genetic Risks, 1393

Schizophrenia and Manic Depressive Disorder, 1394

Schizophrenia and Primitive Mental States, 1395

Schizophrenia in a Molecular Age, 1396

Schizophrenia.com, 3584, 3586

Schizophrenia: A Handbook for Families, 3555

Schizophrenia: From Mind to Molecule, 1397

Schizophrenia: Straight Talk for Family and Friends, 1398

Schizophrenic Biologic Research Center, 1412

Schizophrenics Anonymous Forum, 1415

Schneider Institute for Health Policy, 3440

School Personnel, 1200

School of Nursing, UCLA, 3441

Schools and Services for Children with Autism Spectrum Disorders, 700

Schools for Children With Autism Spectrum Disorders, 625

Sciacca Comprehensive Service Development for MIDAA, 4321

Sciacca Comprehensive Services Development, 2667

Science Directorate-American Psychological Association, 3302

The Science of Addiction: From Neurobiology to Treatment, 148

Science of Prevention: Methodological Advances from Alcohol and Substance Research, 140

Scientific Foundations of Cognitive Theory and Therapy of Depression, 2992

Scinet, 4504

Screening for Brain Dysfunction in Psychiatric Patients, 3338

Screening for Mental Health, 2668

Searcy Hospital, 3739

Seasonal Affective Disorder and Beyond: Light Treatment for SAD and Non-SAD Conditions, 902

Secretariat, 1796

Section for Psychiatric and Substance Abuse Services (SPSPAS), 103

Seelig and Company: Child Welfare and Behavioral Healthcare, 4322

Selecting Effective Treatments: a Comprehensive, Systematic, Guide for Treating Mental Disorders, 2845

Selective Mutism Foundation, 274, 385

Self Help Magazine, 950

Self-Help Brochures, 1646

Self-Help and Psychology Magazine, 3587

Self-Starvation, 1040

Selfish Brain: Learning from Addiction, 141

Seminole Community Mental Health Center, 3804

Senator Garrett Hagedorn Psychiatric Hospital, 3952

Sense of Belonging: Including Students with Autism in Their School Community, 672

Sepracor Pharmaceuticals, 4656

Sequoyah Adolescent Treatment Center, 3956

Seroquel, 4723

Servisource, 4618

Seven Points of Alcoholics Anonymous, 142

Severe Stress and Mental Disturbance in Children, 3152

Sex Education: Issues for the Person with Autism, 626, 648

Sex Murder and Sex Aggression: Phenomenology Psychopathology, Psychodynamics and Prognosis, 3017

Sex, Drugs, Gambling and Chocolate: Workbook for Overcoming Addictions, 143

Sexual Abuse and Eating Disorders, 3003

Sexual Aggression, 1453

Sexual Disorders, 1463

Sexual Dysfunction: Guide for Assessment and Treatment, 3339

Sexuality and People with Disabilities, 1454

Shades of Hope Treatment Center, 4079

Sharing & Caring for Consumers, Families Alliance for the Mentally Ill, 2156

Shelley, The Hyperative Turtle, 459

Sheppard Pratt Health Plan, 4323

Sheppard Pratt Health System, 1939

Sheppard Pratt at Ellicott City, 3899

Shire Richwood, 4657

Shorter Term Treatments for Borderline Personality Disorders, 3040

Shrinktank, 1465

Shueman and Associates, 4324

Shy Children, Phobic Adults: Nature and Trea tment of Social Phobia, 318, 2945

Siblings & Offspring Group Alliance for the Mentally Ill, 2090

Siblings of Children with Autism: A Guide for Families, 627

Sid W Richardson Institute for Preventive Medicine of the Methodist Hospital, 924

Sidran Institute, 3720, 963, 967, 970, 1263, 1311, 1328

Sidran Traumatic Stress Institute, 1788

Siemens Health Services Corporation, 4505

Sigmund Freud Archives (SFA), 2669

Signs of Suicide Risk, 1533

Silver Hill Hospital, 3787

SilverPlatter Information, 4619

Simon & Schuster, 3721

Six County, 2061

Skills Training Manual for Treating Borderline Personality Disorder, Companion Workbook, 3614

Skills Training for Children with Behavior Disorders, 842

Skills Unlimited, 3448

Skypek Group, 2503, 4325, 4506

Sleep Disorder, 1490

Sleep Disorders Sourcebook, Second Edition, 1478

Sleep Disorders Unit of Beth Israel Hospital, 3916

SleepDisorders.com, 1487

Sleepnet.com, 1489

Sls Residential, 4507

SmokeFree TV: A Nicotine Prevention Video, 228

Smooth Sailing, 3309

So Help Me God: Substance Abuse, Religion and Spirituality, 2919

So What are Dads Good For, 1648

Social Anxiety Disorder: A Guide, 319

Social Phobia: Clinical and Research Perspectives, 2946

Social Phobia: From Shyness to Stage Fright, 320

Social Security, 1642

Social Skills Training for Children and Adolescents with Asperger Syndrome and Social-Communications Problems, 530

Social Work, 3310

Social Work Abstracts, 3311

Social Work Dictionary, 2846

Social Work Research, 3312

Social Work in Education, 3313

Social-Emotional Dimension Scale, 3340

Society for Adolescent Psychiatry Newsletter, 3314

Society for Industrial and Organizational Psychology, 3589

Society for Pediatric Psychology (SPP), 2670

Society for Personality Assessment, 2671

Society for Psychophysiological Research, 2672

Society for Women's Health Research, 2673

Society for the Advancement of Social Psychology (SASP), 2674

Society for the Psychological Study of Social Issues (SPSSI), 2675

Society of Behavioral Medicine, 2676

Society of Multivariate Experimental Psychology (SMEP), 2677

Society of Teachers of Family Medicine, 2678

Solutions Step by Step - Substance Abuse Treatment Videotape, 3508

Solutions Step by Step: Substance Abuse Treatment Manual, 2920

Solvay Pharmaceuticals, 4658

Somatization, Physical Symptoms and Psychological Illness, 3075

Somatoform Dissociation: Phenomena, Measurem ent, and Theoretical Issues, 3076

Somatoform and Factitious Disorders, 3077

Somatoform and Factitious Disorders (Review of Psychiatry), 1348

Somebody Somewhere, 628

Somerset Pharmaceuticals, 4659

Something Fishy Music and Publishing, 1082

Sometimes I Drive My Mom Crazy, But I Know She's Crazy About Me, 460

Son-Rise Autism Treatment Center of America, 696

Son-Rise Program at the Option Institute Autism Treatment Center of America, 559

Sonata, 4724

Sonia Shankman Orthogenic School, 3848

Soon Will Come the Light, 629

Souls Self Help Central, 256

The Source Newsletter, 521

South Beach Psychiatric Center, 3997

South Carolina Alliance for the Mentally Ill, 2096, 2097

South Carolina Department of Alcohol and Other Drug Abuse Services, 2431

South Carolina Department of Mental Health, 2432

South Carolina Department of Social Services, 2433

South Carolina Family Support Network, 2098

South Carolina State Hospital, 4050

South Coast Medical Center, 3771

South Dakota Department of Human Services: Division of Mental Health, 2434

South Dakota Department of Social Services Office of Medical Services, 2435

South Dakota Human Services Center, 2436, 4052

South Florida Evaluation and Treatment Center, 3805

South Florida State Hospital, 3806

South King County Alliance for the Mentally Ill, 2157

South Mississippi State Hospital, 3936

Southeast Louisiana Hospital, 3886

Southeast Missouri Mental Health Center, 3940

Southern Illinois University School of Medicine, 3443

Southern Illinois University School of Medicine: Department of Psychiatry, 3442

Southern Nevada Adult Mental Health Services, 2379, 3945

Southern Virginia Mental Health Institute, 4096

Southwest Behavioral Health Services, 3743

Southwest Counseling & Development Services, 1963

Southwestern Pennsylvania Alliance for the Mentally Ill, 2079

Southwestern State Hospital, 3819

Southwestern Virginia Mental Health Institute, 4097

Spanish Support Group Alliance for the Mentally Ill, 2158

The Special Education Consultant Teacher, 2858

Special Education Rights and Responsibilities, 497, 1644

Specialized Alternatives for Families & Youth of America (SAFY), 4326

Specialized Therapy Associates, 4327

Spokane Mental Health, 2159

Spouses & Partners' Group Alliance for the Mentally Ill, 2091

Spring Grove Hospital Center, 3900

Spring Harbor Hospital, 3890

Spring Lake Ranch, 4086

Springer Publishing Company, 1455

Springer Science & Business Media, 646

Springer Science and Business Media, 3722

Springer-Verlag New York, 3078

Springfield Hospital Center, 3901

St. Anthony Behavioral Medicine Center, Behavioral Medicine, 4328

St. Elizabeth's Hospital, 3789

St. Francis Medical Center, 3444

St. Joseph Behavioral Medicine Network, 3445

St. Lawrence Psychiatric Center, 3998

St. Louis Behavioral Medicine Institute, 3446

St. Luke's-Roosevelt Hospital, 1062

St. Martin's Press, 3723, 2744

St. Mary's Home for Boys, 4027

St. Peter Regional Treatment Center, 3931

Stamford: Appleton & Lange, 2823

Standford School of Medicine, 747

Standing in the Spaces: Essays on Clinical Process, Trauma, and Dissociation, 3061

Star Systems Corporation, 4508

Starlite Recovery Center, 4080

Starting Place, 3807

Starving to Death in a Sea of Objects, 1041

State Correctional Institution at Waymart, 4038

State Hospital North, 3823

State Hospital South, 3824

State University of New York Press, 1231

State University of New York at Stony Brook, 2033

State of Rhode Island Department of Mental Health, Retardation and Hospitals, 2428

State of Vermont Developmental Disabilities Services, 2462

Step Workbook for Adolescent Chemical Dependency Recovery, 3615

Stepfamily Information, 1679, 1682, 3575

Stepfamily in Formation, 3591

Stephens Systems Services, 4509

Stepping Stones Recovery Center, 3849

Stigma and Mental Illness, 1399

Still a Dad, 1647

Stonington Institute, 3447

Stop Biting Nails, 1162

Stop Me Because I Can't Stop Myself: Taking Control of Impulsive Behavior, 1143

Stop Obsessing: How to Overcome Your Obsessions and Compulsions, 321

Stop Walking on Eggshells, 1268

Stories of Depression: Does this Sound Like You?, 903

Storm In My Brain, 920

A Story of Bipolar Disorder (Manic-Depressive Illness) Does this Sound Like You?, 717

Stoughton Family Counseling, 2172

Straight Talk About Autism with Parents and Kids, 673

Straight Talk About Substance Use and Violence, 229

Strange Behavior Tales of Evolutionary Neurolgy, 2970

Strategic Advantage, 4510

Strategic Marketing: How to Achieve Independence and Prosperity in Your Mental Health Practice, 2847

Strattera, 4725

Stress, 349

Stress Incredible Facts, 350

Stress Management Research Associates, 4620

Stress Management Training: Group Leader's Guide, 3616

Stress Owner's Manual: Meaning, Balance and Health in Your Life, 3617

Stress Response Syndromes: Personality Styles and Interventions, 29

Stress in Hard Times, 351

Stress-Related Disorders Sourcebook, 322

Structured Adolescent Pscyhotherapy Groups, 3153

Structured Interview for DSM-IV Personality (SIDP-IV), 1269

Struggling with Life: Asperger's Syndrome, 529

Stuck on Fast Forward: Youth with Attention Deficit/Hyperactivity Disorder, 461

Substance Abuse & Mental Health Services Adminsitration, 135

Substance Abuse & Mental Health Services Adminstration (SAMHSA), 2221

Substance Abuse Mental Health Services Administration, 2187

Substance Abuse Treatment and the Stages of Change: Selecting and Planning Interventions (Guilford Substance Abuse Series), 144

Substance Abuse and Learning Disabilities: Peas in a Pod or Apples and Oranges?, 2921

Substance Abuse and Mental Health Services Administration, 2222, 254, 2186
Substance Abuse: A Comprehensive Textbook, 2922
Substance Abuse: Information for School Coun selors, Social Workers, Therapists, and Counselors, 145
Suburban Research Associates, 4329
Succeeding in College with Attention Deficit Disorders: Issues and Strategies for Students, Counselors and Educators, 462
Success Day Training Program, 3448
Sue Krause and Associates, 4330
Suicidal Patient: Principles of Assesment, Treatment, and Case Management, 1512
Suicide From a Psychological Prespective, 3090
Suicide Over the Life Cycle, 1513
Suicide Prevention Action Network USA (SPANUSA), 1498
Suicide Prevention Help, 1525
Suicide Talk: What To Do If You Hear It, 1516
Suicide and Suicide Prevention, 1530
Suicide: Fast Fact 3, 1517
Suicide: Who Is at Risk?, 1518
SumTime Software®, 4511
Sun Microsystems, 4512
SunGard Pentamation, 4513
Sunburst Media, 1140
Suncoast Residential Training Center, 762, 1156
Suncoast Residential Training Center/Developmental Services Program, 104, 275, 716, 833, 870, 1132, 1244, 1290, 1367, 3808
Supervised Lifestyles, 4621
Support Coalition Human Rights & Psychiatry Home Page, 3561
Support Transgendered, 1460
Support and Information on Sex Reassignement, 1466
Supporting Stepfamilies: What Do the Children Feel, 1660
Supportive Systems, 4331
Supports Intensity Scale, 2848
Surmontil, 4726
Survey & Analysis Branch, 1940
Survival Guide for College Students with ADD or LD, 463
Survival Strategies for Parenting Your ADD Child, 464
Surviving & Prospering in the Managed Mental Health Care Marketplace, 2849
Surviving Schizophrenia: A Manual for Families, Consumers and Providers, 1400
Surviving an Eating Disorder: Perspectives and Strategies, 1042
Surviving the Emotional Trauma of Divorce, 53
Survivors of Loved Ones' Suicides, 41
Survivors of Loved Ones' Suicides (SOLOS), 17, 40, 1521
Suzie Brown Intervention Maze, 2850
Sweetwater Health Enterprises, 2504, 4514
Symbyax, 4727
Symptoms of Depression, 2993
Synergistic Office Solutions (SOS Software), 4515
Synthon Pharmaceuticals, 4660
Syracuse University, Facilitated Communication Institute, 596, 650, 666, 668

Systems Advocacy, 1789

T

TASC, 4332
TASH, 573, 601
TEACCH, 651
TOPS Club, 998
Take Charge: Handling a Crisis and Moving Forward, 1308
Takeda Pharmaceuticals North America, 4661
Taking Charge of ADHD: Complete, Authoritative Guide for Parents, 465
Taming Bipolar Disorders, 733
Tarrant County Mental Health: Mental Retardation Services, 2451
Taunton State Hospital, 3917
Taylor & Francis, 121, 602
Taylor & Francis Group, 3724
Taylor & Francis Publishing, 3260
Taylor Hardin Secure Medical Facility, 3740
Taylor Trade Publishing, 412
Taylor and Francis, 3243
Teach & Reach: Tobacco, Alcohol & Other Drug Prevention, 146
Teaching Behavioral Self Control to Students, 3018
Teaching Buddy Skills to Preschoolers, 2851
Teaching Children with Autism: Strategies to Enhance Communication, 630
Teaching Goal Setting and Decision-Making to Students with Developmental Disabilities, 2852
Teaching Practical Communication Skills, 2853
Teaching Problem Solving to Students with Mental Retardation, 2854
Teaching Self-Management to Elementary Students with Developmental Disabilities, 2855
Teaching Students with Severe Disabilities in Inclusive Settings, 2856
Teaching and Mainstreaming Autistic Children, 631
Technical Support Systems, 4622
Teen Dramas, 1641
Teen Guide to Staying Sober, 147
Teen Image, 1057
Teen Relationship Workbook, 1613
Teen Stress!, 352
Teenagers with ADD and ADHD, 2nd Edition: A Guide for Parents and Professionals, 466
Teenagers with ADD: A Parent's Guide, 467
Teens and Alcohol: Gallup Youth Survey Major Issues and Trends, 2923
Teens and Drinking, 193
Teens and Suicide, 3091
Teenwire, 1683
Telepad Corporation, 4623
Temper Tantrums: What Causes Them and How Can You Respond?, 1673
Tempus Software, 4516
Ten Simple Solutions To Panic, 323
Ten Steps for Steps, 1681, 3590
Tender Hearts, 18, 74
Tennessee Alliance for the Mentally Ill, 2105
Tennessee Association of Mental Health Organization, 2106

Tennessee Commission on Children and Youth, 2442
Tennessee Department of Health, 2443
Tennessee Department of Health: Alcohol and Drug Abuse, 2444
Tennessee Department of Human Services, 2445
Tennessee Department of Mental Health and Developmental Disabilities, 2446
Tennessee Mental Health Consumers' Association, 2107
Tennessee Voices for Children, 2108
Terrell State Hospital, 4081
Territorial Apprehensiveness (TERRAP) Programs, 276
Territorial Apprehensiveness Programs (TERRAP), 387
Test Collection at ETS, 3341
Testing Automatic Thoughts with Thought Records, 3509
Texas Alliance for the Mentally Ill, 2119
Texas Commission on Alcohol and Drug Abuse, 2452
Texas Counseling Association, 2120
Texas Department of Aging and Disability Services: Mental Retardation Services, 2453
Texas Department of Family and Protective Services, 2454
Texas Department of State Health Services, 2452
Texas Federation of Families for Children's Mental Health, 2121
Texas Health & Human Services Commission, 2455
Texas Psychological Association, 2122
Texas Society of Psychiatric Physicians, 2123
Textbook of Anxiety Disorders, 324
Textbook of Child and Adolescent Psychiatry, 3154
Textbook of Family and Couples Therapy: Clinical Applications, 2857
Textbook of Pediatric Neuropsychiatry, 3155
Thames Valley Programs, 1853
Then Things Every Child with Autism Wishes Y ou Knew, 633
Theory and Technique of Family Therapy, 2859
Therapeutic Communities for Addictions: Reading in Theory, Research, and Practice, 2924
Therapeutic Communities of America, 2679
Therapeutic Resources, 3725, 790
Therapist Directory, 3579
Therapist's Workbook, 3618
Therapy for Adults Molested as Children: Beyond Survival, 1455
Thesaurus of Psychological Index Terms, 2860
Thinking In Pictures, Expanded Edition: My L Life with Autism, 634
Thirteen Steps to Help Families Stop Fightin Solve Problems Peacefully, 1614
Thomas B Finan Center, 3902
Thomson ResearchSoft, 4517
Three Spheres: Psychiatric Interviewing Primer, 2861
Three Springs, 4058
Three Springs LEAPS, 4058
3m Health Information Systems, 4533
Thresholds Psychiatric Rehabilitation, 1790
Through the Eyes of a Child, 3156
Through the Patient's Eyes, 2862

Tics and Tourette Syndrome: A Handbook for Parents and Professionals, 1552
Time Warner Bookmark, 3726
Time Warner Books, 285, 878
Tinley Park Mental Health Center, 3850
Today's Parent Online, 1684
Tofranil, 4728
Tolvon, 4729
Tools of the Trade: A Therapist's Guide to Art Therapy Assessments, 2863
Topamax, 4730
Topeka Institute for Psychoanalysis, 3449
Tormenting Thoughts and Secret Rituals: The Hidden Epidemic of Obsessive-Compulsive Disorder, 1201
Torrance State Hospital, 4039
Total Quality Management in Mental Health and Mental Retardation, 2864
Touched with Fire: Manic-Depressive Illness and The Artistic Temperament, 1514
Touching Tree, 1209
Tourette Syndrome, 1553, 1569
Tourette Syndrome Association, 1541, 1560, 1561, 1562, 1563, 1564, 1571, 1572
Tourette Syndrome Plus, 1570
Tourette Syndrome and Human Behavior, 1554
Tourette's Syndrome, Tics, Obsession, Compulsions: Developmental Psychopathology & Clinical Care, 1555
Tourette's Syndrome: The Facts, Second Edition, 1556
Tourette's Syndrome: Tics, Obsessions, Compulsions, 1557
Towers Perrin Integrated Heatlh Systems Consulting, 4334
Training Behavioral Healthcare Professionals, 3451
Training Behavioral Healthcare Professionals: Higher Learning in an Era of Managed Care, 3450
Training Families to do a Successful Intervention: A Professional's Guide, 2865
Transforming Trauma: EMDR, 3066
The Transition House, 3809
Transition Matters-From School to Independence, 702, 2866
Transition from School to Post-School Life for Individuals with Disabilities, 30
Transitions Mental Health Rehabilitation, 3851
Transvestites and Transsexuals: Toward a Theory of Cross-Gender Behavior, 3012
Tranxene, 4731
Trauma Resource Area, 978, 1329
Trauma Response, 3067
The Trauma Spectrum: Hidden Wounds and Human Resiliency, 3065
Trauma Treatment Manual, 1354
Traumatic Events & Mental Health, 3068
Traumatic Incident Reduction Association, 4624
Traumatic Incident Reduction Workshop, 3195
Traumatic Stress: Effects of Overwhelming Experience on Mind, Body and Society, 1309
Treating Alcohol Dependence: a Coping Skills Training Guide, 3619
Treating Alcoholism, 149
Treating Anxiety Disorders, 2947
Treating Anxiety Disorders with a Cognitive, 2948

Treating Complex Cases: Cognitive Behavioral Therapy Approach, 2867
Treating Depressed Children: A Therapeutic Manual of Proven Cognitive Behavior Techniques, 2994, 3157
Treating Depression, 2995
Treating Difficult Personality Disorders, 3041
Treating Eating Disorders, 1043
Treating Intellectually Disabled Sex Offenders: A Model Residential Program, 1456
Treating Panic Disorder and Agoraphobia: A Step by Step Clinical Guide, 2949
Treating Schizophrenia, 1403
Treating Substance Abuse: Part 1, 2925
Treating Substance Abuse: Part 2, 2926
Treating Tourette Syndrome and Tic Disorders : A Guide for Practitioners, 1558
Treating Trauma Disorders Effectively, 1317
Treating the Aftermath of Sexual Abuse: a Handbook for Working with Children in Care, 3158
Treating the Alcoholic: Developmental Model of Recovery, 2927
Treating the Tough Adolescent: Family Based Step by Step Guide, 3159
Treatment Plans and Interventions for Depression and Anxiety Disorders, 329, 905
Treatment for Chronic Depression: Cognitive Behavioral Analysis System of Psychotherapy (CBASP), 906
Treatment of Children with Mental Disorders, 34, 476, 649, 845
Treatment of Complicated Mourning, 2868
Treatment of Multiple Personality Disorder, 969
Treatment of Obsessive Compulsive Disorder, 3024
Treatment of Recurrent Depression, 2996
Treatment of Stress Response Syndromes, 31
Treatment of Suicidal Patients in Managed Care, 3092
Treatments of Psychiatric Disorders, 2869
TriZetto Group, 4518
Triavil, 4732
Trichotillomania Learning Center, 1133, 1149, 1150, 1151, 1152
Trichotillomania: A Guide, 330
Trichotillomania: Overview and Introduction to HRT, 1152
Triplet Connection, 20
Triumph Over Fear: a Book of Help and Hope for People with Anxiety, Panic Attacks, and Phobias, 331
Troubled Teens: Multidimensional Family Therapy, 3160
Trust After Trauma: A Guide to Relationships for Survivors and Those Who Love Them, 1310
Tucket Pub, 311
Turbo-Doc EMR, 4519
Turning Point of Tampa, 3810
Twelve-Step Facilitation Handbook, 150
Twenty-Four Hours a Day, 151
Twin Town Treatment Centers, 3772
Twin Valley Behavioral Healthcare, 4017
Twin Valley Psychiatric System, 4018

U

UCLA Department of Psychiatry & Biobehavioral Sciences, 1839
UCLA Neuropsychiatric Institute and Hospital, 3452
UCSF-Department of Psychiatry, Cultural Competence, 3453
UNI/CARE Systems, 4520
UNISYS Corporation, 4625
UNITE, 75
UNITE Inc Grief Support, 21
US DHHS, Administration for Children & Families, PCMR, 2217
US Department of Health & Human Services, 2181
US Department of Health & Human Services: Indian Health Service, 2223
US Department of Health and Human Services Bureau of Primary Health, 2225
US Department of Health and Human Services Planning and Evaluation, 2224
US Department of Health and Human Services: Office of Women's Health, 2226
US Veterans Administration: Mental Health and Behavioral Sciences Services, 2227
USA Today, 3592
USC Psychiatry and Psychology Associates, 3454
USC School of Medicine, 3455
UT Southwestern Medical Center, 750, 773
Ulster County Mental Health Department, 3456
Ultimate Stranger: The Autistic Child, 635
Under the Rug: Substance Abuse and the Mature Woman, 2928
Understanding & Managing the Defiant Child, 848
Understanding Autism, 636
Understanding Dissociative Disorders and Addiction, 195, 970
Understanding Dissociative Disorders: A Guid e for Family Physicians and Healthcare Workers, 971
Understanding Girls with Attention Deficit Hyperactivity Disorder, 468
Understanding Post Traumatic Stress Disorder and Addiction, 1311
Understanding Psychiatric Medications in the Treatment of Chemical Dependency and Dual Diagnoses, 2929
Understanding Schizophrenia: Guide to the New Research on Causes & Treatment, 1404
Understanding and Preventing Suicide: New Perspectives, 1515
Understanding and Teaching Emotionally Disturbed Children and Adolescents, 3161
Understanding and Treating the Hereditary Psychiatric Spectrum Disorders, 486, 849, 1210, 1565
Understanding the Defiant Child, 487
Underwood Books, 3727, 464
Union County Psychiatric Clinic, 3457
Uniquity, 3620
United Advocates for Children of California, 1840
United Behavioral Health, 4335
United Families for Children's Mental Health, 1592, 1791, 1929
United States Psychiatric Rehabilitation Organization (USPRA), 2680

United Way of Connecticut, 203
Universal Behavioral Service, 3861, 4521, 4626
University Behavioral Healthcare, 3458
University Memory and Aging Center, 819
University Pavilion Psychiatric Services, 3811
University of California, 1833
University of California Press, 3728, 1345
University of California at Davis Psychiatry and Behavioral Sciences Department, 3459
University of Chicago Press, 3729, 3055
University of Cincinnati College of Medical Department of Psychiatry, 3460
University of Colorado Health Sciences Center, 3461
University of Connecticut Health Center, 3462
University of Illinois at Chicago, 1781
University of Iowa Hospital, 3463
University of Iowa Hospitals & Clinics, 1908
University of Iowa, Mental Health: Clinical Research Center, 1908
University of Kansas Medical Center, 3464
University of Kansas School of Medicine, 3465
University of Louisville School of Medicine, 3466
University of Maryland Medical Systems, 3467
University of Maryland School of Medicine, 3468
University of Massachusetts Medical Center, 3469
University of Miami - Department of Psychology, 3470
University of Michigan, 3471
University of Minnesota Fairview Health Systems, 3472
University of Minnesota Press, 3730, 1008, 1030
University of Minnesota, Family Social Science, 3473
University of Missouri, 1979
University of New Mexico, School of Medicine Health Sciences Center, 3474
University of North Carolina School of Social Work, 3475
University of North Carolina School of Social Work, Behavioral Healthcare, 4336
University of North Carolina, School of Medicine, 3476
University of Pennsylvania, 748
University of Pennsylvania Health System, 3477
University of Pennsylvania Weight and Eating Disorders Program, 1063
University of Pennsylvania, Department of Psychiatry, 3478
University of Pittsburgh Medical Center, 2080
University of South Florida, 1589, 3308, 3433
University of Tennessee Medical Group: Department of Medicine and Psychiatry, 3479
University of Texas Harris County Psychiatric Center, 4082
University of Texas Medical Branch Managed Care, 3480
University of Texas Southwestern Medical Center, 2124
University of Texas, Southwestern Medical Center, 3481

University of Texas-Houston Health Science Center, 3482
University of Texas: Mental Health Clinical Research Center, 925
University of Utah Neuropsychiatric, 3483
University of Virginia, 2677
University of Virginia Health System/UVHS, 2139
University of Wisconsin Center for Health Policy and Program Evaluation, 2479
Until Tomorrow: A Family Lives with Autism, 637
Uplift, 2178
Upper Shore Community Mental Health Center, 3903
Ups & Downs: How to Beat the Blues and Teen Depression, 3162
Using Computers In Educational and Psycholog ical Research, 2870
Utah Commission on Criminal and Juvenile Justice, 2456
Utah Department of Health, 2457
Utah Department of Health: Health Care Financing, 2458
Utah Department of Human Services, 2459
Utah Department of Human Services: Division of Substance Abuse And Mental Health, 2460
Utah Department of Mental Health, 2461
Utah Parent Center, 2129, 643
Utah Psychiatric Association, 2130
Utah State Hospital, 4084

V

Valeant Pharmaceuticals International, 4662
Valium, 4733
Value Health, 4337
ValueOptions, 1922, 4338
ValueOptions Jacksonville Service Center, 4339
Values Clarification for Counselors, 2871
Vanderbilt University: John F Kennedy Center for Research on Human Development, 2109
Vanderveer Group, 4340
Vann Data Services, 4522
Vasquez Management Consultants, 4341
Vedder Price, 4342
Velocity Healthcare Informatics, 4523
VeriCare, 4343
VeriTrak, 4344
Verispan, 4345
Veritas Villa, 3999
Vermont Alliance for the Mentally Ill, 2134
Vermont Department for Children and Families Economic Services Division (ESD), 2463
Vermont Department of Health: Division of Mental Health Services, 2464
Vermont Employers Health Alliance, 2135
Vermont Federation of Families for Children's Mental Health, 2136
Vermont State Hospital, 4087
VersaForm Systems Corporation, 4524
Via Christi Research, 3871
Viagra, 4734
Victims of Dementia: Service, Support, and Care, 798
Victor School, 3918
Viking Adult, 871

Vintage, 634
Vintage Books A Division Of Random House, 1510
Virginia Beach Community Service Board, 2144, 4346, 4627
Virginia Commonwealth University, Medical College, 3360
Virginia Department of Medical Assistance Services, 2465
Virginia Department of Mental Health, Mental Retardation and Substance Abuse Services (DMHMRSAS), 2466
Virginia Department of Social Services, 2467
Virginia Federation of Families, 2145
Virginia Federation of Families for Children's Mental Health, 2146
Virginia Office of the Secretary of Health and Human Resources, 2468
Virtual Software Systems, 4525
VocalTec, 4449
Voice of the Retarded, 1792
Voices From Fatherhood: Fathers, Sons and ADHD, 469
Voices of Depression, 939
Vyvanse, 4735

W

W.W. Norton, 148
W.W. Norton & Company, 1138, 1391, 1452
WW Norton, 3731
Waco Center for Youth, 4083
Wake Forest University, 3484
Walden House Transitional Treatment Center, 3773
Walter P Carter Center, 3904
Walter P Ruther Psychiatric Hospital, 3927
Wang Software, 4526
Warren Grant Magnuson Clinical Center, 1793
Warren State Hospital, 4040
Warwick Medical & Professional Center, 2143
Washington Advocates for the Mentally Ill, 2160
Washington County Alliance for the Mentally Ill, 2092
Washington Department of Alcohol and Substance Abuse: Department of Social and Health Service, 2469
Washington Department of Social & Health Services, 2470
Washington Department of Social and Health Services: Mental Health Division, 2471
Washington Institute for Mental Illness Research and Training, 2161
Washington State Psychological Association, 2162
Washington State University, Spokane, 2161
Washington University - Saint Louis, 809
Water Balance in Schizophrenia, 1405
Watson Pharmaceuticals, 4663
Watson Wyatt Worldwide, 4347
Way Back Inn-Grateful House, 3852
Wayne University-University of Psychiatric Center-Jefferson: Outpatient Mental Health for Children, Adolescents and Adults, 3485
We Insist on Natural Shapes, 999
Web of Addictions, 258
WebMD, 3593

Webman Associates, 4348
Weirton Medical Center, 4105
Well Mind Association, 4628
WellPoint Behavioral Health, 4349
Wellbutrin, 4736
Wellness Councils of America, 2681
Wellness Integrated Network, 4527
Wells Center, 3853
Wernersville State Hospital, 4041
West Central Georgia Regional Hospital, 3820
West Jefferson Medical Center, 3486
West Virginia Alliance for the Mentally Ill, 2167
West Virginia Bureau for Behavioral Health and Health Facilities, 2472
West Virginia Department of Health & Human Resources, 2473, 2474
West Virginia Department of Health and Human Resources, 2472
West Virginia Department of Welfare Bureau for Children and Families, 2474
West Virginia Division of Criminal Justice Services (DCJS), 2475
Westboro State Hospital, 3919
Westchester Alliance for the Mentally Ill, 2034
Westchester Task Force on Eating Disorders, 2035
Western Mental Health Institute, 4059
Western Missouri Mental Health Center, 3941
Western New York Children's Psychiatric Center, 4000
Western North Carolina Families (CAN), 2042
Western Psychiatric Institute and Clinic, 3487
Western State Hospital, 3878, 4098, 4102
Westlund Child Guidance Clinic, 3928
What Do These Students Have in Common?, 921
What Makes Ryan Tic?, 1559
What Makes Ryan Tick?, 470
What Psychotherapists Should Know About Disability, 2872
What Should I Tell My Child About Drinking?, 230
What Works When with Children and Adolescents: A Handbook of Individual Counseling Techniques, 1615
What to Do When You Worry Too Much: A Kid's Guide to Overcoming Anxiety, 332
What to Do When You're Scared and Worried: A Guide for Kids, 333
What to do When a Friend is Depressed: Guide for Students, 922
Wheaton Franciscan Healthcare: Elmbrook Memo rial, 4109
When A Friend Dies, 32
When Anger Hurts: Quieting The Storm Within, 1145
When Food Is Love, 1044
When Nothing Matters Anymore: A Survival Guide for Depressed Teens, 907
When Once Is Not Enough: Help for Obsessive Compulsives, 1202
When Parents Have Problems: A Book for Teens and Older Children with an Abusive, Alcoholic, or Mentally Ill Parent, 152
When Perfect Isn't Good Enough: Strategies for Coping with Perfectionism, 1203
When Snow Turns to Rain, 638

When Someone You Care About Abuses Drugs and Alcohol: When to Act, What to Say, 196
Where to Start and What to Ask: An Assessmen t Handbook, 2873
Where to Start and What to Ask: Assessment Handbook, 2874
Whidbey Island Alliance for the Mentally Ill, 2163
White Oaks Companies of Illinois, 3854
Who Gets PTSD? Issues of Posttraumatic Stress Vulnerability, 1312
Why Haven't I Been Able to Help?, 197
Why Isn't My Child Happy? Video Guide About Childhood Depression, 934
Why Won't My Child Pay Attention?, 488
WidowNet, 77
WilData Systems Group, 4391
Wiley Europe and Jossey-Bass Publications, 3450
Wiley, John & Sons, 328
William M Mercer, 4350
William Morrow & Company, 1398
William R Sharpe, Jr Hospital, 4106
William S Hall Psychiatric Institute, 4051
William S Hein & Company, 3280
Williams & Wilkins, 3263
Williamson County Council on Alcohol and Drug Prevention, 2447
Willmar Regional Treatment Center, 3932
Willough Healthcare System, 3812
Willow Crest Hospital, 4023
Windhorse Associates, 1794
Wing of Madness: A Depression Guide, 951, 3594
Winnebago Mental Health Institute, 4110
Winter Blues, 908
Winter's Flower, 639
Wisconsin Alliance for the Mentally Ill, 2173
Wisconsin Association of Family and Child Agency, 2174
Wisconsin Bureau of Health Care Financing, 2480
Wisconsin Department of Health and Family Services, 2481
Wisconsin Family Ties, 2175
Wisconsin Psychiatric Institute and Clinic, 2169
Without Reason, 640
A Woman Doctor's Guide to Depression, 2978
Woman's Journal, Special Edition for Use in the Criminal Justice System, 153
Women and Depression, 935
Women with Attention Deficit Disorder, 471
Women's Counselling & Referral Education Cen tre, 1795
Women's Mental Health Services: Public Health Perspective, 2875
Women's Support Services, 1854
Woodbine House, 3732, 466, 467, 590, 599, 638, 1544
Woodlands, 4528
Woodlands Behavioral Healthcare Network, 1964
Woodridge Hospital, 4060
WordPerfect Corporation, 4629
Wordsworth, 3488
Work Group for the Computerization of Behavioral Health, 4529
Workbook: Mental Retardation, 2876
Working Press, 4351
Working Together, 1058

Working with Self-Harming Adolescents: A Collaborative, Strengths-Based Therapy Approach, 3163
Working with the Core Relationship Problem in Psychotherapy, 2877
World Federation for Mental Health, 1796, 3315
World Federation for Mental Health Newsletter, 3315
World Health College, 1688
World Scientific Publishing Company, 1093
World Service Office, 1067
The World of Perversion: Psychoanalysis and the Impossible Absolute of Desire, 1231
WorldatWork, 2682
Worldwide Healthcare Solutions: IBM, 4530
Worry Control Workbook, 334
Writing Behavioral Contracts: A Case Simulation Practice Manual, 2878
Writing Psychological Reports: A Guide for Clinicians, 2879
Wrong Planet, 536
www.1000deaths.com, 41
www.aa.org, 232
www.aacap.org, 3510
www.aan.com, 802, 3511
www.aane.org, 674
www.aap.org, 491
www.aapb.org, 3512
www.aasmnet.org, 1479
www.abcparenting.com, 1640
www.abecsw.org, 3513
www.about.com, 3514
www.aboutteensnow.com/dramas, 1641
www.abpsi.org, 3515
www.aca-usa.org, 233
www.adaa.org, 361
www.add.about.com, 492
www.add.org, 493
www.addictionresourceguide.com, 234
www.additudemag.com, 494
www.addvance.com, 495
www.adhdnews.com.ssi.htm, 1642
www.adhdnews.com/Advocate.htm, 496, 1643
www.adhdnews.com/sped.htm, 497, 1644
www.adultchildren.org, 235
www.agelessdesign.com, 803
www.ahaf.org/alzdis/about/adabout.htm, 804
www.aim-hq.org, 362
www.Al-Anon-Alateen.org, 1638
www.al-anon.alateen.org, 236
www.alcoholism.about.com/library, 237
www.algy.com/anxiety/files/barlow.html, 363
www.alivealone.org, 43
www.alt.support.eating.disord, 1070
www.alz.co.uk, 805
www.alzforum.org, 806
www.alzheimersbooks.com/, 807
www.alzheimersupport.Com, 808
www.ama-assn.org, 3516
www.americasdoctor.com, 3517
www.ani.ac, 675
www.anred.com, 1071
www.apa.org, 364, 3518
www.apa.org/practice/traumaticstress.html, 1318
www.apa.org/pubinfo/anger.html, 1153
www.apna.org, 3519
www.appi.org, 3520
www.apsa.org, 3521
www.aspennj.org, 676

www.aspergerinfo.com, 532
www.aspergers.com, 533
www.aspergersyndrome.org, 534
www.aspiesforfreedom.com, 535
www.assc.caltech.edu, 3522
www.athealth.com, 44
www.autism-society.org, 677
www.autism.org, 678
www.autismresearchinstitute.org, 679
www.autismservicescenter.org, 680
www.autismspeaks.org, 681
www.autisticservices.com, 682
www.babycenter.com/rcindex.html, 498
www.bcm.tmc.edu/civitas/caregivers.htm,
 1319
www.befrienders.org, 938
www.bereavedparentsusa.org, 45
www.biostat.wustl.edu, 809
www.blarg.net/~charlatn/voices, 939, 3523
www.bpso.org, 756, 3524
www.bpso.org/nomania.htm, 757, 3525
www.cape.org, 3526
www.cfc-efc.ca/docs/00000095.htm, 1645
www.cfsny.org, 46, 238, 365, 499, 683, 758,
 1154
www.CHADD.org, 489, 1639
www.chadd.org, 3527
www.climb-support.org, 47
www.closetoyou.org/eatingdisorders, 1072
www.cnn.com/Health, 3528
www.compassionatefriends.org, 48
www.compuserve.com, 3529
www.couns.uiuc.edu, 1646
www.counseling.com, 3530
www.counselingforloss.com, 49, 3531
www.cs.uu.nl/wais/html/na-bng/alt.support.ab
 use-partners.html, 1458
www.csaac.org, 684
www.cyberpsych.org, 50, 366, 500, 685,
 759, 810, 850, 940, 973, 1073, 1114, 1155,
 1211, 1272, 1320, 1418, 1480, 1522, 3532
www.dbsalliance.org, 760
www.death-dying.com, 51
www.Depressedteens.Com, 936
www.divorceasfriends.com, 52
www.divorcecentral.com, 53
www.divorcedfather.com, 1647
www.divorceinfo.com, 54
www.divorcemag.com, 55
www.DivorceNet.com, 42
www.divorcesupport.com, 56
www.doitnow.org/pages/pubhub.hmtl, 239
www.dstress.com/guided.htm, 367
www.duanev/family/dads.html, 1648
www.edap.org, 1074
www.education.indiana.edu/cas/adol/adol.htm
 l, 1649
www.elderlyplace.com, 811
www.emdr.com, 941, 1459
www.ericps.crc.uiuc.edu/npin/index.html,
 1650
www.ericps.crc.uiuc.edu/npin/library/texts.
 html, 1651
www.factsforhealth.org, 368, 1321, 3533
www.fairlite.com/ocd/, 1212
www.fathermag.com, 1652
www.fathers.com, 1653
www.feat.org, 686
www.firelily.com/gender/sstgfaq, 1460
www.flyingsolo.com, 1654
www.fmsf.com, 974
www.freedomfromfear.org, 369
www.freedomvillageusa.com, 1655

www.friendsforsurvival.org, 57
www.fsbassociates.com/fsg/whydivorce.html,
 1656
www.geocities.com, 3534
www.geocities.com/enchantedforest/1068,
 761, 1657, 3535
www.goaskalice.columbia.edu, 3536
www.goodwill-suncoast.org, 370, 762, 1156
www.grasphelp.org, 58
www.griefnet.org, 59
www.grieftalk.com/help1.html, 3537
www.guidetopsychology.com, 371
www.gurze.com, 1075
www.habitsmart.com/cogtitle.html, 812, 3538
www.health-center.com/mentalhealth/
 schizophrenia/default.htm, 1419
www.health.nih.gov, 1115
www.healthanxiety.org, 372
www.healthfinder.gov, 1116
www.healthgate.com/, 3539
www.healthtouch.com, 3540
www.healthy.net, 3541
www.healthyminds.org, 373
www.healthyplace.com/Communities/, 1076
www.helix.com, 3542
www.home.clara.net/spig/guidline.htm, 1658
www.hometown.aol.com/DrgnKprl/BPCAT.h
 tml, 1659
www.hopkinsmedicine.org/epigen, 1420
www.human-nature.com/odmh, 3543
www.ianrpubs.unl.edu/family/nf223.htm,
 1660
www.icisf.org, 374, 1322
www.Ifred.Org, 937
www.iidc.indiana.edu, 687
www.infotrieve.com, 3544
www.intelihealth.com, 375, 1117, 3545
www.interlog.com/~calex/ocd, 1213
www.isst-D.Org, 975
www.jacsweb.org, 240
www.jobstresshelp.com, 376
www.jointogether.org, 241
www.kidshealth.org/kid/feeling/index.html,
 1661
www.kidsource.com/kidsource/pages/parentin
 g, 1662
www.kidsource.com/nedo/, 1077
www.kidspeace.org, 1118
www.klis.com/chandler/pamphlet/bipolar/
 bipolarpamphlet.html, 1663
www.klis.com/chandler/pamphlet/bipolar/bipo
 l arpamphlet.htm, 1664
www.klis.com/chandler/pamphlet/dep/, 942
www.klis.com/chandler/pamphlet/panic/,
 1665
www.krinfo.com, 3546
www.ladders.org, 688
www.LD-ADD.com, 490
www.lexington-on-line.com, 377
www.lexington-on-line.com/, 1214
www.lollie.com/about/suicide.html, 1523
www.lollie.com/blue/suicide.html, 3547
www.maapservices.org, 689
www.madd.org, 242
www.magicnet.net/~hedyyumi/child.html,
 1666
www.manicdepressive.org, 763
www.mayoclinic.com, 1215
www.mayohealth.com, 1119
www.mayohealth.org/mayo, 3548
www.mayohealth.org/mayo/common/htm/,
 813
www.mbpexpert.com, 1098

www.med.jhu.edu/drada/creativity.html, 3549
www.med.nyu.edu/Psych/index.html, 3550
www.med.yale.edu, 764
www.medinfosource.com, 3551
www.medscape.com, 3552
www.medweb.emory.edu/MedWeb/, 3553
www.members.aol.com/AngriesOut, 1157
www.members.aol.com/dswgriff, 3554
www.members.aol.com/dswgriff/suicide.html,
 1524
www.members.aol.com/leonardjk/USA.htm,
 1421
www.members.tripod.com/~suicideprevention
 / index, 1525
www.mentalhealth.com, 243, 814, 1232,
 1273, 1323, 1351, 1422, 1461, 1481, 1526,
 1566
www.mentalhealth.com/book, 3555
www.mentalhealth.com/p20-grp.html, 3556
www.mentalhealth.com/story, 3557
www.mentalhealth.org, 1158
www.mentalhealth.org/publications/allpubs/,
 1667
www.mentalhealth.Samhsa.Gov, 378, 690,
 765
www.mentalhealth.samhsa.gov, 244
www.mentalhealth.smahsa.gov, 815
www.mentalhelp.net, 1078
www.mentalhelp.net/guide/schizo.htm, 1423
www.mentalhelp.net/psyhelp/chap7, 1159
www.metanoia.org/suicide/, 1527, 3558
www.mgl.ca/~chovil, 1424
www.mhsanctuary.com/borderline, 1274
www.mhselfhelp.org, 60, 245, 691, 766, 1160
www.mhsource.com, 3559
www.mhsource.com/, 3560
www.mhsource.com/
 advocacy/narsad/order.html, 1425
www.mhsource.com/advocacy/
 narsad/newsletter.html, 1426
www.mhsource.com/advocacy/narsad
 /narsadfaqs.html, 1427
www.mhsource.com/advocacy/narsad/
 studyops.html, 1428
www.mhsource.com/narsad.html, 1429
www.miminc.org, 767
www.mindfreedom.org, 3561
www.mindstreet.com/training.html, 816
www.mirror-mirror.org/eatdis.htm, 1079,
 3562
www.misschildren.org, 61
www.missfoundation.org, 62
www.moodswing.org/bdfaq.html, 768, 3563
www.msbp.com, 1099
www.muextension.missouri.edu/xpor/hesguide
 /, 1668
www.munchausen.com, 1100
www.naadac.org, 246
www.nami.org, 379, 501, 692, 769
www.naminys.org, 1430
www.naphs.org, 3564
www.naswdc.org/, 3565
www.nationalshareoffice.com, 63
www.naturalchild.com/home, 1669
www.Ncadi.Samhsa.Gov, 231
www.nccbh.org, 247
www.ncptsd.org, 1324
www.ndmda.org/justmood.htm, 3566
www.necc.org, 693
www.nhlbi.nih.gov/about/ncsdr, 1482
www.Nia.Nih.Gov/Alzheimers, 801
www.niaaa.nih.gov, 248
www.nichcy.org, 502, 1670

www.nida.nih.gov, 249
www.nida.nih.gov/drugpages, 250
www.nimh.nih.gov, 3567
www.nimh.nih.gov/anxiety/anxiety/ocd, 1216
www.nimh.nih.gov/publicat/adhd.cfm, 503
www.nimh.nih.gov/publicat/depressionmenu.c
fm, 943
www.nimh.nih.gov/publicat/ocdmenu.cfm,
1217, 1275
www.nimh.nih.gov/publicat/schizoph.htm,
1431
www.nimh.nih.gov/publist/964033.htm, 944
www.ninds.nih.gov, 817
www.nlm.nih.gov, 1120
www.nlm.nih.gov/medlineplus/sleepdisorders.
html, 1483
www.nmha.org, 3568
www.nnfr.org/curriculum/topics/sep_div.html,
1671
www.noah-health.org/en/bns/disorders/
alzheimer.html, 818
www.nofas.org, 251
www.nospank.org/toc.htm, 1672
www.npadnews.com, 380
www.npin.org/pnews/pnews997/, 1673
www.nursece.com/OCD.htm, 1218
www.ocdhope.com/gdlines.htm, 1219, 1276
www.ocfoundation.org, 1220
www.oclc.org, 3569
www.ohioalzcenter.org/facts.html, 819
www.oneaddplace.com, 504
www.oznet.ksu.edu/library/famlf2/, 1674,
3570
www.pace-custody.org, 3571
www.panicattacks.com.au, 381
www.panicdisorder.about.com, 382
www.paperchase.com, 3572
www.parentcity.com/read/library, 1675
www.parenthoodweb.com, 1676, 3573
www.parenthoodweb.com/, 1677
www.personal.psu.edu/faculty, 1678
www.pomc.com, 65
www.positive-way.com/step.htm, 1679, 3575
www.priory.com/sex.htm, 1463
www.psych.org, 3576
www.psych.org/clin_res/pg_dementia.cfm,
821
www.psychcrawler.com, 3578
www.psychology.com/therapy.htm, 3579
www.psychologyinfo.com/depression, 947
www.psycom.net/depression.central.grief.html
, 67
www.psycom.net/depression.central.html,
948, 3580
www.psycom.net/depression.central.suicide.
html, 1530
www.pta.org/commonsense, 1680
www.ptsdalliance.org, 1327
www.queendom.com/selfhelp/depression/
depression.html, 949
www.rainbows.org, 68
www.rcpsych.ac.uk/info/help/memory, 823
www.realtionshipjourney.com, 69
www.recovery-inc.com, 1434, 3581
www.resourcesnyc.org, 695
www.reutershealth.com, 3582
www.sadd.org, 253
www.safecrossingsfoundation.org, 70
www.samhsa.gov, 254
www.save.org, 1531, 3583
www.schizophrenia.com, 1435, 3584
www.schizophrenia.com/ami, 3585
www.schizophrenia.com/discuss/, 1436

www.schizophrenia.com/newsletter, 1437,
3586
www.schizophrenia.com/newsletter/buckets/
success.html, 1438
www.selectivemutismfoundation.org, 385
www.selfhelpmagazine.com/articles/stress,
386
www.shpm.com, 950, 3587
www.shpm.com/articles/depress, 3588
www.shrinktank.com, 1465
www.sidran.org, 978, 1328
www.sidran.org/trauma.html, 1329
www.sidsalliance.org, 71
www.siop.org, 3589
www.sleepdisorders.about.com, 1486
www.sleepdisorders.com, 1487
www.sleepfoundation.org, 1488
www.sleepnet.com, 1489
www.smartrecovery.org, 255
www.sni.net/trips/links.html, 1330
www.something-fishy.com, 1082
www.son-rise.org, 696
www.soulselfhelp.on.ca/coda.html, 256
www.spig.clara.net/guidline.htm, 72
www.stepfamily.org/tensteps.htm, 1681,
3590
www.stepfamilyinfo.org/sitemap.htm, 1682,
3591
www.stopbitingnails.com, 1162
www.talhost.net/sleep/links.htm, 1490
www.teenwire.com/index.asp, 1683
www.terraphouston.com, 387
www.thenadd.org, 73, 388, 507, 697, 772,
1163
www.todaysparent.com, 1684
www.tourette-syndrome.com, 1569
www.tourettesyndrome.net, 1570
www.trauma-pages.com, 1331
www.tripletconnection.org, 74
www.tsa-usa.com, 1571
www.tsa-usa.org, 1572
www.unhooked.com, 257
www.unitegriefsupport.org, 75
www.usatoday.com, 3592
www.users.aol.com:80/jimams/, 1685
www.users.aol.com:80/jimams/answers1,
1686
www.users.lanminds.com/~eds/, 1354
www.utexas.edu, 76
www.utsouthwestern.edu, 773
www.vcc.mit.edu/comm/samaritans/brochure.
html, 1532
www.vvc.mit.edu/comm/samaritans/warning.
html, 1533
www.webmd.com, 3593
www.well.com, 258
www.wholefamily.com/kidteencenter/, 1687
www.widownet.org, 77
www.wingofmadness.com, 951, 3594
www.worldcollegehealth.org, 1688
www.wrongplanet.net, 536
www.xs4all.nl/~rosalind/cha-assr.html, 1466
www.zarcrom.com/users/alzheimers, 824
www.zarcrom.com/users/yeartorem, 825
www2.mc.duke.edu/pcaad, 1689
Wyeth, 4664
Wyoming Alliance for the Mentally Ill, 2179
Wyoming Department of Family Services,
2482
Wyoming Department of Health: Division of
Health Care Finance, 2483
Wyoming Mental Health Division, 2484
Wyoming State Government, 2484

Wyoming State Hospital, 4111

X

XI Tech Corporation, 4531
Xanax, 4737

Y

YAI/National Institute for People with
Disabilities, 3196
Yale Mood Disorders Research Program, 751
Yale University Department of Psychiatry,
926
Yale University School of Medicine, 764
Yale University School of Medicine: Child
Study Center, 3489
Yale University: Depression Research
Program, 926
Year to Remember, 825
Yeshiva University: Soundview-Throgs
Neck Community Mental Health Center,
2036
Yesterday's Tomorrow, 909
You Can Beat Depression: Guide to
Prevention and Recovery, 910
You Can Free Yourself From Alcohol &
Drugs: Work a Program That Keeps You
in Charge, 154
You Mean I'm Not Lazy, Stupid or Crazy?,
472
You've Just Been Diagnosed...What Now?,
745
Young Adult Institute and Workshop (YAI),
1593, 1797
Your Brain on Drugs, 155
Your Drug May Be Your Problem: How and
Why to Stop Taking Pyschiatric
Medications, 2930
Youth Services International, 1594, 1798
Youth Violence: Prevention, Intervention,
and Social Policy, 3164
Youth with Impulse-Control Disorders: On
the Spur of the Moment (Helping Youth
with Mental, Physical, & Social
Disabilities), 1146
Yssociation for Psychological Type, 2683

Z

Zero to Three, 1595, 1799
Zoloft, 4738
Zy-Doc Technologies, 4532
Zyprexa, 4739

Alabama

Alabama Alliance for the Mentally Ill, 1800
Alabama Department of Human Resources, 2231
Alabama Department of Mental Health and Mental Retardation, 2232
Alabama Department of Public Health, 2233
Alabama Disabilities Advocacy Program, 2234
Association of State and Provincial Psychology Boards, 2591
Behavioral Health Systems, 4139, 2595
Birmingham Psychiatry, 1801
Daniel and Yeager Healthcare Staffing Solutions, 3369
Electronic Healthcare Systems, 4413
Horizons School, 1802
Mental Health Board of North Central Alabama, 1803
Mental Health Center of North Central Alabama, 1804
National Alliance on Mental Illness: Alabama, 1805
The Kennion Group Inc, 4333

Alaska

Alaska Alliance for the Mentally Ill, 1806
Alaska Council on Emergency Medical Services, 2235
Alaska Department of Health & Social Services, 2236
Alaska Division of Mental Health and Developmental Disabilities, 2237
Alaska Health and Social Services Division of Behavioral Health, 2238
Alaska Mental Health Board, 2239
Center for Loss in Multiple Birth (CLIMB), 8
Mental Health Association in Alaska, 1807, 2240
National Alliance on Mental Illness: Alaska, 1808

Arizona

Action Healthcare Management, 4117
American Council on Alcoholism, 83
American Psychological Association Division of Independent Practice (APADIP), 2561
Anasazi Software, 4365
Annual Santa Fe Psychiatric Symposium, 3186
Arizona Alliance for the Mentally Ill, 1809
Arizona Center For Mental Health PHD, 4129
Arizona Department of Health Services, 2241
Arizona Department of Health Services: Behavioral Services, 2242
Arizona Department of Health Services: Child Fatality Review, 2243
Arizona Department of Health: Substance Abuse, 2244
Assist Technologies, 4370
BetaData Systems, 4378
CARF: Commission on Accreditation of Rehabilitation Facilities, 2488

Commission on Accreditation of Rehabilitation Facilities, 2603
Community Partnership of Southern Arizona, 1810
Contact Behavioral Health Services, 4165
Devereux Arizona Treatment Network, 1811
Ethos Consulting, 4188
Life Development Institute, 1745
Managed Care Consultants, 4254
Mental Health Association of Arizona, 1812
Mentally Ill Kids in Distress, 1581, 1750
MphasiS(BPO), 4475
National Alliance on Mental Illness: Arizona, 1813
Navajo Nation K'E Project, 1814
Navajo Nation K'E Project: Chinle, 1815
Navajo Nation K'E Project: Tuba City, 1816
Navajo Nation K'E Project: Winslow, 1817
Northern Arizona Regional Behavioral Health Authority, 2245
Pinal Gila Behavioral Health Association, 4293
Professional Horizons, Mental Health Service, 3423
The M.I.S.S. Foundation, 19
WorldatWork, 2682

Arkansas

Arkansas Alliance for the Mentally Ill, 1818
Arkansas Department Health & Human Services, 2246
Arkansas Division of Children & Family Service, 2247
Arkansas Division on Youth Services, 2248
Arkansas State Mental Hospital, 2249
Centers for Mental Healthcare Research, 4154
Mental Health Council of Arkansas, 2250
National Alliance on Mental Illness: Arkansas, 1819
National Child Support Network, 1583, 1760
Star Systems Corporation, 4508

California

AMCO Computers, 4356
ASP Software, 4357
Academy of Managed Care Providers, 4115
Adult Children of Alcoholics World Services Organization, 198
Agilent Technologies, 4362
Alliance For Community Care, 4123
American Association of Mental Health Professionals in Corrections (AAMHPC), 2524
American Board of Examiners of Clinical Social Work Regional Offices, 2486
American Holistic Health Association, 1699
American Society on Aging, 2572
Arthur S Shorr and Associates, 4130
Assistance League of Southern California, 1820
Association for Birth Psychology, 2580
Association for Humanistic Psychology, 2583
Association for Pre- & Perinatal Psychology and Health, 2584
Autism Research Institute, 512, 543
Barbanell Associates, 4132

Behaviordata, 4376
Berkowitz Chassion and Sklar, 4140
Bipolar Disorders Clinic, 747
Breining Institute College for the Advanced Study of Addictive Disorders, 3355
Business Objects, 4381
California Alliance for the Mentally Ill, 1821
California Association of Marriage and Family Therapists, 1822
California Association of Social Rehabilitation Agencies, 1823
California Department of Alcohol and Drug Programs, 2228
California Department of Alcohol and Drug Programs: Resource Center, 2251
California Department of Corrections and Reh abilitation, 2252
California Department of Education: Healthy Kids, Healthy California, 2253
California Department of Health Services: Medicaid, 2254
California Department of Health Services: Medi-Cal Drug Discount, 2255
California Department of Mental Health, 2256
California Health Information Association, 1824
California Hispanic Commission on Alcohol Drug Abuse, 2257
California Institute for Mental Health, 1825, 2258
California Institute of Behavioral Sciences, 3357
California Mental Health Directors Association, 2259
California Psychiatric Association (CPA), 1826
California Psychological Association, 1827
California Women's Commission on Addictions, 2260
Calnet, 1828
Cardiff Software: Vista, 4385
Center for Attitudinal Healing (CAH), 1715
Chartman Software, 4389
Children's Health Council, 2600
Cocaine Anonymous, 202
College Health IPA, 4158
Community Resource Council, 1829
CoolTalk, 4398
Cornucopia Software, 4399
Council of Behavioral Group Practice, 2608
Creative Computer Applications, 4400
DML Training and Consulting, 4174
EAP Technology Systems, 4410
Echo Group, 4411
Essi Systems, 4187
Families Anonymous, 1729
Families for Early Autism Treatment, 550
Family Violence & Sexual Assault Institute, 1731
First Consulting Group, 4194
First Data Bank, 4419
Five Acres: Boys and Girls Aid Society of Los Angeles County, 1830
Freedom To Fly, 4197
Friends for Survival, 36, 1519
Full Circle Programs, 4198
Gamblers Anonymous, 1148
Garner Consulting, 4200
Gelbart and Associates, 4420
GenSource Corporation, 4421
Gold Coast Alliance for the Mentally Ill, 1831

Grief Recovery After Substance Passing (GRASP), 10, 88
HSA-Mental Health, 4426
Healing for Survivors, 1734
Health Services Agency: Mental Health, 1832
HealthLine Systems, 4431
Healthline Systems, 4434
HeartMath, 4219
Horizon Management Services, 4222
Human Behavior Associates, 4225
Innovative Health Systems/SoftMed, 4446
Institute for Advancement of Human Behavior, 3191
Institute for Behavioral Healthcare, 3384
Institute for the Advancement of Human Behavior (IAHB), 2617
Institute of HeartMath, 2618
International Transactional Analysis Association (ITAA), 2624
Just Say No International, 1628
Langley Porter Psych Institute at UCSF Parnassus Campus, 3388
Langley Porter Psychiatric Institute at UCSF Parnassus Campus, 1833
Legacy Consulting Insurance Services, 4242
Lexical Technologies, 4452
Lifespan Care Management Agency, 4245
M/MGMT Systems, 4453
Managed Health Network, 4255
Maniaci Insurance Services, 4258
Marijuana Anonymous, 206
Marin Institute, 4259
Masters of Behavioral Healthcare Management, 3396
Mental Health and Aging Network (MHAN) of the American Society on Aging (ASA), 1748
Nar-Anon Family Group, 207
Narcotics Anonymous, 208
Nation Alliance on Mental Illness: California, 1834
National Association of Mental Illness: California, 1835
National Association to Advance Fat Acceptance (NAAFA), 991
National Health Foundation, 1836
National Youth Crisis Hotline, 1630
Nightingale Vantagemed Corporation, 4481
Northern California Psychiatric Society, 1837
O-Anon General Service Office (OGSO), 996
Optimum Care Corporation, 4282
Oracle Corporation, 4486
Orange County Psychiatric Society, 1838
P and W Software, 4488
PRISMED Corporation, 4489
PSIMED Corporation, 4287
Parents Helping Parents, 1586, 1776
Pepperdine University, Graduate School of Education and Psychology, 3419
Phobics Anonymous, 355
Postpartum Support International, 868
Practice Management Resource Group, 4296
Psy Care, 4307
Psychological Center, 3428
Raintree Systems, 4499
Rational Recovery, 210
Research Center for Severe Mental Illnesses, 1785
School of Nursing, UCLA, 3441
Shueman and Associates, 4324
Sun Microsystems, 4512
Thomson ResearchSoft, 4517

Training Behavioral Healthcare Professionals: Higher Learning in an Era of Managed Care, 3450
Training Behavioral Healthcare Professionals, 3451
TriZetto Group, 4518
Trichotillomania Learning Center, 1133, 1149
Turbo-Doc EMR, 4519
UCLA Department of Psychiatry & Biobehavioral Sciences, 1839
UCLA Neuropsychiatric Institute and Hospital, 3452
UCSF-Department of Psychiatry, Cultural Competence, 3453
USC Psychiatry and Psychology Associates, 3454
USC School of Medicine, 3455
United Advocates for Children of California, 1840
United Behavioral Health, 4335
University of California at Davis Psychiatry and Behavioral Sciences Department, 3459
Valeant Pharmaceuticals International, 4662
VeriCare, 4343
VeriTrak, 4344
VersaForm Systems Corporation, 4524
Watson Pharmaceuticals, 4663
Watson Wyatt Worldwide, 4347
We Insist on Natural Shapes, 999
WellPoint Behavioral Health, 4349
Wellness Integrated Network, 4527
Working Press, 4351

Colorado

Adolescent and Family Institute of Colorado, 1841
American Association for Protecting Children, 2515
American Psychology- Law Society (AP-LS), 2563
Asian Pacific Development Center for Human Development, 3351
Association for Applied Psychophysiology & Biofeedback, 2577
Association for the Advancement of Psycholog y, 2589
Behavioral Health Advisor, 4375
Behavioral Health Care, 4134
CAFCA, 4143
CHINS UP Youth and Family Services, 1842
Clinical Nutrition Center, 4393
Colorado Department of Health Care Policy and Financing, 2261
Colorado Department of Human Services (CDHS), 2262
Colorado Department of Human Services: Alcohol and Drug Abuse Division, 2263
Colorado Division of Mental Health, 2264
Colorado Health Networks-Value Options, 1843
Colorado Medical Assistance Program Information Center, 2265
Colorado Traumatic Brain Injury Trust Fund Program, 2266
Craig Counseling & Biofeedback Services, 1844
Denver County Department of Social Services, 2267
El Paso County Human Services, 2268
Employee Benefit Specialists, 4184

Federation of Families for Children's Mental Health, 1845
Integrated Behavioral Health Consultants, 2620
John Maynard and Associates, 4236
Medcomp Software, 4461
Medical Group Management Association, 2628
Mental Health Association of Colorado, 1846
Micromedex, 4473
Milliman, Inc, 4271
National Academy of Neuropsychology (NAN), 2631
National Alliance on Mental Illness: Colorad o, 1847
PRO Behavioral Health, 1775, 4285
Pragmatix, 4297
University of Colorado Health Sciences Center, 3461

Connecticut

Aetna-US HealthCare, 4120
American Academy of Clinical Psychiatrists, 2510
American Academy of Psychiatry & Law Annual Conference, 3169
American Academy of Psychiatry and the Law (AAPL), 2512
American Academy of Psychoanalysis Preliminary Meeting, 3170
American Academy of Psychoanalysis and Dynam ic Psychiatry, 2513
Annual Summit on International Managed Care Trends, 3187
Casey Family Services, 4151
Connecticut Department of Mental Health and Addiction Services, 2269
Connecticut Department of Children and Families, 2270
Connecticut Families United for Children's Mental Health, 1848
Connecticut National Association of Mentally Ill, 1849
Family & Community Alliance Project, 1850
Gaynor and Associates, 4201
Infoline, 203
Institute of Living Anxiety Disorders Center, 1740
Largesse, The Network for Size Esteem, 987
Mental Health Association: Connecticut, 1851
National Alliance on Mental Illness: Connect icut, 1852
Obsessive-Compulsive Foundation, 1206
Sarmul Consultants, 4318
Stonington Institute, 3447
Thames Valley Programs, 1853
University of Connecticut Health Center, 3462
Value Health, 4337
Women's Support Services, 1854
Yale Mood Disorders Research Program, 751
Yale University School of Medicine: Child Study Center, 3489
Yale University: Depression Research Program, 926

Delaware

Astra Zeneca Pharmaceuticals, 4632
Coventry Health Care of Iowa, 4170
Delaware Alliance for the Mentally Ill, 1855
Delaware Department of Health & Social Services, 2271
Delaware Division of Child Mental Health Services, 2272
Delaware Division of Family Services, 2273
Delaware Guidance Services for Children and Youth, 1856
Mental Health Association of Delaware, 1857
National Alliance on Mental Illness: Delaware, 1858

District of Columbia

AAMR: American Association on Mental Retardation, 1690
Administration for Children and Families, 2180
Administration for Children, Youth and Families, 2181
Administration on Aging, 2182
Administration on Developmental Disabilities US Department of Health & Human Services, 2183
Alliance of Genetic Support Groups, 1694
American Academy of Child and Adolescent Psychiatry (AACAP): Annual Meeting, 3167
American Academy of Child & Adolescent Psychiatry, 2509
American Academy of Child and Adolescent Psychiatry, 1573, 1695, 3347, 3347
American Association of Health Plans, 2521
American Association of Homes & Services for the Aging Annual Convention, 3174
American Association of Homes and Services for the Aging, 2523
American Association of Retired Persons, 2527
American Association of Suicidology, 1492
American Association on Intellectual and Dev elopmental Disabilities Annual Meeting, 3175
American Association on Mental Retardation (AAR), 2528
American Health Care Association, 2543
American Health Care Association Annual Convention, 3181
American Managed Behavioral Healthcare Association, 1700, 4126, 2546, 2546
American Pharmacists Association, 2554
American Psychologial Association: Division of Family Psychology, 2559
American Psychological Association, 1704, 2560
American Psychological Association: Applied Experimental and Engineering Psychology, 2562
American Public Human Services Association, 84
Association for Psychological Science, 2586
Association of Black Psychologists, 2590
Association of Black Psychologists Annual Convention, 3189
Association of Maternal and Child Health Programs (AMCHP), 2185

Bazelon Center for Mental Health Law, 1708, 2594
California Department of Health and Human Services, 2274
Center For Mental Health Services, 6, 391
Center for Mental Health Services, 1335, 1358, 1717, 1717
Center for Mental Health Services Knowledge, 87, 265, 393, 393, 548, 707, 779, 1085, 1103, 1126
Center for the Advancement of Health, 4153
Change for Good Coaching and Counseling, 984
Community Action Partnership, 2605
DC Alliance for the Mentally Ill, 1860
DC Commission on Mental Health Services, 2275
DC Department of Human Services, 2276
DC Department of Mental Health, 2191
Department of Health and Human Services/OAS, 1861
Equal Employment Opportunity Commission, 2192
Family Advocacy & Support Association, 1730, 1862
George Washington University, 3379
Gerontoligical Society of America, 2613
HSP Verified, 4206
Hays Group, 4207
Health & Medicine Counsel of Washington DDNC Digestive Disease National Coalition, 2277
Health Service Providers Verified, 2616
Health Systems Research, 4212
Health and Human Services Office of Assistant Secretary for Planning & Evaluation, 2195
Jacobs Institute of Women's Health, 3385
Kushner and Company, 4240
Managed Health Care Association, 2626
NASW JobLink, 4273
National Alliance on Mental Illness: Distric t of Columbia, 1863
National Association For Childrens Behavioral Health, 2632
National Association of Protection and Advocacy Systems, 1755
National Association of Psychiatric Health Systems, 2638
National Association of Social Workers, 1873, 2025, 2640, 2640
National Association of State Alcohol and Drug Abuse Directors, 91
National Business Coalition Forum on Health (NBCH), 2642
National Coalition for the Homeless, 2643
National Committee for Quality Assurance, 2644
National Council on Aging, 2646
National Criminal Justice Association, 2647
National Dissemination Center for Children with Disabilities, 398, 1584
National Gay and Lesbian Task Force, 1105
National Organization on Disability, 1769
National Organization on Fetal Alcohol Syndrome, 100
National Register of Health Service Providers in Psychology, 2500
National Register of Health Service Provider s in Psychology, 2654
National Technical Assistance Center for Children's Mental Health, 1585, 1773

Parents and Friends of Lesbians and Gays, 1108
Parents, Families and Friends of Lesbians and Gays, 1109
Pharmaceutical Care Management Association, 2657
President's Committee on Mental Retardation, 2217
Presidential Commission on Employment of the Disabled, 2218
Psychology of Religion, 2663
Public Health Foundation, 2220
SAMHSA'S National Mental Health Information Center, 869, 958, 1173, 1173, 1228, 1242, 1289, 1342, 1366, 1444, 1474, 1497, 1540
SAMHSA's National Mental Health Information Center, 15, 101, 273, 273, 401, 557, 715, 787, 959, 997, 1089, 1110, 1131, 1174, 1229, 1243
Samhsa's National Mental Health Information Center, 558
Society for Women's Health Research, 2673
Society for the Psychological Study of Social Issues (SPSSI), 2675
Substance Abuse and Mental Health Services Administration: Center for Mental Health Services, 2222
Suicide Prevention Action Network USA (SPANUSA), 1498
Therapeutic Communities of America, 2679
US Department of Health and Human Services Planning and Evaluation, 2224
US Department of Health and Human Services: Office of Women's Health, 2226
US Veterans Administration: Mental Health and Behavioral Sciences Services, 2227
Zero to Three, 1595, 1799

Florida

Andrew and Associates, 4366
Association for Women in Psychology, 2588
Association of Mental Health Librarians (AMHL), 1707
Behavioral Medicine and Biofeedback Consultants, 3353
Best Buddies International (BBI), 1709
Broward County Healthcare Management, 4141
CLARC Services, 4383
Career Assessment & Planning Services, 85, 263, 705, 705, 828, 1124, 1165, 1236, 1281, 1333, 1356
Cenaps Corporation, 2489
Center for Applications of Psychological Type, 2598
Century Financial Services, 4155
Columbia Hospital M/H Services, 4161
Comprehensive Care Corporation, 4163
CompuLab Healthcare Systems Corporation, 4395
Daniel Memorial Institute, 3368
Department of Human Services For Youth & Families, 1864
Developmental Disabilities Nurses Association, 2610
Eclipsys Corporation, 4412
Emedeon Practice Services, 4414
FPM Behavioral Health: Corporate Marketing, 4191

Facts Services, 4417
Family Network on Disabilities of Florida, 1865
Florida Alcohol and Drug Abuse Association, 1866
Florida Department Health and Human Services: Substance Abuse Program, 2278
Florida Department of Children and Families, 2279
Florida Department of Health and Human Services, 2280
Florida Department of Mental Health and Rehabilitative Services, 2281
Florida Federation of Families for Children's Mental Health, 1867
Florida Health Care Association, 1868
Florida Health Information Management Association, 1869
Florida Medicaid State Plan, 2282
Florida National Alliance for the Mentally Ill, 1870
Food Addicts Anonymous, 1064
Gorski-Cenaps Corporation Training & Consultation, 2614
Health Management Associates, 4211
HealthSoft, 4432
Juniper Healthcare Containment Systems, 4238
Managed Care Concepts, 4253
Med Advantage, 2497, 2627
Medai, 4460
Medware, 4467
Mental Health Association of West Florida, 1871
Mental Health Corporations of America, 2629
Micro Design International, 4471
National Alliance on Mental Illness: Florida, 1872
Parent Child Center, 3416
Psychological Assessment Resources, 4494
Psychometric Software, 4496
Research Center for Children's Mental Health, Department of Children and Family, 3433
Research and Training Center for Children's Mental Health, 1589
Skypek Group, 4325, 4506, 2503, 2503
Somerset Pharmaceuticals, 4659
Suncoast Residential Training Center/Developmental Services Program, 104, 275, 716, 716, 833, 870, 1132, 1244, 1290, 1367
Synergistic Office Solutions (SOS Software), 4515
Tempus Software, 4516
UNI/CARE Systems, 4520
United Families for Children's Mental Health, 1592, 1791
University of Miami - Department of Psychology, 3470
ValueOptions Jacksonville Service Center, 4339
Vann Data Services, 4522
Youth Services International, 1594, 1798

Georgia

Adam Software, 4360
American Board of Professional Psychology (ABPP), 2530
Behavioral Health Partners, 4137
Calland and Company, 4148
Cameron and Associates, 4149
Centers for Disease Control & Prevention, 2188
Emory University School of Medicine, Psychology and Behavior, 3375
Emory University: Psychological Center, 3376
First Horizon Pharmaceutical, 4637
Fowler Healthcare Affiliates, 4196
Georgia Association of Homes and Services for Children, 1874
Georgia Department of Human Resources, 2283
Georgia Department of Human Resources: Division of Public Health, 2284
Georgia Division of Mental Health Developmental Disabilities and Addictive Diseases (MHDDAD), 2285
Georgia National Alliance for the Mentally Ill, 1875
Georgia Parent Support Network, 1876
Georgia Psychological Society First Annual Conference, 3190
Grady Health Systems: Central Fulton CMHC, 1877
Healthport, 4435
IMNET Systems, 4439
Inhealth Record Systems, 4444
Integrated Computer Products, 4448
Interim Physicians, 4231
Locumtenens.com, 3391
MCG Telemedicine Center, 4247, 3392
MSI International, 4250
McKesson HBO and Company, 4263
Medical College of Georgia, 3397
Medical Doctor Associates, 3402
Murphy-Harpst-Vashti, 4272
National Alliance on Mental Illness: Georgia, 1878
National Center for HIV, STD and TB Prevention, 2198
National Families in Action, 4477
Optio Software, 4485
REC Management, 4315
Solvay Pharmaceuticals, 4658
Strategic Advantage, 4510
William M Mercer, 4350

Hawaii

Hawaii Alliance for the Mentally Ill, 1879
Hawaii Department of Adult Mental Health, 2286
Hawaii Department of Health, 2287
Hawaii Families As Allies, 1880
John A Burns School of Medicine Department of Psychiatry, 3387
NAMI Hawaii, 1881
National Alliance on Mental Illness: Hawaii, 1882

Idaho

Ascent, 4368
College of Southern Idaho, 4160, 3362
Department of Health and Welfare: Medicaid Division, 2288
Department of Health and Welfare: Community Rehab, 2289
Healthwise, 4217
Idaho Alliance for the Mentally Ill, 1883
Idaho Bureau of Maternal and Child Health, 2290
Idaho Bureau of Mental Health and Substance Abuse, Division of Family & Community Service, 2291
Idaho Department of Health & Welfare, 2292
Idaho Department of Health and Welfare: Family and Child Services, 2293
Idaho Mental Health Center, 2294
National Alliance on Mental Illness: Idaho, 1884

Illinois

AAMA Annual Conference, 3165
AMA's Annual Medical Communications Conferen ce, 3166
Abbott Laboratories, 4630
Akzo Nobel, 4631
Allendale Association, 1885
Alzheimer's Association National Office, 775
American Academy of Medical Administrators, 2511
American Academy of Pediatrics, 1574, 1696
American Academy of Sleep Medicine, 1468
American Association of Health Care Consultants Annual Fall Conference, 3173
American Association of Healthcare Consultants, 2522
American Board of Psychiatry and Neurology (ABPN), 2531
American College of Healthcare Executives, 2534, 3178, 3348, 3348
American College of Psychiatrists, 2537
American College of Psychiatrists Annual Meeting, 3179
American College of Women's Health Physicians, 3349
American Health Information Management Association Annual Exhibition and Conference, 2544, 3182
American Hospital Association: Section for Psychiatric and Substance Abuse, 2545
American Medical Association, 2547
American Medical Software, 4363
Aon Consulting Group, 4128
Baby Fold, 1886
Bereaved Parents of the USA, 5
CBI Group, 4145
Center for the Study of Adolescence, 1059
Chaddock, 1887
Chicago Child Care Society, 1888
Children's Home Association of Illinois, 1889
Christian Association for Psychological Studies, 2601
Coalition of Illinois Counselors Organization, 1890
College of Dupage, 4159
ComPsych, 4162
Community Service Options, 1725
Compassionate Friends, 35
DD Fischer Consulting, 4173
Depression & Bi-Polar Support Alliance, 855
Depression & BiPolar Support Alliance, 708
Depression and Bi-Polar Alliance, 858
Dorenfest Group, 4178

Dupage County Health Department, 4180
Eating Disorders Research and Treatment
Program, 1061
Family Service Association of Greater Elgin
Area, 1891
HPN Worldwide, 4205
Haymarket Center, Professional
Development, 3381
Healthcare Value Management Group, 4215
Human Resources Development Institute,
1892
Hyde Park Associates, 4227
Illinois Alcoholism and Drug Dependency
Association, 1893, 2295
Illinois Alliance for the Mentally Ill, 1894
Illinois Department of Alcoholism and
Substance Abuse, 2296
Illinois Department of Children and Family
Services, 2297
Illinois Department of Health and Human
Services, 2298
Illinois Department of Human Services:
Office of Mental Health, 2299
Illinois Department of Mental Health and
Drug Dependence, 2300
Illinois Department of Mental Health and
Developmental Disabilities, 2301
Illinois Department of Public Aid, 2302
Illinois Department of Public Health:
Division of Food, Drugs and Dairies/FDD,
2303
Illinois Federation of Families for Children's
Mental Health, 1895
Innovative Data Solutions, 4445
Integrated Business Services, 4447
International Association of Eating Disorders
Professionals, 986
International Society for Traumatic Stress
Studies, 1284
International Society for the Study of
Dissociation, 954
Joint Commission on Accreditation of
Healthcare Organizations, 2495
Larkin Center, 1896
Lifelink Corporation, 4244
Little City Foundation (LCF), 1897
MEDCOM Information Systems, 4454
McHenry County M/H Board, 4456
Medix Systems Consultants, 4466
Mental Health Association in Illinois, 2304
Metropolitan Family Services, 1898
Mihalik Group, 4270
National Alliance on Mental Illness: Illinoi s,
1899
National Association in Women's Health
Professionals, 2634
National Association of Anorexia Nervosa
and Associated Disorders (ANAD), 990
National Treatment Alternative for Safe
Communities, 2655
Northwestern University Medical School
Feinberg School of Medicine, 3412
Perspectives, 4291
Physicians for a National Health Program,
2658
Professional Assistance Center for Education
(PACE), 1780
PsycHealth, 4308
Psychiatric Clinical Research Center, 1781
Pyrce Healthcare Group, 4312
Rainbows, 39, 1631
Recovery, 356, 928, 1414, 1414, 1783
Riveredge Hospital, 3435

SAFE Alternatives, 1271
SPSS, 4502
Saner Software, 4503
Section for Psychiatric and Substance Abuse
Services (SPSPAS), 103
Southern Illinois University School of
Medicine: Department of Psychiatry, 3442
Southern Illinois University School of
Medicine, 3443
TASC, 4332
Takeda Pharmaceuticals North America,
4661
Thresholds Psychiatric Rehabilitation, 1790
Vasquez Management Consultants, 4341
Vedder Price, 4342
Voice of the Retarded, 1792

Indiana

Eli Lilly and Company, 4636
Experior Corporation, 4416
Health Probe, 4430
Indiana Alliance for the Mentally Ill, 1900
Indiana Department of Public Welfare
Division of Family Independence: Food
Stamps/Medicaid/Training, 2305
Indiana Family & Social Services
Administration, 2306
Indiana Family And Social Services
Administration, 2307
Indiana Family and Social Services
Administration: Division of Mental
Health, 2308
Indiana Resource Center for Autism (IRCA),
1901
Indiana University Psychiatric Management,
1902
Medi-Span, 4462
Mental Health Association in Marion County
Consumer Services, 1903
More Advanced Autistic People Services
(MAAPS), 551
More Advanced Persons with Autism and
Asperger's Syndrome (MAAP), 516
National Alliance on Mental Illness: Indiana,
1904
National Association of Nouthetic
Counselors, 2637
Office of Medicaid Policy & Planning
(OMPP), 2309
Psychiatric Associates, 4309, 3426
Psychological Software Services, 4495
Quinco Behavioral Health Systems, 4314
Supportive Systems, 4331
The Indiana Consortium for Mental Health
Services Research (ICMHSR), 2310
Universal Behavioral Service, 4521

Iowa

Control-0-Fax Corporation, 4397
Iowa Alliance for the Mentally Ill, 1905
Iowa Department Human Services, 2311
Iowa Department of Public Health, 2312
Iowa Department of Public Health: Division
of Substance Abuse, 2313
Iowa Division of Mental Health &
Developmental Disabilities: Department
of Human Services, 2314

Iowa Federation of Families for Children's
Mental Health, 1906
Medical Records Solution, 4464
National Alliance on Mental Illness: Iowa,
1907
University of Iowa Hospital, 3463
University of Iowa, Mental Health: Clinical
Research Center, 1908

Kansas

American Academy of Addiction Psychiatry:
Annual Meeting, 3168
Comcare of Sedgwick County, 2315
Division of Health Care Policy, 2316
Kansas Council on Developmental
Disabilities Kansas Department of Social
and Rehabilitation Services, 2317
Kansas Department of Mental Health and
Retardation and Social Services, 2318
Kansas Schizophrenia Anonymous, 1909
Keys for Networking: Kansas Parent
Informati on & Resource Center, 1910
National Alliance on Mental Illness: Kansas,
1911
Preferred Mental Health Management, 4298
Society of Teachers of Family Medicine,
2678
Topeka Institute for Psychoanalysis, 3449
University of Kansas Medical Center, 3464
University of Kansas School of Medicine,
3465

Kentucky

Adanta Group-Behavioral Health Services,
4118
Depressed Anonymous, 927
FACES of the Blue Grass, 1913
FCS, 4190
KY-SPIN, 1914
Kentucky Alliance for the Mentally Ill, 1915
Kentucky Cabinet for Health and Human
Services, 2319
Kentucky Department for Human Support
Services, 2320
Kentucky Department for Medicaid Services,
2321
Kentucky Department of Mental Health and
Mental Retardation, 2322
Kentucky IMPACT, 1916
Kentucky Justice Cabinet: Department of
Juvenile Justice, 2323
Kentucky Psychiatric Association, 1917
National Alliance on Mental Illness: Kentuck
y, 1918
National Anxiety Foundation, 269
Project Vision, 1920
River Valley Behavioral Health, 3201
SPOKES Federation of Families for
Children's Mental Health, 1921
St. Joseph Behavioral Medicine Network,
3445
University of Louisville School of Medicine,
3466

Louisiana

Accreditation Services, 4358
Active Intervention, 3343
Alton Ochsner Medical Foundation,
    Psychiatry Residency, 3346
Family Managed Care, 4192
Louisiana Alliance for the Mentally Ill, 1923
Louisiana Commission on Law Enforcement
    and Administration (LCLE), 2324
Louisiana Department of Health and
    Hospitals: Office of Mental Health, 2325
Louisiana Department of Health and
    Hospitals: Louisiana Office for Addictive
    Disorders, 2326
Louisiana Federation of Families for
    Children's Mental Health, 1924
National Alliance on Mental Illness: Louisia
    na, 1925
SUPRA Management, 2502
West Jefferson Medical Center, 3486

Maine

Advanced Data Systems, 4361
Association of Traumatic Stress Specialists,
    1280
Maine Alliance for the Mentally Ill, 1926
Maine Department Health and Human
    Services Children's Behavioral Health
    Services, 2327
Maine Department of Behavioral and
    Developmental Services, 2328
Maine Office of Substance Abuse:
    Information and Resource Center, 2329
Maine Psychiatric Association, 1927
National Alliance on Mental Illness: Maine,
    1928
United Families for Children's Mental
    Health, 1929

Maryland

Academy of Psychosomatic Medicine, 2505
Agency for Healthcare Research & Quality,
    2507
Agency for Healthcare Research and Quality:
    Office of Communications and
    Knowledge Transfer, 2184
Alzheimer's Disease Education and Referral
    Center, 776
American Association for Geriatric
    Psychiatry, 1697
American Association of Geriatric
    Psychiatry (AAGP), 2520
American Association of Geriatric
    Psychiatry Annual Meetings, 3172
American College Health Association, 2532
American Health Assistance Foundation, 777
American Medical Directors Association,
    2548
American Medical Informatics Association,
    2550
American Nurses Association, 2553
American Society of Addiction Medicine,
    3197
American Society of Health System
    Pharmacists, 2569

American Society of Psychoanalytic
    Physicians (ASPP), 2570
Annie E Casey Foundation, 2573
Annual Meeting & Medical-Scientific
    Conference, 3185
Anxiety Disorders Association of America,
    261
Asher Meadow, 1097
Association of University Centers on
    Disabilities (UACD), 2592
Autism Society of America, 513, 545, 653,
    653
Black Mental Health Alliance (BMHA), 1711
Bonny Foundation, 2596
Center for Health Policy Studies, 4152, 4387,
    3359, 3359
Center for Mental Health Services Homeless
    Programs Branch, 2186
Center for Substance Abuse Treatment, 2187
Centers for Medicare & Medicaid
    Services/CMS: Office of Research,
    Statisctics, Data and Systems, 2330
Centers for Medicare & Medicaid Services,
    2331
Centers for Medicare & Medicaid Services:
    Office of Policy, 2189, 2332
Centers for Medicare and Medicaid Services:
    Office of Financial Management/OFM,
    2333
Chemically Dependent Anonymous, 201
Children and Adults with AD/HD
    (CHADD), 394, 1625
Community Behavioral Health Association
    of Maryland: CBH, 1930
Community Services for Autistic Adults and
    Children, 549
Council on Quality and Leadership, 1727
Counseling Associates, 4168
Docu Trac, 4407
E Services Group, 4409
Epidemiology-Genetics Program in
    Psychiatry, 749
Families Involved Together, 1931
First Candle/SIDS Alliance, 9
Health Resources and Services
    Administration, 1932
Health Systems and Financing Group, 2194
Information Resources and Inquiries Branch,
    2196
International Critical Incident Stress
    Foundation, 267
Johnson, Bassin and Shaw, 4237
KAI Associates, 4239
Magellan Health Service, 4251
Management Recruiters of Washington, DC,
    3394
Maryland Alcohol and Drug Abuse
    Administration, 2334
Maryland Alliance for the Mentally Ill, 1933
Maryland Department of Health and Mental
    Hygiene, 2335
Maryland Department of Human Resources,
    2336
Maryland Division of Mental Health, 2337
Maryland Psychiatric Research Center, 1934
Mental Health Association of Maryland, 1935
National Institutes of Mental Health
    Division of Intramural Research Programs
    (DIRP), 2197
National Alliance on Mental Illness: Marylan
    d, 1936
National Association of Community Health
    Centers, 2636

National Association of School
    Psychologists, 2639, 3409
National Clearinghouse for Alcohol and, 92
National Clearinghouse for Alcohol and
    Drug, 93
National Clearinghouse for Drug & Alcohol,
    2199
National Council for Community Behavioral
    Healthcare, 94, 1761
National Eldercare Services Company, 2648
National Family Caregivers Association, 782
National Federation of Families for Children
    's Mental Health, 1938
National Institute of Alcohol Abuse and
    Alcoholism: Treatment Research Branch,
    2200
National Institute of Alcohol Abuse and
    Alcoholism: Homeless Demonstration and
    Evaluation Branch, 2201
National Institute of Alcohol Abuse and
    Alcoholism: Office of Policy Analysis,
    2202
National Institute of Drug Abuse (NIDA),
    1764
National Institute of Drug Abuse: NIDA,
    2203
National Institute of Mental Health
    Information Resources and Inquiries
    Branch, 517, 865, 993, 993, 1106, 1765
National Institute of Mental Health:
    Schizophrenia Research Branch, 2204
National Institute of Mental Health: Mental
    Disorders of the Aging, 2205
National Institute of Mental Health: Office of
    Science Policy, Planning, and
    Communications, 2206
National Institute of Neurological Disorders
    and Stroke, 783
National Institute of Neurological Disorders
    and Stroke Brain Information Network
    (BRAIN), 518
National Institute on Alcohol Abuse and
    Alcoholism, 96
National Institute on Deafness and Other
    Communication Disorders Information
    Clearinghouse, 519
National Institute on Drug Abuse: Office of
    Science Policy and Communications, 2207
National Institute on Drug Abuse: Division
    of Clinical Neurosciences and Behavioral
    Research, 2208
National Institutes of Health: National Center
    for Research Resources (NCCR), 2209
National Institutes of Mental Health: Office
    on AIDS, 2210
National Library of Medicine, 2211
New Hope Foundation, 1774
Office of Applied Studies, SA & Mental
    Health Services, 2212
Office of Disease Prevention & Health
    Promotion, 2213
Office of National Drug Control Policy, 2214
Office of Program and Policy Development,
    2215
Office of Science Policy OD/NIH, 2216
PSC, 4286
Professional Services Consultants, 4305
Protection and Advocacy Program for the
    Mentally Ill, 2219
Psycho Medical Chirologists, 4310
Samhsa's National Clearinghouse For
    Alcohol And Drug Information, 102
Schizophrenia Research Branch: Division of
    Clinical and Treatment Research, 1411

Sheppard Pratt Health Plan, 4323
Sheppard Pratt Health System, 1939
Sidran Traumatic Stress Institute, 1788
Substance Abuse & Mental Health Services
    Adminstration (SAMHSA), 2221
Survey & Analysis Branch, 1940
US Department of Health & Human
    Services: Indian Health Service, 2223
US Department of Health and Human
    Services Bureau of Primary Health, 2225
United States Psychiatric Rehabilitation
    Organization (USPRA), 2680
University of Maryland Medical Systems,
    3467
University of Maryland School of Medicine,
    3468
Warren Grant Magnuson Clinical Center,
    1793
Yssociation for Psychological Type, 2683

Massachusetts

ABE American Board of Examiners in
    Clinical Social Work, 4112
Advocates for Human Potential, 1692
American Board of Examiners in Clinical
    Social Work, 2485, 2529
American Society of Psychopathology of
    Expression (ASPE), 2571
Analysis Group Economics, 4127
Aries Systems Corporation, 4367
Asperger's Association of New England, 541
Asperger's Association of New England
    (AANE), 510
Associated Counseling Services, 4131
Association for Academic Psychiatry (AAP),
    2574
Autism Research Foundation, 542
Autism Treatment Center of America
    Son-Rise Program, 654
Autism Treatment Center of America: The
    Son -Rise Program, 514
Behavioral Health Care Consultants, 4135
Behavioral Healthcare Center, 3352
Bipolar Clinic and Research Program, 746
Brandeis University/Heller School, 3354
Bridgewell, 1941
Bull HN Information Systems, 4380
CASCAP, 4382
Cambridge Hospital: Department of
    Psychiatry, 3358
Center for Clinical Computing, 4386
Concord Family and Youth Services A
    Division of Justice Resource Institute,
    1942
Dougherty Management Associates Health
    Strategies, 4179
Entropy Limited, 4186
Evaluation Center at HSRI, 4189
Families of Adults Afflicted with Asperger's
    Syndrome (FAAAS), 515
Federation for Children with Special Needs
    (FCSN), 1578, 1732
Glazer Medical Solutions, 4203
HCIA Response, 4423
Hanover Insurance, 4429
Health Care For All(HCFA), 2193
Human Services Research Institute, 1737,
    4226
IBM Global Healthcare Industry, 4437

Jean Piaget Society: Society for the Study of
    Knowledge and Development (JPSSSKD),
    2625
Jewish Family and Children's Services, 1944
Join Together Online, 204
Judge Baker Children's Center, 1743
MEDA, 1065
Magellan Public Solutions, 4252
Massachusetts Alliance for the Mentally Ill,
    1945
Massachusetts Behavioral Health
    Partnership, 1946
Massachusetts Department of Mental Health,
    2338
Massachusetts Department of Public Health,
    2339
Massachusetts Department of Public Health:
    Bureau of Substance Abuse Services, 2340
Massachusetts Department of Social
    Services, 2341
Massachusetts Department of Transitional
    Assistance, 2342
Massachusetts Division of Medical
    Assistance MassHealth Program, 2343
Massachusetts Executive Office of Public
    Safety, 2344
Medical Records Institute, 4463
Mental Health Connections, 4468
Mental Health and Substance Abuse
    Corporations of Massachusetts, 1947
Mental Illness Education Project, 1749
Mercer Consulting, 4267
Mertech, 2498
National Alliance on Mental Illness:
    Massach usetts, 1948
National Empowerment Center, 1762, 4274
National Managed Health Care Congress,
    2649
New England Center for Children, 556
New England Psych Group, 4277
Novartis, 4647
Obsessive Compulsive Foundation, 1171
Parent Professional Advocacy League, 1949
Public Consulting Group, 4311
Refuah, 1784
SADD: Students Against Destructive
    Decisions, 211, 1632
Scheur and Associates, 4320
Schneider Institute for Health Policy, 3440
Screening for Mental Health, 2668
Sepracor Pharmaceuticals, 4656
Son-Rise Program at the Option Institute
    Autism Treatment Center of America, 559
University of Massachusetts Medical Center,
    3469
Wang Software, 4526
Webman Associates, 4348
Windhorse Associates, 1794
Work Group for the Computerization of
    Behavioral Health, 4529
Worldwide Healthcare Solutions: IBM, 4530

Michigan

ACS Healthcare Solutions, 4353
Adult Learning Systems, 4119
Agoraphobics in Motion, 260
American College of Osteopathic
    Neurologists & Psychiatrists, 2536
Ann Arbor Consultation Services
    Performance & Health Solutions, 1950

Association for Behavior Analysis, 2578
Borgess Behavioral Medicine Services, 1951
Boysville of Michigan, 1952
Christian Horizons, 1722
DocuMed, 4408
First Corp-Health Consulting, 4195
Harper House: Change Alternative Living,
    3380
Health Alliance Plan, 4208
Health Decisions, 4210
Inforum, 4443
Justice in Mental Health Organizations, 1953
Lapeer County Community Mental Health
    Center, 1954
Macomb County Community Mental Health,
    1955
Manic Depressive and Depressive
    Association of Metropolitan Detroit, 1956
Metropolitan Area Chapter of Federation of
    Families for Children's Mental Health,
    1957
Michigan Alliance for the Mentally Ill, 1958
Michigan Association for Children with
    Emotional Disorders: MACED, 1959
Michigan Association for Children's Mental
    Health, 1582, 1960
Michigan Department of Community Health,
    2345
Michigan Department of Human Services,
    2346
Michigan State Representative: Co-Chair
    Public Health, 2347
Mississippi Alliance for the Mentally Ill,
    1973
National Alliance on Mental Illness: Michiga
    n, 1961
National Council on Alcoholism and Drug
    Dependence: Greater Detriot Area, 95,
    2348
Northpointe Behavioral Healthcare Systems,
    1962, 4279
Parrot Software, 4490
Posen Consulting Group, 4295
Psychological Diagnostic Services, 3429
Rapid Psychler Press, 2665
Sandra Fields-Neal and Associates, 4317
Save Our Sons And Daughters (SOSAD), 16
Schizophrenics Anonymous Forum, 1415
Southwest Counseling & Development
    Services, 1963
University of Michigan, 3471
Wayne University-University of Psychiatric
    Center-Jefferson: Outpatient Mental
    Health for Children, Adolescents and
    Adults, 3485
Woodlands Behavioral Healthcare Network,
    1964

Minnesota

Allina Hospitals & Clinics Behavioral Health
    Services, 4124
Behavioral Health Services, 4138
CBCA, 4144
CIGNA Behavioral Care, 4146
Centre for Mental Health Solutions:
    Minnesota Bio Brain Association, 1965
Ceridian Corporation, 4388
Corporate Health Systems, 4167
Department of Human Services: Chemical
    Health Division, 2349

Emotions Anonymous International Service Center, 859
HealthPartners, 4213
Healtheast Behavioral Care, 2494
MMHR, 4249
McGladery and Pullen CPAs, 4261
McKesson HBOC, 4457
Minnesota Association for Children's Mental Health, 1966
Minnesota Department of Human Services, 2350
Minnesota Psychiatric Society, 1967
Minnesota Psychological Association, 1968
Minnesota Youth Services Bureau, 2351
NASW Minnesota Chapter, 1969
National Alliance on Mental Illness: Minneso ta, 1970
National Association for Rural Mental Health, 1753
National Multicultural Conference and Summit, 3194
North American Training Institute: Division of the Minnesota Council on Compulsive Gambling, 1971
Pacer Center, 1972
Pearson, 4289
River City Mental Health Clinic, 3434
University of Minnesota Fairview Health Systems, 3472
University of Minnesota, Family Social Science, 3473
Velocity Healthcare Informatics, 4523

Mississippi

Advanced Psychotherapy Association, 2506
Mississippi Alcohol Safety Education Program, 2352
Mississippi Department Mental Health Mental Retardation Services, 2353
Mississippi Department of Human Services, 2354
Mississippi Department of Mental Health: Division of Alcohol and Drug Abuse, 2355
Mississippi Department of Mental Health: Division of Medicaid, 2356
Mississippi Department of Rehabilitation Services: Office of Vocational Rehabilitation (OVR), 2357
Mississippi Families as Allies, 1974
National Alliance on Mental Illness: Mississ ippi, 1975

Missouri

Anorexia Bulimia Treatment and Education Center, 981
CliniSphere version 2.0, 4392
College of Health and Human Services: SE Missouri State, 3361
DST Output, 4403
Depressive and Manic-Depressive Association of St. Louis, 1943, 1976
E-Productivity-Services.Net, 1283
Genelco Software Solutions, 4422
Health Capital Consultants, 4209
Lake Mental Health Consultants, 4241
Mallinckrodt, 4644

Mental Health Association of Greater St. Louis, 1977
Missouri Alliance for the Mentally Ill, 1978
Missouri Department Health & Senior Services, 2358
Missouri Department of Mental Health, 2359
Missouri Department of Public Safety, 2360
Missouri Department of Social Services, 2361
Missouri Department of Social Services: Medical Services Division, 2362
Missouri Division of Alcohol and Drug Abuse, 2363
Missouri Division of Comprehensive Psychiatric Service, 2364
Missouri Division of Mental Retardation and Developmental Disabilities, 2365
Missouri Institute of Mental Health, 1979
Missouri Statewide Parent Advisory Network: MO-SPAN, 1980
National Alliance on Mental Illness: Missour i, 1981
National SHARE Office, 37
Ochester Psychological Service, 3413
Pathways to Promise, 209
Primary Care Medicine on CD, 4493
St. Louis Behavioral Medicine Institute, 3446
Traumatic Incident Reduction Workshop, 3195

Montana

Eastern County Mental Health Center, 3374
Entre Technology Services, 4415
Family Support Network, 1982
Mental Health Association of Montana, 1983
Monatana Department of Human & Community Services, 2229
Montana Alliance for the Mentally Ill, 1984
Montana Department of Health and Human Services: Child & Family Services Division, 2366
Montana Department of Public Health & Human Services: Addictive and Mental Disorders, 2367
Montana Department of Public Health and Human Services: Montana Vocational Rehabilitation Programs, 2368
National Alliance on Mental Illness: Montana, 1985

Nebraska

Department of Health and Human Services Regulation and Licensure, 1986
Mutual of Omaha Companies' Integrated Behavioral Services, 4476
Mutual of Omaha's Health and Wellness Progra ms, 1987
National Alliance on Mental Illness: Nebrask a, 1988
Nebraska Alliance for the Mentally Ill, 1990
Nebraska Department of Health and Human Services (NHHS), 2369
Nebraska Family Support Network, 1991
Nebraska Health & Human Services: Medicaid and Managed Care Division, 2370

Nebraska Health and Human Services Division: Department of Mental Health, 2371
Nebraska Mental Health Centers, 2372
Orion Healthcare Technology, 4487
Pilot Parents: PP, 1588, 1992
Scinet, 4504
Wellness Councils of America, 2681

Nevada

Carson City Alliance for the Mentally Ill Share & Care Group, 1993
National Alliance on Mental Illness: Nevada, 1994
National Council of Juvenile and Family Court Judges, 2645
Nevada Alliance for the Mentally Ill, 1995
Nevada Department of Health & Human Services Health Care Financing and Policy, 2373
Nevada Department of Health and Human Services, 2374
Nevada Division of Mental Health & Developmental Services, 2375
Nevada Employment Training & Rehabilitation Department, 2376
Nevada Principals' Executive Program, 1996
Nevada State Health Division: Bureau of Alcohol & Drug Abuse, 2377
Northern Nevada Adult Mental Health Services, 2378
Southern Nevada Adult Mental Health Services, 2379

New Hampshire

Department of Psychiatry: Dartmouth University, 3370
Echo Management Group, 4181
Helms & Company, 4220
Monadnock Family Services, 1997
National Alliance on Mental Illness: New Ham pshire, 1998
New Hampshire Alliance for the Mentally Ill, 1999
New Hampshire Department of Health & Human Services: Bureau of Community Health Services, 2380
New Hampshire Department of Health and Human Services: Bureau of Developmental Services, 2381
New Hampshire Department of Health and Human Services: Bureau of Behavioral Health, 2382

New Jersey

Aleppos Foundation, 1693
American Society of Group Psychotherapy & Psychodrama, 2568
Apserger Syndrome Education Network of America (ASPEN), 509
Asperger Syndrome Education Network (ASPEN), 540
Association for Advancement of Mental Health, 2000

Association for Children of New Jersey, 2001
Association for the Care of Children's
    Health, 1705
Attention Deficit Disorder Association, 390
Cypruss Communications, 4172
Depression After Delivery, 857
Eating Disorders Association of New Jersey,
    2002
Eisai, 4635
Hoffman-La Roche, 4640
Info Management Associates, 3198
Insurance Management Institute, 4229
InternetPhone, 4449
Janssen, 4641
Jewish Family Service of Atlantic County
    and Cape, 2003
Johnson & Johnson, 4642
Juvenile Justice Commission, 2383
Med Data Systems, 4458
Mellon HR Solutions, 4264
Mental Health Association of New Jersey,
    2004
Merck, 4645
National Alliance on Mental Illness: New Jer
    sey, 2005
National Association for the Mentally Ill of
    New Jersey, 2006
New Jersey Association of Mental Health
    Agencies, 2007
New Jersey Department of Human Services,
    2384
New Jersey Division of Mental Health
    Services, 2385
New Jersey Division of Youth & Family
    Services, 2386
New Jersey Office of Managed Care, 2387
New Jersey Protection and Advocacy, 2008
New Jersey Psychiatric Association, 2009
New Jersey Support Groups, 2010
Organon Schering Plough, 4648
Ortho-McNeil Pharmaceutical, 4649
Pharmacia & Upjohn, 4652
Psychohistory Forum, 2661
Sanofi-Aventis, 4654
Sanofi-Synthelabo, 4655
Specialized Therapy Associates, 4327
Union County Psychiatric Clinic, 3457
University Behavioral Healthcare, 3458
Verispan, 4345
Wyeth, 4664

New Mexico

American College of Mental   Health
    Administration (ACMHA), 2535
Association for Child Psychoanalysts, 2581
Mesa Mental Health, 4269
National Alliance on Mental Illness: New
    Mex ico, 2011
Navajo Nation K'E Project-Shiprock, 2012
New Mexico Alliance for the Mentally Ill,
    2013
New Mexico Behavioral Health
    Collaborative, 2388
New Mexico Department of Health, 2389
New Mexico Department of Human
    Services, 2390
New Mexico Department of Human
    Services: Medical Assistance Division,
    2391

New Mexico Health & Environment
    Department, 2392
New Mexico Kids, Parents and Families
    Office of Child Development: Children,
    Youth and Families Department, 2393
Overeaters Anonymous, 1067
SumTime Software®, 4511
University of New Mexico, School of
    Medicine Health Sciences Center, 3474

New York

AHMAC, 4354
AIMS, 4355
Accumedic Computer Systems, 4359
Ackerman Institute for the Family, 3342
Alcoholics Anonymous (AA): World
    Services, 200
Alcoholics Anonymous (AA): Worldwide, 81
Aldrich and Cox, 4121
Alfred Adler Institute (AAI), 3344
Alliance for the Mentally Ill: Friends &
    Advocates of the Mentally Ill, 2014
American Anorexia/Bulimia Association, 980
American Foundation for Suicide Prevention,
    1493
American Geriatrics Society, 2541
American Group Psychotherapy Association
    Annual Conference, 2542, 3180
American Psychoanalytic Association
    (APsaA), 2558
Andrus Children's Center, 3350
Annual Early Childhood Conference:
    Effective Relationship-Based Practices in
    Promoting Positive Child Outcomes, 3184
Anxiety and Phobia Treatment Center, 262
Association for Advancement of
    Psychoanalysis: Karen Horney
    Psychoanalytic Institute and Center, 2575
Association for Behavioral and Cognitive
    Therapies, 827, 2579
Association for Psychoanalytic Medicine
    (APM), 2585
Association for Research in Nervous and
    Ment al Disease, 2587
Association for the Help of Retarded
    Children, 1576, 1706
Association of the Advancement of Gestalt
    Therapy, 2593
Autism Network International, 511
Autistic Services, 546
Babylon Consultation Center, 2015
Brain Imaging Handbook, 2487
Bristol-Myers Squibb, 4633
CG Jung Foundation for Analytical
    Psychology, 2597
Center for Family Support (CFS), 7, 86, 264,
    264, 392, 547, 706, 778, 829, 854, 953,
    983, 1084, 1102, 1125, 1166, 1224
Center for the Study of Anorexia and
    Bulimia, 1060
Center for the Study of Issues in Public
    Mental Health, 1718
Children's Home of the Wyoming
    Conference, Quality Improvement, 4156
Coalition of Voluntary Mental Health
    Agencies, 1723
Committee for Truth in Psychiatry: CTIP,
    2190
Commonwealth Fund, 2604
Community Access, 1724

Compeer, 2016
Corporate Counseling Associates, 2607
Council on Accreditation (COA) of Services
    for Families and Children, 2492
Council on Size and Weight Discrimination
    (CSWD), 985
Covenant House Nineline, 1626
Creative Health Concepts, 4171
Creative Socio-Medics Corporation, 4401
Downstate Mental Hygiene Association, 3372
Eating Disorder Council of Long Island, 2017
Employee Network, 4185
Facilitated Learning at Syracuse University,
    650
Families Together in New York State, 2018
Finger Lakes Parent Network, 2019
Forest Laboratories, 4638
Freedom From Fear, 266, 860
Gam-Anon Family Groups, 1147
Girls and Boys Town of New York, 1627
HZI Research Center, 4427
Healthcare Association of New York State,
    2020
Heartshare Human Services, 3382
Informix Software, 4442
Institute for Contemporary Psychotherapy,
    1337
Institute for Contemproary Psychotherapy,
    1338
International Center for the Study of
    Psychiatry And Psychology (ISCPP), 2621
International Society of Political
    Psychology, 2623
JM Oher and Associates, 4233
Life Science Associates, 3390
Lifespire, 1580, 1746
McGraw Hill Healthcare Management, 4262
Mental Health Association in Albany
    County, 2021
Mental Health Association in Dutchess
    County, 2022
Mental Health Materials Center (MHMC),
    2630
Mental Health Research Association
    (NARSAD), 861
Metro Intergroup of Overeaters Anonymous,
    2023
NADD Annual Conference & Exhibit Show,
    3192
NARSA: The Mental Health Research
    Associatio n, 1410
NARSAD: The Mental Health Research
    Associati on, 862, 1359
Nathan S Kline Institute for Psychiatric
    Research, 1751, 3407
National Alliance for Research on
    Schizophrenia and Depression, 923, 1360
National Alliance on Mental Illness: New
    Yor k, 2024
National Assocaition for the Dually, 711
National Assocaition for the Dually
    Diagnose d (NADD), 1441
National Association for The Dually
    Diagnose d (NADD), 1362
National Association for the Advancement of
    Psychoanalysis, 2633
National Association for the Dually
    Diagnosed (NADD), 11, 397, 553, 553,
    712, 781, 830, 864, 955, 1086
National Association for the Dually
    Diagnose d (NADD), 270, 989, 1104,
    1104, 1128, 1167, 1225, 1239, 1286, 1339,
    1471, 1537, 1754

National Center for Learning Disabilities, 1758

National Center for Overcoming Overeating, 1066

National Center on Addiction and Substance Abuse at Columbia University, 1759

National GAINS Center for People with Co-Occurring Disorders in the Justice System, 1763

National Medical Health Card Systems, 4478

National Psychological Association for Psychoanalysis (NPAP), 2653

National Resource Center on Homelessness & Mental Illness, 1771

National Self-Help Clearinghouse Graduate School and University Center, 1772

Network Behavioral Health, 4275

New York Association of Psychiatric Rehabilitation Services, 2026

New York Business Group on Health, 2027

New York City Depressive & Manic Depressive Group, 2028

New York Office of Alcohol & Substance Abuse Services, 2394

New York State Alliance for the Mentally Ill, 2029

New York State Department of Health Individual County Listings of Social Services Departments, 2395

New York State Office of Mental Health, 2396

New York University Behavioral Health Programs, 3410

Newbride Consultation, 4278

NineLine, 1520

Obesity Research Center, 1062

Obsessive Compulsive Anonymous, 1170

Obsessive-Compulsive Anonymous, 1205

Orange County Mental Health Association, 2030

Parents United Network: Parsons Child Family Center, 2031

Paris International Corporation, 4288

Parke-Davis Pharmaceutcials, 4650

Pass-Group, 354

Patient Infosystems, 4491

Pfizer, 4651

Porter Novelli, 4294

Postgraduate Center for Mental Health, 3421

Prime Care Consultants, 4299

Project LINK, 2032

Psychiatric Society Of Informatics American Association For Technology In Psychiatry, 2660

Psychology Society (PS), 2662

Resources for Children with Special Needs, 1591, 1787

Right On Programs/PRN Medical Software, 4500

Risk and Insurance Management Society, 2666

Rockland Children's Psychiatric Center, 3437

Salud Management Associates, 4316

Schizophrenic Biologic Research Center, 1412

Sciacca Comprehensive Service Development for MIDAA, 4321

Sciacca Comprehensive Services Development, 2667

Seelig and Company: Child Welfare and Behavioral Healthcare, 4322

Sigmund Freud Archives (SFA), 2669

Sls Residential, 4507

Society for the Advancement of Social Psychology (SASP), 2674

State University of New York at Stony Brook, 2033

Stephens Systems Services, 4509

Success Day Training Program, 3448

Sue Krause and Associates, 4330

Tourette Syndrome Association, 1541, 1560

Towers Perrin Integrated Heatlh Systems Consulting, 4334

Ulster County Mental Health Department, 3456

Westchester Alliance for the Mentally Ill, 2034

Westchester Task Force on Eating Disorders, 2035

YAI/National Institute for People with Disabilities, 3196

Yeshiva University: Soundview-Throgs Neck Community Mental Health Center, 2036

Young Adult Institute and Workshop (YAI), 1593, 1797

Zy-Doc Technologies, 4532

North Carolina

Autism Society of North Carolina, 2037

Barry Associates, 4133

Counseling Services, 3367

East Carolina University Department of Psychiatric Medicine, 3373

Elon Homes for Children, 4182

GlaxoSmithKline, 4639

Habilitation Software, 4428

Managed Healthcare Consultants, 4256

Misys Health Care Systems, 4474

National Alliance on Mental Illness: North Carolina, 2038

National Board for Certified Counselors, 2499

North Carolina Alliance for the Mentally Ill, 2040

North Carolina Department of Human Resources, 2397

North Carolina Division of Mental Health, 2398

North Carolina Division of Social Services, 2399

North Carolina Mental Health Consumers Organization, 2041

North Carolina Substance Abuse Professional Certification Board (NCSAPCB), 2400

Onslow County Behavioral Health, 3414

Synthon Pharmaceuticals, 4660

TEACCH, 651

University of North Carolina School of Social Work, Behavioral Healthcare, 4336

University of North Carolina School of Social Work, 3475

University of North Carolina, School of Medicine, 3476

Wake Forest University, 3484

Western North Carolina Families (CAN), 2042

North Dakota

Meritcare Health System, 4470

National Alliance on Mental Illness: North Dakota, 2043

National Association of Social Workers: North Dakota Chapter, 1859, 1919, 1937, 1937, 1989, 2039, 2044

North Dakota Federation of Families for Children's Mental Health: Region II, 2045

North Dakota Alliance for the Mentally Ill, 2046

North Dakota Department of Human Services: Medicaid Program, 2401

North Dakota Department of Human Services: Mental Health Services Division, 2402

North Dakota Department of Human Services Division of Mental Health and Substance Abuse Services, 2403

North Dakota Federation of Families for Children's Mental Health: Region V, 2047

North Dakota Federation of Families for Children's Mental Health: Region VII, 2048

North Dakota Federation of Families for Children's Mental Health, 2049

Ohio

Alive Alone, 2

Alliance Behavioral Care, 4122

Alliance Behavioral Care: University of Cincinnati Psychiatric Services, 3345

American Neuropsychiatric Association, 2552

Aware Resources, 4372

Bellefaire Jewish Children's Bureau, 4377

Brown Consulting, 4142

ChoiceCare, 4157

Cincom Systems, 4390

Client Management Information System, 4391

Comprehensive Center For Pain Management, 4164

Concerned Advocates Serving Children & Families, 2050

Findley, Davies and Company, 4193

Geauga Board of Mental Health, Alcohol and Drug Addiction Services, 4202

LanVision Systems, 4451

Laurelwood Hospital and Counseling Centers, 3389

Marsh Foundation, 3395

MedPLus, 4459

Medical College of Ohio, Psychiatry, 3398

Mental Health Association of Summit, 2051

Micro Office Systems, 4472

Mount Carmel Behavioral Healthcare, 2052

NEOUCOM-Northeastern Ohio Universities College of Medicine, 3406

National Alliance on Mental Illness: Ohio, 2053

National Association of Social Workers: Ohio Chapter, 2054

National Organization of Parents of Murdered Children, 14

Netsmart Technologies, 4480

Ohio Alliance for the Mentally Ill, 2055

Ohio Association of Child Caring Agencies, 2056
Ohio Community Drug Board, 2404
Ohio Council of Behavioral Healthcare Providers, 2057
Ohio Department of Mental Health, 2058, 2405
Parents of Murdered Children, 38
Penelope Price, 3417
Planned Lifetime Assistance Network of Northeast Ohio, 2059
Positive Education Program, 2060
PsychTemps, 3425
Psychology Department, 3430
QualChoice Health Plan, 4313
RCF Information Systems, 4498
Rosemont Center, 3438
Roxane Laboratories, 4653
SAFY of America, 3439
SAFY of America: Specialized Alternatives for Families and Youth, 2501
SMART-Self Management and Recovery Training, 212
Six County, 2061
Specialized Alternatives for Families & Youth of America (SAFY), 4326
University of Cincinnati College of Medical Department of Psychiatry, 3460
Woodlands, 4528

Oklahoma

Hillcrest Utica Psychiatric Services, 3383
Hogan Assessment Systems, 4436
National Alliance on Mental Illness: Oklahom a, 2062
OK Parents as Partners, 2063
Oklahoma Alliance for the Mentally Ill, 2064
Oklahoma Department of Human Services, 2406
Oklahoma Department of Mental Health and Substance Abuse Service (ODMHSAS), 2407
Oklahoma Healthcare Authority, 2408
Oklahoma Mental Health Consumer Council, 2065, 2409, 4280, 4280
Oklahoma Office of Juvenile Affairs, 2410
Oklahoma Psychiatric Physicians Association, 2066
St. Anthony Behavioral Medicine Center, Behavioral Medicine, 4328

Oregon

Anorexia Nervosa and Related Eating Disorders, 982
Beaver Creek Software, 4374
Deborah MacWilliams, 1336
Interlink Health Services, 4232
Marion County Health Department, 2411
Medipay, 4465
National Alliance on Mental Illness: Oregon, 2067
Nickerson Center, 3411
Northwest Analytical, 4482
Office of Mental Health and Addiction Services Training & Resource Center, 2412
Oregon Alliance for the Mentally Ill, 2068

Oregon Commission on Children and Families, 2413
Oregon Department of Human Resources: Division of Health Services, 2414
Oregon Department of Human Services: Mental Health Services, 2415
Oregon Department of Human Services: Office of Developmental Disabilities, 2416
Oregon Family Support Network, 2069
Oregon Health Policy and Research: Policy and Analysis Unit, 2417
Oregon Psychiatric Association, 2070
People First of Oregon, 2071
Providence Behavioral Health Connections, 4306
Regional Research Institute for Human Services of Portland University, 3432
Research and Training Center on Family Support and Children's Mental Health, 1590, 1786
Riverside Center, 3436

Pennsylvania

ACORN Behavioral Care Management Corporation, 4113
APOGEE, 4114
Access Behavioral Care, 4116
American Association of Chairs of Department s of Psychiatry, 2517
American Association of Directors of Psychiatric Residency Training, 2519
Askesis Development Group, 4369
Association for Hospital Medical Education, 2582
Bipolar Research at University of Pennsylvan ia, 748
CIGNA Corporation, 4147
Cephalon, 4634
Consumer Satisfaction Team, 2491
DB Consultants, 4402
Dauphin County Drug and Alcohol, 2418
Deloitte and Touche LLP Management Consulting, 4175
DeltaMetrics, 4176, 4405
Distance Learning Network, 4406, 3371
Diversified Group Administrators, 4177
Family Services of Delaware County, 4418
GMR Group, 4199
Health Federation of Philadelphia, 2072
Healthcare America, 4214
InfoMC, 4440
International Society of Psychiatric-Mental Health Nurses, 1742
JS Medical Group, 4234
Jefferson Drug/Alcohol, 3386
Kidspeace National Centers, 1629
Learning Disabilities Association of America, 395
Learning Disability Association of America, 1744
MCF Consulting, 4246
MEDecision, 4455
Mayes Group, 4260
Medical College of Pennsylvania, 3399
Mental Health Association of Southeastern Pe nnsylvania (MHASP), 2073
Mental Health Consultants, 3200
Mutual Pharmaceutical Company, 4646
National Alliance on Mental Illness: Pennsyl vania, 2074

National Association of Addiction Treatment Providers, 2635
National Association of Therapeutic Wilderness Camps, 1757
National Mental Health Consumer's, 98, 271, 399, 399, 554, 1340
National Mental Health Consumer's Self-Help, 12, 713, 784, 784, 831, 866, 956, 994, 1087, 1129, 1168, 1226, 1240, 1287, 1364, 1442, 1472
National Mental Health Consumers' Self-Help Clearinghouse, 13, 99, 272, 272, 400, 555, 714, 785, 832, 867, 957, 995, 1088, 1107, 1130, 1169, 1227
North American Society of Adlerian Psychology (NASAP), 2656
One Hundred Top Series, 4281
PMHCC, 4284
Parents Involved Network, 2075
Penn State Hershey Medical Center, 3418
Pennsylvania Alliance for the Mentally Ill, 2076
Pennsylvania Bureau Drug and Alcohol Programs: Monitoring, 2419
Pennsylvania Bureau of Community Program Standards: Licensure and Certification, 2420
Pennsylvania Bureau of Drug and Alcohol Programs: Information Bulletins, 2421
Pennsylvania Chapter of the American Anorexia Bulimia Association, 2077
Pennsylvania Department of Health: Bureau of Drug and Alcohol Programs, 2422
Pennsylvania Department of Public Welfare and Mental Health Services, 2423
Pennsylvania Division of Drug and Alcohol Prevention: Treatment, 2424
Pennsylvania Medical Assistance Programs, 2425
Pennsylvania Society for Services to Children, 2078
Persoma Management, 4290
Philadelphia Health Management, 4292
Pittsburgh Health Research Institute, 3420
Pressley Ridge Schools, 3422
ProMetrics CAREeval, 4301
ProMetrics Consulting & Susquehanna PathFinders, 4302
Psych-Med Association, St. Francis Medical, 3424
SHS Computer Service, 4501
Schafer Consulting, 4319
Shire Richwood, 4657
Siemens Health Services Corporation, 4505
Southwestern Pennsylvania Alliance for the Mentally Ill, 2079
St. Francis Medical Center, 3444
Suburban Research Associates, 4329
SunGard Pentamation, 4513
Systems Advocacy, 1789
UNITE Inc Grief Support, 21
University of Pennsylvania Health System, 3477
University of Pennsylvania Weight and Eating Disorders Program, 1063
University of Pennsylvania, Department of Psychiatry, 3478
University of Pittsburgh Medical Center, 2080
Vanderveer Group, 4340
Virtual Software Systems, 4525
Western Psychiatric Institute and Clinic, 3487
Wordsworth, 3488

XI Tech Corporation, 4531

Rhode Island

American Academy of Addiction Psychiatry (AAAP), 82
East Bay Alliance for the Mentally Ill, 2081
Kent County Alliance for the Mentally Ill, 2082
National Alliance on Mental Illness: Davis Park, 2084
National Alliance on Mental Illness: Rhode Island, 2085
New Avenues Alliance for the Mentally Ill, 2086
Newport County Alliance for the Mentally Ill, 2087
Northern Rhode Island Alliance for the Mentally Ill, 2088
Parent Support Network of Rhode Island, 2089
Rhode Island Council on Alcoholism and Other Drug Dependence, 2230
Rhode Island Department of Human Services, 2426
Rhode Island Division of Substance Abuse, 2427
Siblings & Offspring Group Alliance for the Mentally Ill, 2090
Spouses & Partners' Group Alliance for the Mentally Ill, 2091
State of Rhode Island Department of Mental Health, Retardation and Hospitals, 2428
Washington County Alliance for the Mentally Ill, 2092

South Carolina

Columbia Counseling Center, 3364
Federation of Families of South Carolina, 2093
LRADAC The Behavioral Health Center of the Midlands, 2429
Medical University of South Carolina Institute of Psychiatry, Psychiatry Access Center, 3403
Mental Health Association in South Carolina, 2430
National Alliance on Mental Illness: South Carolina, 2083, 2094
National Mental Health Association: Georgetown County, 2095
Society for Pediatric Psychology (SPP), 2670
South Carolina Alliance for the Mentally Ill, 2096
South Carolina Alliance for the Mentally Ill, 2097
South Carolina Department of Alcohol and Other Drug Abuse Services, 2431
South Carolina Department of Mental Health, 2432
South Carolina Department of Social Services, 2433
South Carolina Family Support Network, 2098

South Dakota

Brookings Alliance for the Mentally Ill, 2099
Huron Alliance for the Mentally Ill, 2100
National Alliance on Mental Illness: South Dakota, 2101
South Dakota Department of Human Services: Division of Mental Health, 2434
South Dakota Department of Social Services Office of Medical Services, 2435
South Dakota Human Services Center, 2436

Tennessee

Alcohol and Drug Council of Middle Tennessee, 2437
American Board of Disability Analysts Annual Conference, 3176
Bridges: Building Recovery & Individual Dreams & Goals Through Education & Support, 2102
Bureau of TennCare: State of Tennessee, 2438
Chattanooga/Plateau Council for Alcohol and Drug Abuse, 2439
Genesis Learning Center (Devereux), 3378
HCA Healthcare, 4204
HMS Healthcare Management Systems, 4424
Jeri Davis Marketing Consultants, 4235
King Pharmaceuticals, 4643
Meharry Medical College, 3404
Memphis Alcohol and Drug Council, 2440
Memphis Business Group on Health, 2103
Middle Tennessee Mental Health Institute, 2441
National Alliance on Mental Illness: Tennessee, 2104
New Day, 4276
Tennessee Alliance for the Mentally Ill, 2105
Tennessee Association of Mental Health Organization, 2106
Tennessee Commission on Children and Youth, 2442
Tennessee Department of Health, 2443
Tennessee Department of Health: Alcohol and Drug Abuse, 2444
Tennessee Department of Human Services, 2445
Tennessee Department of Mental Health and Developmental Disabilities, 2446
Tennessee Mental Health Consumers' Association, 2107
Tennessee Voices for Children, 2108
University of Tennessee Medical Group: Department of Medicine and Psychiatry, 3479
Vanderbilt University: John F Kennedy Center for Research on Human Development, 2109
Williamson County Council on Alcohol and Drug Prevention, 2447

Texas

ACC, 4352
American Association of Community Psychiatrists (AACP), 2516
American College of Psychoanalysts (ACPA), 2538
American Pediatrics Society, 1575, 1702
American Society for Adolescent Psychiatry (ASAP), 2565
American Society for Adolescent Psychiatry: Annual Meeting, 3183
Austin Travis County Mental Health Mental Retardation Center, 4371
Austin Travis County Mental Health: Mental Retardation Center, 2448
Body Logic, 4379
Brown Schools Behavioral Health System, 3356
CSI Software, 4384
Child & Family Center, 846
Children's Mental Health Partnership, 2110
Compu-Care Management and Systems, 4394
Computer Transition Services, 4396
Corphealth, 4166, 3366
Covenant Home Healthcare, 4169
Dallas Federation of Families for Children's Mental Health, 2111
Depression and Bipolar Support Alliance of Houston and Harris County, 2112
Eye Movement Desensitization and Reprocessing International Association (EMDRIA), 1728
Fox Counseling Service, 2113
Group for the Advancement of Psychiatry, 2615
HMS Software, 4425
Harris County Mental Health: Mental Retardation Authority, 2449
Healthcare Vision, 4433
Horizon Behavioral Services, 4221
Horizon Mental Health Management, 4223
Information Management Solutions, 4441
Interface EAP, 4230
International Society for Developmental Psychobiology, 2622
Jewish Family Service of Dallas, 2114
Jewish Family Service of San Antonio, 2115
MADD-Mothers Against Drunk Drivers, 205
Menninger Care Systems, 4265
Menninger Clinic, 1747
Menninger Division of Continuing Education, 3405
Mental Health Association, 2116
Mental Health Association of Greater Dallas, 2450
Mental Health Network, 4266
Mental Health Outcomes, 4469
Meridian Resource Corporation, 4268
National Alliance on Mental Illness: Texas, 2117
OPTAIO-Optimizing Practice Through Assessment, Intervention and Outcome, 4483
PRIMA A D D Corp., 3415
Parent Connection, 2118
Perot Systems, 4492
ProAmerica Managed Care, 4300
Psychological Associates-Texas, 3427
Psychonomic Society, 2664
Reclamation, 1782
Sid W Richardson Institute for Preventive Medicine of the Methodist Hospital, 924
Sweetwater Health Enterprises, 4514, 2504
Tarrant County Mental Health: Mental Retardation Services, 2451
Territorial Apprehensiveness (TERRAP) Programs, 276

Texas Alliance for the Mentally Ill, 2119
Texas Commission on Alcohol and Drug Abuse, 2452
Texas Counseling Association, 2120
Texas Department of Aging and Disability Services: Mental Retardation Services, 2453
Texas Department of Family and Protective Services, 2454
Texas Federation of Families for Children's Mental Health, 2121
Texas Health & Human Services Commission, 2455
Texas Psychological Association, 2122
Texas Society of Psychiatric Physicians, 2123
UT Southwestern Medical Center, 750
University of Texas Medical Branch Managed Care, 3480
University of Texas Southwestern Medical Center, 2124
University of Texas, Southwestern Medical Center, 3481
University of Texas-Houston Health Science Center, 3482
University of Texas: Mental Health Clinical Research Center, 925

Utah

Allies for Youth & Families, 2125
CompHealth Credentialing, 2490
Copper Hills Youth Center, 3365
DMDA/DBSA: Uplift, 2126
DataMark, 4404
Healthwise of Utah, 2127
Human Affairs International, 4224
IHC Behavioral Health Network, 4228
National Alliance on Mental Illness: Utah, 2128
Tender Hearts, 18
Triplet Connection, 20
University of Utah Neuropsychiatric, 3483
Utah Commission on Criminal and Juvenile Justice, 2456
Utah Department of Health, 2457
Utah Department of Health: Health Care Financing, 2458
Utah Department of Human Services, 2459
Utah Department of Human Services: Division of Substance Abuse And Mental Health, 2460
Utah Department of Mental Health, 2461
Utah Parent Center, 2129
Utah Psychiatric Association, 2130

Vermont

Fletcher Allen Health Care, 2131, 3377
IDX Systems Corporation, 4438
National Alliance on Mental Illness: Vermont, 2132
Retreat Healthcare, 2133
State of Vermont Developmental Disabilities Services, 2462
Vermont Alliance for the Mentally Ill, 2134
Vermont Department for Children and Families Economic Services Division (ESD), 2463

Vermont Department of Health: Division of Mental Health Services, 2464
Vermont Employers Health Alliance, 2135
Vermont Federation of Families for Children's Mental Health, 2136

Virginia

Agoraphobics Building Independent Lives, 353
Al-Anon Family Group National Referral Hotline, 199
Alateen and Al-Anon Family Groups, 1624
AmeriChoice, 4125
American Association for Marriage and Family Therapy, 2514
American Association of Pastoral Counselors, 2525
American Association of Pharmaceutical Scientists, 2526
American Association of Psychiatric Services for Children (AAPSC), 1698
American College of Health Care Administrators: ACHCA Annual Meeting, 2533, 3177
American Counseling Association, 2539
American Counseling Association (ACA), 2540
American Medical Group Association, 2549
American Mental Health Counselors Association (AMHCA), 2551
American Network of Community Options and Resources (ANCOR), 1701
American Psychiatric Association, 1703
American Psychiatric Association (APA), 2555
American Psychiatric Nurses Association, 2556
American Psychiatric Press Reference Library CD-ROM, 4364
American Psychiatric Publishing, 2557
American Psychosomatic Society, 2564
American Society for Clinical Pharmacology & Therapeutics, 2566
American Society of Consultant Pharmacists, 2567
Anthem BC/BS of Virginia, 2137
Association for Ambulatory Behavioral Healthcare: Training Conference, 2576, 3188
Child Welfare League of America, 1721
Child Welfare League of America: Washington, 2599
Children and Adolescents with Emotional and Behavioral Disorders, 3360
Clinical Social Work Federation, 2602
Colonial Services Board, 3363
Community Anti-Drug Coalitions of America:, 2606
Council for Learning Disabilities, 1726
Council on Social Work Education, 2493, 2609
Depression & Related Affective Disorders Association (DRADA), 856
Employee Assistance Professionals Association, 4183, 2611
Employee Assistance Society of North America, 2612
Family-to-Family: National Alliance on Mental Illness, 1413

Federation of Families for Children's Mental Health, 1579, 1733
First Hospital Corporation, 2138
Garnett Day Treatment Center, 2139
Healthy Companies, 4218
Institute on Psychiatric Services: American Psychiatric Association, 2619
Lewin Group, 4243
MHM Services, 3199
Managed Networks of America, 4257
Medical College of Virginia, 3400
NAMI, 2140
NAMI National Convention, 3193
National Alliance on Mental Illness, 89, 268, 396, 396, 552, 710, 863, 988, 1238, 1285, 1361, 1470, 1494, 1536, 1752
National Alliance on Mental Illness: Virginia, 2141
National Association Councils on Developmental Disabilities, 780
National Association of Alcholism and Drug Abuse Counselors, 3408
National Association of Alcohol and Drug Abuse Counselors (NAADAC), 90
National Association of State Mental Health Program Directors (NASMHPD), 2641
National Association of State Mental Health Program Directors, 1756
National Mental Health Association, 97, 1363, 1766, 1766, 2650
National Nurses Association, 2651
National Pharmaceutical Council, 2652
National Rehabilitation Association, 1770
Options Health Care, 4283
Parent Resource Center, 2142
Parents Information Network, 1587, 1777
Professional Risk Management Services, 4304, 2659
QuadraMed Corporation, 4497, 3431
Richmond Support Group, 2143
Society for Personality Assessment, 2671
Society of Multivariate Experimental Psychology (SMEP), 2677
Survivors of Loved Ones' Suicides (SOLOS), 17, 40, 1521, 1521
ValueOptions, 1922, 4338
Virginia Beach Community Service Board, 2144, 4346
Virginia Department of Medical Assistance Services, 2465
Virginia Department of Mental Health, Mental Retardation and Substance Abuse Services (DMHMRSAS), 2466
Virginia Department of Social Services, 2467
Virginia Federation of Families, 2145
Virginia Federation of Families for Children's Mental Health, 2146
Virginia Office of the Secretary of Health and Human Resources, 2468
World Federation for Mental Health, 1796

Washington

At Health, 3
AtHealth.Com, 4
Carewise, 4150
Children's Alliance, 1912, 2147
Common Voice for Pierce County Parents, 2148
Good Sam-W/Alliance for the Mentally Ill Family Support Group, 2149

Healthcare in Partnership, 4216
Keane Care, 4450
Kitsap County Alliance for the Mentally Ill, 2150
Lanstat Incorporated, 2496
Mental Health & Spirituality Support Group, 2151
Mental Health Matters, 1127
National Alliance on Mental Illness: Washing ton, 2152
National Eating Disorders Association, 992
NetMeeting, 4479
North Sound Regional Support Network, 2153
Nueva Esperanza Counseling Center, 2154
Occupational Health Software, 4484
Pierce County Alliance for the Mentally Ill, 2155
Sharing & Caring for Consumers, Families Alliance for the Mentally Ill, 2156
South King County Alliance for the Mentally Ill, 2157
Spanish Support Group Alliance for the Mentally Ill, 2158
Spokane Mental Health, 2159
Washington Advocates for the Mentally Ill, 2160
Washington Department of Alcohol and Substance Abuse: Department of Social and Health Service, 2469
Washington Department of Social & Health Services, 2470
Washington Department of Social and Health Services: Mental Health Division, 2471
Washington Institute for Mental Illness Research and Training, 2161
Washington State Psychological Association, 2162
Whidbey Island Alliance for the Mentally Ill, 2163

West Virginia

Autism Services Center, 544, 652
Behavioral Health Management Group, 4136
CAMC Family Medicine Center of Charleston, 2164
Mountain State Parents Children Adolescent Network, 2165
National Alliance on Mental Illness: West Vi rginia, 2166
Process Strategies Institute, 4303
Selective Mutism Foundation, 274
West Virginia Alliance for the Mentally Ill, 2167
West Virginia Bureau for Behavioral Health and Health Facilities, 2472
West Virginia Department of Health & Human Resources (DHHR), 2473
West Virginia Department of Welfare Bureau for Children and Families, 2474
West Virginia Division of Criminal Justice Services (DCJS), 2475

Wisconsin

Alliance for Children and Families, 2508

American Association of Children's Residential Center Annual Conference, 2518, 3171
BOSS Inc, 4373
Bethesda Lutheran Homes and Services, 1710
Bipolar Disorders Treatment Information Center, 704
Bureau of Mental Health and Substance Abuse Services, 2476
Charter BHS of Wisconsin/Brown Deer, 2168
Child and Adolescent Psychopharmacology Information, 2169
Dane County Mental Health Center, 2477
Department of Health and Family Services: Southern Region, 2478
Families United of Milwaukee, 2170
Information Centers for Lithium, Bipolar Disorders Treatment & Obsessive Compulsive Disorder, 1738
Lithium Information Center, 709
MCW Department of Psychiatry and Behavioral Medicine, 4248, 3393
Medical College of Wisconsin, 3401
National Alliance on Mental Illness: Wiscons in, 2171
National Niemann-Pick Disease Foundation, 786
Obsessive Compulsive Information Center, 1172
Phoenix Care Systems, Inc: Willowglen Academ y, 1779
Society for Psychophysiological Research, 2672
Society of Behavioral Medicine, 2676
Stoughton Family Counseling, 2172
TOPS Club, 998
University of Wisconsin Center for Health Policy and Program Evaluation, 2479
Wisconsin Alliance for the Mentally Ill, 2173
Wisconsin Association of Family and Child Agency, 2174
Wisconsin Bureau of Health Care Financing, 2480
Wisconsin Department of Health and Family Services, 2481
Wisconsin Family Ties, 2175

Wyoming

Central Wyoming Behavioral Health at Lander Valley, 2176
National Alliance on Mental Illness: Wyoming, 2177
Uplift, 2178
Wyoming Alliance for the Mentally Ill, 2179
Wyoming Department of Family Services, 2482
Wyoming Department of Health: Division of Health Care Finance, 2483
Wyoming Mental Health Division, 2484

Business Information • Ratings Guides • General Reference • Education • Statistics • Demographics • Health Information • Canadian Information

The Directory of Business Information Resources, 2008

With 100% verification, over 1,000 new listings and more than 12,000 updates, *The Directory of Business Information Resources* is the most up-to-date source for contacts in over 98 business areas – from advertising and agriculture to utilities and wholesalers. This carefully researched volume details: the Associations representing each industry; the Newsletters that keep members current; the Magazines and Journals - with their "Special Issues" - that are important to the trade, the Conventions that are "must attends," Databases, Directories and Industry Web Sites that provide access to must-have marketing resources. Includes contact names, phone & fax numbers, web sites and e-mail addresses. This one-volume resource is a gold mine of information and would be a welcome addition to any reference collection.

"This is a most useful and easy-to-use addition to any researcher's library." –The Information Professionals Institute

Softcover ISBN 978-1-59237-193-8, 2,500 pages, $195.00 | Online Database $495.00

Hudson's Washington News Media Contacts Directory, 2008

With 100% verification of data, Hudson's Washington News Media Contacts Directory is the most accurate, most up-to-date source for media contacts in our nation's capital. With the largest concentration of news media in the world, having access to Washington's news media will get your message heard by these key media outlets. Published for over 40 years, Hudson's Washington News Media Contacts Directory brings you immediate access to: News Services & Newspapers, News Service Syndicates, DC Newspapers, Foreign Newspapers, Radio & TV, Magazines & Newsletters, and Freelance Writers & Photographers. The easy-to-read entries include contact names, phone & fax numbers, web sites and e-mail and more. For easy navigation, Hudson's Washington News Media Contacts Directory contains two indexes: Entry Index and Executive Index. This kind of comprehensive and up-to-date information would cost thousands of dollars to replicate or countless hours of searching to find. Don't miss this opportunity to have this important resource in your collection, and start saving time and money today. Hudson's Washington News Media Contacts Directory is the perfect research tool for Public Relations, Marketing, Networking and so much more. This resource is a gold mine of information and would be a welcome addition to any reference collection.

Softcover ISBN 978-1-59237-393-2, 800 pages, $289.00

Nations of the World, 2007/08 A Political, Economic and Business Handbook

This completely revised edition covers all the nations of the world in an easy-to-use, single volume. Each nation is profiled in a single chapter that includes Key Facts, Political & Economic Issues, a Country Profile and Business Information. In this fast-changing world, it is extremely important to make sure that the most up-to-date information is included in your reference collection. This edition is just the answer. Each of the 200+ country chapters have been carefully reviewed by a political expert to make sure that the text reflects the most current information on Politics, Travel Advisories, Economics and more. You'll find such vital information as a Country Map, Population Characteristics, Inflation, Agricultural Production, Foreign Debt, Political History, Foreign Policy, Regional Insecurity, Economics, Trade & Tourism, Historical Profile, Political Systems, Ethnicity, Languages, Media, Climate, Hotels, Chambers of Commerce, Banking, Travel Information and more. Five Regional Chapters follow the main text and include a Regional Map, an Introductory Article, Key Indicators and Currencies for the Region. As an added bonus, an all-inclusive CD-ROM is available as a companion to the printed text. Noted for its sophisticated, up-to-date and reliable compilation of political, economic and business information, this brand new edition will be an important acquisition to any public, academic or special library reference collection.

"A useful addition to both general reference collections and business collections." –RUSQ

Softcover ISBN 978-1-59237-177-8, 1,700 pages, $155.00

The Directory of Venture Capital & Private Equity Firms, 2008

This edition has been extensively updated and broadly expanded to offer direct access to over 2,800 Domestic and International Venture Capital Firms, including address, phone & fax numbers, e-mail addresses and web sites for both primary and branch locations. Entries include details on the firm's Mission Statement, Industry Group Preferences, Geographic Preferences, Average and Minimum Investments and Investment Criteria. You'll also find details that are available nowhere else, including the Firm's Portfolio Companies and extensive information on each of the firm's Managing Partners, such as Education, Professional Background and Directorships held, along with the Partner's E-mail Address. *The Directory of Venture Capital & Private Equity Firms* offers five important indexes: Geographic Index, Executive Name Index, Portfolio Company Index, Industry Preference Index and College & University Index. With its comprehensive coverage and detailed, extensive information on each company, The Directory of Venture Capital & Private Equity Firms is an important addition to any finance collection.

"The sheer number of listings, the descriptive information and the outstanding indexing make this directory a better value than ...Pratt's Guide to Venture Capital Sources. Recommended for business collections in large public, academic and business libraries." –Choice

Softcover ISBN 978-1-59237-272-0, 1,300 pages, $565/$450 Library | Online Database $889.00

To preview any of our Directories Risk-Free for 30 days, call (800) 562-2139 or fax (518) 789-0556
www.greyhouse.com books@greyhouse.com

Business Information ♦ Ratings Guides ♦ General Reference ♦ Education ♦ Statistics ♦ Demographics ♦ Health Information ♦ Canadian Information

The Encyclopedia of Emerging Industries

*Published under an exclusive license from the Gale Group, Inc.

The fifth edition of the *Encyclopedia of Emerging Industries* details the inception, emergence, and current status of nearly 120 flourishing U.S. industries and industry segments. These focused essays unearth for users a wealth of relevant, current, factual data previously accessible only through a diverse variety of sources. This volume provides broad-based, highly-readable, industry information under such headings as Industry Snapshot, Organization & Structure, Background & Development, Industry Leaders, Current Conditions, America and the World, Pioneers, and Research & Technology. Essays in this new edition, arranged alphabetically for easy use, have been completely revised, with updated statistics and the most current information on industry trends and developments. In addition, there are new essays on some of the most interesting and influential new business fields, including Application Service Providers, Concierge Services, Entrepreneurial Training, Fuel Cells, Logistics Outsourcing Services, Pharmacogenomics, and Tissue Engineering. Two indexes, General and Industry, provide immediate access to this wealth of information. Plus, two conversion tables for SIC and NAICS codes, along with Suggested Further Readings, are provided to aid the user. *The Encyclopedia of Emerging Industries* pinpoints emerging industries while they are still in the spotlight. This important resource will be an important acquisition to any business reference collection.

"This well-designed source...should become another standard business source, nicely complementing Standard & Poor's Industry Surveys. It contains more information on each industry than Hoover's Handbook of Emerging Companies, is broader in scope than The Almanac of American Employers 1998-1999, but is less expansive than the Encyclopedia of Careers & Vocational Guidance. Highly recommended for all academic libraries and specialized business collections." –Library Journal

Hardcover ISBN 978-1-59237-242-3, 1,400 pages, $325.00

Encyclopedia of American Industries

*Published under an exclusive license from the Gale Group, Inc.

The Encyclopedia of American Industries is a major business reference tool that provides detailed, comprehensive information on a wide range of industries in every realm of American business. A two volume set, Volume I provides separate coverage of nearly 500 manufacturing industries, while Volume II presents nearly 600 essays covering the vast array of services and other non-manufacturing industries in the United States. Combined, these two volumes provide individual essays on every industry recognized by the U.S. Standard Industrial Classification (SIC) system. Both volumes are arranged numerically by SIC code, for easy use. Additionally, each entry includes the corresponding NAICS code(s). The *Encyclopedia's* business coverage includes information on historical events of consequence, as well as current trends and statistics. Essays include an Industry Snapshot, Organization & Structure, Background & Development, Current Conditions, Industry Leaders, Workforce, America and the World, Research & Technology along with Suggested Further Readings. Both SIC and NAICS code conversion tables and an all-encompassing Subject Index, with cross-references, complete the text. With its detailed, comprehensive information on a wide range of industries, this resource will be an important tool for both the industry newcomer and the seasoned professional.

"Encyclopedia of American Industries contains detailed, signed essays on virtually every industry in contemporary society. ... Highly recommended for all but the smallest libraries." -American Reference Books Annual

Two Volumes, Hardcover ISBN 978-1-59237-244-7, 3,000 pages, $650.00

Encyclopedia of Global Industries

*Published under an exclusive license from the Gale Group, Inc.

This fourth edition of the acclaimed *Encyclopedia of Global Industries* presents a thoroughly revised and expanded look at more than 125 business sectors of global significance. Detailed, insightful articles discuss the origins, development, trends, key statistics and current international character of the world's most lucrative, dynamic and widely researched industries – including hundreds of profiles of leading international corporations. Beginning researchers will gain from this book a solid understanding of how each industry operates and which countries and companies are significant participants, while experienced researchers will glean current and historical figures for comparison and analysis. The industries profiled in previous editions have been updated, and in some cases, expanded to reflect recent industry trends. Additionally, this edition provides both SIC and NAICS codes for all industries profiled. As in the original volumes, *The Encyclopedia of Global Industries* offers thorough studies of some of the biggest and most frequently researched industry sectors, including Aircraft, Biotechnology, Computers, Internet Services, Motor Vehicles, Pharmaceuticals, Semiconductors, Software and Telecommunications. An SIC and NAICS conversion table and an all-encompassing Subject Index, with cross-references, are provided to ensure easy access to this wealth of information. These and many others make the *Encyclopedia of Global Industries* the authoritative reference for studies of international industries.

"Provides detailed coverage of the history, development, and current status of 115 of "the world's most lucrative and high-profile industries." It far surpasses the Department of Commerce's U.S. Global Trade Outlook 1995-2000 (GPO, 1995) in scope and coverage. Recommended for comprehensive public and academic library business collections." -Booklist

Hardcover ISBN 978-1-59237-243-0, 1,400 pages, $495.00

**To preview any of our Directories Risk-Free for 30 days, call (800) 562-2139 or fax (518) 789-0556
www.greyhouse.com books@greyhouse.com**

The Directory of Mail Order Catalogs, 2008

Published since 1981, *The Directory of Mail Order Catalogs* is the premier source of information on the mail order catalog industry. It is the source that business professionals and librarians have come to rely on for the thousands of catalog companies in the US. Since the 2007 edition, *The Directory of Mail Order Catalogs* has been combined with its companion volume, *The Directory of Business to Business Catalogs*, to offer all 13,000 catalog companies in one easy-to-use volume. Section I: Consumer Catalogs, covers over 9,000 consumer catalog companies in 44 different product chapters from Animals to Toys & Games. Section II: Business to Business Catalogs, details 5,000 business catalogs, everything from computers to laboratory supplies, building construction and much more. Listings contain detailed contact information including mailing address, phone & fax numbers, web sites, e-mail addresses and key contacts along with important business details such as product descriptions, employee size, years in business, sales volume, catalog size, number of catalogs mailed and more. Three indexes are included for easy access to information: Catalog & Company Name Index, Geographic Index and Product Index. *The Directory of Mail Order Catalogs*, now with its expanded business to business catalogs, is the largest and most comprehensive resource covering this billion-dollar industry. It is the standard in its field. This important resource is a useful tool for entrepreneurs searching for catalogs to pick up their product, vendors looking to expand their customer base in the catalog industry, market researchers, small businesses investigating new supply vendors, along with the library patron who is exploring the available catalogs in their areas of interest.

"This is a godsend for those looking for information." –Reference Book Review

Softcover ISBN 978-1-59237-202-7, 1,700 pages, $350/$250 Library | Online Database $495.00

Sports Market Place Directory, 2008

For over 20 years, this comprehensive, up-to-date directory has offered direct access to the Who, What, When & Where of the Sports Industry. With over 20,000 updates and enhancements, the *Sports Market Place Directory* is the most detailed, comprehensive and current sports business reference source available. In 1,800 information-packed pages, *Sports Market Place Directory* profiles contact information and key executives for: Single Sport Organizations, Professional Leagues, Multi-Sport Organizations, Disabled Sports, High School & Youth Sports, Military Sports, Olympic Organizations, Media, Sponsors, Sponsorship & Marketing Event Agencies, Event & Meeting Calendars, Professional Services, College Sports, Manufacturers & Retailers, Facilities and much more. The Sports Market Place Directory provides organization's contact information with detailed descriptions including: Key Contacts, physical, mailing, email and web addresses plus phone and fax numbers. *Sports Market Place Directory* provides a one-stop resources for this billion-dollar industry. This will be an important resource for large public libraries, university libraries, university athletic programs, career services or job placement organizations, and is a must for anyone doing research on or marketing to the US and Canadian sports industry.

"Grey House is the new publisher and has produced an excellent edition...highly recommended for public libraries and academic libraries with sports management programs or strong interest in athletics." -Booklist

Softcover ISBN 978-1-59237-348-2, 1,800 pages, $225.00 | Online Database $479.00

Food and Beverage Market Place, 2008

Food and Beverage Market Place is bigger and better than ever with thousands of new companies, thousands of updates to existing companies and two revised and enhanced product category indexes. This comprehensive directory profiles over 18,000 Food & Beverage Manufacturers, 12,000 Equipment & Supply Companies, 2,200 Transportation & Warehouse Companies, 2,000 Brokers & Wholesalers, 8,000 Importers & Exporters, 900 Industry Resources and hundreds of Mail Order Catalogs. Listings include detailed Contact Information, Sales Volumes, Key Contacts, Brand & Product Information, Packaging Details and much more. *Food and Beverage Market Place* is available as a three-volume printed set, a subscription-based Online Database via the Internet, on CD-ROM, as well as mailing lists and a licensable database.

"An essential purchase for those in the food industry but will also be useful in public libraries where needed. Much of the information will be difficult and time consuming to locate without this handy three-volume ready-reference source." –ARBA

3 Vol Set, Softcover ISBN 978-1-59237-198-3, 8,500 pages, $595 | Online Database $795 | Online Database & 3 Vol Set Combo, $995

The Grey House Performing Arts Directory, 2007

The Grey House Performing Arts Directory is the most comprehensive resource covering the Performing Arts. This important directory provides current information on over 8,500 Dance Companies, Instrumental Music Programs, Opera Companies, Choral Groups, Theater Companies, Performing Arts Series and Performing Arts Facilities. Plus, this edition now contains a brand new section on Artist Management Groups. In addition to mailing address, phone & fax numbers, e-mail addresses and web sites, dozens of other fields of available information include mission statement, key contacts, facilities, seating capacity, season, attendance and more. This directory also provides an important Information Resources section that covers hundreds of Performing Arts Associations, Magazines, Newsletters, Trade Shows, Directories, Databases and Industry Web Sites. Five indexes provide immediate access to this wealth of information: Entry Name, Executive Name, Performance Facilities, Geographic and Information Resources. *The Grey House Performing Arts Directory* pulls together thousands of Performing Arts Organizations, Facilities and Information Resources into an easy-to-use source – this kind of comprehensiveness and extensive detail is not available in any resource on the market place today.

"Immensely useful and user-friendly ... recommended for public, academic and certain special library reference collections." –Booklist

To preview any of our Directories Risk-Free for 30 days, call (800) 562-2139 or fax (518) 789-0556
www.greyhouse.com books@greyhouse.com

Business Information ♦ Ratings Guides ♦ General Reference ♦ Education ♦
Statistics ♦ Demographics ♦ Health Information ♦ Canadian Information

Softcover ISBN 978-1-59237-138-9, 1,500 pages, $185.00 | Online Database $335.00

New York State Directory, 2007/08

The New York State Directory, published annually since 1983, is a comprehensive and easy-to-use guide to accessing public officials and private sector organizations and individuals who influence public policy in the state of New York. *The New York State Directory* includes important information on all New York state legislators and congressional representatives, including biographies and key committee assignments. It also includes staff rosters for all branches of New York state government and for federal agencies and departments that impact the state policy process. Following the state government section are 25 chapters covering policy areas from agriculture through veterans' affairs. Each chapter identifies the state, local and federal agencies and officials that formulate or implement policy. In addition, each chapter contains a roster of private sector experts and advocates who influence the policy process. The directory also offers appendices that include statewide party officials; chambers of commerce; lobbying organizations; public and private universities and colleges; television, radio and print media; and local government agencies and officials.

"This comprehensive directory covers not only New York State government offices and key personnel but pertinent U.S. government agencies and non-governmental entities. This directory is all encompassing... recommended." -Choice

New York State Directory - Softcover ISBN 978-1-59237-190-7, 800 pages, $145.00
New York State Directory with *Profiles of New York* – 2 Volumes, Softcover ISBN 978-1-59237-191-4, 1,600 pages, $225.00

The Grey House Homeland Security Directory, 2008

This updated edition features the latest contact information for government and private organizations involved with Homeland Security along with the latest product information and provides detailed profiles of nearly 1,000 Federal & State Organizations & Agencies and over 3,000 Officials and Key Executives involved with Homeland Security. These listings are incredibly detailed and include Mailing Address, Phone & Fax Numbers, Email Addresses & Web Sites, a complete Description of the Agency and a complete list of the Officials and Key Executives associated with the Agency. Next, *The Grey House Homeland Security Directory* provides the go-to source for Homeland Security Products & Services. This section features over 2,000 Companies that provide Consulting, Products or Services. With this Buyer's Guide at their fingertips, users can locate suppliers of everything from Training Materials to Access Controls, from Perimeter Security to BioTerrorism Countermeasures and everything in between – complete with contact information and product descriptions. A handy Product Locator Index is provided to quickly and easily locate suppliers of a particular product. This comprehensive, information-packed resource will be a welcome tool for any company or agency that is in need of Homeland Security information and will be a necessary acquisition for the reference collection of all public libraries and large school districts.

"Compiles this information in one place and is discerning in content. A useful purchase for public and academic libraries." –Booklist

Softcover ISBN 978-1-59237-196-6, 800 pages, $195.00 | Online Database $385.00

The Grey House Safety & Security Directory, 2008

The Grey House Safety & Security Directory is the most comprehensive reference tool and buyer's guide for the safety and security industry. Arranged by safety topic, each chapter begins with OSHA regulations for the topic, followed by Training Articles written by top professionals in the field and Self-Inspection Checklists. Next, each topic contains Buyer's Guide sections that feature related products and services. Topics include Administration, Insurance, Loss Control & Consulting, Protective Equipment & Apparel, Noise & Vibration, Facilities Monitoring & Maintenance, Employee Health Maintenance & Ergonomics, Retail Food Services, Machine Guards, Process Guidelines & Tool Handling, Ordinary Materials Handling, Hazardous Materials Handling, Workplace Preparation & Maintenance, Electrical Lighting & Safety, Fire & Rescue and Security. Six important indexes make finding information and product manufacturers quick and easy: Geographical Index of Manufacturers and Distributors, Company Profile Index, Brand Name Index, Product Index, Index of Web Sites and Index of Advertisers. This comprehensive, up-to-date reference will provide every tool necessary to make sure a business is in compliance with OSHA regulations and locate the products and services needed to meet those regulations.

"Presents industrial safety information for engineers, plant managers, risk managers, and construction site supervisors..." –Choice

Softcover ISBN 978-1-59237-205-8, 1,500 pages, $165.00

The Grey House Transportation Security Directory & Handbook

This is the only reference of its kind that brings together current data on Transportation Security. With information on everything from Regulatory Authorities to Security Equipment, this top-flight database brings together the relevant information necessary for creating and maintaining a security plan for a wide range of transportation facilities. With this current, comprehensive directory at the ready you'll have immediate access to: Regulatory Authorities & Legislation; Information Resources; Sample Security Plans & Checklists; Contact Data for Major Airports, Seaports, Railroads, Trucking Companies and Oil Pipelines; Security Service Providers; Recommended Equipment & Product Information and more. Using the *Grey House Transportation Security Directory & Handbook*, managers will be able to quickly and easily assess their current security plans; develop contacts to create and maintain new security procedures; and source the products and services necessary to adequately maintain a secure environment. This valuable resource is a must for all Security Managers at Airports, Seaports, Railroads, Trucking Companies and Oil Pipelines.

> *"Highly recommended. Library collections that support all levels of readers, including professionals/practitioners; and schools/organizations offering education and training in transportation security." -Choice*

Softcover ISBN 978-1-59237-075-7, 800 pages, $195.00

The Grey House Biometric Information Directory

This edition offers a complete, current overview of biometric companies and products – one of the fastest growing industries in today's economy. Detailed profiles of manufacturers of the latest biometric technology, including Finger, Voice, Face, Hand, Signature, Iris, Vein and Palm Identification systems. Data on the companies include key executives, company size and a detailed, indexed description of their product line. Information in the directory includes: Editorial on Advancements in Biometrics; Profiles of 700+ companies listed with contact information; Organizations, Trade & Educational Associations, Publications, Conferences, Trade Shows and Expositions Worldwide; Web Site Index; Biometric & Vendors Services Index by Types of Biometrics; and a Glossary of Biometric Terms. This resource will be an important source for anyone who is considering the use of a biometric product, investing in the development of biometric technology, support existing marketing and sales efforts and will be an important acquisition for the business reference collection for large public and business libraries.

> *"This book should prove useful to agencies or businesses seeking companies that deal with biometric technology. Summing Up: Recommended. Specialized collections serving researchers/faculty and professionals/practitioners." -Choice*

Softcover ISBN 978-1-59237-121-1, 800 pages, $225.00

The Environmental Resource Handbook, 2007/08

The Environmental Resource Handbook is the most up-to-date and comprehensive source for Environmental Resources and Statistics. Section I: Resources provides detailed contact information for thousands of information sources, including Associations & Organizations, Awards & Honors, Conferences, Foundations & Grants, Environmental Health, Government Agencies, National Parks & Wildlife Refuges, Publications, Research Centers, Educational Programs, Green Product Catalogs, Consultants and much more. Section II: Statistics, provides statistics and rankings on hundreds of important topics, including Children's Environmental Index, Municipal Finances, Toxic Chemicals, Recycling, Climate, Air & Water Quality and more. This kind of up-to-date environmental data, all in one place, is not available anywhere else on the market place today. This vast compilation of resources and statistics is a must-have for all public and academic libraries as well as any organization with a primary focus on the environment.

> *"...the intrinsic value of the information make it worth consideration by libraries with environmental collections and environmentally concerned users." –Booklist*

Softcover ISBN 978-1-59237-195-2, 1,000 pages, $155.00 | Online Database $300.00

The Rauch Guide to the US Adhesives & Sealants, Cosmetics & Toiletries, Ink, Paint, Plastics, Pulp & Paper and Rubber Industries

The Rauch Guides save time and money by organizing widely scattered information and providing estimates for important business decisions, some of which are available nowhere else. Within each Guide, after a brief introduction, the ECONOMICS section provides data on industry shipments; long-term growth and forecasts; prices; company performance; employment, expenditures, and productivity; transportation and geographical patterns; packaging; foreign trade; and government regulations. Next, TECHNOLOGY & RAW MATERIALS provide market, technical, and raw material information for chemicals, equipment and related materials, including market size and leading suppliers, prices, end uses, and trends. PRODUCTS & MARKETS provide information for each major industry product, including market size and historical trends, leading suppliers, five-year forecasts, industry structure, and major end uses. Next, the COMPANY DIRECTORY profiles major industry companies, both public and private. Information includes complete contact information, web address, estimated total and domestic sales, product description, and recent mergers and acquisitions. *The Rauch Guides* will prove to be an invaluable source of market information, company data, trends and forecasts that anyone in these fast-paced industries.

"An invaluable and affordable publication. The comprehensive nature of the data and text offers considerable insights into the industry, market sizes, company activities, and applications of the products of the industry. The additions that have been made have certainly enhanced the value of the Guide." –Adhesives & Sealants Newsletter of the Rauch Guide to the US Adhesives & Sealants Industry

Paint Industry: Softcover ISBN 978-1-59237-127-3 $595 | Plastics Industry: Softcover ISBN 978-1-59237-128-0 $595 | Adhesives and Sealants Industry: Softcover ISBN 978-1-59237-129-7 $595 | Ink Industry: Softcover ISBN 978-1-59237-126-6 $595 | Rubber Industry: Softcover ISBN 978-1-59237-130-3 $595 | Pulp and Paper Industry: Softcover ISBN 978-1-59237-131-0 $595 | Cosmetic & Toiletries Industry: Softcover ISBN 978-1-59237-132-7 $895

Research Services Directory: Commercial & Corporate Research Centers

This ninth edition provides access to well over 8,000 independent Commercial Research Firms, Corporate Research Centers and Laboratories offering contract services for hands-on, basic or applied research. Research Services Directory covers the thousands of types of research companies, including Biotechnology & Pharmaceutical Developers, Consumer Product Research, Defense Contractors, Electronics & Software Engineers, Think Tanks, Forensic Investigators, Independent Commercial Laboratories, Information Brokers, Market & Survey Research Companies, Medical Diagnostic Facilities, Product Research & Development Firms and more. Each entry provides the company's name, mailing address, phone & fax numbers, key contacts, web site, e-mail address, as well as a company description and research and technical fields served. Four indexes provide immediate access to this wealth of information: Research Firms Index, Geographic Index, Personnel Name Index and Subject Index.

"An important source for organizations in need of information about laboratories, individuals and other facilities." –ARBA

Softcover ISBN 978-1-59237-003-0, 1,400 pages, $465.00

International Business and Trade Directories

Completely updated, the Third Edition of *International Business and Trade Directories* now contains more than 10,000 entries, over 2,000 more than the last edition, making this directory the most comprehensive resource of the worlds business and trade directories. Entries include content descriptions, price, publisher's name and address, web site and e-mail addresses, phone and fax numbers and editorial staff. Organized by industry group, and then by region, this resource puts over 10,000 industry-specific business and trade directories at the reader's fingertips. Three indexes are included for quick access to information: Geographic Index, Publisher Index and Title Index. Public, college and corporate libraries, as well as individuals and corporations seeking critical market information will want to add this directory to their marketing collection.

"Reasonably priced for a work of this type, this directory should appeal to larger academic, public and corporate libraries with an international focus." –Library Journal

Softcover ISBN 978-1-930956-63-6, 1,800 pages, $225.00

TheStreet.com Ratings Guide to Health Insurers

TheStreet.com Ratings Guide to Health Insurers is the first and only source to cover the financial stability of the nation's health care system, rating the financial safety of more than 6,000 health insurance providers, health maintenance organizations (HMOs) and all of the Blue Cross Blue Shield plans – updated quarterly to ensure the most accurate information. The Guide also provides a complete listing of all the major health insurers, including all Long-Term Care and Medigap insurers. Our *Guide to Health Insurers* includes comprehensive, timely coverage on the financial stability of HMOs and health insurers; the most accurate insurance company ratings available–the same quality ratings heralded by the U.S. General Accounting Office; separate listings for those companies offering Medigap and long-term care policies; the number of serious consumer complaints filed against most HMOs so you can see who is actually providing the best (or worst) service and more. The easy-to-use layout gives you a one-line summary analysis for each company that we track, followed by an in-depth, detailed analysis of all HMOs and the largest health insurers. The guide also includes a list of TheStreet.com Ratings Recommended Companies with information on how to contact them, and the reasoning behind any rating upgrades or downgrades.

> *"With 20 years behind its insurance-advocacy research [the rating guide] continues to offer a wealth of information that helps consumers weigh their healthcare options now and in the future." -Today's Librarian*

Issues published quarterly, Softcover, 550 pages, $499.00 for four quarterly issues, $249.00 for a single issue

TheStreet.com Ratings Guide to Life & Annuity Insurers

TheStreet.com Safety Ratings are the most reliable source for evaluating an insurer's financial solvency risk. Consequently, policy-holders have come to rely on TheStreet.com's flagship publication, *TheStreet.com Ratings Guide to Life & Annuity Insurers*, to help them identify the safest companies to do business with. Each easy-to-use edition delivers TheStreet.com's independent ratings and analyses on more than 1,100 insurers, updated every quarter. Plus, your patrons will find a complete list of TheStreet.com Recommended Companies, including contact information, and the reasoning behind any rating upgrades or downgrades. This guide is perfect for those who are considering the purchase of a life insurance policy, placing money in an annuity, or advising clients about insurance and annuities. A life or health insurance policy or annuity is only as secure as the insurance company issuing it. Therefore, make sure your patrons have what they need to periodically monitor the financial condition of the companies with whom they have an investment. The TheStreet.com Ratings product line is designed to help them in their evaluations.

> *"Weiss has an excellent reputation and this title is held by hundreds of libraries. This guide is recommended for public and academic libraries." -ARBA*

Issues published quarterly, Softcover, 360 pages, $499.00 for four quarterly issues, $249.00 for a single issue

TheStreet.com Ratings Guide to Property & Casualty Insurers

TheStreet.com Ratings Guide to Property and Casualty Insurers provides the most extensive coverage of insurers writing policies, helping consumers and businesses avoid financial headaches. Updated quarterly, this easy-to-use publication delivers the independent, unbiased TheStreet.com Safety Ratings and supporting analyses on more than 2,800 U.S. insurance companies, offering auto & homeowners insurance, business insurance, worker's compensation insurance, product liability insurance, medical malpractice and other professional liability insurance. Each edition includes a list of TheStreet.com Recommended Companies by type of insurance, including a contact number, plus helpful information about the coverage provided by the State Guarantee Associations.

> *"In contrast to the other major insurance rating agencies...Weiss does not have a financial relationship worth the companies it rates. A GAO study found that Weiss identified financial vulnerability earlier than the other rating agencies." -ARBA*

Issues published quarterly, Softcover, 455 pages, $499.00 for four quarterly issues, $249.00 for a single issue

TheStreet.com Ratings Consumer Box Set

Deliver the critical information your patrons need to safeguard their personal finances with *TheStreet.com Ratings' Consumer Guide Box Set*. Each of the eight guides is packed with accurate, unbiased information and recommendations to help your patrons make sound financial decisions. TheStreet.com Ratings Consumer Guide Box Set provides your patrons with easy to understand guidance on important personal finance topics, including: *Consumer Guide to Variable Annuities, Consumer Guide to Medicare Supplement Insurance, Consumer Guide to Elder Care Choices, Consumer Guide to Automobile Insurance, Consumer Guide to Long-Term Care Insurance, Consumer Guide to Homeowners Insurance, Consumer Guide to Term Life Insurance,* and *Consumer Guide to Medicare Prescription Drug Coverage*. Each guide provides an easy-to-read overview of the topic, what to look out for when selecting a company or insurance plan to do business with, who are the recommended companies to work with and how to navigate through these often-times difficult decisions. Custom worksheets and step-by-step directions make these resources accessible to all types of users. Packaged in a handy custom display box, these helpful guides will prove to be a much-used addition to any reference collection.

Issues published twice per year, Softcover, 600 pages, $499.00 for two biennial issues

TheStreet.com Ratings Guide to Stock Mutual Funds

TheStreet.com Ratings Guide to Stock Mutual Funds offers ratings and analyses on more than 8,800 equity mutual funds – more than any other publication. The exclusive TheStreet.com Investment Ratings combine an objective evaluation of each fund's performance and risk to provide a single, user-friendly, composite rating, giving your patrons a better handle on a mutual fund's risk-adjusted performance. Each edition identifies the top-performing mutual funds based on risk category, type of fund, and overall risk-adjusted performance. TheStreet.com's unique investment rating system makes it easy to see exactly which stocks are on the rise and which ones should be avoided. For those investors looking to tailor their mutual fund selections based on age, income, and tolerance for risk, we've also assigned two component ratings to each fund: a performance rating and a risk rating. With these, you can identify those funds that are best suited to meet your - or your client's – individual needs and goals. Plus, we include a handy Risk Profile Quiz to help you assess your personal tolerance for risk. So whether you're an investing novice or professional, the *Guide to Stock Mutual Funds* gives you everything you need to find a mutual fund that is right for you.

"There is tremendous need for information such as that provided by this Weiss publication. This reasonably priced guide is recommended for public and academic libraries serving investors." -ARBA

Issues published quarterly, Softcover, 655 pages, $499 for four quarterly issues, $249 for a single issue

TheStreet.com Ratings Guide to Exchange-Traded Funds

TheStreet.com Ratings editors analyze hundreds of mutual funds each quarter, condensing all of the available data into a single composite opinion of each fund's risk-adjusted performance. The intuitive, consumer-friendly ratings allow investors to instantly identify those funds that have historically done well and those that have under-performed the market. Each quarterly edition identifies the top-performing exchange-traded funds based on risk category, type of fund, and overall risk-adjusted performance. The rating scale, A through F, gives you a better handle on an exchange-traded fund's risk-adjusted performance. Other features include Top & Bottom 200 Exchange-Traded Funds; Performance and Risk: 100 Best and Worst Exchange- Traded Funds; Investor Profile Quiz; Performance Benchmarks and Fund Type Descriptions. With the growing popularity of mutual fund investing, consumers need a reliable source to help them track and evaluate the performance of their mutual fund holdings. Plus, they need a way of identifying and monitoring other funds as potential new investments. Unfortunately, the hundreds of performance and risk measures available, multiplied by the vast number of mutual fund investments on the market today, can make this a daunting task for even the most sophisticated investor. This Guide will serve as a useful tool for both the first-time and seasoned investor.

Editions published quarterly, Softcover, 440 pages, $499.00 for four quarterly issues, $249.00 for a single issue

TheStreet.com Ratings Guide to Bond & Money Market Mutual Funds

TheStreet.com Ratings Guide to Bond & Money Market Mutual Funds has everything your patrons need to easily identify the top-performing fixed income funds on the market today. Each quarterly edition contains TheStreet.com's independent ratings and analyses on more than 4,600 fixed income funds – more than any other publication, including corporate bond funds, high-yield bond funds, municipal bond funds, mortgage security funds, money market funds, global bond funds and government bond funds. In addition, the fund's risk rating is combined with its three-year performance rating to get an overall picture of the fund's risk-adjusted performance. The resulting TheStreet.com Investment Rating gives a single, user-friendly, objective evaluation that makes it easy to compare one fund to another and select the right fund based on the level of risk tolerance. Most investors think of fixed income mutual funds as "safe" investments. That's not always the case, however, depending on the credit risk, interest rate risk, and prepayment risk of the securities owned by the fund. TheStreet.com Ratings assesses each of these risks and assigns each fund a risk rating to help investors quickly evaluate the fund's risk component. Plus, we include a handy Risk Profile Quiz to help you assess your personal tolerance for risk. So whether you're an investing novice or professional, the *Guide to Bond and Money Market Mutual Funds* gives you everything you need to find a mutual fund that is right for you.

"Comprehensive... It is easy to use and consumer-oriented, and can be recommended for larger public and academic libraries." -ARBA

Issues published quarterly, Softcover, 470 pages, $499.00 for four quarterly issues, $249.00 for a single issue

TheStreet.com Ratings Guide to Banks & Thrifts

Updated quarterly, for the most up-to-date information, *TheStreet.com Ratings Guide to Banks and Thrifts* offers accurate, intuitive safety ratings your patrons can trust; supporting ratios and analyses that show an institution's strong & weak points; identification of the TheStreet.com Recommended Companies with branches in your area; a complete list of institutions receiving upgrades/downgrades; and comprehensive coverage of every bank and thrift in the nation – more than 9,000. TheStreet.com Safety Ratings are then based on the analysts' review of publicly available information collected by the federal banking regulators. The easy-to-use layout gives you: the institution's TheStreet.com Safety Rating for the last 3 years; the five key indexes used to evaluate each institution; along with the primary ratios and statistics used in determining the company's rating. *TheStreet.com Ratings Guide to Banks & Thrifts* will be a must for individuals who are concerned about the safety of their CD or savings account; need to be sure that an existing line of credit will be there when they need it; or simply want to avoid the hassles of dealing with a failing or troubled institution.

"Large public and academic libraries most definitely need to acquire the work. Likewise, special libraries in large corporations will find this title indispensable." -ARBA

Issues published quarterly, Softcover, 370 pages, $499.00 for four quarterly issues, $249.00 for a single issue

**To preview any of our Directories Risk-Free for 30 days, call (800) 562-2139 or fax (518) 789-0556
www.greyhouse.com   books@greyhouse.com**

TheStreet.com Ratings Guide to Common Stocks

TheStreet.com Ratings Guide to Common Stocks gives your patrons reliable insight into the risk-adjusted performance of common stocks listed on the NYSE, AMEX, and Nasdaq – over 5,800 stocks in all – more than any other publication. TheStreet.com's unique investment rating system makes it easy to see exactly which stocks are on the rise and which ones should be avoided. In addition, your patrons also get supporting analysis showing growth trends, profitability, debt levels, valuation levels, the top-rated stocks within each industry, and more. Plus, each stock is ranked with the easy-to-use buy-hold-sell equivalents commonly used by Wall Street. Whether they're selecting their own investments or checking up on a broker's recommendation, TheStreet.com Ratings can help them in their evaluations.

"Users... will find the information succinct and the explanations readable, easy to understand, and helpful to a novice." -Library Journal

Issues published quarterly, Softcover, 440 pages, $499.00 for four quarterly issues, $249.00 for a single issue

TheStreet.com Ratings Ultimate Guided Tour of Stock Investing

This important reference guide from TheStreet.com Ratings is just what librarians around the country have asked for: a step-by-step introduction to stock investing for the beginning to intermediate investor. This easy-to-navigate guide explores the basics of stock investing and includes the intuitive TheStreet.com Investment Rating on more than 5,800 stocks, complete with real-world investing information that can be put to use immediately with stocks that fit the concepts discussed in the guide; informative charts, graphs and worksheets; easy-to-understand explanations on topics like P/E, compound interest, marked indices, diversifications, brokers, and much more; along with financial safety ratings for every stock on the NYSE, American Stock Exchange and the Nasdaq. This consumer-friendly guide offers complete how-to information on stock investing that can be put to use right away; a friendly format complete with our "Wise Guide" who leads the reader on a safari to learn about the investing jungle; helpful charts, graphs and simple worksheets; the intuitive TheStreet.com Investment rating on over 6,000 stocks — every stock found on the NYSE, American Stock Exchange and the NASDAQ; and much more.

"Provides investors with an alternative to stock broker recommendations, which recently have been tarnished by conflicts of interest. In summary, the guide serves as a welcome addition for all public library collections." -ARBA

Issues published quarterly, Softcover, 370 pages, $499.00 for four quarterly issues, $249.00 for a single issue

TheStreet.com Ratings' Reports & Services

- Ratings Online — An on-line summary covering an individual company's TheStreet.com Financial Strength Rating or an investment's unique TheStreet.com Investment Rating with the factors contributing to that rating; available 24 hours a day by visiting www.thestreet.com/tscratings or calling (800) 289-9222.
- Unlimited Ratings Research — The ultimate research tool providing fast, easy online access to the very latest TheStreet.com Financial Strength Ratings and Investment Ratings. Price: $559 per industry.

Contact TheStreet.com for more information about Reports & Services at www.thestreet.com/tscratings or call (800) 289-9222

TheStreet.com Ratings' Custom Reports

TheStreet.com Ratings is pleased to offer two customized options for receiving ratings data. Each taps into TheStreet.com's vast data repositories and is designed to provide exactly the data you need. Choose from a variety of industries, companies, data variables, and delivery formats including print, Excel, SQL, Text or Access.

- Customized Reports - get right to the heart of your company's research and data needs with a report customized to your specifications.
- Complete Database Download – TheStreet.com will design and deliver the database; from there you can sort it, recalculate it, and format your results to suit your specific needs.

Contact TheStreet.com for more information about Custom Reports at www.thestreet.com/tscratings or call (800) 289-9222

The Value of a Dollar 1600-1859, The Colonial Era to The Civil War

Following the format of the widely acclaimed, *The Value of a Dollar, 1860-2004, The Value of a Dollar 1600-1859, The Colonial Era to The Civil War* records the actual prices of thousands of items that consumers purchased from the Colonial Era to the Civil War. Our editorial department had been flooded with requests from users of our *Value of a Dollar* for the same type of information, just from an earlier time period. This new volume is just the answer – with pricing data from 1600 to 1859. Arranged into five-year chapters, each 5-year chapter includes a Historical Snapshot, Consumer Expenditures, Investments, Selected Income, Income/Standard Jobs, Food Basket, Standard Prices and Miscellany. There is also a section on Trends. This informative section charts the change in price over time and provides added detail on the reasons prices changed within the time period, including industry developments, changes in consumer attitudes and important historical facts. This fascinating survey will serve a wide range of research needs and will be useful in all high school, public and academic library reference collections.

"The Value of a Dollar: Colonial Era to the Civil War, 1600-1865 will find a happy audience among students, researchers, and general browsers. It offers a fascinating and detailed look at early American history from the viewpoint of everyday people trying to make ends meet. This title and the earlier publication, The Value of a Dollar, 1860-2004, complement each other very well, and readers will appreciate finding them side-by-side on the shelf." -Booklist

Hardcover ISBN 978-1-59237-094-8, 600 pages, $145.00 | Ebook ISBN 978-1-59237-169-3 www.gale.com/gvrl/partners/grey.htm

The Value of a Dollar 1860-2004, Third Edition

A guide to practical economy, *The Value of a Dollar* records the actual prices of thousands of items that consumers purchased from the Civil War to the present, along with facts about investment options and income opportunities. This brand new Third Edition boasts a brand new addition to each five-year chapter, a section on Trends. This informative section charts the change in price over time and provides added detail on the reasons prices changed within the time period, including industry developments, changes in consumer attitudes and important historical facts. Plus, a brand new chapter for 2000-2004 has been added. Each 5-year chapter includes a Historical Snapshot, Consumer Expenditures, Investments, Selected Income, Income/Standard Jobs, Food Basket, Standard Prices and Miscellany. This interesting and useful publication will be widely used in any reference collection.

"Business historians, reporters, writers and students will find this source... very helpful for historical research. Libraries will want to purchase it." –ARBA

Hardcover ISBN 978-1-59237-074-0, 600 pages, $145.00 | Ebook ISBN 978-1-59237-173-0 www.gale.com/gvrl/partners/grey.htm

Working Americans 1880-1999
Volume I: The Working Class, Volume II: The Middle Class, Volume III: The Upper Class

Each of the volumes in the *Working Americans* series focuses on a particular class of Americans, The Working Class, The Middle Class and The Upper Class over the last 120 years. Chapters in each volume focus on one decade and profile three to five families. Family Profiles include real data on Income & Job Descriptions, Selected Prices of the Times, Annual Income, Annual Budgets, Family Finances, Life at Work, Life at Home, Life in the Community, Working Conditions, Cost of Living, Amusements and much more. Each chapter also contains an Economic Profile with Average Wages of other Professions, a selection of Typical Pricing, Key Events & Inventions, News Profiles, Articles from Local Media and Illustrations. The *Working Americans* series captures the lifestyles of each of the classes from the last twelve decades, covers a vast array of occupations and ethnic backgrounds and travels the entire nation. These interesting and useful compilations of portraits of the American Working, Middle and Upper Classes during the last 120 years will be an important addition to any high school, public or academic library reference collection.

"These interesting, unique compilations of economic and social facts, figures and graphs will support multiple research needs. They will engage and enlighten patrons in high school, public and academic library collections." –Booklist

Volume I: The Working Class Hardcover ISBN 978-1-891482-81-6, 558 pages, $145.00 | Volume II: The Middle Class Hardcover ISBN 978-1-891482-72-4, 591 pages, $145.00 | Volume III: The Upper Class Hardcover ISBN 978-1-930956-38-4, 567 pages, $145.00 | Ebooks www.gale.com/gvrl/partners/grey.htm

Working Americans 1880-1999 Volume IV: Their Children

This Fourth Volume in the highly successful *Working Americans* series focuses on American children, decade by decade from 1880 to 1999. This interesting and useful volume introduces the reader to three children in each decade, one from each of the Working, Middle and Upper classes. Like the first three volumes in the series, the individual profiles are created from interviews, diaries, statistical studies, biographies and news reports. Profiles cover a broad range of ethnic backgrounds, geographic area and lifestyles – everything from an orphan in Memphis in 1882, following the Yellow Fever epidemic of 1878 to an eleven-year-old nephew of a beer baron and owner of the New York Yankees in New York City in 1921. Chapters also contain important supplementary materials including News Features as well as information on everything from Schools to Parks, Infectious Diseases to Childhood Fears along with Entertainment, Family Life and much more to provide an informative overview of the lifestyles of children from each decade. This interesting account of what life was like for Children in the Working, Middle and Upper Classes will be a welcome addition to the reference collection of any high school, public or academic library.

Hardcover ISBN 978-1-930956-35-3, 600 pages, $145.00 | Ebook ISBN 978-1-59237-166-2 www.gale.com/gvrl/partners/grey.htm

**To preview any of our Directories Risk-Free for 30 days, call (800) 562-2139 or fax (518) 789-0556
www.greyhouse.com books@greyhouse.com**

Working Americans 1880-2003 Volume V: Americans At War

Working Americans 1880-2003 Volume V: Americans At War is divided into 11 chapters, each covering a decade from 1880-2003 and examines the lives of Americans during the time of war, including declared conflicts, one-time military actions, protests, and preparations for war. Each decade includes several personal profiles, whether on the battlefield or on the homefront, that tell the stories of civilians, soldiers, and officers during the decade. The profiles examine: Life at Home; Life at Work; and Life in the Community. Each decade also includes an Economic Profile with statistical comparisons, a Historical Snapshot, News Profiles, local News Articles, and Illustrations that provide a solid historical background to the decade being examined. Profiles range widely not only geographically, but also emotionally, from that of a girl whose leg was torn off in a blast during WWI, to the boredom of being stationed in the Dakotas as the Indian Wars were drawing to a close. As in previous volumes of the *Working Americans* series, information is presented in narrative form, but hard facts and real-life situations back up each story. The basis of the profiles come from diaries, private print books, personal interviews, family histories, estate documents and magazine articles. For easy reference, *Working Americans 1880-2003 Volume V: Americans At War* includes an in-depth Subject Index. The Working Americans series has become an important reference for public libraries, academic libraries and high school libraries. This fifth volume will be a welcome addition to all of these types of reference collections.

Hardcover ISBN 978-1-59237-024-5, 600 pages, $145.00 | Ebook ISBN 978-1-59237-167-9 www.gale.com/gvrl/partners/grey.htm

Working Americans 1880-2005 Volume VI: Women at Work

Unlike any other volume in the *Working Americans* series, this Sixth Volume, is the first to focus on a particular gender of Americans. *Volume VI: Women at Work*, traces what life was like for working women from the 1860's to the present time. Beginning with the life of a maid in 1890 and a store clerk in 1900 and ending with the life and times of the modern working women, this text captures the struggle, strengths and changing perception of the American woman at work. Each chapter focuses on one decade and profiles three to five women with real data on Income & Job Descriptions, Selected Prices of the Times, Annual Income, Annual Budgets, Family Finances, Life at Work, Life at Home, Life in the Community, Working Conditions, Cost of Living, Amusements and much more. For even broader access to the events, economics and attitude towards women throughout the past 130 years, each chapter is supplemented with News Profiles, Articles from Local Media, Illustrations, Economic Profiles, Typical Pricing, Key Events, Inventions and more. This important volume illustrates what life was like for working women over time and allows the reader to develop an understanding of the changing role of women at work. These interesting and useful compilations of portraits of women at work will be an important addition to any high school, public or academic library reference collection.

Hardcover ISBN 978-1-59237-063-4, 600 pages, $145.00 | Ebook ISBN 978-1-59237-168-6 www.gale.com/gvrl/partners/grey.htm

Working Americans 1880-2005 Volume VII: Social Movements

Working Americans series, Volume VII: Social Movements explores how Americans sought and fought for change from the 1880s to the present time. Following the format of previous volumes in the Working Americans series, the text examines the lives of 34 individuals who have worked -- often behind the scenes --- to bring about change. Issues include topics as diverse as the Anti-smoking movement of 1901 to efforts by Native Americans to reassert their long lost rights. Along the way, the book will profile individuals brave enough to demand suffrage for Kansas women in 1912 or demand an end to lynching during a March on Washington in 1923. Each profile is enriched with real data on Income & Job Descriptions, Selected Prices of the Times, Annual Incomes & Budgets, Life at Work, Life at Home, Life in the Community, along with News Features, Key Events, and Illustrations. The depth of information contained in each profile allow the user to explore the private, financial and public lives of these subjects, deepening our understanding of how calls for change took place in our society. A must-purchase for the reference collections of high school libraries, public libraries and academic libraries.

Hardcover ISBN 978-1-59237-101-3, 600 pages, $145.00 | Ebook ISBN 978-1-59237-174-7 www.gale.com/gvrl/partners/grey.htm

Working Americans 1880-2005 Volume VIII: Immigrants

Working Americans 1880-2007 Volume VIII: Immigrants illustrates what life was like for families leaving their homeland and creating a new life in the United States. Each chapter covers one decade and introduces the reader to three immigrant families. Family profiles cover what life was like in their homeland, in their community in the United States, their home life, working conditions and so much more. As the reader moves through these pages, the families and individuals come to life, painting a picture of why they left their homeland, their experiences in setting roots in a new country, their struggles and triumphs, stretching from the 1800s to the present time. Profiles include a seven-year-old Swedish girl who meets her father for the first time at Ellis Island; a Chinese photographer's assistant; an Armenian who flees the genocide of his country to build Ford automobiles in Detroit; a 38-year-old German bachelor cigar maker who settles in Newark NJ, but contemplates tobacco farming in Virginia; a 19-year-old Irish domestic servant who is amazed at the easy life of American dogs; a 19-year-old Filipino who came to Hawaii against his parent's wishes to farm sugar cane; a French-Canadian who finds success as a boxer in Maine and many more. As in previous volumes, information is presented in narrative form, but hard facts and real-life situations back up each story. With the topic of immigration being so hotly debated in this country, this timely resource will prove to be a useful source for students, researchers, historians and library patrons to discover the issues facing immigrants in the United States. This title will be a useful addition to reference collections of public libraries, university libraries and high schools.

Hardcover ISBN 978-1-59237-197-6, 600 pages, $145.00 | Ebook ISBN 978-1-59237-232-4 www.gale.com/gvrl/partners/grey.htm

To preview any of our Directories Risk-Free for 30 days, call (800) 562-2139 or fax (518) 789-0556
www.greyhouse.com books@greyhouse.com

The Encyclopedia of Warrior Peoples & Fighting Groups

Many military groups throughout the world have excelled in their craft either by fortuitous circumstances, outstanding leadership, or intense training. This new second edition of *The Encyclopedia of Warrior Peoples and Fighting Groups* explores the origins and leadership of these outstanding combat forces, chronicles their conquests and accomplishments, examines the circumstances surrounding their decline or disbanding, and assesses their influence on the groups and methods of warfare that followed. Readers will encounter ferocious tribes, charismatic leaders, and daring militias, from ancient times to the present, including Amazons, Buffalo Soldiers, Green Berets, Iron Brigade, Kamikazes, Peoples of the Sea, Polish Winged Hussars, Teutonic Knights, and Texas Rangers. With over 100 alphabetical entries, numerous cross-references and illustrations, a comprehensive bibliography, and index, the *Encyclopedia of Warrior Peoples and Fighting Groups* is a valuable resource for readers seeking insight into the bold history of distinguished fighting forces.

"Especially useful for high school students, undergraduates, and general readers with an interest in military history." –Library Journal

Hardcover ISBN 978-1-59237-116-7, 660 pages, $135.00 | Ebook ISBN 978-1-59237-172-3 www.gale.com/gvrl/partners/grey.htm

The Encyclopedia of Invasions & Conquests, From the Ancient Times to the Present

This second edition of the popular *Encyclopedia of Invasions & Conquests*, a comprehensive guide to over 150 invasions, conquests, battles and occupations from ancient times to the present, takes readers on a journey that includes the Roman conquest of Britain, the Portuguese colonization of Brazil, and the Iraqi invasion of Kuwait, to name a few. New articles will explore the late 20th and 21st centuries, with a specific focus on recent conflicts in Afghanistan, Kuwait, Iraq, Yugoslavia, Grenada and Chechnya. In addition to covering the military aspects of invasions and conquests, entries cover some of the political, economic, and cultural aspects, for example, the effects of a conquest on the invade country's political and monetary system and in its language and religion. The entries on leaders – among them Sargon, Alexander the Great, William the Conqueror, and Adolf Hitler – deal with the people who sought to gain control, expand power, or exert religious or political influence over others through military means. Revised and updated for this second edition, entries are arranged alphabetically within historical periods. Each chapter provides a map to help readers locate key areas and geographical features, and bibliographical references appear at the end of each entry. Other useful features include cross-references, a cumulative bibliography and a comprehensive subject index. This authoritative, well-organized, lucidly written volume will prove invaluable for a variety of readers, including high school students, military historians, members of the armed forces, history buffs and hobbyists.

"Engaging writing, sensible organization, nice illustrations, interesting and obscure facts, and useful maps make this book a pleasure to read." –ARBA

Hardcover ISBN 978-1-59237-114-3, 598 pages, $135.00 | Ebook ISBN 978-1-59237-171-6 www.gale.com/gvrl/partners/grey.htm

Encyclopedia of Prisoners of War & Internment

This authoritative second edition provides a valuable overview of the history of prisoners of war and interned civilians, from earliest times to the present. Written by an international team of experts in the field of POW studies, this fascinating and thought-provoking volume includes entries on a wide range of subjects including the Crusades, Plains Indian Warfare, concentration camps, the two world wars, and famous POWs throughout history, as well as atrocities, escapes, and much more. Written in a clear and easily understandable style, this informative reference details over 350 entries, 30% larger than the first edition, that survey the history of prisoners of war and interned civilians from the earliest times to the present, with emphasis on the 19th and 20th centuries. Medical conditions, international law, exchanges of prisoners, organizations working on behalf of POWs, and trials associated with the treatment of captives are just some of the themes explored. Entries are arranged alphabetically, plus illustrations and maps are provided for easy reference. The text also includes an introduction, bibliography, appendix of selected documents, and end-of-entry reading suggestions. This one-of-a-kind reference will be a helpful addition to the reference collections of all public libraries, high schools, and university libraries and will prove invaluable to historians and military enthusiasts.

"Thorough and detailed yet accessible to the lay reader.
Of special interest to subject specialists and historians; recommended for public and academic libraries." - Library Journal

Hardcover ISBN 978-1-59237-120-4, 676 pages, $135.00 | Ebook ISBN 978-1-59237-170-9 www.gale.com/gvrl/partners/grey.htm

The Encyclopedia of Rural America: the Land & People

History, sociology, anthropology, and public policy are combined to deliver the encyclopedia destined to become the standard reference work in American rural studies. From irrigation and marriage to games and mental health, this encyclopedia is the first to explore the contemporary landscape of rural America, placed in historical perspective. With over 300 articles prepared by leading experts from across the nation, this timely encyclopedia documents and explains the major themes, concepts, industries, concerns, and everyday life of the people and land who make up rural America. Entries range from the industrial sector and government policy to arts and humanities and social and family concerns. Articles explore every aspect of life in rural America. *Encyclopedia of Rural America*, with its broad range of coverage, will appeal to high school and college students as well as graduate students, faculty, scholars, and people whose work pertains to rural areas.

"This exemplary encyclopedia is guaranteed to educate our
highly urban society about the uniqueness of rural America. Recommended for public and academic libraries." -Library Journal

Two Volumes, Hardcover, ISBN 978-1-59237-115-0, 800 pages, $195.00

To preview any of our Directories Risk-Free for 30 days, call (800) 562-2139 or fax (518) 789-0556
www.greyhouse.com books@greyhouse.com

The Religious Right, A Reference Handbook

Timely and unbiased, this third edition updates and expands its examination of the religious right and its influence on our government, citizens, society, and politics. From the fight to outlaw the teaching of Darwin's theory of evolution to the struggle to outlaw abortion, the religious right is continually exerting an influence on public policy. This text explores the influence of religion on legislation and society, while examining the alignment of the religious right with the political right. A historical survey of the movement highlights the shift to "hands-on" approach to politics and the struggle to present a unified front. The coverage offers a critical historical survey of the religious right movement, focusing on its increased involvement in the political arena, attempts to forge coalitions, and notable successes and failures. The text offers complete coverage of biographies of the men and women who have advanced the cause and an up to date chronology illuminate the movement's goals, including their accomplishments and failures. This edition offers an extensive update to all sections along with several brand new entries. Two new sections complement this third edition, a chapter on legal issues and court decisions and a chapter on demographic statistics and electoral patterns. To aid in further research, *The Religious Right*, offers an entire section of annotated listings of print and non-print resources, as well as of organizations affiliated with the religious right, and those opposing it. Comprehensive in its scope, this work offers easy-to-read, pertinent information for those seeking to understand the religious right and its evolving role in American society. A must for libraries of all sizes, university religion departments, activists, high schools and for those interested in the evolving role of the religious right.

" Recommended for all public and academic libraries." - Library Journal

Hardcover ISBN 978-1-59237-113-6, 600 pages, $135.00 | Ebook ISBN 978-1-59237-226-3 www.gale.com/gvrl/partners/grey.htm

From Suffrage to the Senate, America's Political Women

From Suffrage to the Senate is a comprehensive and valuable compendium of biographies of leading women in U.S. politics, past and present, and an examination of the wide range of women's movements. Up to date through 2006, this dynamically illustrated reference work explores American women's path to political power and social equality from the struggle for the right to vote and the abolition of slavery to the first African American woman in the U.S. Senate and beyond. This new edition includes over 150 new entries and a brand new section on trends and demographics of women in politics. The in-depth coverage also traces the political heritage of the abolition, labor, suffrage, temperance, and reproductive rights movements. The alphabetically arranged entries include biographies of every woman from across the political spectrum who has served in the U.S. House and Senate, along with women in the Judiciary and the U.S. Cabinet and, new to this edition, biographies of activists and political consultants. Bibliographical references follow each entry. For easy reference, a handy chronology is provided detailing 150 years of women's history. This up-to-date reference will be a must-purchase for women's studies departments, high schools and public libraries and will be a handy resource for those researching the key players in women's politics, past and present.

"An engaging tool that would be useful in high school, public, and academic libraries
looking for an overview of the political history of women in the US." –Booklist

Two Volumes, Hardcover ISBN 978-1-59237-117-4, 1,160 pages, $195.00 | Ebook ISBN 978-1-59237-227-0
www.gale.com/gvrl/partners/grey.htm

An African Biographical Dictionary

This landmark second edition is the only biographical dictionary to bring together, in one volume, cultural, social and political leaders – both historical and contemporary – of the sub-Saharan region. Over 800 biographical sketches of prominent Africans, as well as foreigners who have affected the continent's history, are featured, 150 more than the previous edition. The wide spectrum of leaders includes religious figures, writers, politicians, scientists, entertainers, sports personalities and more. Access to these fascinating individuals is provided in a user-friendly format. The biographies are arranged alphabetically, cross-referenced and indexed. Entries include the country or countries in which the person was significant and the commonly accepted dates of birth and death. Each biographical sketch is chronologically written; entries for cultural personalities add an evaluation of their work. This information is followed by a selection of references often found in university and public libraries, including autobiographies and principal biographical works. Appendixes list each individual by country and by field of accomplishment – rulers, musicians, explorers, missionaries, businessmen, physicists – nearly thirty categories in all. Another convenient appendix lists heads of state since independence by country. Up-to-date and representative of African societies as a whole, An African Biographical Dictionary provides a wealth of vital information for students of African culture and is an indispensable reference guide for anyone interested in African affairs.

"An unquestionable convenience to have these concise, informative biographies gathered into
one source, indexed, and analyzed by appendixes listing entrants by nation and occupational field." –Wilson Library Bulletin

Hardcover ISBN 978-1-59237-112-9, 667 pages, $135.00 | Ebook ISBN 978-1-59237-229-4 www.gale.com/gvrl/partners/grey.htm

American Environmental Leaders, From Colonial Times to the Present

A comprehensive and diverse award winning collection of biographies of the most important figures in American environmentalism. Few subjects arouse the passions the way the environment does. How will we feed an ever-increasing population and how can that food be made safe for consumption? Who decides how land is developed? How can environmental policies be made fair for everyone, including multiethnic groups, women, children, and the poor? *American Environmental Leaders* presents more than 350 biographies of men and women who have devoted their lives to studying, debating, and organizing these and other controversial issues over the last 200 years. In addition to the scientists who have analyzed how human actions affect nature, we are introduced to poets, landscape architects, presidents, painters, activists, even sanitation engineers, and others who have forever altered how we think about the environment. The easy to use A–Z format provides instant access to these fascinating individuals, and frequent cross references indicate others with whom individuals worked (and sometimes clashed). End of entry references provide users with a starting point for further research.

"Highly recommended for high school, academic, and public libraries needing environmental biographical information." –Library Journal/Starred Review

Two Volumes, Hardcover ISBN 978-1-59237-119-8, 900 pages $195.00 | Ebook ISBN 978-1-59237-230-0
www.gale.com/gvrl/partners/grey.htm

World Cultural Leaders of the Twentieth & Twenty-First Centuries

World Cultural Leaders of the Twentieth & Twenty-First Centuries is a window into the arts, performances, movements, and music that shaped the world's cultural development since 1900. A remarkable around-the-world look at one-hundred-plus years of cultural development through the eyes of those that set the stage and stayed to play. This second edition offers over 120 new biographies along with a complete update of existing biographies. To further aid the reader, a handy fold-out timeline traces important events in all six cultural categories from 1900 through the present time. Plus, a new section of detailed material and resources for 100 selected individuals is also new to this edition, with further data on museums, homesteads, websites, artwork and more. This remarkable compilation will answer a wide range of questions. Who was the originator of the term "documentary"? Which poet married the daughter of the famed novelist Thomas Mann in order to help her escape Nazi Germany? Which British writer served as an agent in Russia against the Bolsheviks before the 1917 revolution? A handy two-volume set that makes it easy to look up 450 worldwide cultural icons: novelists, poets, playwrights, painters, sculptors, architects, dancers, choreographers, actors, directors, filmmakers, singers, composers, and musicians. *World Cultural Leaders of the Twentieth & Twenty-First Centuries* provides entries (many of them illustrated) covering the person's works, achievements, and professional career in a thorough essay and offers interesting facts and statistics. Entries are fully cross-referenced so that readers can learn how various individuals influenced others. An index of leaders by occupation, a useful glossary and a thorough general index complete the coverage. This remarkable resource will be an important acquisition for the reference collections of public libraries, university libraries and high schools.

"Fills a need for handy, concise information on a wide array of international cultural figures."-ARBA

Two Volumes, Hardcover ISBN 978-1-59237-118-1, 900 pages, $195.00 | Ebook ISBN 978-1-59237-231-7
www.gale.com/gvrl/partners/grey.htm

Political Corruption in America: An Encyclopedia of Scandals, Power, and Greed

The complete scandal-filled history of American political corruption, focusing on the infamous people and cases, as well as society's electoral and judicial reactions. Since colonial times, there has been no shortage of politicians willing to take a bribe, skirt campaign finance laws, or act in their own interests. Corruption like the Whiskey Ring, Watergate, and Whitewater cases dominate American life, making political scandal a leading U.S. industry. From judges to senators, presidents to mayors, *Political Corruption in America* discusses the infamous people throughout history who have been accused of and implicated in crooked behavior. In this new second edition, more than 250 A–Z entries explore the people, crimes, investigations, and court cases behind 200 years of American political scandals. This unbiased volume also delves into the issues surrounding Koreagate, the Chinese campaign scandal, and other ethical lapses. Relevant statutes and terms, including the Independent Counsel Statute and impeachment as a tool of political punishment, are examined as well. Students, scholars, and other readers interested in American history, political science, and ethics will appreciate this survey of a wide range of corrupting influences. This title focuses on how politicians from all parties have fallen because of their greed and hubris, and how society has used electoral and judicial means against those who tested the accepted standards of political conduct. A full range of illustrations including political cartoons, photos of key figures such as Abe Fortas and Archibald Cox, graphs of presidential pardons, and tables showing the number of expulsions and censures in both the House and Senate round out the text. In addition, a comprehensive chronology of major political scandals in U.S. history from colonial times until the present. For further reading, an extensive bibliography lists sources including archival letters, newspapers, and private manuscript collections from the United States and Great Britain. With its comprehensive coverage of this interesting topic, *Political Corruption in America: An Encyclopedia of Scandals, Power, and Greed* will prove to be a useful addition to the reference collections of all public libraries, university libraries, history collections, political science collections and high schools.

"...this encyclopedia is a useful contribution to the field. Highly recommended." - CHOICE
"Political Corruption should be useful in most academic, high school, and public libraries." Booklist

Hardcover ISBN 978-1-59237-297-3, 500 pages, $135.00

**To preview any of our Directories Risk-Free for 30 days, call (800) 562-2139 or fax (518) 789-0556
www.greyhouse.com books@greyhouse.com**

Religion and Law: A Dictionary

This informative, easy-to-use reference work covers a wide range of legal issues that affect the roles of religion and law in American society. Extensive A–Z entries provide coverage of key court decisions, case studies, concepts, individuals, religious groups, organizations, and agencies shaping religion and law in today's society. This *Dictionary* focuses on topics involved with the constitutional theory and interpretation of religion and the law; terms providing a historical explanation of the ways in which America's ever increasing ethnic and religious diversity contributed to our current understanding of the mandates of the First and Fourteenth Amendments; terms and concepts describing the development of religion clause jurisprudence; an analytical examination of the distinct vocabulary used in this area of the law; the means by which American courts have attempted to balance religious liberty against other important individual and social interests in a wide variety of physical and regulatory environments, including the classroom, the workplace, the courtroom, religious group organization and structure, taxation, the clash of "secular" and "religious" values, and the relationship of the generalized idea of individual autonomy of the specific concept of religious liberty. Important legislation and legal cases affecting religion and society are thoroughly covered in this timely volume, including a detailed Table of Cases and Table of Statutes for more detailed research. A guide to further reading and an index are also included. This useful resource will be an important acquisition for the reference collections of all public libraries, university libraries, religion reference collections and high schools.

Hardcover ISBN 978-1-59237-298-0, 500 pages, $135.00

Human Rights in the United States: A Dictionary and Documents

This two volume set offers easy to grasp explanations of the basic concepts, laws, and case law in the field, with emphasis on human rights in the historical, political, and legal experience of the United States. Human rights is a term not fully understood by many Americans. Addressing this gap, the new second edition of *Human Rights in the United States: A Dictionary and Documents* offers a comprehensive introduction that places the history of human rights in the United States in an international context. It surveys the legal protection of human dignity in the United States, examines the sources of human rights norms, cites key legal cases, explains the role of international governmental and non-governmental organizations, and charts global, regional, and U.N. human rights measures. Over 240 dictionary entries of human rights terms are detailed—ranging from asylum and cultural relativism to hate crimes and torture. Each entry discusses the significance of the term, gives examples, and cites appropriate documents and court decisions. In addition, a Documents section is provided that contains 59 conventions, treaties, and protocols related to the most up to date international action on ethnic cleansing; freedom of expression and religion; violence against women; and much more. A bibliography, extensive glossary, and comprehensive index round out this indispensable volume. This comprehensive, timely volume is a must for large public libraries, university libraries and social science departments, along with high school libraries.

> *"...invaluable for anyone interested in human rights issues ... highly recommended for all reference collections."*
> *- American Reference Books Annual*

Two Volumes, Hardcover ISBN 978-1-59237-290-4, 750 pages, $225.00

The Comparative Guide to American Elementary & Secondary Schools, 2008

The only guide of its kind, this award winning compilation offers a snapshot profile of every public school district in the United States serving 1,500 or more students – more than 5,900 districts are covered. Organized alphabetically by district within state, each chapter begins with a Statistical Overview of the state. Each district listing includes contact information (name, address, phone number and web site) plus Grades Served, the Numbers of Students and Teachers and the Number of Regular, Special Education, Alternative and Vocational Schools in the district along with statistics on Student/Classroom Teacher Ratios, Drop Out Rates, Ethnicity, the Numbers of Librarians and Guidance Counselors and District Expenditures per student. As an added bonus, *The Comparative Guide to American Elementary and Secondary Schools* provides important ranking tables, both by state and nationally, for each data element. For easy navigation through this wealth of information, this handbook contains a useful City Index that lists all districts that operate schools within a city. These important comparative statistics are necessary for anyone considering relocation or doing comparative research on their own district and would be a perfect acquisition for any public library or school district library.

"This straightforward guide is an easy way to find general information.
Valuable for academic and large public library collections." –ARBA

Softcover ISBN 978-1-59237-223-2, 2,400 pages, $125.00 | Ebook ISBN 978-1-59237-238-6 www.gale.com/gvrl/partners/grey.htm

The Complete Learning Disabilities Directory, 2008

The Complete Learning Disabilities Directory is the most comprehensive database of Programs, Services, Curriculum Materials, Professional Meetings & Resources, Camps, Newsletters and Support Groups for teachers, students and families concerned with learning disabilities. This information-packed directory includes information about Associations & Organizations, Schools, Colleges & Testing Materials, Government Agencies, Legal Resources and much more. For quick, easy access to information, this directory contains four indexes: Entry Name Index, Subject Index and Geographic Index. With every passing year, the field of learning disabilities attracts more attention and the network of caring, committed and knowledgeable professionals grows every day. This directory is an invaluable research tool for these parents, students and professionals.

"Due to its wealth and depth of coverage, parents, teachers and others… should find this an invaluable resource." -Booklist

Softcover ISBN 978-1-59237-207-2, 900 pages, $145.00 | Online Database $195.00 | Online Database & Directory Combo $280.00

Educators Resource Directory, 2007/08

Educators Resource Directory is a comprehensive resource that provides the educational professional with thousands of resources and statistical data for professional development. This directory saves hours of research time by providing immediate access to Associations & Organizations, Conferences & Trade Shows, Educational Research Centers, Employment Opportunities & Teaching Abroad, School Library Services, Scholarships, Financial Resources, Professional Consultants, Computer Software & Testing Resources and much more. Plus, this comprehensive directory also includes a section on Statistics and Rankings with over 100 tables, including statistics on Average Teacher Salaries, SAT/ACT scores, Revenues & Expenditures and more. These important statistics will allow the user to see how their school rates among others, make relocation decisions and so much more. For quick access to information, this directory contains four indexes: Entry & Publisher Index, Geographic Index, a Subject & Grade Index and Web Sites Index. *Educators Resource Directory* will be a well-used addition to the reference collection of any school district, education department or public library.

"Recommended for all collections that serve elementary and secondary school professionals." –Choice

Softcover ISBN 978-1-59237-179-2, 800 pages, $145.00 | Online Database $195.00 | Online Database & Directory Combo $280.00

Profiles of New York | Profiles of Florida | Profiles of Texas | Profiles of Illinois | Profiles of Michigan | Profiles of Ohio | Profiles of New Jersey | Profiles of Massachusetts | Profiles of Pennsylvania | Profiles of Wisconsin | Profiles of Connecticut & Rhode Island | Profiles of Indiana | Profiles of North Carolina & South Carolina | Profiles of Virginia | Profiles of California

The careful layout gives the user an easy-to-read snapshot of every single place and county in the state, from the biggest metropolis to the smallest unincorporated hamlet. The richness of each place or county profile is astounding in its depth, from history to weather, all packed in an easy-to-navigate, compact format. Each profile contains data on History, Geography, Climate, Population, Vital Statistics, Economy, Income, Taxes, Education, Housing, Health & Environment, Public Safety, Newspapers, Transportation, Presidential Election Results, Information Contacts and Chambers of Commerce. As an added bonus, there is a section on Selected Statistics, where data from the 100 largest towns and cities is arranged into easy-to-use charts. Each of 22 different data points has its own two-page spread with the cities listed in alpha order so researchers can easily compare and rank cities. A remarkable compilation that offers overviews and insights into each corner of the state, each volume goes beyond Census statistics, beyond metro area coverage, beyond the 100 best places to live. Drawn from official census information, other government statistics and original research, you will have at your fingertips data that's available nowhere else in one single source.

"The publisher claims that this is the 'most comprehensive portrait of the state of Florida ever published,' and this reviewer is inclined to believe it...Recommended. All levels." –Choice on Profiles of Florida

Each Profiles of... title ranges from 400-800 pages, priced at $149.00 each

America's Top-Rated Cities, 2008

America's Top-Rated Cities provides current, comprehensive statistical information and other essential data in one easy-to-use source on the 100 "top" cities that have been cited as the best for business and living in the U.S. This handbook allows readers to see, at a glance, a concise social, business, economic, demographic and environmental profile of each city, including brief evaluative comments. In addition to detailed data on Cost of Living, Finances, Real Estate, Education, Major Employers, Media, Crime and Climate, city reports now include Housing Vacancies, Tax Audits, Bankruptcy, Presidential Election Results and more. This outstanding source of information will be widely used in any reference collection.

"The only source of its kind that brings together all of this information into one easy-to-use source. It will be beneficial to many business and public libraries." –ARBA

Four Volumes, Softcover ISBN 978-1-59237-349-9, 2,500 pages, $195.00 | Ebook ISBN 978-1-59237-233-1
www.gale.com/gvrl/partners/grey.htm

America's Top-Rated Smaller Cities, 2008/09

A perfect companion to *America's Top-Rated Cities*, *America's Top-Rated Smaller Cities* provides current, comprehensive business and living profiles of smaller cities (population 25,000-99,999) that have been cited as the best for business and living in the United States. Sixty cities make up this 2004 edition of America's Top-Rated Smaller Cities, all are top-ranked by Population Growth, Median Income, Unemployment Rate and Crime Rate. City reports reflect the most current data available on a wide-range of statistics, including Employment & Earnings, Household Income, Unemployment Rate, Population Characteristics, Taxes, Cost of Living, Education, Health Care, Public Safety, Recreation, Media, Air & Water Quality and much more. Plus, each city report contains a Background of the City, and an Overview of the State Finances. *America's Top-Rated Smaller Cities* offers a reliable, one-stop source for statistical data that, before now, could only be found scattered in hundreds of sources. This volume is designed for a wide range of readers: individuals considering relocating a residence or business; professionals considering expanding their business or changing careers; general and market researchers; real estate consultants; human resource personnel; urban planners and investors.

"Provides current, comprehensive statistical information in one easy-to-use source... Recommended for public and academic libraries and specialized collections." –Library Journal

Two Volumes, Softcover ISBN 978-1-59237-284-3, 1,100 pages, $195.00 | Ebook ISBN 978-1-59237-234-8
www.gale.com/gvrl/partners/grey.htm

Profiles of America: Facts, Figures & Statistics for Every Populated Place in the United States

Profiles of America is the only source that pulls together, in one place, statistical, historical and descriptive information about every place in the United States in an easy-to-use format. This award winning reference set, now in its second edition, compiles statistics and data from over 20 different sources – the latest census information has been included along with more than nine brand new statistical topics. This Four-Volume Set details over 40,000 places, from the biggest metropolis to the smallest unincorporated hamlet, and provides statistical details and information on over 50 different topics including Geography, Climate, Population, Vital Statistics, Economy, Income, Taxes, Education, Housing, Health & Environment, Public Safety, Newspapers, Transportation, Presidential Election Results and Information Contacts or Chambers of Commerce. Profiles are arranged, for ease-of-use, by state and then by county. Each county begins with a County-Wide Overview and is followed by information for each Community in that particular county. The Community Profiles within the county are arranged alphabetically. *Profiles of America* is a virtual snapshot of America at your fingertips and a unique compilation of information that will be widely used in any reference collection.

A Library Journal Best Reference Book *"An outstanding compilation." –Library Journal*

Four Volumes, Softcover ISBN 978-1-891482-80-9, 10,000 pages, $595.00

To preview any of our Directories Risk-Free for 30 days, call (800) 562-2139 or fax (518) 789-0556
www.greyhouse.com books@greyhouse.com

The Comparative Guide to American Suburbs, 2007/08

The Comparative Guide to American Suburbs is a one-stop source for Statistics on the 2,000+ suburban communities surrounding the 50 largest metropolitan areas – their population characteristics, income levels, economy, school system and important data on how they compare to one another. Organized into 50 Metropolitan Area chapters, each chapter contains an overview of the Metropolitan Area, a detailed Map followed by a comprehensive Statistical Profile of each Suburban Community, including Contact Information, Physical Characteristics, Population Characteristics, Income, Economy, Unemployment Rate, Cost of Living, Education, Chambers of Commerce and more. Next, statistical data is sorted into Ranking Tables that rank the suburbs by twenty different criteria, including Population, Per Capita Income, Unemployment Rate, Crime Rate, Cost of Living and more. *The Comparative Guide to American Suburbs* is the best source for locating data on suburbs. Those looking to relocate, as well as those doing preliminary market research, will find this an invaluable timesaving resource.

> *"Public and academic libraries will find this compilation useful...The work draws together figures from many sources and will be especially helpful for job relocation decisions." – Booklist*

Softcover ISBN 978-1-59237-180-8, 1,700 pages, $130.00 | Ebook ISBN 978-1-59237-235-5 www.gale.com/gvrl/partners/grey.htm

The American Tally: Statistics & Comparative Rankings for U.S. Cities with Populations over 10,000

This important statistical handbook compiles, all in one place, comparative statistics on all U.S. cities and towns with a 10,000+ population. *The American Tally* provides statistical details on over 4,000 cities and towns and profiles how they compare with one another in Population Characteristics, Education, Language & Immigration, Income & Employment and Housing. Each section begins with an alphabetical listing of cities by state, allowing for quick access to both the statistics and relative rankings of any city. Next, the highest and lowest cities are listed in each statistic. These important, informative lists provide quick reference to which cities are at both extremes of the spectrum for each statistic. Unlike any other reference, *The American Tally* provides quick, easy access to comparative statistics – a must-have for any reference collection.

> *"A solid library reference." -Bookwatch*

Softcover ISBN 978-1-930956-29-2, 500 pages, $125.00 | Ebook ISBN 978-1-59237-241-6 www.gale.com/gvrl/partners/grey.htm

The Asian Databook: Statistics for all US Counties & Cities with Over 10,000 Population

This is the first-ever resource that compiles statistics and rankings on the US Asian population. *The Asian Databook* presents over 20 statistical data points for each city and county, arranged alphabetically by state, then alphabetically by place name. Data reported for each place includes Population, Languages Spoken at Home, Foreign-Born, Educational Attainment, Income Figures, Poverty Status, Homeownership, Home Values & Rent, and more. Next, in the Rankings Section, the top 75 places are listed for each data element. These easy-to-access ranking tables allow the user to quickly determine trends and population characteristics. This kind of comparative data can not be found elsewhere, in print or on the web, in a format that's as easy-to-use or more concise. A useful resource for those searching for demographics data, career search and relocation information and also for market research. With data ranging from Ancestry to Education, *The Asian Databook* presents a useful compilation of information that will be a much-needed resource in the reference collection of any public or academic library along with the marketing collection of any company whose primary focus in on the Asian population.

> *"This useful resource will help those searching for demographics data, and market research or relocation information… Accurate and clearly laid out, the publication is recommended for large public library and research collections." -Booklist*

Softcover ISBN 978-1-59237-044-3, 1,000 pages, $150.00

The Hispanic Databook: Statistics for all US Counties & Cities with Over 10,000 Population

Previously published by Toucan Valley Publications, this second edition has been completely updated with figures from the latest census and has been broadly expanded to include dozens of new data elements and a brand new Rankings section. The Hispanic population in the United States has increased over 42% in the last 10 years and accounts for 12.5% of the total US population. For ease-of-use, *The Hispanic Databook* presents over 20 statistical data points for each city and county, arranged alphabetically by state, then alphabetically by place name. Data reported for each place includes Population, Languages Spoken at Home, Foreign-Born, Educational Attainment, Income Figures, Poverty Status, Homeownership, Home Values & Rent, and more. Next, in the Rankings Section, the top 75 places are listed for each data element. These easy-to-access ranking tables allow the user to quickly determine trends and population characteristics. This kind of comparative data can not be found elsewhere, in print or on the web, in a format that's as easy-to-use or more concise. A useful resource for those searching for demographics data, career search and relocation information and also for market research. With data ranging from Ancestry to Education, *The Hispanic Databook* presents a useful compilation of information that will be a much-needed resource in the reference collection of any public or academic library along with the marketing collection of any company whose primary focus in on the Hispanic population.

> *"This accurate, clearly presented volume of selected Hispanic demographics is recommended for large public libraries and research collections."-Library Journal*

Softcover ISBN 978-1-59237-008-5, 1,000 pages, $150.00

Ancestry in America: A Comparative Guide to Over 200 Ethnic Backgrounds

This brand new reference work pulls together thousands of comparative statistics on the Ethnic Backgrounds of all populated places in the United States with populations over 10,000. Never before has this kind of information been reported in a single volume. Section One, Statistics by Place, is made up of a list of over 200 ancestry and race categories arranged alphabetically by each of the 5,000 different places with populations over 10,000. The population number of the ancestry group in that city or town is provided along with the percent that group represents of the total population. This informative city-by-city section allows the user to quickly and easily explore the ethnic makeup of all major population bases in the United States. Section Two, Comparative Rankings, contains three tables for each ethnicity and race. In the first table, the top 150 populated places are ranked by population number for that particular ancestry group, regardless of population. In the second table, the top 150 populated places are ranked by the percent of the total population for that ancestry group. In the third table, those top 150 populated places with 10,000 population are ranked by population number for each ancestry group. These easy-to-navigate tables allow users to see ancestry population patterns and make city-by-city comparisons as well. This brand new, information-packed resource will serve a wide-range or research requests for demographics, population characteristics, relocation information and much more. *Ancestry in America: A Comparative Guide to Over 200 Ethnic Backgrounds* will be an important acquisition to all reference collections.

"This compilation will serve a wide range of research requests for population characteristics ... it offers much more detail than other sources." –Booklist

Softcover ISBN 978-1-59237-029-0, 1,500 pages, $225.00

Weather America, A Thirty-Year Summary of Statistical Weather Data and Rankings

This valuable resource provides extensive climatological data for over 4,000 National and Cooperative Weather Stations throughout the United States. Weather America begins with a new Major Storms section that details major storm events of the nation and a National Rankings section that details rankings for several data elements, such as Maximum Temperature and Precipitation. The main body of Weather America is organized into 50 state sections. Each section provides a Data Table on each Weather Station, organized alphabetically, that provides statistics on Maximum and Minimum Temperatures, Precipitation, Snowfall, Extreme Temperatures, Foggy Days, Humidity and more. State sections contain two brand new features in this edition – a City Index and a narrative Description of the climatic conditions of the state. Each section also includes a revised Map of the State that includes not only weather stations, but cities and towns.

"Best Reference Book of the Year." –Library Journal

Softcover ISBN 978-1-891482-29-8, 2,013 pages, $175.00 | Ebook ISBN 978-1-59237-237-9 www.gale.com/gvrl/partners/grey.htm

Crime in America's Top-Rated Cities

This volume includes over 20 years of crime statistics in all major crime categories: violent crimes, property crimes and total crime. *Crime in America's Top-Rated Cities* is conveniently arranged by city and covers 76 top-rated cities. Crime in America's Top-Rated Cities offers details that compare the number of crimes and crime rates for the city, suburbs and metro area along with national crime trends for violent, property and total crimes. Also, this handbook contains important information and statistics on Anti-Crime Programs, Crime Risk, Hate Crimes, Illegal Drugs, Law Enforcement, Correctional Facilities, Death Penalty Laws and much more. A much-needed resource for people who are relocating, business professionals, general researchers, the press, law enforcement officials and students of criminal justice.

"Data is easy to access and will save hours of searching." –Global Enforcement Review

Softcover ISBN 978-1-891482-84-7, 832 pages, $155.00

The Complete Directory for People with Disabilities, 2008

A wealth of information, now in one comprehensive sourcebook. Completely updated, this edition contains more information than ever before, including thousands of new entries and enhancements to existing entries and thousands of additional web sites and e-mail addresses. This up-to-date directory is the most comprehensive resource available for people with disabilities, detailing Independent Living Centers, Rehabilitation Facilities, State & Federal Agencies, Associations, Support Groups, Periodicals & Books, Assistive Devices, Employment & Education Programs, Camps and Travel Groups. Each year, more libraries, schools, colleges, hospitals, rehabilitation centers and individuals add *The Complete Directory for People with Disabilities* to their collections, making sure that this information is readily available to the families, individuals and professionals who can benefit most from the amazing wealth of resources cataloged here.

"No other reference tool exists to meet the special needs of the disabled in one convenient resource for information." –Library Journal

Softcover ISBN 978-1-59237-194-5, 1,200 pages, $165.00 | Online Database $215.00 | Online Database & Directory Combo $300.00

The Complete Learning Disabilities Directory, 2008

The Complete Learning Disabilities Directory is the most comprehensive database of Programs, Services, Curriculum Materials, Professional Meetings & Resources, Camps, Newsletters and Support Groups for teachers, students and families concerned with learning disabilities. This information-packed directory includes information about Associations & Organizations, Schools, Colleges & Testing Materials, Government Agencies, Legal Resources and much more. For quick, easy access to information, this directory contains four indexes: Entry Name Index, Subject Index and Geographic Index. With every passing year, the field of learning disabilities attracts more attention and the network of caring, committed and knowledgeable professionals grows every day. This directory is an invaluable research tool for these parents, students and professionals.

"Due to its wealth and depth of coverage, parents, teachers and others... should find this an invaluable resource." -Booklist

Softcover ISBN 978-1-59237-207-2, 900 pages, $145.00 | Online Database $195.00 | Online Database & Directory Combo $280.00

The Complete Directory for People with Chronic Illness, 2007/08

Thousands of hours of research have gone into this completely updated edition – several new chapters have been added along with thousands of new entries and enhancements to existing entries. Plus, each chronic illness chapter has been reviewed by a medical expert in the field. This widely-hailed directory is structured around the 90 most prevalent chronic illnesses – from Asthma to Cancer to Wilson's Disease – and provides a comprehensive overview of the support services and information resources available for people diagnosed with a chronic illness. Each chronic illness has its own chapter and contains a brief description in layman's language, followed by important resources for National & Local Organizations, State Agencies, Newsletters, Books & Periodicals, Libraries & Research Centers, Support Groups & Hotlines, Web Sites and much more. This directory is an important resource for health care professionals, the collections of hospital and health care libraries, as well as an invaluable tool for people with a chronic illness and their support network.

"A must purchase for all hospital and health care libraries and is strongly recommended for all public library reference departments." –ARBA

Softcover ISBN 978-1-59237-183-9, 1,200 pages, $165.00 | Online Database $215.00 | Online Database & Directory Combo $300.00

The Complete Mental Health Directory, 2008/09

This is the most comprehensive resource covering the field of behavioral health, with critical information for both the layman and the mental health professional. For the layman, this directory offers understandable descriptions of 25 Mental Health Disorders as well as detailed information on Associations, Media, Support Groups and Mental Health Facilities. For the professional, The Complete Mental Health Directory offers critical and comprehensive information on Managed Care Organizations, Information Systems, Government Agencies and Provider Organizations. This comprehensive volume of needed information will be widely used in any reference collection.

"... the strength of this directory is that it consolidates widely dispersed information into a single volume." –Booklist

Softcover ISBN 978-1-59237-285-0, 800 pages, $165.00 | Online Database $215.00 | Online & Directory Combo $300.00

The Comparative Guide to American Hospitals, Second Edition

This new second edition compares all of the nation's hospitals by 24 measures of quality in the treatment of heart attack, heart failure, pneumonia, and, new to this edition, surgical procedures and pregnancy care. Plus, this second edition is now available in regional volumes, to make locating information about hospitals in your area quicker and easier than ever before. The Comparative Guide to American Hospitals provides a snapshot profile of each of the nations 4,200+ hospitals. These informative profiles illustrate how the hospital rates when providing 24 different treatments within four broad categories: Heart Attack Care, Heart Failure Care, Surgical Infection Prevention (NEW), and Pregnancy Care measures (NEW). Each profile includes the raw percentage for that hospital, the state average, the US average and data on the top hospital. For easy access to contact information, each profile includes the hospital's address, phone and fax numbers, email and web addresses, type and accreditation along with 5 top key administrations. These profiles will allow the user to quickly identify the quality of the hospital and have the necessary information at their fingertips to make contact with that hospital. Most importantly, *The Comparative Guide to American Hospitals* provides easy-to-use Regional State by State Statistical Summary Tables for each of the data elements to allow the user to quickly locate hospitals with the best level of service. Plus, a new 30-Day Mortality Chart, Glossary of Terms and Regional Hospital Profile Index make this a must-have source. This new, expanded edition will be a must for the reference collection at all public, medical and academic libraries.

> *"These data will help those with heart conditions and pneumonia make informed decisions about their healthcare and encourage hospitals to improve the quality of care they provide. Large medical, hospital, and public libraries are most likely to benefit from this weighty resource."*-Library Journal

Four Volumes Softcover ISBN 978-1-59237-182-2, 3,500 pages, $325.00 | Regional Volumes $135.00 |
Ebook ISBN 978-1-59237-239-3 www.gale.com/gvrl/partners/grey.htm

Older Americans Information Directory, 2007

Completely updated for 2007, this sixth edition has been completely revised and now contains 1,000 new listings, over 8,000 updates to existing listings and over 3,000 brand new e-mail addresses and web sites. You'll find important resources for Older Americans including National, Regional, State & Local Organizations, Government Agencies, Research Centers, Libraries & Information Centers, Legal Resources, Discount Travel Information, Continuing Education Programs, Disability Aids & Assistive Devices, Health, Print Media and Electronic Media. Three indexes: Entry Index, Subject Index and Geographic Index make it easy to find just the right source of information. This comprehensive guide to resources for Older Americans will be a welcome addition to any reference collection.

> *"Highly recommended for academic, public, health science and consumer libraries..."* –Choice

1,200 pages; Softcover ISBN 978-1-59237-136-5, $165.00 | Online Database $215.00 | Online Database & Directory Combo $300.00

The Complete Directory for Pediatric Disorders, 2008

This important directory provides parents and caregivers with information about Pediatric Conditions, Disorders, Diseases and Disabilities, including Blood Disorders, Bone & Spinal Disorders, Brain Defects & Abnormalities, Chromosomal Disorders, Congenital Heart Defects, Movement Disorders, Neuromuscular Disorders and Pediatric Tumors & Cancers. This carefully written directory offers: understandable Descriptions of 15 major bodily systems; Descriptions of more than 200 Disorders and a Resources Section, detailing National Agencies & Associations, State Associations, Online Services, Libraries & Resource Centers, Research Centers, Support Groups & Hotlines, Camps, Books and Periodicals. This resource will provide immediate access to information crucial to families and caregivers when coping with children's illnesses.

> *"Recommended for public and consumer health libraries."* –Library Journal

Softcover ISBN 978-1-59237-150-1, 1,200 pages, $165.00 | Online Database $215.00 | Online Database & Directory Combo $300.00

The Directory of Drug & Alcohol Residential Rehabilitation Facilities

This brand new directory is the first-ever resource to bring together, all in one place, data on the thousands of drug and alcohol residential rehabilitation facilities in the United States. The Directory of Drug & Alcohol Residential Rehabilitation Facilities covers over 1,000 facilities, with detailed contact information for each one, including mailing address, phone and fax numbers, email addresses and web sites, mission statement, type of treatment programs, cost, average length of stay, numbers of residents and counselors, accreditation, insurance plans accepted, type of environment, religious affiliation, education components and much more. It also contains a helpful chapter on General Resources that provides contact information for Associations, Print & Electronic Media, Support Groups and Conferences. Multiple indexes allow the user to pinpoint the facilities that meet very specific criteria. This time-saving tool is what so many counselors, parents and medical professionals have been asking for. *The Directory of Drug & Alcohol Residential Rehabilitation Facilities* will be a helpful tool in locating the right source for treatment for a wide range of individuals. This comprehensive directory will be an important acquisition for all reference collections: public and academic libraries, case managers, social workers, state agencies and many more.

> *"This is an excellent, much needed directory that fills an important gap..."* –Booklist

Softcover ISBN 978-1-59237-031-3, 300 pages, $135.00

**To preview any of our Directories Risk-Free for 30 days, call (800) 562-2139 or fax (518) 789-0556
www.greyhouse.com books@greyhouse.com**

The Directory of Hospital Personnel, 2008

The Directory of Hospital Personnel is the best resource you can have at your fingertips when researching or marketing a product or service to the hospital market. A "Who's Who" of the hospital universe, this directory puts you in touch with over 150,000 key decision-makers. With 100% verification of data you can rest assured that you will reach the right person with just one call. Every hospital in the U.S. is profiled, listed alphabetically by city within state. Plus, three easy-to-use, cross-referenced indexes put the facts at your fingertips faster and more easily than any other directory: Hospital Name Index, Bed Size Index and Personnel Index. *The Directory of Hospital Personnel* is the only complete source for key hospital decision-makers by name. Whether you want to define or restructure sales territories... locate hospitals with the purchasing power to accept your proposals... keep track of important contacts or colleagues... or find information on which insurance plans are accepted, *The Directory of Hospital Personnel* gives you the information you need – easily, efficiently, effectively and accurately.

"Recommended for college, university and medical libraries." -ARBA

Softcover ISBN 978-1-59237-286-7, 2,500 pages, $325.00 | Online Database $545.00 | Online Database & Directory Combo, $650.00

The Directory of Health Care Group Purchasing Organizations, 2008

This comprehensive directory provides the important data you need to get in touch with over 800 Group Purchasing Organizations. By providing in-depth information on this growing market and its members, *The Directory of Health Care Group Purchasing Organizations* fills a major need for the most accurate and comprehensive information on over 800 GPOs – Mailing Address, Phone & Fax Numbers, E-mail Addresses, Key Contacts, Purchasing Agents, Group Descriptions, Membership Categorization, Standard Vendor Proposal Requirements, Membership Fees & Terms, Expanded Services, Total Member Beds & Outpatient Visits represented and more. Five Indexes provide a number of ways to locate the right GPO: Alphabetical Index, Expanded Services Index, Organization Type Index, Geographic Index and Member Institution Index. With its comprehensive and detailed information on each purchasing organization, *The Directory of Health Care Group Purchasing Organizations* is the go-to source for anyone looking to target this market.

"The information is clearly arranged and easy to access...recommended for those needing this very specialized information." –ARBA

1,000 pages; Softcover ISBN 978-1-59237-287-4, $325.00 | Online Database, $650.00 | Online Database & Directory Combo, $750.00

The HMO/PPO Directory, 2008

The HMO/PPO Directory is a comprehensive source that provides detailed information about Health Maintenance Organizations and Preferred Provider Organizations nationwide. This comprehensive directory details more information about more managed health care organizations than ever before. Over 1,100 HMOs, PPOs, Medicare Advantage Plans and affiliated companies are listed, arranged alphabetically by state. Detailed listings include Key Contact Information, Prescription Drug Benefits, Enrollment, Geographical Areas served, Affiliated Physicians & Hospitals, Federal Qualifications, Status, Year Founded, Managed Care Partners, Employer References, Fees & Payment Information and more. Plus, five years of historical information is included related to Revenues, Net Income, Medical Loss Ratios, Membership Enrollment and Number of Patient Complaints. Five easy-to-use, cross-referenced indexes will put this vast array of information at your fingertips immediately: HMO Index, PPO Index, Other Providers Index, Personnel Index and Enrollment Index. *The HMO/PPO Directory* provides the most comprehensive data on the most companies available on the market place today.

"Helpful to individuals requesting certain HMO/PPO issues such as co-payment costs, subscription costs and patient complaints. Individuals concerned (or those with questions) about their insurance may find this text to be of use to them." -ARBA

Softcover ISBN 978-1-59237-204-1, 600 pages, $325.00 | Online Database, $495.00 | Online Database & Directory Combo, $600.00

Medical Device Register, 2008

The only one-stop resource of every medical supplier licensed to sell products in the US. This award-winning directory offers immediate access to over 13,000 companies - and more than 65,000 products – in two information-packed volumes. This comprehensive resource saves hours of time and trouble when searching for medical equipment and supplies and the manufacturers who provide them. Volume I: The Product Directory, provides essential information for purchasing or specifying medical supplies for every medical device, supply, and diagnostic available in the US. Listings provide FDA codes & Federal Procurement Eligibility, Contact information for every manufacturer of the product along with Prices and Product Specifications. Volume 2 - Supplier Profiles, offers the most complete and important data about Suppliers, Manufacturers and Distributors. Company Profiles detail the number of employees, ownership, method of distribution, sales volume, net income, key executives detailed contact information medical products the company supplies, plus the medical specialties they cover. Four indexes provide immediate access to this wealth of information: Keyword Index, Trade Name Index, Supplier Geographical Index and OEM (Original Equipment Manufacturer) Index. *Medical Device Register* is the only one-stop source for locating suppliers and products; looking for new manufacturers or hard-to-find medical devices; comparing products and companies; know who's selling what and who to buy from cost effectively. This directory has become the standard in its field and will be a welcome addition to the reference collection of any medical library, large public library, university library along with the collections that serve the medical community.

"A wealth of information on medical devices, medical device companies... and key personnel in the industry is provide in this comprehensive reference work... A valuable reference work, one of the best hardcopy compilations available." -Doody Publishing

Two Volumes, Hardcover ISBN 978-1-59237-206-5, 3,000 pages, $325.00

**To preview any of our Directories Risk-Free for 30 days, call (800) 562-2139 or fax (518) 789-0556
www.greyhouse.com books@greyhouse.com**

Canadian Almanac & Directory, 2008

The Canadian Almanac & Directory contains sixteen directories in one – giving you all the facts and figures you will ever need about Canada. No other single source provides users with the quality and depth of up-to-date information for all types of research. This national directory and guide gives you access to statistics, images and over 100,000 names and addresses for everything from Airlines to Zoos - updated every year. It's Ten Directories in One! Each section is a directory in itself, providing robust information on business and finance, communications, government, associations, arts and culture (museums, zoos, libraries, etc.), health, transportation, law, education, and more. Government information includes federal, provincial and territorial - and includes an easy-to-use quick index to find key information. A separate municipal government section includes every municipality in Canada, with full profiles of Canada's largest urban centers. A complete legal directory lists judges and judicial officials, court locations and law firms across the country. A wealth of general information, the *Canadian Almanac & Directory* also includes national statistics on population, employment, imports and exports, and more. National awards and honors are presented, along with forms of address, Commonwealth information and full color photos of Canadian symbols. Postal information, weights, measures, distances and other useful charts are also incorporated. Complete almanac information includes perpetual calendars, five-year holiday planners and astronomical information. Published continuously for 160 years, *The Canadian Almanac & Directory* is the best single reference source for business executives, managers and assistants; government and public affairs executives; lawyers; marketing, sales and advertising executives; researchers, editors and journalists.

Hardcover ISBN 978-1-59237-220-1, 1,600 pages, $315.00

Associations Canada, 2008

The Most Powerful Fact-Finder to Business, Trade, Professional and Consumer Organizations
Associations Canada covers Canadian organizations and international groups including industry, commercial and professional associations, registered charities, special interest and common interest organizations. This annually revised compendium provides detailed listings and abstracts for nearly 20,000 regional, national and international organizations. This popular volume provides the most comprehensive picture of Canada's non-profit sector. Detailed listings enable users to identify an organization's budget, founding date, scope of activity, licensing body, sources of funding, executive information, full address and complete contact information, just to name a few. Powerful indexes help researchers find information quickly and easily. The following indexes are included: subject, acronym, geographic, budget, executive name, conferences & conventions, mailing list, defunct and unreachable associations and registered charitable organizations. In addition to annual spending of over $1 billion on transportation and conventions alone, Canadian associations account for many millions more in pursuit of membership interests. *Associations Canada* provides complete access to this highly lucrative market. *Associations Canada* is a strong source of prospects for sales and marketing executives, tourism and convention officials, researchers, government officials - anyone who wants to locate non-profit interest groups and trade associations.

Hardcover ISBN 978-1-59237-277-5, 1,600 pages, $315.00

Financial Services Canada, 2008/09

Financial Services Canada is the only master file of current contacts and information that serves the needs of the entire financial services industry in Canada. With over 18,000 organizations and hard-to-find business information, Financial Services Canada is the most up-to-date source for names and contact numbers of industry professionals, senior executives, portfolio managers, financial advisors, agency bureaucrats and elected representatives. Financial Services Canada incorporates the latest changes in the industry to provide you with the most current details on each company, including: name, title, organization, telephone and fax numbers, e-mail and web addresses. *Financial Services Canada* also includes private company listings never before compiled, government agencies, association and consultant services - to ensure that you'll never miss a client or a contact. Current listings include: banks and branches, non-depository institutions, stock exchanges and brokers, investment management firms, insurance companies, major accounting and law firms, government agencies and financial associations. Powerful indexes assist researchers with locating the vital financial information they need. The following indexes are included: alphabetic, geographic, executive name, corporate web site/e-mail, government quick reference and subject. *Financial Services Canada* is a valuable resource for financial executives, bankers, financial planners, sales and marketing professionals, lawyers and chartered accountants, government officials, investment dealers, journalists, librarians and reference specialists.

Hardcover ISBN 978-1-59237-278-2, 900 pages, $315.00

Directory of Libraries in Canada, 2008/09

The Directory of Libraries in Canada brings together almost 7,000 listings including libraries and their branches, information resource centers, archives and library associations and learning centers. The directory offers complete and comprehensive information on Canadian libraries, resource centers, business information centers, professional associations, regional library systems, archives, library schools and library technical programs. *The Directory of Libraries in Canada* includes important features of each library and service, including library information; personnel details, including contact names and e-mail addresses; collection information; services available to users; acquisitions budgets; and computers and automated systems. Useful information on each library's electronic access is also included, such as Internet browser, connectivity and public Internet/CD-ROM/subscription database access. The directory also provides powerful indexes for subject, location, personal name and Web site/e-mail to assist researchers with locating the crucial information they need. *The Directory of Libraries in Canada* is a vital reference tool for publishers, advocacy groups, students, research institutions, computer hardware suppliers, and other diverse groups that provide products and services to this unique market.

Hardcover ISBN 978-1-59237-279-9, 850 pages, $315.00

✳ **To preview any of our Directories Risk-Free for 30 days, call (800) 562-2139 or fax (518) 789-0556**
www.greyhouse.com   books@greyhouse.com

Canadian Environmental Directory, 2008 /09

The Canadian Environmental Directory is Canada's most complete and only national listing of environmental associations and organizations, government regulators and purchasing groups, product and service companies, special libraries, and more! The extensive Products and Services section provides detailed listings enabling users to identify the company name, address, phone, fax, e-mail, Web address, firm type, contact names (and titles), product and service information, affiliations, trade information, branch and affiliate data. The Government section gives you all the contact information you need at every government level – federal, provincial and municipal. We also include descriptions of current environmental initiatives, programs and agreements, names of environment-related acts administered by each ministry or department PLUS information and tips on who to contact and how to sell to governments in Canada. The Associations section provides complete contact information and a brief description of activities. Included are Canadian environmental organizations and international groups including industry, commercial and professional associations, registered charities, special interest and common interest organizations. All the Information you need about the Canadian environmental industry: directory of products and services, special libraries and resource, conferences, seminars and tradeshows, chronology of environmental events, law firms and major Canadian companies, *The Canadian Environmental Directory* is ideal for business, government, engineers and anyone conducting research on the environment.

Softcover ISBN 978-1-59237-224-9, 900 pages, $315.00

Canadian Parliamentary Guide, 2008

An indispensable guide to government in Canada, the annual *Canadian Parliamentary Guide* provides information on both federal and provincial governments, courts, and their elected and appointed members. The Guide is completely bilingual, with each record appearing both in English and then in French. The Guide contains biographical sketches of members of the Governor General's Household, the Privy Council, members of Canadian legislatures (federal, including both the House of Commons and the Senate, provincial and territorial), members of the federal superior courts (Supreme, Federal, Federal Appeal, Court Martial Appeal and Tax Courts) and the senior staff for these institutions. Biographies cover personal data, political career, private career and contact information. In addition, the Guide provides descriptions of each of the institutions, including brief historical information in text and chart format and significant facts (i.e. number of members and their salaries). The Guide covers the results of all federal general elections and by-elections from Confederations to the present and the results of the most recent provincial elections. A complete name index rounds out the text, making information easy to find. No other resources presents a more up-to-date, more complete picture of Canadian government and her political leaders. A must-have resource for all Canadian reference collections.

Hardcover ISBN 978-1-59237-310-9, 800 pages, $184.00